S0-CDW-944

Cancer Patient Follow-Up

Cancer Patient Follow-Up

FRANK E. JOHNSON, M.D.
Professor of Surgery
St. Louis University Health Sciences Center;
Chief of Surgery Service
Department of Veterans Affairs Medical Center
St. Louis, Missouri

KATHERINE S. VIRGO, Ph.D.
Associate Professor of Surgery
St. Louis University Health Sciences Center;
Statistician/Clinical Research Coordinator
Department of Veterans Affairs Medical Center
St. Louis, Missouri

Associate Editors

STEPHEN B. EDGE, M.D.
Chief, Breast Department
Division of Surgical Oncology, Roswell Park Cancer Institute;
Associate Professor of Surgery, State University of New York
Buffalo, New York

CARLOS A. PELLEGRINI, M.D.
Professor and Chairman, Department of Surgery
University of Washington Medical School
Seattle, Washington

GRAEME J. POSTON, M.S., F.R.C.S.
Consultant Surgical Oncologist, Royal Liverpool University Hospital;
Lecturer in Surgery, Liverpool University
Liverpool, United Kingdom

STIMSON P. SCHANTZ, M.D.
Staff Surgeon, Head and Neck Service
Department of Surgery, Memorial Sloan-Kettering Cancer Center;
Associate Professor of Surgery, Cornell University Medical Center
New York, New York

NAOKI TSUKAMOTO, M.D.
Director, National Kyushu Cancer Center
Fukuoka, Japan

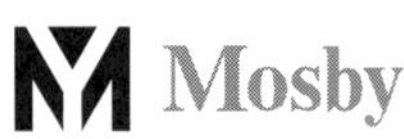

St. Louis Baltimore Boston Carlsbad Chicago Minneapolis New York Philadelphia Portland
London Milan Sydney Tokyo Toronto

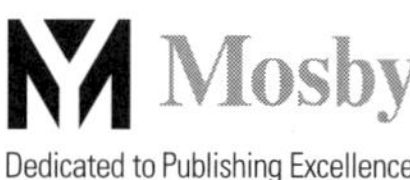

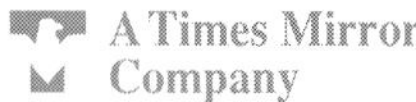

Vice President and Publisher: Anne S. Patterson
Editor: Susie Baxter
Developmental Editor: Ellen Baker Geisel
Project Manager: Patricia Tannian
Book Design Manager: Gail Morey Hudson
Manufacturing Manager: David Graybill
Cover Designer: Teresa Breckwoldt

Printed in the United States of America
Composition by Accu-Color, Inc.
Printing/binding by Maple-Vail Book Mfg Group

Mosby–Year Book, Inc.
11830 Westline Industrial Drive
St. Louis, Missouri 63146

Library of Congress Cataloging in Publication Data

Cancer patient follow-up / [edited by] Frank E. Johnson, Katherine S. Virgo: associate editors, Stephen B. Edge ... [et al.].
p. cm.
Includes bibliographical references and index.
ISBN 0-8151-4925-5
1. Cancer--Treatment. 2. Cancer--Relapse--Prevention. 3. Cancer --Patients--Long-term care. I. Johnson, Frank E., 1943- .
II. Virgo, Katherine S.
[DNLM: 1. Neoplasms. 2. Follow-up Studies. QZ 200 C21536367 1997]
RC270.8.C367 1997
616.99' 406--dc21
DNLM/DLC
for Library of Congress 96-50270
CIP

97 98 99 00 01 / 9 8 7 6 5 4 3 2 1

To

OUR FAMILIES

whose support made the creation of this book feasible

To

OUR COLLEAGUES

whose research findings we incorporated in writing this book

To

OUR PATIENTS

whose care this book is intended to improve

Contributors

NADEEM R. ABU-RUSTUM, M.D.
Fellow, Gynecology Service
Department of Surgery
Memorial Sloan-Kettering Cancer Center
New York, New York

PETER E. ANDERSEN, M.D.
Assistant Professor of Otolaryngology, Head and Neck Surgery
Oregon Health Sciences University
Portland, Oregon

BENJAMIN O. ANDERSON, M.D.
Assistant Professor of Surgical Oncology
University of Washington School of Medicine;
Affiliate Investigator, Division of Clinical Research
Fred Hutchinson Cancer Research Center
Seattle, Washington

FREDERICK R. APPELBAUM, M.D.
Director
Clinical Research Division
Fred Hutchinson Cancer Research Center;
Professor of Medicine
University of Washington School of Medicine
Seattle, Washington

MARK A. ARREDONDO, M.D.
Associate Professor of Surgery
Division of Surgical Oncology
Medical College of Ohio
Toledo, Ohio

RICHARD R. BARAKAT, M.D.
Assistant Attending Surgeon
Gynecology Service, Department of Surgery
Memorial Sloan-Kettering Cancer Center;
Assistant Professor of Obstetrics and Gynecology
Cornell University Medical College
New York, New York

LINDA M. BAVISOTTO, M.D.
Assistant Professor in the Medical Oncology Division
Department of Medicine
University of Washington Medical Center
Seattle, Washington

RICHARD H. BELL, Jr., M.D.
Professor and Vice-Chairman
Department of Surgery
University of Washington School of Medicine;
Chief of the Surgical Service
Department of Veterans Affairs
Puget Sound Health Care System
Seattle, Washington

PATRICK I. BORGEN, M.D.
Chief of the Breast Service
Department of Surgery
Memorial Sloan-Kettering Cancer Center;
Assistant Professor of Surgery
Cornell University Medical College
New York, New York

MURRAY F. BRENNAN, M.D.
Chairman
Department of Surgery
Memorial Sloan-Kettering Cancer Center;
Professor of Surgery
Cornell University Medical College
New York, New York

JAMES D. BRUCKNER, M.D.
Assistant Professor of Orthopaedic Surgery
University of Washington Medical School
Seattle, Washington

DAVID J. BRUINVELS, M.D.
General Surgery Resident
Leiden University Hospital
Leiden, The Netherlands

DAVID R. BYRD, M.D.
Chief of Surgical Oncology and Assistant Professor
University of Washington School of Medicine;
Director of the Melanoma Center
University of Washington Medical Center
Seattle, Washington

HIROKAZU CHUMAN, M.D.
Chief, Department of Bone and Soft Tissue
National Kyushu Cancer Center
Fukuoka-City, Japan

RICHARD E. CLARK, M.A., M.D., F.R.C.P., F.R.C.Path
Senior Lecturer and Consultant Hematologist
Department of Hematology
Royal Liverpool University Hospital
Liverpool, United Kingdom

DANIEL G. COIT, M.D.
Associate Professor of Surgery
Cornell University Medical College;
Associate Attending Surgeon
Memorial Sloan-Kettering Cancer Center
New York, New Yrok

KEVIN C. P. CONLON, M.B., M.Ch., F.R.C.S.I.
Assistant Professor of Surgery
Cornell University;
Director, Endosurgical Program
Assistant Attending Surgeon
Memorial Sloan-Kettering Cancer Center
New York, New York

ERNEST U. CONRAD III, M.D.
Associate Professor of Orthopaedic Surgery
University of Washington School of Medicine;
Director, Sarcoma Service
University of Washington;
Director, Bone Tumor Clinic at Children's Hospital
Seattle, Washington

JOHN P. CURTIN, M.D.
Director of the Gynecologic Oncology Fellowship
Memorial Sloan-Kettering Cancer Center;
Assistant Professor of Obstetrics and Gynecology
Cornell University Medical College
New York, New York

MYRON S. CZUCZMAN, M.D.
Department of Hematologic Oncology and Bone Marrow Transplantation
Roswell Park Cancer Institute;
Assistant Professor of Medicine
State University of New York
Buffalo, New York

GUIDO DALBAGNI, M.D.
Assistant Attending Surgeon
Memorial Sloan-Kettering Cancer Center;
Assistant Professor of Urology
Cornell University Medical College
New York, New York

ROBERT J. DOWNEY, M.D.
Director of Surgical Critical Care
Division of Thoracic Surgery and Critical Care
Memorial Sloan-Kettering Cancer Center;
Assistant Professor of Surgery
Cornell University Medical College
New York, New York

STEPHEN B. EDGE, M.D.
Chief, Breast Department
Division of Surgical Oncology
Roswell Park Cancer Institute;
Associate Professor of Surgery
State University of New York
Buffalo, New York

WILLIAM J. ELLIS, M.D.
Assistant Professor of Urology
University of Washington School of Medicine
Seattle, Washington

WARREN E. ENKER, M.D.
Vice-Chairman, Department of Surgery
Beth Israel Medical Center;
Chief, Division of Colorectal Surgery
Professor of Surgery
Albert Einstein College of Medicine
New York, New York

WILLIAM R. FAIR, M.D.
Chief of Urologic Surgery
Director of the Prostate Diagnostic Center
Memorial Sloan-Kettering Cancer Center;
Professor of Urology
Cornell University Medical College
New York, New York

YUMAN FONG, M.D.
Assistant Professor of Surgery
Memorial Sloan-Kettering Cancer Center;
Assistant Professor of Cell Biology and Anatomy
Cornell University Medical College
New York, New York

SHIN FUJITA, M.D., Ph.D.
Staff Surgeon
National Cancer Center Hospital
Tokyo, Japan

TAKASHI FUKUTOMI, M.D.
Chief, Breast Cancer Surgical Division
National Cancer Center Hospital
Tokyo, Japan

ROBERT J. GINSBERG, M.D.
Professor of Surgery
Cornell University Medical College;
Chief of the Thoracic Service
Memorial Sloan-Kettering Cancer Center
New York, New York

BARBARA A. GOFF, M.D.
Assistant Professor
Department of Obstetrics and Gynecology
University of Washington School of Medicine
Seattle, Washington

PAUL J. GOODFELLOW, Ph.D.
Associate Professor, Department of Surgery and Genetics
Washington University School of Medicine
St. Louis, Missouri

JULIE R. GRALOW, M.D.
Instructor
Department of Medicine
Division of Oncology
University of Washington School of Medicine;
Affiliate Investigator
Division of Clinical Research
Fred Hutchinson Cancer Research Center
Seattle, Washington

BENJAMIN E. GREER, M.D.
Professor and Director
Department of Obstetrics and Gynecology
University of Washington School of Medicine
Seattle, Washington

JOSE G. GUILLEM, M.D., M.P.H.
Assistant Professor of Surgery
Cornell University Medical College;
Staff Surgeon, Colorectal Service, Department of Surgery
Memorial Sloan-Kettering Cancer Center
New York, New York

W. SCOTT HELTON, M.D.
Associate Professor of Surgery
University of Washington Medical Center
Seattle, Washington

HARRY W. HERR, M.D.
Assistant Attending Surgeon
Urology Service
Department of Surgery
Memorial Sloan-Kettering Cancer Center;
Professor of Urology
Cornell University Medical College
New York, New York

MICHAEL J. HERSHMAN, M.Sc., M.S., F.R.C.S.
Head of Colorectal Surgery
Director of the M.A.S.T.E.R. (Minimal Access Surgery Training, Education and Research) Unit
Royal Liverpool University Hospital
Liverpool, United Kingdom

CELESTIA S. HIGANO, M.D.
Associate Professor, Division of Oncology
Department of Medicine
University of Washington School of Medicine;
Adjunct Associate Professor
Department of Urology
Associate in Clinical Research
Fred Hutchinson Cancer Research Center
Seattle, Washington

ROBERT P. HUBEN, M.D.
Chief, Department of Urologic Oncology
Roswell Park Cancer Institute;
Associate Professor, Department of Urology
State University of New York
Buffalo, New York

YUKITO ICHINOSE, M.D.
Chief, Department of Chest Surgery
National Kyushu Cancer Center;
Lecturer
Kyushu University
Fukuoka, Japan;
Visiting Scientist, Department of Cell Biology
M.D. Anderson Hospital and Tumor Institute

JOHN A. JOHNKOSKI, M.D.
Resident, Cardiothoracic Surgery
University of Washington
Seattle, Washington

FRANK E. JOHNSON, M.D.
Professor of Surgery
St. Louis University Health Sciences Center;
Chief of Surgical Service
Department of Veterans Affairs Medical Center
St. Louis, Missouri

ANDREW SIMPSON JONES, M.D., F.R.C.S.
Professor of Otolaryngology, Head and Neck Surgery
University of Liverpool;
Royal Liverpool University Hospital
Liverpool, United Kingdom

TADAO KAKIZOE, M.D.
Director, National Cancer Center Hospital
Tokyo, Japan

TOSHIHARU KAMURA, M.D., Ph.D.
Associate Professor of Gynecology and Obstetrics
Kyushu University;
Chief of Gynecologic Oncology
Fukuoka, Japan

MARTIN S. KARPEH, Jr., M.D.
Assistant Attending Surgeon
Gastric and Mixed Tumor Service
Memorial Sloan-Kettering Cancer Center;
Assistant Professor of Surgery
Cornell University Medical College
New York, New York

HOWARD M. KARPOFF, M.D.
Research Fellow, Hepatic Oncology Laboratory
Memorial Sloan-Kettering Cancer Center
New York, New York

HITOSHI KATAI, M.D., Ph.D.
Vice-Head Surgeon
Gastric Division, Department of Surgical Oncology
National Cancer Center Hospital
Tokyo, Japan

JOB KIEVIT, M.D.
Professor of Clinical Decision Analysis
Head, Medical Decision Making Unit
Associate Professor of Surgery
Leiden University Hospital
Leiden, The Netherlands

ANDREW N. KINGSNORTH, B.Sc.(Hons), M.B.B.S., M.S., F.R.C.S.
Reader in Surgery
Royal Liverpool University Hospital
Liverpool, United Kingdom;
Professor of Surgery
Plymouth Postgraduate Medical School
Plymouth, United Kingdom

TAIRA KINOSHITA, M.D., Ph.D.
Head Surgeon, Department of Surgical Oncology
National Cancer Center Hospital East
Kashiwa, Japan

WUI-JIN KOH, M.D.
Associate Professor of Radiation Oncology
Adjunct Associate Professor of Obstetrics and Gynecology
University of Washington School of Medicine
Seattle, Washington

TOMOO KOSUGE, M.D.
Head of the Hepatopancreatobiliary Unit
Department of Oncological Surgery
National Cancer Center Hospital;
Lecturer, Department of Surgery
University of Tokyo
Tokyo, Japan

LORRIE A. LANGDALE, M.D.
Associate Professor of Surgery
University of Washington;
Director of Surgical Critical Care
Veterans Affairs Medical Center
Seattle, Washington

PAUL H. LANGE, M.D.
Professor and Chairman
Department of Urology
School of Medicine
University of Washington Medical Center
Seattle, Washington

SAM J. LEINSTER, B.Sc., M.D., F.R.C.S.
Lecturer in Surgery
Welsh National School of Medicine;
Professor of Surgery
University of Liverpool;
Honorary Consultant Surgeon
Royal Liverpool University Hospital
Liverpool, United Kingdom

ELLIS G. LEVINE, M.D.
Chief of the Breast Department
Division of Medicine
Roswell Park Cancer Institute;
Associate Professor of Medicine
State University of New York
Buffalo, New York

JONATHAN J. LEWIS, M.D., Ph.D.
Assistant Attending Surgeon
Gastric and Mixed Tumor Service
Memorial Sloan-Kettering Cancer Center;
Assistant Professor of Surgery
Cornell University Medical College
New York, New York

THOM R. LOREE, M.D., F.A.C.S.
Assistant Professor of Surgery
State University of New York at Buffalo
Roswell Park Cancer Institute
Buffalo, New York

ETHEL L. MACINTOSH, M.D.
Surgical Oncology Fellow
Department of Surgical Oncology
Roswell Park Cancer Institute
Buffalo, New York

DAVID G. MALONEY, M.D., Ph.D.
Assistant Member
Fred Hutchinson Cancer Research Center;
Assistant Professor of Medicine
Division of Oncology
University of Washington School of Medicine
Seattle, Washington

NAEL MARTINI, M.D.
Attending Thoracic Surgeon
Memorial Sloan-Kettering Cancer Center;
Professor of Surgery
Cornell University Medical College
New York, New York

KEIICHI MARUYAMA, M.D., Ph.D.
Head of the Gastric Division
Department of Surgical Oncology
National Cancer Center Hospital
Tokyo, Japan

PETER McCULLOCH, M.D., F.R.C.S.Ed.
Senior Lecturer in Surgery
Department of Surgery
University of Liverpool;
Consultant Surgeon, Department of General Surgery
Aintree Hospitals Trust
Liverpool, United Kingdom

NEAL J. MEROPOL, M.D.
Medical Co-Director, Gastrointestinal Oncology
Roswell Park Cancer Institute;
Assistant Professor of Medicine
State University of New York
Buffalo, New York

YOSHIHIRO MORIYA, M.D., Ph.D.
Head, Colorectal Division
National Cancer Center Hospital
Tokyo, Japan

ARTHUR SUN MYINT, F.R.C.P.(Edin), F.R.C.S., F.R.C.R.
Consultant in Clinical Oncology
Department of Radiotherapy and Oncology
Clatterbridge Centre for Oncology;
Lecturer, Radiation Oncology Department
Royal Liverpool University Hospital
Liverpool, United Kingdom

TADASHI NAKASHIMA, M.D.
Director of Head and Neck Surgery
National Kyushu Cancer Center;
Assistant Professor of Otolaryngology
Kyushu University School of Medicine
Fukuoka, Japan

HECTOR R. NAVA, M.D.
Research Assistant Professor of Surgery
State University of New York;
Associate Chief of Surgical Oncology
Chief of Endoscopy
Roswell Park Cancer Institute
New York, New York

RICHARD J. O'DONNELL, M.D.
Acting Instructor
Department of Orthopaedics
University of Washington Medical School
Seattle, Washington

BRIAN J. O'HEA, M.D.
Breast Fellow
Memorial Sloan-Kettering Cancer Center;
Assistant Professor of Surgery
Department of Surgery
State University of New York
Stony Brook, New York

JUN OKAMURA, M.D.
Staff Member
Section of Pediatrics
National Kyushu Cancer Center
Fukuoka, Japan

RICHARD D. PAGE, Ch.M., F.R.C.S.(C.Th.)
Honorary Lecturer, Department of Surgery
University of Liverpool;
Consultant in Cardiothoracic Surgery
The Cardiothoracic Centre
Liverpool, United Kingdom

CARLOS A. PELLEGRINI, M.D.
The Henry N. Harkins Professor and Chairman
Department of Surgery
University of Washington Medical School
Seattle, Washington

RAYMOND P. PEREZ, M.D.
Assistant Professor
State University of New York at Buffalo;
Departments of Solid Tumor Oncology and Investigational Therapeutics
Division of Medicine
Roswell Park Cancer Institute
Buffalo, New York

NICHOLAS J. PETRELLI, M.D.
Professor of Surgery
State University of New York at Buffalo;
Chair of Surgical Oncology
Roswell Park Cancer Institute
Buffalo, New York

GRAEME J. POSTON, M.B., M.S., F.R.C.S. (England), F.R.C.S. (Edin)
Consultant Surgical Oncologist
Royal Liverpool University Hospital;
Lecturer, Department of Surgery
Liverpool University;
Director of Surgery
The Liverpool Cancer Centre
Liverpool, United Kingdom

DIANE M. RADFORD, M.D.
Assistant Professor, Divisions of Surgery and Human Molecular Genetics
Department of Surgery
Washington University School of Medicine
St. Louis, Missouri

DEREK RAGHAVAN, M.B.B.S., Ph.D., F.R.A.C.P., F.A.C.P.
Chief, Departments of Solid Tumor Oncology and Investigational Therapeutics
Roswell Park Cancer Institute;
Professor of Medicine and Urology
State University of New York
Buffalo, New York

MIGUEL A. RODRIGUEZ-BIGAS, M.D.
Assistant Professor of Surgery
State University of New York at Buffalo;
Associate Chief
Colorectal Surgery Department
Roswell Park Cancer Institute
Buffalo, New York

VALERIE W. RUSCH, M.D.
Attending Surgeon
Memorial Sloan-Kettering Cancer Center;
Professor of Surgery
Cornell University Medical College
New York, New York

PAUL RUSSO, M.D.
Assistant Attending Surgeon
Memorial Sloan-Kettering Cancer Center;
Assistant Professor of Surgery
Cornell University Medical College
New York, New York

TAKAO SAITO, M.D.
Chief, Department of Gastroenterological Surgery
National Kyushu Cancer Center
Fukuoka, Japan

TAKESHI SANO, M.D., Ph.D.
Head Surgeon, Gastric Division
Department of Surgical Oncology
National Cancer Center Hospital
Tokyo, Japan

MITSURU SASAKO, M.D., Ph.D.
Head, Gastric Division
Department of Surgical Oncology
National Cancer Center Hospital
Tokyo, Japan

STIMSON P. SCHANTZ, M.D.
Associate Professor
Cornell University Medical College;
Director, Cancer Prevention
Department of Surgery
Chief, Head and Neck Research Laboratory
Memorial Sloan-Kettering Cancer Center;
New York, New York

YOUSUKE SEO, M.D.
Chief of Staff of the Operating Room
National Kyushu Cancer Center
Fakuota, Japan

JOEL SHEINFELD, M.D.
Assistant Attending Member, Urology Service
Memorial Sloan-Kettering Cancer Center;
Assistant Professor, Department of Urology
Cornell University Medical College
New York, New York

KAZUAKI SHIMADA, M.D.
Surgical Staff, Hepatopancreaticobiliary Division
National Cancer Center Hospital
Tokyo, Japan

MURIEL F. SIADAK, P.A.-C
Director, Physician Assistant Service
Manager, Long-Term Follow-up Program
Fred Hutchinson Cancer Research Center
Seattle, Washington

MIKA N. SINANAN, M.D., Ph.D.
Assistant Professor of Surgery
University of Washington Medical School
Seattle, Washington

JUDY L. SMITH, M.D.
Department of Surgical Oncology
Roswell Park Cancer Institute;
Assistant Professor of Surgery
State University of New York
Buffalo, New York

TAKAHIKO SONODA, M.D.
Chief, Department of Gynecology
National Cancer Center Hospital
Tokyo, Japan

JAMES E. SPELLMAN, Jr., M.D.
Assistant Professor of Surgery
State University of New York at Buffalo;
Attending Physician
Departments of Molecular Medicine and Surgical Oncology
Roswell Park Cancer Institute
Buffalo, New York

DAVID J. STRAUS, M.D.
Associate Attending Physician
Memorial Sloan-Kettering Cancer Center;
Associate Professor of Clinical Medicine
Cornell University Medical College
New York, New York

KEITH M. SULLIVAN, M.D.
Professor of Medicine
University of Washington Medical School;
Director, Long-Term Follow-up Program
Fred Hutchinson Cancer Research Center
Seattle, Washington

CAROL J. SWALLOW, M.D., Ph.D.
Assistant Professor in the Department of Surgery
University of Toronto;
Attending Physician,
Departments of Surgery and Surgical Oncology
Mount Sinai Hospital and
Princess Margaret Hospital
Toronto, Ontario, Canada

THOMAS K. TAKAYAMA, M.D.
Acting Instructor and Urologic Oncology Fellow
Department of Urology
University of Washington Medical School
Seattle, Washington

HALUK TEZCAN, M.D.
Division of Medicine
Roswell Park Cancer Institute;
Assistant Professor of Medicine
State University of New York
Buffalo, New York

MICHAEL GRAHAM THOMAS, M.B.B.S., B.Sc., M.S., F.R.C.S., F.R.C.S.(Ed), F.R.C.S.(Gen)
Consultant Senior Lecturer
Department of Surgery
University of Bristol;
Honorary Consultant Surgeon
Bristol Royal Infirmary
Bristol, United Kingdom

JOHN A. THOMPSON, M.D.
Associate Professor of Medicine
Division of Medical Oncology
University of Washington Medical School
Seattle, Washington

NAOKUNI UIKE, M.D.
Chief, Department of Hematology
National Kyushu Cancer Center
Fukuoka, Japan

JOHN D. URSCHEL, M.D., F.R.C.S.C, F.R.C.S. ED
Chief of Thoracic Surgery
Roswell Park Cancer Institute
Buffalo, New York

KATHERINE S. VIRGO, Ph.D., M.B.A.
Associate Professor, Department of Surgery
St. Louis University Health Sciences Center;
Statistician, Surgical Service
Department of Veterans Affairs Medical Center
St. Louis, Missouri

ERNEST A. WEYMULLER, Jr., M.D.
Professor and Chairman
Department of Otolaryngology–Head and Neck Surgery
University of Washington Medical School
Seattle, Washington

JOHN WINSTANLEY, B.D.S., M.D., F.R.C.S.
Consultant in Surgical Oncology
Royal Liverpool and Broadgreen University Hospitals;
Honorary Clinical Lecturer
Department of Surgery
University of Liverpool Medical School
Liverpool, United Kingdom

DOUGLAS E. WOOD, M.D.
Head, Section of General Thoracic Surgery
Surgical Director, Lung Transplantation
Assistant Professor of Surgery
University of Washington;
Chief of Cardiothoracic Surgery
Veteran's Affairs Puget Sound Health Care System
Seattle, Washington

AKIFUMI YAMAMOTO, M.D.
Head, Dermatology Division
National Cancer Center Hospital;
Visiting Assistant Professor
Department of Dermatology
Gifu University School of Medicine
Tokyo, Japan

JUNJI YAMAMOTO, M.D.
Staff, Department of Surgery
National Cancer Center Hospital
Tokyo, Japan

SUSUMU YAMASAKI, M.D.
Staff, Department of Surgery
National Cancer Center Hospital
Tokyo, Japan

Foreword

Fifteen years ago, when we wrote a book devoted to the same subject as this one, the follow-up management of patients following initial treatment for cancer was the ugly neglected stepchild in the oncology family.[1] Once primary therapy was completed, there was little available to influence outcome and little attention was paid to this phase of management. The dramatic change within 15 years is proved by this splendid scholarly volume written by world-renowned experts. The ugly duckling has turned into a much-sought-after princess. It would be satisfying but untrue to think that the magic kiss of our book wrought the conversion of the unattractive child into the current popular superstar. The truth is that, however measured, our book attracted little attention. Our objective was to provide the many types of generalists and specialists a sense of order in both choice and timing of diagnostic tests and treatment following primary tumor therapy. Perhaps the most important result of our book was to excite the interest of one of our best surgical residents of that time, Frank Johnson, who continued his training in oncology and is the chief editor of this remarkable volume. The product of his efforts far exceeds anything previously attained by his teacher.

Logical decisions in the follow-up management for any specific tumor require an understanding of the biology of that tumor. For this reason each chapter in this volume addresses not merely what tests to perform at what time period following treatment, but the basic cellular and clinical features of the tumor. With less disciplined editors this might have provided license to rewrite a routine textbook of oncology. Wisely they have maintained their focus primarily on those aspects of the tumor that affect its recurrence characteristics.

The remarkable basic science advances in oncology during the past 15 years since we wrote our manual are reflected in the complete change in recommended follow-up clinical protocols. Scarcely a page of our 15-year-old book is now appropriately current. As I read the scientifically sophisticated chapters of this book in manuscript form, I began to keep tally of the new diagnostic and therapeutic techniques that have come into prominence in these 15 short years.

Some of these stem from advances in technology, such as computed tomography, magnetic resonance imaging, and positron emission tomography. Others grew from revolutionary discoveries in immunology and cellular biology. These include tumor markers, monoclonal antibodies, and immune enhancers. The most recent burst of new discoveries applicable to oncology involve genetics, which seems to overflow from every line within this book, from subclassification of what previously was considered a single tumor, to determining risks in a given patient. Such tautological reclassification is reminiscent of the nineteenth century but now is based on chromosomal architecture.

The editors of this book invited each chapter author to predict the future in his or her assigned subject. As the author of the foreword, I will assume I have a similar invitation to make some observations on the future course of follow-up care of patients following completion of their initial therapy.

Returning to the analogy that this area of oncology is the glamour girl of the closing years of the twentieth century, we must be aware that the ever-changing gowns and baubles that decorate this charmer are extremely expensive. Like the cautious father of the Prince Charming trying to attract her attention, I would warn that our purse is not without bottom and that those who pursue her had better be certain that the cost is justified by performance. In the dizzy excitement of scientific advances in genetics, cellular biology, immunology, or in the technology of digital imaging, it is easy to forget that those who pay the bill will only support what will improve length or quality of survival of a patient for whom the exciting discoveries are being applied. Oncologists will be challenged to justify by clinical outcome analysis their exciting but expensive forms of tumor detection or treatment. Health care payors will demand solid evidence that early detection of a recurrent tumor of a specific type will improve survival. Is there justification, for example, in spending health insurance money except for general moral support of a patient with oat-cell carcinoma of the lung, or the majority of pancreatic tumors? Whether the payors be private or government insurers, it is predictable they will increase rationing of payment for follow-up diagnostic tests and therapeutic care of those dying patients.

So long as payors are also willing to fund promising cost-benefit research in a few highly organized centers, such questions are reasonable. Indeed, they will force a sense of discipline on the almost profligate use of health care funds for management of cancer patients in the follow-up period in the commercial marketplace of most community and many academic hospitals. Test selection, timing, and sequencing will have to be justified if they are to be funded. This will lead—like it or not—to approved protocols or practice guidelines. Justification for such management will have to be based on objective data documenting increased quality-adjusted life years of a treated sample of patients compared to adequate controls.

Fifteen years ago we lamented that very little hard data were available to support the advised management protocols on which our book was based. They were produced by serious students of each tumor but were based on recalled personal experience plus study of historical reviews. Although the situation is somewhat better at the present time, I would judge that at least half of the recommendations contained in this current book for patient management lack a base of hard scientific data. The uncompromising logic of economics will provide additional incentive for prompt accumulation of such data.

Finally, I will admit to a weakness. As I read and was dazzled by the startling new approaches to the management of patients with recurrent tumors so magnificently documented in this volume and compared it with the much simpler diagnostic and therapeutic techniques we advocated 15 years ago, I wondered, "How many patients currently are cured or comforted with modern techniques that would have unduly suffered if managed by those available 15 years ago?" I have no answer to this sobering question.

Of one prediction I am certain: this is the first edition of what is going to be an ongoing series of subsequent publications. The field is changing so fast, and the stakes are so high, in terms not only of costs but the far more important goals of length and quality of human life, that this will be an important milestone in the field of oncology.

Ben Eiseman, M.D.

REFERENCE

1. Eiseman B, Robinson W, Steele G. Follow up of the cancer patient. New York: Thieme and Stratton, Inc., 1982.

Preface

There are currently few well-accepted standards for cancer patient follow-up. Similarly, few publications document patient benefit from surveillance in terms of extended survival time or improved quality of life. This book is intended to provide clinicians with guidance regarding the follow-up of cancer patients after treatment by compiling in one publication the strategies recommended by acknowledged experts. Displaying these strategies in a standardized format should encourage comparative analysis and consensus building, laying the foundation for clinical trials and the eventual establishment of evidence-based guidelines. We hope this book will stimulate discussion and promote rational change in the field.

Current actual cancer patient surveillance strategies of practicing clinicians and the factors influencing variability in current practice are reviewed in 19 organ-specific chapters. Both currently available and promising new diagnostic tests are evaluated, including those based on molecular biological concepts. The effect of recurrence of the index neoplasm or a new primary neoplasm on prognosis is examined. Concluding each chapter are three to four counterpoints from distinguished authors at major cancer centers in the United States, the United Kingdom, and Japan. These counterpoints highlight similarities and differences in follow-up strategies both across cancer centers and across countries. The follow-up recommendations provided by experts at each institution are summarized in standardized tables throughout. The tables display years after treatment on the horizontal axis and surveillance modalities (office visits and tests) on the vertical axis. Each entry in each column depicts the total number of times per year the surveillance modality is performed. (The publisher has also included a comprehensive grid at the end of each chapter.) Standardization by means of these tables and grids should facilitate comparisons across strategies.

One difficulty encountered in publishing a book of this type was in the selection of cancers that could feasibly be included in this first edition. Cancer sites such as the thyroid gland, uterine cervix, eye, and brain, although excluded from the current edition, are candidates for inclusion in the next edition. Standardization of the table for displaying follow-up recommendations, although seemingly straightforward, was a second problem area. Although authors from different countries generally use common terminology as it relates to diagnostic testing, interpretation often differs regarding what the test includes. Achieving a balance between simplicity and comprehensiveness in displaying follow-up recommendations was also problematic. Through trial and error, compromise, and dialogue, we developed a table format that we believe addresses these issues and is simple, understandable, and comprehensive.

We take great personal satisfaction in the completion of this project, especially as it is one so long overdue. Special thanks are extended to Dr. Ben Eiseman for his input and guidance. We also wish to express our gratitude to Ms. Mary Ellen Kissling, who served as editorial assistant on the project. She accomplished the mammoth task of copyediting all manuscripts, ensuring consistency in style and format throughout, with grace, skill, and good humor—a rare blend. The book could not have been completed without her hard work and attention to detail.

Frank E. Johnson
Katherine S. Virgo

Contents

Detailed Contents

SECTION I

Concepts

CHAPTER 1

Overview

St. Louis University Health Sciences Center ▪ St. Louis
Department of Veterans Affairs Medical Center

Frank E. Johnson

HISTORY

For millennia, humans have struggled to understand disease processes. Some with particular insight (or at least clinical success) became shamans, medicine men, or healers. Often these individuals also sought to divine the future while dealing with nonmedical issues, leading to dual roles as necromancers, astrologers, or soothsayers. They commonly solicited the intervention of supernatural forces to benefit their clients or patients, blending the function of priest with that of healer. Some, like the barber-surgeons of England, began their evolution into medical practitioners as tradesmen. Eventually, after many false starts, the occupation of physician developed and became a full-time enterprise. A chief function of physicians, like that of their predecessors, has traditionally been to anticipate future developments for their patients. In earlier times, before effective therapies were available, this was perhaps the most important contribution to be made to the patient, and it remains important today. This book deals with an outgrowth of that function—how to detect and manage illness in patients who have had potentially curative treatment for cancer.[1] In general, the success of physicians' ministrations has been closely related to their understanding of pathophysiology.[2] Physicians now look back on the diagnostic and therapeutic maneuvers of previous generations of doctors and shake their heads at the futility of those efforts. Like other diseases, cancer has been managed by many strategies that now seem outlandish.[1] Undoubtedly, the future will bring deeper knowledge of pathological processes, which will make current efforts seem inadequate as well.

Cancer, in all its forms, has been poorly understood, feared, and usually fatal. This disease, now thought to be a heterogeneous group of related disorders, was often diagnosed in the past on the basis of macroscopic features such as mass, relentless growth, and metastatic spread. However, the invention of the microscope in the seventeenth century and the resultant flowering of microscopic pathology led to greatly improved diagnostic criteria. For the first time, neoplastic diseases could be clearly and unequivocally separated from other disorders such as syphilis, which can mimic clinical aspects of cancer. Modern understanding of the genetic basis of cancer is likely to supplant microscopic, morphological criteria with quantitative ones based on DNA structure, offering the prospect that knowledge of the malignant process will soon be far more precise. With better understanding of pathophysiology and the natural history of disease has come the ability to link a disease process such as cancer and the consequences of its initial treatment with subsequent events, such as recurrence or new primary cancer development.

Until recently, cure of most neoplasms was rare. Thus cancer patient follow-up was usually an exercise in palliative care delivered to symptomatic patients with a short life expectancy. In the nineteenth century, with the advent of modern surgery, cures became possible with some regularity for the first time.[3] This created a population of cancer patients with unique attributes—they had survived treatment carried out with curative intent, had a realistic prospect of having been cured, and were more or less asymptomatic. By the twentieth century the natural history of this then-novel patient population had become clearer and indicated that these patients were more vulnerable than the population at large to certain types of cancer.

Although instances of multiple primary cancers of a single organ were generally considered medical curiosities and reported as single instances until well into the twentieth century, inklings of genetic predisposition to cancer began to occur.[4] In addition, many authors recognized that cancer in one organ might serve as a marker for the later development of cancer in another site. It is instructive to realize that major medical textbooks[5,6] written earlier in this century make little mention of the phenomenon of second primary neoplasms in patients treated for common carcinomas, such as those of the breast, upper aerodigestive tract, and large intestine. Many common cancers, and a number of uncommon ones as well, are now known to be markers for the development of synchronous or metachronous new carcinomas (in the same or other organs). Since patients who were successfully treated for cancer of one organ can have a second cancer arise in the remaining portion of that organ, the concept of organ-specific surveillance arose. For example, it was realized early in the twentieth century that cure of cancer in one breast could be followed by the development of cancer in the contralateral breast[7] and that the second cancer could also be treated with curative potential.

Thus the detection of new organ-specific cancers became enshrined in clinical practice. These two goals, detection of recurrence of the index lesion and detection of second primary tumors, have been the foundation of surveillance strategies. Patients with recurrent cancers such as testicular carcinoma and Hodgkin's disease can often be cured, and even those with incurable recurrences of most sorts of cancer can often receive effective palliation. With certain other tumors, unfortunately, presymptomatic detection of recurrence is currently of little practical value. Effective therapy is not available, which calls into question whether active surveillance is beneficial.[8] Chapters 5 through 23 in this text discuss what is known about the surveillance of patients after potentially curative treatment of cancers in various organs, focusing primarily on the detection of recurrence of the index malignancy and the detection of new organ-specific cancers. One can only agree with Lewis Thomas, who wrote, "I wish there were some formal courses in medical school on Medical Ignorance; textbooks as well, although they would have to be very heavy volumes. We have a long way to go."[1]

The steady progress in medical understanding and care of cancer patients has been aided by improvements in diagnostic testing and medical record documentation. It is instructive to read today the fragmentary histories, physical examinations, and diagnostic tests upon which important clinical decisions were based in the past.[9] Not surprisingly, treatment outcomes were difficult to predict and often poor. Record keeping is now intimately linked with that most revolutionary invention, the computer, which permits better documentation of, and easier access to, clinical parameters. Medical record keeping is an underappreciated area that has greatly improved the ability to analyze data on clinical patient care. This humble sort of effort, based on countless retrospective reviews of patient records, has led to continuous improvements in patient care and has improved physicians' ability to discern the future for patients of all sorts, including those treated for cancer. This, in turn, has helped shape strategies for follow-up after cancer therapy.

The evolution of surveillance strategies for patients after cancer treatment has been further aided by the introduction of staging systems. Staging helps clinicians to assess prognosis in individual patients and to differentiate patients with the same tumor type on the basis of differing prognoses. Early staging systems were independently adopted by several specialty societies, but by 1977 the American Joint Committee on Cancer had agreed on rules for tumor, nodes, metastases (TNM) staging for all common solid tumors. More recently the American Joint Committee on Cancer and the International Union Against Cancer have reached an international consensus on staging criteria,[10] and further refinements are inevitable. Staging is an important part of cancer therapy because it allows clinicians to tailor treatment on the basis of prognosis.

Once the causal role of environmental and genetic factors in carcinogenesis became clear, preventive measures were integrated into posttreatment follow-up efforts. For decades physicians during follow-up appointments have advised lung cancer patients to stop smoking, skin cancer patients to minimize sun exposure, and so on. Physicians now know that diet, obesity, and other modifiable risk factors exist for certain cancers and can counsel patients appropriately. Many different sorts of drugs, such as retinoids, tamoxifen, and finasteride, are being tested in clinical trials aimed at preventing common cancers.[11] If these chemopreventive regimens are found to be effective, monitoring of intermediate endpoints and drug toxicities will provide new justification for follow-up in large populations of cancer patients. How follow-up strategies should be modified to accommodate chemoprevention regimens is not known.

Initiatives to develop consensus among physicians are becoming more important as information about medical matters proliferates, particularly when controversy persists despite such efforts. Surveillance strategies for patients after potentially curative treatment often differ greatly among experts,[12-14] the costs of surveillance can vary widely,[15-18] and the effectiveness of various strategies has been poorly documented in almost every instance. A goal of this book is to describe and discuss the detailed, organ-specific surveillance strategies recommended by acknowledged experts. Presenting these various strategies should help build consensus and lay the foundation for thorough analysis.

The rationales, opinions, and current practice plans of the many contributors to the organ site–specific chapters in this book should not be construed as defining the optimal practice for a given patient, but rather should aid clinicians in their efforts to help patients. To make the contributors' recommendations more understandable, guidelines are summarized in tables. These display, in a relatively standardized way, the main points made by individual authors. Simplifying and codifying the complexities of the clinical art in this way is a Procrustean approach, but this appears to be the best alternative. Others have also found this method worthwhile.[12-14,18-23] For the most part the follow-up of patients with advanced disease treated for palliation is not dealt with here. Such patients are commonly symptomatic, unlike the patient who has been cured of the index lesion. Furthermore, such patients are always at hazard for the development of symptoms, unlike patients treated with curative intent, a fraction of whom can be expected to live indefinitely without recurrence. This text does not deal with treatment of recurrence, since that topic is discussed extensively in other books. Generally, heroic measures are required for cure, and noncurative treatments are often controversial as well. Similarly, management of a new primary cancer is not discussed, as this topic is satisfactorily covered in other reference works. Since the data on which many of the current recommendations are based are scant and deeply flawed, it is hoped that the opinions, attitudes, and prejudices offered in this book will stimulate the proper design and implementation of clinical trials.

GOALS OF SURVEILLANCE

Consider the problem of neoplasms of high TNM stage at the time of initial treatment. Despite exciting successes, treatment of advanced cancers is often followed by failure. The detection of recurrent disease often leads to secondary treatment. In the case of surgically treated sarcomas of the extremities, skin cancers, and other neoplasms in which local recurrence may be easy to discover, secondary surgical therapy can be curative. Modern medical management even permits salvage therapy for some patients with deeply seated cancers. In similar fashion, radiation treatment when surgery has failed and surgical treatment when radiation has failed can benefit some cancer patients. Most clinicians believe that earlier detection of recurrence might be associated with a more favorable treatment outcome. Thus the concept of surveillance after potentially curative treatment of cancers has become widely accepted, although not often substantiated by well-designed clinical trials. Methods for early detection of tumor recurrence have improved markedly over the years. A complicating factor is that adjuvant chemotherapy and radiation therapy have established a firm niche in the therapeutic plan for patients with many common tumors. Surgery itself can be considered adjuvant therapy in organ-conserving treatment of breast cancer, for example. How adjuvant therapy should affect posttreatment surveillance strategies is almost completely unknown.

A secondary gain inherent in any surveillance strategy, and one not commonly considered in assessing the utility of follow-up management plans, is the detection of other medically significant conditions.[16] The patient who receives a chest x-ray as a method of detecting pulmonary metastases from breast cancer may have tuberculosis detected instead; gallstones may be observed on a computed tomographic scan after colon cancer surgery. Similarly, the patient who returns for an office visit after melanoma treatment may have a breast cancer detected, even though melanoma is not known to be a marker of high risk for breast cancer. Tabulation of the benefits of surveillance should consider unanticipated advantages such as these.

Another important benefit of postoperative surveillance is psychological in nature.[19] Undoubtedly some patients derive comfort from receiving a clean bill of health from their doctor after a clinic visit, since fear of recurrent cancer is so common (and so often well warranted). Little has been written about the psychological benefits to the patient of receiving posttreatment surveillance, although one recent, well-controlled trial of surveillance after breast cancer treatment did not find an impact on quality of life resulting from intensive surveillance when compared with a nonintensive strategy.[24] Such surveillance has psychological disadvantages as well. Most clinicians are only dimly aware of how their patients feel about undergoing the battery of tests that constitute surveillance, since the feared recurrence may be detected by any of the surveillance tests used.[25] The optimal management of a patient who has undergone potentially curative treatment for cancer requires considerable clinical wisdom. The physician must synthesize knowledge, insight into patient concerns,[26] and, to a growing extent, the ability to maneuver within externally imposed guidelines. Each practitioner must rely on personal conscience, and this is not easily described in a textbook.

The editors believe this book will foster the design and promulgation of rational posttreatment surveillance strategies for the common cancers that can be treated with curative intent. Discussion of other neoplasms, such as primary brain tumors,[8] has been left out because they are rarely cured. Moreover, early detection of recurrent disease or new primary disease may be futile, since salvage therapies are not very effective. Perhaps future editions of this book will encompass such neoplasms. The rare neoplasms are also not covered. Appropriate follow-up of small bowel carcinoma, for example, although important to the unfortunate individual with this condition, does not seem to warrant discussion for several reasons. First, there is little literature from which to draw. Second, the number of patients at risk is small. Third, the financial implications for society at large are limited. However, the follow-up of patients with very early neoplasia, such as superficial bladder cancer, in situ breast carcinoma, and TNM stage I invasive prostatic carcinoma, is discussed in the chapters dealing with these organ sites.

LIMITATIONS OF SURVEILLANCE

The reliable possibility of cure after cancer therapy represented a milestone in medicine, one that has important socioeconomic implications. This positive outcome was strongly desired, in spite of expense, by physicians and patients. The success of surgery was shortly followed by the development of ionizing radiation as a reliable treatment tool.[27] Effective systemic therapy has been available since 1896[28] but largely consisted of hormonal ablative treatments until the introduction of toxic drugs such as nitrogen mustard into clinical medicine after World War II.[29] Although systemic therapy for common solid tumors made relatively scant progress until recently, chemotherapy for upper aerodigestive tract carcinoma,[30] breast carcinoma,[31] large bowel carcinoma,[32] and other common cancers is now incorporated into standard care. Again, a fraction of patients receiving chemotherapy are long-term disease-free survivors in unmaintained remission, now thought of as cured. This subset of patients forms a population in which screening for new primary cancers or recurrence of the index neoplasm has been vigorously pursued. The screening of these patients has been aided by more powerful diagnostic tests, the increase of which has been dramatic in clinical use in this century. An example is the discovery of ionizing radiation. One hundred years ago this was an untapped resource in medical diagnosis.[33] How would physicians today cope with the loss of diagnostic radiographs, computed tomographic scans, nuclear medicine images, and the like from the practice of medicine? It is difficult to imagine. Similarly, who can visualize how clinical practice would have developed without radioimmunoassays, metabolic studies employing radioisotopes, and the many similar laboratory tests employing radioactive material that have been developed in this century?

The profusion of tests and their obvious utility in many clinical situations have led to a dilemma. How can clinicians best select which tests to order for their patients who have received treatment for cancer and who are now seemingly well? How often should tests be ordered? Which ones are likely to provide useful new information and which are not? How does the information affect clinical decision making and patient outcomes? Clinicians now employ these tests in their patients treated with curative intent for cancer, usually without rigorous prior demonstration of the usefulness of the tests[20] and often with little knowledge of the costs involved.

For example, many factors are now known to indicate an increasing risk of treatment failure, even if initial therapy was administered with curative intent. There is an apparent rationale favoring increased surveillance in such patients. It is unclear whether more intensive surveillance is cost effective in terms of lives saved or improved. In addition, quality of life has been investigated rather little. Russell[34] has provided a scholarly analysis of this issue for carcinoma of the cervix, a neoplasm for which the Papanicolaou (Pap) test has been well established as an effective screening tool. Her analysis concerns primary screening of patients without prior cancer, but the message can be applied to cancer patient follow-up. The Pap test detects premalignant lesions and intraepithelial neoplasia as well as invasive cancer and permits detection and treatment before symptoms appear. It has been extensively validated and has substantially reduced the death rate from cervical cancer in populations receiving screening, as compared with similar populations not screened. Soon after the Pap test was validated, experts advised annual screening, but subsequent analyses of the implications of this policy have led to modifications. One area of concern is test sensitivity. No test detects a disorder infallibly, and the Pap test is no exception. Overreliance on this single test can lead to a false sense of security. False-positive test results also occur. Although false positives are uncommon, a consequence of frequent testing is that the more often Pap smears are done, the more likely one test is to be falsely positive. This results in further testing to prove that cancer does not, in fact, exist. Even more serious is the possibility that active treatment could be carried out on the basis of a false-positive result, with medical risks, increased costs, and unnecessary hysterectomy in some instances. A further problem occurs when the Pap test discloses a premalignant lesion. Under these circumstances active treatment may not be warranted because invasive cancer does not inevitably arise. In fact, regression of cytologic dysplasia is common.

The value of surveillance for cervical cancer is indisputable, but how often should screening be carried out? A large impact on the death rate from cervical cancer is achieved by screening adult women every 10 years. This is improved by more frequent screening, but at ever-increasing marginal cost and ever-decreasing marginal gain in life expectancy.[15] For example, Pap testing every 3 years is estimated to increase mean life expectancy by only 1.5 days, as compared with testing every 4 years.[34] This leads to a consideration of costs. Patients, insurance companies, health care policymakers, and physicians view this issue somewhat differently for obvious reasons. Assuming a cost of $75 per Pap test, screening every 3 years for every woman from 20 to 74 years old in the United States would cost about $2 billion per year, while annual screening would cost $6 billion per year. Such sums warrant scrutiny, and this text aims to provide a basis for cost-benefit analysis of current practice for many different organ site–specific cancers.

Surveillance testing provides a diagnosis only, and costs of active treatment must be factored into any rational analysis. For cervical cancer, Eddy[16] calculates that Pap testing every 4 years saves 1 year of life at a cost of about $10,000, while annual screening costs about $40,000 per year of life saved, as compared with a policy of no screening. However, when annual surveillance is compared with surveillance every 2 years, the cost per additional year of life saved by the more intensive strategy exceeds $1 million. Such considerations are causing changes in health care policy. Society, if it behaves rationally, should not neglect the small risk that detectable and curable cancer may exist in certain patient groups, but should avoid excessive diagnostic testing and treatment. Society cannot rationally afford to squander its resources in low-benefit, high-cost enterprises, particularly when these disrupt patients' lives needlessly and impose risks.

Physicians are increasingly being forced to realize that the dramatic advances in diagnostic testing have implications for clinical medicine and for medical economics.[15,16,35] Computed tomographic scans, sonograms, and other modern imaging tests can provide remarkable anatomical detail. Deeply seated lesions can be detected before they produce any clinical disease. It is common for abnormalities in serological tumor markers, endoscopy, and the like to antedate clinical disease, but these tests are all expensive. The profusion of medical information can also make clinical decision making ambiguous. What is the physician to do, for example, when a breast cancer patient given potentially curative treatment several years earlier has an abnormal bone scan, but plain x-ray films show no lesion? It is easy to see how such information could harm patients. Toxic therapy might be given needlessly if the breast cancer had not actually recurred. Crippling complications might develop if cancer had recurred but therapy was withheld.

Paradoxically, advances in diagnosis can make the physician's work more difficult and the patient's decision making more confusing. Some of the confusion dwells in documenting the anatomical distribution of cancer and defining the value of cancer treatment. The images produced by the modern diagnostic armamentarium can be spectacular and compelling. A sufficiently abnormal image may prompt a flurry of diagnostic and therapeutic interventions that sometimes yield few benefits and may in fact be detrimental. Black and Welch[35] point out that the apparent incidence and prevalence of a disease increase as ability to detect the disease improves. In the case of tumor marker substances in blood or other body fluids, abnormalities are loosely related to tumor size. For diagnostic imaging tests the size of the radiographic abnormality correlates highly with diagnostic sensitivity and specificity. With improved imaging tests, smaller and smaller abnormalities can be reliably detected. A cycle may develop in which some form of new imaging technique decreases the threshold for detection of cancer, which yields a higher percentage of positive diagnoses in a given population. This is taken as providing an improvement in clinical management, which reinforces the increased use of the imaging test. These considerations are important when deciding how to follow cancer patients after primary treatment.

The assessment of diagnostic accuracy, which rests on such concepts as sensitivity and specificity, uses short-term pathological interpretation to validate tests. This assessment commonly incorporates neither the long-term clinical implications of the diagnosis nor the effects of therapies. Addressing these considerations requires different types of evidence, which are generally more difficult to come by. Nonetheless, more sensitive tests usually replace less sensitive ones, even though some of the cancers detected by very sensitive tests are of unknown natural history and have unknown responses to treatment. An example of this is cervical intraepithelial neoplasia, the detection of which is greatly aided by the Pap test. Frequent Pap testing established this diagnosis in many women and led them to receive hysterectomies until it became clear that equivalent survival could be achieved with lesser ablative procedures.

The simple example of cervical cancer shows how shifting perceptions of cancer prevalence and unclear documentation of therapeutic effectiveness can prompt increased diagnostic testing and excessive treatment.[35] It illustrates how improved diagnostic tests may not help the clinician reach a decision about how the newly detectable, subclinical disease should best be treated. Because the incidence and prevalence of detected disease increase as the sensitivity of testing methods increase, patient outcomes often appear to improve because of noncomparability with historical controls. This seeming gain in treatment outcome further reinforces the initial trend toward an intensive testing strategy prompted by improved test sensitivity. As the example of Pap testing shows, this can lead to increased treatment intensity and even greater use of the diagnostic tests. In addition, the establishment of a cancer diagnosis is not always accompanied by the development of clinical disease[36] and certainly does not establish whether a patient will benefit from a therapeutic intervention. Clinical trials can help avoid these problems. Large-scale clinical trials of screening in high-risk groups for breast cancer, lung cancer, and the like have often yielded results not favoring frequent testing, as discussed in more detail elsewhere in this text.

Stage migration is another distorting influence that can be attributed to imaging tests, creating an illusion of increased survival for patients at all stages of cancer.[37] Stage migration is the change in TNM stage that results from improved staging techniques. The detection of an occult adrenal metastasis by computed tomographic scan in a patient with apparent TNM stage I lung cancer generally removes that patient from consideration for curative treatment. This phenomenon eventually improves the reported outcome for therapy of TNM stage I lung cancer by eliminating futile treatment in such individuals. It also improves outcomes in TNM stage IV patients, since asymptomatic individuals with small tumor burdens do significantly better than those with symptoms and large tumor burdens.

Cancers are currently defined in terms of microscopic morphological criteria. Thus the prevalence of cancer increases with the ability to sample large amounts of tissue. Increasingly sophisticated imaging techniques can be so sensitive as to call into question what is meant by the term "cancer."[36] An excellent example of this is found in the field of breast cancer. Before mammography, breast cancer was generally diagnosed clinically because a breast mass was discovered. However, breast cancers detected by screening mammography are often so small as to be impalpable. In addition, they often are in situ lesions, the natural history of which is not clear. The ever lower threshold for breast cancer detection helps explain the increased prevalence of cancer on mammographic screening and the increase in the percentage of carcinomas in situ among breast cancers detected via mammography. This illustrates the fact, relatively unappreciated until recently, that clinically occult cancer is present in many apparently healthy people.[35,36,38] What should clinicians do about such abnormalities that are detected during surveillance of patients who have been treated for cancer? Some answers may be found in this text. Where answers do not exist, the editors hope this text will help clarify issues and promote research designed to provide answers.

The advances in surveillance are changing clinicians' notions about the prevalence of cancer. They also alter perceptions of the natural history of disease and the response of cancer to treatment. Unfortunately, in selecting tests and treatments to offer patients, physicians are rarely able to rely on the results of well-controlled, prospective clinical trials, which are expensive and difficult to carry out. Rather, physicians must usually depend on less rigorous sources of guidance, such as consensus development panels, traditions imparted during medical school and residency training, and knowledge of nonscientific issues, such as patient preference and the constraints of third-party payors.

Common sources of bias in deciding on the value of diagnostic and therapeutic interventions are lead time and length bias,[35] both of which are discussed at greater length elsewhere. Some of the confusion resulting from improvements in diagnostic testing will undoubtedly persist, since medicine remains an art as well as a science. However, some confusion can be eliminated by thinking through the implications of diagnosis of tiny neoplasms of uncertain significance. Stratification of diagnostic certainty (according to tumor size and adjusting for the sensitivity and specificity of a given method of detection) could make estimation of disease prevalence more independent of the continually evolving imaging methodologies. Historical comparisons to assess the utility of newly introduced tests and treatment strategies could be made more reliable by minimizing lead time and length bias, but this is easier said than done.

The incidence and prevalence of many diseases can be expected to increase as advances continue in imaging modalities, molecular genetic tools, and other diagnostic methods. Some of these increases can be predicted.[36] When diseases are detected during cancer patient follow-up, physicians must resist the temptation to treat them in novel ways with potentially harmful and expensive therapies. They must also expect that improved diagnostic techniques will be accompanied by seeming improvements in patient outcomes owing to lead time and length biases, stage migration, and similar factors. Because of these and other complexities, well-controlled, randomized clinical trials will be needed more than ever in the coming decades. The insights from such trials are likely to be great, and the time, effort, and money expended should be rewarded with improved patient management.

COSTS OF SURVEILLANCE

The decision to implement a screening program of any sort is ideally founded on a judgment that its benefits and savings exceed its risks and costs. The information needed to arrive at this judgment is, unfortunately, difficult to obtain. Cost containment has become a pervasive and controversial issue, particularly in wealthy countries where access to sophisticated and expensive follow-up modalities can impose a crushing financial burden on society, individuals, corporations, and insurers. Three methods of assessing relationships among costs, savings, risks, and benefits have been particularly influential, all requiring interdisciplinary research. Cost-effectiveness analysis focuses on a measure of effect, such as survival time, and attempts to describe the costs, savings, and risks of a specific intervention. Included in the analysis is an estimate of opportunities forfeited because certain resources consumed by the surveillance scheme are not available for other uses. Cost-utility analysis is an extension of this technique, used to factor in several measures of effect simultaneously. The measures are given relative weights to arrive at a global measure of the intervention. This is called the utility. The best-known utility measure is the quality-adjusted life year, a simultaneous measure of duration of life and quality of life. The cost-benefit analysis reckons the costs and utility of an intervention, derived from a cost-utility analysis, by attaching a price value to the unit of utility. Other considerations such as legal and ethical issues can also be factored in, with attendant increases in complexity; this is often termed a medical technology assessment.[39]

This text supplies, where possible, a factual basis for discussion of costs, benefits, and rationales of the various diagnostic options. Current estimates of costs and charges of various surveillance tests in the United States are provided, which should serve as a guideline for estimates of future costs and charges, as well as for estimates of these values in other countries. The costs of cancer patient follow-up, about which surprisingly little is known, are the topic of Chapter 3, and overall considerations of factors that should influence the design of surveillance strategies are introduced in Chapters 2 and 4. Much is written in scattered form on these topics throughout the medical literature, and this book organizes these data into a more coherent unit.

The discussions outlined in this text are not intended to serve as rigid practice parameters, yet it seems likely that opinions of acknowledged experts representing prestigious institutions will be treated as de facto consensus statements. Perhaps this is inevitable because guidelines and current practice patterns of societies or institutions have been regarded as consensus statements in the past. Nonetheless, the tentative nature of many of the recommendations is obvious, since in many instances rigorous comparison of alternative strategies for follow-up has not been conducted with prospective, controlled trials. Counterbalancing this is the fact that the referring or primary physician, who is often responsible for follow-up care, bears a heavy burden, yet may not realize the optimal follow-up plan for the patient. The individual responsible for follow-up wants to detect recurrence and new primary tumors but is not always familiar with the nuances of costs versus benefits. In addition, there are practical problems regarding what questions to ask during office visits and the constraints imposed by society, insurance companies, managed care firms, and the like. Thus the conscientious physician needs to know a great deal about follow-up for practical reasons, and this book is aimed at providing guidance in a clinical arena where practice patterns vary widely.

FUTURE OF SURVEILLANCE

Although the bulk of this text deals with organ site–specific surveillance strategies and focuses on clinical issues, the final section touches on two topics expected to increase in importance. The first is the implications of molecular medicine for cancer patient follow-up. Genetic testing can now reliably predict the development of certain types of cancer. Testing for relevant oncogenes and tumor suppressor genes in peripheral blood leukocytes,[40] feces,[41] sputum,[42] pancreatic juice,[43] and other specimens can already quantify future cancer risk or diagnose subclinical cancer. Textbooks outlining gene-level diagnostic tests in clinical medicine have begun to appear.[44] None of these techniques are in common use, but undoubtedly they will rapidly enter clinical practice once they are shown to be sensitive, specific, and affordable.

They will probably be quickly embraced by physicians and patients, since in most cases obtaining diagnostic specimens is safe, comfortable, and convenient. This will predictably result in dilemmas in patient care, as discussed earlier. What will occur when a patient being followed after lung cancer surgery turns up with molecular evidence of cancer in DNA in the sputum, for example, but no lesions on chest x-ray or bronchoscopy? Similar problems were encountered in earlier surveillance efforts like the Lung Cancer Detection Demonstration Project, when sputum cytological examination was positive but chest x-ray was unrevealing. What about the traditional follow-up tests? Will the revolution in molecular medicine render them irrelevant? Will gene-level treatments that can cure advanced cancer emerge? Such developments seem possible.

The last part of this text deals with decision analytical techniques for evaluating cancer patient follow-up strategies. Computer simulation is used to identify categories of patients who may benefit from follow-up and treatment of recurrence. It is also an inexpensive method of assessing the expected outcome of controlled randomized trials. This method is particularly applicable to the study of cancer patient follow-up because the required sample size for prospective randomized clinical trials dictates a budget often deemed too large to be fundable by any one agency.

REFERENCES

1. Thomas L. Medicine as a very old profession. In: Wyngaarden JB, Smith LH, editors. Textbook of medicine. Philadelphia: WB Saunders Company, 1988:9-12.
2. Thomas L. Becoming a doctor. In: Thomas L. The fragile species. New York: Collier Books, 1992:7-15.
3. Wangensteen OH, Wangensteen SD. The rise of surgery from empiric craft to scientific discipline. Minneapolis: University of Minnesota Press, 1978:567-72.
4. Bacon HE. Anus–rectum–sigmoid colon: diagnosis and treatment. Philadelphia: JB Lippincott Company, 1941:557-70.
5. Cecil RL, Loeb RF, Gutman AB, McDermott W, Wolff HG, editors. Textbook of medicine. 10th ed. Philadelphia: WB Saunders Company, 1959.
6. Bell ET. Tumors. In: Bell ET, editor. Textbook of pathology. 3rd ed. Philadelphia: Lea & Febiger, 1938:232-371.
7. Ewing J. Epithelial and other tumors of the breast. In: Ewing J. Neoplastic diseases. 3rd ed. Philadelphia: WB Saunders Company, 1928:546.
8. Torres CF, Rebsamen S, Silber JH, et al. Surveillance scanning of children with medulloblastoma. N Engl J Med 1994;330:892-5.
9. Halstead WS. The results of operations for the cure of cancer of the breast performed at the Johns Hopkins from June 1889 to January 1894. Arch Surg 1894;20:497-555.
10. American Joint Committee on Cancer, Beahrs OH, Henson DE, Robert VP, Kennedy BJ, editors. Manual for staging of cancer. 4th ed. Philadelphia: JB Lippincott Company, 1992.
11. Lippman SM, Benner SE, Hong WK. Cancer chemoprevention. J Clin Oncol 1994;12:851-73.
12. Vignati PV, Roberts PL. Preoperative evaluation and postoperative surveillance for patients with colorectal carcinoma. Surg Clin North Am 1993;73:67-84.
13. Vernava AM, Longo WE, Virgo KS, Coplin MA, Wade TP, Johnson FE. Current follow-up strategies after resection of colon cancer. Dis Colon Rectum 1994;37:573-83.
14. Langevin JM, Wong WD. What is appropriate follow-up for the patient with colorectal cancer? Can J Surgery 1985;28:424-8.
15. IARC Working Group. Screening for squamous cervical cancer: duration of low risk after negative results of cervical cytology and its implications for screening policies. Br Med J 1986;293:659-64.
16. Eddy DM. Screening for cervical cancer. Ann Intern Med 1990;113:214-26.
17. Moertel CG, Fleming TR, Macdonald JS, Haller DG, Laurie JA, Tangen C. An evaluation of the carcinoembryonic antigen (CEA) test for monitoring patients with resected colon cancer. JAMA 1993;270:943-7.
18. Virgo KS, Vernava AM, Longo WE, McKirgan LW, Johnson FE. Cost of patient follow-up after potentially curative colon cancer treatment. JAMA 1995;273:1837-41.
19. Naunheim KS, Virgo KS, Coplin MA, Johnson FE. Clinical surveillance testing after lung cancer operations. Ann Thorac Surg 1995;60:1612-6.
20. Loomer L, Brockschmidt JK, Muss HB, Saylor G. Postoperative follow-up of patients with early breast cancer: patterns of care among clinical oncologists and a review of the literature. Cancer 1991;67:55-60.
21. Fischer DS, editor. Follow-up of cancer. New Haven: American Cancer Society, Connecticut Division, Inc., 1990.
22. Favia G, D'Amico DF, editors. Il follow-up immediato e a distanza del malato neoplastico operato. Padova: Liviana Editrice spa, 1989.
23. Eiseman B, Robinson WA, Steele G. Follow-up of the cancer patient. New York: Thieme-Stratton, 1982.
24. GIVIO investigators. Impact of follow-up testing on survival and health-related quality of life in breast cancer patients. JAMA 1994;271:1587-92.
25. Lampic C, Wennberg A, Schill J, Brodin O, Glimelius B, Sjoden P. Anxiety and cancer-related worry of cancer patients at routine follow-up visits. Acta Oncol 1994;33:119-25.
26. Kassirer JP. Incorporating patients' preferences into medical decisions. N Engl J Med 1994;330:1895-6.
27. Morgan KZ. History of damage and protection from ionizing radiation. In: Morgan KZ, Turner JE. Principles of radiation protection: a textbook of health physics. New York: John Wiley & Sons, Inc, 1967:1-75.
28. Beatson GT. On the treatment of inoperable cases of carcinoma of the mamma: suggestions for a new method of treatment. Lancet 1896;2:104-7.
29. DeVita VT. The evolution of therapeutic research in cancer. N Engl J Med 1978;298:907-10.
30. Department of Veterans Affairs Laryngeal Cancer Study Group. Induction chemotherapy plus radiation compared with surgery plus radiation in patients with advanced laryngeal cancer. N Engl J Med 1991;324:1685-90.
31. Wood WC, Budman DR, Korzun AH, et al. Dose and dose intensity of adjuvant chemotherapy for stage II, node-positive breast carcinoma. N Engl J Med 1994;330:1253-9.
32. Moertel CG, Fleming TR, Macdonald JS, et al. Levamisole and fluorouracil for adjuvant therapy of resected colon carcinoma. N Engl J Med 1990;322:352-8.
33. Roentgen WC. On a new kind of rays (translation). Br J Radiol 1931;4:32.
34. Russell LB. Screening for cervical cancer. In: Educated guesses: making policy about medical screening tests. Los Angeles: University of California Press, 1994:6-24.
35. Black WD, Welch HG. Advances in diagnostic imaging and overestimations of disease prevalence and the benefits of therapy. N Engl J Med 1993;328:1237-43.
36. Harach HR, Franssila KO, Wasenius V. Occult papillary carcinoma of the thyroid: a "normal" finding in Finland: a systematic autopsy study. Cancer 1985;56:531-8.
37. Feinstein AR, Sosin DN, Wells CK. Will Rogers phenomenon: stage migration and new diagnostic techniques as a source of misleading statistics for survival in cancer. N Engl J Med 1985;312:1604-8.

38. Montie JE, Wood DP, Pontes E, Boyett JM, Levin HS. Adenocarcinoma of the prostate in cystoprostatectomy specimens removed for bladder cancer. Cancer 1989;63:381-5.
39. Habbema JDF, Van Ineveld BM, DeKoning HJ. A cost-effectiveness approach to breast cancer screening. In: Miller AB, Chamberlain J, Day NE, Hakama M, Prorak PC, editors. Cancer screening. Cambridge: Cambridge University Press, 1991.
40. Krontiris TG, Devlin B, Karp DD, Robert NJ, Risch N. An association between the risk of cancer and mutation in the HRASI minisatellite locus. N Engl J Med 1993;329:517-23.
41. Sidransky D, Tokino T, Hamilton SR, et al. Identification of oncogene mutations in the stool of curable colorectal tumors. Science 1992;256:102-5.
42. Mao L, Hruban RH, Boyle J, Tockman M, Sidransky D. Detection of oncogene mutations in sputum precedes diagnosis of lung cancer. Cancer Res 1994;54:1634-7.
43. Tada M, Ornata M, Kawai S, et al. Detection of ras gene mutations in pancreatic juice and peripheral blood of patients with pancreatic adenocarcinoma. Cancer Res 1993;53:2472-4.
44. Bernstam VA. Handbook of gene level diagnostics in clinical practice. Boca Raton, Florida: CRC Press, 1992.

CHAPTER 2

Assessment of Surveillance Test Performance and Cost

St. Louis University Health Sciences Center ▪ St. Louis Department of Veterans Affairs Medical Center

KATHERINE S. VIRGO AND FRANK E. JOHNSON

For several reasons, surveillance test performance and costs are important considerations for a book summarizing the state of the art in cancer patient management after completion of primary treatment. The first reason is the growing concern about more efficient use of limited resources, made more apparent by the health reform debate. Second is the expanding role of "gatekeepers," who wield increasing control over the cost of health care. Third is the push for clinicians to develop guidelines, adherence to which could subsequently be tied to reimbursement.

Given such issues and the high cost of cancer patient care, one would expect to see a plethora of articles assessing strategies to increase efficacy, efficiency, and cost effectiveness, but few exist. One reason for the shortage of articles may be that the appropriate patient management strategy after curative treatment is not well delineated for many cancers. Many articles on cancer patient follow-up suggest strategies based on inadequate sample size or on no data at all. Few proposed patient management strategies are based on the results of large retrospective analyses of secondary datasets or prospective, randomized, clinical trials.

Another reason for the shortage of articles may be that few clinicians sufficiently understand epidemiological and cost analysis methodologies. Therefore this chapter reviews the tools needed to weigh alternative follow-up strategies. The epidemiology section describes how to determine whether screening for disease is appropriate in a given population, assess the performance of individual diagnostic tests, compare performance across diagnostic tests, and decide whether further diagnostic testing is required. The economics section specifies how to calculate and compare the costs and benefits of individual diagnostic tests or entire follow-up strategies.

EPIDEMIOLOGICAL PRINCIPLES FOR EVALUATING DIAGNOSTIC TEST PERFORMANCE IN SCREENING FOR DISEASE

Overview

Epidemiology is the study of the frequency and determinants of disease and injury in human populations.[1] While clinical medicine focuses on the delivery of medical care to patients, epidemiology analyzes why different populations have differing incidences and prevalences of disease. Incidence refers to the probability that individuals without disease will develop disease over a given time period and is calculated as the number of new cases of disease divided by the population at risk. Prevalence refers to the number of people in a population who already have the disease and is calculated as the number of existing cases of disease divided by the total population. Clinical epidemiology focuses on the application of epidemiological principles to the practice of clinical medicine. This section of Chapter 2 uses basic principles of epidemiology to assess diagnostic test performance in screening for disease.

Screening

Asymptomatic patients rarely seek care unless participating in a regular surveillance program. When symptoms do appear, patients often delay seeking care for an extended period, by which time it is too late for curative treatment. It is generally believed that early detection through screening tests improves the probability of cure and reduces the probabilities of both death and disability.

Screening is the use of tests or examinations to distinguish asymptomatic individuals with a high probability of disease from asymptomatic individuals with a low probability of disease. Some screening programs are designed to identify individuals who might not have disease now but have a high probability of developing it in the future. Screening tests are usually quick, minimally invasive, and inexpensive. Screening or surveillance is generally performed among populations who have not previously been diagnosed with the disease under evaluation. However, the term "surveillance" is also used to refer to the follow-up of patients after primary treatment of disease to detect, as in the case of cancer, recurrences or second primaries. Although the term "screening" is used throughout this section, the same concepts apply to both screening and surveillance.

Diagnostic Test Characteristics

Validity

Important characteristics of screening tests are validity, reliability, and yield. Validity refers to the ability of a test to distinguish between those who have disease and those who do

Table 2-1 Derivation of sensitivity and specificity

	DISEASE CATEGORY	
SCREENING TEST RESULT	DISEASE PRESENT	DISEASE ABSENT
Positive	*a* (TP)	*b* (FP)
Negative	*c* (FN)	*d* (TN)

Sensitivity = $a / (a + c)$ = TP / (TP + FN).
Specificity = $d / (b + d)$ = TN / (FP + TN).

not. The two measures of validity are sensitivity and specificity. Sensitivity, often referred to as the true-positive rate (TPR), measures the ability of the test to identify those who actually have disease. Sensitivity is calculated as the percentage of all patients with disease who screen positive for disease. Specificity, also referred to as the true-negative rate (TNR), measures the ability of the test to identify those who do not have disease. Specificity is calculated as the percentage of all patients without disease who screen negative for disease.[1]

Table 2-1 depicts the derivation of sensitivity and specificity.[2] Patients who are correctly predicted by the diagnostic test of interest to have disease are referred to as true positives (TP), and those who are correctly predicted to be disease free are referred to as true negatives (TN). Patients falsely predicted to have disease are false positives (FP), and those falsely predicted to be disease free are false negatives (FN). Once the sensitivity and specificity of a diagnostic test are known, clinicians can use these estimates to revise the estimates of the probability of disease that were made before the diagnostic test was ordered (pretest probability). According to a principle known as Bayes' theorem, posttest probability can be calculated as:

$$P_r = \frac{(P_i)\,(\text{Sensitivity})}{(P_i)\,(\text{Sensitivity}) + (1 - P_i)\,(100\% - \text{Specificity})}$$

where P_r is the posttest probability and P_i is the pretest probability. Tabular and graphic expressions of Bayes' theorem are also available, such as Bayes' nomogram and Benish's tables, which permit one to look up the posttest probability once the pretest probability, sensitivity, and specificity are known.[3,4]

Sensitivity and specificity are derived by comparing the results from the test in question (the index test) with those of a definitive test (a gold standard test). Irrespective of the results of the screen (positive or negative), in most cases every person screened must be tested using the gold standard to establish or rule out disease.[5,6] The optimal test would be 100% specific and 100% sensitive. Unfortunately, this is not observed in practice because sensitivity and specificity usually are inversely related. In other words, sensitivity can be improved, but only at the expense of specificity, and specificity can be improved, but only at the expense of sensitivity.

The relationship between sensitivity and specificity can be understood by viewing the range of diagnostic test results that can be considered either normal or abnormal, as depicted by the overlapping bell-shaped curves in Figure 2-1. If the range of overlapping values is 20 to 40 and the line distinguishing normal from abnormal test results is drawn so that 20 and above is considered abnormal, the screening intervention will have high sensitivity because all patients with diagnostic test results in the 20 and above range will be treated as positives. However, the intervention will have low specificity because many of the results treated as positive will turn out to be FPs. Alternatively, if the line distinguishing normal from abnormal test results is redrawn so that 40 and above is considered abnormal and all other values are considered normal, the screening intervention will have low sensitivity and high specificity because all patients with diagnostic test results in the 39 and below range will be treated as negatives.

Other factors that influence measurement of the validity of a test are the severity of disease and the presence of comorbid conditions. With some diagnostic tests, such as the serological test for syphilis, the probability of an FN is very high in the early or very late stages of disease.[1] The presence of comorbid conditions and drugs taken for these conditions can also greatly influence diagnostic test results.

In addition to a diagnostic test's sensitivity and specificity, the test's ability to discriminate correctly between the presence and absence of disease depends on the prevalence of disease. The greater the prevalence of disease, the greater the predictive value (PV) of a positive test, which is the probability that a positive test result is accurately predicting disease. As prevalence approaches zero, the PV of a positive test approaches zero. The PV of a positive test is calculated as $a / (a + b)$ or TP / (TP + FP). According to Bayes' theorem of conditional probabilities, the PV of a positive test can also be calculated as (sensitivity × prevalence) / [(sensitivity × prevalence) + (1 - specificity) × (1 - prevalence)].[7] The PV of a negative test is $d / (c + d)$ or TN / (FN + TN). According to Vecchio,[8] the prevalence of a disease must be at least 15% to 20% to reach an acceptable PV (70% to 80%).

Reliability

The second important characteristic of screening tests is reliability or precision. Reliability measures whether the same test administered more than once to the same person will produce the same results repetitively. The two types of vari-

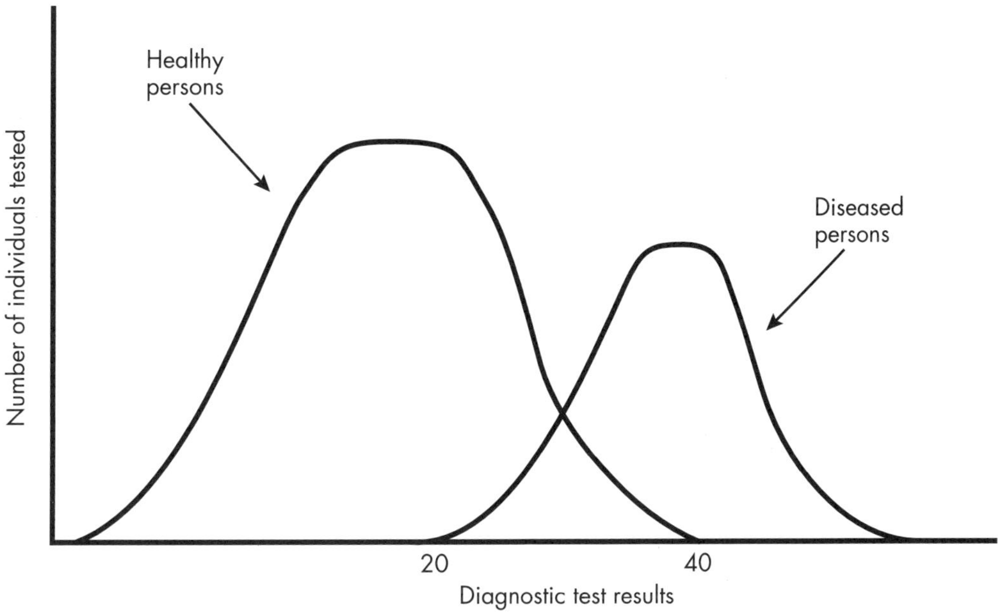

Figure 2-1 Distribution of diagnostic test results.

ation that can occur are variation in the method itself and variation related to the person(s) interpreting the results. Variation in method can be due to mechanical fluctuations (fluctuations in the testing apparatus) or fluctuations in the substance being measured by the diagnostic test. Variation caused by interpretation of the results can be classified into two types. Intraobserver variation is variation occurring when one person interprets the results differently on different occasions. Interobserver variation is variation across different persons interpreting the results.[9] Such variation can be substantially reduced through training seminars and use of independent observations on a subsample of cases.

Yield

The third important characteristic of screening tests is yield, which refers to the number of cases with previously undiagnosed disease that are detected and treated as a result of the screen. Yield is affected by the sensitivity of the diagnostic test, the prevalence of unrecognized disease, whether the screening is multiphasic (multiple diagnostic tests were administered), screening frequency, and the number of persons screening positive who actually receive treatment.[1] The effect of sensitivity on yield is that if few TPs are identified, the other factors become immaterial because yield will be low. If the prevalence of unrecognized disease is low because of such factors as high availability of medical care or recent screening of the population, the yield will be low.

The ability to identify risk factors for the disease and, using these, to reduce the number of individuals who must be screened will increase yield. Another way to increase yield is through multiphasic screening, in which a variety of tests are used to screen for multiple conditions in one visit.

Frequency of Screening

On the issue of screening frequency, the literature is not clear. Frequency should be dictated by the natural history of the disease, the incidence of disease, and risk factors. Whether a patient with identified disease will consent to treatment is determined by whether the patient believes there is a serious threat to health, feels vulnerable, and decides that seeking treatment will be beneficial.[1]

Likelihood Ratios

A way to measure the performance of a diagnostic test that has not yet been discussed is the use of likelihood ratios. To understand likelihood ratios, which are a type of odds ratio, one must understand the difference between probability and odds. Probability ranges from zero to one and measures the likelihood that a particular outcome will occur. A value close to zero indicates little chance of occurrence; a value close to one indicates a large chance of occurrence. If an experiment is conducted n times and the event of interest occurs m times, the probability of that event occurring is calculated as m/n.[10] Sensitivity and specificity are both measures of the probabilities that specific events will occur.

Odds are ratios of two probabilities and are calculated as the probability of an event/(1 - the probability of an event).[7] One can also work backwards and calculate probability from odds using the following equation: odds/(1 + odds). Likelihood ratios measure how much more likely it is that a diagnosis will be made in the presence of disease than in the absence of disease and can be defined for any number of test results over the entire range of possible values. For positive and negative test results the respective likelihood ratios are sensitivity/(1 - specificity) and (1 - sensitivity)/specificity.[11]

Use of likelihood ratios has the advantage of placing more weight on very high and very low test results than on borderline results when the odds that a disease is really present are being determined. In comparison to sensitivity and specificity measures, likelihood ratios also have the advantage that diagnostic test performance is quantified as one measure rather than two. A disadvantage of likelihood ratios is that the conversion from probability to odds and back again can be difficult.

Requirements for Establishing a Screening Program

Several major prerequisites for establishing a screening program have been identified by Wilson and Jungner.[12] Among these are that the health problem be important, that the disease have either a latent stage or an early treatable stage, that a diagnostic test acceptable to the population be available, that the natural history of the condition be sufficiently understood, that treatment be available for identified cases, that curatively treatable cases be clearly identifiable, and that screening be cost effective.

Receiver Operating Characteristic Curve

Once the need for a screening program is established and the appropriate diagnostic test is selected, the next step is to clarify how test results will be interpreted. Complicating the situation is that such factors as age, sex, race, and nutrition can influence laboratory test results. For example, what is normal for a 70-year-old male may not be normal for a 25-year-old female. Although what is considered normal can vary by patient, the distribution of clinical measurements for an individual is generally represented by a normally distributed (bell-shaped) curve.[13] The dispersion of values around the mean in a normal distribution is due to random variation alone.

In addition to variation among subjects in what is normal and abnormal, the cutoff between normal and abnormal for a given diagnostic test can be varied given the goals of the screening intervention. If the goal is to identify, for example, 95% of all cases of disease, the range of values constituting an abnormal test result can be expanded until this goal is reached. Unfortunately, doing so causes the number of false-positive results to increase, thus decreasing specificity, since sensitivity and specificity are inversely related. Similarly, if the goal is to identify 95% of all persons without disease, the range of values constituting a normal test result can be expanded until this goal is reached. However, increased specificity is achieved at the expense of decreased sensitivity.

When diagnostic test results by patient are depicted graphically for both healthy and diseased individuals (Figure 2-1), there is usually a range of values that is clearly normal and another that is clearly abnormal. However, there is also a range of values that could easily represent either normal or abnormal results, as depicted by the overlapping bell-shaped curves. Figure 2-1 shows how the selected cutoff between normal and abnormal determines the sensitivity and specificity of a test.

Receiver operating characteristic (ROC) curves are used to depict the trade-off between TPR, or sensitivity, and FPR, or 1 - specificity.[14] Unlike the limited information provided by a single estimate of sensitivity and specificity for one possible cutoff point between normal and abnormal, ROC curves are more useful because they depict the complete range of possible TPR/FPR trade-offs corresponding to all possible cutoffs between normal and abnormal. Derived from signal detection theory, ROC curves plot sensitivity on the vertical axis and 1 - specificity on the horizontal axis (Figure 2-2).[15] For all points along the 45-degree line, sensitivity equals 1 - specificity. Points on this line have no impact on the probability of disease. The probability of disease increases for points above the 45-degree line and decreases for points below the line. The points on the curve are calculated as sensitivity/(1 - specificity). Each point on the curve represents a different selected cutoff point between normal and abnormal. The perfect curve would extend straight from the origin to the upper left-hand corner and then over to the upper right-hand corner, maximizing the area under the curve (AUC).[16] The AUC is considered an index of diagnostic performance.[17] If two tests are being compared statistically, the test with the greater AUC is considered the better test.[18-23] A perfect diagnostic test has an AUC of 1.0. Some authors consider the AUC concept, and ROC curve analysis in general, not very useful because prevalence is not incorporated.[2]

ROC curve analysis can also be used to identify the appropriate cutoff point between normal and abnormal.[24,25] Clinicians generally use the "upper limit of normal" provided by the laboratory. Sox et al.[24] suggest that the ROC curve method is better, but its use is severely limited by the time needed to perform the analysis.

Thresholds for Treatment

Once it has been decided whether a test is normal or abnormal, the next issue is whether sufficient testing has been completed to make a diagnosis. If no further testing is required, treatment can begin. The goal here is to determine the point at which acquisition of additional information would have no effect on the diagnosis. Major determining factors in this decision are the probability of disease and the penalty for being wrong. If the probability of disease is high and the margin for error is wide, the willingness to make a diagnosis will also be high. However, if the probability of disease is low and the margin for error is slim, the need for more information will be high and the willingness to make a diagnosis will be low.

A term commonly used to describe the dividing line between a decision to treat or not to treat is the treatment threshold. The treatment threshold, p^*, is the probability of disease at which the clinician is indifferent between treating and withholding treatment.[24] If the probability of disease for a given patient is above the treatment threshold, treatment will be selected because the acquisition of more information will not change the diagnosis. If the probability of disease is

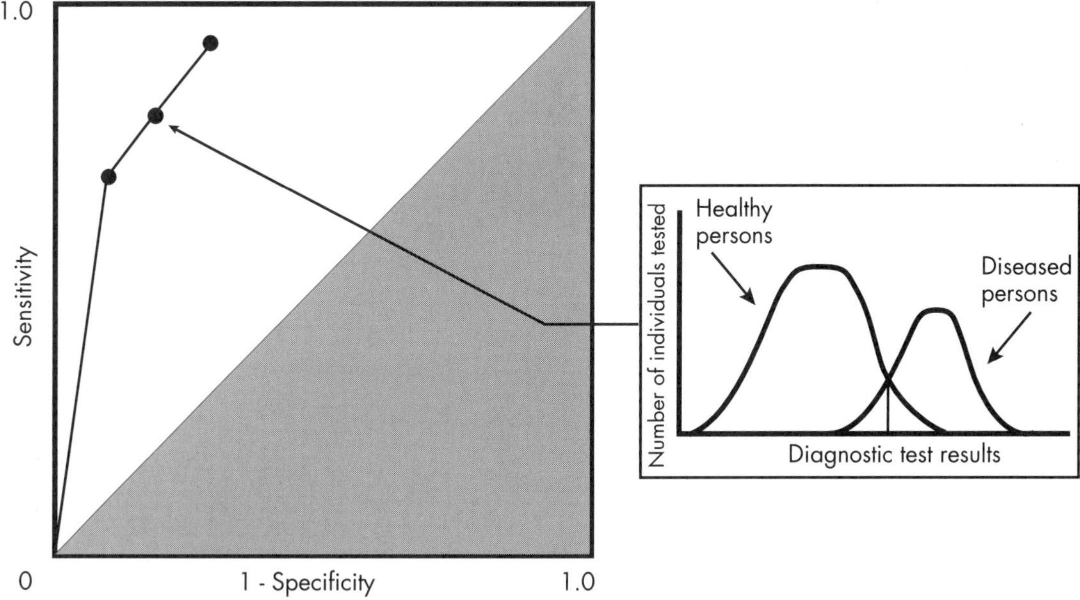

Figure 2-2 Receiver operating characteristics curve depicting the trade-off between sensitivity and 1 - specificity. (From Sox HC, Blatt MA, Higgins HC, Marton KI. Medical decision making. Boston: Butterworths, 1988.)

below the treatment threshold, treatment will be withheld and more testing may be ordered (or no action may be taken).

The treatment threshold can be depicted graphically with the probability of disease on the horizontal axis and the expected utility of the treatment on the vertical axis (Figure 2-3). Utility is defined here as the value or the level of well-being an individual assigns to a given option. The treatment threshold is calculated by solving for p^* in the following equation:

$$\frac{p^*}{1 - p^*} = \frac{U[D\text{-}T\text{-}] - U[D\text{-}T\text{+}]}{U[D\text{+}T\text{+}] - U[D\text{+}T\text{-}]}$$

where U = utility, D- = absence of disease, D+ = presence of disease, T- = withholding treatment, T+ = providing treatment, $U[D\text{-}T\text{-}]$ = the utility of withholding treatment in the absence of disease, $U[D\text{-}T\text{+}]$ = the utility of providing treatment in the absence of disease, $U[D\text{+}T\text{+}]$ = the utility of providing treatment in the presence of disease, and $U[D\text{+}T\text{-}]$ = the utility of withholding treatment in the presence of disease. The line defined by the points *A, C,* and *E* in Figure 2-3 represents the utility of withholding treatment irrespective of whether disease is present or absent. The line defined by the points *B, C,* and *D* represents the utility of providing treatment irrespective of whether disease is present or absent. The point of intersection between these two lines is the treatment threshold. At this point the utilities of the two choices are equal.

The above equation can also be rephrased in terms of costs and benefits, still solving for the treatment threshold, p^*. The difference in utility between treating and not treating patients without disease can be considered a cost, *C*, because no benefit derives from treating these patients. Similarly, the difference between treating and not treating patients with disease can be considered a benefit, *B*. The previous equation would then be simplified to $p^* = C/(C + B)$.[24]

Thresholds for Testing

Up to this point only the threshold between treating and withholding treatment has been discussed. There are two other thresholds: the no-treatment-test threshold and the treatment-test threshold.[26] The no-treatment-test threshold, p_1, is the probability of disease at which there is indifference between no treatment and further diagnostic testing. The treatment-test threshold, p_2, is the probability of disease at which there is indifference between treatment and further diagnostic testing. A third line can be plotted on Figure 2-3 to depict these testing thresholds (Figure 2-4). The testing thresholds are calculated as follows:

$$p_1 = \frac{p^* \times \text{FPR} - p^* \times (U[\text{Test}] / (U[D\text{-}T\text{-}] - U[D\text{-}T\text{+}]))}{p^* \times \text{FPR} + (1 - p^*) \times \text{TPR}}$$

$$p_2 = \frac{p^* \times \text{TNR} + p^* \times (U[\text{Test}] / (U[D\text{-}T\text{-}] - U[D\text{-}T\text{+}]))}{p^* \times \text{TNR} + (1 - p^*) \times \text{FNR}}$$

where FPR = the false positive rate or 1 - specificity, FNR = the false negative rate or 1 - sensitivity, TNR = the true negative rate or specificity, TPR = the true positive rate or sensitivity, and U [Test] represents the net utility of the diagnostic test as determined by the patient's assessment of the test regarding such factors as cost, potential side effects, unpleasantness, and reassurance provided by having the test performed.[24] (The remaining variables have already been defined.)

Below p_1, treatment is never preferred because the infor-

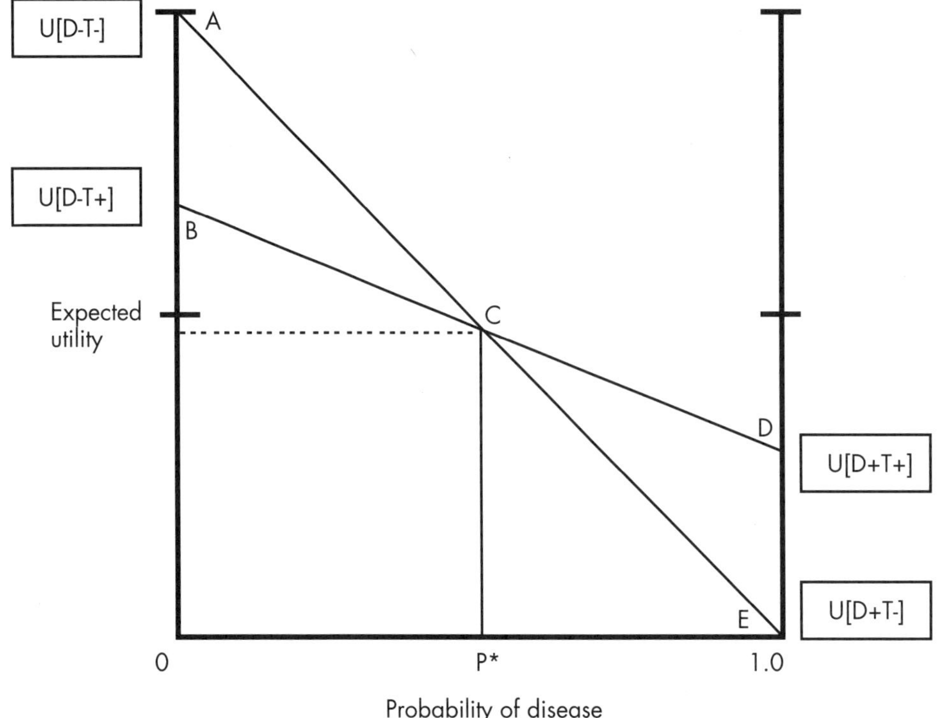

Figure 2-3 Treatment threshold or the point of intersection between providing treatment and withholding treatment–irrespective of whether disease is present or absent. (From Sox HC, Blatt MA, Higgins MC, Marton KI. Medical decision making. Boston: Butterworths, 1988.)

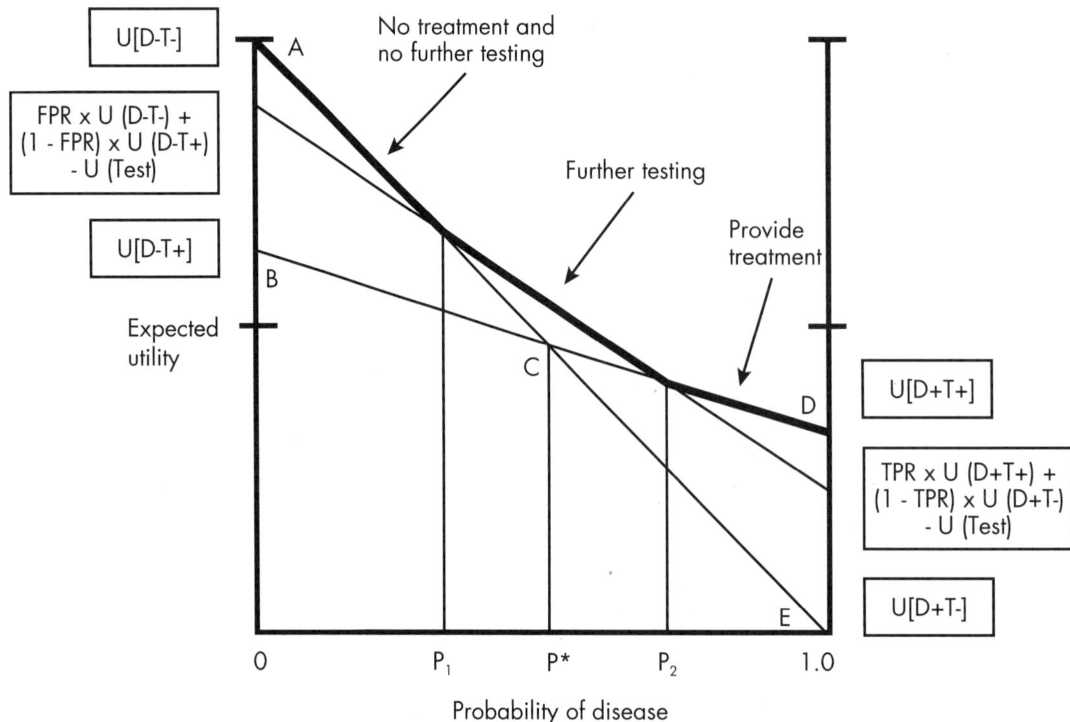

Figure 2-4 Depiction of the no-treatment-test threshold, p_1, and the treatment-test threshold, p_2. (From Sox HC, Blatt MA, Higgins MC, Marton KI. Medical decision making. Boston: Butterworths, 1988.)

mation to be gained from additional testing would not increase the probability of disease sufficiently to cross the treatment threshold. Above p_2, treatment is always preferred because the information gained from additional testing would not decrease the probability of disease sufficiently to cross the treatment threshold. Only for the range of disease probabilities between p_1 and p_2 could an abnormal test result influence disease probability enough to cross the treatment threshold and change patient management.

The same analysis developed in the discussion of treatment thresholds and expanded in the discussion of testing thresholds can be expanded still further to permit choosing among two or more diagnostic tests or selecting combinations of diagnostic tests. For a more in-depth discussion of these topics, refer to Sox et al.[24] For an application of threshold analysis to cases where a single diagnostic test provides information about more than one event, specifically the case of computed tomography in providing information about both mediastinal and hilar metastases in lung cancer, see Nease et al.[27] For an adaptation of Bayes' nomogram to threshold analysis, see Glasziou.[28]

ECONOMIC PRINCIPLES OF FOLLOW-UP EVALUATION

Overview of Cost Analysis

Clinicians, health administrators, and other decision makers in the health field are faced with the problem of appropriating limited resources to cover an ever-growing number of health needs. For what illnesses should every patient be automatically screened? How much follow-up is sufficient after primary treatment of a condition? If personnel dollars are short, where should cuts be made and what trade-offs should decision makers be willing to make? The need to clarify the decision-making process and promote efficiency is the reason that economic evaluation (also known as efficiency evaluation) methodologies were developed. The three most widely used methods for assessing the relative merit of alternative courses of action are cost-effectiveness analysis (CEA), cost-benefit analysis (CBA), and utility analysis.[29,30] This section of the chapter provides an overview of these methods, followed by a discussion of concepts common to all three. The differences among the methods are discussed in detail in subsequent sections.

Briefly, CEA places priorities on alternative expenditures without requiring that the dollar value of life and health be assessed.[31] Some benefits are measured in nonmonetary units. CEA is usually the method of choice unless there is no single, quantifiable unit by which alternatives can be compared, in which case CBA is the method of choice.

CBA requires the valuation of all outcomes in economic terms, including lives or years of life and morbidity.[32-34] This analysis, which is often viewed as a subset of CEA, assumes a goal of economic efficiency. Economic efficiency is defined as providing each unit of output at minimum possible cost.[35] In CBA, total costs minus total benefits equals net benefit.

Utility analysis or cost-utility analysis is very similar to CEA and is often treated as a special type of CEA. The main difference with utility analysis is that benefits must be converted into quality adjusted life years (QALYs), a measure of years of life gained from an intervention that is then weighted to reflect the quality of life in each year.[36]

Subjectivity is important in any type of economic evaluation. Different analysts performing basically the same analysis can easily reach very different conclusions. This can be confusing to the novice. However, the variation in conclusions is tied directly to differences in the assumptions made in the design of the evaluation. Different conclusions do not imply that one analysis is correct and the other incorrect. They just imply that different assumptions were made.

Selection of Perspective

A first step in any economic evaluation is selecting the perspective from which the analysis will be performed. Such analyses are generally performed from a societal perspective, but other, narrower perspectives often apply, such as the provider's perspective, the payor's perspective, or the patient's perspective. Which perspective is selected guides the identification of costs and benefits. For example, an insurance company will evaluate a new health prevention from a payor's perspective with respect to the change in total future costs, whereas a societal perspective would assign some inherent value to illness prevented.

Specification of the Problem

The second step is specifying the problem, objective(s), and alternatives. This would seem obvious at first glance. However, if the problem is not well delineated, the range of alternatives selected to address the problem may be too narrow, ignoring important alternatives. For example, if in the case of cancer patients the problem is defined as the suffering undergone by current patients, only treatment alternatives will be considered. However, if the problem is defined as affecting both current and future patients, options such as delaying or preventing the onset of disease will also be considered in the analysis.

Production Function

The third step is describing the production function. In economics, the production function is the relationship between the output of a good or service and the inputs required to produce it. The goal of this step is to specify the resources that would be used under each of the alternatives, the way in which the resources would be combined, and the expected result. Completion of this step will allow the analyst to begin calculating costs and benefits. Complexity is not synonymous with accuracy, although models often become complex quickly.

Warner and Luce[29] mention six issues that must be considered in the development of the production model. First, economies of scale may exist that cause fewer and fewer inputs to be required as sample size increases to produce the same level of output per person. In other words, an intervention that cost $25,000 for 1,000 patients may cost only $35,000 for 5,000 patients. Second, if technological change is occurring or is expected, this must be built into the model. If, while future costs of cancer patient follow-up using currently available diagnostic tests are being projected, preliminary results are published of a new follow-up methodology that may replace one or more of the existing tests, the effect of substituting this test must be factored into the analysis. Third, market characteristics may affect the inputs required to produce a given output, causing the required inputs to vary by geographical location. For example, geographical differences in pay rates for health care personnel or variation in the supply of personnel may cause an intervention to be more expensive in one city than in another. Fourth, populations may differ in compliance with an intervention. More costly follow-up mechanisms may then be required to achieve the desired effect. Fifth, efficiency cannot always be assumed. The fact that a task has always been done one way does not mean that way is the most efficient. Sixth, some inputs are unique to a particular facility. If attempting to model an intervention at one facility after an existing one at a second facility, one must ensure that all the inputs are available or can be made available at the first facility.

Once the production function is specified, costs and benefits can be calculated. Costs can be direct, indirect, or intangible. Direct costs are defined as variable costs plus fixed (overhead) costs. In the health sector, the terms "direct medical costs" and "direct nonmedical costs" are often used. Direct medical costs are the costs directly related to the provision of care and usually involve monetary transactions, such as physicians' fees, nurses' salaries, drug purchases, equipment purchases, and independent laboratory processing fees. Direct nonmedical costs are costs incurred in the process of seeking care, such as the patient's costs of transportation to the hospital or clinic, parking costs, hotel costs if the patient cannot return home each evening because of distance, the costs of special equipment in the home to accommodate a disabled family member, and child care costs.[37]

Indirect costs are defined as the costs of foregone opportunities. These include the costs of morbidity and mortality. The indirect costs of morbidity are typically measured as time lost from work and the resulting wages foregone or production losses. In addition, morbidity includes the costs associated with an increased risk of complications. Similarly, the indirect costs of mortality can be measured as time lost from work, since premature death causes permanent removal from the work force.

Intangible costs are defined as the psychological costs of illness such as pain, suffering, and grief. These are the most difficult costs to measure.

Benefits can also be divided into the three categories of direct, indirect, or intangible. Benefits are often considered savings in costs. Direct benefits are tangible savings in health resource utilization, such as decreased length of stay or diagnostic test utilization. Indirect benefits are earnings not lost, such as the avoidance of premature death or disability. Intangible benefits include the avoidance of pain, discomfort, and grief not only by the patient, but by family and friends as well. Depending on the perspective from which the analysis is performed, an item may be a cost in one analysis but a benefit (that is, a cost averted) in another.

The next three sections describe in greater depth the types of economic evaluation. CEA is presented first.

Cost-Effectiveness Analysis

To understand CEA, one needs to understand the term "cost-effective." To be cost effective, an intervention must be worth the money required to conduct it. "Cost-effective" is not always synonymous with "inexpensive" or "technically efficient," although the term is often used in this fashion. Cost effectiveness is based on the concept of opportunity cost. The real cost of an intervention or treatment is the value of the alternative uses of the same resources.[29]

The goal in CEA is to determine which alternative intervention or treatment yields the greatest benefits for the lowest cost. There is no requirement that costs and benefits be measured in the same units. Some benefits are measured in nonmonetary units, such as years of life saved or disability days avoided. Indirect economic benefits are generally ignored. Unlike CBA, CEA does not allow a comparison of interventions or treatments with different outcome measures. In addition, it does not generate sufficient results to determine what dollar value per year of life saved is an acceptable level of investment.

The steps in CEA are:

1. Define the problem and the objective(s) to be attained.
2. Identify alternative solutions.
3. Identify the costs of solving the problem under each alternative and all relevant benefits.
4. Compare the alternatives on the basis of prespecified criteria and select the best alternative.

Although CEA is considered simpler than CBA because benefits do not need to be expressed in monetary terms, CEA has its share of methodological problems. The first difficulty arises if there is more than one benefit and different units of measure apply to each benefit. The benefits are not additive and therefore must be analyzed separately. The next problem is how to interpret the results if the separate analyses produce contrary results. A third difficulty in CEA arises when costs and benefits accrue over a period longer than 1 year. Both costs and benefits would need to be discounted to present value. This can easily be achieved for costs, as explained in the CBA section below. The problem arises in discounting benefits, since these are not measured in monetary terms.

Cost-Benefit Analysis

Cost-Benefit Analysis Versus Cost-Effectiveness Analysis

CBA was previously considered a superior analysis to CEA because of its simplicity in valuing all costs and benefits in dollars. CBA is now considered inferior to CEA by some researchers, because it ignores the noneconomic aspects of a program or intervention. The steps in CBA are[38]:

1. Define the problem and the objective(s) to be attained.
2. Identify alternative solutions.

3. Identify the costs of solving the problem under each alternative and all relevant benefits.
4. Assign monetary values to the costs and benefits.
5. Discount future streams of costs and benefits to net present value if costs and benefits accrue over a period longer than 1 year.
6. Compare total present values.
7. Interpret the results.

The first three steps are identical to those in CEA. However, the assignment of monetary values to all costs and benefits represents a major difference between CBA and CEA. As discussed in more detail in a subsequent section, CBA requires that a dollar value be assigned to life years saved. This issue has been quite controversial over the years.

The next step is to discount all future streams of costs and benefits to their net present value if costs and benefits accrue over a period longer than 1 year. Discounting is particularly important if one of the alternatives being compared has future costs and benefits and the other does not. The concept of discounting derives from the fact that time makes a difference. A dollar received today is worth more than a dollar to be received next year because a dollar received today could be invested and earn interest, so that by next year it would be worth \$1.05, assuming a 5% interest rate. On the other hand, a dollar to be received next year is worth only \$.95 today, assuming the same rate of interest. The equation for calculating the present value is:

$$PV = FV/(1 + r)^t$$

where PV = present value, FV = costs or benefits to be incurred in the future, r = discount rate, and t = number of years into the future when the costs or benefits are expected to be incurred. The selection of the appropriate discount rate should be a function of the rate of inflation, the perspective of the analysis, and the political process as a means of reflecting social values.[39]

The last two steps in the analysis are to compare present values and interpret the results. A benefit-cost ratio can be calculated as the present value of total benefits divided by the present value of total costs. In comparing two interventions, the intervention with the highest benefit-cost ratio would be considered as returning greater benefit per dollar of cost. The difference between the present value of total benefits and the present value of total costs (the net benefit) is another measure commonly used to compare interventions.

Valuation of Life

A controversial issue that often comes up in CBA is how to estimate the value of human life in dollar terms.[40,41] This is an extremely difficult task. A number of methodologies have been suggested in the literature, with no single method considered the most correct. The two major approaches for valuing life are the willingness-to-pay approach and the human capital approach. Factors to consider in valuing life include income potential, age, quality of life, number of dependents, productivity, personal preference (religion), and personal habits.

The willingness-to-pay approach is based on how much a person is willing to pay to avoid sacrificing lives. The two methods of valuing lives under the willingness-to-pay approach are the questionnaire method and the risk premium method. The questionnaire method is self-explanatory in that it entails surveying individuals to determine their willingness to pay. The problem with the questionnaire method is that respondents have little incentive to answer truthfully. However, it is easy to obtain data in the format required for analysis because the analyst has control over design of the instrument.

In contrast to the questionnaire method in which individuals are surveyed regarding their willingness to pay, the risk premium method entails observing actual behavior. For example, if people work in riskier jobs, do they really get paid more and what does that say about how they value life? Often people assume high-risk jobs because they have few job opportunities elsewhere. Other examples of high-risk behavior include smoking, drinking alcohol, and eating hazardous foods. While activities that increase the risk of certain death are generally intolerable to individuals, activities that increase the risk of uncertain death are apparently not.[42]

An alternative method for valuing life is the human capital approach, which is productivity based and ignores the costs associated with the pain and suffering avoided by averting illness and prolonging life. The term "human capital" refers to the fact that individuals, like capital equipment, can be expected to yield productive activity over their lifetimes that can be valued at their wage rate.[43] There are three methods of valuing human life under the human capital approach: discounted future earnings, discounted consumption, and discounted net production. The discounted future earnings method involves discounting to present value all earnings that would be realized as a result of the prolongation of life or the avoidance of a disabling illness. The advantages of the discounted earnings method are that it is reasonably objective and easy to compute. The discounted consumption method calculates a person's value of life by estimating a person's lifetime consumption of goods and services and discounting it back, resulting in a conservative estimate of the value of life. The discounted net production method, a method often used in malpractice suits, combines discounted consumption with discounted earnings. The problem with this method is that the result may be a negative number because the present value of an individual's future consumption may be more than the present value of an individual's future earnings. Of all the human capital approach methodologies, the discounted net production method clearly results in the lowest estimate of the value of life.

Utility Analysis

Utility Analysis Versus Cost-Effectiveness Analysis

Utility analysis or cost-utility analysis is similar to CEA and is often treated as a special type of CEA. Relevant benefits include final outcomes, such as years of life saved or disability days averted. The difference is that in utility analysis these benefits must be converted into QALYs or, as some have suggested, healthy-years equivalents.[44,45] Therefore some benefits that would be included in a CEA, such as cases found or patients correctly treated, cannot be considered in a utility analysis because they cannot be converted into QALYs. The difference between years of life saved and QALYs saved relates to the quality of life of the patient whose life was saved. Having one's life saved and being in a wheelchair should be valued much differently from having one's life saved and being healthy. The results of utility analyses are usually expressed as cost per QALY gained.

There are several circumstances in which utility analysis has particular applicability. These circumstances are (1) if quality of life is an important outcome; (2) if both morbidity and mortality are affected by the intervention and the preference is for a single outcome combining both effects; and (3) if multiple alternative programs are being compared with a wide variety of outcome measures, since the use of utility analysis would simplify the evaluation by converting all outcomes to one unit of measure.[30]

Utility Values for Health States

The most time-consuming task in a utility analysis is determining utility values for health states. Utility is broadly defined in economics as the value an individual assigns to a given option. In health care it is generally defined as the level of well-being experienced in a given health state. While these values could be estimated or possibly obtained from the literature, the best way to determine utility values for health states is to measure them directly.[46] There are different schools of thought on what populations should be used to measure utilities. One approach is to identify a population with the condition of interest and measure the population's utility for the condition. The analyst needs to keep in mind that patients have a tendency to exaggerate the disutility of their conditions. The second approach is to identify a population without the condition, provide a scenario of what the life of a patient with the condition is like, and measure the population's utility for the condition. The methodological difficulty with the second approach is determining how much detail to provide, what media to use to describe the condition, and how to describe the condition without biasing the result. It is suggested that the level of detail be kept to a minimum and that a balanced presentation of the condition be provided, showing both positive and negative implications of the condition.

Utilities are generally measured on a scale from zero to one, with one representing healthy and zero representing dead. Health states often viewed as worse than death, such as dementia and coma, are assigned negative values.[47] The three methods currently in use for measuring utility values are the rating scale, standard gamble, and time trade-off.[48] The rating scale method is normally depicted as a line on a page segmented into gradations by multiples of 10. A single chronic health state or multiple chronic health states and a single age of onset of illness are described to the individual whose utility for the various health states is being measured. A state of perfect health and a state of death are also described to the individual as points of reference. The individual is asked to select from among the various health states the most preferred and least preferred, which become the ends of the scale. The individual is then asked to locate the chronic health states relative to each other on the scale.

The standard gamble method is generally displayed as two circles, one representing a chronic health state and the other representing the gamble as a pie graph.[49-51] The individual is given a choice between two alternatives. The first alternative is a definite probability of living in a particular chronic health state for life. The second alternative, or the gamble, depicts the individual returning to normal health and living for an additional number of years or dying immediately. For the gamble, the probability of perfect health is initially set at 100% and the probability of death is set at zero. After the individual makes a choice, the probabilities are changed to 100% probability of death and zero probability of perfect health, the pie graph is changed accordingly, and the question is posed again. This process continues until the individual is indifferent between living in the chronic health state for life and the gamble. This indifference point is the individual's utility for the health state.

In the time trade-off method the patient is given a choice between living in a given health state for a given period followed by death versus being healthy for a shorter period followed by death.[52] After the individual makes a choice, the times are varied, and the process repeats continuously until an indifference point is reached. That indifference point is the individual's utility for the health state.

Converting Utilities to Quality-Adjusted Life Years

Irrespective of the method used to calculate utilities, the final step in a utility analysis is to convert these utilities into QALYs and interpret the results. Assume a group's utility for lung cancer averages 0.45 and a new follow-up strategy has been demonstrated to result in a 1.5-year increase in survival over the status quo. The group's QALYs would be 0.68 (0.45×1.5). The analyst would then calculate the cost of the follow-up strategy per QALY, discount costs and benefits to net present value if costs and benefits accrue over a period longer than 1 year, and use these data to determine if the new strategy was worth the investment.[31,53,54]

The use of QALYs is not without criticism. It has been suggested that QALYs discriminate against the elderly, equity issues are disregarded, and the resulting quality-of-life scores are biased.[44,55-59]

Sensitivity Analysis

No matter which method of cost analysis is chosen, certain assumptions must be made in relation to causation. These assumptions should be carefully delineated. In addition, the analyst needs to determine how sensitive the results of the cost analysis are to the assumptions made. For example, if there is known imprecision in any of the estimates used, both conservative and liberal alternative estimates should be constructed and the sensitivity of the results to the varying estimates should be tested.

There are three major forms of sensitivity analysis: simple sensitivity analysis, extreme scenarios, and probabilistic sensitivity analysis. Simple sensitivity analysis involves varying one or more of the assumptions on which the economic evaluation is based to determine the effect on the results. The extreme scenarios approach consists of analyzing the extremes of the distribution of costs and effectiveness and determining whether the results hold up under the most optimistic and pessimistic assumptions. Probabilistic sensitivity analysis assigns ranges and distributions to variables, using computer programs to select values at random from each range and measure the effects. This approach can handle a large number of variables and basically generates confidence intervals for each option.[60] Irrespective of the type of sensitivity analysis conducted, the goal is to measure whether large variations in the assumptions result in significant variations in the results of the cost evaluation. If significant variations are not the result, more confidence can be placed in the study's results. If significant variations are the result, an attempt should be made either to reduce uncertainty or to improve the accuracy of crucial variables.[30]

SUMMARY

This chapter provides a review of the tools needed to assess and compare the performance of diagnostic tests, to determine thresholds for diagnostic testing and treating, and to calculate the total costs of cancer patient follow-up. These tools allow the clinician to gather data, thus permitting more informed decision making regarding the composition of the chosen strategy. The concepts presented here lay the groundwork for the next chapter, which applies cost-evaluation methodology to the management of cancer patients, assigning dollar values to the follow-up strategies suggested in subsequent chapters. This chapter also lays the foundation for Chapter 4, which discusses clinical, legal, economic, and ethical issues that affect decisions about the composition of follow-up strategies.

REFERENCES

1. Mausner JS, Kramer S. Epidemiology—an introductory text. 2nd ed. Philadelphia: WB Saunders Company, 1985.
2. Fisher LD, van Belle G. Biostatistics: a methodology for the health sciences. New York: John Wiley & Sons, Inc, 1993.
3. Benish WA. Graphic and tabular expressions of Bayes' theorem. Med Decis Making 1987;7:104-6.
4. Fagan TJ. Nomogram for Bayes' formula. N Engl J Med 1975;293:257.
5. Matchar DB, Simel DL, Geweke JF, Feussner JR. A Bayesian method for evaluating medical test operating characteristics when some patients' conditions fail to be diagnosed by the reference standard. Med Decis Making 1990;10:102-11.
6. Irwig L, Glasziou PP, Berry G, Chock C, Mock P, Simpson JM. Efficient study designs to assess the accuracy of screening tests. Am J Epidemiol 1994;140:759-69.
7. Fletcher RH, Fletcher SW, Wagner EH. Clinical epidemiology: the essentials. 2nd ed. Baltimore: Williams & Wilkins, 1988.
8. Vecchio TJ. Predictive value of a single diagnostic test in unselected populations. N Engl J Med 1966;274:1171-3.
9. Friedman GD. Primer of epidemiology. 2nd ed. New York: McGraw-Hill Book Company, 1980.
10. Woolson RF. Statistical methods for the analysis of biomedical data. New York: John Wiley & Sons, Inc, 1987.
11. Knottnerus JA, Leffers P. The influence of referral patterns on the characteristics of diagnostic tests. J Clin Epidemiol 1992;45:1143-54.
12. Wilson JM, Jungner F. Principles and practice of screening for disease. Geneva: World Health Organization, Public Health Papers; 1968: No. 34.
13. Feinstein AR. Clinical epidemiology: the architecture of clinical research. Philadelphia: WB Saunders Company, 1985.
14. Metz CE. Basic principles of ROC analysis. Semin Nucl Med 1978;8:283-98.
15. Swets JA. Signal detection and recognition by human observers. New York: John Wiley & Sons, Inc, 1964.
16. Centor RM. Signal detectability: the use of ROC curves and their analysis. Med Decis Making 1991;11:102-6.
17. van der Schouw YT, Straatman H, Verbeek AL. ROC curves and the areas under them for dichotomized tests: empirical findings for logistically and normally distributed diagnostic test results. Med Decis Making 1994;14:374-81.
18. Hanley JA, McNeil BJ. The meaning and use of the area under a receiver operating characteristic (ROC) curve. Radiology 1982;143:29-36.
19. Hanley JA, McNeil BJ. A method of comparing the areas under receiver operating characteristic curves derived from the same cases. Radiology 1983;148:839-43.
20. Metz CE, Kronman HB. Statistical significance tests for binormal ROC curves. J Math Psych 1980;22:218-43.
21. Moise A, Clement B, Ducimetiere P, Bourassa MG. Comparison of receiver operating curves derived from the same population: a bootstrapping approach. Comput Biomed Res 1985;18:125-31.
22. DeLong ER, DeLong DM, Clarke-Pearson DL. Comparing the areas under two or more correlated receiver operating characteristic curves: a nonparametric approach. Biometrics 1985;44:837-45.
23. McClish DK. Comparing the areas under more than two independent ROC curves. Med Decis Making 1987;7:149-55.
24. Sox HC, Blatt MA, Higgins MC, Marton KI. Medical decision making. Boston: Butterworths, 1988.
25. Pasanen PA, Eskelinen M, Partanen K, Pikkarainen P, Penttila I, Alhava E. Receiver operating characteristic (ROC) curve analysis of the tumour markers CEA, CA 50, and CA 242 in pancreatic cancer: results from a prospective study. Br J Cancer 1993;67:852-5.
26. Pauker SG, Kassirer JP. The threshold approach to clinical decision making. N Engl J Med 1980;302:1109-17.
27. Nease RF, Owens DK, Sox HC. Threshold analysis using diagnostic tests with multiple results. Med Decis Making 1989;9:91-103.
28. Glasziou P. Threshold analysis via the Bayes' nomogram. Med Decis Making 1991;11:61-2.
29. Warner KE, Luce BR. Cost-benefit and cost-effectiveness analysis in health care. Ann Arbor, Michigan: Health Administration Press, 1982.
30. Drummond MF, Stoddart GL, Torrance GW. Methods for the economic evaluation of health care programmes. Oxford: Oxford Medical Publications, 1987.
31. Weinstein MC. Foundations of cost-effectiveness analysis for health and medical practices. N Engl J Med 1977;296:716-21.
32. Dasgupta AK, Pearce DW. Cost-benefit analysis: theory and practice. London: Macmillan, 1972.
33. Mishan EJ. Cost-benefit analysis. London: George Allen and Unwin, 1975.
34. Sugden R, Williams AH. The principles of practical cost-benefit analysis. Oxford: Oxford University Press, 1979.
35. Eastaugh SR. Medical economics and health finance. Dover, Massachusetts: Auburn House Publishing Company, 1981.

36. Robinson R. Cost-utility analysis. Br Med J 1993;307:859-62.
37. Strom BL. Pharmacoepidemiology. New York: Churchill Livingstone, 1989.
38. Rapoport J, Robertson RL, Stuart B. Understanding health economics. Rockville, Maryland: Aspen Systems Corporation, 1982.
39. Krahn M, Gafni A. Discounting in the economic evaluation of health care interventions. Med Care 1993;31:403-18.
40. Muller A, Reutzel TJ. Willingness to pay for reduction in fatality risk: an exploratory survey. Am J Public Health 1984;74:808-12.
41. Zeckhauser R. Procedures for valuing lives. Public Policy 1975;23:419-64.
42. Jacobs P. The economics of health and medical care. Rockville, Maryland: Aspen Publishers, Inc, 1987.
43. Robinson R. Cost-benefit analysis. Br Med J 1993;307(b):924-6.
44. Mehrez A, Gafni A. Quality adjusted life years and healthy year equivalents. Med Decis Making 1989;9:142-9.
45. Mehrez A, Gafni A. Healthy-years equivalents versus quality-adjusted life years. Med Decis Making 1993;13:287-92.
46. Sackett DL, Torrance GW. The utility of different health states as perceived by the general public. J Chron Dis 1978;31:697-704.
47. Patrick DL, Starks HE, Cain KC, Uhlmann RF, Pearlman RA. Measuring preferences for health states worse than death. Med Decis Making 1994;14:9-18.
48. Torrance GW. Social preferences for health states: an empirical evaluation of three measurement techniques. Socio Econ Plan Sci 1976;10:129-36.
49. von Neumann J, Morgenstern O. Theory of games and economic behavior. New York: John Wiley & Sons, Inc, 1953.
50. Sonnenberg FA. U-maker 1.0 [computer program]. Microcomputer utility assessment program. New Brunswick, New Jersey, 1993.
51. Gafni A. The standard gamble method: what is being measured and how it is interpreted. Health Serv Res 1994;29:207-24.
52. Torrance GW, Thomas WH, Sackett DL. A utility maximization model for evaluation of health care programmes. Health Serv Res 1972;7:118-33.
53. Weinstein MC. Principles of cost-effective resource allocation in health care organizations. Int J Technol Assess Health Care 1990;6:93-103.
54. Johannesson M, Pliskin JS, Weinstein MC. A note on QALYs, time tradeoff, and discounting. Med Decis Making 1994;14:188-93.
55. Carr-Hill R. Assumptions of the QALY procedure. Soc Sci Med 1989;29:469-77.
56. Carr-Hill R. Allocating resources to health care: is the QALY a technical solution to a political problem? Int J Health Serv 1991;21:351-63.
57. Loomes G, McKenzie L. The use of QALYs in health care decision making. Soc Sci Med 1989;28:299-308.
58. Wagstaff A. QALYs and the equity-efficiency trade-off. J Health Econ 1991;10:21-41.
59. Johannesson M, Pliskin JS, Weinstein MC. Are healthy-years equivalents an improvement over quality-adjusted life years? Med Decis Making 1993;13:281-6.
60. Robinson R. Cost-effectiveness analysis. Br Med J 1993;307(c):793-5.

CHAPTER 3

Costs of Surveillance After Potentially Curative Treatment for Cancer

St. Louis University Health Sciences Center ▪ St. Louis Department of Veterans Affairs Medical Center

KATHERINE S. VIRGO AND FRANK E. JOHNSON

Cancer patient follow-up is a neglected research topic. Few practice guidelines have been widely accepted, attempts at measuring costs have been weak, and the potential exists for unrestrained costs.[1] Among the estimated 1 to 2 million new primary cancers projected to be diagnosed in the United States this year (including 800,000 squamous and basal cell carcinomas of the skin),[2] the majority will be treated with curative intent and enter follow-up programs. The percentage of patients undergoing resection who will develop recurrence within 5 years varies widely by the site of cancer. Few of these recurrences are curatively treated. A small percentage develop second primary cancers each year, a risk that is relatively constant over at least the first 5 years after treatment. Many second primary cancers can be treated with curative intent.

Various surveillance programs following curative treatment of many solid tumors such as breast and colon have been advocated, but little has been written about postoperative surveillance for cancers such as those of lung. Textbooks rarely discuss surveillance in detail. Few published analyses suggest that intensive follow-up practices actually benefit patients by lengthening survival or improving quality of life. Prospective studies have been conducted, but rarely has a randomized controlled trial design been used to compare outcomes of varying intensities of follow-up. Because of the lack of objective data, physicians often adopt the surveillance regimen specific to their residency training program without questioning the impact on patient survival. Although this practice is not surprising, it is difficult to justify, particularly in an environment increasingly dominated by managed care. With 53.3 million people currently enrolled in managed care systems in the United States,[3] cost effectiveness has become the yardstick for determining whether these patients will be allowed access to high-cost or highly used health care services. Increasing emphasis on the practice of evidence-based medicine[4-6] and the implementation of medical practice guidelines will further restrict the current tendency of physicians to follow patients intensively.

With disagreement over the appropriate frequency of follow-up and no solid data on which to base surveillance strategies, it is not surprising that few attempts have been made to ascertain the costs associated with cancer patient follow-up. Because of their sheer magnitude the costs of screening, diagnosis, and treatment of the primary malignancy are frequently analyzed, whereas the costs of posttreatment surveillance are rarely mentioned and are generally treated as nonsignificant. In an attempt to fill this void, this chapter has two objectives. The first is to summarize in one source the past 15 years of literature in the field, which clearly shows that little research has been conducted and methodology is not standardized. The second is to provide per-patient cost data for every 5-year follow-up strategy discussed in this book across all 19 cancer sites. Although many assumptions are made in calculating these cost estimates, the data represent a conservative starting point for understanding how expensive cancer patient follow-up can be and how minor modifications in strategy can result in major modifications in cost.

METHODS

Literature Review

A Medline search of the literature for the years 1982 to 1996 was performed to identify citations measuring the cost of posttreatment surveillance for cancer patients. Articles were eliminated if they examined only the period of follow-up after relapse, focused on the follow-up of patients with benign tumors, or simply compared alternative ways of carrying out a specific diagnostic test. Another exclusion criterion was lack of per-patient cost or charge data. If only nationwide totals were provided and insufficient data were available to calculate costs or charges on a per-patient level, the article was excluded. Also eliminated were many studies that were described as cost-effectiveness or cost-benefit analyses but were mere statements that follow-up can be expensive and lacked objective data or formal analyses to substantiate such statements. In general, articles that focused on the cost of follow-up after a positive test result were also eliminated because only a small portion of the follow-up period (usually less than 6 months) was examined. A notable exception was the article by Moertel et al.,[7] which analyzed a full 5 years of follow-up after a positive test result and provided convincing evidence that carcinoembryonic antigen testing is highly cost ineffective for the follow-up of patients with colorectal cancer because it is expensive and seldom leads to cures. If more than three published articles were identified for a cancer site, an attempt was made to summarize results across articles.

Cost Analyses

Nationwide average charges for 1992 associated with the strategies recommended in this text for the follow-up of 19 different cancers for the 5-year period after treatment were computed for an individual cancer patient. The charges associated with alternative strategies recommended in the counterpoints to each chapter were also computed. Charge data were obtained from the 1992 Part B Medicare Annual Data file[8] and the first quarter 1992 Hospital Outpatient Bill file.[9] Average allowed charges nationwide for physician services were extracted from the Part B Medicare Annual Data file, which contains Medicare Part B data categorized by Current Procedural Terminology (CPT) code and place of service (such as inpatient hospital, outpatient hospital, or office). With substantial assistance from the Office of Research and Development of the Health Care Financing Administration, corresponding nationwide average facility charges were extracted from the Hospital Outpatient Bill file.

A difficult task in calculating the total surveillance charges was the appropriate assignment of recommended tests to CPT codes. Although the CPT coding system is now highly specific, many gray areas existed in 1992 (the most recent year for which facility charge data were available). We thank the authors of the cancer-specific chapters and counterpoints for their assistance in this task.

Physician charges and, where applicable, facility charges were summed to obtain a nationwide average charge per test or visit. Unfortunately, for anoscopy and intravenous pyelography, no facility charge data were available for 1992 because of the low volume of these procedures. Since only physician fees were available, the total charges for follow-up strategies using these modalities are conservative. This difficulty affects only the follow-up of patients with anal cancer or urinary bladder cancer.

No additional charges were assessed for examinations considered part of the history and physical examination, such as pelvic examination for patients with breast, ovarian, or endometrial cancers and digital rectal examination for patients with anal or prostate cancers, although charges for the office visit itself were calculated. Charges for tests unrelated to the follow-up of the primary malignancy, such as general health screening, were also excluded. If alternative modalities were recommended as equal substitutes for one another, total charges for the strategy were recalculated using each modality. Similarly, if certain diagnostic tests were indicated for only certain subsets of the population, total charges were calculated for each subset individually. Subsets were generally defined by tumor stage, histology, treatment of primary tumor, gender, age, or tumor marker levels.

Calculating total charges of follow-up for patients with soft tissue cancers was somewhat problematic because tumor site varies among patients and charges vary by site for common testing modalities such as ultrasound, x-ray, magnetic resonance imaging (MRI), and computed tomography (CT). Since none of the site-specific charges were applicable to all patients, an average charge was calculated across all possible sites for each modality.

Many assumptions were necessary to achieve consistency across the follow-up strategies recommended by the many authors in this text. Unless otherwise specified, it was assumed that computed tomography of the abdomen did not automatically imply computed tomography of the pelvis. Similarly, it was assumed that authors who specified sigmoid-oscopy actually meant sigmoidoscopy (examination of the rectum, sigmoid colon, and a portion of the descending colon) and authors who specified proctosigmoidoscopy actually meant proctosigmoidoscopy (examination of the rectum and sigmoid colon). In the case of liver function tests, a full panel of tests was assumed unless the author specified only certain tests.

A best-case scenario was assumed in calculating charges. For example, it was assumed that patients were healthy and that additional workup based on either symptoms or positive test results was not required. Further, it was assumed that each patient survived for 5 years, since the purpose of the analysis was to measure the cost of the initial 5 years of follow-up. It is true that many cancer patients do not live for 5 years after treatment, but this assumption can be easily relaxed. The result would be a table of follow-up costs for every combination of tumor, nodes, metastases (TNM) stage and projected years of survival. Indirect costs, such as time lost from work, transportation charges, and child or adult care charges, were not factored into this analysis. Similarly, treatment costs for second primary cancers, recurrences of the initial primary cancer, and other conditions detected during surveillance were ignored, although they may impose massive additional expenses for individual patients. Under these assumptions the resulting cost estimates should be considered very conservative and constitute baseline estimates of follow-up costs. All costs assumed away in this analysis would be considered add-ons to the estimates presented. Medicare-allowed charges were held constant at the 1992 level as charges were totaled over the 5-year period for each of the strategies and compared across strategies within each site. Total Medicare-allowed charges were converted to an actual charge proxy using a conversion ratio of 1.62, which was calculated from actual submitted Medicare charges for 1992.[8,9] Variation in charges between each main chapter and each counterpoint was then reanalyzed.

RESULTS

Literature Review

A total of 27 articles analyzing posttreatment surveillance costs were identified (Table 3-1).[1,7,10-34] Unfortunately, there was little standardization in methodology across articles. As is obvious from the frequency of question marks in the cost/charge column of Table 3-1, one of the first difficulties in interpreting the literature is discerning the meaning of the term "costs" from the information regarding cost analyses in the methods section of these articles. In most cases the data were scanty. It was usually unclear whether costs or charges were the focus of the analysis. Comparing the results of various studies was extremely difficult. In the economics literature, costs are generally defined as resources expended to produce a given unit of output. These resources typically include such items as personnel, supplies, capital equipment, and overhead. Charges are typically defined as the price paid by purchasers of the output and usually equal the cost of producing the output plus some percentage profit. In the case of health services these purchasers are patients or third-party payors such as insurance companies. Since costs are the more difficult data to obtain, it was assumed that the term "costs" generally referred to charges unless otherwise indicated.

An exception to the assumption above was made for studies conducted in countries with national health insurance. One might presume that a national health insurance system would not bill itself for more than the cost of a given service (i.e., there would be no profit margin), and therefore it could be assumed that the data reported in these studies referred to costs. However, many of these countries also have private hospitals operating within their borders. Therefore, unless the article specifically stated that the data were derived from the national health insurance system, the data were not interpreted as costs.

Minimal documentation of cost analysis methodology in the literature leads to another problem, which is lack of information regarding the source of cost or charge data. In approximately one third of the articles it was unclear whether the data were for a single facility, regional data, or nationwide data. Without information on the data source, generalizability of the cost or charge estimates was questionable.

Furthermore, in half of the articles the year associated with the cost or charge data was not identified. Without this information it is difficult to inflate the figures to the current year, since it is unclear which year is the baseline. For the articles written by individuals from outside the United States, an additional problem caused by the lack of year identification is selection of an appropriate exchange rate for conversion to a common currency (U.S. dollars). For the five articles presenting cost or charge data in other than U.S. dollars,[15,22,23,28,32] the exchange rate as of July 8, 1996, was used for conversion.[35] The applicable U.S. dollar exchange rates were 0.6437 for the British pound, 1.5268 for the German mark, and 1533.75 for the Italian lire.

Unfortunately, the shortage of articles precluded a definitive analysis of the cost of cancer patient follow-up by site for most cancer sites from the literature alone. The breast (eight articles)[10,18-24] and the colon and rectum (10 articles)[1,7,27-34] were the only sites discussed in more than three articles. The literature on these sites is discussed in detail here. For purposes of assimilating the literature, all costs or charges were inflated to 1996 dollars using the medical care component of the Consumer Price Index.[36] Since, as previously mentioned, many articles did not identify the year associated with the data, the date 2 years preceding publication of the article was assumed. For example, if the publication date was 1995, 1993 data were assumed. Although Table 3-1 lists all articles presenting even 1 year of follow-up cost or charge data, for purposes of analysis only articles with data for the full 5-year period were included. If greater than 5 years of data were available but the 5-year period could not be extracted, these articles were also excluded.

For breast cancer, after two articles were excluded[10,18] and all charges were inflated to 1996 levels, total charges for routine follow-up ranged from $692[22] to $4,187.[18] The average charge for the routine follow-up of breast cancer was $1,940 (after the Medicare charge data of Kattlove et al.[24] were converted to an actual charge proxy). Only one article[22] addressed the issue of cost per recurrence detected, and none addressed the issues of cost per operable recurrence or cost per recurrence curatively treated. Cost per recurrence detected, inflated to 1996 levels, was $3,393 for ultrasound, $2,288 for chest x-ray, $2,327 for unilateral mammography, and $4,656 for bilateral mammography.

For colorectal cancer, after exclusion of two articles[27,33] and inflation of all charges to 1996 levels, total charges for routine follow-up ranged from $789[31] to $33,111[1] (after converting Medicare-allowed charge data to an actual charge proxy). The average charge for the routine follow-up of colorectal cancer was $8,165 (when only the least and most intensive follow-up strategies reviewed by Virgo et al.[1] were included) and $8,752 (when all 18 articles reviewed by Virgo et al.[1] were included). Four articles addressed the issue of cost per recurrence detected,[7,28,31,34] two articles addressed the issue of cost per operable recurrence,[28,34] and one article addressed the issue of cost per recurrence curatively treated.[34] Estimates of the cost per recurrence detected, inflated to 1996 levels, ranged from $15,166[34] to $665,520[7] and averaged $259,767. The two estimates of cost per operable recurrence, inflated to 1996 levels, ranged from $40,346 to $791,057 and averaged $415,702. The one estimate of cost per recurrence curatively treated, inflated to 1996 levels, was $66,824.

Cost Analyses

Tables 3-2 through 3-20 display nationwide average Medicare-allowed charges for 1992 associated with the strategies recommended in this text for the follow-up of 19 different cancers for the 5-year posttreatment period. For each follow-up strategy an actual charge proxy (applicable to non-Medicare patients) is also presented. For no cancer site was there total agreement across all follow-up strategies recommended, although consensus was nearly achieved for endometrial

Text continued on p. 44.

Table 3-1 Cancer patient follow-up cost literature

AUTHOR(S)	PUBLICATION YEAR	N	CANCER(S)	COST/CHARGE
MULTIPLE CANCERS				
Pauwels et al.[10]	1986	N/A	Breast, lung, prostate	Costs?
Riley and Lubitz[11] in Scheffler and Andrews	1989	11,469	All	Medicare charges averaged over the years preceding death
Baker et al.[12] in Scheffler and Andrews	1989	125,832	All	Medicare charges in 1984 dollars
LYMPHOMA				
Pera et al.[13]	1987	126	Lymphoma	Charges for a Texas medical center
GASTRIC CANCER				
D'Amico et al.[14]	1989	82	Gastric	Costs? Converted from Italian lire as of 3/86
TESTICULAR CANCER				
Ellis et al.[15]	1984	106	Testicular	Costs? Converted from British pounds using a 1996 exchange rate of £ .6427 = $1
Ciatto et al.[16]	1986	253	Testicular seminoma	Costs? Converted from Italian lire
Berdel et al.[17]	1987	138	Testicular, Stage IIb-IV NSGCT in CR	Costs? Converted from German marks
BREAST CANCER				
Horton[18]	1984	N/A	Breast	1983 charges for a New York medical center

N/A, Not available; *CT,* computed tomography; *KUB,* x-ray of kidneys, ureter, and bladder; *CXR,* chest x-ray; *EGD,* esophagogastroduodenoscopy; *US,* ultrasound; *HIDA,* N'N'-(2,6-dimethylphenyl) carbamoylmethyl iminodiacetic acid; *BE,* barium enema; *AFP,* alpha-fetoprotein; *HCG,* human chorionic gonadotropin; *NSGCT,* nonseminoma germ cell tumor; *CR,* complete remission; *CBC,* complete blood count; *LFTs,* liver function tests; *FOBT,* fecal occult blood test; *CEA,* carcinoembryonic acid; *ESR,* erythrocyte sedimentation rate; *XR,* x-ray; *DM,* Deutsche mark; *MRI,* magnetic resonance imaging; *CE,* cost effectiveness; *QALY,* quality-adjusted life year; *HIAA,* Health Insurance Association of America; *ALP,* alkaline phosphatase.

*Cost data as shown in this table are prior to inflation to 1996 levels.

5-YR FOLLOW-UP PROTOCOL	5-YR FOLLOW-UP COST PER PATIENT*	COST PER RECURRENCE DETECTED*	COST PER OPERABLE RECURRENCE*
Bone scans = 8	$1,600[a]	$16,000	Not available
Not prespecified	Age 65-74 = $3,590[b] Age 75-84 = $4,605[b] Age 85+ = $3,635[b]	Not available	Not available
Not prespecified	$2,890[b,c]	Not available	Not available
No set frequency of follow-up prespecified; averages per patient: abdominal and pelvic CT = 5.3, KUB = 6.6, lymphangiogram = 0.10	With CT = $3,479[d] With KUB and lymphangiogram = $870[d]	Not available	Not available
Office visits, blood, and urine tests = 11 each; CXR, EGD, liver US, and abdominal CT = 7 each; gastric scan with HIDA and BE as needed.	$3,750	Not available	Not available
Office visits, CXR, AFP, and beta-HCG = 22; abdominal CT = 3; if CXR clear, CT of thorax = 3	$4,661[e]	$233,028[f]	Not available
Office visits and CXR = 9 each	$450[g]	$4,600[g,h]	Not available
Office visits, CXR, AFP, beta-HCG, CBC, LFTs = 12 each; Abdominal = CT = 10	$2,720	$18,000	Not available
Stages I and II: office visits = 16; blood tests and CXR = 3 each; Pap smear, mammography, and FOBT = 6 each Stage III: office visits = 21; blood tests, CXR, Pap smear, and FOBT = 7 each; mammography = 6, bone scan = 5 Stage IV: office visits = 22; blood tests and skeletal XR = 11 each; CXR, Pap smear, and FOBT = 6 each; bone scan and CEA = 1 each	Stages I and II = $1,755 Stage III = $4,511 Stage IV = $4,195	Not available	Not available

Continued.

Table 3-1 Cancer patient follow-up cost literature–cont'd

AUTHOR(S)	PUBLICATION YEAR	N	CANCER(S)	COST/CHARGE
Schapira and Urban[19,20]	1991; 1993	N/A	Breast	Charges? in 1990 dollars, adjusted for losses under the assumption of a constant recurrence rate of 0.076/yr, and discounted by 5% over the 5-yr period
Schapira and Urban[19,20]				
Hannisdal et al.[21]	1993	430	Breast	Costs in 1990; converted from Norwegian kronen
Von Christa Wieland-Schneider et al.[22]	1994	420	Breast	Costs? Converted from German marks at 1996 exchange rate of DM 1.5268 = $1
Mapelli et al.[23]	1995	N/A	Breast	1. Costs? To the Italian national health service 2. Charges to patients from self-employed physicians 3. Charges? To the private voluntary/integrative health insurance funds All figures converted from Italian lire at 1996 exchange rate of 1533.75 lire = $1
Kattlove et al.[24]	1995	N/A	Breast	1993 Medicare charges for Southern California
LUNG CANCER				
Walsh et al.[25]	1995	358	Lung	1987-1994 charges for a Texas medical center
Virgo et al.[26]	1996	N/A	Lung	1992 Medicare charges and an actual charge proxy
COLORECTAL CANCER				
Sandler et al.[27]	1984	N/A	Colorectal	1982 charges for a North Carolina hospital

5-YR FOLLOW-UP PROTOCOL	5-YR FOLLOW-UP COST PER PATIENT	COST PER RECURRENCE DETECTED	COST PER OPERABLE RECURRENCE
Minimal: office visits = 18 and mammography = 5 Intensive: office visits, blood tests, and CEA = 18 each; mammography, CXR and bone scan = 5	Minimal = $1,025 No discount = $1,116 No recurrence adjustment or discount = $1,330 Intensive = $5,735 No discount = $6,247 No recurrence adjustment or discount = $7,390	Not available	Not available
Office visits, LFTs, ESR, and CBC = 13 each; CXR, pelvic XR, lumbar spine XR, upper femur XR, and bone scan = 5 each	$507[i] $1206[j]	Not available	Not available
Office visits = 7, CXR = 6.6, abdominal US = 6.3, and mammography = 5.8	$558	US = $2,738 CXR = $1,846 Mammography: 1-sided = $1,878 2-sided = $3,757	Not available
Basic: office visits = 14 and mammography = 5 Intensive: office visits and blood tests = 14; CXR = 10; bone scan, liver US, and mammography = 5	Basic No. 1 = $347 Basic No. 2 = $593 Basic No. 3 = $1,006 Intensive No. 1 = $1,104 Intensive No. 2 = $3,024 Intensive No. 3 = $2,649	Not available	Not available
Routine: office visits = 20 and mammography = 5 Intensive: office visits = 20; mammography, bone scan, liver US, CXR, and blood tests = 5 each	Routine = $1,140 Intensive = $3,200	Not available	Not available
Not prespecified	No recurrence = $4,379 per yr over 4-5 yr Palliatively treated recurrence = $10,306 per yr over 18.3 mo Curatively treated recurrence = $15,072 per yr over 27.7 mo	Not available	Not available
Multiple protocols recommended in the literature	Medicare: least intensive = $946; most intensive = $5,645 Actual charges: least intensive = $1,533; most intensive= $9,145	Not available	Not available
No recurrence: CEA = 23[k]; with recurrence: CEA = 12[k]	No recurrence = $715[k]; with recurrence = $3,002[k]	$24,779	Not available

Continued.

Table 3-1 Cancer patient follow-up cost literature—cont'd

AUTHOR(S)	PUBLICATION YEAR	N	CANCER(S)	COST/CHARGE
Saviano[28]	1989	N/A	Rectal	Costs? Converted from Italian lire at a 1996 conversion rate of 1533.75 lire = $1
Kievit and van de Velde[29]	1990	N/A	Colon	1988 Costs? Converted from Dutch guilders
Rocklin et al.[30]	1990	65	Colorectal	Costs? For a West Virginia university hospital as of 1988
Ransohoff et al.[31]	1991	N/A	Colorectal	Physician charges discounted at 5%
Moertel et al.[7]	1993	1017	Colorectal	Lab tests: average charge data from 5 major labs; endoscopies: median national charges from 1991 HIAA data; Other: rough estimates of charges derived from third-party payors and providers
Muller et al.[32]	1994	598	Colorectal	Charges from national tariff schedule for physician services; converted from German marks at 1996 exchange rate of DM 1.5268 = $1
Bruinvels[33]	Thesis, 1995	N/A	Colorectal	Costs at a university hospital in Leiden; converted from Dutch guilders at 1994 exchange rate of Dfl 1.80 = $1

5-YR FOLLOW-UP PROTOCOL	5-YR FOLLOW-UP COST PER PATIENT	COST PER RECURRENCE DETECTED	COST PER OPERABLE RECURRENCE
CEA = 28; US = 14; CXR, CT, and MRI = 7	CEA = $913; US = 639; CXR = $94; CT = $1,878; MRI = $4,173	CEA = $1,984; US = $4,258; CXR = $854; CT = $9,389; MRI = $20,864	CEA = $10,139; US = $15,974; CXR = $7,824; CT = $125,183; MRI = $277, 751
Office visits, blood tests, CXR, and colonoscopy; Frequencies not available beyond 2 yr	Without CEA = $714; with CEA = $1,254 Including diagnosis and treatment costs: without CEA = $1,839; with CEA = $3,377 Marginal CE of CEA = $86,277/ QALY saved	Not available	Not available
Tested: office visits, CEA, LFTs, and CXR = 14 each; colonoscopy or BE and proctosigmoidoscopy = 7 each Recommended: office visits, CEA, and CXR = 18 each; colonoscopy = 9	Tested: with BE and Proctosig-moidoscopy = $5,586; with colonoscopy = $8,925 Recommended: $10,989	Not available	Not available
1. Colonoscopy = 3 2. Colonoscopy = 2 3. Colonoscopy = 1	1. $1,500 2. $1,000 3. $500	If colonoscopy 100% effective and risk for mortality from cancer without examinations = 1.25% 1. $248,476[l] 2. $165,650[l] 3. $99,390[l]	Not available
Office visits, blood tests, and CXR = 13 each; colonoscopy or colon XR and proctosig-moidoscopy = 3 each; CEA (optional) averaged 6.5	After a positive CEA = $621; including treatment costs = $1,415	$500,000	Not available
Office visits, blood tests, CEA, CA 19-9, and FOBT = 9 each; CXR, abdominal US, and colonoscopy = 7 each	$2,086	Not available	Not available
No follow-up Minimal follow-up: office visits = 5 Intensive follow-up No. 1: office visits and CEA = 13 each; colonoscopy = 2 Intensive follow-up No. 2: office visits, ALP, CEA, and FOBT = 14 each; colonoscopy, CXR, and liver US = 10 each	Minimal or no follow-up = $3,250[b,i] Intensive follow-up No. 1 or No. 2 = $4,500[b,i] Marginal CE: minimal follow-up = $300/yr; intensive follow-up No. 1 = $8,333/yr; intensive follow-up No. 2 = $6,721/yr	Not available	Not available

Continued.

Table 3-1 Cancer patient follow-up cost literature–cont'd

AUTHOR(S)	PUBLICATION YEAR	N	CANCER(S)	COST/CHARGE
Virgo et al.[1]	1995	N/A	Colorectal	1992 Medicare charges and actual charge proxy
Audisio et al.[34]	1996	505	Colorectal	Costs? For a private hospital in Italy; converted from Italian lire

[a]Four-year follow-up only.
[b]Includes positive test evaluation and treatment costs and may include nursing home and home health care costs.
[c]Includes costs unrelated to cancer care.
[d]Twenty-month follow-up only.
[e]Three-year follow-up only.
[f]Applies to seminoma patients only.
[g]Includes travel costs and costs associated with time lost from work.
[h]Cost per intrathoracic metastasis detected in year 1 after treatment only.
[i]Eight-year follow-up.
[j]Calculated for asymptomatic patients from the author's suggested strategy and cost data.
[k]Two-year follow-up only.
[l]Cost per death prevented.

Table 3-2 Head and neck carcinoma (Chapter 5): total 5-year follow-up charges*

	MEDICARE CHARGES ($)	ACTUAL CHARGES ($)†
MSKCC PRIMARY (TABLE 5-7)	2,621.60	4,247.00
Patients at risk for hypothyroidism	2,887.10	4,677.10
JAPAN COUNTERPOINT (TABLES 5-8 AND 5-9)		
Patients with high cure rates of disease	3,192.88	5,172.47
And high SCCAg titer at initial treatment	3,548.32	5,748.28
And nasopharyngeal carcinoma (MRI not available)	5,781.16	9,365.48
And nasopharyngeal carcinoma (MRI available)	7,204.16	11,670.74
And both high SCCAg titer at initial treatment and nasopharyngeal carcinoma (MRI not available)	6,136.60	9,941.29
And both high SCCAg titer at initial treatment and nasopharyngeal carcinoma (MRI available)	7,559.60	12,246.55
Patients with poor prognosis	4,703.36	7,619.45
And high SCCAg titer at initial treatment	5,058.80	8,195.26
And nasopharyngeal carcinoma (MRI not available)	7,291.64	11,812.46
And nasopharyngeal carcinoma (MRI available)	8,714.64	14,117.72
And both high SCCAg titer at initial treatment and nasopharyngeal carcinoma (MRI not available)	7,647.08	12,388.27
And both high SCCAg titer at initial treatment and nasopharyngeal carcinoma (MRI available)	9,070.08	14,693.53
RPCI COUNTERPOINT (TABLE 5-13)	2,621.60	4,247.00
Patients at risk for hypothyroidism	2,887.10	4,677.10
UK COUNTERPOINT (TABLE 5-12)	3,093.66	5,011.73
UWMC COUNTERPOINT (TABLE 5-14)	1,632.50	2,644.65

SCCAg, Squamous cell carcinoma antigen; *MRI,* magnetic resonance imaging. Throughout Tables 3-2 to 3-20, *MSKCC,* Memorial Sloan-Kettering Cancer Center; *RPCI,* Roswell Park Cancer Institute; *UK,* United Kingdom; *UWMC,* University of Washington Medical Center.
*Using 1992 charge data.
†Medicare-allowed charges × 1.62 conversion ratio.

5-YR FOLLOW-UP PROTOCOL	5-YR FOLLOW-UP COST PER PATIENT	COST PER RECURRENCE DETECTED	COST PER OPERABLE RECURRENCE
Multiple protocols recommended in the literature	Medicare: least intensive = $561; most intensive = $16,492 Actual charges: least intensive = $910; most intensive = $26,717	Not available	Not available
Office visits, CEA, and US = 11; CXR and colonoscopy = 5	$5,400	$13,581	$36,130

Table 3-3 Esophageal carcinoma (Chapter 6): total 5-year follow-up charges*

	MEDICARE CHARGES ($)	ACTUAL CHARGES ($)†
UWMC PRIMARY (TABLE 6-1)	718.30	1,163.65
JAPAN COUNTERPOINT (TABLE 6-6)	26,279.52	42,572.82
MSKCC COUNTERPOINT (TABLES 6-2, 6-3, AND 6-4)		
Patients receiving standard community care and considered at low risk of recurrence	1,734.48	2,809.86
Patients in clinical trials or institutions engaged in studies of staging and cancer biology	19,376.88	31,390.55
Patients at high risk of local recurrence	20,991.44	34,006.13
RPCI COUNTERPOINT (TABLE 6-9)	19,527.32	31,634.26
UK COUNTERPOINT (TABLE 6-7)	718.30	1,163.65

*Using 1992 charge data.
†Medicare-allowed charges × 1.62 conversion ratio.

Table 3-4 Gastric carcinoma (Chapter 7): total 5-year follow-up charges*

	MEDICARE CHARGES ($)	ACTUAL CHARGES ($)†
RPCI PRIMARY (TABLE 7-4)	20,052.68	32,485.34
JAPAN COUNTERPOINT (TABLES 7-10 AND 7-12)		
Patients with early gastric cancer	4,948.75	8,016.98
Patients with advanced gastric cancer	13,342.96	21,615.60
MSKCC COUNTERPOINT (TABLES 7-6, 7-7, AND 7-8)		
Low-risk patients	4,658.35	7,546.53
Intermediate-risk patients	6,744.11	10,925.46
High-risk patients	2,623.39	4,249.90
UK COUNTERPOINT (TABLE 7-13)		
With carcinoembryonic antigen	18,552.75	30,055.46
With CA 72.4	18,565.23	30,075.67
UWMC COUNTERPOINT (TABLE 7-14)	6,488.60	10,511.53

*Using 1992 charge data.
†Medicare-allowed charges × 1.62 conversion ratio.

Table 3-5 Colorectal carcinoma (Chapter 8): total 5-year follow-up charges*

	MEDICARE CHARGES ($)	ACTUAL CHARGES ($)†
RPCI PRIMARY (TABLE 8-1)		
Patients with colon cancer	15,225.08	24,664.63
Patients with rectal cancer	15,726.78	25,477.38
JAPAN COUNTERPOINT (TABLE 8-3)		
Nonintensive follow-up (with colonoscopy)	10,708.91	17,348.43
Nonintensive follow-up (with barium enema)	7,398.31	11,985.26
Intensive follow-up (with colonoscopy)	21,035.98	34,078.29
Intensive follow-up (with barium enema)	17,404.08	28,194.61
MSKCC COUNTERPOINT (TABLE 8-2)	3,661.36	5,931.40
After sphincter-sparing procedures for rectal cancer	7,750.76	12,556.23
UK COUNTERPOINT (TABLES 8-4 AND 8-5)		
Patients with colon cancer	3,945.02	6,390.94
And presenting as an emergency	4,887.59	7,917.90
Patients with rectal cancer	6,803.10	11,021.02
And an isolated elevation of carcinoembryonic antigen levels	10,573.38	17,128.87
UWMC COUNTERPOINT (TABLES 8-6, 8-7, AND 8-8)		
Patients with colon cancer	7,129.72	11,550.15
Patients with rectal cancer	8,156.65	13,213.78
Patients with increased risk of recurrence	9,908.10	16,051.11

*Using 1992 charge data.
†Medicare-allowed charges × 1.62 conversion ratio.

Table 3-6 Anal carcinoma (Chapter 9): total 5-year follow-up charges*

	MEDICARE CHARGES ($)	ACTUAL CHARGES ($)†
UWMC PRIMARY (TABLE 9-3)	11,805.28‡	19,124.55‡
Patients with high-grade and stage III-IV tumors (MRI not available)	13,368.97‡	21,657.73‡
Patients with high-grade and stage III-IV tumors (MRI available)	13,776.79‡	22,318.40‡
JAPAN COUNTERPOINT (TABLES 9-5 AND 9-6)		
Patients with adenocarcinoma	4,456.79	7,220.00
And advanced cancer	5,226.09	8,466.27
Patients with squamous cell carcinoma	6,463.59	10,471.02
And advanced cancer (MRI not available)	7,232.89	10,470.89
And advanced cancer (MRI available)	7,451.79	12,071.90
And recurrence suspected	15,718.40‡	25,463.81‡
And both advanced cancer (MRI not available) and recurrence suspected	16,488.34‡	26,711.12‡
And both advanced cancer (MRI available) and recurrence suspected	16,707.24‡	27,065.73‡
MSKCC COUNTERPOINT (TABLE 9-4)	9,064.26‡	14,684.10‡
Patients at high risk of persistent or locally recurrent disease	13,158.24‡	21,316.35‡
RPCI COUNTERPOINT (TABLE 9-7)	2,840.21	4,601.14
Patients with stage III or IV tumors	3,609.51	5,847.41
UK COUNTERPOINT (TABLE 9-8)	12,146.09‡	19,676.66‡

MRI, Magnetic resonance imaging.
*Using 1992 charge data.
†Medicare-allowed charges × 1.62 conversion ratio.
‡Totals are conservative because facility charge estimates are used for anoscopy.

Table 3-7 Pancreatic carcinoma (Chapter 10): total 5-year follow-up charges*

	MEDICARE CHARGES ($)	ACTUAL CHARGES ($)†
RPCI PRIMARY (TABLE 10-3)	3,853.99	6,243.46
JAPAN COUNTERPOINT (TABLE 10-6)	25,241.23	40,891.62
MSKCC COUNTERPOINT (TABLE 10-5)	2,129.13	3,449.19
UK COUNTERPOINT (TABLE 10-7)	2,566.23	4,157.30
UWMC COUNTERPOINT (TABLE 10-8)	1,602.24	2,595.62

*Using 1992 charge data.
†Medicare-allowed charges × 1.62 conversion ratio.

Table 3-8 Hepatobiliary carcinoma (Chapter 11): total 5-year follow-up charges*

	MEDICARE CHARGES ($)	ACTUAL CHARGES ($)†
MSKCC PRIMARY (TABLES 11-5 AND 11-6)		
Patients with HCC	10,802.45	17,499.98
Patients with cholangiocarcinoma or gallbladder cancer	6,256.65	10,135.78
Patients with T1 gallbladder cancer	8,417.03	13,635.59
JAPAN COUNTERPOINT (TABLES 11-9 AND 11-10)		
Patients with HCC	15,398.60	24,945.73
Patients with cholangiocarcinoma or gallbladder cancer	12,216.01	19,789.94
RPCI COUNTERPOINT (TABLES 11-13 AND 11-14)		
Patients with HCC	18,359.46	29,742.32
And elevated AFP preoperatively	19,029.06	30,827.07
And elevated CEA preoperatively	19,216.86	31,131.31
And AFP and CEA elevated preoperatively	19,886.46	32,216.06
Patients with cholangiocarcinoma or gallbladder cancer	7,326.27	11,868.55
And elevated CEA preoperatively	7,783.55	12,609.34
And elevated CA 19-9 preoperatively	7,800.19	12,636.30
And CEA and CA 19-9 elevated preoperatively	8,257.47	13,377.09
UK COUNTERPOINT (TABLES 11-11 AND 11-12)		
Patients with HCC	7,267.92	11,774.04
Patients with cholangiocarcinoma or gallbladder cancer	1,381.20	2,237.54
UWMC COUNTERPOINT (TABLES 11-16, 11-18, AND 11-19)		
Patients with recurrent HCC	8,839.11	14,319.36
And cirrhosis	9,622.71	15,588.80
Patients with persistent or recurrent HCC following nonresectional ablative techniques	8,706.01	14,103.74
And persistently elevated AFP and increased attenuation by CT	9,103.03	14,746.91
Patients with cholangiocarcinoma or gallbladder cancer	1,013.32	1,641.57

HCC, Hepatocellular carcinoma; *AFP,* alpha-fetoprotein; *CEA,* carcinoembryonic antigen; *CT,* computed tomography.
*Using 1992 charge data.
†Medicare-allowed charges × 1.62 conversion ratio.

Table 3-9 Bronchogenic carcinoma (Chapter 12): total 5-year follow-up charges*

	MEDICARE CHARGES ($)	ACTUAL CHARGES ($)†
MSKCC PRIMARY (TABLE 12-2)	2,142.22	3,470.40
JAPAN COUNTERPOINT (TABLES 12-3 AND 12-7)		
Clinical trial intensive follow-up protocol	23,823.94	38,594.77
And sputum cytology for patients with resected squamous cell carcinoma and for either current or former smokers	24,032.89	38,933.27
Patients not enrolled in clinical trials	2,980.16	4,827.86
RPCI COUNTERPOINT (TABLE 12-8)	2,142.22	3,470.40
UWMC COUNTERPOINT (TABLE 12-9)	1,734.48	2,809.86

*Using 1992 charge data.
†Medicare-allowed charges × 1.62 conversion ratio.

Table 3-10 Soft tissue sarcoma (Chapter 13): total 5-year follow-up charges*

	MEDICARE CHARGES ($)	ACTUAL CHARGES ($)†
UWMC PRIMARY (TABLES 13-7 AND 13-8)		
Patients at low risk	12,563.16	20,352.31
Patients at high risk	18,471.15	29,923.26
JAPAN COUNTERPOINT (TABLES 13-18, 13-19, AND 13-20)		
Patients with low-grade sarcomas		
And superficial or small lesions	2,956.08	4,788.85
And deeply seated or large primary lesions	18,663.62	30,235.06
Patients with high-grade sarcomas	33,149.20	53,701.70
MSKCC COUNTERPOINT (TABLES 13-11, 13-12, AND 13-13)		
Patients with extremity sarcomas <5 cm	1,244.10	2,015.44
Patients with low-grade extremity sarcomas ≥5 cm	1,244.10	2,015.44
Patients with high-grade extremity sarcomas		
≥5 cm and ≤10 cm	2,097.80	3,398.44
>10 cm	3,282.80	5,318.14
Patients with retroperitoneal, gastrointestinal, or visceral sarcomas	26,477.28	42,893.19
RPCI COUNTERPOINT (TABLES 13-22 AND 13-23)		
Patients with extremity soft tissue sarcoma	8,069.28	13,072.23
Patients with intraabdominal and retroperitoneal soft tissue sarcoma	24,460.94	39,626.72
UK COUNTERPOINT (TABLE 13-21)	3,306.90	4,919.77

*Using 1992 charge data.
†Medicare-allowed charges × 1.62 conversion ratio.

Table 3-11 Cutaneous melanoma (Chapter 14): total 5-year follow-up charges*

	MEDICARE CHARGES ($)	ACTUAL CHARGES ($)†
MSKCC PRIMARY (TABLES 14-1, 14-2, AND 14-3)		
Patients with negative nodes		
And primary tumor <1 mm	1,048.20	1,698.08
And primary tumor 1-4 mm	1,648.12	2,669.96
And primary tumor >4 mm	1,832.88	2,969.27
Patients with positive nodes	1,807.04	2,927.40
JAPAN COUNTERPOINT (TABLES 14-4, 14-5, 14-6, AND 14-7)		
Patients with negative nodes		
And primary tumor ≤1.5 mm	1,427.13	2,311.96
And primary tumor 1.51-3 mm	1,949.53	3,158.25
And primary tumor >3 mm	3,865.39	6,261.93
Patients with positive nodes	6,913.17	11,199.32
RPCI COUNTERPOINT (TABLES 14-11 AND 14-12)		
Patients with negative nodes		
And primary tumor <1 mm	1,284.64	2,081.11
And primary tumor ≥1 mm	2,569.28	4,162.23
Patients with positive nodes	2,569.28	4,162.23
UK COUNTERPOINT (TABLES 14-8, 14-9, AND 14-10)		
Patients with negative nodes		
And primary tumor <0.76 mm	65.30	105.79
And primary tumor ≥0.76 mm	1,150.48	1,863.79
Patients with positive nodes	1,807.04	2,927.40

*Using 1992 charge data.
†Medicare-allowed charges × 1.62 conversion ratio.

Continued.

Table 3-11 Cutaneous melanoma (Chapter 14): total 5-year follow-up charges*–cont'd

	MEDICARE CHARGES ($)	ACTUAL CHARGES ($)†
UWMC COUNTERPOINT (TABLES 14-13 AND 14-14)		
Patients with negative nodes		
And primary tumor <1 mm	918.60	1,488.13
And primary tumor ≥1 mm	1,375.70	2,228.63
Patients with positive nodes	1,375.70	2,228.63

Table 3-12 Breast carcinoma (Chapter 15): total 5-year follow-up charges*

	MEDICARE CHARGES ($)	ACTUAL CHARGES ($)†
RPCI PRIMARY (TABLE 15-1)	1,856.69	3,022.43
JAPAN COUNTERPOINT (TABLES 15-8, 15-9)		
Node-negative patients (except those with grade 3 histology and/or positive p53 expression)	6,022.30	9,756.12
Node-positive patients (and node-negative patients excluded above)	6,693.26	10,843.07
And with tumors ≥10 cm	8,265.56	13,390.20
And with tumors ≥4 cm with c-*erb*B-2 positive expression and/or grade 3 histology	8,265.56	13,390.20
MSKCC COUNTERPOINT (TABLE 15-3)	2,709.86	4,389.97
UK COUNTERPOINT (TABLE 15-10)	936.55	1,517.21
UWMC COUNTERPOINT (TABLE 15-11)	2,207.96	3,576.90
Intermediate- and high-risk patients	2,498.96	4,048.32

*Using 1992 charge data.
†Medicare-allowed charges × 1.62 conversion ratio.

Table 3-13 Ovarian carcinoma (Chapter 16): total 5-year follow-up charges*

	MEDICARE CHARGES ($)	ACTUAL CHARGES ($)†
RPCI PRIMARY (TABLE 16-3)	1,518.72	2,460.33
JAPAN COUNTERPOINT (TABLES 16-6 AND 16-7)		
Patients with early-stage, low-risk disease	4,508.85	7,304.34
Patients with high-risk, advanced disease	19,061.76	30,880.05
MSKCC COUNTERPOINT (TABLES 16-4 AND 16-5)		
Patients with epithelial tumors after bilateral adnexectomy	1,044.80	1,692.58
And previously abnormal CA-125 levels	1,518.72	2,460.33
Patients with retained adnexae	1,044.80	1,692.58
And previously abnormal CA-125 levels	1,518.72	2,460.33
And with germ cell tumors and previously abnormal levels of beta-HCG or AFP	1,669.92	2,705.27
And low-malignant potential tumors or well-differentiated tumors confined to the ovary	3,101.50	5,024.43
And both previously abnormal CA-125 levels, with germ cell tumors, and previously abnormal levels of beta-HCG or AFP	2,143.84	3,473.02
And both previously abnormal CA-125 levels and low-malignant potential tumors or well-differentiated tumors confined to the ovary	3,575.42	5,792.18
And both with germ cell tumors, previously abnormal levels of beta-HCG or AFP, and low-malignant potential tumors or well-differentiated tumors confined to the ovary	3,726.62	6,037.12
UWMC COUNTERPOINT (TABLE 16-8)	1,613.64	2,614.09

HCG, Human chorionic gonadotropin; AFP, alpha-fetoprotein.
*Using 1992 charge data.
†Medicare-allowed charges × 1.62 conversion ratio.

Table 3-14 Endometrial carcinoma (Chapter 17): total 5-year follow-up charges*

	MEDICARE CHARGES ($)	ACTUAL CHARGES ($)†
UWMC PRIMARY (TABLE 17-8)	560.65	908.26
Patients with elevated CA-125 at time of initial treatment or with known extrauterine disease	797.61	1,292.14
JAPAN COUNTERPOINT (TABLE 17-19)	4,945.72	8,011.34
MSKCC COUNTERPOINT (TABLE 17-9)	560.65	908.26
Patients with elevated CA-125 at time of initial treatment or with known extrauterine disease	797.61	1,292.14
RPCI COUNTERPOINT (TABLE 17-21)	560.65	908.26
Patients with elevated CA-125 at time of initial treatment or with known extrauterine disease	797.61	1,292.14

*Using 1992 charge data.
†Medicare-allowed charges × 1.62 conversion ratio.

Table 3-15 Prostate carcinoma (Chapter 18): total 5-year follow-up charges*

	MEDICARE CHARGES ($)	ACTUAL CHARGES ($)†
RPCI PRIMARY (TABLE 18-2)	1,351.00	2,188.62
JAPAN COUNTERPOINT (TABLE 18-8)	2,837.06	4,596.03
MSKCC COUNTERPOINT (TABLE 18-4)	1,139.04	1,845.24
UWMC COUNTERPOINT (TABLE 18-9)	1,100.99	1,783.60

*Using 1992 charge data.
†Medicare-allowed charges × 1.62 conversion ratio.

Table 3-16 Testicular carcinoma (Chapter 19): total 5-year follow-up charges*

	MEDICARE CHARGES ($)	ACTUAL CHARGES ($)†
RPCI PRIMARY (TABLES 19-4 AND 19-5)		
Patients with stage A testicular cancer	11,864.42	19,220.36
Patients with stage B or C testicular cancer	10,586.00	17,149.32
JAPAN COUNTERPOINT (TABLES 19-12, 19-13, AND 19-14)		
Patients with stage I seminoma treated by prophylactic retroperitoneal irradiation		
With computed tomography	5,766.47	9,341.68
With ultrasound	3,307.85	5,358.70
Patients with stage I NSGCT without RPLND		
With computed tomography	11,208.04	18,157.03
With ultrasound	6,582.44	10,663.56
Patients with stage II seminoma and NSGCT		
With computed tomography	10,555.04	17,099.16
With ultrasound	5,929.44	9,605.69
Patients with stage III seminoma and NSGCT		
With computed tomography	10,999.30	17,818.86
With ultrasound	6,373.70	10,325.39

RPLND, Retroperitoneal lymph node dissection; *NSGCT,* nonseminoma germ cell tumor.
*Using 1992 charge data.
†Medicare-allowed charges × 1.62 conversion ratio..

Continued.

Table 3-16 Testicular carcinoma (Chapter 19): total 5-year follow-up charges*—cont'd

	MEDICARE CHARGES ($)	ACTUAL CHARGES ($)†
MSKCC COUNTERPOINT (TABLES 19-6, 19-7, 19-8, AND 19-9)		
Patients with stage I NSGCT		
N0	14,885.55	24,114.60
N1 or N2 with no adjuvant chemotherapy	14,885.55	24,114.60
All other stage I NSGCT	27,395.07	44,380.02
Patients with stage II N1, N2b, or N3 NSGCT after RPLND	4,621.14	7,486.25
Patients with stage III NSGCT after RPLND and adjuvant chemotherapy	4,213.48	6,825.84
And teratoma detected in the retroperitoneum	10,468.24	16,958.55
Patients with stage I, IIA, or III seminoma	12,031.93	19,491.73
UWMC COUNTERPOINT (TABLES 19-15, 19-16, 19-17, 19-18, AND 19-19)		
Patients with stage I testicular cancer after orchiectomy alone	28,347.27	45,922.58
Patients with stage I or II testicular cancer after RPLND	7,067.10	11,448.71
Patients with stage II testicular cancer after adjuvant chemotherapy	11,449.17	18,547.66
Patients with stage III testicular cancer after chemotherapy with complete response	12,138.18	19,663.86
Patients with seminoma after orchiectomy and radiation therapy	12,031.93	19,491.73

Table 3-17 Urinary bladder carcinoma (Chapter 20): total 5-year follow-up charges*

	MEDICARE CHARGES ($)	ACTUAL CHARGES ($)†
MSKCC PRIMARY (TABLES 20-1 AND 20-2)		
Patients with superficial bladder tumors	13,818.26‡	22,385.58‡
After cystectomy		
With IVP	15,990.11‡	25,903.97‡
With renal ultrasound	17,278.73	27,991.54
And receiving an orthotopic internal reservoir to the urethra		
With IVP	16,948.97‡	27,457.33‡
With renal ultrasound	18,237.59	29,544.90
JAPAN COUNTERPOINT (TABLES 20-3 AND 20-4)		
Patients with superficial bladder tumors	12,108.24‡	19,615.34‡
After cystectomy	14,105.05‡	22,850.18‡
And receiving an orthotopic internal reservoir to the urethra	16,097.13‡	26,077.35‡
RPCI COUNTERPOINT (TABLES 20-5 AND 20-6)		
Patients with superficial bladder tumors	11,253.23‡	18,230.23‡
After cystectomy	3,099.21‡	5,020.72‡
And receiving an orthotopic internal reservoir to the urethra	3,989.58‡	6,463.12‡
UWMC COUNTERPOINT (TABLES 20-7 AND 20-8)		
Patients with superficial bladder tumors		
Except papilloma TaG1	8,044.53‡	13,032.13‡
Papilloma TaG1	6,465.11‡	10,473.47‡
After cystectomy		
With IVP	18,749.45‡	30,374.10‡
With renal ultrasound	20,038.07	32,461.66

IVP, Intravenous pyelography.
*Using 1992 charge data.
†Medicare-allowed charges × 1.62 conversion ratio.
‡Totals are conservative because facility charge data are not available for intravenous pyelogram.

Table 3-18 Renal cell carcinoma (Chapter 21): total 5-year follow-up charges*

	MEDICARE CHARGES ($)	ACTUAL CHARGES ($)†
MSKCC PRIMARY (TABLE 21-1)		
Patients with P1 tumors	653.00	1,057.86
And undergoing partial nephrectomy	882.60	1,429.81
And with VHL disease	18,713.80	30,316.36
And both undergoing partial nephrectomy and with VHL disease	18,943.40	30,688.31
Patients with P2 or P3 tumors	1,509.00	2,444.58
And undergoing partial nephrectomy	1,738.60	2,816.53
And with VHL disease	19,569.80	31,703.08
And both undergoing partial nephrectomy and with VHL disease	19,799.40	32,075.31
JAPAN COUNTERPOINT (TABLES 21-2 AND 21-3)		
Patients with P1 tumors after radical nephrectomy		
With ultrasound	2,584.35	4,186.65
With computed tomography	4,318.95	6,996.70
Patients with P1 tumors after partial nephrectomy		
With ultrasound	4,892.25	7,925.45
With computed tomography	6,626.85	10,735.50
Patients with P2 or P3 tumors after radical nephrectomy or P4 tumors after resections of metastases simultaneous with or subsequent to radical nephrectomy		
With ultrasound	3,576.45	5,793.85
With computed tomography	6,467.45	10,477.27
RPCI COUNTERPOINT (TABLE 21-4)		
Patients with T1 tumors	579.04	938.05
Patients with T2 or T3 tumors	1,318.08	2,135.29
UWMC COUNTERPOINT (TABLE 21-5)		
Patients with T1 or T2 N- tumors	2,688.29	4,355.03
And <50% residual renal mass postoperatively	2,695.37	4,366.50
Patients with T1 or T2 N+ tumors	5,071.46	8,215.77
And <50% residual renal mass	5,078.54	8,227.24
Patients with T3 or T4 tumors	5,071.46	8,215.77
And <50% residual renal mass	5,078.54	8,227.24
And N+	5,802.97	9,400.82
And both <50% residual renal mass and N+	5,810.05	9,412.28

VHL, von Hippel-Lindau.
*Using 1992 charge data.
†Medicare-allowed charges × 1.62 conversion ratio.

Table 3-19 Lymphoma (Chapter 22): total 5-year follow-up charges*

	MEDICARE CHARGES ($)	ACTUAL CHARGES ($)†
UWMC PRIMARY (TABLE 22-3)		
Patients with aggressive NHL	2,532.70	4,102.98
And treated with mediastinal or neck irradiation	2,665.45	4,318.03
And abnormal LDH and beta-2 microglobulin levels in absence of detectable disease		
With computed tomography	13,128.30	21,267.85
With MRI	16,128.30	26,127.85
And both treated with mediastinal or neck irradiation and with abnormal LDH and beta-2 microglobulin levels in absence of disease		
With computed tomography	13,261.05	21,482.91
With MRI	16,261.05	26,342.91

NHL, Non-Hodgkin's lymphoma; *LDH*, lactic dehydrogenase; *MRI*, magnetic resonance imaging.
*Using 1992 charge data.
†Medicare-allowed charges 3 1.62 conversion ratio.

Continued.

Table 3-19 Lymphoma (Chapter 22): total 5-year follow-up charges*—cont'd

	MEDICARE CHARGES ($)	ACTUAL CHARGES ($)†
UWMC PRIMARY (TABLE 22-3)		
Patients with Hodgkin's lymphoma	2,246.96	3,640.08
And treated with mediastinal or neck irradiation	2,379.71	3,855.14
And abnormal LDH and beta-2 microglobulin levels in absence of detectable disease		
With computed tomography	12,842.56	20,804.95
With MRI	15,842.56	25,664.95
And both treated with mediastinal or neck irradiation and with abnormal LDH and beta-2 microglobulin levels in absence of disease		
With computed tomography	12,975.31	21,020.01
With MRI	15,975.31	25,880.01
JAPAN COUNTERPOINT (TABLE 22-7)		
Patients with aggressive NHL	2,751.85	4,458.00
And treated with mediastinal or neck irradiation	2,884.60	4,673.05
And abnormal LDH and beta-2 microglobulin levels in absence of detectable disease		
With computed tomography	13,347.45	21,622.87
With MRI	16,347.45	26,482.87
And both treated with mediastinal or neck irradiation and with abnormal LDH and beta-2 microglobulin levels in absence of disease		
With computed tomography	13,480.20	21,837.93
With MRI	16,480.20	26,697.93
Patients with Hodgkin's lymphoma	2,466.11	3,995.10
And treated with mediastinal or neck irradiation	2,598.86	4,210.16
And abnormal LDH levels in absence of detectable disease		
With computed tomography	13,061.71	21,159.97
With MRI	16,061.71	26,019.97
And both treated with mediastinal or neck irradiation and with abnormal LDH levels in absence of disease		
With computed tomography	13,194.46	21,375.03
With MRI	16,194.46	26,235.03
MSKCC COUNTERPOINT (TABLES 22-4, 22-5, AND 22-6)		
Patients with NHL		
Low-grade	18,206.18	29,494.01
Intermediate-grade	18,022.66	29,196.71
High-grade	18,389.70	29,791.31
Patients with Hodgkin's lymphoma	16,767.08	27,162.67
And female patients over age 30 after mantle irradiation	17,113.84	27,724.42

Continued.

Table 3-19 Lymphoma (Chapter 22): total 5-year follow-up charges*—cont'd

	MEDICARE CHARGES ($)	ACTUAL CHARGES ($)†
RPCI COUNTERPOINT (TABLE 22-9)		
Patients with NHL	1,918.22	3,107.51
And treated with mediastinal or neck irradiation	2,050.97	3,322.57
And with elevated beta-2 microglobulin levels pretreatment	2,225.80	3,605.79
And abnormal LDH and beta-2 microglobulin levels in absence of detectable disease		
With computed tomography	10,715.47	17,359.06
With MRI	13,715.47	22,219.06
And both treated with mediastinal or neck irradiation and with elevated beta-2 microglobulin levels pretreatment	2,358.55	3,820.85
And both treated with mediastinal or neck irradiation and with abnormal LDH and beta-2 microglobulin levels in absence of disease		
With computed tomography	10,848.22	17,574.12
With MRI	13,848.22	22,434.12
And both with elevated beta-2 microglobulin levels pretreatment and with abnormal LDH and beta-2 microglobulin levels in absence of disease		
With computed tomography	11,023.05	17,857.34
With MRI	14,023.05	22,717.34
And both treated with mediastinal or neck irradiation, with abnormal LDH and beta-2 microglobulin levels in absence of disease, and with elevated beta-2 microglobulin levels pretreatment		
With computed tomography	11,155.80	18,072.40
With MRI	14,155.80	22,932.40
Patients with Hodgkin's lymphoma	1,987.38	3,219.55
And treated with mediastinal or neck irradiation	2,120.13	3,434.61
And abnormal LDH and beta-2 microglobulin levels in absence of detectable disease		
With computed tomography	10,784.63	17,471.10
With MRI	13,784.63	22,331.10
And both treated with mediastinal or neck irradiation and with abnormal LDH and beta-2 microglobulin levels in absence of disease		
With computed tomography	10,917.38	17,686.16
With MRI	13,917.38	22,546.16
UK COUNTERPOINT (TABLE 22-8)	1,683.44	2,727.17
Patients with residual chest, abdominal, or pelvic masses	6,273.84	10,163.61

Table 3-20 Stem cell transplantation (Chapter 23): total 5-year follow-up charges*

	MEDICARE CHARGES ($)	ACTUAL CHARGES ($)†
UWMC PRIMARY (TABLES 23-5 AND 23-6)		
Adult male patients	4,316.49	6,992.71
And with chronic myelogenous leukemia	5,228.59	8,470.31
Adult female patients	4,414.39	7,151.31
And with chronic myelogenous leukemia	5,326.49	8,628.91
And total body irradiation recipient, >35 years of age	4,847.84	7,853.50
And both with chronic myelogenous leukemia and total body irradiation recipient, >35 years of age	5,759.94	9,331.10
Children <8 years of age	3,785.29	6,132.17
Children ≥8 years of age		
Males	3,975.79	6,440.78
Females	3,983.29	6,452.93
JAPAN COUNTERPOINT (TABLE 23-10)		
Males		
With computed tomography	108,513.85	175,792.12
With MRI	134,586.40	218,029.66
Females		
With computed tomography	108,611.75	175,950.72
With MRI	134,684.30	218,188.26
MSKCC COUNTERPOINT (TABLES 23-7, 23-8, AND 23-9)		
Patients with NHL		
Low-grade	18,206.18	29,494.01
Intermediate-grade	18,022.66	29,196.71
High-grade	18,389.70	29,791.31
Patients with Hodgkin's lymphoma	16,767.08	27,162.67
And female patients over age 30 after mantle irradiation	17,113.84	27,724.42
RPCI COUNTERPOINT (TABLE 23-13)		
Adult male patients	3,266.29	5,291.40
And with chronic myelogenous leukemia	4,178.39	6,769.00
Adult female patients	3,312.04	5,365.52
And with chronic myelogenous leukemia	4,224.14	6,843.12
And total body irradiation recipient, >35 years of age	3,745.49	6,067.71
And both with chronic myelogenous leukemia and total body irradiation recipient, >35 years of age	4,657.59	7,545.31
UK COUNTERPOINT (TABLE 23-12)		
Males	1,954.54	3,166.36
Females	2,350.54	3,807.88

MRI, magnetic resonance imaging; *NHL*, non-Hodgkin's lymphoma.
*Using 1992 charge data.
†Medicare-allowed charges × 1.62 conversion ratio.

cancer, with three of four authors in agreement. It was even uncommon for any two authors in this text to agree on one follow-up strategy for a given cancer site. This is not to say that the recommended strategies for all remaining sites were in no way similar, as an examination of charge ranges reveals, although the majority varied substantially.

As a demonstration of the similarity across strategies, the range of total Medicare-allowed charges was narrowest for bronchogenic carcinoma ($1,246), thin node-negative cutaneous melanoma ($1,362), intermediate-thickness node-negative cutaneous melanoma ($1,419), head and neck carcinoma ($1,560), and prostate carcinoma ($1,736). Other cancers with low variation across recommendations include P2 or T2 renal carcinoma ($2,258), thick node-negative cutaneous melanoma ($2,715), ovarian carcinoma ($3,464), and P3 or T3 renal carcinoma ($3,753).

The range of total Medicare-allowed charges for cancer patient follow-up was broadest after stem cell transplantation where charges for males varied by $106,559 and for females by $106,261. The ranges of charges for esophageal ($25,561) and pancreatic cancer ($23,638) were also high but were nowhere near stem cell transplantation. For both of these cancers, differences between follow-up intensity in Japan and in the United States accounted for the large variation in charges. Excluding the Japanese counterpoint, follow-up charges for pancreatic cancer varied by approximately $2,300. The average range of charges across all 19 sites was $14,534 (standard deviation [s.d.] = $24,939). When stem cell transplantation was classified as an outlier and excluded from the analysis, the average range of charges was $8,409 (s.d. = $6,625).

The magnitude of the difference in total Medicare-allowed charges by site was then examined. The charge differential for stem cell transplantation was 56-fold for males and 46-fold for females, while for esophageal cancer the differential was 37-fold. For thin node-negative cutaneous melanomas the magnitude of the charge differential was also high (22-fold), although the range of charges was only $1,362. Other cancer sites with high charge differentials included pancreatic (16-fold), cholangiocarcinoma or gallbladder (12-fold), non-Hodgkin's lymphoma (NHL) (11-fold), Hodgkin's lymphoma (10-fold), and soft tissue carcinoma (10-fold). Twenty-one percent of cancer sites had low charge differentials (≤ two-fold). These sites included bronchogenic carcinoma, intermediate-thickness node-negative cutaneous melanoma, head and neck carcinoma, superficial bladder carcinoma, stage II or B testicular carcinoma, testicular seminoma, and rectal carcinoma. An additional six sites (18.8%) had three-fold differences, and five (15.6%) had four-fold differences. The average charge differential across all 19 sites was 10 (s.d. = 13) and 7 (s.d. = 7) when stem cell transplantation was treated as an outlier.

When Medicare-allowed charges were converted to an actual charge proxy using a conversion ratio of 1.62, the range of actual charges was $172,626 for males after stem cell transplantation and $172,143 for females, $41,409 for esophageal cancer, $38,296 for pancreatic cancer, $2,046 for thin node-negative cutaneous melanoma, and $2,018 for bronchogenic cancer. The average range of actual charges across all sites was $23,540 (s.d. = $40,404) and, when stem cell transplantation was treated as an outlier, $13,617 (s.d. = $10,738).

Not surprisingly, strategies using frequent endoscopy, nuclear medicine scans, computed tomography, and magnetic resonance imaging over the 5-year period were at the high end of the cost distribution. Regimens that consisted mainly of some combination of office visits, complete blood count, liver function tests, tumor markers, and chest x-ray were the least expensive. The lowest cost approaches consisted of only one or two types of tests. Across all cancer sites the strategy with the greatest frequency of either visits or any single test was the Japanese strategy for the follow-up of patients after stem cell transplantation. Over the 5-year follow-up period, 40 to 45 office visits are recommended. Other strategies with high frequencies of office visits or any single test include the Japanese strategy for the follow-up of head and neck cancer patients with a poor prognosis, which recommends 40 office visits, the Japanese strategy for the follow-up of esophageal cancer patients with 36 office visits and 36 squamous cell antigen titers, and the University of Washington Medical Center (UWMC) strategy for patient follow-up after stem cell transplantation with 32 office visits. The most intensive 5-year strategy across the greatest number of tests was the Japanese strategy for the management of patients after stem cell transplantation with 40 to 45 office visits recommended in conjunction with electroencephalogram, computed tomography of the brain or magnetic resonance imaging, chest x-ray, electrocardiogram, echocardiogram, and pulmonary function tests for a total of 325 total visits and tests. Other high-intensity strategies include the Japanese strategy for the follow-up of pancreatic cancer with 272 visits and tests and the Japanese strategy for the management of endometrial cancer with 218 visits and tests. It is worth noting that total charges for the Japanese strategy for endometrial cancer patient surveillance were not particularly high ($4,946). This was due to the predominance of low-cost blood tests and tumor markers as opposed to more expensive radiological or nuclear medicine tests.

The charge figures quoted here can be considered conservative in today's economy since they were derived from 1992 data. These figures can easily be updated to 1996 levels by using the medical care component of the Consumer Price Index. Since 1960 this component has never been negative.[36] The medical care component increased 5.94% in 1993, 4.76% in 1994, and 4.5% in 1995. A 10-year (1985-1995) average increase in the medical care component of 6.86% was used as an estimated increase for 1996. Pancreatic cancer is used as an example to illustrate the effect of incorporating these increases. The 1996 updated Medicare-allowed charge figures are $4,776 for Roswell Park Cancer Institute (RPCI), $2,639 for Memorial Sloan-Kettering Cancer Center (MSKCC), $1,985 for UWMC, $31,282 for Japan, and $3,180 for the United Kingdom for a range of $29,297. The 1996 updated actual charge figures are $7,737 for RPCI, $4,274 for MSKCC, $3,217 for UWMC, $50,679 for Japan, and $5,152 for the United Kingdom for a range of $47,462.

COMMENT

Few attempts have been made to measure the relevant costs associated with many medical practices, and cancer patient follow-up is no exception. As this analysis indicates, charges for follow-up can vary widely. Although variation in the range of charges for follow-up depends largely on site, variation as high as 56-fold within sites cannot easily be justified in this era of cost containment and health care reform. The problem is an especially interesting one because little is known about how outcomes vary when components of the follow-up strategy are altered, and optimal follow-up testing intervals are rarely defined by well-designed trials. For most cancers no one strategy has been established as more efficacious than any other in terms of survival and quality of life, yet the surveillance of cancer patients has achieved considerable consensus (e.g., lung cancer).[26]

As this chapter has shown, cost analyses of postoperative cancer surveillance have rarely been conducted over the past 15 years. The existing literature has often provided insufficient data for rigorous interpretation of results and comparison to other studies. Because this book summarizes the recommendations of major cancer centers throughout the United States, Japan, and the United Kingdom for the follow-up of 19 major cancer sites after treatment, it has provided an excellent opportunity to use one methodology to estimate costs and thereby facilitate comparisons across strategies. Although many assumptions were made in calculating cost estimates, the data represent a conservative starting point for understanding how expensive cancer patient follow-up can be and how minor modifications in strategy can result in major modifications in cost. As explained in detail in Chapter 2, such analyses should ideally incorporate not only the direct costs of follow-up as approximated in this chapter, but also the indirect costs such as time lost from work, transportation costs, and child and adult care costs. Quality-of-life data should also be examined, since such data are practically nonexistent in this field.[37] Quality of life may be either directly or indirectly affected by the intensity of the follow-up regimen.

One limitation of the current analysis is that actual cancer patients were not followed prospectively to estimate costs. Although several strategies included in the literature review are based on actual patient data, a large prospective study would allow one to collect data on the costs of many factors assumed away in many analyses, such as diagnosis and treatment costs for patients with symptoms or positive test results.

A second limitation is that this chapter mainly examines follow-up after resection, unless a strategy was provided by the chapter author or counterpoint author for follow-up after nonoperative therapy. Many patients are treated with chemotherapy or radiation therapy and are followed intensively after therapy. The cost ramifications of current follow-up practice for this large patient population may be even greater than for curatively treated patients with much less potential for improving survival.

The cost differentials among surveillance strategies identified in this chapter will be increasingly difficult to sustain in the current competitive medical practice environment in which cost containment is such a dominant force. Even in instances in which the variation in costs is moderate, such as prostate cancer or bronchogenic carcinoma, the number of patients with these diagnoses is large and therefore the total costs associated with each annual cohort of newly diagnosed patients are staggering. Research in the form of clinical trials is clearly needed to compare intensities of follow-up and determine if higher costs are substantiated by improved quality of life and longer survival.

REFERENCES

1. Virgo KS, Vernava AM, Longo WE, McKirgan LW, Johnson FE. Cost of patient follow-up after potentially curative colorectal cancer treatment. JAMA 1995;273:1837-41.
2. Parker SL, Tong T, Bolden S, Wingo PA. Cancer statistics 1996. CA Cancer J Clin 1996;65:5-27.
3. Kosecoff JB. Fundamentals of HMOs, PHOs, PSOs, PSNs and other emerging network structures: what are they and how do they differ? Presentation at the annual meetings of the Association for Health Services Research, June 9-11, 1996, Atlanta, GA.
4. Bero L, Rennie D. The Cochrane Collaboration: preparing, maintaining, and disseminating systematic reviews of the effects of health care. JAMA 1995;274:1935-8.
5. Robinson A. Research, practice, and the Cochrane Collaboration. Can Med Assn J 1995;152:883-9.
6. Chalmers I, Haynes B. Reporting, updating, and correcting systematic reviews of the effects of health care. Br Med J 1994;309:862-5.
7. Moertel CG, Fleming TR, MacDonald JS, Haller DG, Laurie JA, Tangen C. An evaluation of the carcinoembryonic antigen (CEA) test for monitoring patients with resected colon cancer. JAMA 1993;270:943-7.
8. Health Care Financing Administration. Part B Medicare Annual Data (BMAD) file, 1992a.
9. Health Care Financing Administration. Medicare Hospital Outpatient Bill (HOP) file, 1992b.
10. Pauwels EK, Schütte HE, Arndt JW, van Langevelde A. Bone scintigraphy in oncology: an update with emphasis on efficacy and cost-effectiveness. Diag Imag Clin Med 1986;55:314-20.
11. Riley GF, Lubitz J. Longitudinal patterns in Medicare costs for cancer decedents. In: Scheffler RM, Andrews NC, editors. Cancer care and cost: DRGs and beyond. Ann Arbor, Michigan: Health Administration Press, 1989.
12. Baker MS, Kessler LG, Smucker RC. Site-specific treatment costs for cancer: an analysis of the Medicare continuous history sample file. In: Scheffler RM, Andrews NC, editors. Cancer care and cost: DRGs and beyond. Ann Arbor, Michigan: Health Administration Press, 1989.
13. Pera A, Capek M, Shirkhoda A. Lymphangiography and CT in the follow-up of patients with lymphoma. Radiology 1987;164:631-3.
14. D'Amico, Bassi N, Ranzato R. Cost-benefit of follow-up after total gastrectomy. Hepatogastroenterology 1989;36:266-72.
15. Ellis M, Hartley L, Sikora K. Value of follow up in testicular cancer. Br Med J 1984;289:1423.
16. Ciatto S, Cionini L, Pacini P. Cost-effectiveness of chest x-ray follow-up of patients treated for seminoma of the testis. Tumori 1986;72:405-8.
17. Berdel WE, Clemm C, Hartenstein R, et al. Benefit and costs of follow-up programs in nonseminomatous germ cell tumors of the stages IIb-IV: the Munich experience. Oncology 1987;44:273-8.
18. Horton J. Follow-up of breast cancer patients. Cancer 1984;53:790-7.
19. Schapira DV, Urban N. A minimalist policy for breast cancer surveillance. JAMA 1991;265:380-2.
20. Schapira DV. Breast cancer surveillance—a cost-effective strategy. Breast Cancer Res Treat 1993;25:107-11.
21. Hannisdal E, Gundersen S, Kvaloy S, et al. Follow-up of breast cancer patients stage I-II: a baseline strategy. Eur J Cancer 1993;29A:992-7.
22. Von Christa Wieland-Schneider EV, Kauczor H, Thelen M. Nachsorge des mammakarzinoms. Fortschr Röntgenstr 1994;160:513-7.
23. Mapelli V, Dirindin N, Grilli R. Economic evaluation of diagnostic follow-up after primary treatment for breast cancer: results of the working group on economic-organizational aspects of follow-up. Ann Oncol 1995;6:S61-4.
24. Kattlove H, Liberati A, Keeler E, Brook RH. Benefits and costs of screening and treatment for early breast cancer: development of a basic benefit package. JAMA 1995;273:142-8.
25. Walsh GL, O'Connor M, Willis KM, et al. Is follow-up of lung cancer patients following resection medically indicated and cost effective? Ann Thorac Surg 1995;60:1563-72.
26. Virgo KS, Naunheim KS, McKirgan LW, Kissling ME, Lin JC, Johnson FE. Cost of patient follow-up after potentially curative lung cancer treatment. J Thorac Cardiovasc Surg 1996;112:356-63.

27. Sandler RS, Freund DA, Herbst CA, Sandler DP. Cost effectiveness of postoperative carcinoembryonic antigen monitoring in colorectal cancer. Cancer 1984;53:193-8.
28. Saviano MS. Costi e benefici nel follow-up dopo amputazione addomino-perineale del retto per cancro. Minerva Med 1989;80:1225-31.
29. Kievit J, van de Velde CJ. Utility and cost of carcinoembryonic antigen monitoring in colon cancer follow-up evaluation. Cancer 1990;65:2580-7.
30. Rocklin MS, Slomski CA, Watne AL. Postoperative surveillance of patients with carcinoma of the colon and rectum. Am Surg 1990;56:22-7.
31. Ransohoff DF, Lang CA, Kuo HS. Colonoscopic surveillance after polypectomy: considerations of cost effectiveness. Ann Intern Med 1991;114:177-82.
32. Müller JM, Tübergen D, Zieren U. Nachsorge beim kolo-rektalen Karzinom: eine daten- und patientenorientierte Bewertung. Zentralbl Chir 1994;119:65-74.
33. Bruinvels DJ. Follow of patients with colorectal cancer. Doctoral thesis. Leiden, Netherlands, 1995.
34. Audisio RA, Setti-Carraro P, Segala M, Capko D, Andreoni B, Tiberio G. Follow-up in colorectal cancer patients: a cost-benefit analysis. Ann Surg Oncol 1996;3:349-57.
35. Currency trading. Wall Street Journal, July 8, 1996.
36. U.S. Bureau of Labor Statistics. Consumer Price Index, detailed report, multiple years.
37. Ladurie ML, Ranson-Bitker B. Quality of life following resection for lung cancer. In: Delarue NC, Eschapasse H, editors. International trends in general thoracic surgery, vol 1: lung cancer. Philadelphia: WB Saunders, 1985.

CHAPTER 4

How Are Surveillance Strategies Chosen?

St. Louis University Health Sciences Center ▪ St. Louis Department of Veterans Affairs Medical Center

FRANK E. JOHNSON

PATIENT, PHYSICIAN, AND SOCIETAL CONCERNS

How physicians reach clinical decisions of any sort is difficult to decipher, and decisions about cancer patient care are no exception. Guidelines formulated by groups of experts, such as the American Cancer Society and Consensus Conferences of the National Institutes of Health, have probably been influential,[1] but the extent of their influence cannot be measured easily. The controlled clinical trial is accepted as the most persuasive type of evidence, but such trials are expensive, time consuming, and hard to carry out.[2] Many trials deal with the best way to achieve cure, but few deal with posttreatment surveillance.[3] The clinician typically devises a follow-up strategy for each patient based on many factors, conscious as well as unconscious. There is clear evidence that early detection of certain types of cancer has a large impact on survival. Detection of disease in asymptomatic patients during routine evaluation was a strong predictor of outcomes for lung, prostate, and cervix cancers in the Seattle Longitudinal Assessment of Cancer Study.[4] Unfortunately, prompt evaluation of symptoms only weakly predicted long-term survival. These and other data provide empirical evidence that surveillance of asymptomatic individuals at high risk for cancer can be beneficial.

At this point it is worthwhile to distinguish screening from early detection. Screening tests usually provide only clues that may possibly indicate cancer in an apparently well population but do not usually result in the diagnosis of cancer. An abnormal fecal occult blood test, for example, is often due to a benign disorder. Early detection requires a definitive test that is almost always more invasive—a biopsy. Surveillance after primary cancer treatment typically relies more on screening tests than on tests requiring direct tissue sampling. Ideal screening tests should be simple, minimally invasive, quick to administer, accurate, reproducible, inexpensive, quantitative, acceptable to patients, and directed at a disorder with a distinct preclinical phase. The disorder should be one for which an effective intervention exists.[4] Major patient concerns are comfort and convenience. Physicians are more concerned with test specificity, sensitivity, and safety. Society is concerned with costs and outcomes. In a sense, patient and physician concerns are difficult to separate because the physician is morally bound to design and carry out a management plan for the patient that is in the patient's best interest. Nonetheless, physicians are only dimly aware of many patient and societal concerns. For example, physicians often ignore the logistical difficulties patients experience in complying with the requested posttreatment surveillance tests.

In addition, modern methods of decision analysis[5] reveal that patients and physicians view possible outcomes of medical management differently. It is becoming clearer that cost-benefit or cost-utility analysis, although complicated to carry out, may be too simplistic and that a more global view of health care outcome analysis may be preferable. The analysis should simultaneously take into account the overall health of an entire population (rather than an individual patient), the clinical outcome for each specific patient, the degree of patient satisfaction with possible or actual outcomes, and costs to patients and society. This is a tall order and likely to be warranted for only a few problems because of the difficulty in carrying it out. The current tendency in medicine to seek standardization, consensus building, and codification of practice promises to run afoul of differences among patients, especially when decisions involve major differences among possible strategies and corresponding differences among possible outcomes. Physicians should ideally honor patient preferences,[6] but there are obvious pitfalls of unconventional patient choices. Resistance must be expected from those who pay the bills when patient preferences involve excessive cost. In the future, many more analyses of patient preference can be anticipated, using tools from game theory such as the standard gamble, analog scales, and time trade-off methods.[5,6] When possible, patients should actively participate in medical decision making, and this is usually possible once the hurly-burly of cancer treatment has died down and emotions are no longer at flood tide.

Kassirer[6] has identified a number of attributes of "utility-sensitive" decisions (those strongly influenced by how patients value various possible outcomes). Such decisions arise when the possible choices involve large differences in possible outcomes, possible risks of intervention, trade-offs between near- and long-term events, small differences in outcomes in spite of large differences among interventions, and variations among patients in attaching values to specific possible outcomes or processes. Because considerations based on cost and effectiveness are increasing in prominence, it is becoming more important to identify what the patient values in life so that he or she is not shortchanged by impersonal, intrusive rules. This shift toward cost- and outcome-based decision making makes it increasingly important to assess patients' preferences and is a new reason for a close and trusting patient-physician relationship.

One would think that a major factor shaping clinical strategy after potentially curative treatment for cancer should be patient input. However, some patients are naive about the pathophysiology of cancer and rely on the physician's judgment. Other patients are highly motivated, intelligent, and aware of the natural history of cancer and risks and benefits of therapy; they may be more aggressive in planning their own posttreatment surveillance strategy. The subject of how patients' wishes and fears should and do affect clinical management has been studied relatively little.

Other pertinent concerns include the expense of follow-up, which can be considerable, as outlined in Chapter 3. This is particularly true for lesions for which modern medicine has some effective therapy, such as a second primary lesion arising in the same organ as the index lesion. Treatment costs are certainly a concern, particularly for the uninsured or underinsured individual being asked to undergo extensive tests in spite of feeling well. Currently, in Western industrial societies, the cost of follow-up is often largely assumed by entities other than the patient, creating a situation for these entities referred to as moral hazard. As a result, patients are willing to undergo more extensive and expensive postoperative surveillance testing than they might if costs were directly assessed to them. Physicians and patients also have concern about the inconvenience and periodic emotional upheaval associated with frequent surveillance testing. Thus patient choices can sway a physician in the direction of more intensive or less intensive surveillance.

Physicians' concerns primarily center on test validity. For a test to be valid, it must have high reproducibility (precision) and accuracy (concordance with a known standard). Precision evaluation requires testing multiple batches of identical samples on the same machine and evaluating machine-to-machine variation using multiple analytical machines. Estimation of test linearity requires measurement of the analyte of interest at varying concentrations. Run-to-run precision determination requires testing of known standards at several time points. Often the estimates of the analyte require comparison with reference methods to ensure comparability, since the test methodology may involve a different type of chemical reaction. These multiple validation procedures are usually carried out by the instrument manufacturer before introduction into the market, leaving more complicated issues, such as defining sensitivity, specificity, and predictive power, for clinicians to confirm. This can be difficult because both biological and analytical factors contribute to variability, even for an individual patient.

The critical difference between final test results is the degree of change needed to be considered clinically meaningful. This can be expressed as $K\,(X^2 + Y^2)^{1/2}$, where X is the coefficient of test variation resulting from analytical variability, Y is the coefficient of test variation resulting from biological variability, and K is a constant that is chosen on the basis of the probability level desired.[7] Analytical variability is commonly calculated rigorously, but biological variability, which is the degree of fluctuation of a test result in a single patient measured at various times, is often not evaluated.[7] Decision analysis theory can help root out such sources of irrationality in decision making. Biological variability probably will be more carefully documented in the future.

As physicians devise surveillance strategies, they often fail to consider the unpleasantness of undergoing testing. For about 20% of patients the clinic visit itself generates anxiety.[8] Some patients fear venipuncture, and others dread the claustrophobic feelings encountered during computed tomography scanning. More invasive tests often involve pain, which can be a real barrier. Patients' adherence to recommended surveillance schemes is often poor, probably related to these factors.[9] On the other hand, some patients suffer such anxiety about their cancer that they request, even demand, frequent surveillance. Coping with these difficult-to-quantify considerations is a matter of concern to physicians, particularly in the current climate of shrinking physician autonomy. When quality of life has been looked at in well-designed trials of more-intensive versus less-intensive follow-up for cancer patients,[3] the frequency of testing seems to have little impact on quality of life but patients do want regular follow-up by their physicians. This preference may simply reflect the trust patients have in modern medicine, particularly because little accurate information exists on the risks, benefits, and costs of various follow-up strategies. Certainly, patients cannot be expected to have detailed knowledge of this area. Alternatively, patients may derive emotional benefit from posttreatment follow-up, since this is what they have come to expect. Detrimental effects of frequent testing can also come into play, since patients may fear the discovery of cancer relapse every time testing is performed or a clinic visit occurs. Psychological benefit is also likely when tests do not reveal disease recurrence. A minimalist approach to cancer patient surveillance may not be achievable in wealthy societies, since patients and physicians frequently seek information from diagnostic tests to evaluate symptoms or physical signs, even though physicians are well aware of test limitations, such as low sensitivity, low specificity, and high cost. Controversies about costs and benefits continue to appear in the scientific literature. It is not surprising that patients, appropriately concerned with their own welfare, expect (and receive) intensive follow-up.[10,11]

There is little doubt that testing often reveals recurrent cancer before it is clinically apparent. It is less clear whether recurrence of the index lesion can be managed successfully, and even more doubtful whether such recurrences can be detected in a cost-effective way.[12] Well-designed, randomized clinical trials are very persuasive and may alter the way physicians practice, but the practical problems in carrying them out[2] have led to a rapid expansion in outcomes research. This sort of research typically involves sifting information stored in extremely large computer-based data sets to discern how a medical intervention received by patients with a given condition is linked with various outcomes. The goal is to find out what intervention works best for which patients. Dominant forces behind this kind of retrospective data analysis have been industry and government officials who want to encourage physicians to use the most cost-effective treatments. The perception that physicians, bureaucrats, and accountants often cannot determine which medical maneuvers work best[13] has led to the idea that searching the medical records maintained by government agencies, insurance companies, and hospitals could generate a next-best idea of how well medical interventions pay off, avoiding costly, cumbersome, prospective, clinical trials. Use of administrative data to conduct medical research clearly has large advantages in terms of the number of evaluable patients, availability of information about cost, representativeness of the population studied, and substantial freedom from biases affecting randomized trials.[2] Equally clearly, research using these techniques cannot easily discern and analyze the reasons a particular physician chose a particular medical intervention for a particular patient. Even the harshest critics of this research technique concede that it is often the only way to obtain information on uncommon conditions, uncommon treatments, or special populations of patients. Advocates insist that such retrospective research has a long record of producing results—far longer than randomized controlled trials—and is clearly better than nothing, which is what would be available if prospective trials were relied on to address every issue of interest.[13] In the field of surveillance after primary cancer treatment, secondary analysis of prospectively collected data can yield compelling data.[12] The statistical tool of metaanalysis, which has been available for nearly a century, has experienced explosive growth recently. This technique allows many small studies, each with little statistical power and often with conflicting results, to be considered together. It promises to resolve nettlesome questions at the interface of medicine and social policy.[14,15]

Another common method of affecting medical decisions is the generation of practice guidelines, which are used to limit inappropriate or harmful medical practice, reduce geographic variation in medical practice patterns, and eliminate waste. This is a powerful and broad-based trend in modern medicine.[16] The main motivation underlying this process is undoubtedly financial, but guidelines are also considered vehicles of physician education. Many methods of developing guidelines exist,[17] and many different yardsticks can be used to evaluate the success of these guidelines.[18] There is growing concern that the promulgation of guidelines could harm patient care.[18] Enforcement schemes, which inflict punishment on physicians who do not follow such guidelines, are of particular concern, since guidelines cannot define optimal care for all patients under all circumstances. When guidelines become more detailed, comprehensibility is often sacrificed to specificity. As generalizability decreases, cumbersomeness increases. If "cookbook" medicine replaces sound medical judgment—a fear often expressed—it is inconceivable that any cookbook of clinical guidelines will have enough recipes to encompass the complexities of human life and human disease.[19] The impulse to codify medical care can easily leave out approaches that are in a patient's best interests. Guidelines may be used as statements of the standard of care in medicolegal cases, tending to compel physicians to avoid valuable management options not spelled out in the cookbook. Parmley[19] also points out that guidelines are relatively conservative documents that cannot reflect late-breaking evidence of benefit or harm resulting from treatment decisions and are useful only if applied with wisdom and flexibility. Guidelines are particularly likely to be used in cancer patient follow-up, but stringent enforcement offers the prospect of harm to patients, paradoxically increased costs, and unfair legal or administrative judgments against physicians who deviate from them.[18] The limited literature to date suggests that clinical guidelines do improve clinical practice,[1] but the improvement is often disappointingly small.[20] Increasingly, physician concerns are being superseded by the financial aspects of modern medical care, in which cost-benefit analyses are paramount, and authoritative opinions from experienced physicians may count less than the formula prescribed by impersonal committees constructing practice parameters.

ETHICAL AND LEGAL ISSUES

Physicians, particularly in the United States but to an increasing extent in other countries, must be concerned with medicolegal issues. Everyone knows of patients who seem impossible to satisfy and from whom lawsuits may arise. Busy clinicians always have poor results of therapy in some instances, whether this is measured in terms of cosmesis, function, wound pain, or in other ways. One way to avoid medicolegal concerns is to obtain appropriate consultation when patients have suboptimal treatment outcomes, with the hope that responsibility for the poor outcome will be diffused among many individuals and with the expectation that the consultants will endorse the correctness of the treatment plan undertaken. In the United States, fear of being sued has assumed legendary proportions, not easily comprehended by practitioners in other countries, where lawsuits are much less common. Undoubtedly, defensive medicine plays a role in the decision making of individual physicians caring for their patients, and this includes posttreatment cancer surveillance.

An interesting opinion regarding the intensity of surveillance has been promulgated by Steele,[21] who believes that, at least for patients with colorectal cancer, follow-up should be conditioned by the setting in which it occurs. According to this concept, individuals who practice medicine in an arena where clinical research trials are available should assiduously search for eligible patients through relatively intensive follow-up testing. On the other hand, physicians in non-research-oriented institutions may do more harm to their patients, for example, by invasive testing to detect recurrent colorectal carcinoma in an asymptomatic, yet incurable, status. Such patients may best be suited for a low-intensity surveillance strategy. This has an appealing rationale, but does not seem to be widely accepted. In settings where patient care costs are of less concern to individual practitioners, as in the Department of Defense or the Department of Veterans Affairs, issues of cost containment are easier to overlook.

The effect of fear of a lawsuit on surveillance strategies is not well documented,[22] but a considerable amount of current testing is undoubtedly defensive maneuvering by physicians eager to avoid legal entanglements with their patients, should recurrence or a new primary cancer occur. Although they are unpopular topics, often considered by physicians only subconsciously and without much discussion with patient or family, the implications of patient age, projected life span, and comorbid conditions must also be incorporated into any rational analysis of surveillance strategy. While surveillance is often rather extensive, invasive, risky, and uncomfortable, such as after potentially curative surgery for colon cancer, the intensity is likely to be diminished when the patient has other major comorbid conditions. To some extent, this clashes with ethical and medicolegal concerns, since withholding of otherwise-indicated surveillance testing for elderly patients may be considered age discrimination and thus opens a physician to a lawsuit. Nonetheless, it seems to be common practice among physicians.

DURATION OF SURVEILLANCE

Intensity of surveillance typically diminishes with time. Recurrence of many solid tumors (for example, of the pancreas, lung, or stomach) past 5 years from the point of primary treatment is rare. This is the rationale for considering patients who are disease free after 5 years to be cured of their initial lesion. However, as more patients are cured of their primary cancer, the specter of new primary neoplasms in the same organ or other organs continues to justify surveillance in most instances. Patients with melanoma may develop a second primary melanoma elsewhere in their body; breast cancer patients, unless bilateral mastectomies have been carried out, remain at risk for second primary breast cancer; and so on. Lifelong follow-up is appropriate for most cancers, even after the risk of recrudescence of the index neoplasm has faded into insignificance.

The length of follow-up bears a strong relationship to the type of disease being followed. Those with breast cancer, melanoma, and low-grade sarcoma are likely to be at risk for recurrence of the primary disease for many years, even decades. The risk of recurrence of other cancers decreases dramatically if a patient survives free of disease for several years. For example, patients with colorectal cancer, head and neck cancer, and other aggressive solid tumors have a small chance of primary recurrence if they are free of evident disease at the 5-year point following treatment. Those who retain any of the original organ after primary treatment, however, are generally at risk for separate new (metachronous) cancers arising in the remaining fragment of the organ harboring the index neoplasm. Occasionally, the organ can be fully ablated at the primary treatment. An example of this is a patient with ulcerative colitis and cancer who has had a total proctocolectomy. Since all large bowel mucosa has been removed, the patient can be considered free of risk of second primary colorectal carcinoma.

SECONDARY BENEFITS OF FOLLOW-UP

Depression, guilt, fear of death, and a sense of vulnerability[23] are common patient emotions after the rigors of initial therapy are past. A traditional role of the physician providing posttreatment surveillance is to offer a nonthreatening, nonjudgmental outlet for these feelings. Patients are known to value such an outlet. With time, if cancer does not recur, the depression and feelings of loneliness and isolation tend to diminish. In addition, follow-up should assess the sequelae of treatment. This could include regular testing for pernicious anemia in the patient who has undergone a gastrectomy and is receiving vitamin B_{12} therapy, assessment of higher integrative function in patients who have undergone prophylactic brain radiation for small cell lung cancer, and similar situations. The possibility of late effects of treatment also warrants surveillance in some instances. Sterility, pulmonary fibrosis, and cardiomyopathy following chemotherapy, accelerated coronary artery disease following mediastinal radiation therapy, and wound problems after surgery are examples of this. Delayed neoplasms caused by surgery, radiation, and chemotherapy may also warrant follow-up.[24-26] A dose-response relationship exists between chemotherapy and radiation dose and subsequent complications, but whether intensively treated patients deserve more frequent follow-up to detect late effects of therapy is virtually uninvestigated. In addition to the cancer-specific aspects of surveillance, physician input is important in assessing the full return of the patient to good health, ensuring follow-through with rehabilitation plans, and evaluating posttreatment concerns, such as wound healing, on a regular basis.

HOW TUMOR CHARACTERISTICS SHOULD AFFECT POSTTREATMENT SURVEILLANCE

The likelihood of recurrence of the index neoplasm for which the patient underwent the original treatment can usually be assessed. Among the most powerful predictors of primary tumor recurrence are tumor, nodes, metastases (TNM) stage and tumor grade. In most types of neoplasms, stage is a more powerful predictor of primary tumor recurrence than grade, but both are well accepted. Local recurrence is more likely in patients with microscopically involved surgical margins, as discussed in greater detail elsewhere in this book. Other, less well-established risk factors for recurrence include surface markers, DNA ploidy, and nucleic acid replication rate. Patients with vascular, perineural, and lymphatic involvement generally have a poorer outlook than patients who do not, and these patients are likely to warrant increased surveillance. An important, but difficult to quantify, risk factor for recurrence of the primary tumor is adequacy of surgical technique.[27] Patients with close surgical margins may need closer follow-up to facilitate salvage treatment of recurrence, but this is not a settled issue.[28] TNM stage–specific variation in surveillance strategy has been documented for a number of tumors.[22,29] However, the variation appears to be only moderate and presumably reflects the difficulty busy clinicians have in integrating multiple parameters in the design of surveillance strategies for individual patients.

PRIMARY PREVENTION AND ADJUVANT THERAPY

A relative newcomer on the list of indications for posttreatment surveillance in the cancer patient is primary cancer prevention. This discipline is in its infancy, although physicians have long advised their patients to avoid practices, such as smoking and sun exposure, that led to the original cancer. If a patient has known risk factors, such as smoking or excessive radiation exposure, the clinician may be inclined to increase the intensity of surveillance, but the yield of such policies has often been disappointingly small when studied carefully.

Chemopreventive agents are now receiving clinical trials for cancers of the upper airway digestive tract, lung, breast, colon, bladder, cervix, and other organs.[30] Most of the interventions are not in widespread use, and all require evaluation of drug toxicities and measurement of intermediate endpoints to determine efficacy in individual patients. The future seems promising for this area of treatment, which undoubtedly will justify some degree of surveillance in large numbers of patients.

Adjuvant chemotherapy and radiation therapy after surgical treatment have established firm niches in patient management for many common cancers, including those of the breast, colon, and upper aerodigestive tract. In some instances the role of surgery itself has assumed a secondary or adjuvant role. An example of this is a patient receiving minimal surgery for breast cancer when the primary treatment is radiation therapy. How modern multimodality treatment should alter surveillance practices is almost completely unknown. This is due in part to ignorance of the actual practice patterns of clinicians managing patients with cancers of any sort and in part to the many different forms of adjuvant therapy for each individual tumor type. In this area, where data are lacking and the variables are so numerous, a rational policy probably cannot be devised currently. Modern techniques of decision analysis[5,6] are likely to prove valuable, however. Computer modeling, which has demonstrated power to predict such complex phenomena as the behavior of national economies, chemical reactions, and the weather, is likely to prove valuable in medical decision making as well. As is often the case, help may also arrive from a more profound understanding of the cancer process itself. As discussed in Chapter 24, it seems likely that molecular biological techniques will be able not only to predict the development of new primary cancers in patients who have undergone treatment for one index neoplasm, but also to detect recurrence. Indeed, preclinical diagnosis of neoplasms, such as multiple endocrine neoplasia type II, is already available, circumventing many of the more expensive, invasive, and nonspecific tests still used outside the research setting.

Some tumors can be treated primarily by chemotherapy, radiation, or surgery. An example of this is a well-localized lymphoma of the stomach, for which all of the main treatment modalities have been used as single therapies, although combination therapy is common as well. Breast and prostate cancers are also good examples, since either primary surgical treatment or primary radiation treatment is commonly used for both types of cancer. There is little empirical evidence suggesting that follow-up strategies should vary by the type of primary treatment, if delivered with curative intent, or whether adjuvant therapy is employed. In part this represents the difficulty of mounting comparative clinical trials, and in part it represents a lack of identification of surveillance as an area worthy of investigation.

HOW INNOVATIONS IN MODERN CANCER CARE MAY AFFECT FOLLOW-UP

Two new areas that may affect the practice of cancer patient follow-up are managed care and minimally invasive surgery. In managed care settings more and more guidelines are being promulgated by diverse regulatory bodies, ranging from insurance companies to health maintenance organizations to the federal government, all of which restrict physicians' autonomy. This has probably affected the pattern of care in countries where socialized medicine has been adopted with fixed budgets and seemingly limitless demands for medical attention. Health care executives have been forced to search for evidence that a given policy pays off in terms of patient benefit before writing it into patient care guidelines. Although this has not been well documented, strategies appear to vary appreciably from one health care setting (such as Department of Veterans Affairs hospitals) to others (such as private hospitals). Eddy,[31] an influential analyst of clinical decision-making theory, proposes that cost control in medicine will lead to rationing of services. The costs of health care, measured as a fraction of the gross domestic product of any country, cannot rise indefinitely. The rewards to those who can reduce costs are so large, and the adverse consequences to an economy of continued failure to do so are so severe, that the imposition of effective cost-control measures can be taken as inevitable. The greater the delay in instituting such measures, the deeper the cuts will eventually have to be. It will not be possible to control costs by increased managerial efficiency and elimination of wasteful medical practices alone, indicating that rationing is unavoidable. Whether quality of care can be maintained, irrespective of rationing, is open to question.[31]

Scientific advances may help maintain medical care quality. Genetic testing, for example, holds promise as a way to detect cancer in apparently healthy people, which could render expensive traditional surveillance schemes obsolete. Molecular genetic testing may allow us to discriminate between patients who deserve particularly vigorous surveillance and those who do not. However, gene-based screening must take into account the large number of possible variations in each pertinent allele and the relative risk of cancer associated with each. Because gene-based diagnostic testing carries with it the aura of infallibility, a positive test result can have shattering consequences. Patients may become uninsurable, undergo prophylactic excision of the organ at risk, refrain from childbearing, or suffer grave psychological stress. Thus, it will be crucial not to interpret a harmless genetic polymorphism as a dangerous mutation.[32]

The National Center for Human Genome Research at the National Institutes of Health has addressed the important issue of genetic testing and has issued a statement defining several fundamental questions that should be answered before such testing for common cancer risk genes is offered to high-risk individuals or the general public as accepted medical practice.[33] These questions include: How many mutations of each gene conferring risk exist? What is the clinical cancer risk associated with each? What is the frequency of false-positive and false-negative test results? How can technical quality of genetic testing be ensured? How are clinicians and patients to use the test results—in other words, what interventions can be carried out to prevent or treat cancer in affected populations? How can patients be educated about the implications of DNA testing to ensure that consent for testing is informed? How is genetic counseling to be given? How can discrimination against those found to harbor cancer risk genes be avoided? The insurance industry, for obvious reasons, is very interested in this topic, although at present insurers do not carry out such tests themselves.[34] Already the political process is working to modify the outcomes flowing from genetic testing.[32] The National Center for Human Genome Research has begun to gather information and establish methods to carefully introduce the powerful tools of genetic testing into clinical practice.[33]

Rationing of care given to asymptomatic cancer patients after primary therapy will probably be easier for the general public to accept, at least at first glance, than rationing of care intended for symptomatic, ill individuals. Justification of any diagnostic or therapeutic intervention should ideally be considered by reference to widely agreed-upon assumptions. This will restrict the tendency for pressure groups to petition health care providers for special treatment and will introduce rationality, rather than political tactics, into the decision-making process. The following assumptions and criteria might best govern a future care-rationing process[35]:

1. The financial resources available to provide health care to a population are limited.
2. Because financial resources are limited, when deciding about the appropriate use of treatments, it is both valid and important to consider the financial costs of the treatments.
3. Because financial resources are limited, it is necessary to set priorities.
4. As a consequence of priority setting, not every treatment that might have some benefit can be covered by shared resources.
5. The objective of health care is to maximize the health of the population served, subject to the available resources.
6. The priority a treatment should receive should not depend on whether the particular individuals who would receive treatment are the physician's personal patients.
7. Determining the priority of a treatment will require estimating the magnitudes of its benefits, harms, and costs.
8. To the greatest extent possible, estimates of benefits, harms, and costs should be based on empirical evidence. A corollary is that when empirical evidence contradicts subjective judgments, empirical evidence should take priority.
9. Before being promoted for use, a treatment should satisfy three criteria. There should be convincing evidence that, compared with no treatment, the treatment improves health outcomes. Compared with no treatment, its beneficial effects on health outcomes should outweigh any harmful effects on health outcomes. Compared with the next best alternative treatment, the treatment should represent a good use of resources in the sense that it satisfies principle number 5.
10. Any judgments about benefits, harms, and costs should reflect, to the greatest extent possible, the preferences of the individuals who will actually receive the treatments.
11. In determining whether a treatment satisfies the criteria of principle number 9, the burden of proof should be on those who are promoting the use of the treatment.

The trend toward less invasive surgery will also have implications for follow-up. There is a clear tendency to document the outcomes of less radical surgery for melanoma in order to prove that results are good. Endoscopic surgery for early large bowel cancer would not have achieved popularity without good documentation of outcomes. The same is likely to hold true for laparoscopic surgery, which is in vogue. Sizeable trials, not always well controlled, are being carried out to assess this issue, and a consensus is evolving that the same surgical objectives (wide local excision, adequate lymphadenectomy, and the like) should be demanded of laparoscopic procedures as of standard surgical procedures. The emergence of limited surgery as therapy for a number of cancers seems likely to continue and even accelerate. Limited surgery for breast cancer has replaced radical mastectomy for all practical purposes, and local excisions of selected rectal cancers and endoscopic surgery for transitional cell carcinoma of the bladder are well established. Others are likely to arise. There is little evidence that follow-up for patients treated with limited surgery should be different from that offered patients treated with more radical conventional surgery. The conventional belief is that factors related to tumor biology (such as grade, stage,[36] and patient performance status) should determine follow-up, irrespective of the type of surgery.

SUMMARY

Medical care today is better than ever, but its very success breeds new problems, and posttreatment cancer surveillance is no exception. Rising health care costs affect the economy at large, resulting in pressure to contain them. New ways to analyze the benefits of care result in changes in the delivery of care. Better understanding of pathological processes promises to improve surveillance and introduce new and fascinating questions. Physicians will require a close relationship with their patients and a clear appreciation of societal desires to reap the benefits of these trends for their patients, while avoiding the inevitable hazards.

REFERENCES

1. Grimshaw JM, Russell IT. Effect of clinical guidelines on medical practice: a systematic review of rigorous evaluations. Lancet 1993;342:1317-22.
2. Romano PS, Roos LL, Luft HS, Jollis JG, Doliszny K. Ischemic Heart Disease Patient Outcomes Research Team. A comparison of administrative versus clinical data: coronary artery bypass surgery as an example. J Clin Epidemiol 1994;47:249-60.
3. GIVIO Investigators. Impact of follow-up testing on survival and health-related quality of life in breast cancer patients. JAMA 1994;271:1587-92.
4. Greenwald HP. Early detection: the key to survival? In: Greenwald HP. Who survives cancer? Berkeley: University of California Press, 1992:119-46.
5. O'Meara JJ, McNutt RA, Evans AT, Moore SW, Downs SM. A decision analysis of streptokinase plus heparin as compared with heparin alone for deep-vein thrombosis. N Engl J Med 1994;330:1864-9.
6. Kassirer JP. Incorporating patients' preferences into medical decisions. N Engl J Med 1994;330:1895-6.
7. Gion M, Cappelli G, Mione R, et al. Variability of tumor markers in the follow-up of patients radically resected for breast cancer. Tumour Biol 1993;14:325-33.
8. Lampic C, Wennberg A, Schill J, Brodin O, Glimelius B, Sjoden P. Anxiety and cancer-related worry of cancer patients at routine follow-up visits. Acta Oncol 1994;33:119-25.
9. Myers RE, Bralow SP, Goldstein R, Jacobs M, Wolf TA, Engstrom PF. Surveillance for colorectal neoplasia: is patient adherence following treatment a problem? Cancer Detect Prev 1993;17:609-17.
10. Schapira DV, Urban M. A minimalist policy for breast cancer surveillance. JAMA 1991;265:380-2.
11. Wertheimer MD. Against minimalism in breast cancer follow-up. JAMA 1991;265;396-7.
12. Moertel CG, Fleming TR, MacDonald JS, Haller DG, Laurie JA, Tangen C. An evaluation of the carcinoembryonic antigen (CEA) test for monitoring patients with resected colon cancer. JAMA 1993;270:943-7.
13. Anderson C. Measuring what works in health care. Science 1994;263:1080-1.
14. Mann CC. Can meta-analysis make policy? Science 1994;266:960-2.
15. Bruinvels DJ, Stiggelbout AM, Kievit J, van Houwelingen HC, Habbema DF, van de Velde JH. Follow-up of patients with colorectal cancer: a meta-analysis. Ann Surg 1994;219:174-82.
16. Woolf SH. Practice guidelines: a new reality in medicine I. Recent developments. Arch Intern Med 1990;150:1811-8.
17. Woolf SH. Practice guidelines: a new reality in medicine II. Methods of developing guidelines. Arch Intern Med 1992;152:946-52.
18. Woolf SH. Practice guidelines: a new reality in medicine III. Impact on patient care. Arch Intern Med 1993;153:2646-55.
19. Parmley WW. Clinical practice guidelines. Does the cookbook have enough recipes? JAMA 1994;272:1374-5.
20. Grilli R, Apolone G, Marsoni S, Nicolucci A, Zola P, Liberati A. The impact of patient management guidelines on the care of breast, colorectal, and ovarian cancer patients in Italy. Med Care 1991;29:50-63.
21. Steele G. Follow-up plans after treatment of primary colon and rectum cancer. World J Surg 1991;15:583-8.
22. Naunheim KS, Virgo KS, Coplin MA, Johnson FE. Clinical surveillance testing after lung cancer operations. Ann Thorac Surg 1995;60:1612-6.
23. Shanfield SB. On surviving cancer: psychological considerations. Compr Psychiatry 1980;21:128-34.
24. Brady MS, Garfein CF, Petrek JA, Brennan MF. Post-treatment sarcoma in breast cancer patients. Ann Surg Oncol 1994;1:66-72.
25. Gralla RJ, Weiss RB, Vogelzang NJ, et al. Adverse effects of treatment. In: DeVita VT, Hellman S, Rosenberg SA, editors. Cancer. 4th ed. Philadelphia: JB Lippincott Company, 1993:2338-416.
26. Stewart FW, Treves N. Lymphangiosarcoma in postmastectomy lymphedema. Cancer 1948;1:64-81.
27. Balch CM, Durant JR, Bartolucci AA. The impact of surgical quality control in multi-institutional group trials involving adjuvant cancer treatments. Ann Surg 1983;198:164-7.
28. Warren WH, Faber LP. Segmentectomy versus lobectomy in patients with stage I pulmonary carcinoma. Five-year survival and patterns of intrathoracic recurrence. J Thorac Cardiovasc Surg 1994;107:1087-93.
29. Johnson FE, Longo WE, Vernava AM, Wade TP, Coplin MA, Virgo KS. How tumor stage affects surgeons' surveillance strategies after colon cancer surgery. Cancer 1995;76:1325-9.
30. Lippman SM, Benner SE, Hong WK. Cancer chemoprevention. J Clin Oncol 1994;12:851-73.
31. Eddy DM. Health system reform. Will controlling costs require rationing services? JAMA 1994;272:324-8.
32. Nowak R. Genetic testing set for take-off. Science 1994;265:464-7.
33. National Advisory Council for Human Genome Research. Statement on use of DNA testing for presymptomatic identification of cancer risk. JAMA 1994;271:785.
34. Lowden J. Genetic testing. Science 1994;265:1509-10.
35. Eddy DM. Principles for making difficult decisions in difficult times. JAMA 1994;271:1792-8.
36. American Joint Committee on Cancer, Beahrs OH, Henson DE, Robert VP, Kennedy BJ, editors. Manual for staging of cancer. 4th ed. Philadelphia: JB Lippincott Company, 1992.

SECTION II

Current Practice

CHAPTER 5

Head and Neck Carcinoma

Memorial Sloan-Kettering Cancer Center

STIMSON P. SCHANTZ AND PETER E. ANDERSEN

About 50,000 new cases of cancer of the head and neck were diagnosed in the United States in 1996.[1] This represents less than 5% of the overall new cancer diagnoses in the United States.[2] Worldwide, however, head and neck cancer is the sixth most common human malignancy.[3] The geographical distribution of these cases is nonuniform, with areas of high incidence in China, the Indian subcontinent, and parts of Europe.[1]

Cancer of the head and neck does not refer to a single histological diagnosis or organ of origin. Rather, it refers to malignant tumors arising from the upper aerodigestive tract, salivary glands, thyroid and parathyroid glands, paranasal sinuses, and the skin of the head and neck. Because of this heterogeneity, a wide spectrum of etiologies, disease presentations, and clinical characteristics must be considered when caring for these patients. However, the term "head and neck cancer" usually refers to squamous carcinomas arising from the mucosal surfaces of the upper aerodigestive tract. These tumors make up greater than 95% of the cases of head and neck cancer.[2] For the remainder of this chapter, "head and neck cancer" refers to these cases unless otherwise stated.

Because of the relatively small number of cases of head and neck cancer in the United States, the economic consequences of follow-up are relatively small. To the individual patient, however, the impact of this disease can be enormous. Radical surgery and radiation therapy can leave the patient with permanent cosmetic deformities and functional deficits. This may result in social isolation and psychiatric illness. In fact, the sequelae of treatment often prevent a previously employed person from returning to work after treatment.

ETIOLOGY

In contrast to other more common solid malignancies, the etiology of head and neck cancer is known in the vast majority of cases. Greater than 95% of patients have a prior history of tobacco or alcohol abuse.[4,5] The relative risk of developing head and neck cancer is strongly correlated with the intensity and duration of use of these substances, and their concomitant use results in a synergistic increase in the risk of developing head and neck cancer.[6] The effects of concomitant abuse of alcohol and tobacco are shown in Figure 5-1.

Etiological agents for other types of head and neck cancer are known, but these account for a small number of head and neck cancers in general. There is not the striking correlation as is identified with tobacco and alcohol use and the development of squamous cancer of the upper aerodigestive tract. Examples of such agents are ionizing radiation exposure and differentiated thyroid carcinoma, sun exposure and development of skin cancer, hardwood dust exposure and adenocarcinoma of the ethmoid sinus, and exposure to nickel compounds and development of squamous carcinoma of the paranasal sinuses.[7,8]

STAGING

The American Joint Committee on Cancer (AJCC) and International Union Against Cancer (UICC) have agreed on a uniform staging system for head and neck cancer based on the tumor, nodes, metastases (TNM) classification. This staging system is presented in Tables 5-1 through 5-6.[9] As shown in the tables, the staging system for the primary tumor varies according to the site of origin. The staging of regional lymphatics in the neck and the overall clinical staging rules, however, are consistent across primary sites.

TREATMENT

An in-depth discussion of the treatment of head and neck cancer is beyond the scope of this chapter. Some generalizations, however, can be made. The treatment of a particular patient must be individualized according to the stage and location of the tumor. Other patient factors such as overall medical condition, distance from the patient's home to the treating center, and patient motivation are also important.

In general, head and neck cancer is treated with surgery, radiation therapy, or a combination of both. Early stage lesions may be treated with surgical excision or radiation therapy as a single modality; high-stage lesions are generally treated with surgical excision followed by postoperative radiation therapy.[10-14] When the treatment modality is chosen, various factors must be considered, such as the efficacy of the treatment, its morbidity, and the length of treatment. For example, early stage squamous carcinoma of both the oral cavity and glottic larynx can be equally well treated with

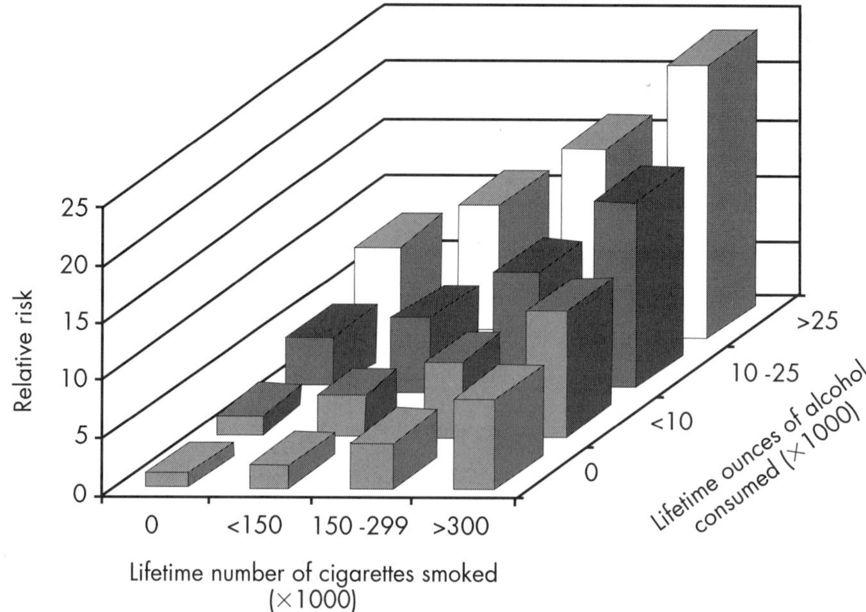

Figure 5-1 Effect of lifetime alcohol and tobacco consumption on the risk of developing head and neck cancer. (Data from Burch JD, Howe GR, Miller AB, Semencle R. Tobacco, alcohol, asbestos, and nickel in the etiology of cancer of the larynx: a case-control study. J Natl Cancer Inst 1981;67:1219-24.)

Table 5-1 AJCC/UICC staging system for oral cavity primary tumors

T STAGE	DESCRIPTION
TX	Primary tumor cannot be assessed
T0	No evidence of primary tumor
Tis	Carcinoma in situ
T1	Tumor 2 cm or less in greatest dimension
T2	Tumor more than 2 cm but not more than 4 cm in greatest dimension
T3	Tumor more than 4 cm in greatest dimension
T4	Massive tumor, invades adjacent structures (through cortical bone, into deep [extrinsic] muscle of tongue, maxillary sinus, skin)

Data from American Joint Committee on Cancer, Beahrs OH, Henson DE, Robert VP, Kennedy BJ, editors. Manual for staging of cancer. 4th ed. Philadelphia: JB Lippincott Company, 1992:2-48.

Table 5-2 AJCC/UICC staging system for oropharyngeal primary tumors

T STAGE	DESCRIPTION
TX	Primary tumor cannot be assessed
T0	No evidence of primary tumor
Tis	Carcinoma in situ
T1	Tumor 2 cm or less in greatest dimension
T2	Tumor more than 2 cm but not more than 4 cm in greatest dimension
T3	Tumor more than 4 cm in greatest dimension
T4	Massive tumor, invades adjacent structures (through cortical bone, soft tissues of neck, into deep [extrinsic] muscle of tongue)

Data from American Joint Committee on Cancer, Beahrs OH, Henson DE, Robert VP, Kennedy BJ, editors. Manual for staging of cancer. 4th ed. Philadelphia: JB Lippincott Company, 1992:2-48.

surgery or radiation therapy.[15-18] In the case of tongue cancer the treatment of choice is usually surgery because treatment can be completed in only a few days and the functional consequences of partial glossectomy are minimal. However, the use of radiation therapy to treat a small tongue cancer will induce permanent xerostomia, leaving the patient at risk for dental decay and osteoradionecrosis of the mandible, and use up a valuable treatment alternative if the patient happens to suffer a recurrence or develop a second primary tumor. On the other hand, the treatment of early glottic cancer is usually radiation therapy, primarily because the voice quality is superior to that following partial laryngectomy; this outweighs the inconvenience of radiation therapy. In patients with advanced disease the results of surgery or radiation therapy as single-modality treatment are inferior to combination therapy.[19] There is no advantage in survival or disease control in using preoperative as compared with postoperative radiation therapy.[20] Therefore most head and neck oncologists prefer surgical resection followed by postoperative radiation therapy. Surgical resection is technically easier in the nonirradiated patient, and there is no radiation dose limitation because of concern about healing.

Table 5-3 AJCC/UICC staging system for laryngeal primary tumors

T STAGE	DESCRIPTION
TX	Primary tumor cannot be assessed
T0	No evidence of primary tumor
Tis	Carcinoma in situ
SUPRAGLOTTIS	
T1	Tumor limited to one subsite of the supraglottis with normal vocal cord mobility
T2	Tumor invades more than one subsite of the supraglottis or glottis with normal vocal cord mobility
T3	Tumor limited to the larynx with vocal cord fixation and/or invades the postcricoid area, medial wall of the pyriform sinus, or preepiglottic tissues
T4	Tumor invades through the thyroid cartilage and/or extends to other tissues beyond the larynx
GLOTTIS	
T1	Tumor limited to the vocal cord(s) with normal mobility
T2	Tumor extends to the supraglottis and/or subglottis, and/or with impaired vocal cord mobility
T3	Tumor limited to the larynx with vocal cord fixation
T4	Tumor invades through the thyroid cartilage and/or extends to other tissues beyond the larynx
SUBGLOTTIS	
T1	Tumor limited to the subglottis
T2	Tumor extends to the vocal cord(s) with normal or impaired mobility
T3	Tumor limited to the larynx with vocal cord fixation
T4	Tumor invades through the cricoid or thyroid cartilage and/or extends to other tissues beyond the larynx

Data from American Joint Committee on Cancer, Beahrs OH, Henson DE, Robert VP, Kennedy BJ, editors. Manual for staging of cancer. 4th ed. Philadelphia: JB Lippincott Company, 1992:2-48.

PROGNOSIS

The prognosis of patients with head and neck cancer is intimately related to the stage of disease and its location. In general, patients with stage I or II disease have a 60% to 95% survival rate, depending on the location of the primary tumor.[21,22] Stage I cancer of the glottic larynx has a 90% to 95% cure rate,[17,18] and similar-stage oral cavity lesions have a cure rate of approximately 80%.[10,15,16] Advanced-stage lesions (stages III and IV) have much lower cure rates, approximately 10% to 50%.[19,23] Again, the location is critical, with advanced lesions of the larynx having a better cure rate than similarly staged lesions of the oral cavity, oropharynx, and hypopharynx.[10-14] A common adverse prognostic indicator is the presence of cervical lymph node metastasis, which decreases the cure rate by 50% when compared with a similar lesion without lymph node metastasis.[24]

Table 5-4 AJCC/UICC staging system for hypopharyngeal primary tumors

T STAGE	DESCRIPTION
TX	Primary tumor cannot be assessed
T0	No evidence of primary tumor
Tis	Carcinoma in situ
T1	Tumor limited to one subsite of hypopharynx
T2	Tumor invades more than one subsite of hypopharynx or an adjacent site, without fixation of hemilarynx
T3	Tumor invades more than one subsite of hypopharynx or an adjacent site, with fixation of hemilarynx
T4	Tumor invades adjacent structures (cartilage or soft tissues of neck)

Data from American Joint Committee on Cancer, Beahrs OH, Henson DE, Robert VP, Kennedy BJ, editors. Manual for staging of cancer. 4th ed. Philadelphia: JB Lippincott Company, 1992:2-48.

Table 5-5 AJCC/UICC staging system for the regional lymphatics

N STAGE	DESCRIPTION
NX	Regional lymph nodes cannot be assessed
N0	No regional lymph node metastasis
N1	Metastasis in a single ipsilateral lymph node, 3 cm or less in greatest dimension
N2a	Metastasis in a single ipsilateral lymph node more than 3 cm but not more than 6 cm in greatest dimension
N2b	Metastasis in multiple ipsilateral lymph nodes, none more than 6 cm in greatest dimension
N2c	Metastasis in bilateral or contralateral lymph nodes, none more than 6 cm in greatest dimension
N3	Metastasis in a lymph node more than 6 cm in greatest dimension

Data from American Joint Committee on Cancer, Beahrs OH, Henson DE, Robert VP, Kennedy BJ, editors. Manual for staging of cancer. 4th ed. Philadelphia: JB Lippincott Company, 1992:2-48.

Table 5-6 AJCC/UICC clinical staging system

	N STAGE					
T STAGE	0	1	2A	2B	2C	3
1	I	III	IV	IV	IV	IV
2	II	III	IV	IV	IV	IV
3	III	III	IV	IV	IV	IV
4	IV	IV	IV	IV	IV	IV

Data from American Joint Committee on Cancer, Beahrs OH, Henson DE, Robert VP, Kennedy BJ, editors. Manual for staging of cancer. 4th ed. Philadelphia: JB Lippincott Company, 1992:2-48.
Any T, Any N, M1 = Stage IV.

DEVELOPMENT OF A SECOND PRIMARY TUMOR

Second primary squamous carcinomas often develop in previously treated patients. The term "field cancerization" has been proposed for this by Slaughter et al.[25] Because of chronic exposure to environmental carcinogens in these patients, it is thought that even normal-appearing mucosa accumulates a substantial amount of genetic damage. Thus these patients are at increased risk for developing another distinct squamous carcinoma for the remainder of their lives.[26]

The current strategy for follow-up in patients with head and neck cancer evolved along with knowledge of the clinical behavior of this disease. Most disease recurrences become manifest in the first 2 to 3 years after treatment. Therefore, follow-up intensity is greatest during this period. However, even if a patient is cured of the index tumor, developing a second primary malignancy remains a risk. Thus follow-up is required for the remainder of the patient's life.

The lifetime risk for development of a second primary tumor is approximately 10% to 40%, with a higher risk seen in patients who continue to use alcohol and tobacco.[27,28] In fact, second primary tumors are the chief cause of treatment failure and death in patients who have early-stage disease when initially seen.[29] In addition, certain sites are predisposed to the development of a second primary, depending on the location of the index tumor. Patients with an index tumor of the larynx have a higher risk of developing a second primary in the lung,[30] while those with an index tumor in the oral cavity have a higher risk of developing a second primary in the hypopharynx or esophagus.[31]

OBJECTIVES OF FOLLOW-UP CARE

The goals for follow-up care of head and neck cancer patients are several fold. The first and most obvious is the early detection and treatment of any recurrence of the index tumor, be it local, regional, or distant. Unfortunately, treatment of recurrent disease in these patients has a low success rate.[23] However, recurrent disease detected by routine follow-up examination has been shown to have a higher cure rate than disease detected by the patient who does not receive routine follow-up care.[32] The second goal is the detection of a second primary tumor. Treatment of these lesions results in acceptable cure rates, depending on the stage and location of the lesion.[21] The third goal is the detection and treatment of functional disabilities relating to the primary treatment. Such disabilities may include problems with speech, swallowing, cosmesis, teeth and gums, and shoulder function.[33]

An emerging area of interest is the prevention of second primary tumors in this patient population. This usually takes the form of aggressive counseling and treatment regarding the cessation of alcohol and tobacco use and, more recently, the use of chemopreventive agents such as cis-retinoic acid. These issues are discussed in detail in later sections.

FOLLOW-UP CARE

Follow-up care of the head and neck cancer patient begins at discharge from the hospital after completion of treatment. The schedule of follow-up routinely used on the Head and Neck Service of Memorial Sloan-Kettering Cancer Center is shown in Table 5-7.

Table 5-7 Follow-up of patients with head and neck cancer*: Memorial Sloan-Kettering Cancer Center

	YEAR				
	1	2	3	4	5
Office visit	12	6	4	2	1-2
Chest x-ray	1-2	1-2	1-2	1-2	1-2
Thyroid function	†	†	†	†	†

*Further diagnostic studies may be used at any time when indicated by physical examination or patient complaints.
†Performed at 6- to 12-month intervals in patients who are at risk for hypothyroidism.

This schedule has arisen from the empirical observation that most tumor recurrences (80%) occur in the first 2 years following completion of therapy.[23] The risk of a second primary tumor is approximately 3% per year and continues for the rest of the patient's life.[28] In addition, most functional problems are evident early in the posttreatment phase and can be addressed. It is less likely that new functional problems will develop as the time from treatment progresses. The schedule of follow-up routinely used on the Head and Neck Service at Memorial Sloan-Kettering generally requires visits every month for the first year, every 2 months for the second year, every 3 months for the third year, and every 6 months for the fourth year. Subsequently, follow-up visits are scheduled every 6 to 12 months for the remainder of the patient's life. This schedule is used for all patients with head and neck cancer regardless of treatment modality.

Each follow-up visit should consist of a standard evaluation. The evaluation discussed below is generally applicable to all patients with head and neck cancer. It can be tailored to an individual patient's situation. For example, particular care should be given to the site of a previous primary tumor, and follow-up care may differ depending on the treatment employed (more attention to dental care may be necessary in the patient treated with radiation therapy, for example). The patient's weight should be checked and compared with weight at previous visits. This is an effective and comprehensive measure for detecting problems with the patient's swallowing function and nutritional status. The patient should be questioned regarding alcohol and tobacco use, changes in swallowing or voice, pain, hemoptysis, or any other concerns.

Physical examination should consist of a comprehensive evaluation of the head and neck region, with particular attention to the site of the patient's tumor. The neck should be palpated for regional adenopathy. All mucosal surfaces of the head and neck should be visualized. A headlight is invaluable for this purpose. The larynx and pharynx should be examined with either the laryngeal mirror or a flexible fiberoptic laryngoscope. An important part of the examination is the bimanual palpation of structures in the oral cavity and oropharynx to detect submucosal lesions that are not visible.

In the absence of any symptom or physical finding, the routine use of blood chemistries and radiographs is not necessary beyond a chest radiograph at 6- to 12-month intervals. The issue of thyroid function tests is an interesting one. Treatment with irradiation of the thyroid gland or surgical resection requiring hemithyroidectomy (that is, total laryngectomy) results in hypothyroidism in approximately 30% of patients. The combination of both treatment modalities results in biochemical hypothyroidism in approximately 50% of patients.[34] This hypothyroidism is often not clinically appreciated. Therefore it is appropriate to check thyroid function at 6- to 12-month intervals in patients who, by virtue of their treatment, are at risk for hypothyroidism and to institute appropriate therapy when indicated. The routine use of panendoscopy or barium esophogram in the absence of any suspicious physical finding or patient complaint has a low yield and is not cost effective.[35,36]

Other areas of concern during posttreatment follow-up in patients with head and neck cancer include speech and swallowing rehabilitation, dental prophylaxis and restoration, shoulder function, and psychological issues relating to treatment sequelae. In this regard it is valuable to have an integrated team of medical professionals to which the head and neck oncologist can refer patients when necessary. The degree of speech and swallowing dysfunction varies greatly from patient to patient, depending on the particular surgical treatment and whether radiation therapy was administered. In patients for whom this is an issue, the assistance of a speech pathologist familiar with patients who have had head and neck cancer is invaluable. In cases where extensive dental extractions are necessary or where resection of the palate or mandible is required, a maxillofacial prosthodontist can often provide prosthetic rehabilitation that can improve speech and swallowing. Patients who have received radiation therapy of the oral cavity are at increased risk of caries and osteoradionecrosis of the mandible as a result of the therapy. These patients require frequent fluoride prophylaxis and regular dental visits to prevent premature loss of dentition and to detect early problems with osteoradionecrosis. Problems with neck and shoulder strength or mobility can be substantially ameliorated with a program of physical therapy. Often, simple instruction in range-of-motion exercises by the surgeon is adequate, but if not, referral to a physical therapist can be extremely helpful. Finally, many patients have psychological problems as a result of therapy. Therapy for head and neck cancer frequently results in severe problems with function and cosmesis. Some patients become depressed and withdraw from society.[37,38] The head and neck oncologist must be aware of these reactions and detect them early. If the treating oncologist cannot provide the necessary psychological care, prompt referral to a psychiatrist experienced in dealing with cancer patients is warranted.

Fortunately, pain control is usually not a major issue in head and neck cancer patients beyond the immediate posttherapy period. In fact, the occurrence of pain that requires medication in a patient who was previously pain free should alert the clinician to the possibility of cancer recurrence. Unfortunately, in the few patients who do have chronic pain as a result of treatment, it is often difficult to control. This pain usually takes the form of chronic oral and pharyngeal pain in patients who have received radiation therapy, shoulder pain after radical neck dissection, and occasionally neuralgia-like pain in those requiring the sacrifice of cranial nerves. Often, significant elements such as psychological problems contribute to the severity of the pain. After recurrence of cancer has been ruled out, patients suffering from uncontrolled pain commonly benefit from treatment by a physician skilled in managing chronic pain syndromes.

SMOKING AND ALCOHOL CESSATION

Beyond detection of disease recurrence or the development of a second primary cancer, a major goal of follow-up care in the patient with head and neck cancer is the cessation of tobacco and alcohol abuse. In addition to the increased risk of developing a second primary in patients who continue to smoke and drink, there is evidence of increased rates of treatment failure.[39]

Many physicians do not inquire about the use of tobacco and do not attempt to intervene in this regard.[40] Effective strategies to quit smoking do exist[41,42]; however, many physicians do not use them, since most former smokers quit on their own. While two thirds of smokers who attempt to quit are initially successful, only 20% are abstinent after 1 year. Strategies that have proved successful include group therapy, hypnosis, acupuncture, behavioral modification, nicotine replacement (nicotine gum or transdermal patch), and the use of clonidine.

Reasons for nonintervention by physicians include not wanting to irritate the patient, believing that smoking is irrelevant to the current medical problem, and feeling pessimistic about effectiveness. Studies show, however, that physician intervention improves the chances that a patient will ultimately quit smoking.[43,44] In addition, premalignant changes in the mucosa of tobacco users often regress after cessation of tobacco use.[44] In many respects the above discussion applies to alcohol cessation as well.

CHEMOPREVENTION

The high rate of second primary development in patients with head and neck cancer and the concept of field cancerization that is thought to occur in these patients[25] make this population ideal for the use of chemopreventive agents.[45] This is the subject of active research and several clinical trials are under way. The active agents under investigation that show the most promise are retinoids.

Oral leukoplakia has been shown to regress during treatment with retinoids. Hong et al.[46] treated 44 patients with oral leukoplakia with either 13-cis-retinoic acid (1 to 2 mg/kg/day for 3 months) or a placebo. In the treated arm, lesions decreased in size in 67% of patients, versus 10% in the placebo arm. After cessation of therapy, however, lesions recurred in 56% of patients. In another study from the same group,[47] 70 patients with leukoplakia were treated with an induction phase of 13-cis-retinoic acid (1.5 mg/kg/day for 3 months) and then were randomly selected to receive either low-dose 13-cis-retinoic acid (0.5 mg/kg/day) or beta-carotene (30 mg/day) for 9 months. The response rate to induction was 55%. During low-dose maintenance therapy the group receiving 13-cis-retinoic acid maintained response rates better than those in the beta-carotene group (92% versus 45%). These studies show that treatment with retinoids can cause regression of oral premalignant lesions. Response is durable as long as therapy is continued; however, if treatment stops, a significant number of lesions will return.

Retinoids also appear to prevent the development of second primary tumors in patients with prior head and neck cancer. Hong et al.[48] treated 103 patients with 13-cis-retinoic acid (50-100 mg/m^2) or a placebo for 12 months. After a median follow-up of 32 months, the rate of second primary tumor development in the treatment arm was 4% versus 24% in the placebo arm. After a median of 54 months of follow-up in the same patients, the rate of second primary development was 14% in the treatment group versus 31% in the placebo group. A multiinstitutional study is in progress to validate the usefulness of 13-cis-retinoic acid in the prevention of second primary tumors in patients with head and neck cancer.

Treatment with 13-cis-retinoic acid has significant toxicity. The compound is teratogenic and is contraindicated if there is any possibility of pregnancy. Frequent toxicities include cheilitis, pruritus, xerostomia, conjunctivitis, hepatic toxicity, hypercholesterolemia, and hypertriglyceridemia. Toxicities were noted in 40% of patients, forcing withdrawal of the drug in 18% in one trial.[47] While these studies are interesting and promising, use of this drug should currently be restricted to the environment of a controlled trial.

CONCLUSION

Squamous carcinoma of the head and neck is a relatively uncommon neoplasm in the United States. Worldwide, however, it is a major health problem. The major etiologies of the disease are tobacco and alcohol abuse. Because of the wide range of anatomical structures involved, treatment varies widely from patient to patient. In general, early-stage disease is treated with surgery or radiation therapy as a single modality, whereas patients with advanced disease require combination therapy. Cure rates vary according to disease stage and site but generally approximate 50% to 60%.

Posttreatment follow-up is dominated by clinical and laboratory examination. Careful clinical examination and use of newer instruments, such as the flexible nasopharyngoscope, detect disease recurrence and second primaries in the vast majority of patients. Routine use of panendoscopy and advanced radiologic procedures is not cost effective unless indicated by clinical suspicion or patient complaint.

The clinician must be concerned not only with the status of the tumor but also with any functional or cosmetic consequences of the treatment. In this regard an integrated team approach to the management of these patients is vital. This team should include a speech pathologist, dentists, a maxillofacial prosthodontist, and a psychiatrist.

The high incidence of second primaries in patients with head and neck cancer mandates routine follow-up for the remainder of the patients' lives. A chest x-ray should be obtained every 6 to 12 months. The clinician should be aware of these patients' tendencies to develop hypothyroidism as a result of their therapy.

The cessation of tobacco and alcohol abuse is vital to patient well-being. There is evidence that those patients who continue to smoke and drink have a much higher incidence of second primary cancers and may even respond less successfully to the treatment of their index lesion. The treating physician should take the lead in the effort to stop the use of these substances, since studies have shown that the intervention of a physician improves patients' chances of being long-term abstainers. Many effective treatment strategies exist to assist patients in smoking and alcohol cessation.

FUTURE PROSPECTS

Research into the molecular genetics of head and neck cancer has identified multiple areas in the genome of the tumor that are commonly altered. These changes may consist of either point mutations, such as those present in the p53 gene, or deletions of chromosomal segments.[49,50] This has raised the possibility that, if the status of a particular set of genetic markers is known in a tumor, the patient could be screened for recurrence by examining these markers in exfoliated cells obtained through expectoration.[51] Using such an approach, p53 mutations corresponding to those present in tumors were found in the preoperative saliva of five of seven patients with head and neck cancer.[52] These results are exciting but must be viewed with caution, since it is known that the histologically normal epithelium of the upper aerodigestive tract in patients with head and neck cancer can also harbor mutations in the p53 gene.[53] These mutations may be identical to those present in the tumor and may be a source of false-positive results. Through the use of multiple genetic markers a profile for an individual tumor may be developed that may decrease the incidence of false-positive results. These discoveries, however, are not yet ready for clinical use, although they may be in the near future.

Current research suggests that agents such as 13-cis-retinoic acid may cause regression of premalignant lesions and prevent second primary cancers. Initial studies have been promising but require validation in the large clinical trials that are ongoing. Until these studies are complete, these agents must be considered experimental and their use should be limited to the setting of a clinical trial.

REFERENCES

1. Parker S, Tong T, Bolden S, Wingo PA. Cancer statistics, 1996. CA Cancer J Clin 1996;65:5-27.

2. Muir C, Weiland L. Upper aerodigestive tract cancers. Cancer 1995;75:147-53.
3. Parkin DM, Muir CS, Laara E. Global burden of cancer. Lyon: World Health Organization, International Agency for Research on Cancer, Biennial Report;1986-87:11.
4. Brugere J, Guenel P, LeClerc A, Rodriquez J. Differential effects of tobacco and alcohol in cancer of the larynx, pharynx, and mouth. Cancer 1986;57:391-5.
5. Wynder E, Stellman S. Comparative epidemiology of tobacco-related cancers. Cancer Res 1977;37:4608-22.
6. Flanders WD, Rothman KJ. Interaction of alcohol and tobacco in laryngeal cancer. Am J Epidemiol 1982;115:371.
7. Blitzer PH. Epidemiology of head and neck cancer. Semin Oncol 1988;15:2-9.
8. Gerin M, Siemiatycki J, Nadon L, Dewar R, Krewski D. Cancer risks due to occupational exposure to formaldehyde: results of a multi-site case-control study in Montreal. Int J Cancer 1989;44:53-8.
9. American Joint Committee on Cancer, Beahrs OH, Henson DE, Robert VP, Kennedy BJ, editors. Manual for staging of cancer. 4th ed. Philadelphia: JB Lippincott Company, 1992:2-48.
10. Spiro RH. Squamous cancer of the tongue. CA Cancer J Clin 1985;35:252-6.
11. Million RR, Cassisi NJ, Wittes RE. Cancer of the head and neck. In: DeVita VT Jr, Hellman S, Rosenberg SA, editors. Cancer: principles and practice of oncology. Philadelphia: JB Lippincott Company, 1985:407-96.
12. Mendenhall WM, Parsons JT, Devine JW, Cassisi NJ, Million RR. Squamous cell carcinoma of the pyriform sinus treated with surgery and/or radiotherapy. Head Neck Surg 1987;10:88-92.
13. Fu KK, Eisenberg L, Dedo HH, Phillips TL. Results of integrated management of supraglottic carcinoma. Cancer 1977;40:2874-81.
14. Kaplan MJ, Johns ME, Clark DA, Cantrell RW. Glottic carcinoma: the roles of surgery and irradiation. Cancer 1984;53:2641-8.
15. Shaha AR, Spiro FH, Shah JP, Strong EW. Squamous carcinoma of the floor of the mouth. Am J Surg 1984;148:455-9.
16. Mazeron JJ, Grimard L, Raynal M, Haddad E, Piedbois P, Martin M. Iridium-192 Curietherapy for T1 and T2 epidermoid carcinomas of the floor of the mouth. Int J Radiat Oncol Biol Phys 1990;18:1299-306.
17. Mendenhall WM, Parsons JT, Stringer SP, Cassisi NJ, Million FF. T1-T2 vocal cord carcinoma: a basis for comparing the results of radiotherapy and surgery. Head Neck Surg 1988;10:373-7.
18. Harwood AR. Cancer of the larynx: the Toronto experience. J Otolaryngol Suppl 1982;11:1-21.
19. Goffinet DR, Fee WE, Goode RL. Combined surgery and postoperative irradiation in the treatment of cervical lymph nodes. Arch Otolaryngol 1984;110:736-8.
20. Tupchong L, Scott CB, Blitzer PH, et al. Randomized study of preoperative versus postoperative radiation therapy in advanced head and neck carcinoma: long-term follow-up of RTOG study 73-03. Int J Radiat Oncol Biol Phys 1991;20:21-8.
21. Cooper JS, Pajak TF, Rubin P, et al. Second malignancies in patients who have head and neck cancer: incidence, effect on survival, and implications based on the RTOG experience. Int J Radiat Oncol Biol Phys 1989;17:449-56.
22. Lippman SM, Hong WK. Retinoid chemoprevention of upper aerodigestive tract carcinogenesis. In: DeVita VT Jr, Hellman S, Rosenberg SA, editors. Important advances in oncology. Philadelphia: JB Lippincott Company, 1992:93-107.
23. Vikram B, Strong EW, Shah JP, Spiro R. Failure in the neck following multimodality treatment for advanced head and neck cancer. Head Neck Surg 1984;6:724-9.
24. Shah JP. Cancer of the upper aerodigestive tract. In: Alfonso AE, Gardner B, editors. The practice of cancer surgery. New York: Appleton-Century-Crofts, 1982.
25. Slaughter DP, Southwick HW, Smejkal W. "Field cancerization" in oral stratified squamous epithelium: clinical implications of multicentric origin. Cancer 1953;6:963-8.
26. Spitz MR, Hsu TC, Schantz SP. Genetic and environmental interactions as risks for aerodigestive cancers. Adv Exp Med Biol 1992;320:31-4.
27. Hong WK, Bromer RH, Amato DA, et al. Patterns of relapse in locally advanced head and neck cancer patients who achieved complete remission after combined modality therapy. Cancer 1985;56:1242-5.
28. Wynder E, Mushinsk M, Spivak J. Tobacco and alcohol consumption in relation to the development of multiple primary cancers. Cancer 1977;40:1872-8.
29. Lippman SM, Hong WK. Second malignant tumors in head and neck squamous cell carcinoma: the overshadowing threat for patients with early-stage disease. Int J Radiat Oncol Biol Phys 1989;17:691-4.
30. McDonald S, Haie C, Rubin P, Nelson D, Divers L. Second malignant tumors in patients with laryngeal carcinoma: diagnosis, treatment, and prevention. Int J Radiat Oncol Biol Phys 1989;17:457-65.
31. Jovanovic A, Van Der Tol I, Schulten E, et al. Risk of multiple primary tumors following oral squamous cell carcinoma. Int J Cancer 1994;56:320-3.
32. De Visscher A, Manni J. Routine long-term follow-up in patients treated with curative intent for squamous cell carcinoma of the larynx, pharynx, and oral cavity. Arch Otolaryngol Head Neck Surg 1994;120:934-9.
33. Nahum AM, Mullally W, Marmor L. A syndrome resulting from radical neck dissection. Arch Otolaryngol 1961;74:82-6.
34. Posner MR, Ervin TJ, Miller D, et al. Incidence of hypothyroidism following multimodality treatment for advanced squamous cell cancer of the head and neck. Laryngoscope 1984;94:451-4.
35. Atkins J, Keane W, Young K, Rowe L. Value of panendoscopy in determination of second primary cancer: a study of 451 cases of head and neck cancer. Arch Otolaryngol 1984;110:533-4.
36. Leipzig B, Zellmer J, Klug D. The role of endoscopy in evaluating patients with head and neck cancer: a multi-institutional prospective study. Arch Otolaryngol 1985;111:589-94.
37. Nordlight S. Facial disfigurement and psychiatric sequelae. NY State J Med 1979;79:1382-4.
38. Breitbart W, Holland J. Psychological aspects of head and neck cancer. Semin Oncol 1988;15:61-9.
39. Browman GP, Wong G, Hodson I, et al. Influence of cigarette smoking on the efficacy of radiation therapy in head and neck cancer. N Engl J Med 1993;328:159-63.
40. Schwarz J. Review and evaluation of smoking cessation methods: the United States and Canada, 1978-1985. Washington (DC): U.S. Department of Health and Human Services, National Cancer Institute;1987:NIH 87-2940.
41. Cullen J. Strategies to stop smoking. Cancer Prevention 1989;May:1-12.
42. Fiore M, Pierce J, Remington P, Fiore B. Cigarette smoking: the clinician's role in cessation, prevention, and public health. Dis Mon 1990;35:183-242.
43. Russell M, Wilson C, Taylor C, Backer C. Effect of general practitioner's advice against smoking. Br Med J 1979;2:231-5.
44. Gupta PC, Mehta FS, Pindborg JJ, et al. Intervention study for primary prevention of oral cancer among 36,000 Indian tobacco users. Lancet 1986;1:1235-9.
45. Shillitoe E, Schantz S, Spitz M, Hecht S. Environmental carcinogenesis and its prevention: the head and neck cancer model. Cancer Res 1993;53:2189-91.
46. Hong WK, Endicott J, Itri L, et al. 13-Cis retinoic acid in the treatment of oral leukoplakia. N Engl J Med 1986;315:1501-5.
47. Lippman SM, Batsakis JG, Toth BB, et al. Comparisons of low-dose isotretinoin with beta carotene to prevent oral carcinogenesis. N Engl J Med 1993;328:15-20.
48. Hong WK, Lippman SM, Itri LM, et al. Prevention of second primary tumors with isotretinoin in squamous cell carcinoma of the head and neck. N Engl J Med 1990;323:795-801.

49. Brennan JA, Boyle JO, Koch WM, et al. Association between cigarette smoking and mutation of the p53 gene in squamous cell carcinoma of the head and neck. N Engl J Med 1995;332:712-7.
50. Lydiatt WM, Davidson BJ, Shah J, Schantz SP, Chaganti RS. The relationship of loss of heterozygosity to tobacco exposure and early recurrence in head and neck squamous cell carcinomas. Am J Surg 1994;168:437-40.
51. Sidransky D, Boyle J, Koch W. Molecular screening prospects for a new approach. Arch Otolaryngol Head Neck Surg 1993;119:1187-90.
52. Boyle JO, Mao L, Brennan JA, et al. Gene mutations in saliva as molecular markers for head and neck squamous cell carcinomas. Am J Surg 1994;168:429-32.
53. Nees M, Homann N, Discher H, et al. Expression of mutated in p53 occurs in tumor-distant epithelia of head and neck cancer patients: a possible molecular basis for the development of multiple tumors. Cancer Res 1993;53:4189-96.
54. Burch JD, Howe GR, Miller AB, Semencle R. Tobacco, alcohol, asbestos, and nickel in the etiology of cancer of the larynx: a case-control study. J Natl Cancer Inst 1981;67:1219-24.

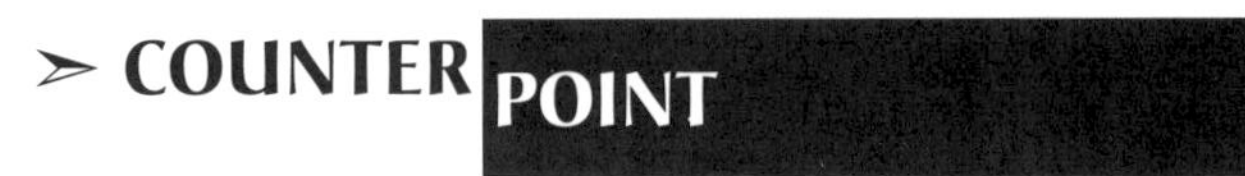

National Kyushu Cancer Center, Japan

TADASHI NAKASHIMA

I agree with the follow-up methodology described by Schantz and Andersen. Following are additional data concerning etiology and the follow-up schedule at National Kyushu Cancer Center.

Head and neck cancer is diagnosed in approximately 15,000 new patients per year (4% of overall new cancer patients) in Japan, making it the seventh most common malignancy in the country.[1] Squamous cell carcinoma is the most common histological type, and the oral cavity is the most common site, followed by the larynx and hypopharynx.

Carcinomas of the maxillary sinus represent approximately 7% of head and neck cancers in Japan. This percentage is probably greater than those for other countries in this text. Tobacco and alcohol abuse is an etiological factor in carcinomas of the maxillary sinus, supraglottic larynx, oropharynx, and hypopharynx. The presence of maxillary sinusitis correlates significantly with the high incidence of maxillary sinus carcinoma. However, because of improved nutrition and hygiene, as well as early diagnosis and treatment of maxillary sinusitis, the incidence of maxillary carcinoma has decreased dramatically.

TREATMENT OF HEAD AND NECK CANCER

In Japan radiation therapy is the preferred treatment of most early-stage lesions of the head and neck. Early glottic laryngeal cancer, early oropharyngeal cancer, and nasopharyngeal cancer of any T category are treated by radiation therapy alone as a first choice. In cases of early-stage tongue cancer, implant radiation therapy combined with external irradiation is also a treatment option. In advanced head and neck cancer, combination therapy consisting of surgery and preoperative or postoperative radiation therapy is performed.

Table 5-8 Follow-up of patients with head and neck cancer (patients with relatively high cure rates*): National Kyushu Cancer Center, Japan

	YEAR				
	1	2	3	4	5
Office visit	12	6	4	4	4
Chest x-ray	2	2	2	2	2
Complete blood count	6	6	0	0	0
Liver function tests	6	6	0	0	0
SCCAg†	6	6	0	0	0
Computed tomography/magnetic resonance imaging of the maxillofacial area‡	2	2	0	0	0

SCCAg, Squamous cell carcinoma–related antigen.
*Such as glottic laryngeal cancer.
†Performed in patients whose titer of SCCAg was high at the time of initial treatment.
‡Performed for nasopharyngeal cancer patients. Test selection based on availability. Magnetic resonance imaging also performed when deemed necessary by the radiologist for diagnosing recurrence.

DEVELOPMENT OF A SECOND PRIMARY TUMOR

Occurrence of a second primary cancer in the head and neck is not uncommon in Japan. The synchronous or metachronous occurrence of multiple upper aerodigestive tract cancers, such as esophageal cancer, is observed frequently.[2-4] The prevalence of heavy smoking and heavy drinking is extremely high among patients with multiple esophageal cancers and among those with concurrent head and neck cancers. Although both tobacco and alcohol contribute to the risk of second cancers, the effect of smoking is more pronounced.[5]

Since family aggregation has been frequently observed among patients with either esophageal cancer or head and neck cancer, genetic factors might also play an important role in the occurrence.[6,7] A family history of upper aerodigestive cancer seems to predispose patients with head and neck cancer or esophageal cancer to second primary cancers.

For early diagnosis of second lesions, routine panendoscopy, including laryngoscopy, esophagoscopy, and bronchoscopy, has been reported to be most useful.[4,8] Esophagoscopy with Lugol dye staining and biopsy is useful for the accurate diagnosis of early concomitant esophageal cancers.[9]

FOLLOW-UP CARE

The follow-up care of patients with head and neck cancer begins at discharge from the hospital and should continue for at least 5 years. The schedule of follow-up is generally divided into two groups according to the site of origin of head and neck cancers. Patients with relatively high cure rates of disease, such as glottic laryngeal cancer, are followed up in the same manner as scheduled by Schantz and Andersen for

Table 5-9 Follow-up of patients with head and neck cancer (patients with poor prognosis at any stage*): National Kyushu Cancer Center, Japan

	YEAR				
	1	2	3	4	5
Office visit	12	12	6	6	4
Chest x-ray	2	2	2	2	2
Complete blood count	6	6	0	0	0
Liver function tests	6	6	0	0	0
SCCAg†	6	6	0	0	0
Computed tomography/magnetic resonance imaging of the maxillofacial area‡	2	2	0	0	0
Neck ultrasonography§	4	0	0	0	0

SCCAg, Squamous cell carcinoma–related antigen.
*Such as cancers of the hypopharynx or the tongue.
†Performed in patients whose titer of SCCAg was high at the time of initial treatment.
‡Performed for patients with nasopharyngeal cancer. Test selection based on availability. Magnetic resonance imaging also performed when deemed necessary by the radiologist for diagnosing recurrence.
§Performed for patients with neck node adenopathy.

the first 3 years (Table 5-8). For years 4 and 5, however, they are followed up quarterly. Beyond 5 years they are followed up every 6 to 12 months for the remainder of life.

In contrast, patients with a poor prognosis, such as those with cancers of the hypopharynx or tongue (at any stage), are carefully monitored in the first year (Table 5-9). They visit the clinic once or twice a month for the first 6 months. Monthly visits are continued through the second year. Bimonthly visits are required for the third and fourth years, followed by quarterly visits for the fifth year.

At each follow-up visit, physical examination of the primary organ and palpation for abnormal neck lymph nodes are carefully done. In patients with laryngeal cancer whose local findings are not easily visualized by a laryngeal mirror, flexible fiberoptic examination is performed at each follow-up visit. In the first year of follow-up for such cancers as those of the tongue, supraglottis, and hypopharynx, neck lymph nodes are also examined using ultrasonography at 3-month intervals. Chest radiographs are examined at 6-month intervals for life, if not examined elsewhere.

In the first 2 years of follow-up monitoring of maxillofacial areas for patients with nasopharyngeal or paranasal sinus cancer, evaluation by computed tomographic scans is done at 6-month intervals if necessary. When there is evidence of recurrence, magnetic resonance imaging is also performed according to the radiologist's suggestion. Routine blood studies involving complete blood cell counts and liver function tests are performed bimonthly for 2 years. In patients whose titer of squamous cell carcinoma–related antigen (SCCAg)[10] was high at the time of initial treatment, SCCAg is repeatedly examined in the first 2 years.

Physicians at National Kyushu Cancer Center also refer patients to medical professionals for shoulder dysfunction, psychological problems, or dental prophylaxis and restoration when necessary. For postoperative voice rehabilitation in patients after a laryngectomy for advanced laryngeal cancer or hypopharyngeal cancer, a voice-training group in the hospital offers lessons in esophageal speech or use of a hand-held electrolarynx.

REFERENCES

1. Kakizoe T, editor. Figures on cancer in Japan. Tokyo: Figures on Cancer in Japan Publishing Committee, 1993.
2. Cohn AM, Peppard SB. Multiple primary malignant tumors of the head and neck. Am J Otolaryngol 1980;1:411-7.
3. Shapshay SM, Hong WK, Fried MP, et al. Simultaneous carcinomas of the esophagus and upper aerodigestive tract. Otolaryngol Head Neck Surg 1980;8:373-7.
4. Abemayor E, Moore DM, Hanson DG. Identification of synchronous esophageal tumors in patients with head and neck cancer. J Surg Oncol 1988;38:94-6.
5. Day GL, Blot WJ, Shore RE, et al. Second cancers following oral and pharyngeal cancers: role of tobacco and alcohol. J Natl Cancer Inst 1994;86:131-7.
6. Coffin CM, Rich SS, Dehner LP. Family aggregation of nasopharyngeal carcinoma and other malignancies. Cancer 1991;68:1323-8.
7. Ghadirian P. Family history of esophageal cancer. Cancer 1985;56:2112-6.
8. Weaver A, Fleming SM, Knechtges TC, et al. Triple endoscopy: a neglected essential in head and neck cancer. Surgery 1979;86:493-6.
9. Ina H, Shibuya H, Ohashi I, Kitagawa M. The efficacy of concomitant early esophageal cancer in male patients with oral and oropharyngeal cancer: screening results using Lugol dye endoscopy. Cancer 1994;73:2038-41.
10. Kato H, Torigoe T. Radioimmunoassay for tumor antigen of human cervical squamous cell carcinoma. Cancer 1977;40:1621-8.

➢ COUNTERPOINT

Royal Liverpool University Hospital, UK

ANDREW SIMPSON JONES

In the United Kingdom, head and neck cancer accounts for only a small proportion of human malignancies. In 1986, there were 1,784 new cancers of the larynx and 2,787 new cancers of the lip, oral cavity, and pharynx.[1] In 1989, 861 patients died of laryngeal cancer and 1,716 died of cancers of the lip, oral cavity, and pharynx.[1]

Head and neck cancer is predominantly a disease of men and of urban areas.[2] The main causes of head and neck squamous cell carcinoma are smoking[3,4] and alcohol consumption.[4,5] Alcohol intake alone may be a relatively unimportant cause of head and neck cancer but in combination with smoking is synergistic.[5] Other factors such as poor dentition and dietary factors may also increase the risk of oral cancer, but the effects are small when compared with those of smoking.[4] Workers in certain industries may be exposed to an increased risk of head and neck cancer. For example, the risk of laryngeal cancer is higher in individuals working with asbestos, textiles, woods, and leather, as well as those involved in the manufacture of plastic products, rubber products, pesticides, and sulfuric acid.[6]

The Mersey region of Great Britain illustrates the fact that head and neck cancer is more common in large industrial areas. The region has a population of 2.4 million, with a standardized reporting ratio for laryngeal cancer of 127% for males and 161% for females and for oral cavity and pharyngeal cancers of 149% for males and 127% for females.

Squamous cell carcinoma is by far the most common histological type.[7] The University of Liverpool Head and Neck Database contains details of 4,688 patients with malignant tumors of the head and neck collected over a 30-year period. Of these, 80% are of squamous cell histology. Lymphomas form 5% of the series, malignant salivary tumors 4%, undifferentiated carcinomas 3%, sarcomas 1%, and thyroid tumors also 1%. The remaining 6% include such tumors as neuroendocrine carcinomas. Most head and neck squamous cell carcinomas are differentiated, with 37% well differentiated, 36% moderately differentiated, and only 27% poorly differentiated.

The major head and neck sites are the larynx, oral cavity, hypopharynx, and oropharynx, which together account for 90% of head and neck squamous cell carcinomas. The Liverpool database contains 3,596 patients with squamous cell carcinoma, of which 36% occurred in the larynx, 21% in the oral cavity, 18% in the hypopharynx, and 15% in the oropharynx. Interestingly, differences exist in the contribution of various subsites to the total number of cancers in a certain site. For example, in laryngeal cancer a well-known variation in proportion exists between glottic and supraglottic cancers. In Sweden supraglottic cancers are fairly unusual, whereas in Liverpool the ratio of supraglottic to glottic cancers is equal,[8] each constituting 42% of the total number of laryngeal cancers. Similarly, regional differences exist between the proportion of postcricoid cancer and pyriform fossa cancer in the hypopharyngeal site. Postcricoid cancer is relatively unusual in most of the world but is much more common in certain areas, particularly Northern Europe. In Liverpool postcricoid cancer forms 41% of cases of hypopharyngeal cancer and 43% of cases of pyriform fossa tumors.

PROGNOSIS

Head and neck squamous cell carcinoma, in general, has a good prognosis compared with cancers of other sites. The 5-year, tumor-specific survival for all head and neck squamous cell carcinomas on the Liverpool database is 50% (95% confidence intervals of 48% to 53%). Survival varies widely among various sites; tumor-specific 5-year survival for previously untreated laryngeal carcinoma is 67% at 5 years, for oral cavity cancer 47%, and for oropharyngeal cancer 43%. Hypopharyngeal cancer has the worst prognosis with 26% survival at 5 years. These figures are in broad agreement with those of other authors.[9-17]

The pattern of spread of head and neck tumors is different for different sites, determined largely by the type of underlying tissue.[18,19] In the larynx the pattern of invasion of cancer has been well studied[20] and is determined by structures that resist tumor spread and those that do not. For example, in the larynx, nonossified cartilage, the hyoepiglottic ligament, and the conus elasticus resist tumor spread effectively, whereas ossified cartilage, the thyroepiglottic ligament, the cricothyroid membrane, and the ventricular cavity all allow tumors to spread relatively easily. In the oral cavity, tumors spread with great ease through the muscle planes of the tongue[18] and, of great practical importance, invade the mandible by direct extension, particularly in edentulous patients.[21] In oropharyngeal cancer, tumors extend eccentrically and preferentially into lymphoid tissue. In the hypopharynx the spread of tumors is not controlled by well-defined, anatomical structures in the same way as tumors of the larynx. Laterally based pyriform fossa cancer tends to extend through the thyroid cartilage and thyrohyoid membrane, producing a contiguous mass in the neck and frequently invading the thyroid gland. Medially based pyriform fossa cancer tends to invade through the aryepiglottic fold into the paraglottic space. Cricothyroid cancer, on the other hand, extends down the cervical esophagus and frequently invades into the trachea anteriorly.[19]

Nearly all head and neck cancers drain into the regional lymph nodes of the neck, which are accessible for radical and potentially curative treatment. The incidence of lymph node metastases depends mainly on the size and site of the primary tumor. Glottic cancers tend not to produce lymph node metastases until late, whereas pyriform fossa cancers almost always have lymph node metastases early in the disease process. The depth of infiltration of the primary tumor is probably more important in predicting the probability of cervical node metastasis than the actual size.[22]

Of particular prognostic importance is the presence or absence of extranodal spread and, of course, the number of nodes invaded.[23] Free metastases outside lymph nodes within the neck are an especially poor prognostic sign.[24] The lymph nodes of the neck that are important in tumor spread are the deep cervical nodes. These may be divided into five regions[25]: submandibular nodes, upper, middle, and deep cervical nodes (jugular chain), and the supraclavicular and posterior triangle nodes. The spread of tumor to the various nodes can be predicted based on the site of the primary cancer.[26] The upper deep cervical nodes are most frequently involved by oral tumors; mouth cancer frequently involves the submandibular nodes; and hypopharyngeal cancer frequently involves the lower deep cervical nodes. Supraclavicular and posterior triangle nodes are relatively infrequently involved. It should be noted, however, that the upper deep cervical nodes are by far the most common site for neck node metastases.

A particular therapeutic problem is the involvement of mediastinal nodes in postcricoid and subglottic cancer. In such instances the chances of curing disease are slight.

EVALUATION

Assessment of head and neck cancer is crucial to the treatment of this complex and challenging condition. A full history must be taken and a thorough head and neck examination carried out. Approximately 5% of patients present with a node in the neck, but the primary site is usually evident at the time of examination.[27] Following the physical examination, computed tomography or magnetic resonance imaging of the head and neck region should be carried out. Scanning is important because it provides a permanent record of the lesion. In laryngeal cancer, scanning is of particular value in visualizing the preepiglottic space[28] and magnetic resonance imaging is particularly valuable in detecting cartilage invasion.[29] Moreover, magnetic resonance imaging appears to be superior to other methods in the evaluation of tumor invasion of the mandible.[30] Examination of the neck has been the subject of much scrutiny. Nodes in deep parts of the neck can be palpated only when the examiner is experienced and the nodes are 1 cm or more in diameter.[31] Conversely, nodes of 2 cm in diameter may be normal in some individuals. It is not surprising therefore that approximately one fourth of neck cancers are incorrectly staged by physical examination.[32] Scanning of the neck by computed tomography or magnetic resonance imaging of the neck at least modestly increases the accuracy of detection of metastases,[33] particularly in short, muscular, or previously treated necks. A node detected by scanning should be sampled by fine-needle aspiration to obtain a cytological diagnosis. Following scanning the patient should have a full panendoscopy, including bronchoscopy and esophagoscopy. The full extent of tumor should be assessed by inspection and palpation, if possible, and a biopsy should be taken. Performing panendoscopy is important because the incidence of synchronous second primary tumors is approximately 1%. Head, neck, and lung sites are the most common.[34]

Distant metastases should be sought. In a T1 cancer with no neck nodes, a chest radiograph will suffice. In patients with high-volume disease in whom radical treatment is planned, a chest computed tomographic scan and liver ultrasound should be carried out.[35] A bone scan may be ordered if appropriate on clinical grounds.

TREATMENT

Curative treatment for head and neck carcinoma takes the form of irradiation, surgery, or a combination of the two. Historically, treatment of head and neck cancer has been marred by rivalry between radiotherapists and surgeons. Exclusively single-modality treatment has been used until quite recently.[36] This may have been due partly to a belief by each discipline that its treatment was superior and partly to a nihilistic attitude that treatment modality does not affect survival.[37] In the United Kingdom early laryngeal cancer is almost always treated with irradiation[38,39] and radiation therapy is also used for early cancers of the oropharynx[40] and hypopharynx.[41,42] While frequently used for small tumors in the treatment of mouth cancer,[43] irradiation has become less popular because small tumors of the oral cavity can be removed by surgery with little morbidity, whereas irradiation leaves the mouth at least partially crippled by xerostomia.

In Liverpool surgery is now the primary treatment modality for all mouth cancers, bulky T3 and T4 laryngeal cancers,[44] T3 or T4 hypopharyngeal cancers, and T3 or T4 oropharyngeal cancers. In all cases other than small oral cancers, postoperative radiation therapy is administered, and such combined treatment has been shown to improve local control.[45] Such adjuvant radiation therapy is administered postoperatively.[46] The role of chemotherapy in end-stage disease is well known, but up to now its role in prolonging survival as an adjuvant to irradiation or surgery has not been proved.[47]

Billroth[48] was the first to suggest that a patient could have cancer twice. In 1964 Ju[49] studied the results of 2,700 postmortem examinations. Of these, 340 patients had died of neoplasms of the head and neck. Second primary neoplasms, excluding carcinoma of the prostate, occurred in only 6% of the general autopsy group but in 15.5% of patients with head and neck cancer. Other authors noted different second primary cancer rates, ranging from 7.5%[50] to 14%.[51]

In a recent study carried out by the Department of Otolaryngology of Royal Liverpool University Hospital,[34] the records of 3,436 patients with squamous cell carcinoma of the head and neck were examined. The actuarial second primary rate was 9.1% at 30 years, and the median time to presentation of a second tumor was 36 months. Second tumors were more likely to occur in male patients younger than 60 years of age at the time of diagnosis of the index tumor and in laryngeal and oral cavity index tumors. Patients with a small index tumor mass at the time of diagnosis had a greater chance of a second primary tumor, presumably because they lived long enough for such an event to occur. The most common sites for second primary tumors were in the head and neck (50%) and the lung (34%); nearly all were squamous cell carcinomas. The development of a second primary tumor significantly affected survival. The 15-year survival rate from the time of diagnosis of the index tumor was 20% for those who developed a second primary tumor, compared with 44% for those who did not. The total tumor-specific, 5-year survival for patients who developed a second primary tumor (from the date of diagnosis of this second primary tumor) was 26%. The 5-year survival rate for those patients who developed a second primary tumor of the head and neck region (from the time of diagnosis of the second tumor) was 31%, compared with an overall 5-year survival rate in patients with a head and neck cancer of 48%. This demonstrates that treatment of the second primary tumor in the head and neck region is therapeutically rewarding.

Of particular interest is that radiation therapy to the index tumor was not associated with an increased risk of a second primary tumor and did not adversely affect survival.[34] The work of Hong et al.[52,53] is well known, but long-term treatment with 13-cis-retinoic acid has many problems. The drug is potentially toxic, particularly because it raises serum lipid

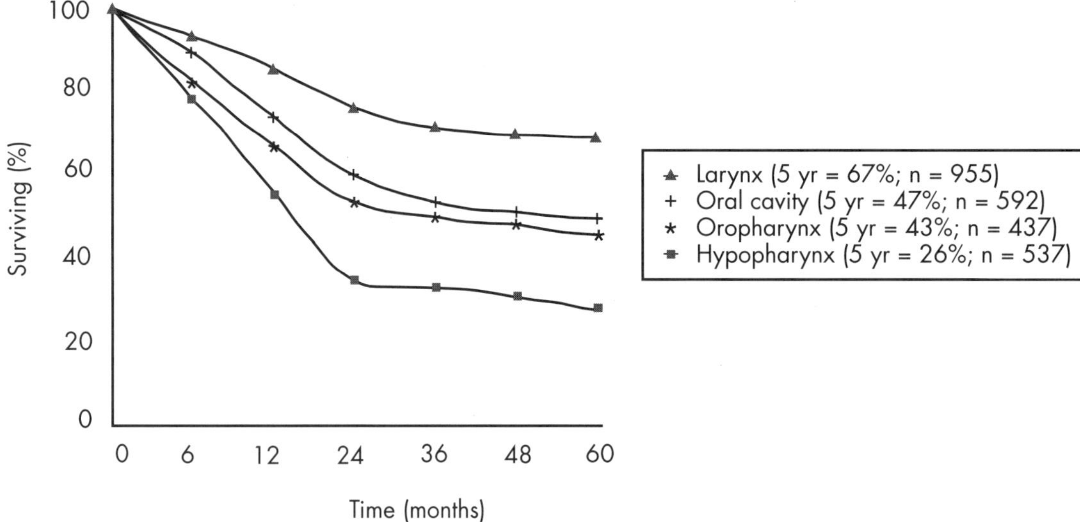

Figure 5-2 Tumor-specific 5-year survival for previously untreated squamous cell carcinoma of the four main head and neck sites. (Data from University of Liverpool Head and Neck Database.)

levels and may therefore be associated with an increased cardiovascular mortality. The Department of Otolaryngology of Royal Liverpool University Hospital has adopted a pragmatic approach toward patients who have had second primary cancers; this approach consists of daily administration of 30 mg beta-carotene. Although less effective than cis-retinoic acid, beta-carotene is nontoxic.[54]

SURVIVAL

In follow-up of patients with head and neck cancer, physicians need to be aware of the dynamics of survival. The University of Liverpool database contains the details of 3,596 patients with head and neck squamous cell carcinomas. When the tumor-specific actuarial survival is calculated, the 5-year survival is 50% (95% confidence intervals of 48% to 52%). After 5 years the tumor-specific survival decreases by only 2% over the next 7 years. Twenty percent of all deaths occur in the first 6 months, 46% within the first year, 68% within the first 18 months, and 76% within 2 years. Eighty-eight percent of all deaths have occurred by 3 years and 94% by 4 years. Thus, three fourths of the patients who are going to die of cancer die within 2 years of diagnosis. Some malignant tumors behave differently. Adenoid cystic carcinoma and mucosal malignant melanoma, for example, can have very long natural histories, with deaths occurring 20 years after diagnosis. The rare small cell neuroendocrine carcinoma, on the other hand, has a short natural history.

The 5-year survival rates for squamous cell carcinomas of the four main sites (larynx, oral cavity, hypopharynx, and oropharynx) are shown in Figure 5-2. The index cancer is not, of course, the only cause of death in patients with head and neck tumors. For example, the 5-year, tumor-specific death rate for laryngeal cancer is 33% and an additional 22% of patients die of other causes, mainly cardiovascular disease and second primary tumors, particularly carcinoma of the lung. Thus the observed survival rate of such patients is 45% at 5 years (Figure 5-3). In hypopharyngeal cancer the difference is even more pronounced, with a 5-year, tumor-specific survival rate of 26% and an observed survival rate of half this amount (Figure 5-4). To further illustrate the fate of patients, the outcome at 5 years for a group of patients with T1-3 N0 squamous cell carcinoma of the larynx is shown in Table 5-10, and the outcome for a group of patients with T1-3 N1-2 hypopharyngeal squamous cell carcinoma is shown in Table 5-11. Both groups were treated by primary irradiation with surgical salvage if necessary.

The Liverpool experience is not unique. Boysen et al.[55] reported in 1985 that 85% of recurrences in their patients with head and neck cancer occurred within 2 years and only 5% occurred after 3 years.

FOLLOW-UP

The follow-up of patients with head and neck cancer is fairly uniform. The University of Liverpool Head and Neck Cancer Unit uses primarily the same follow-up system described by Schantz and Andersen for Memorial Sloan-Kettering Cancer Center (Table 5-12). In his unit in Amsterdam, Snow[56] employs a similar pattern of follow-up. The main reason for following patients after the fifth year is the detection of second primary tumors, the treatment of which, if they occur in the head and neck region, can be particularly rewarding.[34] Early detection of recurrence in a patient having an early glottic carcinoma treated by irradiation may allow treatment by vertical hemilaryngectomy rather than by total laryngectomy.[57] At every follow-up visit a full history is taken and the neck is examined. Weighing the patient is particularly important and should be carried out at every visit. A complete blood count, serum biochemistry (including calcium), and thyroid

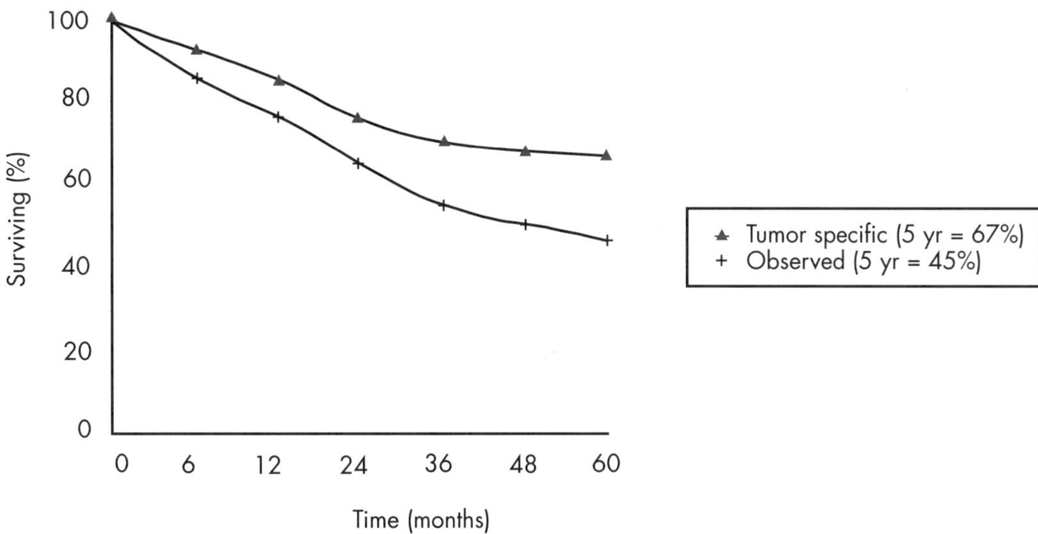

Figure 5-3 Observed and tumor-specific 5-year survival for laryngeal squamous cell carcinoma. (Data from University of Liverpool Head and Neck Database.)

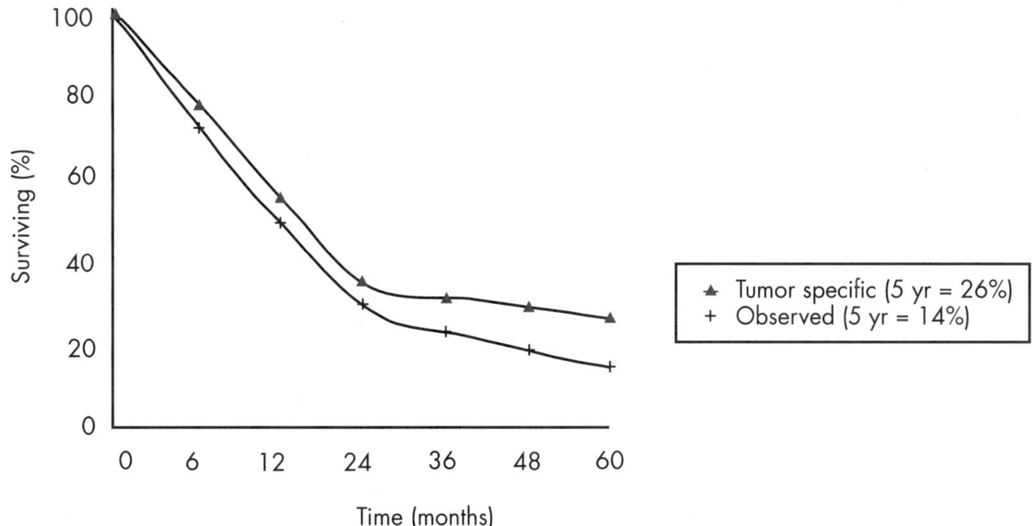

Figure 5-4 Observed and tumor-specific 5-year survival for hypopharyngeal squamous cell carcinoma. (Data from University of Liverpool Head and Neck Database.)

Table 5-10 Fate at 5 years of 320 patients suffering from T1-3 N0 carcinoma of the larynx treated with irradiation and salvage surgery if necessary

ALIVE	DIED OF ORIGINAL CANCER	DIED OF OTHER CAUSES	DIED OF SECOND CANCER
54%	13%	27%	6%

Data from the University of Liverpool Head and Neck Database.

Table 5-11 Fate at 5 years of 119 patients suffering from T1-3 N1-2 carcinoma of the hypopharynx treated with irradiation and salvage surgery as necessary

ALIVE	DIED OF ORIGINAL CANCER	DIED OF OTHER CAUSES	DIED OF SECOND CANCER
20%	48%	29%	3%

Data from the University of Liverpool Head and Neck Database.

Table 5-12 Follow-up of patients with head and neck cancer: Royal Liverpool University Hospital, UK

	YEAR				
	1	2	3	4	5
Office visit	12	6	4	3	2
Chest x-ray	2	2	2	1	1
Complete blood count	2	2	2	1	1
Erythrocyte sedimentation rate	2	2	2	1	1
Electrolytes	2	2	2	1	1
Liver function tests*	2	2	2	1	1
Serum calcium	2	2	2	1	1
Thyroid function	2	2	2	1	1

*Includes measurement of total protein, albumin, globulin, bilirubin, gamma-glutamyltransferase, and alanine aminotransferase.

function test are performed biannually for the first 3 years and annually thereafter. These and other tests are, of course, ordered at any time if clinically indicated. A particular problem in follow-up treatment of head and neck cancer patients is the detection of early lung second primary tumors. After the head and neck region, the lung is the most common site for such tumors and early detection is important. Chest x-ray examination is carried out at 6-month intervals at Royal Liverpool University Hospital for the first 3 years and at yearly intervals thereafter. However, it is well known that routine chest radiographs do not affect survival in patients with carcinoma of the lung.[58,59] More aggressive attempts to detect lung tumors by fiberoptic bronchoscopy and sputum cytology every 6 months for patients treated for laryngeal cancer show that a higher number of cases of lung cancer are diagnosed at the stage when they may be curable, compared with when less aggressive follow-up techniques are used.[60] The number of patients likely to benefit would be small, however, and in the Liverpool series the second primary tumor rate was 9.1%, of which one third were in the lung. This implies that over a 30-year period approximately 100 patients with carcinoma of the lung would be expected, of which only a minority would be suitable for treatment with curative intent. The logistical and economic implications of performing bronchoscopy and cytology every 6 months in a large number of patients are hard to reconcile in a large unit. Therefore Royal Liverpool University Hospital does not carry out this type of follow-up.

Patients who have undergone extensive surgery require considerable support. When appropriate, patients are seen by a speech therapist who has an interest in swallowing difficulties. Such therapy is of course continued between follow-up visits. Input from other professionals, including prosthodontists, physiotherapists, pain specialists, support nurses, and social workers, is frequently necessary.

Prevention of second primary tumors is important, although in the Liverpool series they developed in only 9.1% of patients. To have a second primary tumor, one must survive the index tumor and other causes of death. The majority of patients with head and neck cancer do not survive beyond 5 years. Among the few long-term survivors, second cancers commonly develop. In 1984 Vikram[61] studied 98 previously untreated patients with advanced head and neck squamous cell carcinoma who were then treated with surgery and postoperative radiation therapy and compared these with a group of historical control subjects. He found that the control rate above the clavicles was improved but that patients tended to die of distant metastases and, in particular, second primary tumors, the latter occurring at a rate of 6% of patients per year.

Every effort must be made to reduce the patient's risk of a second primary tumor, particularly after the first 2 years of follow-up. This risk is greater if the patient continues to smoke.[62] Therefore helping the patient desist from this habit is important.

Patients should be encouraged to moderate alcohol intake and eat a normal, well-balanced diet. Chemoprevention, particularly with cis-retinoic acid, has not been proved to improve overall survival and is itself toxic. At Royal Liverpool University Hospital a pragmatic policy of giving beta-carotene to high-risk patients is followed, such as for the young patient with oral cavity cancer who is almost certainly cured of the index tumor.[54]

As discussed previously, the pattern of follow-up of head and neck cancer patients is remarkably uniform across most centers and demonstrates a balance between the practical and the ideal. Although most physicians would like to follow up on their patients as closely as possible, it is unlikely that survival could be markedly improved by more vigorous follow-up, so that the system described here is considered satisfactory.

REFERENCES

1. Office of Population Censuses and Surveys. Cancer statistics registrations, 1986. HMSO 1991.
2. Wake M. The urban/rural divide in head and neck cancer: the effect of atmospheric pollution. Clin Otolaryngol 1993;18:298-302.
3. Krajina Z, Kulcar Z, Konic-Carnellutti V. Epidemiology of laryngeal cancer. Laryngoscope 1975;85:1155-61.
4. Marshall JR, Graham S, Haughey BP, et al. Smoking, alcohol, dentition and diet in the epidemiology of oral cancer. Eur J Cancer B Oral Oncol 1992;28B:9-15.
5. Rothman KJ, Cann CI, Flanders D, Fried MP. Epidemiology of laryngeal cancer. Epidemiol Rev 1980;2:195-209.
6. Maier H, De Vries N, Snow GB. Occupational factors in the aetiology of head and neck cancer. Clin Otolaryngol 1991;16:406-12.
7. Batsakis JK. Tumours of the head and neck. 2nd ed. Baltimore: Williams & Wilkins, 1979:1-573.
8. Stell PM. Prognosis in laryngeal carcinoma: tumour factors. Clin Otolaryngol 1990;15:69-81.
9. Mendenhall WM, Parsons JT, Stringer SP, Cassisi NJ. Vocal cord carcinoma: a basis for comparing the results of radiotherapy and surgery. Head Neck Surg 1988;10:373-7.
10. Mendenhall WM, Parsons JT, Stringer SP, Cassisi NJ. Stage T3 squamous cell carcinoma of the glottic larynx: a comparison of laryngectomy and irradiation. Int J Radiat Oncol Biol Phys 1992;23:725-32.

11. Weem S, Mendenhall WM, Parsons JT, Cassisi NJ. Squamous cell carcinoma of the supraglottic larynx treated with surgery and/or radiation therapy. Int J Radiat Oncol Biol Phys 1987;13:1483-7.
12. Mendenhall WM, Parsons JT, Devine JW, Cassisi NJ. Squamous cell carcinoma of the pyriform sinus treated with surgery and/or radiotherapy. Head Neck Surg 1987;10:88-92.
13. Hibbert J, Marks NJ, Winter PJ. Carcinomas and their relation to clinical strategy. Clin Otolaryngol 1983;8:197-203.
14. Pukunder J, Karhuketo T, Pentilla M, Pertrovaara H, Karma P. Radical surgery for lingual cancer. Clin Otolaryngol 1990;15:229-34.
15. Decroix Y, Ghossein NA. Experience of the Curie Institute in treatment of cancer of the mobile tongue. I. Treatment policies and result. Cancer 1981;47:496-502.
16. Pachelo-Ojeda L, Marandas P, Julieron M, Lusinchi A, Malmelle G, Luboinski B. Salvage surgery by composite resection for epidermoid carcinoma of the tonsillar region. Arch Otolaryngol Head Neck Surg 1992;118:181-4.
17. Mendenhall WM, Parsons JT, Cassisi NJ, Million RR. Squamous cell carcinoma of the tonsillar area treated with radical irradiation. Radiother Oncol 1987;10:23-30.
18. Cachin Y. Perspectives on cancer of the head and neck. In: Cancer of the head and neck. 2nd ed. Myers EN, Suen JY, editors. New York: Churchill Livingstone, 1989:1-16.
19. Stell PM, Maran AG. Head and neck surgery. London: William Heinemann Medical Books Ltd, 1978:1-456.
20. Kleinasser O. Tumours of the larynx and hypopharynx. Stuttgart: Georg Thieme Verlag, 1988:1-349.
21. McGregor IA, McGregor FM. Cancer of the face and mouth: pathology and management for surgeons. Edinburgh: Churchill Livingstone, 1986.
22. Mohit-Tabatabai MA, Sobel HJ, Rush BF, et al. Relation of thickness of floor of mouth stage I and II cancers to regional metastasis. Am J Surg 1986;152:351-3.
23. Snow GB, Annyas AA, Van Slooten EA, et al. Prognostic factors of neck node metastasis. Clin Otolaryngol 1982;7:185-92.
24. Violaris NS, O'Neill D, Helliwell TR, Caslin AW, Roland NJ, Jones AS. Soft tissue cervical metastases of squamous cell carcinoma of the head and neck. Clin Otolaryngol 1994;19:394-9.
25. Shah JP, Strong E, Spiro RH, Vikram B. Neck dissection: current status and future possibilities. Clin Bull 1981;11:25-33.
26. Jones AS, Roland NJ, Field JK, Phillips DE. The level of cervical lymph node metastases: their prognostic relevance and relationship with head and neck squamous cell carcinoma primary sites. Clin Otolaryngol 1994;19:63-9.
27. Jones AS, Cook JA, Phillips DE, Roland NJ. Squamous cell carcinoma presenting as an enlarged cervical lymph node. Cancer 1993;72:1756-61.
28. Gerritsen GJ, Valk J, van Velzen DJ, et al. Computed tomography: a mandatory investigational procedure for the T-staging of advanced laryngeal cancer. Clin Otolaryngol 1986;11:307-16.
29. Castelijns JA, Gerritsen GJ, Kaiser MC, et al. MRI of normal or cancerous laryngeal cartilages: histopathologic correlation. Laryngoscope 1987;97:1085-93.
30. Ator GA. Abemayor E, Lufkin RB. Evaluation of mandibular tumor invasion with magnetic resonance imaging. Arch Otolaryngol Head Neck Surg 1990;116:454-9.
31. Salp L, Pradier RN, Marchetta FC, et al. Fallibility of palpation in the diagnosis of metastases to cervical nodes. Surg Gynecol Obstet 1964;118:989-90.
32. Ali S, Tiwari RM, Snow GB. False-positive and false-negative neck nodes. Head Neck Surg 1985;8:78-82.
33. van den Brekel MW, Stel HV, Castelijns JA, et al. Cervical lymph node metastases: assessment of radiologic criteria. Radiology 1990;177:379-84.
34. Jones AS, Morar P, Phillips DE, Field JK, Husband D, Helliwell TR. Second primary tumours in head and neck squamous carcinoma. Cancer. In press.
35. Dinkel E, Mundinger A, Schopp D, Grosser G, Hauesstein KH. Diagnostic imaging in metastatic lung disease. Lung 1990;168 Suppl:1129-36.
36. Martin HE. The history of lingual cancer. Am J Surg 1940;48:703-16.
37. Till JE, Bruce WR, Elwan A, et al. A preliminary analysis of end results for cancer of the larynx. Laryngoscope 1975;85:259-75.
38. Lederman M. Radiotherapy of cancer of the larynx. J Laryngol Otol 1970;84:867-96.
39. Viani L, Dammeijer P, Jones AS, Dalby JE, Stell PM. Recurrence after radiotherapy for glottic carcinoma. Cancer 1991;76:577-84.
40. Viani L, Dammeijer P, Jones AS, Dalby JE, Stell PM. Recurrence of oropharyngeal carcinoma after radiotherapy. J Laryngol Otol 1991;105:24-8.
41. Jones AS. The management of early hypopharyngeal cancer: primary radiotherapy and salvage surgery. Clin Otolaryngol 1992;17:545-9.
42. Jones AS, McRae RD, Phillips DE, Hamilton J, Field JK, Husband D. The treatment of node negative squamous cell carcinoma of the post-cricoid region. J Laryngol Otol 1995;199:114-9.
43. Jones AS, Khan H. Patterns and treatment of recurrence following radiotherapy for carcinoma of the oral cavity. Clin Otolaryngol 1993;18:14-8.
44. Jones AS, Cook JA, Phillips DE, Soler-Lluch E. Treatment of T3 carcinoma of the larynx by surgery or radiotherapy. Clin Otolaryngol 1992;17:433-6.
45. Vikram B, Strong W, Shah JP, Spiro R. Failure at the primary site following multimodality treatment in advanced head and neck cancer. Head Neck Surg 1984;6:720-3.
46. Montravadi RV, Skolnik EM, Applebaum EL. Complications of postoperative and pre-operative radiation therapy in head and neck cancer. Arch Otolaryngol 1981;107:690-3.
47. Stell PM. Adjuvant chemotherapy in head and neck cancer. Clin Otolaryngol 1990;15:193-5.
48. Billroth T. Die allgemeine chirurgische pathologie und therapie, in 51 vorlesungen. In: Handbuch für studirende und ärtze. 14th ed. Reimer G, editor. Berlin: 1889:908.
49. Ju DM. A study of the behaviour of cancer of the head and neck during the late and terminal phases. Am J Surg 1964;108:552-7.
50. Marchetta FC, Sako K, Camp E. Multiple malignancies in patients with head and neck cancer. Am J Surg 1965;110:537-41.
51. De Vries N, Snow GB. Multiple primary tumours in laryngeal cancer. J Laryngol Otol 1986;100:915-8.
52. Hong WK, Endicott J, Itri LM, Doos W, Batsakis JG, Bell R. 13 Cis-retinoic acid in the treatment of oral leukoplakia. N Engl J Med 1986;315:1501-5.
53. Hong WK, Lippman SM, Itri LM, Karp DD, Lee JS, Byers RM. Prevention of second primary tumors with isotretinoin in squamous cell carcinoma of the head and neck. N Engl J Med 1990;323:795-801.
54. Garswal HS, Schantz S. Emerging role of beta-carotene and antioxidant nutrients in prevention of oral cancer. Arch Otolaryngol Head Neck Surg 1995;121:141-4.
55. Boysen M, Natvig K, Winther FO, Tausjo J. Value of routine follow-up in patients treated for squamous cell carcinoma of the head and neck. J Otolaryngol 1985;14:211-4.
56. Snow GB. Evaluation and staging. In: Multimodal therapy for head and neck cancer. Snow GB, Clark JR, editors. Stuttgart: George Thieme Verlag, 1992:2-22.
57. Croll GA, van den Broek P, Tiwari RM, et al. Vertical partial laryngectomy for recurrent glottic carcinoma after irradiation. Head Neck Surg 1985;7:390-3.
58. Fontana R, Sanderson D, Woolner L, et al. Lung cancer screening: the Mayo program. J Occup Med 1986;28:746-50.
59. Taylor WF, Fontana RS, Uhlenhopp MA, et al. Some results of screening for early lung cancer. Cancer 1981;47:1114-20.
60. Rodriquez E, Castella J, Puzo C. Lung cancer in patients with tracheostomy due to cancer of the larynx. Respiration 1984;46:323-7.
61. Vikram B. Changing patterns of failure in advanced head and neck cancer. Arch Otolaryngol 1984;110:564-5.
62. Moore C. Smoking and cancer of the mouth, pharynx and larynx. JAMA 1965;191:283-6.

➢ COUNTERPOINT

Roswell Park Cancer Institute

THOM R. LOREE

The follow-up recommendations and principles for cancers of the head and neck described by Schantz and Andersen are widely accepted and followed. At Roswell Park Cancer Institute, the approach is identical to that employed at Memorial Sloan-Kettering Cancer Center (Table 5-13). The authors correctly state that squamous cell carcinoma accounts for the majority of head and neck malignancies. For nonsquamous histological types the same follow-up strategy is usually followed. The most notable exception to this strategy concerns differentiated thyroid cancer, which is usually more indolent than squamous cancer. Recurrence of differentiated thyroid cancer is not usually as ominous an event as recurrence of squamous cancer. However, the time interval during which the patient is at risk for recurrent disease is quite long for differentiated thyroid cancer.[1] These observations suggest that the frequency of visits can be reduced in these patients, perhaps to three or four times a year for the first several years after treatment and then once or twice per year for the remainder of the patient's life. Such a schedule allows appropriate monitoring of thyroid hormone replacement and thyroid-stimulating hormone suppression therapy, as well as thyroglobulin and radioactive iodine screening when such follow-up screening is indicated.

Adenoid cystic carcinoma, an uncommon lesion of salivary gland origin, also has a unique behavior in that the risk of recurrence appears to be constant for the remainder of the patient's life.[2] Therefore follow-up for these should be lifelong, but the optimal follow-up strategy is unknown.

REFERENCES

1. Shah JP, Loree TR, Dharker D, Strong EW, Begg C, Vlamis V. Prognostic factors in differentiated carcinoma of the thyroid gland. Am J Surg 1992;164:658-61.
2. Spiro RH, Thaler HT, Hicks WF, Kher UA, Huvos AH, Strong EW. The importance of clinical staging of minor salivary gland carcinoma. Am J Surg 1991;162:330-6.

Table 5-13 Follow-up of patients with head and neck cancer*: Roswell Park Cancer Institute

	YEAR				
	1	2	3	4	5
Office visit	12	6	4	2	1-2
Chest x-ray	1-2	1-2	1-2	1-2	1-2
Thyroid function tests	†	†	†	†	†

*The follow-up strategy I recommend is identical to the strategy recommended by Schantz and Andersen of Memorial Sloan-Kettering Cancer Center. Further diagnostic studies may be used at any time when indicated by physical examination or patient complaints.
†Performed at 6- to 12-month intervals in patients who are at risk for hypothyroidism.

➢ COUNTERPOINT

University of Washington Medical Center

ERNEST A. WEYMULLER, JR.

Schantz and Andersen have provided an excellent summary of generally accepted follow-up practices for patients with head and neck cancer. Table 5-7 indicates the traditional follow-up recommendations for the frequency of office visits and chest x-ray, although both are open to question. In this era of cost containment, physicians must question the yield or utility of each entity that introduces additional costs. Experience suggests it is reasonable to adjust the frequency of office visits (Table 5-14) according to the clinical aggressiveness of the tumor, the treatment modality used, and the convenience for the patient (such as the patient's geographical proximity to the follow-up institution).

Similarly, the utility of chest x-rays must be seriously questioned. The incidence of second primary lung tumors in a group of patients with an incident cancer of the head and neck is constant at 1% to 2% a year throughout the follow-up period. Unfortunately, by the time the tumor can be seen on chest x-ray, the likelihood of cure is minimal. Thus it is important that physicians reassess the utility of this modality. They should consider either eliminating all follow-up with regard to the chest or modifying follow-up.

Screening the chest for metastatic disease from the original primary tumor is not a rational exercise, since it most often identifies an untreatable condition. Screening for second primary cancers, however, does make sense if the screening modality will identify that new lesion at a treatable phase. With this in mind, physicians must consider the utility of annually performing flexible fiberoptic bronchoscopy or computed tomography of the chest. Since the incidence of a second primary tumor in the lung is the same throughout the rest of the patient's life, analysis of the utility of this endeavor must include consideration of repetitive examinations for the remainder of the patient's life. The following discussion focuses on some additional issues that might be appropriately addressed in an expanded consideration of multiinstitutional trials.

Table 5-14 Follow-up of patients with head and neck cancer: University of Washington Medical Center

	YEAR				
	1	2	3	4	5
Office visit	6-8	6-8	4	3	2

STAGING

Staging of head and neck cancer is an area worthy of continued attention and improvement. The TNM system has proved its value over time and provides a good framework for reporting results and prognostication for the individual patient. However, the TNM system is inadequate for the statistical demands of multiinstitutional trials. Without a better framework for the clinical study of head and neck cancer, future trials will probably fail to achieve statistically significant results.

For the purpose of discussion, it is suggested that T stage is not an effective prognostic variable except in early-stage disease (T1 and T2, N0). The suggestion that T stage is inadequate as a prognostic variable is indicated by both univariate and multivariate analysis. Vikram et al.[1] reviewed 107 patients treated with combined therapy and found that "the recurrence rate was no higher in patients with T3 or T4 primaries than in those with T1 or T2 primaries. . . . The patients whose margins were microscopically involved by cancer had more recurrences than the patients whose margins were not involved" (p. 722). Similarly, in a multivariate study Jones and Weissler[2] found that T stage was not a predictor of locoregional recurrence or survival and was insignificant in comparison to margin status and nodal disease.

Alternatives to T Stage

The common alternatives for providing staging information are narrative reports or drawings. The narrative format can be presented as text or coded (TNM system). When presented as TNM data, reports have the inherent weaknesses discussed previously. When staging information is presented in written form or as a drawing, it cannot easily be standardized or collated for computer analysis. The range of options to replace T staging is wide.

At one end of the spectrum is the system used by the national tumor data bank of the National Cancer Institute. The Surveillance, Epidemiology, and End Results (SEER) system categorizes patients into three categories of disease: local, regional, and distant. Data in the Northwest SEER data bank were analyzed to assess the value of this system. The three stages provided distinct separation of the three levels of disease with a confidence level of $p = .001$.[3]

Slightly more detailed than the American Joint Committee on Cancer stage I to IV system is the T and N Integer system methodology. This system has the appeal of simplicity and familiarity, since it expands the TNM system to create seven classes of staging. When analyzed with respect to oral cavity cancer, it provided a somewhat better separation of prognostic groups.[4] Certainly this modification of the TNM system is worthy of further evaluation.

At the other end of the tumor staging spectrum is a format that would render all T information in more precise anatomical terms. The appeal of this method is that it may more accurately describe each tumor clinically and radiographically and provide a format for computer-based integrated reporting of preoperative imaging, final preoperative staging, and the extent of surgical extirpation. By this method, three successive aspects of patient evaluation and treatment could be categorized and computer coded for subsequent analysis. Surgical staging and operative data could be stratified along with other clinical, pathological, and tumor data. This would permit analysis of more uniform subsets of patients and perhaps allow a more confident assessment of the therapeutic intervention under analysis. If this system were considered to have potential value, it would require prospective evaluation and comparison with the TNM system.[5]

PROGNOSIS

Emerging information will refine physicians' understanding of the multiple factors that influence prognosis in the head and neck cancer patient. Generally these factors may be considered under the headings of the biological aggressiveness of the tumor and the comorbid health status of the host. The intensity of patient follow-up and the selection of multiple modalities of treatment may soon hinge on such data. In addition, as indicated in the recent publication by Deleyiannis et al.,[3] intervention in patients who have documented medical comorbidity may affect survival as much as treatment of the tumor itself.

Biological Indicators of Tumor Aggressiveness

When the physician is dealing with smaller tumors of the oral cavity, there appears to be good reason to include a measure of tumor depth and microvascular invasion (in analysis of the primary resection). Spiro et al.[6] demonstrated a direct association between tumor depth and cervical metastasis. Both Close et al.[7] and O'Brien et al.[8] showed that microvascular invasion in the resected specimen of oral cavity tumors was associated with a significantly higher incidence of cervical metastasis in T1 and T2 oral tumors.

Cellular markers of biological aggressiveness appear to have great potential but represent an area of unresolved debate. Tumor differentiation is one aspect of pathological analysis that has not shown any relationship to locoregional control.[1,2,9] Other forms of tumor analysis are likewise clouded by uncertainty. Welkoborsky et al.[10] evaluated 40 laryngeal cancer patients treated by surgery with clear margins and found strong correlation between recurrence and numerous parameters including proliferating cell nuclear antigen (PCNA), Ki67, DNA content, and tumor front grade. T stage had no value in predicting recurrence ($p = .17$) or survival ($p = .21$). In contrast, Resnick et al.[11] used multivariate analysis to evaluate patients with laryngeal cancer with clear surgical margins and found no correlation between lymph node metastasis or survival and the presence of PCNA, Ki67, or aneuploidy. The authors did find that advanced T stage and the presence of cervical metastases predicted poor survival.

Tumor angiogenesis has been recognized as a predictor of metastasis and survival in breast cancer.[12] Two recently published analyses of patients with head and neck cancer emphasize the uncertainty of this parameter as a prognostic predictor. Dray et al.[13] found no correlation of microvessel counts with subsequent recurrence or survival. In contrast, Williams et al.[14] found a high correlation ($p < .0001$) between angiogenesis and recurrence. Both series were based on multivariate analysis of T1 through T3, N0 cohorts. In a related study Hughes et al.[15] demonstrated that expression of the potent angiogenic peptide bFGF is associated with development of more aggressive biological behavior in squamous carcinomas.

Host Health Status Data

Host data include health status information accumulated during the pretreatment evaluation of the patient. A recent analysis of the head and neck cancer population in the Northwest SEER registry defined alcohol consumption as a highly significant predictor of survival. This detailed study of 649 patients with head and neck cancer revealed a distinct prognostic gradient based on severity of alcohol-related comorbidity that was independent of tumor stage.[3]

The impact of general health status on the survival of laryngeal cancer patients was defined by Piccirillo et al.,[16] who demonstrated a profound negative effect of comorbid health status on the survival of patients with laryngeal cancer. Also to be included in the evaluation of medical comorbidity is the patient's nutritional status. Mick et al.[17] found weight loss to be the most significant predictor of survival in a prospective analysis of outcomes in a chemoradiation trial.

The search for immunological markers to monitor, prognosticate, and hopefully control head and neck cancer has been, until recently, nonrevealing. In 1987 Schantz and Goepfert[18] found that low natural killer cell activity interacted with positive nodal status, radiation, and surgery to give the worst prognosis. Wolf et al.[19] have found a significant correlation between disease-free survival and elevated T4/T8 ratios and low percentage of T8 cells, which remains after adjusting for tumor stage, T class, N class, and tumor site. In 1990 Clayman et al.[20] demonstrated a strong association (p <.001) between C1qBM and serum immunoglobulin A and survival in patients with head and neck cancer. This finding was limited to patients with stage IV disease and thus is considered nonspecific by the investigators.

Four recent studies of patients with head and neck cancer have demonstrated a correlation between blood transfusion and tumor recurrence.[2,21-23] In one study this relationship was independent of margin status, although the highest probability of recurrence was associated with a combination of positive margins, transfusion, and histologically positive cervical nodes.[2] With respect to the contention that poor data confound multiinstitutional studies, it is ironic that one of the few studies arguing that transfusion does not affect locoregional control in head and neck cancer is based on information collected in the Intergroup Trial (0034).[24] In a study of patients with head and neck cancer, McCulloch et al.[25] recently reported that preoperative hematocrit was the single laboratory value with prognostic implications irrespective of the transfusion status of the patient.

FOLLOW-UP CARE

The discussion presented by Schantz and Andersen of the details and objectives of follow-up care summarizes the accepted methods for patients with head and neck cancer. In particular, their emphasis on an integrated team is worth reiteration. Patients with head and neck cancer present a spectrum of therapeutic challenges during and after treatment.

Imaging

As treatment and imaging undergo continuous changes, some additional commentary seems appropriate. The management of patients using concomitant chemotherapy and radiation therapy with curative intent is influencing the selection of modalities for patient follow-up. In particular, lesions of the skull base, tongue, posterior oropharynx, and hypopharynx when treated with chemoradiation are not effectively followed up with traditional modalities. In this setting, follow-up with computed tomography or magnetic resonance imaging on a scheduled basis seems most appropriate. At the University of Washington Medical Center we obtain a baseline computed tomographic scan approximately 3 months after completion of therapy and repeat the procedure every 6 months for at least 2 years as recommended by Wolf et al.[26] Bailet et al.[27] have provided new information regarding the efficacy of positron emission tomography in this challenging group of patients who have deep tumors that cannot be effectively analyzed with traditional techniques. The combination of imaging and needle aspiration cytology to provide follow-up information will become more prominent in the near future.

FUTURE PROSPECTS

When responding to the question of whether multiinstitutional trials are needed or feasible, one must come to grips with the statistical concerns associated with the analysis of outcomes in patients with head and neck cancer. Head and neck cancer is relatively uncommon, occurring in a population of generally debilitated patients. Patients with early disease generally do well regardless of treatment selection. The most challenging clinical issues relate to patients with moderately advanced tumors in whom treatment with conventional therapy (surgery plus radiation) results in major functional deficits.

Physicians are thus confronted with designing studies comparing organ preservation and standard therapy in a small but complex patient pool. Because of the numerous prognostic variables listed above and the perhaps incalculable variance introduced by surgery itself, one could conclude that a clinical study of head and neck cancer is not feasible.[28]

The issues that should be addressed in multiinstitutional trials include early tumors, advanced but resectable tumors, imaging, and molecular biology. Regarding these issues, several questions can be raised. First, given that both surgery and radiation have equal cure rates, which modality is more cost effective? Which offers the better quality of life? Furthermore, what is the best way to manage the N0 neck? Does combined therapy improve survival (as distinct from locoregional control as an end point)? Does concomitant chemoradiation therapy offer equal locoregional control and survival at all sites in the head and neck? Can positron emission tomography (or other scans) improve follow-up, and will that translate into improved survival? Finally, can physicians use improved analysis of tumor specimens to select therapy and reduce the impact of treatment to a minimum?

To end on a favorable note, I believe that future progress lies in carefully crafted studies of tightly defined study populations. Before those studies are initiated, physicians must refine the stratification of study patients with a new and more precise set of outcome predictors. As indicated by Capron[29] in his discussion of the ethics of human experimentation, "The need for knowledge extends beyond the discovery and perfection of new diagnostic and therapeutic methods from human gene therapy to artificial organs to effective cancer cures to encompass, perhaps even more importantly, the development of means to validate and calibrate existing therapies" (p. 127).

REFERENCES

1. Vikram B, Strong EW, Shah JP, Spiro R. Failure at the primary site following multimodality treatment in advanced head and neck cancer. Head Neck Surg 1984;6:720-3.
2. Jones KR, Weissler MC. Blood transfusion and other risk factors for recurrence of squamous cell carcinoma of the head and neck. Arch Otolaryngol Head Neck Surg 1991;116:304-9.
3. Deleyiannis FW, Thomas DB, Vaughan TL. The prognostic importance of classifying the severity of alcohol abuse in head and neck cancer. J Natl Cancer Inst. In press.
4. Snyderman CH, Wagner RL. Superiority of the T and N integer score (TANIS) staging system for squamous cell carcinoma of the oral cavity. Otolaryngol Head Neck Surg 1995;112:691-4.
5. Weymuller EA Jr, Ahmad K, Casiano RR, et al. Surgical reporting instrument designed to improve outcome data in head and neck cancer trials. Ann Otol Rhinol Laryngol 1994;103:499-509.
6. Spiro RH, Spiro JD, Strong EW. Surgical approach to squamous carcinoma confined to the tongue and the floor of the mouth. Head Neck Surg 1986;9:27-31.
7. Close LG, Burns DK, Reisch J, Schaefer SD. Microvascular invasion in cancer of the oral cavity and oropharynx. Arch Otolaryngol Head Neck Surg 1987;113:1191-5.
8. O'Brien CJ, Lahr CJ, Soong SJ, et al. Surgical treatment of early-stage carcinoma of the oral tongue—would adjuvant treatment be beneficial? Head Neck Surg 1986;8:401-8.
9. Griffin TW, Pajak TF, Gillespie BW, et al. Predicting the response of head and neck cancers to radiation therapy with a multivariate modelling system: an analysis of RTOG head and neck registry. Int J Radiat Oncol Biol Phys 1984;10:481-7.
10. Welkoborsky HJ, Hinni M, Dienes HP, Mann WJ. Predicting recurrence and survival in patients with laryngeal cancer by means of DNA cytometry, tumor front grading, and proliferation markers. Ann Otol Rhinol Laryngol 1995;104:503-10.
11. Resnick JM, Uhlman D, Niehans G, et al. Cervical lymph node status and survival in laryngeal carcinoma: prognostic factors. Ann Otol Rhinol Laryngol 1995;104:685-94.
12. Weidner N. Tumor angiogenesis and metastasis—correlation in invasive breast carcinoma. N Engl J Med 1991;324:1-8.
13. Dray TG, Hardin NJ, Sofferman RA. Angiogenesis as a prognostic marker in early head and neck cancer. Ann Otol Rhinol Laryngol 1995;104:724-9.
14. Williams JK, Carlson GW, Cohen C, Derose PB, Hunter S, Jurkiewicz MJ. Tumor angiogenesis as a prognostic factor in oral cavity tumors. Am J Surg 1994;168:373-80.
15. Hughes CJ, Reed JA, Cabal R, Huvos AG, Albino AP, Schantz SP. Increased expression of basic fibroblast growth factor in squamous carcinogenesis of the head and neck is less prevalent following smoking cessation. Am J Surg 1994;168:381-5.
16. Piccirillo JF, Wells CK, Sasaki CT, Feinstein AR. New clinical severity staging system for cancer of the larynx: five-year survival rates. Ann Otol Rhinol Laryngol 1994;103:83-92.
17. Mick R, Vokes EE, Weichselbaum RR, Panje WR. Prognostic factors in advanced head and neck cancer patients undergoing multimodality therapy. Otolaryngol Head Neck Surg 1991;105:62-73.
18. Schantz SP, Goepfert H. Multimodality therapy and distant metastases: the impact of natural killer cell activity. Arch Otolaryngol Head Neck Surg 1987;113:1207-13.
19. Wolf GT, Schmaltz S, Hudson J, et al. Alteration in T-lymphocyte subpopulations in patients with head and neck cancer. Arch Otolaryngol Head Neck Surg 1987;113:1200-6.
20. Clayman GL, Savage HE, Ainslie N, Liu FJ, Schantz SP. Serologic determinants of survival in patients with squamous cell carcinoma of the head and neck. Am J Surg 1990;160:434-8.
21. Jackson RM, Rice DH. Blood transfusions and recurrence in head and neck cancer. Ann Otol Rhinol Laryngol 1989;98:171-3.
22. Johnson JT, Taylor FH, Thearle PB. Blood transfusion and outcome in stage III head and neck carcinoma. Arch Otolaryngol Head Neck Surg 1987;113:307-10.
23. Woolley AL, Nagikyan ND, Gates GA, Haughey BH, Schectmar KB, Goldenberg JL. Effect of blood transfusion on recurrence of head and neck carcinoma: retrospective review and meta-analysis. Ann Otol Rhinol Laryngol 1992;101:724-30.
24. Schuller DE, et al. The effect of peri-operative blood transfusion on survival in head and neck cancer. Arch Otolaryngol Head Neck Surg. In press.
25. McCulloch TM, VanDaele DJ, Hillel A. Blood transfusion as a risk factor for death in stage III and IV operative laryngeal cancer. Department of Veterans Affairs Laryngeal Cancer Study Group. Arch Otolaryngol Head Neck Surg 1995;121:1227-35.
26. Wolf GT, Fisher SG. Effectiveness of salvage neck dissection for advanced regional metastases when induction chemotherapy and radiation are used for organ preservation. Laryngoscope 1992;102:934-9.
27. Bailet JW, Abemayor E, Jabour BA, Hawkins RA, Ho C, Ward PH. Positron emission tomography: a new, precise imaging modality for detection of primary head and neck tumors and assessment of cervical adenopathy. Laryngoscope 1992;102:281-7.
28. Weymuller EA Jr. Moratorium on multi-institutional head and neck cancer trials [editorial]. Head Neck 1994;16:529-30.
29. Capron AM. Human experimentation. In: Veatch RM, editor. Medical ethics. Boston: Jones & Bartlett Publishers, 1989.

Table 5-15 Follow-up of patients with head and neck cancer by institution

YEAR/PROGRAM	OFFICE VISIT	CXR	TFT	CBC	LFT
Year 1					
Memorial Sloan-Kettering[a]	12	1-2	[b]		
Roswell Park[c]	12	1-2	[b]		
Univ Washington	6-8				
Japan: National Kyushu I[d]	12	2		6	6
Japan: National Kyushu II[g]	12	2		6	6
UK: Royal Liverpool	12	2	2	2	2[i]
Year 2					
Memorial Sloan-Kettering[a]	6	1-2	[b]		
Roswell Park[c]	6	1-2	[b]		
Univ Washington	6-8				
Japan: National Kyushu I[d]	6	2		6	6
Japan: National Kyushu II[g]	12	2		6	6
UK: Royal Liverpool	6	2	2	2	2[i]
Year 3					
Memorial Sloan-Kettering[a]	4	1-2	[b]		
Roswell Park[c]	4	1-2	[b]		
Univ Washington	4				
Japan: National Kyushu I[d]	4	2			
Japan: National Kyushu II[g]	6	2			
UK: Royal Liverpool	4	2	2	2	2[i]
Year 4					
Memorial Sloan-Kettering[a]	2	1-2	[b]		
Roswell Park[c]	2	1-2	[b]		
Univ Washington	3				
Japan: National Kyushu I[d]	4	2			
Japan: National Kyushu II[g]	6	2			
UK: Royal Liverpool	3	1	1	1	1[i]
Year 5					
Memorial Sloan-Kettering[a]	1-2	1-2	[b]		
Roswell Park[c]	1-2	1-2	[b]		
Univ Washington	2				
Japan: National Kyushu I[d]	4	2			
Japan: National Kyushu II[g]	4	2			
UK: Royal Liverpool	2	1	1	1	1[i]

CA++ calcium
CBC complete blood count
CT computed tomography
CXR chest x-ray
ELE electrolytes
ESR erythrocyte sedimentation rate
LFT liver function tests
MAXILL maxillofacial
MRI magnetic resonance imaging
SCCAG squamous cell carcinoma antigen
TFT thyroid function tests
US ultrasound

SCCAG	MAXILL CT/MRI	ESR	ELE	SERUM CA^{++}	NECK US
6[e]	2[f]				
6[e]	2[f]				4[h]
		2	2	2	
6[e]	2[f]				
6[e]	2[f]				
		2	2	2	
		2	2	2	
		1	1	1	
		1	1	1	

a Further diagnostic studies may be used at any time when indicated by physical examination or patient complaints.
b Performed at 6- to 12-month intervals in patients at risk for hypothyroidism.
c Further diagnostic studies may be used at any time when indicated by physical examination or patient complaints.
d For patients with relatively high cure rates of disease, such as glottic laryngeal cancer.
e Performed in patients whose titer of SCCAg was high at initial treatment.
f Performed for patients with nasopharyngeal cancer. Test selection based on availability. Magnetic resonance imaging also performed when deemed necessary by the radiologist for diagnosing recurrence.
g For patients with poor prognosis at any stage, such as cancers of the hypopharynx or the tongue.
h Performed for patients with neck node adenopathy.
i Includes measurement of total protein, albumin, globulin, bilirubin, gamma-glutamyltransferase, and alanine aminotransferase.

CHAPTER 6

Esophageal Carcinoma

University of Washington Medical Center

DOUGLAS E. WOOD AND CARLOS A. PELLEGRINI

The diagnosis of esophageal cancer carries a grim prognosis for almost all patients despite aggressive surgical resection and neoadjuvant and adjuvant chemotherapy and radiation. The incidence of esophageal carcinoma varies widely across geographical locations. Worldwide, esophageal cancer is estimated to be the seventh most frequent malignancy in the world after cancers of the stomach, lung, breast, colon, uterine, cervix, and oropharynx.[1]

The incidence of adenocarcinoma of the esophagus and gastric cardia is increasing at a faster rate than that of any other malignancy and has surpassed squamous cell carcinoma of the esophagus among white males younger than age 50 in North America.[2] From 1976 to 1987 primary esophageal adenocarcinoma increased at an average annual rate of 9.4% for white males.[2] It has been speculated that the decrease in gastric acidity resulting from the use of potent H_2 receptor agonists and proton pump inhibitors,[3] as well as other drugs that relax the lower esophageal sphincter,[4] is related to the increased incidence of Barrett's esophagus and esophageal carcinoma. However, this issue is far from settled and the ultimate reasons for the increased incidence in adenocarcinoma of the esophagus remain unclear.

Carcinoma of the esophagus has a 5-year survival rate of 6%.[5] This low survival is due both to delayed presentation and to the propensity of esophageal cancer to spread through submucosal lymphatics, invade local intrathoracic structures, and metastasize. For patients with limited disease undergoing treatment with curative intent, surgical resection remains the procedure of choice. However, resectability rates range from 24% to 59%, with a 5-year survival rate after esophagectomy of 13% to 35%.[6-8]

Two strategies have evolved to improve results after resection. Skinner et al.[6,9] favor a radical en bloc esophagectomy, and several Japanese groups perform esophagectomy combined with radical lymph node dissections in the neck, thorax, and abdomen.[10-12] The second strategy is the use of neoadjuvant protocols involving preoperative chemotherapy, radiation therapy, or combined chemoradiotherapy. The rationale of neoadjuvant therapy is to improve resectability by decreasing tumor size and microscopic local tumor extension, to sterilize regional lymph node metastases, and to sterilize microscopic metastatic disease.

Despite aggressive surgical techniques and multimodality therapy, 5-year survival rates for patients who have undergone surgical resection remain disappointingly low. Exceptions are subsets of patients with early tumors and no lymph node metastases and those with complete pathological responses after neoadjuvant chemoradiotherapy. Thus recurrence after initial treatment is common. A rational and cost-effective follow-up must be predicated on the knowledge of the pattern of recurrent disease, the potential for salvage treatment with curative intent, and the indications for and efficacy of palliative treatments of cancer recurrence.

TUMOR RECURRENCE

Recurrences are defined here as local, regional, or distant. Local recurrences can be divided into intramural recurrences at the anastomosis or disease in the bed of the resected esophageal cancer. An esophageal resection should include a 10 cm margin, since these tumors tend to propagate upward via the submucosal lymphatics. Intramural recurrences are more common in patients who have undergone limited longitudinal resection of the esophagus. Recurrence in the bed of the resected tumor is considered to represent an incomplete surgical resection. A regional recurrence is defined as disease in the lymphatic drainage area of the esophagus within the neck, mediastinum, or upper abdomen. Distant recurrence is defined as hematogenous metastasis to other organs. Although locoregional and distant recurrences are by far the most common patterns of failure after resection for esophageal carcinoma, second primary malignancies in the esophageal remnant must also be considered when formulating a rational follow-up plan.

PATTERNS OF RECURRENCE AND EFFICACY OF TREATMENT

Although the results after surgical resection, radiation therapy, or multimodality therapy are poor because of high rates of local, regional, and distant metastatic recurrence, little has been written about the patterns of recurrence, detection of recurrent disease, or treatment of esophageal tumor recurrence. Four large series from Japan provide the only systematic analyses of recurrent esophageal cancer.[13-16] Isono et al.[14] analyzed 147 cases of recurrence after resection for esophageal cancer. In this series, the incidence of lymph node recurrence was 42%, distant metastasis 40%, esophageal remnant 7.5%, other local recurrence 6.5%, and peritoneal recurrence 3.4%. Morita et al.[13] showed that recurrence rates were high even in early-stage esophageal cancer and in the absence of lymph node metastasis at the time of primary resection.

Local Recurrence

Both Hzuka et al.[15] and Isono et al.[14] provide evidence that local recurrence is more common when the primary cancer infiltrates through the adventitia and into surrounding mediastinal structures, which occurred in 4% to 24% of patients. The mean disease-free interval for these patients was 6.1 months (range 4 to 9 months), and the mean survival after recurrence was 4.2 months (range 1 to 7 months).[14] Four patients with mediastinal recurrences discovered 17 to 60 months after esophagectomy have been treated by Hzuka et al.,[15] three with radiation and one with surgery. Three of these patients died 2 to 30 months after radiation treatment, with one patient living 4 years after resection for mediastinal recurrence. Despite aggressive therapy by this Japanese group, patients with local mediastinal recurrence have a negligible chance of long survival.

Isolated recurrence in the esophageal stump is uncommon, occurring in 3% to 7.5% of patients with recurrent disease in three of the Japanese series.[13-15] Recurrence in the esophageal remnant is thought to be caused by unrecognized submucosal extension, skip lesions, or in some cases a presumed second primary tumor, as evidenced by two patients in the series by Isono et al.,[14] with recurrence in the esophageal remnant at 16 and 17 years postoperatively. The average disease-free interval was 18 months in that series,[14] with an average survival after esophageal stump recurrence of only 5.6 months. However, all three of the patients of Hzuka et al.[15] with local esophageal recurrence underwent surgery or radiation, and all patients were alive 2 to 7 years after treatment of their recurrence. In five cases of esophageal repeat resection for local esophageal recurrence at Massachusetts General Hospital, there was only one 5-year survivor, with one dying of mediastinal recurrence 3 years after the repeat resection and the others dying of mediastinal or metastatic disease 6 to 18 months postoperatively.[17]

Regional Recurrence

Regional lymph node metastasis is the only site of recurrence in 40% to 50% of patients with recurrent disease, and another 23% have combined regional and distant metastatic recurrent disease.[13,14] Regional lymph node recurrence is more common in patients with involvement of lymph nodes at the time of surgery or with evidence of lymphatic invasion in the primary tumor.[16] The median interval from primary surgery to lymphatic regional recurrence is 18.3 months for stage I disease, 16.2 months for stage II disease, and 8.5 months for stage III disease, with an overall median interval to lymphatic recurrence of 13 months.[13] Although Hzuka et al.[15] have reported two patients with lymph node recurrences treated with surgery or radiation, survival after regional lymph node recurrence is only anecdotal, with a mean survival of 8.4 months.[14]

Distant Recurrence

Distant metastatic disease is present in 95% of patients who die of esophageal cancer.[18] The most common site is lung, followed by liver and bone. These sites account for the vast majority of instances. Distant metastatic disease is more common when vascular invasion of the primary tumor or lymph node metastases has occurred at the time of primary resection.[13] It occurs significantly later than regional lymph node recurrence, ranging from 4 to 52 months with a mean of 17 months. However, the survival period after diagnosis of distant recurrence is uniformly poor, with a mean survival of 4 months.[14]

Second Primary Malignancy

There are few data regarding the occurrence of second primary tumors within the esophagus after previous esophageal resection. In two patients of Isono et al.[14] recurrence in the remnant esophagus 16 and 17 years after esophageal resection was presumed to be new primary disease. An esophageal remnant is certainly at risk for a new squamous cell primary long after a primary curative resection, particularly in patients with multiple aerodigestive tract squamous cancers. All columnar epithelium should be excised during esophagectomy for adenocarcinomas arising in Barrett's esophagus. Technical difficulties resulting in residual Barrett's esophagus will result in an incidence of a new esophageal cancer approximately 30 to 40 times that in the general population.[19,20]

DETECTION AND TREATMENT OF RECURRENCE

Multiple modalities are available for the detection of recurrent local, regional, or metastatic disease. Many esophageal surgeons take a nihilistic approach after esophageal resection, performing little or no follow-up. This approach is based on the rationale that most recurrence is either extensive mediastinal disease or distant disease for which no cure is possible and with a very short survival duration. Other surgeons recommend routine use of chest roentgenograms, bone scintigrams, computed tomography of the abdomen, and abdominal ultrasonography to detect early lymphangitic and hematogenous recurrent disease.[13] However, no effective therapy for extensive regional or distant disease has been established, so it seems unlikely that these investigations would significantly change the patients' treatment or natural history. Treatment in these cases remains primarily palliative, with surgery, radiation, or chemotherapy directed at relief of symptoms such as pain, airway obstruction, or tracheoesophageal fistula.

The only instance of recurrence with a reasonable possibility of curative therapy is a local esophageal recurrence in the esophageal stump. Such patients usually have progressive dysphagia 6 months to 3 years postoperatively. This should incite further investigation, preferably with esophagoscopy

Table 6-1 Follow-up of patients with esophageal cancer: University of Washington Medical Center

	YEAR				
	1	2	3	4	5
Office visit	3	3	2	2	1
Esophagoscopy	*	*	*	*	*
Chest computed tomography	*	*	*	*	*
Abdominal computed tomography	*	*	*	*	*

*Performed as needed for patients with a high risk of local esophageal recurrence or a remnant of Barrett's esophagus.

and biopsy. In three small reports such patients have a potential for long-term survival after repeat resection or radiation treatment.[14,15,17] There is no evidence that routine radiological studies, nuclear scans, serum cancer screening panels, or carcinoembryonic antigen levels provide early detection of treatable recurrent disease. Routine follow-up esophagoscopy would be the only modality likely to discover asymptomatic and potentially curable disease. In patients with a close proximal margin or a remnant of Barrett's esophagus, routine postoperative esophagoscopy may be warranted but is not cost effective on a routine basis because of the low incidence of isolated esophageal recurrences. History and physical examination alone remain the most sensitive and cost-effective follow-up modalities for patients with esophageal cancer.

Many in vitro studies have examined the molecular biological features of esophageal carcinogenesis and the roles of a variety of oncogenes, tumor suppressor genes, gene mutations in tumor lines, and serum levels of tumor-related antigens. Levels of epidermal growth factor receptor, p21 oncoprotein, and p53 tumor suppressor gene are elevated in a high percentage of esophageal cancers.[21,22] Molecular markers may identify individuals with premalignant lesions at high risk for the development of esophageal cancer and may improve the accuracy of cytology in diagnosis and surveillance. These markers may also be useful in predicting prognosis and tailoring aggressive therapy. However, studies have not yet produced breakthroughs in earlier recognition of esophageal cancer or detection of treatable recurrence. Serum levels of carcinoembryonic antigen, CA 19-9, and CA 50 do not have close correlation with clinicopathologic parameters and have not proved useful in the diagnosis of esophageal cancer recurrence.

FOLLOW-UP PROTOCOL

Given the time course of the development of recurrent disease and the prognosis and natural history of recurrent esophageal carcinoma, a rational and cost-effective follow-up protocol seems straightforward. Patients should undergo a careful history and physical examination directed at eliciting symptoms of a local esophageal recurrence or early symptoms of mediastinal or metastatic disease. Since most recurrences occur in the first 2 years postoperatively, examinations should take place every 4 months for the first 2 years after surgery (Table 6-1). Curable local recurrences and symptomatic metastatic disease can still occur after that time, but the follow-up interval can increase to every 6 months for years 3 and 4, and annually after that. In patients with a close esophageal margin an esophagoscopy for anastomotic surveillance at the same interval may be warranted. Patients with residual Barrett's esophagus should continue to be followed by routine endoscopic surveillance techniques as established for the columnar-lined esophagus.[23] Routine radiological or blood tests have not shown any advantage in detecting asymptomatic recurrence after esophageal resection.

CONCLUSION

Esophageal cancer is a common and deadly cancer whose poor prognosis is due to a high rate of locoregional and metastatic disease. Recurrences are usually manifested as regional or systemic disease within 6 to 18 months of surgery. Since effective treatment for these recurrences is rare, extensive testing is not warranted. Occasionally a careful history and physical examination detect early esophageal stump recurrence or a second primary tumor that should be confirmed by esophagoscopy and biopsy. These patients may still be candidates for an attempt at curative repeat resection or radiation. Surveillance endoscopy should be considered for a patient with a high risk of local esophageal recurrence or a remnant of Barrett's esophagus. Because of the extreme rarity of a treatable recurrence with current diagnostic and treatment regimens, even large multiinstitutional trials are unlikely to show different outcomes among various protocols of esophageal cancer follow-up.

REFERENCES

1. Parkin DM, Laara E, Muir CS. Estimates of worldwide frequency of sixteen major cancers in 1980. Int J Cancer 1988;41:184-97.
2. Blot WJ, Devesa SS, Kneller RW, Fraumeni JF Jr. Rising incidence of adenocarcinoma of the esophagus and gastric cardia. JAMA 1991;265:1287-9.
3. Cancer Surveillance System Newsletter. Epidemiology of gastroesophageal reflux and gastric cardia adenocarcinoma. Vol. 2, No. 2. Seattle: Fred Hutchinson Cancer Research Center, 1993.
4. Wang HH, Hsieh HC, Antonioli DA. Rising incidence of esophageal adenocarcinoma and use of pharmaceutical agents that relax the lower esophageal sphincter. Cancer Causes Control 1994;5:573-8.
5. Boring CC, Squires TS, Tong T. Cancer statistics, 1991. CA Cancer J Clin 1991;41:19-39.
6. Skinner DB, Little AG, Ferguson MK, Soriano A, Staszak VM. Selection of operation for esophageal cancer based on staging. Ann Surg 1986;204:391-401.
7. Akiyama H, Tsurumaru M, Kawamura T, Ono Y. Principles of surgical treatment for carcinoma of the esophagus: analysis of lymph node involvement. Ann Surg 1981;194:438-46.
8. Matthews HR, Powell DJ, McConkey CC. Effect of surgical experience on the results of resection for oesophageal carcinoma. Br J Surg 1986;73:621-3.
9. Skinner DB. En bloc resection for neoplasms of the esophagus and cardia. J Thorac Cardiovasc Surg 1983;85:59-71.
10. Kato H, Tachimori Y, Watanabe H. Evaluation of the treatment of thoracic esophageal carcinoma by the pattern of recurrence. J Jpn Surg Soc 1988;89:1468-70.

11. Kato H, Watanabe H, Tachimori Y, Iizuka T. Evaluation of neck lymph node dissection for thoracic esophageal carcinoma. Ann Thorac Surg 1991;51:931-5.
12. Kakegawa T, Yamana H, Fujita H, Shirozu G. Recent surgical treatment of thoracic esophageal carcinoma. Jpn J Thorac Surg 1991;44:1132-40.
13. Morita M, Kuwano H, Ohno S, Furusawa M, Sugimachi K. Characteristics and sequence of the recurrent patterns after curative esophagectomy for squamous cell carcinoma. Surgery 1994;116:1-7.
14. Isono K, Onada S, Okuyama K, Sato H. Recurrence of intrathoracic esophageal cancer. Jpn J Clin Oncol 1985;15:49-60.
15. Hzuka T, Kato H, Watanabe H. One-hundred-and-two 5-year survivors of esophageal carcinoma after resective surgery. Jpn J Clin Oncol 1985;15:369-75.
16. Sugimachi K, Inokuchi K, Kuwano H, Kai H, Okamura T, Okudaira Y. Patterns of recurrence after curative resection for carcinoma of the thoracic part of the esophagus. Surg Gynecol Obstet 1983;157:537-40.
17. Mathisen DJ. Personal communication.
18. Japanese Pathological Society. The annual of the pathological autopsy cases in Japan. 1970-1980.
19. Spechler SJ, Robbins AH, Rubins HB, et al. Adenocarcinoma and Barrett's esophagus: an overrated risk? Gastroenterology 1984;87:927-33.
20. Cameron AJ, Ott BJ, Payne WS. The incidence of adenocarcinoma in columnar-lined (Barrett's) esophagus. N Engl J Med 1985;313:857-9.
21. Roth JA. The cell and molecular biology of esophageal cancer. Chest Surg Clin North Am 1994;12:205-16.
22. Casson AG. Esophageal cancer: biology. In: Pearson FG, Deslaurier J, Ginsberg RJ, Hiebert CA, McNeally MF, Urschel HC Jr, editors. Esophageal surgery. New York: Churchill-Livingston, 1995: 539-51.
23. Levine DS, Haggitt RC, Blount PL, Rabinovitch PS, Rusch VM, Reid BJ. An endoscopic biopsy protocol can differentiate high-grade dysplasia from early adenocarcinoma in Barrett's esophagus. Gastroenterology 1993;105:40-50.

➢ COUNTERPOINT

Memorial Sloan-Kettering Cancer Center

VALERIE W. RUSCH

Wood and Pellegrini clearly describe why elaborate methods of follow-up after resection for esophageal carcinoma are generally considered inappropriate. Most esophageal carcinomas are diagnosed when already locally advanced and are associated with a poor prognosis despite complete resection. Carcinomas at an early enough stage to be cured by surgery are infrequent and are usually seen in endoscopic surveillance programs for high-risk patient populations. No curative therapy currently exists for distant metastatic disease, and salvage treatment or repeat resection for locoregional recurrence is rarely successful. Therefore surgical resection is often viewed as simply the best palliation for a malignancy with poor prognosis, long-term survival is seen as fortuitous, and salvage therapy is considered futile. In this context, frequent or invasive types of follow-up appear cost ineffective. Designing the optimal approach to follow-up after resection for esophageal carcinoma is especially difficult because unlike some other solid tumors, including germ cell tumors and breast and ovarian cancers, esophageal cancer has no serum marker. Accurate follow-up may require serial endoscopies and multiple radiographic examinations in addition to clinical assessment.

What could be the goals of follow-up after resection for esophageal carcinoma? Potential objectives include the early detection of local recurrence in high-risk patients (such as those with residual Barrett's esophagus or multifocal squamous dysplasia or carcinoma in situ) and the early detection of new primary cancers in patients cured of an early esophageal carcinoma (for example, other tobacco-related malignancies in patients who have had squamous cell carcinoma of the esophagus). A better understanding of the natural history of the disease and patterns of relapse after surgical resection is also an important objective. Finally, a careful evaluation of overall survival, progression-free survival, and sites of relapse in patients entered in clinical trials evaluating new therapies and the ability to correlate molecular biological abnormalities with clinical outcome could also help to improve outcome. Although 10 years ago these objectives would have been theoretical, recent changes in epidemiology, treatment, and ways of studying biology now make them clinically relevant. However, not all of these objectives are relevant to every patient with esophageal cancer.

As discussed by Wood and Pellegrini, salvage therapy for regional recurrence is rarely effective because the tumor often involves the mediastinum too extensively to allow complete resection and may be the prelude to systemic relapse. Purely local recurrences confined to the wall of the gastric or esophageal remnant are infrequent and result from inadequate initial resections.[1,2] Patients with early-stage adenocarcinomas in Barrett's esophagus in whom the Barrett's segment is incompletely excised and patients with multifocal early squamous cell carcinomas who do not undergo complete thoracic esophagectomy are two patient groups at risk.[3] Although the recent development of surveillance programs for patients with Barrett's esophagus has increased the number of patients with early-stage adenocarcinoma undergoing surgical resection,[4] experience with the management of local recurrences remains anecdotal. Endoscopic surveillance techniques established for Barrett's esophagus with the frequency of endoscopy based on the severity of dysplasia are probably warranted for this small subset of patients.[5]

Experience with patients cured of early-stage cancers of the lung and the head and neck has shown the need for close follow-up because these patients have a 15% to 40% risk of new tobacco-related malignancies.[6-8] However, follow-up for the detection of new nonesophageal malignancies is not relevant to most North American patients because so few are cured of esophageal carcinoma. An epidemiological dichotomy based on histology is also emerging.[9] The number of adenocarcinomas of the gastroesophageal junction arising from Barrett's esophagus has risen dramatically. It is hypothesized that this is related to increased use of H_2 blockers and other medications that relax the gastroesophageal sphincter.[10,11] In contrast to patients in high-incidence areas such as China, Japan, Iran, and South Africa, where squamous cell carcinomas predominate and are thought to be caused by

Table 6-2 Follow-up of patients with esophageal cancer (standard community care): Memorial Sloan-Kettering Cancer Center

	YEAR				
	1	2	3	4	5
Office visit	3	3	2	2	1
Chest x-ray	3	3	2	2	1
Esophagoscopy	*	*	*	*	*
Chest computed tomography	*	*	*	*	*
Abdominal computed tomography	*	*	*	*	*

*Performed as clinically indicated.

Table 6-3 Follow-up of patients with esophageal cancer (patients at high risk for local recurrence): Memorial Sloan-Kettering Cancer Center

	YEAR				
	1	2	3	4	5
Office visit	3	3	2	2	1
Chest x-ray	3	3	2	2	1
Esophagoscopy	3	2	2	1	*
Chest computed tomography	3	2	2	1	*
Abdominal computed tomography	3	2	2	1	*

*Performed as clinically indicated.

smoking, alcohol, and nutritional deficiencies,[12] patients with esophageal adenocarcinoma are not at an increased risk for second primary nonesophageal cancers. Therefore, patients who merit surveillance for second primary malignancies include those whose tobacco or alcohol use places them at risk and whose early-stage squamous cell carcinoma is potentially cured by resection.

Follow-up to achieve a better understanding of the natural history of disease and patterns of relapse after resection is still an important objective. Systematic clinicopathological correlation in patients undergoing resection for non–small cell lung cancer led in 1986 to the development of a revised international staging system for selecting patients for resection.[13] This staging system has also been pivotal in clinical trials of combined modality therapy for stage III non–small cell lung cancer because it stratifies patients into relatively homogeneous groups. Using data on survival and patterns of relapse obtained since 1986, another revision of the lung cancer staging system is under way. However, with few exceptions, similar data are not available for esophageal carcinoma. The surgical literature focuses on surgical technique and operative mortality and morbidity,[14] reports overall survival without respect to stage, and does

Table 6-4 Follow-up of patients with esophageal cancer (patients in clinical trials or institutions engaged in studies of staging and cancer biology): Memorial Sloan-Kettering Cancer Center

	YEAR				
	1	2	3	4	5
Office visit	3	3	2	2	1
Chest x-ray	3	3	2	2	1
Chest computed tomography	3	2	2	1	*
Abdominal computed tomography	3	2	2	1	*
Bone scan	2	2	*	*	*
Esophagoscopy	2	2	*	*	*

*Performed as clinically indicated.

not analyze patterns of relapse. When sites of relapse are reported, they are usually classified only as local or locoregional and distant, without specifying which distant organs are involved.[15-17]

The current staging system for esophageal carcinoma engenders confusion and controversy because it does not clearly define regional nodes and equates involvement of nodes not immediately adjacent to the primary tumor with metastatic disease. The discrepancy between the gastric cancer staging system, which contains N2 classification, and the esophageal staging system, which does not, creates particular confusion for the staging of tumors of the gastroesophageal junction, which theoretically can be classified according to either system. Data exist to support the distinction among the current T stages but are insufficient to correlate nodal involvement precisely with survival and sites of relapse.[18] As with non–small cell lung cancer, this information must be acquired and the staging system modified to allow a more rational selection of patients for surgical resection or combined modality treatment. Unfortunately, it cannot be acquired through history and physical examination alone. To determine accurately when and where patients relapse requires serial chest roentgenograms, computed tomographic scans of the chest and upper abdomen, and bone scans.

Similar arguments can be made in favor of more extensive follow-up of patients entered in clinical trials of combined modality therapy. In the treatment of most solid tumors, improvements occur in small increments and specific determinations of progression-free survival, overall survival, and sites of relapse are essential for analyzing trial end points and developing novel approaches to therapy. Similarly, the investigation of the molecular genetic abnormalities associated with the development and progression of a cancer requires precise correlation with pathological stage and clinical course. The characterization of molecular genetic abnormalities in the context of clinical outcome and sites of relapse is the key to developing future therapies or methods of early detection that could reduce the current high mortality of esophageal carcinoma. Such an approach is already under investigation to define which patients with Barrett's esophagus may be at risk for progression from dysplasia to invasive carcinoma.[19-21]

The selection of a follow-up protocol must be tailored to the individual patient, the etiology and stage of the tumor, and the patient's risk for recurrence. A patient who has undergone a complete resection of high-grade dysplasia in a Barrett's esophagus is different from a patient who has had resection of a T3N1 squamous cell carcinoma of the midesophagus, and both of these are different from a patient who has had an incomplete resection of multifocal early squamous cell carcinoma of the esophagus. In an era dominated by concerns about medical economics, the follow-up protocol outlined by Wood and Pellegrini represents a rational, inexpensive approach for the North American clinician performing occasional esophageal resections. However, it does not take into account the broader spectrum of patients with esophageal cancer being seen worldwide today and their varying needs. More important, it does not consider that improved outcomes derive from a better understanding of the natural history and biology of esophageal carcinoma and that these in turn are predicated on accurate evaluation of sites and times of relapse. Institutions whose caseload permits statistically meaningful analysis of treatment results and surgeon participation in clinical trials must consider a more systematic study of the disease, including more extensive follow-up tests. Such an approach is surely justified for a malignancy currently associated with an overall mortality of 90%.

Three separate algorithms for follow-up can be envisioned based on tumor stage, histology and etiology, and objectives of the surgeon or institution (Tables 6-2 to 6-4). Table 6-2 outlines standard community care, as suggested by Wood and Pellegrini. This would be appropriate for patients who are considered at low risk for local recurrence and are not involved in clinical trials. Table 6-3 outlines a follow-up plan that could lead to early detection of a local recurrence. Table 6-4 outlines the most extensive follow-up program and is consistent with the guidelines used in most cooperative group clinical trials of treatment for thoracic malignancies. This approach aims to assess the benefit of new treatment regimens by identifying the sites and dates of recurrence accurately.

REFERENCES

1. Tam PC, Siu KF, Cheung HC, Ma L, Wong J. Local recurrences after subtotal esophagectomy for squamous cell carcinoma. Ann Surg 1987;205:189-94.
2. Sagar PM, Johnston D, McMahon MJ, Dixon MF, Quirke P. Significance of circumferential resection margin involvement after oesophagectomy for cancer. Br J Surg 1993;80:1386-8.
3. Misumi A, Harada K, Murakami A, et al. Early diagnosis of esophageal cancer: analysis of 11 cases of esophageal mucosal cancer. Ann Surg 1989;210:732-9.
4. Yu E, Souhami L, Guerra J, Clark B, Gingras C, Fava P. Accelerated fractionation in inoperable non-small cell lung cancer: a phase I/II study. Cancer 1993;71:2727-31.
5. Levine DS, Haggitt RC, Blount PL, Rabinovitch PS, Rusch VW, Reid BJ. An endoscopic biopsy protocol can differentiate high-grade dysplasia from early adenocarcinoma in Barrett's esophagus. Gastroenterology 1993;105:40-50.
6. Thomas P, Rubinstein L. Cancer recurrence after resection: T1 N0 non-small cell lung cancer. Lung Cancer Study Group. Ann Thorac Surg 1990;49:242-7.
7. Thomas PA Jr, Rubinstein L. Malignant disease appearing late after operation for T1 N0 non-small-cell lung cancer. Lung Cancer Study Group. J Thorac Cardiovasc Surg 1993;106:1053-8.
8. Shons AR, McQuarrie DG. Multiple primary epidermoid carcinomas of the upper aerodigestive tract. Arch Surg 1985;120:1007-9.
9. Powell J, McConkey CC. Increasing incidence of adenocarcinoma of the gastric cardia and adjacent sites. Br J Cancer 1990;62:440-3.
10. Wang HH, Hsieh CC, Antonioli DA. Rising incidence rate of esophageal adenocarcinoma and use of pharmaceutical agents that relax the lower esophageal sphincter (United States). Cancer Causes Control 1994;5:573-8.
11. Lerut T, Coosemans W, Van Raemdonck D, et al. Surgical treatment of Barrett's carcinoma: correlations between morphologic findings and prognosis. J Thorac Cardiovasc Surg 1994;107:1059-66.
12. Gao YT, McLaughlin JK, Blot WJ, et al. Risk factors for esophageal cancer in Shanghai, China. I. Role of cigarette smoking and alcohol drinking. Int J Cancer 1994;58:192-6.
13. Mountain CF, Greenberg SD, Fraire AE. Tumor stage in non-small cell carcinoma of the lung. Chest 1991;99:1258-60.
14. Katlic MR, Wilkins EW Jr, Grillo HC. Three decades of treatment of esophageal squamous carcinoma at the Massachusetts General Hospital. J Thorac Cardiovasc Surg 1990;99:929-38.
15. Giuli R, Gignoux M. Treatment of carcinoma of the esophagus. Retrospective study of 2,400 patients. Ann Surg 1980;192:44-52.
16. Galandiuk S, Hermann RE, Cosgrove DM, Gassman JJ. Cancer of the esophagus: the Cleveland Clinic experience. Ann Surg 1986;203:101-8.
17. Vigneswaran WT, Trastek VF, Pairolero PC, Deschamps C, Daly RC, Allen MS. Transhiatal esophagectomy for carcinoma of the esophagus. Ann Thorac Surg 1993;56:838-46.
18. Lerut T, De Leyn P, Coosemans W, Van Raedonck D, Scheys I, LeSaffre E. Surgical strategies in esophageal carcinoma with emphasis on radical lymphadenectomy. Ann Surg 1992;216:583-90.
19. Moore JH, Lesser EJ, Erdody DH, Natale RB, Orringer MB, Beer DG. Intestinal differentiation and p53 gene alterations in Barrett's esophagus and esophageal adenocarcinoma. Int J Cancer 1994;56:487-93.
20. Blount PL, Meltzer SJ, Yin J, Huang Y, Krasna MJ, Reid BJ. Clonal ordering of 17p and 5q allelic losses in Barrett dysplasia and adenocarcinoma. Proc Natl Acad Sci U S A 1993;90:3221-5.
21. Huang Y, Boynton RF, Blount PL, et al. Loss of heterozygosity involves multiple tumor suppressor genes in human esophageal cancers. Cancer Res 1992;52:6525-30.

➢ COUNTERPOINT

National Kyushu Cancer Center, Japan

TAKAO SAITO

In Japan, aggressive surgery consisting of esophagectomy and three-field lymph node dissection including the neck, thorax, and abdomen is commonly performed for curatively resectable, advanced cancer of the esophagus. This procedure is considered to partially prevent the most frequent type of recurrence, lymph node metastasis, and data are accumulating to support this.[1,2] However, the rate of distant organ recurrence is still high in patients who receive three-field lymph node dissection. On the other hand, endoscopic mucosal resection is performed for a so-called early cancer confined to the mucosa without lymph node metastasis and the recurrence rate is low.[3]

Early detection and treatment are the usual policy for postoperative recurrences of esophageal cancer at National Kyushu Cancer Center and the First Department of Surgery at Oita Medical University in Japan. Most patients who undergo curative surgery for advanced cancer are seen every month for the first 2 years and then every 3 months until the fifth year for routine examinations including computed tomographic scans to detect early recurrences.[4] Early treatment is also recommended for such recurrences. Surgery is often performed for recurrences in the remnant esophagus, recurrent nodes in the neck, or a single lesion in a distant organ. Chemoradiation therapy is performed for both locoregional recurrences and distant lesions. For patients who receive endoscopic mucosal resection, an endoscopic observation schedule using staining with Lugol's solution is followed.

Physicians at National Kyushu Cancer Center and Oita Medical University have used multiple modalities, including surgery, for recurrent esophageal cancer, based on the strategy of early detection and early treatment, and the outcome shows the efficacy of these treatments. Concurrent chemoradiation therapy including cisplatin contributes to improvement. The results and follow-up protocol are described below.

FOLLOW-UP, EARLY DETECTION, AND TREATMENT

At the First Department of Surgery at Oita Medical University in Japan, 90 patients underwent curative resection for squamous cell carcinoma. The standard surgical procedure was a transthoracic subtotal esophagectomy with regional lymphadenectomy. Three-field lymph node dissection, including peritracheobronchial and lower cervical nodes,[5] and postoperative concurrent chemoradiation therapy were added after 1986.

Patients were followed at 1-month intervals for the first 2 years, at 3-month intervals until the fifth year, and annually thereafter. A careful history and physical examination and measurement of squamous cell carcinoma antigen (SCCAg, a tumor marker for squamous cell carcinoma) were performed at that time. Neck, chest, and abdominal computed tomographic scans were performed every 6 months for the first 2 years and then annually until the fifth year. Chest roentgenography, bone scintigraphy, and esophagoscopy were performed once a year until the fifth year.

Patients with a recurrence underwent chemotherapy or radiation therapy (or both) and, as required, surgery. Chemotherapy regimens used were cisplatin, vindesine, and pepleomycin[6] or cisplatin and 5-fluorouracil. Surgery was indicated for lymph node recurrences in the neck and hematogenous recurrences limited to a single focus in a distant organ.

PATTERNS OF RECURRENCE AND DISEASE-FREE INTERVALS

In this series recurrence was detected in 51 of 90 patients (56.7%) and patterns were classified into local, lymph node, hematogenous, pleural, and esophageal remnant. Since there were often more than two types of recurrences in the same patient, 77 recurrences were recorded in 51 patients. The incidence of recurrence was as follows: local, 6.7% of 90 patients; lymph node, 26.7%; hematogenous, 41.1%; pleural, 6.7%; and esophageal remnant, 4.4%. The pattern of recurrence was also divided into single and multiple. Multiple recurrences were designated when there were more than two types of recurrences in the same patient synchronously (within 6 months). According to this classification, 56 recurrences, including five asynchronous ones, were noted in 51 patients. The incidence of multiple recurrence was 17.8% of 90 patients (16 recurrences), while that of single recurrence was 44.4% (40 recurrences).

The mean disease-free interval after surgery was 13 months; in 84.3% of patients recurrence took place within 2 years. The disease-free interval differed depending on the patterns of recurrence. The mean was greater than 2 years in cases of esophageal remnant recurrence, between 1 and 2 years for lymph node, hematogenous, and pleural recurrences, and less than 1 year for local recurrence.

The tumor, nodes, metastases (TNM) stage of primary tumors is related to recurrence rates and disease-free intervals. The recurrence rate was less than 20% in TNM stages 0 and I and 25% in stage IIa, while it was 70% to 90% in stages IIb through IV. The mean of the disease-free interval was greater than 2 years for stages 0 and I, between 1 and 2 years for stages II and III, and 6 months for stage IV. Hematogenous recurrence was predominant in early-stage tumors. Recurrence was noted in 8 of 39 patients with stages 0 through IIa tumors, and in 7 there was a hematogenous pattern.

EFFICACY OF TREATMENT

Treatment including chemoradiation therapy or surgery or both was given to 32 of 51 patients with recurrences. The remaining 19 were cared for in other hospitals and not given any particular treatment. Treatment was given for 41 recurrences in 32 patients at relatively early stages. There were single recurrences in 24 patients, two asynchronous recurrences in seven patients, and three asynchronous recurrences in one patient. Of the 41 recurrences, 32 were treated with chemoradiation, five with surgery and chemoradiation, and four with surgery alone.

Chemoradiation therapy was performed for one local recurrence, 10 lymph node recurrences, nine hematogenous recurrences, one pleural recurrence, three esophageal remnant recurrences, and eight multiple recurrences. Surgery with or without chemoradiation therapy was performed for three lymph node recurrences (three modified radical neck dissections) and six hematogenous recurrences (one nephrectomy, one pulmonary lobectomy, two extirpations of brain tumors, one resection of the bone, and one resection of the skin).

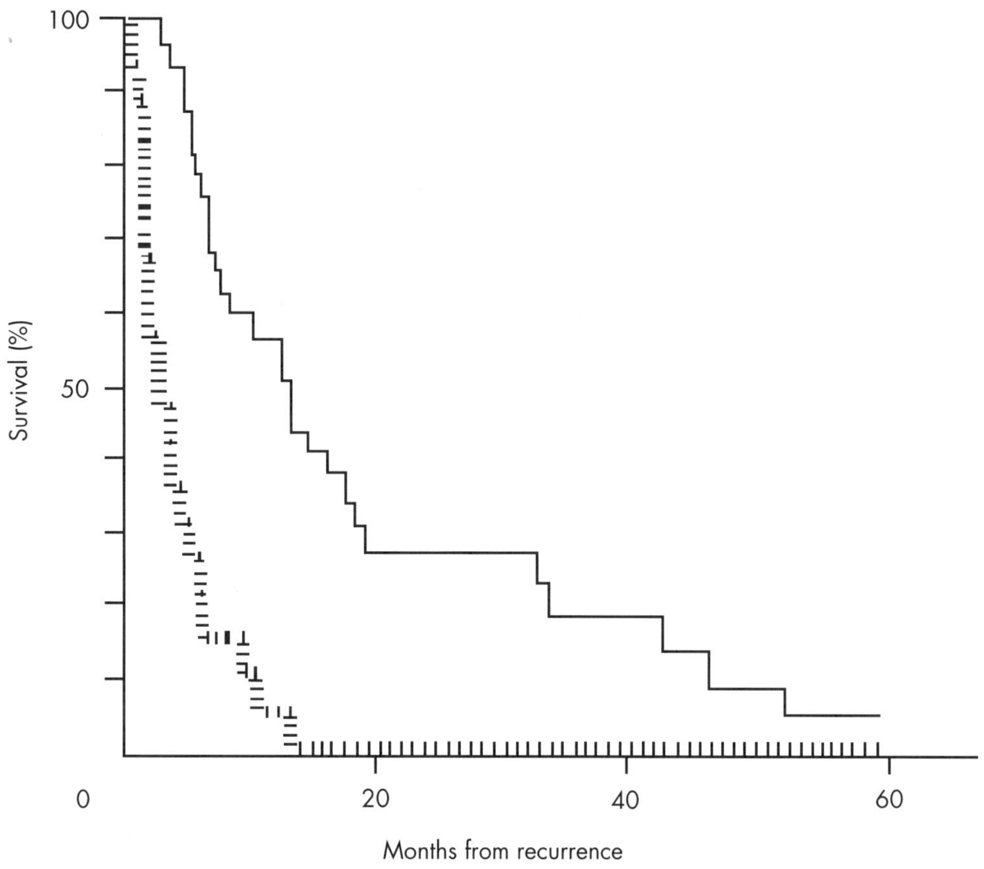

Figure 6-1 Survival after recurrence. There was a statistically significant difference between the treated group *(solid line)* and the untreated group *(broken line)* (mean = 21 versus 3 months, $p < .0001$).

Survival after recurrence in the treated group was significantly better than that of the untreated group (mean = 21 versus 3 months, $p < .0001$; median = 12 versus 2 months), as shown in Figure 6-1. Survival rates at 1, 2, and 5 years were 50%, 26.7%, and 4.4% in the treated group, respectively, and 5.6%, no survival, and no survival in the untreated group, respectively. Longer survival times were especially noted for lymph node recurrence (17 versus 3 months in the treated and untreated groups, respectively, $p < .01$) and for hematogenous recurrence (13 versus 3 months, $p < .01$). Two- and 5-year survival rates were 14.7% and 7.4%, respectively, for those with lymph node recurrence, and rates were 21.8% and no survival for those with a hematogenous recurrence. The best result was noted in the case of esophageal remnant recurrence, with a mean survival duration of 32 months and 50% 2-year survival rates.

Survival after recurrence also differed among TNM stages of primary tumors. The mean survival duration was 51 months in stage 0 through II tumors. However, it was only 7 months in stage IV tumors, even when patients with recurrent tumors were treated.

Response to chemoradiation therapy was evaluated in 32 of 41 recurrences. The response rate was 37.5%, with five complete responses and seven partial responses (Table 6-5). The rate was better in cases of a single recurrence than in multiple recurrences (41.7% versus 25%). Patients with a remnant esophageal recurrence responded well (three of three recurrences), and the response rate was 30% in the case of lymph node recurrence and 22.2% in the case of a hematogenous recurrence. Surgery resulted in no relapse for five of nine recurrences in eight patients (three lymph node recurrences and two hematogenous recurrences). Mean survival time from recurrence was 3 years 4 months (1 year 10 months to 7 years 10 months). One patient required nephrectomy for a renal metastasis and survived until the second recurrence in the brain 1 year 10 months later. The other patient treated by pulmonary lobectomy for recurrence in the lung has survived for 2 years 6 months and is living at this writing.

PREDICTION OF RECURRENCES

Recurrence in lymph nodes and distant organs commonly follows curative resection of esophageal cancer. Prediction of recurrence in lymph nodes and distant organs before surgery might allow not only more appropriate treatment for primary tumors but also a more effective follow-up study for recurrent diseases. Physicians at National Kyushu Cancer Center and the First Department of Surgery at Oita Medical University reported that lymph node recurrence following

Table 6-5 Response to chemotherapy and/or radiation for recurrences of esophageal cancer

	NUMBER OF RECURRENCES						
	TOTAL	CR	PR	NC	PD	NE	RESPONSE RATE (%)
All recurrences	32*	5	7	12	6	2	37.5
Single recurrence	24*	5	5	10	2	2	41.7
Local	1	1	0	0	0	0	
Lymph node	10	0	3	5	1	1	
Hematogenous	9	1	1	5	1	1	
Pleural	1	1	0	0	0	0	
Remnant esophagus	3	2	1	0	0	0	
Multiple recurrences	8	0	2	2	4	0	25.0

CR, Complete response; *PR,* partial response; *NC,* no change; *PD,* progressive disease; *NE,* no evaluation.
*Of 41 recurrences in 32 patients, 32 were treated with chemoradiation and nine with surgery plus chemoradiation.

curative resection of esophageal cancer is associated with stemline heterogeneity of cellular DNA content,[7] while hematogenous recurrence is related to amplification of the hst-1 gene.[8] In an attempt to predict these two types of recurrences preoperatively, univariate and multivariate analyses for clinical prognostic factors combined with these two biological factors were made. The results indicated that hst-1 gene amplification and stemline heterogeneity of DNA content are the most important independent predictors of hematogenous and lymph node recurrences, respectively.[9] Thus these markers may be useful for predicting two types of recurrences clinically.

FOLLOW-UP PROTOCOL

As shown previously, the trials suggest that early detection and early treatment can improve survival time of patients with recurrence of esophageal cancer. Based on these results the follow-up protocol prescribed at National Kyushu Cancer Center aims at detecting recurrences at an early stage (Table 6-6).

Definite differences exist between the follow-up protocol used by Wood and Pellegrini and the one I use. The major differences are concerned with hospital visit intervals and diagnostic tests used for detecting recurrence. Since the rate of recurrence is extremely high and the disease-free interval is short, an extensive follow-up schedule with more frequent hospital visits is required. To detect recurrences in mediastinal or abdominal lymph nodes or in the liver, bone, or lung in the early, clinically inapparent stages, tests such as computed tomography, chest radiography, or bone scintigraphy are also needed.

Patients should undergo a careful history and physical examination to detect early symptoms of recurrence, as described by Wood and Pellegrini. Monthly examinations should take place for the first 2 years after surgery. Patients should be examined every 3 months for years 3, 4, and 5, and annually thereafter. The serum SCCAg level often rises with recurrence and changes with treatment in some patients. SCCAg levels should be measured at the same intervals as

Table 6-6 Follow-up of patients with esophageal cancer: National Kyushu Cancer Center, Japan

	YEAR				
	1	2	3	4	5
Office visit	12	12	4	4	4
SCCAg	12	12	4	4	4
Neck computed tomography	2	2	1	1	1
Chest computed tomography	2	2	1	1	1
Abdominal computed tomography	2	2	1	1	1
Chest x-ray	1	1	1	1	1
Bone scan	1	1	1	1	1
Esophagoscopy	1	1	1	1	1

SCCAg, Squamous cell carcinoma antigen.

the history and physical examination. Computed tomography is the best test available to detect recurrences in the chest, abdomen, and neck. Patients should be followed by routine computed tomographic scans every 6 months for the first 2 years and annually thereafter. Chest radiography and bone scintigraphy should be performed once a year to detect lung and bone recurrences, respectively. Patients should undergo annual esophagoscopy to detect recurrences in the remnant esophagus until at least the fifth year after surgery. Patients with TNM stage 0 tumors can be followed with endoscopy in addition to history and physical examinations every 3 months for the first 2 years and at an annual interval thereafter because the likelihood of recurrence is low. Patients with endoscopic mucosal resection for in situ cancer should undergo endoscopic follow-up at the same intervals.

CONCLUSION

In the series described here, 90 patients who underwent transthoracic subtotal esophagectomy with three-field lymph node dissection and postoperative chemoradiation therapy with curative intent were followed with the goal of early detection and treatment of recurrence. Recurrence was detected in 51 patients (56.7%) and chemoradiation therapy with or without surgery was indicated for 41 recurrences in 32 patients. Concurrent chemotherapy, including cisplatin and radiation, was effective in some cases for those with lymph node, hematogenous, and esophageal remnant recurrences. Surgery often resulted in cure for those with recurrences in neck lymph nodes or with a single focus in a distant organ.

Survival rates 2 and 5 years from the time of recurrence were 26.7% and 4.4%, respectively, with a mean survival of 21 months in the treated group. The response rate for chemoradiation therapy was 37.5% in 41 evaluated recurrences. Surgery resulted in a mean survival of 3 years 4 months from the time of recurrence in eight patients. Overall 5-year survival from surgery for primary esophageal tumors was 9.2% in a total of 51 patients with recurrence. These results suggest that early detection and early treatment can extend survival time for patients with postoperative recurrence of esophageal cancer.

Since recurrences are detected within 2 years of surgery in most cases and occur widely in lymph nodes, distant organs, and local regions such as the mediastinum or esophageal remnant, frequent follow-up with extensive testing is considered necessary. A careful history and physical examination and, if possible, measurement of SCCAg levels should be performed every month for the first 2 years and every 3 months until the fifth year. Patients should periodically undergo such tests as neck, chest, and abdominal computed tomography, chest radiography, bone scintigraphy, and esophagoscopy, regardless of the presence or absence of symptoms.

REFERENCES

1. Kato H, Watanabe H, Tachimori Y, Iizuka T. Evaluation of neck lymph node dissection for thoracic esophageal carcinoma. Ann Thorac Surg 1991;51:931-5.
2. Isono K, Sato H, Nakayama K. Results of a nationwide study on the three-field lymph node dissection of esophageal cancer. Oncology 1991;48:411-20.
3. Makuuchi H, Machimura T, Mizutani K, et al. Endoscopic mucosal resection for early carcinomas of esophagus. In: Takahashi T, editor. Recent advances in management of digestive cancers. Tokyo: Springer-Verlag, 1993:94-7.
4. Morita M, Kuwano H, Ohno S, Furusawa M, Sugimachi K. Characteristics and sequence of the recurrent patterns after curative esophagectomy for squamous cell carcinoma. Surgery 1994;116:1-7.
5. Saito T, Shimoda K, Shigemitsu Y, Kinoshita T, Miyahara M, Kobayashi M. Extensive lymphadenectomy for thoracic esophageal carcinoma: a two-stage operation for high-risk patients. Surg Today 1994;24:610-5.
6. Saito T, Shigemitsu U, Kinoshita T, et al. Cisplatin, vindesine, pepleomycin and concurrent radiation therapy following esophagectomy with lymph adenectomy for patients with an esophageal carcinoma. Oncology 1993;50:293-7.
7. Kaketani K, Saito T, Kuwahara A, et al. DNA stemline heterogeneity in esophageal cancer accurately identified by flow cytometric analysis. Cancer 1993;72:3564-70.
8. Chikuba K, Saito T, Uchino S, et al. High amplification of the hst-1 gene correlates with hematogenous recurrence after curative resection of oesophageal carcinoma. Br J Surg 1995;82:364-7.
9. Saito T, Chikuba K, Uchino S, et al. Prediction of postoperative organ and lymph node recurrences of esophageal cancer. Bologna: Monduzzi Editore, 1996.

➢ COUNTER POINT

The Cardiothoracic Centre, National Health Service Trust, UK

RICHARD D. PAGE

In the United Kingdom esophageal cancer accounts for around 6,000 deaths each year. As in the United States, the overall incidence is increasing because of the increase in adenocarcinoma arising in the gastric cardia and distal esophagus.[1,2] The incidence of squamous cell carcinoma is static and currently accounts for about two thirds of esophageal carcinomas. The disease is more common in males, the elderly, and those from poorer socioeconomic groups.

Although not one of the most common cancers, because of its severity and aggressiveness esophageal cancer has economic implications somewhat out of proportion to its incidence. In only about 10% of cases is a long-term cure possible.[3] Operative treatment of patients, whether for cure or palliation, often involves lengthy surgery and hospitalization, with an ongoing need for care after discharge. Patients not suitable for surgery also consume significant medical resources for both specific treatment (radiation therapy and chemotherapy) and general care in both the hospital and the community.

PATTERNS OF RECURRENCE AND DIAGNOSIS

The British experience of recurrent esophageal cancer is similar to that detailed by Wood and Pellegrini. After surgical resection of the primary tumor the majority of patients die of locoregional or distant metastases, with a variety of clinical presentations, depending on the anatomical site involved.

It is important to be aware that many patients being treated for esophageal cancer have symptoms not attributable to recurrence of their tumor. This may cause management problems. Especially after surgical excision of the esophagus with reconstruction, a number of patients have difficulty returning to a normal diet. Because of the relatively small caliber of the stomach after reconstruction with a gastric tube, patients often report being unable to tolerate large meals. This condition usually improves with time, or the patients adapt to it by eating smaller meals more frequently. In a small number of patients a pyloroplasty or pyloromyotomy may be appropriate if this has not already been carried out at the original operation. Esophagectomy usually results in removal of both vagus nerve trunks in the thorax, which can lead to poor gastric peristalsis and delayed emptying.[4]

Dysphagia may occur because of benign anastomotic stricture. This usually arises within 3 months after surgery and is easily dealt with in most cases by dilatation at endoscopy. Tumor recurrence at the anastomosis or in regional lymph nodes should be excluded by endoscopic biopsy or computed tomography of the chest, especially when the condition does not respond to dilatation. Reflux of gastric contents into the esophagus may be a factor leading to nonmalignant strictures, and patients may report heartburn and waterbrash. Medical therapy helps to alleviate these symptoms, which usually settle with time. Aspiration causing respiratory symptoms is uncommon in the absence of tumor recurrence.

In a minority of cases surgical revision of the anastomosis is necessary. Previously undiagnosed tumor recurrence may become immediately obvious at operation. In this situation attempts at resection are unlikely to be beneficial.

Weight loss resulting from poor nutritional intake in the absence of dysphagia may be monitored by a period of supervised nutrition in the hospital. Adequate oral feeding can usually be established. Occasionally, enteral tube feeding or parenteral nutrition is needed to establish an adequate intake. In the absence of any unrelated disease or intestinal malabsorption, if weight loss and deterioration continue, tumor recurrence can be diagnosed with confidence.

ROUTINE SURVEILLANCE AFTER PRIMARY TREATMENT

Patients who undergo resection or radical radiation therapy for esophageal carcinoma survive for a mean period of 12 to 18 months.[5] Therefore they should be examined relatively frequently for 2 years after surgery to detect and treat recurrence should it occur. Also, patients who experience symptoms after primary treatment not attributable to recurrence of their tumor need to be seen regularly. Patients are monitored clinically every 3 months for 2 years. In the absence of problems they are then reviewed annually (Table 6-7).

As is the practice of Wood and Pellegrini at the University of Washington Medical Center, no routine hematological, biochemical, or radiological investigations are deemed necessary in the absence of symptoms. Detecting tumor recurrence before symptoms or physical signs develop does not improve survival time. Any investigations ordered should be dictated by the patient's symptoms.

MANAGEMENT OF A RECURRENT TUMOR

If an esophageal tumor recurs after primary treatment, the mean survival time is slightly more than 4 months.[6] In all cases patients with a recurrent tumor after primary treatment should be managed symptomatically (Table 6-8).

Irradiation, either by external beam radiation therapy or by brachytherapy, is useful for symptomatic locoregional recurrence in the absence of systemic disease, such as anastomotic recurrence or cervical, mediastinal, or retroperitoneal lymph node metastases. Skeletal deposits are also usefully treated with radiation therapy. Appropriate analgesia is indicated for pain, especially when caused by bone and liver metastases. Stenting, brachytherapy, or laser therapy of endoluminal recurrence may provide useful palliation. Stenting may be the only method available for treating a malignant tracheoesophageal fistula.

Table 6-7 Follow-up of patients with esophageal cancer: Cardiothoracic Centre, National Health Service Trust, UK

	YEAR				
	1	2	3	4	5
Office visit	4	4	1	1	1
Esophagoscopy	*	*	*	*	*
Chest x-ray	*	*	*	*	*
Chest computed tomography	*	*	*	*	*

*Performed as clinically indicated.

Symptomatic superficial lesions can be treated by local excision. Cervical lymph node metastases are treated in the first instance by radiation therapy. In select patients, if the metastases recur or fail to respond to radiation therapy and remain painful, they can be treated by wide local excision and if necessary covered with a myocutaneous flap.

Chemotherapy may be given to patients with systemic disease who are in relatively good nutritional status. It can lead to tumor regression and symptomatic relief in up to 30% of cases but rarely extends life by more than a few weeks. For patients whose disease is terminal with widespread metastases, no active treatment beyond supportive therapy and general nursing care is warranted. Narcotic agents and anxiolytic drugs may be useful.

MANAGEMENT OF A NEW PRIMARY NEOPLASM

The advent of an apparently new primary neoplasm at some point after successful treatment of an esophageal neoplasm is unusual. Most surgical approaches to resection of esophageal cancers involve removal of the majority of the organ. The appearance of a tumor in the residual esophagus proximal to the site of anastomosis is more likely to represent a recurrence of the original tumor, usually because of submucosal spread.[7] A tumor of different histological type from the original implies a totally new primary growth. Management of a patient in this unusual circumstance must be individualized. Surgical excision is not likely to be technically possible, and radiation therapy is more likely to be appropriate.

REFERENCES

1. Hesketh PJ, Clapp RW, Doos WG, Spechler SJ. The increasing frequency of adenocarcinoma of the esophagus. Cancer 1989;64:526-30.
2. Powell J, McConkey CC. Increasing incidence of adenocarcinoma of the gastric cardia and adjacent sites. Br J Cancer 1990;62:440-3.
3. Muller JM, Erasmi H, Stelzner M, Ziernen U, Pichlmaier H. Surgical therapy of oesophageal carcinoma. Br J Surg 1990;77:845-57.
4. Morton KA, Karwande SV, Davis RK, Datz FL, Lynch RE. Gastric emptying after gastric interposition for cancer of the esophagus or hypopharynx. Ann Thorac Surg 1991;51:759-63.
5. Wright CD, Mathisen DJ, Wain JC, et al. Evolution of treatment strategies for adenocarcinoma of the esophagus and gastroesophageal junction. Ann Thorac Surg 1994;58:1574-9.

Table 6-8 Management plan for suspected recurrent esophageal carcinoma

			RECURRENCE	
FOLLOW-UP	LIKELY CAUSES	INVESTIGATIONS	NOT CONFIRMED	CONFIRMED
Weight loss	Occult recurrence; nutritional	General health screen	Nutritional support	?Chemotherapy
Dysphagia	Locoregional recurrence; benign fibrous stricture	Endoscopy; computed tomography of the chest	Dilatation; ? operative revision	Radiation therapy; stent; laser therapy
Postprandial fullness	Gastric outlet obstruction	Contrast swallow; endoscopy	Observe; ? operative revision	Radiation therapy
Anemia	Blood loss	Endoscopy	H_2 antagonists	Radiation therapy
Jaundice	Liver metastases; unrelated	Liver ultrasound	Appropriate to diagnosis	Nil specific; ?radiation therapy
Subcutaneous nodules	Skin metastasis	Biopsy	Observe	Radiation therapy; ?wide excision
Bone pain	Bone metastases	Isotope/magnetic resonance imaging	Analgesia	Radiation therapy; analgesia
Acute respiratory distress	Tracheoesophageal fistula	Endoscopy; contrast swallow	Observe; treat as appropriate	Stent

6. Isono K, Onada S, Okuyama K, Sato H. Recurrence of intrathoracic esophageal cancer. Jpn J Clin Oncol 1985;15:49-60.
7. Watanabe H, Iizuka N, Hirata K. Examination of esophageal cancer with intramural skip or separate satellite nodules. Geka Shinrvo 1979;21:1096-9.

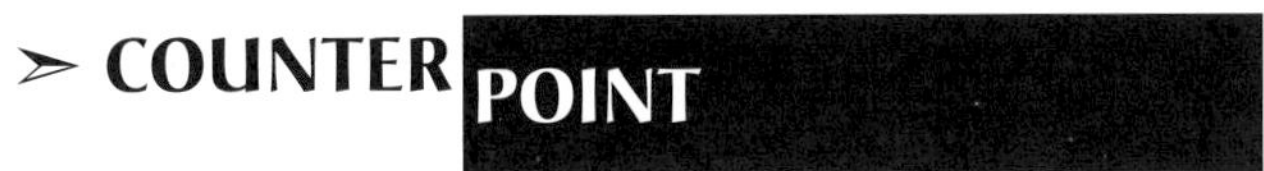

Roswell Park Cancer Institute

Hector R. Nava

In their discussion of the follow-up of carcinoma of the esophagus following surgical resection, Wood and Pellegrini provide an excellent rationale for optimizing the use of diagnostic studies and controlling costs. I would like to offer a somewhat different perspective on the approach and rationale of follow-up at a major cancer center.

A key question is who should be following the patient and with what aim. Should it be the surgeon, the medical oncologist, the gastroenterologist, or the primary care physician? Each of these physicians offers areas of expertise that may be invaluable to the patient. In my experience the primary care physician is an important link in the overall management and should be part of the follow-up team. The majority of patients with esophageal malignancy are old and have innumerable nononcological chronic medical problems (cardiac, pulmonary, and the like) that require close follow-up and management. If ignored, these problems will negatively affect the length of life and, more important, the quality of life of the patient.

The medical oncologist may be part of the follow-up team if the patient has received neoadjuvant chemotherapy or if chemotherapy is to be used after surgery. Since the definitive value of chemotherapy is still to be established, at present the medical oncologist's participation is limited to patients treated under investigational protocols.

The gastroenterologist, who frequently makes the diagnosis and refers the patient to the surgeon, may continue to play a role in the management of long-term complications of esophageal resection, such as dumping syndrome, diarrhea, malabsorption, reflux esophagitis, and stricture, as well as in the diagnosis of anastomotic or intraluminal recurrence. I concur with the recommendation of Wood and Pellegrini that routine endoscopic follow-up is not needed in most cases and should be used only for the management of anastomotic strictures or the diagnosis of recurrences or esophagitis.

The operating surgeon has expertise in the natural behavior of cancer of the esophagus, as well as knowledge of the form of reconstruction and the specifics of each individual operation. The surgeon has an advantage in detecting early postoperative complications, such as leaks, strictures, effusions, and obstructions, and should be in command of the early posthospitalization management until satisfied that the patient is free of surgery-related problems. The patient should also be nutritionally independent and stable, since many of these patients have trouble achieving and sustaining an adequate oral caloric intake and thus require close supervision and frequent nutritional supplementation. This is especially true if the patient is to receive adjuvant radiation therapy or chemotherapy. Long-term jejunostomy tube feedings are often necessary to carry these patients through the effects of the adjuvant therapy. This close follow-up is needed, usually on a monthly basis, for 6 months or more after surgery. Once the nutritional state is stable and normal daily activity is resumed, the follow-up frequency can be diminished to once every 2 to 3 months during the first year, every 3 months during the second year, every 4 months during the third year, and every 6 months thereafter until 5 years have been reached. Beyond 5 years, physicians at Roswell Park Cancer Institute examine patients on a yearly basis with a focus on detecting metachronous cancer.

Although effective treatment for recurrent or metastatic disease may not exist, it is important in some cases to detect recurrence as early as possible, since physicians may be able to intervene with palliative therapies (radiation) to diminish the impact of recurrent disease on the patient's quality of life. A good example of this is the patient with spinal metastases who may become paraplegic if diagnosis and treatment are delayed. Another example is anastomotic recurrence or other forms of locoregional disease that may require endoscopic laser therapy or radiation for palliation of obstruction. Although there are no studies that measure the actual impact of these palliative treatments on the group as a whole, early management of some recurrent disease delays tumor progression and maintains a reasonable quality of life for quite some time.

Most patients have the optimistic expectation that, if they should have recurrent disease, early detection will give them a better chance for remission or cure. As is well described by Wood and Pellegrini, cure is rarely possible. Unfortunately, physicians may be responsible for creating that illusion by attempting to provide patients with a positive view that will enhance their daily lives rather than a pessimistic view of waiting for inevitable death, which degrades quality of life.

Emphasis during follow-up visits should be on obtaining a good clinical history of a patient's eating habits, caloric consumption, and episodes of dysphagia, regurgitation, aspiration, or vomiting. Careful questioning will detect symptoms of dumping, malabsorption, or food intolerance that may respond to dietary changes or digestive enzyme supplementation. Episodes of dysphagia or regurgitation suggest a stricture that will require investigation by barium swallow or endoscopy. Protruding sutures or staples that cause symptoms can be easily removed endoscopically, and anastomotic strictures usually respond to a single session of balloon or Savary dilatation.

Table 6-10 Follow-up of patients with esophageal cancer by institution

YEAR/PROGRAM	OFFICE VISIT	ESOPH	CHEST CT	ABD CT	CBC
Year 1					
Memorial Sloan-Kettering I[a]	3	[b]	[b]	[b]	
Memorial Sloan-Kettering II[c]	3	3	3	3	
Memorial Sloan-Kettering III[d]	3	2	3	3	
Roswell Park	12	[b]	4[e]	4[e]	13[e]
Univ Washington	3	[f]	[f]	[f]	
Japan: National Kyushu	12	1	2	2	
UK: Cardiothoracic Centre	4	[b]	[b]		
Year 2					
Memorial Sloan-Kettering I[a]	3	[b]	[b]	[b]	
Memorial Sloan-Kettering II[c]	3	2	2	2	
Memorial Sloan-Kettering III[d]	3	2	2	2	
Roswell Park	4-6	[b]	2	2	4-6
Univ Washington	3	[f]	[f]	[f]	
Japan: National Kyushu	12	1	2	2	
UK: Cardiothoracic Centre	4	[b]	[b]		

ABD CT abdominal computed tomography
CBC complete blood count
CHEST CT chest computed tomography
CXR chest x-ray
ESOPH esophagoscopy
LFT liver function tests
NECK CT neck computed tomography
SCCAG squamous cell carcinoma antigen

The clinical history should include investigation of new pains, especially in joints or bones, followed by a thorough physical examination. If present, such pain increases the degree of suspicion and indicates the need for radiography, bone scanning, and other procedures. Other areas of importance during the physical examination should include careful examination for lymphadenopathy, especially in the supraclavicular areas (Virchow's node). The presence of suspect lymph nodes may indicate the need for a complete metastatic workup and fine-needle aspiration. Pleural or pericardial effusions, hepatomegaly, abdominal masses, ascites, and the presence of Blumer's shelf are physical findings that may be detected before symptoms appear. Stool examination for occult blood may be an early indication of local recurrence, other nonmalignant pathological conditions, or a metachronous gastrointestinal neoplasia (colon polyps or carcinoma).

Although I have not heard of litigation against physicians for delaying diagnosis of recurrent or metastatic disease in esophageal cancer, taking a nihilistic approach to the follow-up of these patients is not prudent. Also, when patients are entered on a neoadjuvant or adjuvant treatment protocol, closer follow-up is required, since delay in the diagnosis of recurrent or metastatic disease will affect the results of the study. Table 6-9 presents the routines used in the follow-up of patients with esophageal cancer at Roswell Park Cancer Institute.

Table 6-9 Follow-up of patients with esophageal cancer: Roswell Park Cancer Institute

	YEAR				
	1	2	3	4	5
Office visit	12	4-6	2-4	2-4	2-4
Complete blood count	13*	4-6	2-4	2-4	2-4
Liver function tests	13*	4-6	2-4	2-4	2-4
Chest x-ray	7*	4-6	2-4	2-4	2-4
Abdominal computed tomography	4*	2	1	1	1
Chest computed tomography	4*	2	1	1	1
Barium swallow	1*,†	†	†	†	†
Bone scan	1*,†	†	†	†	†
Esophagoscopy	†	†	†	†	†

*Includes one test performed at baseline.
†Performed as clinically indicated.

LFT	CXR	BARIUM SWALLOW	BONE SCAN	SCCAG	NECK CT
	3				
	3				
	3		2		
13[e]	7[e]	1[b,e]	1[b,e]		
	1		1	12	2
	b				
	3				
	3				
	3		2		
4-6	4-6	b	b		
	1		1	12	2
	b				

a Standard community care.
b Performed as clinically indicated.
c Patients at high risk for local recurrence.
d Patients in clinical trials or institutions engaged in studies of staging and cancer biology.
e Includes one test performed at baseline.
f Performed as needed for patients with a high risk of local esophageal recurrence or a remnant of Barrett's esophagus.

Continued.

Table 6-10 Follow-up of patients with esophageal cancer by institution—cont'd

YEAR/PROGRAM	OFFICE VISIT	ESOPH	CHEST CT	ABD CT	CBC
Year 3					
Memorial Sloan-Kettering I[a]	2	[b]	[b]	[b]	
Memorial Sloan-Kettering II[c]	2	2	2	2	
Memorial Sloan-Kettering III[d]	2	[b]	2	2	
Roswell Park	2-4	[b]	1	1	2-4
Univ Washington	2	[f]	[f]	[f]	
Japan: National Kyushu	4	1	1	1	
UK: Cardiothoracic Centre	1	[b]	[b]		
Year 4					
Memorial Sloan-Kettering I[a]	2	[b]	[b]	[b]	
Memorial Sloan-Kettering II[c]	2	1	1	1	
Memorial Sloan-Kettering III[d]	2	[b]	1	1	
Roswell Park	2-4	[b]	1	1	2-4
Univ Washington	2	[f]	[f]	[f]	
Japan: National Kyushu	4	1	1	1	
UK: Cardiothoracic Centre	1	[b]	[b]		
Year 5					
Memorial Sloan-Kettering I[a]	1	[b]	[b]	[b]	
Memorial Sloan-Kettering II[c]	1	[b]	[b]	[b]	
Memorial Sloan-Kettering III[d]	1	[b]	[b]	[b]	
Roswell Park	2-4	[b]	1	1	2-4
Univ Washington	1	[f]	[f]	[f]	
Japan: National Kyushu	4	1	1	1	
UK: Cardiothoracic Centre	1	[b]	[b]		

LFT	CXR	BARIUM SWALLOW	BONE SCAN	SCCAG	NECK CT
	2				
	2				
	2		[b]		
2-4	2-4	[b]	[b]		
	1		1	4	1
	[b]				
	2				
	2				
	2		[b]		
2-4	2-4	[b]	[b]		
	1		1	4	1
	[b]				
	1				
	1				
	1		[b]		
2-4	2-4	[b]	[b]		
	1		1	4	1
	[b]				

CHAPTER 7

Gastric Carcinoma

Roswell Park Cancer Institute

NEAL J. MEROPOL AND JUDY L. SMITH

In the United States there were an estimated 24,000 new cases of gastric cancer and 14,000 deaths from this disease in 1994.[1] At least 90% of primary gastric cancers are adenocarcinomas. Leiomyosarcoma and lymphoma are the only other histological types that account for more than 1% of cases. Little is known about current follow-up practices after gastric resection. In this chapter we attempt to present rational guidelines for the follow-up of patients with gastric adenocarcinoma after surgical resection, based on available surveillance methods and the natural history of this disease.

POTENTIAL BENEFITS OF SURVEILLANCE

Approximately 50% of patients with gastric adenocarcinoma have their tumor resected with curative intent, and decisions about follow-up for these patients are challenging.[2] The benefits of a surveillance program may take several forms.

Survival

The main argument for follow-up after a potentially curative operation is that such a program could improve patient survival. This generally requires effective salvage therapy. Treatment begun when the patient is still asymptomatic may result in a better outcome than therapy begun after symptoms develop, when the disease would have been identified even without a routine surveillance program. Early detection of second primary malignancies may also increase the survival of patients at high risk.

Quality of Life

A second potential reason for follow-up of asymptomatic patients is that early identification of relapse could improve quality, if not quantity, of life.

Economics

The costs associated with surveillance may play a role in determining an optimal follow-up schedule. This is the case particularly when the other benefits of surveillance are marginal.

Research

Intensive postoperative surveillance may be an important component in evaluating a new follow-up tool or may be necessary to gather data regarding patterns of failure. In prospective clinical research trials, patients are asked to give appropriate informed consent for participation.

This chapter provides a framework for the development of rational surveillance guidelines following definitive treatment for primary gastric adenocarcinoma. This framework should permit modification of guidelines as methods of surveillance evolve and outcomes of treatment intervention improve.

GASTRIC CANCER STAGING AND SURVIVAL

The first issue that arises with regard to follow-up is whether there is a subset of patients with a prognosis so favorable that surveillance is unnecessary. The tumor, nodes, metastases (TNM) staging system for gastric cancer (Table 7-1) stratifies patients by risk level.[3] As shown in Figure 7-1, stage correlates well with survival.[3] However, even the most favorable stage (minimally invasive, node negative) carries a 40% risk of death during the first 5 years, although not all the deaths are the result of gastric carcinoma. Nevertheless, if postoperative surveillance is beneficial, all patients who undergo potentially curative treatment have a recurrence risk that warrants participation. It is notable that the Japanese experience suggests a more favorable outcome for early-stage disease than is reported in Western studies. Sano et al.[4] reported a 1.4% death rate from recurrent disease in 1,475 patients with early gastric cancer. Interestingly, 6.6% of the patients who had undergone resection died of other causes, half of which were other cancers, which suggests shared risk factors or heritable predispositions for multiple malignancies. Whether the apparent global differences in prognosis for early-stage gastric cancer reflect a biological heterogeneity in this disease is not known.

Follow-up of gastric cancer should continue until survival approximates that of age-matched control subjects. This does not occur until 8 years after curative surgical therapy.[5] However, the slopes of the survival curves are not constant over this time period. Rather, approximately 80% of deaths occur during the first 3 years, after which the risk of relapse gradually decreases. Based on these data, follow-up should continue at least until year 8 but should be most intensive during the initial 3 years of highest risk.

Table 7-1 TNM staging system of gastric cancer

PRIMARY TUMOR (T)

TX	Primary tumor cannot be assessed
T0	No evidence of primary tumor
Tis	Carcinoma in situ; intraepithelial tumor without invasion of the lamina propria
T1	Tumor invades lamina propria or submucosa
T2	Tumor invades the muscularis propria or the subserosa
T3	Tumor penetrates the serosa (visceral peritoneum) without invasion of adjacent structures
T4	Tumor invades adjacent structures

REGIONAL LYMPH NODES (N)

NX	Regional lymph node(s) cannot be assessed
N0	No regional lymph node metastasis
N1	Metastasis in perigastric lymph node(s) within 3 cm of the edge of the primary tumor
N2	Metastasis in perigastric lymph node(s) more than 3 cm from the edge of the primary tumor, or in lymph nodes along the left gastric, common hepatic, splenic, or celiac arteries

DISTANT METASTASIS (M)

MX	Presence of distant metastasis cannot be assessed
M0	No distant metastasis
M1	Distant metastasis

STAGE GROUPING

Stage 0	Tis	N0	M0
Stage IA	T1	N0	M0
Stage IB	T1	N1	M0
	T2	N0	M0
Stage II	T1	N2	M0
	T2	N1	M0
	T3	N0	M0
Stage IIIA	T2	N2	M0
	T3	N1	M0
	T4	N0	M0
Stage IIIB	T3	N2	M0
	T4	N1	M0
Stage IV	T4	N2	M0
	Any T	Any N	M1

From American Joint Committee on Cancer, Beahrs OH, Henson DE, Hutter RVP, Kennedy BJ, editors: Manual for staging of cancer. Philadelphia: JB Lippincott Company, 1992.

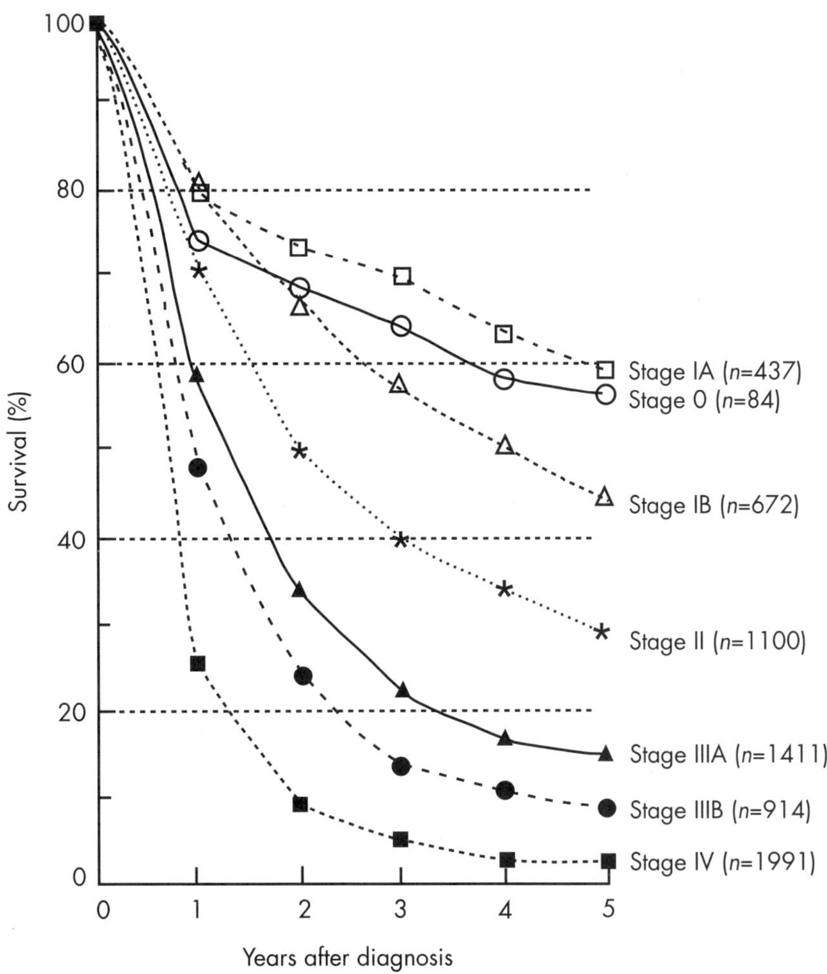

Figure 7-1 Survival for patients with stomach cancer by pathological stages diagnosed in 1982. (From American Joint Committee on Cancer, Beahrs OH, Henson DE, Hutter RVP, Kennedy BJ, editors: Manual for staging of cancer. Philadelphia: JB Lippincott Company, 1992.)

Table 7-2 Gastric adenocarcinoma patterns of failure (%)

	BRUCKNER AND STABLEIN[*8]	CLARKE ET AL.[*9]	DUPONT ET AL.[6]	SONS AND BORCHARD[12]	STOUT[10]	WARWICK[7]	WISBECK ET AL.[11]
Number of patients	232	195	348	117	143	176	85
Abdominal wall		3			<1		
Adrenal glands		15	15	10		5	
Biliary		5				2	
Bone							
Any bone, marrow	6	12	1	9	11		19
Ribs						2	
Vertebrae						<1	
Brain, meninges		3	<1	2	<1	1	2
Bronchial nodes, thoracic, mediastinum		10				9	19
Diaphragm			6	4		2	
Esophagus			7				
Heart, pericardium		2	1	1			5
Intestines			16[†]			4	
Kidneys, bladder		10	3/3	7		3	
Liver	38	51	54	27	49	38	39
Lungs, pleura	9	24	22	9	33	12/8	34/25
Lymph nodes							
Cervical, supraclavicular nodes					8		
Perigastric lymph nodes		88[‡]				36	
Retroperitoneal lymph nodes						28	
Mesentery						9	
Omentum			26			13	
Ovaries			3		14	1	
Pancreas	21		29	3		7	
Peritoneum	40	22	24	17	43[§]	20	47
Prostate						<1	
Skin		1	<1				
Spleen			13	2		2	
Thyroid			1	<1			
Uterus						1	

*All data are based on autopsy series except Bruckner and Stablein[8] and Clarke et al.[9]
†Sixteen percent duodenum, 16% colon, 13% small bowel.
‡Includes retroperitoneal lymph nodes.
§Includes omentum and mesentery.

PATTERNS OF FAILURE

Once a surveillance interval is chosen, patterns of failure guide the choice of detection methods. Gastric cancer has four patterns of spread and relapse: local, lymphatic, hematogenous, and peritoneal. Autopsy series provide the most complete assessment of metastatic disease sites. Several large reports that describe patterns of spread are summarized in Table 7-2.[6-12]

Local extension to adjacent structures such as the liver, pancreas, or diaphragm may render curative therapy impossible and are also sites of relapse in patients rendered free of disease by initial treatment. Several investigators have reported on the specific problem of local relapse in the gastric bed, gastric remnant, or duodenal stump following subtotal gastrectomy. In fact, distant metastases are uncommon in the absence of locoregional relapse. Reports detailing patterns of local recurrence are listed in Table 7-3.[8,13-16] The tendency toward locoregional relapse appears to diminish with more extensive primary dissections, but a randomized trial comparing relapse patterns based on initial procedure has not been successfully conducted.[17-19]

Distant metastasis may follow several patterns. Lymphatic spread may result in recurrence in regional or more distant (for example, mediastinal or supraclavicular) nodal sites. The hematogenous route leads to relapse in organs such as the liver, lung, or bone. Subclinical peritoneal seeding may ultimately produce symptomatic peritoneal carcinomatosis. The most common sites of distant metastases are hepatic (27% to 51% of cases), pulmonary or pleural (9% to 34%), intrathoracic or mediastinal (9% to 19%), and bone (1% to 19%). Intraabdominal or retroperitoneal relapse is frequent. Sites include lymph nodes (28% to 88%), peritoneum (17% to

Table 7-3 Local recurrence patterns in gastric cancer (%)

	BRUCKNER AND STABLEIN[8]	LANDRY ET AL.[16]	MCNEER ET AL.[13]	PAPACHRISTOU AND FORTNER*[15]	THOMSON AND ROBINS[14]
Number of patients	71	88	92	86	28
Total local	10	56	81	32	
Gastric remnant		38	50		46†
Duodenal stump			10		
Gastric bed		31	21		46
Distant only			15		
Local only	1	24			
Total distant		76			

*Only gastric cardia primary tumors included.
†Includes duodenal stump recurrences.

47%), omentum (13% to 26%), pancreas (3% to 29%), adrenal glands (5% to 15%), ovaries (3% to 14%), genitourinary organs (3% to 10%), and spleen (2% to 13%). Sites with metastases occurring in less than 5% of cases include the diaphragm, biliary system, uterus, central nervous system, abdominal wall, heart or pericardium, thyroid, and skin.

METHODS OF SURVEILLANCE

History and Physical Examination

Although least sensitive and specific, the history and physical examination of patients are also the least expensive and invasive screening measures. An interval history may provide a suggestion of relapse through the development of symptoms related to local recurrence or metastases. Patients may relate the development of adenopathy, hepatomegaly, bone pain, or dysphagia. In addition, more nonspecific symptoms may be present, such as weight loss, anorexia, nausea, or diffuse abdominal pain. A new symptom of any kind must alert the physician to recurrence, since relapse occurs in the majority of patients and multiple patterns of spread are common.

A directed physical examination may also be the first indicator of relapse in an asymptomatic patient or confirm suspicion in a patient with symptoms. This evaluation should include attention to weight; skin and scleral color; lymph nodes (especially supraclavicular); abdominal, rectal, and pelvic examinations (Blumer's shelf); and testing of stool for occult blood.

Esophagogastroduodenoscopy

Local recurrence may be detected endoscopically. Endoscopy is more sensitive and specific than barium contrast study and permits immediate biopsy of suspect lesions. In addition, endoscopic ultrasound may help guide decisions about resectability of recurrent disease, although this would not be a component of routine surveillance.

Computed Tomography

Given the high incidence of intraabdominal recurrence in gastric cancer, computed tomography may be used to evaluate the liver, gastric bed, mesentery, retroperitoneal lymph nodes, and pelvis. The frequency of such evaluations must be tempered by the recognition that curable disease is not likely to be identified. The role of magnetic resonance imaging of the abdomen has not been defined. It is likely to be complementary in specific situations when an inconclusive computed tomographic scan has been obtained. Current studies are comparing the specificity and sensitivity of these scanning methods in evaluating hepatic metastases from solid tumors.

Serological Surveillance

Since the identification of tumor-associated antigens and the development of monoclonal antibodies against them, several serum tumor markers have been studied in gastric cancer. Elevated levels of carcinoembryonic antigen (CEA) are commonly present in the serum of patients with gastric cancer. Unfortunately, the sensitivity of this assay is low. For patients with gastric cancer the reported sensitivity for CEA has ranged from 25% to 59%.[20-22] In 410 patients with benign gastrointestinal diseases, Heptner et al.[20] reported a false-positive rate for CEA of 10.5%. False-positive results may also occur in smokers and in patients with pulmonary infections. In a retrospective analysis of CEA monitoring following colorectal cancer surgery, a false-positive rate of 16% was largely responsible for a lack of overall benefit in postoperative screening.[23]

Other circulating tumor antigens in gastric cancer are CA 19-9 and TAG-72. CA 19-9 is a sialylated form of the Lewis^a blood group antigen that is present in patients with a variety of malignancies. Numerous studies have evaluated its utility in the detection of gastric cancer. The sensitivity of CA 19-9 for gastric cancer ranges from 28% to 62% in various reports.[20,22,24-26] Unfortunately, this marker also has a low specificity, with false-positive rates greater than 20% in some reports.[20,24,26]

The TAG-72 antigen is a high–molecular weight, mucin-like glycoprotein present on a variety of epithelial neoplasms, particularly adenocarcinomas.[27] Two distinct epitopes on TAG-72 are recognized by monoclonal antibodies B72.3 and CC49. These antibodies have been combined in a sequential assay for the detection of circulating levels of TAG-72 in patients with gastric cancer. This radioimmunoassay, named

CA 72-4, has a false-positive rate of less than 5%; however, the sensitivity remains low, ranging from 59% to 71%.[20,28] Given a high specificity, this assay may prove valuable in combination with other tumor markers that increase sensitivity.[28] At present the CA 72-4 assay remains investigational.

Monoclonal Antibody Imaging

Imaging of the abdomen and pelvis using monoclonal antibody-radionuclide conjugates has recently become possible. A high level of specificity has been reported for an antibody scan using a TAG-72 monoclonal antibody, B72.3, in patients with abdominopelvic, extrahepatic metastases from colorectal cancer.[29] This antibody recognizes a glycoprotein antigen present on most adenocarcinomas.[27] The value of this and other monoclonal antibody scans for surveillance is limited by insufficient sensitivity and by the fact that resectable disease is only rarely identified. In addition, the currently available studies use murine monoclonal antibodies, which stimulate a human-anti-mouse antibody response, thereby limiting repeat application. The development of humanized monoclonal antibodies with improved sensitivity may increase the clinical utility of this modality as a surveillance tool.

BOTTOM LINE: TREATMENT OF RECURRENT DISEASE

A detailed discussion of therapy for metastatic gastric cancer is beyond the scope of this chapter. However, the value of postoperative surveillance depends largely on whether intervention will benefit a patient with asymptomatic recurrence. Although numerous series document long-term disease-free survival in patients who have undergone metastasectomy for isolated recurrences of several solid tumors, such data are scant for gastric cancer, probably because it tends to appear in multiple metastatic sites concurrently and because metastases commonly are not resectable. If there is a group of gastric cancer patients who have metastases resectable for cure, it is small and select.

Bruckner et al.[8] reviewed the patterns of failure in the Gastrointestinal Tumor Study Group adjuvant studies and reported that in 71 relapses, 11 (15%) were in the lung only and 12 (17%) were in the liver only. Therefore, within the limits of current ability to detect metastases, at least a small subset of patients might have distant recurrence that is technically resectable. Whether such patients can be identified preoperatively or whether survival in this group would be improved by resection is unknown.

Considering the high frequency of locoregional relapse, the question arises as to whether some of these patients can benefit from surgery. In as many as half of patients undergoing curative resections for gastric cancer the disease recurs at the anastomosis, in the gastric or duodenal stump, or in the esophagus.[13-16] Curative resections are not commonly possible in these patients, although in rare instances survival after resection has exceeded several years.[30] Papachristou and Fortner[30] reported a series of 257 patients who underwent primary resection and were followed until death. The local recurrence rate was 25%, with 80% of these patients also having distant metastases. Forty-six patients with local recurrence were surgically explored with the intent of resection. Thirteen patients underwent resection of gross disease; 10 of these patients had stump recurrences. At the time of the report eight of the patients who had undergone resection had survived for at least 5 years. Interestingly, all of these patients were initially TNM stage I or II. Gunderson and Sosin[31] reported the findings of planned second-look operations in 107 patients after initial gastric surgery. Five patients were potentially rendered disease free by the second procedure, but eight perioperative deaths occurred. Follow-up on the patients who had undergone resection was not included. Based on this experience the authors argued against the routine use of the second-look approach. If there is an advantage of surveillance for local recurrence, it may be in a select subgroup of patients with resectable disease and those with unresectable disease for whom early palliative intervention, such as laser, mechanical dilatation, stenting, or radiation therapy, might be of value.

In terms of systemic therapy for advanced disease, several commonly used chemotherapeutic regimens yield responses in at least one third of patients, with transient complete responses in a small subset. Some patients have palliation of disease-related symptoms, but the impact of treatment on overall survival is likely to be modest.[32] Even with treatment the natural history of metastatic gastric cancer is short, with a median survival of less than 1 year in most reports.[32] Whether early intervention at a time of lower tumor bulk is superior to treatment initiated when symptoms occur is unknown. For patients who have access to clinical trials, early detection may provide an opportunity to participate, whereas awaiting the development of symptoms may compromise eligibility.

The psychological impact of surveillance is also difficult to assess when early identification of recurrence shortens the disease-free interval without having much impact on survival for most patients. Many patients wish to proceed with a follow-up program, not because early detection will benefit them, but because the inability to identify recurrence in those remaining disease free provides an emotional benefit. In fact, given that the median survival of patients with advanced gastric cancer is measured in months, early detection of asymptomatic metastases is not likely to abbreviate the disease-free interval substantially.

SPECIAL ISSUES IN GASTRIC CANCER FOLLOW-UP

Nutrition

Vitamin B_{12} deficiency is common after gastrectomy because of the loss of parietal cell mass. Long-term parenteral vitamin B_{12} replacement is required and is sufficient to maintain normal hematopoiesis. However, hemoglobin level and mean corpuscular volume should be monitored after gastrectomy to detect megaloblastic anemia in patients who are insufficiently repleted.

Other late complications from gastrectomy include anorexia, weight loss or inability to gain weight, dumping syndromes, poor gastric emptying, and marginal ulceration. The frequency of these complications depends in part on the type and extent of resection. These sequelae must be recognized and addressed early to avoid major morbidity.

Second Primary Malignancies

A potential benefit of postsurgical follow-up of gastric cancer is early detection of second primary malignancies, either nongastric or in the gastric remnant. Some individuals have a heritable predisposition toward development of malignancies at various sites. Gastric cancer is associated with hereditary nonpolyposis colon cancer.[33,34] Recently, several DNA repair genes have been identified that are abnormally expressed in patients with hereditary nonpolyposis colon cancer.[35,36] Germline mutations in these genes are likely to identify patients at high risk for the development of malignancies at specific sites. In these patients tumors are characterized by the presence of DNA replication errors manifested as nucleotide microsatellite instability. Interestingly, six of 33 (18%) sporadic gastric carcinomas were found by Peltomaki et al.[33] to show replication errors, suggesting that the affected patients inherited a tendency toward this malignancy. Even without availability of routine screening for such mutations, a family history of malignancies at an early age should raise suspicion of a heritable predisposition. Recognition of such a family history in a patient treated curatively for gastric cancer should heighten awareness that this patient is at increased risk for cancers in other sites and that postoperative follow-up should take this into account. This information is important in long-term follow-up.

Numerous case reports and cohort studies have suggested that gastric surgery for benign disease is a significant risk factor for the development of gastric cancer, which may also apply to recurrence in the gastric remnant after cancer surgery. The increase in risk may begin within the first 5 years postoperatively and extend for at least 20 years.[37] Potential pathogenetic mechanisms include reflux of bile acids and chronic gastric hypoacidity with bacterial overgrowth. Recently an association has been described between *Helicobacter pylori* infection and gastric cancer.[38-40] Whether postgastrectomy patients are at increased risk for *H. pylori* infection or whether gastric cancer patients with the infection are at increased risk of local recurrence is unknown. A cohort study involving 15,983 subjects demonstrated that the greatest risk of gastric cancer after surgery for benign disease occurs 2 to 5 years postoperatively.[37] This period coincides with the highest recurrence rate following gastric surgery for malignancy. Therefore it is possible that some stump recurrences represent second primary malignancies. To be effective, surveillance for local recurrence should be concentrated during the period of highest compounded risk; the cost effectiveness of long-term endoscopic screening after gastrectomy for any cause remains uncertain.

RECOMMENDATIONS

Before embarking on a postoperative surveillance program in gastric cancer, both physician and patient must clearly understand the goals. Given that the number of patients cured of asymptomatic recurrences who would otherwise have died of their disease is small, a case could be made for a surveillance program that includes only minimal follow-up until symptom development. However, considering the potential benefits to a patient of negative results of a surveillance examination and the better palliation obtained when metastasis is found early in a disease with a short natural history, a more extensive program may be appropriate. The follow-up routine should be based on patient preferences whenever possible.

Based on the data presented and the caveats noted, the surveillance approach outlined in Table 7-4 may serve as a guide. These guidelines represent a consensus among medical and surgical oncologists at Roswell Park Cancer Institute. Interval history, physical examination, complete blood count, CEA measurement, and liver function tests should be performed every 3 months during the first 3 years, every 4 months in years 4 and 5, every 6 months from year 5 until 8, and annually thereafter. Chest roentgenograms and abdominal and pelvic computed tomographic scans should be obtained every 6 months in the first 3 years and annually in years 4 to 8. Upper endoscopy should be performed every 6 months for the first year, then annually until year 8. Long-term endoscopic screening may be considered because of the risk of a second primary cancer in the gastric stump.

FUTURE PROSPECTS

An ideal follow-up program for gastric cancer would prolong life and be convenient, inexpensive, and widely available. A prospective, randomized comparison of various follow-up regimens, such as the one presented here, is warranted. Such a clinical trial should address several major end points, including quality of life, survival, and health care costs. A successfully conducted study of gastric cancer follow-up would have important implications for the management of patients with this disease.

Table 7-4 Follow-up of patients with gastric cancer: Roswell Park Cancer Institute

	YEAR				
	1	2	3	4	5
Office visit	4	4	4	3	3
Complete blood count	4	4	4	3	3
Liver function tests	4	4	4	3	3
Chest x-ray	2	2	2	1	1
Abdominal computed tomography	2	2	2	1	1
Esophagogastroscopy	2	1	1	1	1

ACKNOWLEDGMENTS

We wish to thank Marybeth Nelson for research assistance and Lynn Duewiger for expert secretarial support in preparation of this chapter.

REFERENCES

1. Boring CC, Squires TS, Tong T, Montgomery S. Cancer statistics, 1994. CA Cancer J Clin 1994;44:7-26.
2. Weed TE, Neussle W, Ochsner A. Carcinoma of the stomach: why are we failing to improve survival? Ann Surg 1981;193:407-13.
3. American Joint Committee on Cancer, Beahrs OH, Henson DE, Hutter RVP, Kennedy BJ, editors. Manual for staging of cancer. 4th ed. Philadelphia: JB Lippincott Company, 1992.
4. Sano T, Sasako M, Kinoshita T, Maruyama K. Recurrence of early gastric cancer: follow-up of 1475 patients and review of the Japanese literature. Cancer 1993;72:174-8.
5. Serlin O, Keehn R, Higgins G, Harrower H, Mendeloff G. Factors related to survival following resection for gastric carcinoma: analysis of 903 cases. Cancer 1977;40:1318-29.
6. Dupont B Jr, Lee JR, Barton GR, Cohn I Jr. Adenocarcinoma of the stomach: review of 1,497 cases. Cancer 1978;41:941-7.
7. Warwick M. Analysis of one-hundred and seventy-six cases of carcinoma of the stomach submitted to autopsy. Ann Surg 1928;88:216-26.
8. Bruckner H, Stablein D. Sites of treatment failure: gastrointestinal tumor study group analyses of gastric, pancreatic, and colorectal trials. Cancer Treat Symp 1983;2:199-210.
9. Clarke JS, Cruze K, El Farra S, Longmire WP Jr. The natural history and results of surgical therapy for carcinoma of the stomach: an analysis of 250 cases. Am J Surg 1961;102:143-52.
10. Stout P. Pathology of carcinoma of the stomach. Arch Surg 1943;46:807-822.
11. Wisbeck WA, Becker EM, Russell AH. Adenocarcinoma of the stomach: autopsy observations with therapeutic implications for the radiation oncologist. Radiother Oncol 1986;7:13-8.
12. Sons HU, Borchard F. Cancer of the distal esophagus and cardia: incidence, tumorous infiltration and metastatic spread. Ann Surg 1986;203:188-95.
13. McNeer G, VandenBerg H Jr, Donn FY, Bowden L. A critical evaluation of subtotal gastrectomy for the stomach. Ann Surg 1951;134:2-7.
14. Thomson FB, Robins RE. Local recurrence following subtotal resection for gastric carcinoma. Surg Gynecol Obstet 1952;95:341-4.
15. Papachristou DN, Fortner JG. Adenocarcinoma of the gastric cardia: the choice of gastrectomy. Ann Surg 1980;192:58-64.
16. Landry J, Tepper J, Wood W, Moulton E, Koerner F, Sullinger J. Patterns of failure following curative resection of gastric carcinoma. Int J Radiat Oncol Biol Phys 1990;19:1357-62.
17. Shiu M, Papachristou D, Kosloff C, Eliopoulos G. Selection of operative procedure for adenocarcinoma of the midstomach. Ann Surg 1980;192:730-7.
18. Maruyama K, Gunven P, Okabayashi K, Sasako M, Kinoshita T. Lymph node metastases of gastric cancer. Ann Surg 1989;210:596-602.
19. Bunt AM, Hermans J, Boon MC, et al. Evaluation of the extent of lymphadenectomy in a randomized trial of Western- versus Japanese-type surgery in gastric cancer. J Clin Oncol 1994;12:417-22.
20. Heptner G, Domschke S, Domschke W. Comparison of CA 72-4 with CA 19-9 and carcinoembryonic antigen in the serodiagnostics of gastrointestinal malignancies. Scand J Gastroenterol 1989;24:745-50.
21. Cooper MJ, Mackie CR, Skinner DB, Moosa AR. A reappraisal of the value of carcinoembryonic antigen in the management of patients with various neoplasms. Br J Surg 1979;66:120-3.
22. Gupta MK, Arciaga R, Bocci L, Tubbs R, Bukowski R, Deodhar SD. Measurement of a monoclonal-antibody-defined antigen (CA 19-9) in the sera of patients with malignant and nonmalignant diseases. Cancer 1985;56:277-83.
23. Moertel CG, Fleming TR, MacDonald JS, Haller DG, Laurie JA, Tangen C. An evaluation of the carcinoembryonic antigen (CEA) test for monitoring patients with resected colon cancer. JAMA 1993;270:943-7.
24. Marechal F, Berthiot G, Legrand MG, Labre H, Cattan A, Deltour G. CA-50 and CA-19.9 as tumour markers: which is preferable? Anticancer 1990;10:977-82.
25. Jalanko H, Kuusela P, Roberts P, Sipponen P, Haglund C, Makela O. Comparison of a new tumor marker, CA 19-9, with alpha fetoprotein and carcinoembryonic antigen in patients with upper gastrointestinal diseases. J Clin Pathol 1984;37:218-22.
26. Ruibal A, Encabo G, Gefaell R, Martinez-Miralles E, Fort JM, Fernandez-Llamazares J. Clinical interest of serial CA 19.9 determination in differential diagnosis of patients with peptic ulcers and gastric cancer. Bull Cancer 1983;70:438-40.
27. Thor A, Ohuchi N, Szpak CA, Johnston WW, Schlom J. Distribution of oncofetal antigen tumor-associated glycoprotein-72 defined by monoclonal antibody B72.3. Cancer Res 1986;46:3118-24.
28. Gero EJ, Colcher D, Ferrnoi P, et al. CA 72-4 radioimmunoassay for the detection of the TAG-72 carcinoma-associated antigen in serum of patients. J Clin Lab Anal 1989;3:360-9.
29. Collier BD, Abdel-Nabi H, Doerr RJ, et al. Immunoscintigraphy performed with In-111-labeled CYT-103 in the management of colorectal cancer: comparison with CT. Radiology 1992;185:179-86.
30. Papachristou DN, Fortner JG. Local recurrence of gastric adenocarcinomas after gastrectomy. J Surg Oncol 1981;18:47-53.
31. Gunderson LL, Sosin H. Adenocarcinoma of the stomach: areas of failure in a reoperation series (second or symptomatic looks): clinicopathologic correlation and implications for adjuvant therapy. Int J Radiat Oncol Biol Phys 1982;8:1-11.
32. Kelsen D. The use of chemotherapy in the treatment of advanced gastric and pancreas cancer. Semin Oncol 1994;21(7 Suppl):58S-66S.
33. Peltomaki P, Lothe RA, Aaltonen LA, et al. Microsatellite instability is associated with tumors that characterize the hereditary non-polyposis colorectal carcinoma syndrome. Cancer Res 1993;53:5853-5.
34. Lynch HT, Smyrk TC, Watson P, et al. Genetics, natural history, tumor spectrum, and pathology of hereditary nonpolyposis colorectal cancer: an updated review. Gastroenterology 1993;104:1535-49.
35. Fishel R, Lescoe MK, Rao MR, et al. The human mutator gene homolog *MSH2* and its association with hereditary nonpolyposis colon cancer. Cell 1993;75:1027-38.
36. Bronner CE, Baker SM, Morrison PT, et al. Mutation in the DNA mismatch repair gene homologue *hMLH1* is associated with hereditary non-polyposis colon cancer. Nature 1994;368:258-61.
37. Fisher SG, Davis F, Nelson R, Weber L, Goldberg J, Haenszel W. A cohort study of stomach cancer risk in men after gastric surgery for benign disease. J Natl Cancer Inst 1993;85:1303-10.
38. The Eurogast Study Group. An international association between *Helicobacter pylori* infection and gastric cancer. Lancet 1993;341:1359-62.
39. Nightingale TE, Gruber J. *Helicobacter* and human cancer. J Natl Cancer Inst 1994;86:1505-9.
40. Parsonnet J, Friedman GD, Vandersteen DP, et al. *Helicobacter pylori* infection and the risk of gastric carcinoma. N Engl J Med 1991;325:1127-31.

➢ COUNTERPOINT

Memorial Sloan-Kettering Cancer Center

MARTIN S. KARPEH, JR., AND MURRAY F. BRENNAN

The relevant issue in screening asymptomatic patients with gastric carcinoma is to identify patients with localized disease who will benefit most from early therapeutic intervention. Chemotherapy and radiation therapy can provide good palliation in the management of recurrent gastric cancer, but their use in asymptomatic patients should be considered on a case by case basis until more effective agents are developed. Based on these assumptions, the follow-up plan recommended by Meropol and Smith attempts to maximize (within reason) the probability of identifying recurrent disease before symptom onset through frequent visits and routine use of computed tomography and esophagogastroscopy for all patients. However, these follow-up recommendations do not address the fact that the risk and pattern of recurrence vary widely among patients with resected gastric cancer.

In contrast to the generalized follow-up plan of Meropol and Smith, I propose that surveillance be based on the probability of disease recurrence so that diagnostic investigations are focused on asymptomatic patients in whom the probability of finding a potentially resectable local recurrence is reasonably high. The TNM stage of the original tumor, if properly determined, is a powerful prognostic factor that can be used to select patients most likely to benefit from frequent surveillance and early intervention. Reliable data from Western series allow physicians to make fairly sound estimates regarding an individual's chances for long-term survival.[1-3] These data are useful in selecting which asymptomatic patients should, for example, undergo routine yearly endoscopy. Defining risk recurrence directly influences the sensitivity and specificity of all diagnostic methods used in surveillance; this will have an impact on the efficiency and ultimate cost of gastric cancer follow-up.

IMPORTANCE OF pT STAGE IN FOLLOW-UP

The low survival figures for stage I disease published in an American College of Surgeons survey[4] and in the National Cancer Data Base report on gastric cancer[5] reflect the need for better staging in a disease that all too often is viewed at the outset as fatal. Data from other Western centers, including Memorial Sloan-Kettering Cancer Center, have demonstrated 5-year survival rates of more than 85% for stages IA and IB (Table 7-5). Concern for early recurrence will differ significantly depending on which survival figures are used as a basis for follow-up decisions. The American Joint Committee on Cancer (AJCC) staging system clearly stratifies gastric cancer patients into definable risk groups, but in practice the recording of TNM staging is often inaccurate, leading to the potential for widely divergent interpretations of recurrence risk. Of the three components of TNM staging, depth of tumor invasion (pT stage) determined at final histopathological analysis is the most reproducible. The pN stage can vary greatly, depending on the extent of the lymph node dissection, the surgeon's description of lymph node location, and the number of nodes removed and examined.

Recurrences after the complete resection of pT1 or pT2 stomach cancer usually occur after the first 36 months for pT1 tumors and 24 months for pT2 tumors, which is a reasonable disease-free interval in this disease. The possibility of resecting a local recurrence in this group can be viewed with cautious optimism. In contrast, the anastomotic recurrence following resection of a transmural pT3 or pT4 tumor is almost always a harbinger of more extensive peritoneal disease. Tumor depth of invasion is a well-recognized independent prognosticator of patient survival[6-9] with sufficient power to stand alone as a valid measure of risk recurrence. Moreover, the potential for intraobserver variability in determining pT stage is significantly less than is seen in the pN and final AJCC stages. The pT stage of the original tumor is a straightforward, practical measure of recurrence risk that should be applied to the postoperative follow-up algorithm of the patient with gastric cancer.

SURVEILLANCE OF LOW-RISK PATIENTS

Patients with early gastric cancers (defined as pT1 tumors) are at extremely low risk for early recurrence. In practice, these patients are often followed up closely for signs of local recurrence as recommended by Meropol and Smith, although in fact long-term follow-up in this group reveals a pattern of late hematogenous metastasis. Moreover, they are at risk for metachronous cancer in other organs[10] or for death from noncancerous causes. Sano et al.[11] reported the follow-up results of 1,475 patients with early gastric cancer treated at the National Cancer Center Hospital in Tokyo. Excluding operative deaths and deaths from noncurative operations, the death rate from recurrent disease was just 1.4%. Most patients died of either nonmalignant causes or other malignancies. Koga et al.[12] reported 101 late deaths after resection of early gastric cancer, with 63% attributable to nonmalignant causes. Of the remaining 38 deaths (37.4%), 20 were due to recurrent disease, 15 to primary cancers in other organs, and three to new gastric primaries in the residual stomach. Both studies reveal

Table 7-5 Percent of patients surviving 5 years after curative treatment of gastric cancer by AJCC stage

	STAGE					
	IA	IB	II	IIIA	IIIB	IV
American College of Surgeons Survey[4]	59	44	29	15	9	3
National Cancer Data Base[5]	*	43	37	*	18	10
German Gastric Carcinoma Study Group[1]	85	75	55	35	20	10
Memorial Sloan-Kettering Cancer Center†	90	86	49	25	12	‡

*Data not given for subgroups.
†Study period July 1, 1985, through July 1, 1995 (n = 730).
‡Too few patients.

a dominant pattern of hematogenous recurrence in which the liver, lung, and bone were common sites of involvement. Although some of these patients are cured after resection, the long disease-free interval even in Western patients with pT1 tumors negates the need for routine surveillance computed tomography.

The risk of dying from disease in patients with pT1 tumors does not begin to increase until 2 years after resection. Less than 8% of such patients at Memorial Sloan-Kettering Cancer Center died of disease within the first 36 months, with the earliest death occurring at 25 months. In most series 70% of patients with early gastric cancer survive more than 10 years, with most deaths occurring after 5 years.[13] During the first year the patient should be monitored every 3 months for signs and symptoms of anemia, nutritional deficiencies, and post-gastrectomy problems (Table 7-6). A computed tomographic scan should be obtained as a baseline at the first postoperative anniversary and then only as clinically indicated. Beyond the first year the frequency of follow-up visits can be lengthened to every 6 months and then yearly beyond the third year. Because of the low rate of local recurrence, it has been argued that endoscopy should be performed only if symptoms warrant it and should not be performed routinely. In the absence of sufficient data a policy of endoscopy every other year seems reasonable in Western populations, extrapolating from recommendations for colonoscopy in colon cancer.

SURVEILLANCE OF INTERMEDIATE-RISK PATIENTS

Patients with pT2 tumors have a recurrence risk intermediate to that seen in low-risk patients (pT1 tumors) and high-risk patients (pT3/4 tumors). The current definition of pT2 tumors includes lesions with limited invasion of the muscularis propria to those invading to within micrometers of the serosa, making this the most difficult group in which to predict outcome. At Memorial Sloan-Kettering Cancer Center the 5-year survival rate for this intermediate group after curative resection (R0) is greater than 50%, with about half of the disease-related deaths occurring within the first 2 years. These earlier deaths are typically from recurrences of deeper pT2 tumors involving the subserosa, which are more likely to have associated N1 or N2 metastases than lesions limited to the muscularis propria. When more data are available, an argument could be made to place pT2 lesions with invasion limited to the muscularis propria (pT2A) within the low-risk category and deeper pT2 lesions involving the subserosa (pT2B) within the high-risk group.[8]

The relevance of defining risk groups is clear when trying to decide who will benefit from being explored for recurrent disease. In an unpublished review of 114 patients admitted and treated for recurrent gastric cancer at Memorial Sloan-Kettering Cancer Center, 55% underwent resection. The most important factors predicting resectability were the original pT stage of the primary tumor and the presence of a recurrence confined to either the gastric remnant or anastomosis. Only patients whose initial tumor was confined to the mucosa or muscularis propria survived longer than 12 months. It seems reasonable that patients with a localized remnant or anastomotic recurrence should be explored for possible resection if the pT stage of the original lesion is T1 or T2 (that is, patients are in the low- or intermediate-risk group).

Pursuing a more intensive local surveillance program in the intermediate-risk patients may affect the natural history of the disease. The local failure rate is higher than in the low-risk group, while the risk of having concurrent occult distant disease (particularly for pT2A tumors) is much less than that seen in high-risk patients. For this reason the endoscopy schedule should be more frequent in the intermediate-risk group (Table 7-7) than in low-risk patients, in whom the yield will be low, and more frequent than in high-risk patients, in whom the risk of occult metastatic disease is high enough to preclude curative resection.

Table 7-6 Follow-up of patients with gastric cancer (low-risk patients): Memorial Sloan-Kettering Cancer Center

	YEAR				
	1	2	3	4	5
Office visit	4	2	1	1	1
Complete blood count	4	2	1	1	1
Multichannel blood tests*	4	2	1	1	1
Chest x-ray	1	1	1	1	1
Esophagogastroscopy	1	†	1	†	1
Abdominal computed tomography	1	†	†	†	†

*Includes aspartate aminotransferase, albumin, alkaline phosphatase, bilirubin, calcium, creatinine, glucose, lactic dehydrogenase, phosphorus, total protein, blood urea nitrogen, uric acid, sodium, potassium, chloride, and carbon dioxide.
†Performed as clinically indicated.

Table 7-7 Follow-up of patients with gastric cancer (intermediate-risk patients): Memorial Sloan-Kettering Cancer Center

	YEAR				
	1	2	3	4	5
Office visit	4	4	2	2	1
Complete blood count	4	4	2	2	1
Multichannel blood tests*	4	4	2	2	1
Chest x-ray	1	1	1	1	1
Esophagogastroscopy	1	1	1	1	1
Abdominal computed tomography	1	†	†	†	†

*Includes aspartate aminotransferase, albumin, alkaline phosphatase, bilirubin, calcium, creatinine, glucose, lactic dehydrogenase, phosphorus, total protein, blood urea nitrogen, uric acid, sodium, potassium, chloride, and carbon dioxide.
†Performed as clinically indicated.

Hepatic resection of metastases from gastric cancer rarely influences outcome, but long-term survival has been reported in highly selected groups of patients. Ochiai et al.[14] analyzed prognostic factors in 21 patients who underwent liver resection for metastatic gastric cancer. They found that the patients likely to benefit from hepatic resection of metachronous metastases had primary tumors with no serosal invasion and either no lymphatic or vascular invasion or only one of the two. While encouraging, these results apply to too few patients to justify routine computed tomography surveillance of asymptomatic patients with pT2 tumors.

SURVEILLANCE OF HIGH-RISK PATIENTS

Patients with resected pT3 or pT4 gastric cancer are at high risk for recurrence and their tumors are much less likely to be resectable when they do recur than are recurrences in the aforementioned risk groups. It is this advanced T stage group that accounts for more than two thirds of gastric cancer in the United States and that has most heavily influenced the way gastric cancer surveillance is performed. The 25% 5-year survival after R0 resection underscores the need for effective adjuvant chemotherapy for this disease. Recurrences are often in the form of peritoneal metastases distant from the dominant site of recurrence and are almost always multiple. Even when resection is possible, both disease-free survival and overall survival are brief. These patients are at extremely high risk for distant metastases, and while the recurrence may appear radiographically localized, it is often just the tip of the iceberg. Although physicians at Memorial Sloan-Kettering Cancer Center found recurrent tumors to be resectable in 55% of patients, most of the resections were for relief of symptoms and only 29% were complete resections of all gross and microscopic disease. In the experience of this institution, the median survival time of patients after resection of recurrence was only 3.9 months. Peritoneal metastasis was usually present. In contrast to patients with pT2 tumors, 60% to 70% of these high-risk patients die of disease within 2 years of resection.

Resection of recurrent disease is rarely curative in the high-risk group, so that the question of when to begin treatment becomes essential. In our view the decision should be based on the level of symptoms. Surgical resection for obstruction, bleeding, or pain can be effective. Moreover, accumulating data support the use of palliative chemotherapy over best supportive care in symptomatic patients, an approach that may also be more cost effective.[15] For high-risk patients, frequent follow-up for surveillance of treatable symptoms seems the most prudent approach (Table 7-8). The positive impact of frequent normal results of follow-up examinations can go a long way toward enhancing the quality of life.

Until more effective therapies for recurrent gastric cancer are developed, a risk-based approach should be considered preferable as outlined in Tables 7-6 to 7-8, recognizing the differences in recurrence patterns and in the disease-free interval among patients treated for gastric cancers of different pT stages.

Table 7-8 Follow-up of patients with gastric cancer (high-risk patients): Memorial Sloan-Kettering Cancer Center

	YEAR				
	1	2	3	4	5
Office visit	4	4	4	2	1
Complete blood count	4	4	4	2	1
Multichannel blood tests*	4	4	4	2	1
Chest x-ray	1	1	1	1	1
Abdominal computed tomography	1	†	†	†	†
Esophagogastroscopy	†	†	†	†	†

*Includes aspartate aminotransferase, albumin, alkaline phosphatase, bilirubin, calcium, creatinine, glucose, lactic dehydrogenase, phosphorus, total protein, blood urea nitrogen, uric acid, sodium, potassium, chloride, and carbon dioxide.
†Performed as clinically indicated.

REFERENCES

1. Roder JD, Bottcher K, Siewert JR, Busch R, Hermanek P, Meyer HJ. Prognostic factors in gastric carcinoma: results of the German Gastric Carcinoma Study 1992. Cancer 1993;72:2089-97.
2. Siewert JR, Bottcher K, Roder JD, Busch R, Hermanek P, Meyer HJ. Prognostic relevance of systematic lymph node dissection in gastric carcinoma: German Gastric Carcinoma Study Group. Br J Surg 1993;80:1015-8.
3. Sue-Ling HM, Johnston D, Martin IG, et al. Gastric cancer: a curable disease in Britain. Br Med J 1993;307:591-6.
4. Wanebo HJ, Kennedy BJ, Chmiel J, Steele G Jr, Winchester D, Osteen R. Cancer of the stomach: a patient care study by the American College of Surgeons. Ann Surg 1993;218:583-92.
5. Lawrence W Jr, Menck HR, Steele GD Jr, Winchester DP. The National Cancer Data Base report on gastric cancer. Cancer 1995;75:1734-44.
6. Kennedy BJ. TNM classification for stomach cancer. Cancer 1970;26:971-83.
7. Harrison JD, Fielding JW. Prognostic factors for gastric cancer influencing clinical practice. World J Surg 1995;19:496-500.
8. Hermanek P, Wittekind C. News of TNM and its use for classification of gastric cancer. World J Surg 1995;19:491-5.
9. Yu C, Levison DA, Dunn JA, et al. Pathological prognostic factors in the second British Stomach Cancer Group trial of adjuvant therapy in resectable gastric cancer. Br J Cancer 1995;71:1106-10.
10. Houghton PW, Mortensen NJ, Allan A, Williamson RC, Davies JD. Early gastric cancer: the case for long term surveillance. Br Med J 1985;291:305-8.
11. Sano T, Sasako M, Kinoshita T, Maruyama K. Recurrence of early gastric cancer: follow-up of 1475 patients and review of the Japanese literature. Cancer 1993;72:3174-8.
12. Koga S, Kaibara N, Tamura H, Nishidoi H, Kimura O. Cause of late postoperative death in patients with early gastric cancer with special reference to recurrence and the incidence of metachronous primary cancer in other organs. Surgery 1984;96:511-6.
13. Lawrence M, Shiu MH. Early gastric cancer: twenty-eight year experience. Ann Surg 1991;213:327-34.
14. Ochiai T, Sasako M, Mizuno S, et al. Hepatic resection for metastatic tumours from gastric cancer: analysis of prognostic factors. Br J Surg 1994;81:1175-8.
15. Glimelius B, Hoffman K, Graf W, et al. Cost-effectiveness of palliative chemotherapy in advanced gastrointestinal cancer. Ann Oncol 1995;6:267-74.

➢ COUNTERPOINT

National Cancer Center Hospital, Japan

TAKESHI SANO, MITSURU SASAKO, HITOSHI KATAI, TAIRA KINOSHITA, AND KEIICHI MARUYAMA

Despite a gradually decreasing incidence in Japan, gastric carcinoma is still the most common cancer for both sexes. The National Cancer Center Hospital in Tokyo treats 300 new patients with gastric carcinoma every year. The proportion of early gastric cancer has steadily increased and is now approaching 60%. However, there remains a constant proportion of patients with nonresectable tumors at the time of surgery. These trends are observed nationwide and have resulted in a relative decrease in the proportion of patients with curatively resected advanced tumors who are the target of close follow-up. In this counterpoint, recent treatment results and trends in surveillance strategies employed at the National Cancer Center Hospital are discussed.

EARLY GASTRIC CANCER

Surgical Results, Recurrence, and Treatment Options

Early gastric cancers or T1 carcinomas have traditionally been treated by gastrectomy with systematic lymphadenectomy. The follow-up records of 1,475 patients treated at the National Cancer Center Hospital between 1975 and 1989 were examined, and a recurrence rate of 1.4% was reported.[1] The hazard of death from other causes, including other malignancies, far exceeded that of disease recurrence (Figure 7-2). In a review of the Japanese literature on this subject, only 2% of patients with early gastric cancer were found to have recurrence after gastrectomy.

The most important risk factor for recurrence was lymph node involvement. Nearly 10% of patients with early gastric cancer and lymph node metastasis had a recurrence. Other, although less important, statistically significant factors were submucosal tumor invasion and histological type. Hematogenous metastasis, most frequently to the liver, was the predominant mode of recurrence. The mean survival period of those with recurrent disease was 40 months, and 23% died more than 5 years after surgery.

The very low recurrence rate of early gastric cancer, while confirming the effectiveness of radical gastrectomy, also suggests the possibility of introducing less invasive treatments. Based on meticulous pathological examination of more than 2,000 resected specimens of early gastric cancer, physicians at the National Cancer Center Hospital have established criteria for selecting tumors in which lymph node metastasis is not possible (Table 7-9). Endoscopic mucosal resection is now used to treat patients who satisfy all of these criteria.[2] Patients who benefit from endoscopic mucosal resection account for 15% of all patients with early gastric cancer, and

Table 7-9 Criteria for endoscopic mucosal resection at the National Cancer Center Hospital, Japan

Tumors must satisfy all of the following conditions:
1. Tumor invasion confined to the mucosa
2. Tumor diameter less than 3 cm
3. Macroscopically elevated (type 0-I or 0-IIa) or depressed (type 0-IIc) without peptic ulcerative changes
4. Histologically differentiated–type carcinoma (papillary, well- or moderately differentiated adenocarcinoma)

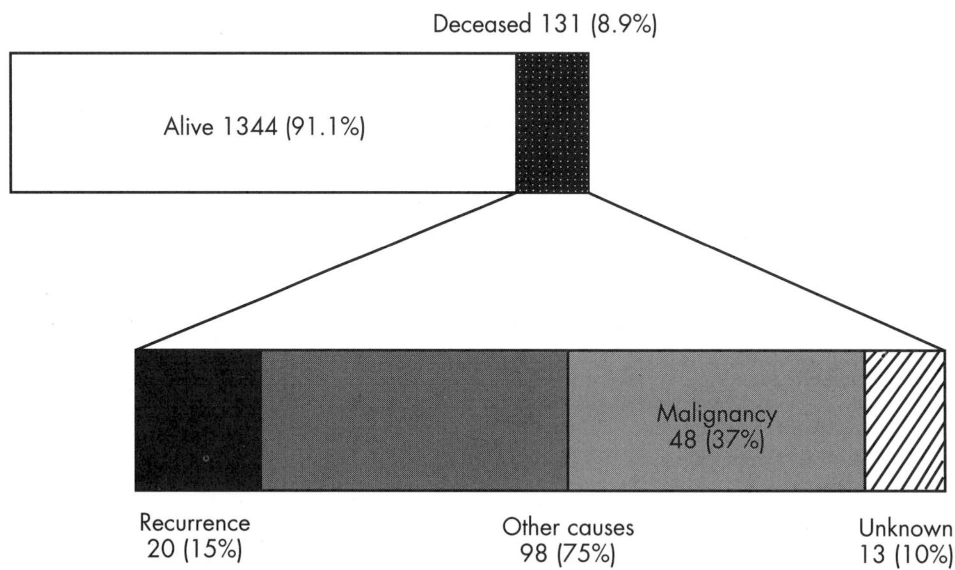

Figure 7-2 Outcomes of curative resection for early gastric cancer (1,475 cases treated at the National Cancer Center Hospital between 1975 and 1989). (Data from Sano T, Sasako M, Kinoshita T, et al. Cancer 1993;72:3174–8.)

this percentage is increasing. Curative wedge resections are also conducted for tumors that meet all of the above criteria except for histological type or tumor size. The use of endoscopic mucosal resection, as well as other treatment options for gastric cancer, is determined for each patient in a weekly consensus conference attended by diagnostic radiologists, endoscopists, and surgeons.

Follow-Up of Early Gastric Cancer

After gastrectomy with histological confirmation of node negativity the possibility of recurrence is remote. The current surveillance strategy at the National Cancer Center Hospital has evolved by consensus among surgeons, gastroenterologists, and medical oncologists and takes into account the favorable natural history of this patient subset. Patients with resected early gastric cancer are seen only once a year at the National Cancer Center Hospital (Table 7-10). In these annual checkups emphasis is placed on detecting other malignant diseases. Chest radiography, abdominal ultrasound, and blood tests, including tumor markers CEA and CA 19-9, are performed. Endoscopic follow-up of the remnant stomach and esophagus is performed every other year because recurrences and new primary lesions in the gastric stump are rare. A barium enema study to look for colorectal cancer, the most common cause of cancer death after early gastric cancer treatment, is recommended.

The finding of nodal metastases (which occur in 10% of all early gastric cancer) at surgery mandates closer follow-up. Ultrasonography is performed to detect hepatic and lymphatic metastases every 6 months for the first 3 years. For pN2 tumor cases, although the incidence is low in early gastric cancer, follow-up focuses on the detection of paraaortic nodal involvement. Computed tomography is the most reliable means of assessing the paraaortic lymph nodes noninvasively. When residual malignant foci in the paraaortic nodes are strongly suspected, additional lymphadenectomy in this area is advocated.

After endoscopic mucosal resection or surgical wedge resection, endoscopic surveillance of the entire gastric mucosa, including the primary site, plays a central role in follow-up. Endoscopy is performed at 1, 3, 6, and 12 months after endoscopic mucosal resection, and annually thereafter. Biopsy of the post-endoscopic mucosal resection scar is essential for detection of possible residual malignant foci. When local recurrence at the primary site is confirmed by biopsy, gastrectomy is the treatment of choice because the recurrent foci may already represent advanced cancer. When follow-up endoscopy finds a second lesion apart from the primary site and the lesion satisfies the aforementioned criteria, another endoscopic mucosal resection is considered. All these options and strategies are explained to the patient before endoscopic mucosal resection.

Follow-up of early gastric cancer should not be discontinued at postoperative year 5, since one fourth of patients with recurrence die more than 5 years after surgery. Death resulting from recurrence is, however, extremely rare after 8 years.

Table 7-10 Follow-up for patients with gastric cancer (early stage): National Cancer Center Hospital, Japan

	YEAR				
	1	2	3	4	5
Office visit	1	1	1	1	1
Chest x-ray	1	1	1	1	1
Abdominal ultrasound*	1	1	1	1	1
Liver function tests	1	1	1	1	1
Kidney function tests	1	1	1	1	1
Glucose	1	1	1	1	1
CEA	1	1	1	1	1
CA 19-9	1	1	1	1	1
Esophagogastroscopy†	1	0	1	0	1

CEA, Carcinoembryonic antigen.
*Performed biannually for the first 3 years if nodal metastases are found at surgery.
†Performed quarterly in year 1 and annually thereafter for patients after endoscopic mucosal resection or surgical wedge resection.

ADVANCED GASTRIC CANCER

Surgical Results and Patterns of Failure

Radical gastrectomy with systematic D2 lymphadenectomy has long been the gold standard of treatment for advanced gastric cancer in Japan. At the National Cancer Center Hospital more extensive nodal dissection, including clearance around the abdominal aorta, has been used in a limited number of cases over the past 10 years. An estimated 20% of tumors satisfying all the conditions listed in Table 7-11 have nodal metastases in the paraaortic area, and an estimated 30% of patients with cancer in the paraaortic nodes can be cured by extensive dissection.

The National Cancer Center Hospital results for 1,994 cases of T2 through T4 carcinomas in which curative resection was attempted have been published.[3] Two important prognostic factors were the depth of tumor invasion (T2 versus T3 and T4) and the extent of lymph node metastasis (Figure 7-3). The histological type of tumor was significantly related to the mode of recurrence. Peritoneal dissemination predominated in undifferentiated-type tumors (signet-ring cell, poorly differentiated, and mucinous carcinomas), while both hepatic and peritoneal metastases were frequently seen in differentiated-type tumors.

Table 7-11 Criteria for paraaortic lymph node dissection at the National Cancer Center Hospital, Japan

Tumors must satisfy all of the following conditions:

1. Macroscopically resectable without peritoneal or distant metastases
2. Negative intraoperative peritoneal lavage cytology
3. T3 or T4, or T1 or T2 associated with N2 lymph node metastasis

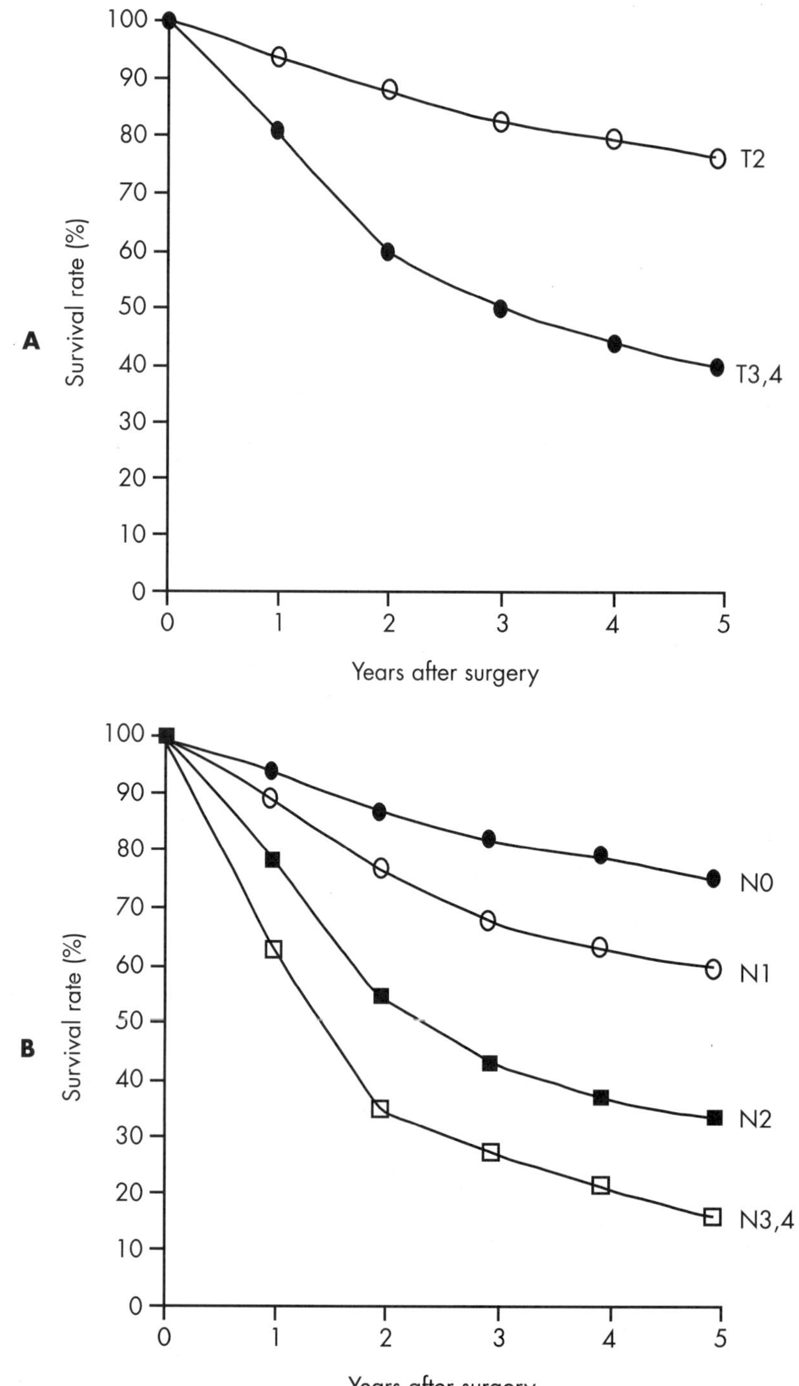

Figure 7-3 Survival curves after curative resection of advanced gastric cancer. **A**, According to serosal penetration. **B**, According to nodal status (by Japanese classification). (Data from the National Cancer Center Hospital, 1967-1986. In: Japanese Research Society for Gastric Cancer: Japanese classification of gastric carcinoma. Tokyo: Kanehara & Co, 1995.)

In sharp contrast to many reports from Western countries,[4] anastomotic or stump recurrence is uncommon among Japanese patients and the incidence has further decreased in recent decades. Preoperative assessment of tumor spread and frequent intraoperative confirmation of cut margins using frozen sections have contributed to this trend. Gastric bed or local recurrence is also uncommon after thorough clearance of regional lymph nodes and peritoneal disease.

Borrmann type 4 or linitis plastica tumors have specific features of recurrence. In addition to the peritoneal dissemi-

Table 7-12 Follow-up of patients with gastric cancer (advanced stage): National Cancer Center Hospital, Japan

	YEAR				
	1	2	3	4	5
Office visit	4	4	2	2	2
Liver function tests	2	2	2	2	2
Kidney function tests	2	2	2	2	2
Glucose	2	2	2	2	2
CEA	2	2	2	2	2
CA 19-9	2	2	2	2	2
Abdominal ultrasound or computed tomography*	2	2	2	2	2
Chest x-ray	2	2	1	1	1
Barium enema	0	1†	1	1	1
Esophagogastroscopy‡	0	1	0	1	0
Intravenous pyelography	§	§	§	§	§

CEA, Carcinoembryonic antigen.
*Computed tomography selected over ultrasound in patients with specific conditions such as suspected paraaortic node recurrence.
†Performed at 24 months.
‡Performed at 24 months and then every 2 years.
§Performed as indicated when retroperitoneal recurrence is suspected in diffuse-type tumors.

nation seen in other types, diffuse sclerosing spread in the retroperitoneal space often obstructs the urinary tracts or rectum. In female patients the ovaries can be involved without other apparent peritoneal disease. Diffuse bone marrow infiltration by signet-ring cell carcinoma is an uncommon but important form of metastasis. Liver metastasis rarely occurs in linitis plastica tumors.

In this series 60% of deaths from recurrence were in the first 2 years after surgery and late recurrence (after 5 years) accounted for less than 9%. In a few exceptional instances the patient died of recurrence after 10 years. All these very late-recurring tumors were undifferentiated-type adenocarcinomas.

Follow-Up of Advanced Gastric Cancer

The basic surveillance schedule for patients with advanced gastric cancer at the National Cancer Center Hospital is shown in Table 7-12. As with early gastric cancer, this represents a consensus among clinicians commonly treating these patients and is based on the analysis of tumor biology and treatment results. Follow-up methods and intervals are, however, highly individualized according to the pathological factors in each patient. Macroscopic tumor type, depth of invasion, nodal status, and histological type are important in determining strategy. For example, in exophytic T2 intestinal-type tumors, surveillance is focused on liver metastasis; in T3 diffuse-type tumors, peritoneal disease is the most probable pattern of failure irrespective of nodal status. Generally, patients return every 3 months for the first 2 years and then every 6 months until at least the end of the fifth year. Subsequently, annual checkups are recommended. Routine surveillance includes chest radiography, ultrasonography, computed tomography of the abdomen, and blood chemistry studies, including such tumor markers as CEA and CA 19-9.

Compared with the recommendations of Roswell Park Cancer Institute, emphasis is placed on the detection of peritoneal disease rather than stump or local recurrence. A barium enema is useful in detecting peritoneal involvement. Esophagogastroscopy is performed only every other year because recurrence or second primary occurrence in the gastric stump is rare.

Intravenous pyelography is ordered when retroperitoneal sclerosing recurrence is suspected in diffuse-type tumors. When available, outpatient bedside ultrasonography facilitates the detection of minimal ascites and mild hydronephrosis.

BENEFITS OF FOLLOW-UP

Although effective salvage therapy is frequently not possible, early detection of recurrence may be beneficial under limited conditions.

Survival Benefits

Surgical treatments for recurrent gastric carcinoma are nearly always for palliative purposes. While these procedures may enhance quality of life, they do not improve survival. The only exception is hepatic resection for liver metastases, which has resulted in long-term survival.[5] Unlike colorectal cancers, however, liver metastases from gastric carcinomas are frequently multiple and associated with concurrent peritoneal disease. Physicians at the National Cancer Center Hospital attempt hepatic resection for recurrent tumors when the primary gastric tumor does not penetrate the gastric serosa and histological study of the primary tumor does not reveal lymphatic or venous capillary invasion.

Systemic treatments, such as chemotherapy or immunotherapy, may be indicated for recurrent tumors. Survival benefits have yet to be demonstrated, however, and such therapies are still considered experimental. Theoretically, early detection of recurrence would allow systemic therapy to begin when tumor volume is minimal, thereby producing maximal therapeutic effects. However, the potential deterioration in a patient's quality of life caused by ineffective therapy must always be considered. The role of molecular biology in the follow-up of gastric cancer is not discussed in this counterpoint because the field has not developed enough to enable prediction of its role in the future.

Psychological Effects

When patients are fully informed of the risk of recurrence, particularly the decreasing risk over time, negative results of periodic checkups are reassuring. When asymptomatic recurrence is detected by surveillance examination, this early diagnosis allows the patient time to make important decisions about, and prepare for, further treatment.

REFERENCES

1. Sano T, Sasako M, Kinoshita T, et al. Recurrence of early gastric cancer: follow-up of 1475 patients and review of the Japanese literature. Cancer 1993;72:3174-8.
2. Sano T, Kobori O, Muto T. Lymph node metastasis from early gastric cancer: endoscopic resection of tumour. Br J Surg 1992;79:241-4.
3. Katai H, Maruyama K, Sasako M, et al. Mode of recurrence after gastric cancer surgery. Dig Surg 1994;11:99-103.
4. Landry J, Tepper JE, Wood WC, Moulton EO, Koerner F, Sullinger J. Patterns of failure following curative resection of gastric carcinoma. Int J Radiat Oncol Biol Phys 1990;19:1357-62.
5. Ochiai T, Sasako M, Mizuno S, et al. Hepatic resection for metastatic tumours from gastric cancer: analysis of prognostic factors. Br J Surg 1994;81:1175-8.
6. Japanese Research Society for Gastric Cancer. Japanese classification of gastric carcinoma. Tokyo: Kanehara & Co, 1995.

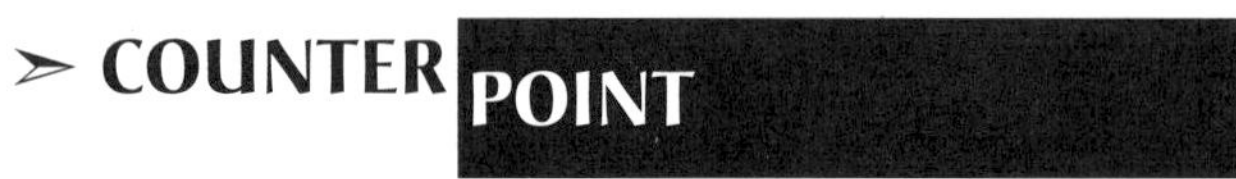

Royal Liverpool University Hospital, UK

Peter McCulloch

SURVEILLANCE: THE PROBLEM

There is no convincing evidence that following patients after potentially curative resection for gastric cancer does any good. It befits the British reputation for skeptical conservatism in cancer treatment to begin with that discouraging but accurate sentence. Despite this, follow-up of these patients is universally practiced by British surgeons. What is the background to this paradox?

Rationale for Surveillance

The reasons for continued follow-up after cancer surgery are (1) to allow accurate audit of the results of treatment, which may help in devising improvements; (2) to detect and treat problems resulting from the surgical procedure such as nutritional difficulties and motility disorders; (3) to detect and treat recurrent disease, whether by attempting eradication or by palliating symptoms; and (4) to provide psychological support and reassurance for the patient. Current practice in Great Britain is informed as much by tradition as by reason. Surgeons and cancer patients find the bond of trust formed by the act of operating, particularly when attempting cure, difficult to break when the cold dictates of logic suggest it. The traditional practice of regular clinic visits is largely a symbolic act of reaffirmed faith, principally fulfilling the fourth objective. In British practice, staging information is often far from complete, so the element of doubt regarding the prognosis remains large for many patients. For between one fourth and one half of those undergoing resection, however, the incurability of the lesion is already clear by the time of discharge from the hospital. In these cases the relationship between patient and surgeon is already changed and the need for frequent follow-up often more pressing, since symptoms of residual disease often need alleviation all too quickly.

Size and Nature of the Problem

In overall size the problem of follow-up for patients with gastric cancer is dwarfed by other major problems in British surgical oncology, such as carcinoma of the breast and colorectum. The disparity in incidence, which is about 2.5 times higher for the breast and 2.8 times higher for the large bowel, is enhanced in follow-up by the difference in prognosis. Despite recent improvements the prognosis for stomach cancer remains dismal in the United Kingdom, largely because of late diagnosis.[1,2] The percentage of patients offered curative resection has increased significantly over the last two decades and now stands at more than 50%,[3] but most surgeons still see a majority of patients with lesions in International Union Against Cancer stages III and IV.[3,4] The cohort of patients likely to return repeatedly to outpatient clinics is therefore a minority within a minority. The economic demands of this relatively small group are likely to be modest but nonetheless require justification. This is difficult to find, simply through the lack of good evidence that surveillance provides benefit.

A minority of previous studies suggest that intensive follow-up will allow resection of up to 20% of recurrent cancers thereby detected.[5-7] Most reports, however, indicate that successful resection with prolonged survival is extremely rare.[8-10] In one of the most careful Western studies, conducted in Heidelberg, Germany, Schlag et al.[11] reported on a 4-year experience of intensive surveillance using CEA, endoscopy, and ultrasound scanning in a population of 132 patients after potentially curative resection. Of 33 early relapses, 15 were detected by surveillance before symptoms ensued. Only one of these patients underwent further surgery, compared with six of the 18 with symptomatic recurrences. In none of the seven reoperations was resection of the recurrent tumor possible. Median survival time from the initial operation was not increased by the detection of asymptomatic recurrence (median 12 months) compared with symptomatic recurrence (median 14 months). Therefore it seems that although physicians may be able to detect 50% of recurrent disease before the patient, they rarely affect the outcome. The psychological effects of detecting asymptomatic disease and the costs of ineffective surveillance are powerful arguments against intensive investigations.

CURRENT PRACTICE AND PHILOSOPHY IN THE UNITED KINGDOM

The diagnosis of gastric cancer is made by various specialists in British practice, usually gastroenterologists, general physicians, geriatricians, and surgeons. Many patients are not referred for surgery (appropriately or not), are turned down for operation, or have a palliative procedure performed. For the cohort who do undergo potentially curative resection and who survive the postoperative period, follow-up in standard British practice emphasizes noninvasive tests.

Frequency of Attendance and Clinical Protocol

The high probability that recurrence, if it occurs, will manifest itself within 2 years of surgery[6] is reflected in the rapidly decreasing frequency of office visits after that time. For the first 2 years most surgeons request reviews every 3 months. This generally comprises a history, physical examination, and blood sampling for analysis of hemoglobin, vitamin B_{12}, folate, calcium, and transaminases. The history concentrates on appetite, weight, and symptoms referable to the upper gastrointestinal tract, particularly early satiety, vomiting, dysphagia, heartburn, epigastric pain on eating, and dumping. Physical examination permits some objective assessment of nutritional status and anemia and may detect recurrent disease directly by the presence of ascites, supraclavicular lymphadenopathy, or masses in the scar, drain site, liver, or epigastrium. Rectal examination occasionally provides the first evidence of peritoneal dissemination, which has a tendency to be most prominent in the pelvis.

Role of Gastroscopy

The sensitivity of clinical assessment after gastrectomy is considerably reduced by the frequency with which gastrectomy itself causes symptoms similar to those of tumor recurrence. The increased risk of development of a second cancer in the remaining gastric mucosa is also well known. For these reasons most British surgeons with a special interest in gastric cancer carry out regular gastroscopy in patients who have had a partial gastrectomy. The intervals vary, but an average would be 3-month intervals in the first year and 6-month intervals in the second and subsequent years. Different clinicians cease endoscopic follow-up at times varying between 2 and 10 years after surgery. In practice only a minority of disease-free patients actually receive this program because many are considered unfit for surgical intervention should a local recurrence or new primary cancer be discovered.

Role of Imaging Studies

Consideration of a patient's fitness for aggressive treatment is even more important in relation to the use of scanning modalities to detect metachronous nodal and hepatic metastases. The situations in which resection for hepatic metastasis is a reasonable option are far rarer for patients with gastric cancer than for those with colorectal disease. This is explained by the great tendency for gastric cancer to behave as a locoregional disease and to recur in either the regional nodes or the remnant stomach and associated tissues, with or without evidence of more distant spread. The rarity of isolated, blood-borne metastatic disease without recurrence locally, in the regional nodes, or in the peritoneum is well documented by postmortem, follow-up, and second-look laparotomy studies.[6,12-17] The list of metastatic sites and frequencies given by Meropol and Smith does not accurately reflect the realities of the metastatic mechanisms that are involved.

In effect, hematogenous metastasis occurs only to the liver, lung, and bone, except in very rare cases. The other forms of metastasis mentioned occur through a combination of direct invasion, lymphatic metastasis, and transcoelomic spread. The importance of the distinction is that isolated hematogenous metastasis, although rare, is potentially treatable by surgery or local radiation therapy but the other, more common forms are not. The criteria that would justify resection of hepatic metastasis are therefore rarely met in cases of gastric cancer.

British surgeons rarely if ever reoperate for nodal metastasis, as is done in some Japanese centers. For these reasons many British specialists do not carry out regular scanning but reserve it for the confirmation of suspected recurrence in patients who have significant new symptoms. Access to sophisticated imaging modalities has always been more limited in Great Britain than in the United States, which has led to the development of restrictive indications for their use. These comments do not apply to major university centers, but the vast majority of British patients with stomach cancer are not treated or followed up in such locations.

Ultrasound in the upper abdomen after surgery is both operator dependent and generally rather insensitive. Therefore computed tomography has been the scanning technique of choice. An important change in this situation has occurred with the introduction of endoscopic ultrasound techniques. These have the greatest accuracy of any currently available procedure in staging the depth of wall invasion by primary gastric cancers.[18,19] They are less accurate for the assessment of lymph node metastasis, suffering from the same problem as other scanning techniques in this regard. There is little or no reported experience in the use of endosonography as a surveillance tool after gastrectomy, but in principle it should have great potential for the early detection of locoregional recurrence.

The literature on computed tomography in the diagnosis and staging of primary stomach cancer shows that it has difficulty in visualizing the primary tumor accurately and in determining direct invasion of the liver or pancreas.[20] Detection of nodal metastasis is more satisfactory, with 51% to 80% accuracy,[21,22] but approximately 40% of patients with clinically normal nodes at laparotomy have some nodal deposits[23,24] and in 23% of those with apparent node involvement by computed tomography the pathological result is negative.[24] Computed tomography can differentiate normal from abnormal nodes only on the basis of size and is therefore unlikely to be any more accurate than surgical assessment. Computed tomography is about 70% accurate for the detection of liver metastasis, but this may have limited value in gastric cancer, since these lesions are usually just one part of a more general dissemination pattern. Computed tomography is of little value in the detection of peritoneal deposits because the size of individual deposits and their location at the plane between organs make them difficult to detect until a late stage. The likely value of computed tomography in surveillance after surgery for gastric cancer patients is therefore limited. It may detect ascites, hepatic metastases, or enlargement of regional nodes but is unlikely to detect unsuspected local recurrence or peritoneal disease. Will magnetic resonance imaging offer any advance? The evidence is scant, but it seems unlikely in view of the findings in other visceral cancers.

Role of Serum Tumor Markers

For much the same reasons as those related to imaging, most British specialists are skeptical of the value of regular estimation of serum CEA or CA 19-9 levels and would use these markers only when recurrence is already suspected, if at all. That only 60% to 70% of gastric cancers secrete CEA adds to the doubts generally felt over the value of this test. The increased sensitivity of CA 19-9 has not been proved to have great value. A recent multicenter observational study of the clinical value of CEA in colorectal cancer follow-up showed that the expected benefits are meager.[25] Aggressive treatment of recurrent colorectal cancer is increasing steadily in frequency and is producing clear survival benefits in a minority of patients, so these results may already be out of date. The chances of effective treatment for recurrent gastric cancer at present are at least as slim as those for colorectal cancer a decade ago. Byrne et al.[26] have described a marker protein (CA 72.4) with greater specificity and sensitivity than either CEA or CA 19-9 in gastric cancer, which may hold promise for the future once an effective treatment can be offered for patients with recurrence.[26] Until that time the main justification for marker studies is the accumulation of detailed information about their accuracy and failings. These data can also be used to evaluate newly introduced markers.

Influence of TNM Stage, Grade, and Other Prognostic Factors on Strategy

Whether the average curative resection in Britain is extensive enough is open to question. The influence of tumor stage and grade on follow-up protocol is limited in such cases, in which the lesion is usually T3. The presence of lymph node metastasis clearly has an adverse effect on prognosis, but its independent effect in a group of serosa-positive cases is not so marked as to indicate a different follow-up strategy. Histological grade is also ignored in the planning of surveillance protocols, since the therapeutic issues involved are likely to be the same regardless of grade. However, the patient with early gastric cancer is a different matter. This condition is being detected with increasing frequency in certain parts of the United Kingdom but generally remains rare. Contrary to the statement by Meropol and Smith, patients with early gastric cancer have an excellent chance of cure from surgical resection, with 5-year survival figures approaching 95% in many international series.[27-30] Naturally, such data influence follow-up strategies. There is a significantly increased risk of a second primary tumor, either in the remnant stomach or elsewhere.[31] Infrequent but prolonged follow-up by gastroscopy with a low threshold for the intensive investigation of symptoms is indicated. Since the overall mortality of survivors after radical resection for early gastric cancer is so low, economic implications of this kind of approach may need to be thought through carefully if the increased follow-up intensity noted by some British authors becomes more widespread. Studies are necessary to determine whether the early results of surveillance can be safely used to predict long-term outcome.

Influence of Adjuvant Therapy

Adjuvant therapy with both radiation therapy and chemotherapy has generally been disappointing in gastric cancer. With the exception of studies from the Gastrointestinal Tumor Study Group and one Spanish group, which reported a significant benefit from adjuvant mitomycin C,[32,33] all large, prospective, randomized trials against placebo or no treatment have shown little or no benefit. For a more detailed discussion see Bleiberg et al.[34] The Japanese approach to chemotherapy differs from that in the West principally in starting treatment very early after surgery, often within a week, and by the adjuvant use of nonspecific immunostimulants such as OK432. British surgeons do not favor any form of adjuvant treatment, which is supported by their oncologist and radiotherapist colleagues.

There is current interest in Great Britain in two trials of newer forms of adjuvant therapy that may have something to offer. A regimen based on infusional 5-fluorouracil with cisplatin and an anthracycline has shown promise in phase II studies in advanced disease.[35] A Japanese protocol using preoperative instillation of mitomycin C adsorbed onto activated carbon to produce a slow-release preparation is also being investigated in patients with T3 tumors.[36] Follow-up for patients in these studies is determined by protocol considerations.

Effect on Prognosis of Recurrence or Second Primary Tumors

Recurrence of any kind usually predicts rapid decline and death. The difference between median durations of disease-free and overall survival is approximately 4 months.[11] The rarity of aggressive intervention in British practice leaves physicians uncertain as to whether there are small subgroups whose survival and quality of life could be improved by further treatment. No effective treatment for peritoneal disease exists. Locoregional recurrence without significant disease elsewhere is unusual but occasionally responds to secondary surgery. Liver metastasis without multifocal recurrent or progressive disease is also rare in gastric cancer and, when technically resectable, is often rendered practically inoperable because of the general condition of the patient. Synchronous primary tumors are found in up to 12.5% of gastric cancers.[37] The development of second primary tumors, in contrast to locally recurrent tumors, is relatively rare in the remnant stomach, but their prognosis is more encouraging. The prognosis essentially depends on the stage of the new primary lesion.

PERSONAL VIEW

As in other countries, follow-up practice varies greatly within Great Britain. I take issue with Meropol and Smith's recommendations for detailed physical examination including rectal examination. The value of findings made on such routine examination is extremely low. Little therapeutic gain, for example, is found in diagnosing Blumer's shelf in an asymptomatic patient. Instead, a rather limited abdominal and cervical examination should by carried out, together with specific examination of any areas where the patient has complaints (Table 7-13). Regular serum chemistry measurements are not recommended, since no evidence of benefit has been found. Regular complete blood counts, on the other hand, are important because of the nutritional problems posed by gastrectomy. Endoscopy has value after total gastrectomy, particularly for cardia cancer. Computed tomography is most likely to be valuable for the detection of hepatic and nodal disease and should be used twice a year for the first 2 years. Regular CEA estimations are also performed if patients had an elevated preoperative level. At present the additional cost of CA 72.4 cannot be justified. As previous comments would suggest, these investigations are omitted when it appears that chemotherapy or further surgery is not an option if recurrence is found.

Table 7-13 Follow-up of patients with gastric cancer*: Royal Liverpool University Hospital, UK

	YEAR				
	1	2	3	4	5
Office visit†	4	4	3	3	3
Complete blood count	4	4	3	3	3
Serum iron level	4	4	3	3	3
Serum vitamin B_{12} level	4	4	3	3	3
Serum folic acid level	4	4	3	3	3
Albumin	4	4	3	3	3
CEA‡	3	3	2	2	2
Esophagogastroscopy	3	3	2	2	2
Abdominal computed tomography	2	2	1	1	1

*These are recommendations based on my practice. They reflect a personal interest in auditing the results of treatment and are therefore in excess of measures that can be justified on the grounds of clinical necessity. Many British surgeons use less intensive follow-up based on the arguments found in this text.
†Includes weight check.
‡Alternatively, serum CA 72.4 level can be measured.

FUTURE PROSPECTS

Place for Multicenter Trials

Trials of different surveillance methods are illogical in the absence of effective treatment for recurrence. In this respect the most important studies must be chemotherapy regimens suitable for the treatment of patients with recurrence. No prospect for surgical salvage without such effective adjuvant therapy is in sight. The potential of endoscopic ultrasonography and magnetic resonance imaging for detecting recurrence should be evaluated by comparison with current best practice techniques. Endoscopic ultrasound for detecting early locoregional recurrence should be studied initially in uncontrolled, prospective audits of the outcome in patients who could be considered for further aggressive treatment if early localized recurrence were detected. If these studies provide evidence of substantially improved sensitivity compared with the current methods of detecting locoregional recurrence, prospective, controlled trials may be appropriate to determine whether improvements in the quality or quantity of life can be achieved by aggressive treatment.

Role of Molecular Biology

As with other forms of cancer, advances in the understanding of the molecular biology of gastric cancer offer the prospect of improved diagnosis and staging and improved treatment. At the moment such progress appears far removed in this disease. Considerable work is being done on the molecular genetics of the cancer, and genes that apparently play a role in the growth pattern, progression, and malignant potential of the tumor have been identified. Whether this knowledge can be turned to clinical advantage remains uncertain. It is possible that the study of genes such as c-met and k-sam in the primary tumor will provide physicians with useful prognostic markers in the near future, but the use of gene therapy or antisense technology to inhibit malignant gastric tumors seems remote at present.

REFERENCES

1. Cunningham D, Hole D, Taggart DJ, Soukop M, Carter DC, McArdle CS. Evaluation of the prognostic factors in gastric cancer: the effect of chemotherapy on survival. Br J Surg 1987;74:715-20.
2. Akoh JA, Sedgwick DM, MacIntyre IM. Improving results in the treatment of gastric cancer: an 11 year audit. Br J Surg 1991;78:349-51.
3. Sue-Ling HM, Johnston D, Martin IG, et al. Gastric cancer: a curable disease in Britain. Br Med J 1993;307:591-6.
4. McCulloch P. Should general surgeons treat gastric cancer? An audit of practice and results, 1980-1985. Br J Surg 1994;81:417-20.
5. Metzger U, Kupffer A, Hollinger A, et al. Tumornachsorge beim radikal operierten magenkarzinom. Ein prospektive studie. In: Haring R, editor. Therapie des magenkarzinoms. Basel, Switzerland: Ed Medizin, 1984:433.
6. Papachristou DN, Fortner JG. Local recurrence of gastric adenocarcinomas after gastrectomy. J Surg Oncol 1981;18:47-53.
7. Suzuki H, Endo M, Nakayama K. A review of the five-year survival rate and clinicopathological factors in stomach cancer treated by surgery alone. Int Adv Surg Oncol 1983;6:271-308.
8. Allum WH, Hockey MS, Fielding JW. Gastric remnant recurrence—detection and implications for the management of gastric cancer. Clin Oncol 1984;10:333-9.
9. Viste A, Rygh AB, Soreide O. Cancer of the stomach—is a follow-up programme of any importance for the patient? Clin Oncol 1984;10:325-32.
10. Wenzl E, Feil W, Schliessel R. Wert einer konsequenten nachsorge beim magenkazinom. Weiner Klin Wschr 1987;12:420-3.
11. Schlag P, Buhl K, Herfarth C. Follow-up care and surgery for recurrent gastric cancer. In: Hotz J, Meyer HJ, Schmoll HJ, editors. Gastric carcinoma. Berlin: Springer-Verlag, 1989:98-104.

12. Warwick M. Analysis of 176 cases of carcinoma of the stomach submitted to autopsy. Ann Surg 1928;88:216-23.
13. Warren S. Studies on tumour metastasis IV: metastases of cancer of the stomach. N Engl J Med 1933;209:825-34.
14. Wisbeck WM, Becher EM, Russell AH. Adenocarcinoma of the stomach: autopsy observations with therapeutic implications for the radiation oncologist. Radiother Oncol 1986;7:13-8.
15. McNeer G, Vandenberg H Jr, Donn FY, Bowden L. A critical evaluation of subtotal gastrectomy for the cure of cancer of the stomach. Ann Surg 1951;134:2.
16. Thomson FB, Robins RE. Local recurrence following subtotal resection for gastric carcinoma. Surg Gynecol Obstet 1952;45:341-4.
17. Gunderson LL, Sosin H. Adenocarcinoma of the stomach: areas of failure in a reoperation series (second or symptomatic look): clinicopathological correlation and implications for adjuvant therapy. Int J Radiat Oncol Biol Phys 1982;8:1-11.
18. Nattermann C, Galbenu-Grunwald R, Nier H, Dancygier H. Endoscopic ultrasound in the TN staging of stomach cancer: a comparison with computerized tomography and conventional ultrasound. Z Gesamte Inn Med 1993;48:60-4.
19. Balbo G, Soldati T, De Paolis P, et al. Endoscopic and intraoperative ultrasonography in staging of stomach neoplasms. Minerva Chir 1992;47:1455-9.
20. Ziegler K, Sanft C, Zimmer T, et al. Comparison of computed tomography, endosonography, and intraoperative assessment in TN staging of gastric carcinoma. Gut 1993;34:604-10.
21. Moss AA, Schnyder P, Marks W, et al. Gastric adenocarcinoma: a comparison of the accuracy and economics of staging by computed tomography and surgery. Gastroenterology 1981;80:45-51.
22. Grote R, Meyer HJ, Milbradt H, Jahne J, Heintz P. Clinical staging of gastric cancer by ultrasound, computed tomography and magnetic resonance tomography. In: Hotz J, Meyer HJ, Schmoll HJ, editors. Gastric carcinoma. Berlin: Springer-Verlag, 1989:41-5.
23. Gunven P, Maruyama K, Okabayashi K, Sasako M, Kinoshita T. Non-ominous micrometastases of gastric cancer. Br J Surg 1991;78:352-4.
24. Madden MV, Price SK, Learmonth GM, Dent DM. Surgical staging of gastric carcinoma: sources and consequences of error. Br J Surg 1987;74:119-21.
25. Moertel CG, Fleming TR, MacDonald JS, Haller DG, Laurie JA, Tangen C. An evaluation of the carcinoembryonic antigen (CEA) test for monitoring patients with resected colon cancer. JAMA 1993;270:943-7.
26. Byrne DJ, Browning MC, Cushieri A. CA72-4: a new tumour marker for gastric cancer. Br J Surg 1990;77:1010-3.
27. Kitaoka H, Yoshikawa K, Hirota T, Itabashi M. Surgical treatment of early gastric cancer. Jpn J Clin Oncol 1984;14:283-93.
28. Oleagoitea JM, Echevarria A, Santidrian JI, Ulacia MA, Hernandez-Calvo J. Early gastric cancer. Br J Surg 1986;73:804-6.
29. Iriyama K, Asakawa T, Koike H, Nishiwake N, Suzuki H. Is extensive lymphadenectomy necessary for surgical treatment of intramucosal carcinoma of the stomach? Arch Surg 1989;124:309-11.
30. Sue-Ling HM, Martin I, Griffith J, et al. Early gastric cancer: 46 cases treated in one surgical department. Gut 1992;33:1318-22.
31. Koga S, Kaibara N, Tamura H, Nishidoi H, Kimura O. Cause of late postoperative death in patients with early gastric cancer, with special reference to recurrence and the incidence of metachronous primary cancer of other organs. Surgery 1984;96:511-6.
32. The Gastrointestinal Tumour Study Group. Controlled trial of adjuvant chemotherapy following curative resection of gastric cancer. Cancer 1982;49:1116-22.
33. Estape J, Grau JJ, Lcobendas F, et al. Mitomycin C as an adjuvant treatment to resected gastric cancer: a 10-year follow-up. Ann Surg 1991;213:219-21.
34. Bleiberg H, Gerard B, Deguiral P. Adjuvant therapy in resectable gastric cancer. Br J Cancer 1992;66:987-91.
35. Hickish TF, Cunningham D. Should induction chemotherapy be considered for all patients with gastric cancer? Eur J Surg Oncol 1994;20:185-6.
36. Hagiwara A, Takahashi T, Kojima O, et al. Prophylaxis with carbon-adsorbed mitomycin against peritoneal recurrence of gastric cancer. Lancet 1992;339:629-31.
37. Moreaux J, Bougaran J. Early gastric cancer: a 25 year surgical experience. Ann Surg 1993;217:347-55.

➢ COUNTER POINT

University of Washington Medical Center

MIKA N. SINANAN AND LORRIE A. LANGDALE

The difficulty in establishing an appropriate regimen for surveillance of patients with gastric adenocarcinoma reflects the insidious and aggressive natural history of this disease, both at original presentation and in patterns of recurrence. Although the incidence of gastric cancer is declining in the West, the majority of patients still have advanced disease at diagnosis. Resection of the primary cancer for cure is a reasonable option in less than 50% of patients, and even in this select group (Figure 7-1) locoregional or metastatic failure is common. Despite aggressive multimodality treatment, only 10% to 30% of patients with gastric cancer are ultimately cured.[1] The limited efficacy of current adjuvant chemotherapeutic regimens[2,3] emphasizes the importance of early diagnosis and complete surgical extirpation at the time of original resection if the quality of life and survival of these patients are to be improved.[4]

Meropol and Smith point out that only two groups of patients, those with isolated, mucosal recurrence after partial gastrectomy for stage I or II disease and those developing a second primary cancer,[5] are amenable to further potentially curative therapy. But these two groups represent only 10% to 15% of patients in whom recurrent disease develops.[3,6] In this small fraction of the at-risk population, treatable recurrent gastric cancer is rarely detectable except at endoscopy. The more diffuse or remote disease that characterizes 90% of recurrences is essentially incurable. Given these grim outcome statistics, physicians must carefully consider who might benefit from an aggressive follow-up protocol and target efforts toward that population.

Meropol and Smith propose a surveillance regimen for patients who initially undergo a complete resection of the primary disease. Their objectives are to improve survival in some patients and with earlier detection to enhance the benefits of palliative treatment in the rest. While they have recommended scaling the stringency of follow-up to the individual patient, being more or less aggressive depending on goals to which the patient and physician have explicitly agreed, their surveillance recommendations (Table 7-4) represent one extreme. Certainly, protocols similar to those they have outlined are widely used today. Unfortunately, like other physicians, they cannot find evidence for any benefit from the likely outcome of such a strategy in most patients, namely in the detection of asymptomatic but incurable recurrent disease.

Using charge estimates of $40 per laboratory test and chest radiograph and $500 for the average abdominopelvic computed tomographic scan (based on values from the University of Washington), these studies alone in the surveillance program outlined by Meropol and Smith would conservatively cost the patient annually $1,400 for the first 3 years, $780 for the subsequent 2 years, and $750 for the last 2 years. Over an 8-year period the total charges of such follow-up would reach $7,260 per patient or $72,600 per potentially resectable recurrence detected, exclusive of endoscopy, clinic, and professional fees. Such a strategy would probably also incur additional charges from false-positive studies, treatment of side effects from the studies, and additional evaluations, including biopsies. On confirmation of recurrence the patient and physician would then need to consider whether palliative treatment is indicated for an asymptomatic patient, potentially adding to the expense, risk, mental anguish, and morbidity of the surveillance strategy—all without proven benefit.

Given the preceding considerations, we propose an alternative surveillance strategy that is targeted at reassuring the asymptomatic patient and detecting potentially curable lesions (Table 7-14). Patients with stages 0 to III disease, who have undergone resection of all macroscopic disease but who also still have some portion of stomach remaining, are followed intensively for 2 years with endoscopy. Despite the grim prognosis, stage III patients are explicitly included so that any patient with a chance of cure is followed. In addition to regular office visits, which assure both patient and physician that new symptoms or signs are not neglected, endoscopic ultrasound is advocated as a key diagnostic study for potentially curable recurrent disease. The increasing availability of this technology and its value in the high-resolution inspection of both gastric remnant wall and adjacent lymph nodes hold great promise.[7,8]

Stage IV or residual macroscopic disease, except in patients enrolled in an adjuvant therapy research trial requiring specific surveillance, is best managed in a supportive fashion with an emphasis on early detection and palliation of symptoms. These patients should not be asked to endure costly and uncomfortable examinations that contribute minimally to the quality of their remaining time. Conversely, once symptoms develop, aggressive surgical palliation may be beneficial in some patients.[9,10] Very few patients with potentially curable recurrence would be missed by such a strategy, while all patients would continue to receive the close clinical support that, in the experience of the University of Washington Medical Center, is of greatest benefit during the follow-up period.

In their analysis Meropol and Smith focus on gastric adenocarcinoma. Follow-up strategies for neoplasms derived from other cell types (lymphoma, carcinoid, and leiomyosarcoma) often benefit from a more aggressive, radiographically oriented surveillance because of improved overall cure rate, survival duration, and a wider range of treatment options for recurrent disease.

Table 7-14 Follow-up of patients with gastric cancer: University of Washington Medical Center

	YEAR				
	1	2	3	4	5
Office visit	4*	3*	1	1	1
Esophagogastroscopy	2	2	0-1	0-1	0-1
Endoscopic ultrasound	2	1	†	†	†

*Frequency of office visits during the first and second years is designed to detect subtle new symptoms that might be indicative of recurrent disease.
†Performed as clinically indicated.

Primary gastric lymphoma constitutes less than 5% of gastric malignancies. Wide local excision to clear margins, the most common treatment in clinical stage IE and IIE patients, is achievable in 50% of patients and has been associated with a 70% to 90% 5-year survival rate that compares favorably with an overall 5-year survival rate of 50% to 60% with this disease.[11] Recurrences, usually detected in the first year of follow-up, are rarely localized to the gastric remnant, but even diffuse disease responds well to chemotherapy.[12,13] Thus early detection of recurrence is important. Surveillance strategies after curative partial gastrectomy for gastric lymphoma should include clinical evaluation, endoscopic studies, and computed tomography of the chest, abdomen, and pelvis on a regular schedule that is most intensive during the first 1 to 2 years after resection. The surveillance plan outlined in Table 7-4 with the addition of computed tomography of the chest for mediastinal recurrence and possibly endoscopic ultrasound for reasons outlined previously[14] seems appropriate. A number of prognostic factors have been identified that may help target follow-up to more appropriate groups.[15]

Gastric carcinoid tumors make up less than 1% of gastric neoplasms but up to 30% of carcinoids.[16] Carcinoids associated with hypertrophy of enterochromaffin cells from hypergastrinemia are generally benign, whereas sporadic carcinoids, those that develop under conditions of normal gastrin levels, are malignant lesions. These have the potential for local extension and metastasis, although they are generally less aggressive than gastric adenocarcinoma.[17] Resection to clear margins with regional lymphadenectomy offers the best chance of cure for these lesions, provided they are regionally localized.[16] Carcinoid syndrome occurs only after hepatic metastases have developed in these patients. After curative resection, options for screening for recurrence include serum and urine chemical markers,[17] endoscopy,[18] computed tomography of the abdomen,[19] and innovative radioisotopic scans that take advantage of the presence of somatostatin receptors found on the tumor cell surface.[20] Chemotherapy and ablative treatment of hepatic and other metastases (including resection in selected patients) may provide effective palliation for years and justify aggressive screening of asymptomatic patients.

Gastric leiomyosarcoma includes several cell types with differing malignant potential and management. For patients with the usual histological features of gastric leiomyosarcoma, surgical opinion has been mixed regarding the benefits of extended resection. Surgery is, however, still preferable to the relatively less effective chemotherapeutic options available. Recent reviews from the Mayo Clinic[21] and elsewhere[22] suggest that conservative resection to clear margins provides equivalent survival to more radical resection and preserves some portion of the stomach for better gastrointestinal function after surgery. In the Mayo Clinic series of 53 patients, 19 (36%) had recurrence and three (6%) had disease isolated to the gastric remnant. Two of the three achieved long-term, disease-free status by repeat resection to clear margins. Given the biological nature of this disease and a pattern of recurrence resembling gastric adenocarcinoma, a surveillance protocol similar to the one outlined in Table 7-14 seems appropriate.

Malignant epithelioid leiomyosarcoma, also termed leiomyoblastoma or epithelioid gastric stromal tumor, is a common variant of leiomyosarcoma that has a less aggressive behavior. These tumors are characterized by round cell morphology and variable anaplastic features that correlate with their malignant potential. Once clearly distinguished from benign variants, malignant lesions with low cytological grade benefit from local resection to clear margins (where feasible) and close follow-up, including radiographic studies and endoscopy (adding endoscopic ultrasonography) as outlined in Table 7-4.[23] Although tumors with high-grade histology usually recur and are generally fatal regardless of treatment, they should still be resected if possible to improve palliation and gain additional time.[24] Like patients with stage IV gastric adenocarcinoma, those with epithelioid leiomyosarcoma are unlikely to benefit from more than clinical surveillance after resection of the primary tumor.

REFERENCES

1. Boring CC, Squires TS, Tong T. Cancer statistics, 1992. CA Cancer J Clin 1992;42:19-38.
2. Hallissey MT, Dunn JA, Ward LC, Allum WH. The second British Stomach Cancer Group trial of adjuvant radiotherapy or chemotherapy in resectable gastric cancer: five-year follow-up. Lancet 1994;343:1309-12.
3. Tabuenca AD, Aitken DR, Ihde JK, Smith J, Garberoglio C. Factors influencing survival in advanced gastric cancer. Am Surg 1993; 59:855-9.
4. Buhl K, Schlag P, Herfarth C. Quality of life and functional results following different types of resection for gastric carcinoma. Eur J Surg Oncol 1990;16:404-9.

Table 7-15 Follow-up of patients with gastric cancer by institution

YEAR/PROGRAM	OFFICE VISIT	CBC	LFT	CXR	ABD CT	ESOPHG	MCBT
Year 1							
Memorial Sloan-Kettering I[a]	4	4		1	1	1	4[b]
Memorial Sloan-Kettering II[c]	4	4		1	1	1	4[b]
Memorial Sloan-Kettering III[d]	4	4		1	1	[e]	4[b]
Roswell Park	4	4	4	2	2	2	
Univ Washington	4[f]					2	
Japan: National Cancer Ctr I[g]	1		1	1		1[h]	
Japan: National Cancer Ctr II[j]	4		2	2	2[k]	[l]	
UK: Royal Liverpool[n]	4[o]	4			2	3	

ABD CT abdominal computed tomography
ABD US abdominal ultrasound
ALB albumin
B12 vitamin B_{12}
CBC complete blood count
CEA carcinoembryonic antigen
CXR chest x-ray
ENDO US endoscopic ultrasound
ESOPHG esophagogastroscopy
GLUC glucose
IVP intravenous pyelography
KFT kidney function test
LFT liver function tests
MCBT multichannel blood tests

5. Maehara Y, Tomisaki S, Emi Y, et al. Clinicopathological features of patients who died with second primary cancer after curative resection for gastric cancer. Anticancer Res 1995;15:1049-53.
6. Moriguchi S, Odaka T, Hayashi Y, et al. Death due to recurrence following curative resection of early gastric cancer depends on age of the patient. Br J Cancer 1991;64:555-8.
7. Rosch T, Lorenz R, Zenker K, et al. Local staging and assessment of resectability in carcinoma of the esophagus, stomach and duodenum by endoscopic ultrasonography. Gastrointest Endosc 1992;38:460-7.
8. Akahoshi K, Misawa T, Fujishima H, Chijiiwa Y, Nawata H. Regional lymph node metastasis in gastric cancer: evaluation with endoscopic US. Radiology 1992;182:559-64.
9. Ekbom GA, Gleysteen JJ. Gastric malignancy: resection for palliation. Surgery 1980;88:476-81.
10. Koga S, Kawaguchi H, Kishimoto H, et al. Therapeutic significance of noncurative gastrectomy for gastric cancer with liver metastasis. Am J Surg 1980;140:356-9.
11. Donohue JH, Habermann TM. The management of gastric lymphoma. Surg Oncol Clin North Am 1993;2:213-32.
12. Rosen CB, van Heerden JA, Martin JK Jr, Wold LE, Ilstrup DM. Is an aggressive surgical approach to the patient with gastric lymphoma warranted? Ann Surg 1987;205:634-40.
13. Jelic S, Kovcin V, Jovanovic V, Opric M, Milanovic N. Primary gastric non-Hodgkin's lymphoma localized to the gastric wall: no adjuvant treatment following radical surgery. Oncology 1994;51:270-2.
14. Fujishima H, Misawa T, Maruoka A, Chijiiwa Y, Sakai K, Nawata H. Staging and follow-up of primary gastric lymphoma by endoscopic ultrasonography. Am J Gastroenterol 1991;86:719-24.
15. Montalban C, Castrillo JM, Abraira V, et al. Gastric B-cell mucosa-associated lymphoid tissue (MALT) lymphoma: clinicopathological study and evaluation of the prognostic factors in 143 patients. Ann Oncol 1995;6:355-62.
16. Modlin IM, Gilligan CJ, Lawton GP, Tang LH, West AB, Darr U. Gastric carcinoids: the Yale experience. Arch Surg 1995;130:250-5.
17. Thomas RM, Baybick JH, Elsayed AM, Sobin LH. Gastric carcinoids: an immunohistochemical and clinicopathologic study of 104 patients. Cancer 1994;73:2053-8.
18. Nakamura S, Iida M, Yao T, Fujishima M. Endoscopic features of gastric carcinoids. Gastrointest Endosc 1991;37:535-8.
19. Picus D, Glazer HS, Levitt RG, Husband JE. Computed tomography of abdominal carcinoid tumors. AJR Am J Roentgenol 1984;143:581-4.
20. Hurst RD, Modlin IM. Use of radiolabeled somatostatin analogs in the identification of and treatment of somatostatin receptor-bearing tumors. Digestion 1993;54(Suppl 1):88-91.
21. Grant CS, Kim CH, Farrugia G, Zinsmeister A, Goellner JR. Gastric leiomyosarcoma: prognostic factors and surgical management. Arch Surg 1991;126:985-9.
22. McGrath PC, Neifeld JP, Lawrence W Jr, Kay S, Horsley JS 3d, Parker GA. Gastrointestinal sarcomas: analysis of prognostic factors. Ann Surg 1987;206:706-10.
23. Persson S, Kindblom LG, Angervall L, Tisell LE. Metastasizing gastric epithelioid leiomyosarcomas (leiomyoblastomas) in young individuals with long-term survival. Cancer 1992;70:721-32.
24. Lee JS, Nascimento AG, Farnell MB, Carney JA, Harmsen WS, Ilstrup DM. Epithelioid gastric stromal tumors (leiomyoblastomas): a study of fifty-five cases. Surgery 1995;118:653-60.

ABD US	KFT	GLUC	CEA	CA 19-9	BARIUM ENEMA	IVP	SERUM IRON, B_{12}, FOLIC ACID, ALB	ENDO US
								2
1[i]	1	1	1	1				
2[k]	2	2	2	2		[m]		
			3[p]				4	

a Low-risk patients.
b Includes aspartate aminotransferase, albumin, alkaline phosphatase, bilirubin, calcium, creatinine, glucose, lactic dehydrogenase, phosphorus, total protein, blood urea nitrogen, uric acid, sodium, potassium, chloride, and carbon dioxide.
c Intermediate-risk patients.
d High-risk patients.
e Performed as clinically indicated.
f Frequency of office visits during the first and second years is designed to detect subtle new symptoms that might be indicative of recurrent disease.
g Patients with early gastric cancer.
h Performed quarterly in year 1 and annually thereafter for patients after endoscopic mucosal resection or surgical wedge resection.
i Performed biannually for the first 3 years if nodal metastases are found at surgery.
j Patients with advanced gastric cancer.
k Computed tomography selected over ultrasound in patients with specific conditions such as suspected paraaortic node recurrence.
l Performed at 24 months and then every 2 years.
m Performed as indicated when retroperitoneal recurrence is suspected in diffuse-type tumors.
n These are recommendations based on this author's practice. They reflect a personal interest in auditing the results of treatment and are therefore in excess of measures that can be justified on the grounds of clinical necessity. Many British surgeons use less intensive follow-up based on the arguments found in this text.
o Includes weight check.
p Alternatively, serum CA 72.4 level can be measured.
q Performed at 24 months.

Continued.

Table 7-15 Follow-up of patients with gastric cancer by institution—cont'd

YEAR/PROGRAM	OFFICE VISIT	CBC	LFT	CXR	ABD CT	ESOPHG	MCBT
Year 2							
Memorial Sloan-Kettering I[a]	2	2		1	[e]	[e]	2[b]
Memorial Sloan-Kettering II[c]	4	4		1	[e]	1	4[b]
Memorial Sloan-Kettering III[d]	4	4		1	[e]	[e]	4[b]
Roswell Park	4	4	4	2	2	1	
Univ Washington	3[f]					2	
Japan: National Cancer Ctr I[g]	1		1	1		[h]	
Japan: National Cancer Ctr II[j]	4		2	2	2[k]	1[l]	
UK: Royal Liverpool[n]	4[o]	4			2	3	
Year 3							
Memorial Sloan-Kettering I[a]	1	1		1	[e]	1	1[b]
Memorial Sloan-Kettering II[c]	2	2		1	[e]	1	2[b]
Memorial Sloan-Kettering III[d]	4	4		1	[e]	[e]	4[b]
Roswell Park	4	4	4	2	2	1	
Univ Washington	1					0-1	
Japan: National Cancer Ctr I[g]	1		1	1		1[h]	1[b]
Japan: National Cancer Ctr II[j]	2		2	1	2[k]	[l]	
UK: Royal Liverpool[n]	3[o]	3			1	2	
Year 4							
Memorial Sloan-Kettering I[a]	1	1		1	[e]	[e]	1[b]
Memorial Sloan-Kettering II[c]	2	2		1	[e]	1	2[b]
Memorial Sloan-Kettering III[d]	2	2		1	[e]	[e]	2[b]
Roswell Park	3	3	3	1	1	1	
Univ Washington	1					0-1	
Japan: National Cancer Ctr I[g]	1		1	1		[h]	
Japan: National Cancer Ctr II[j]	2		2	1	2[k]	1[l]	
UK: Royal Liverpool[n]	3[o]	3			1	2	
Year 5							
Memorial Sloan-Kettering I[a]	1	1		1	[e]	1	1[b]
Memorial Sloan-Kettering II[c]	1	1		1	[e]	1	1[b]
Memorial Sloan-Kettering III[d]	1	1		1	[e]	[e]	1[b]
Roswell Park	3	3	3	1	1	1	
Univ Washington	1					0-1	
Japan: National Cancer Ctr I[g]	1		1	1		1[h]	
Japan: National Cancer Ctr II[j]	2		2	1	2[k]	[l]	
UK: Royal Liverpool[n]	3[o]	3			1	2	

ABD US	KFT	GLUC	CEA	CA 19-9	BARIUM ENEMA	IVP	SERUM IRON, B_{12}, FOLIC ACID, ALB	ENDO US
								1
1[i]	1	1	1	1				
2[k]	2	2	2	2	1[q]	[m]		
			3[p]				4	
								[e]
1[i]	1	1	1	1				
2[k]	2	2	2	2	1	[m]		
			2[p]				3	
								[e]
1[i]	1	1	1	1				
2[k]	2	2	2	2	1	[m]		
			2[p]				3	
								[e]
1[i]	1	1	1	1				
2[k]	2	2	2	2	1	[m]		
			2[p]				3	

CHAPTER 8

Colorectal Carcinoma

Roswell Park Cancer Institute

ETHEL L. MACINTOSH, MIGUEL A. RODRIGUEZ-BIGAS, AND NICHOLAS J. PETRELLI

Short-term follow-up of patients after surgery for colorectal carcinoma is mandatory to assess the initial result and deal with any problems that have arisen in relation to the operation. It is the value of long-term follow-up that has become controversial. The concept of continued clinical follow-up of patients after curative resection of colorectal cancer developed from the belief that patients with recurrent disease could undergo further surgery for potential cure.

In the 1950s Wangensteen[1] proposed second-look laparotomy as a method of potential cure for recurrent colon cancer. Although the morbidity and mortality of this approach were found to negate any potential benefit,[2] many physicians continue routine follow-up programs for colorectal cancer patients in hopes of improving outcomes. Current strategies range from patient education in the symptoms of early recurrence, with instructions to return if any of these develop, to a rigorous routine of frequent physical examinations, serological studies, and radiological investigations.

Colorectal carcinoma is the third leading cause of cancer death in the United States, accounting for approximately 10% of cancer deaths annually. In 1997 there will be an estimated 131,200 new colorectal cancer cases, with approximately 55,000 deaths.[3] The goals of surveillance after curative resection of colorectal carcinoma are to detect early recurrence when it is treatable for cure, to allow analysis of present treatment results, and to detect and treat metachronous colorectal polyps and carcinomas.

Approximately 30% to 44% of patients who have undergone curative colorectal resection have recurrence and die of the disease.[4,5] Most recurrences occur in patients with TNM stage II and III cancers, but patients with stage I lesions also have appreciable risk. Even patients with in situ carcinoma can have metachronous tumors.

Since a relatively small percentage of the population with colorectal cancer benefit from a program of follow-up, it is debated whether the cost of comprehensive follow-up yields comparable benefit. The psychological and medical burdens of follow-up include the distress caused by false-positive test results and that associated with early detection of an incurable recurrence, as well as the morbidity and mortality related to operations performed for other positive test results. From the economic evidence available, aggressive follow-up seems difficult to justify in patients after curative resection for colorectal cancer. The least expensive regimen, in which no follow-up program is instituted and the patient returns only when symptoms occur, also presents a problem because some patients operated on with early recurrence or metastatic disease can be cured.

CURRENT PRACTICE

How can the cost-effectiveness of follow-up schedules be optimized? Physicians must select which patients to follow, what tests to use, and how frequently to perform evaluations. The approach should be logical and based on knowledge of tumor biology. Follow-up should be designed to minimize costs and maximize gain. Aggressive, expensive follow-up protocols may be justified when the recurrent tumor is highly responsive to treatment modalities.

Accurate assessment of the primary tumor stage and identification of patients with occult metastatic disease at the time of initial surgery may be important. High-risk patients may benefit from an intensive follow-up regimen. In some patients overt liver metastases develop within a few months after surgery. In one study, occult hepatic metastases were missed in 16 of 70 patients (23%) undergoing curative resection of the primary tumor.[6] For these patients to be removed from routine follow-up and receive appropriate therapy, their tumors must be accurately staged at the time of initial surgery.

A recent survey of the members of the American Society of Colon and Rectal Surgeons (ASCRS) looked at patterns of follow-up in patients whose colon cancer was treated with potentially curative surgery.[7] The surgeons were asked to respond to a questionnaire regarding nine different follow-up measures, which included office visits, complete blood count, liver function tests, carcinoembryonic antigen (CEA), chest x-ray, bone scan, computed tomography, colonoscopy, and flexible sigmoidoscopy. Separate evaluations were sought for each tumor, nodes, metastases (TNM) stage (I, II, and III) and for each of the first 5 years after operation. Among the members of the ASCRS, office visits, complete blood count, liver function tests, CEA, and chest x-ray examination were used significantly more frequently for patients with TNM stage III. No significant differences across stages were found in the frequency of use of bone scan, computed tomography, colonoscopy, or sigmoidoscopy. The data in this report reflect the general uncertainty about the most appropriate program for postoperative colon cancer surveillance.

Most ASCRS surgeons examined postoperative patients every 3 to 6 months for the first 2 years after surgery, every 6 months during the third and fourth years, and annually thereafter. CEA measurement was the most frequently employed serological test and was generally performed at each office visit. In general, chest radiography and colonoscopy were performed annually. Routine computed tomography and bone scanning were also performed. Opinion regarding the utility of complete blood counts or liver function tests was not uniform. Few ASCRS surgeons discharged patients from follow-up after recovery from the initial procedure, instructing them to return only when symptoms occurred. Surprisingly, the intensity of follow-up did not vary markedly with pathological stage.

In 1987 Foster et al.[8] reported on the follow-up patterns of British surgeons in Wales and Southwest Great Britain. At that time 6% of British surgeons did not carry out routine follow-up and among the remaining 94% the methods used and the frequency of their use varied greatly.

In any follow-up program designed to detect early, asymptomatic recurrence after colorectal resection, the first 2 years would seem to be crucial, since 60% to 80% of recurrences become apparent within 2 years of the initial operation and 90% occur within 4 years. In most reports the median time to recurrence is approximately 22 months.[9-12] The rationale for most follow-up regimens is based on analysis of the timing and sites of likely recurrence. Programs to detect recurrence are typically most intensive during the first 2 years and less rigorous after 5 years. The risk of new primary metachronous lesions has been used to justify lifelong follow-up.

Ovaska et al.[13] examined the effectiveness of follow-up in detecting potentially curable recurrences after surgery in patients with colorectal carcinoma. Cancer recurrence and reoperations with curative intent were significantly more common in the intensively followed group. However, no significant difference in survival was found between the 368 patients enrolled in the intensive follow-up program and the 139 patients who dropped out or who received follow-up care elsewhere. A prospective, randomized study compared an intensive strategy after curative colorectal resection (consisting of physical examination, proctoscopy, blood chemistries, chest x-ray examination, and double-contrast barium enema performed every 3 months for the first 2 years, every 6 months for the following 2 years, and annually thereafter) to a program of the same tests done less frequently (at 3 months, 1 year, and annually thereafter).[13] No difference was found in the rate of curative reoperation when the more intensive follow-up regimen was compared with the less intensive follow-up regimen.

Steele[14] has proposed three possible follow-up schedules, depending on the practicing physician. For those who practice at facilities where protocols are unavailable either for adjuvant therapy or for recurrent cancer, a strategy of no follow-up is suggested unless the patient becomes symptomatic. For those practicing at facilities where a variety of experimental treatment plans are available, an intensive follow-up strategy is recommended. For those who find neither extreme acceptable, a simplified strategy partly dependent on patient symptoms has been proposed. There is no clear agreement nor any consensus among gastroenterologists, radiation oncologists, surgeons, and medical oncologists on the optimal follow-up program for patients with colorectal cancer after curative resection.

Table 8-1 Follow-up of patients with colorectal cancer: Roswell Park Cancer Institute

	YEAR				
	1	2	3	4	5
Office visit	4	4	4	3	3
Complete blood count	2	2	2	1	1
Liver function tests	2	2	2	1	1
CEA	2	2	2	1	1
Chest x-ray	1	1	2	1	0
Colonoscopy	2*	0	0	1	0
Pelvic computed tomography†	2	1	1	1	1
Abdominal computed tomography	1‡,§	1	1	1	1
Rectal ultrasound†	1	1	0	0	0

CEA, Carcinoembryonic antigen.
*Performed once preoperatively and once postoperatively. If there is no preoperative colonoscopy, performed at 6 and 12 months.
†Performed for patients with rectal cancer only.
‡For patients with colon cancer receiving adjuvant therapy, performed at 6 and 12 months.
§Performed twice in year 1 for patients with rectal cancer.

HISTORY AND PHYSICAL EXAMINATION

Since the majority of colorectal cancer recurrences are within the first 3 years after initial treatment, surveillance strategies should be more concentrated during this time period. Clinical evaluation using history and physical examination to elicit symptoms and signs of recurrent colorectal cancer should be performed every 3 months during the first 3 years, every 4 months during years 4 and 5, and annually thereafter (Table 8-1).

CARCINOEMBRYONIC ANTIGEN

CEA was first identified in colorectal cancer tissue in 1965 by Gold and Freedman.[15] CEA is measured with a variety of assays in different laboratories. In general, a serum level greater than 5 ng/ml is considered abnormal. Because interassay discordance is common, however, a single assay system must be used in the follow-up of an individual patient.

CEA levels are elevated in about 50% of patients with colorectal cancer before initial surgery. After curative resection the CEA level should fall to normal levels in 4 to 8 weeks.[16] If this does not occur, incomplete resection is likely. A sustained and progressive rise in CEA levels after colorectal resection is strong evidence for recurrent disease. Unfortunately, 20% to 30% of patients with recurrent disease do not have an elevated CEA level.[17] It has been suggested that CEA is immunogenic, which can result in CEA-anti-CEA complex formation.[18] The presence of these complexes may account in part for spurious low or normal CEA levels in patients with recurrent disease.

The sensitivity and specificity of CEA in detecting recurrent colorectal cancer are approximately 80% and 70%, respectively. In a prospective follow-up study of patients with colon cancer, an elevated CEA level was the initial positive test leading to a diagnosis of recurrent cancer in 67% of patients.[19]

The utility of postoperative monitoring of CEA levels after a potentially curative colorectal cancer resection in patients who had a normal serum CEA before initial surgery has been debated. In 114 node-positive colorectal cancer patients in whom the preoperative CEA was less than 5 ng/ml, CEA, as detected by immunohistochemistry in the primary tumor and lymph nodes, was positive in 109 patients (95.6%).[20] Four of the five patients with negative CEA stains had poorly differentiated tumors. In the follow-up period, 32 patients had recurrences. Forty-four percent of these patients (14 of 32), three of whom had poorly differentiated primary tumors, had a CEA level greater than 5 ng/ml. This suggests that serum CEA is a useful marker in the detection of recurrent disease, despite normal preoperative values.

Armitage et al.[17] have suggested that CEA monitoring is useful only in patients with positive CEA immunohistochemical staining of the original tumor. If this is true, the spectrum of patients followed up with serial CEA levels may ultimately be narrowed to those whose tumors stain positive for CEA.

Several authors have attempted to correlate tumor ploidy with CEA levels.[21-23] Goslin et al.[21] showed that aneuploid carcinomas had a greater CEA output than those with a diploid pattern. In 100 patients, 63 with aneuploid tumors and 37 with diploid tumors, Rognum[23] reported that preoperative CEA levels were significantly higher in the aneuploid group. Subsequently, 14 of 17 recurrences in the aneuploid group were preceded by a rise in CEA, whereas this was seen in only one of eight patients in the diploid group. All patients with aneuploid tumors who had an elevated preoperative CEA level had an elevated CEA level with recurrence. In this report the median time between plasma CEA elevation and clinically manifest recurrence was 5 months in the aneuploid group, suggesting that CEA is a sensitive indicator of relapse in patients with aneuploid tumors but not diploid tumors. Rognum suggested that the determination of serial CEA levels in all patients who had an elevated preoperative CEA or who show an aneuploid tumor pattern will permit the prediction of 60% of tumor recurrences approximately 4 months before overt clinical presentation.

Serial monitoring of CEA levels clearly detects recurrence in some patients earlier than by other diagnostic means, but most patients with recurrence are not treatable for cure. How CEA levels are used to diagnose recurrent disease varies among physicians. Some use a cutoff level on one determination, whereas others require two or three consecutive elevations above a particular value, and still others calculate the slope of the rise to suggest recurrence.[24] Most agree that a single elevated CEA in the postoperative period after potentially curative resection is unreliable in the detection of recurrent disease, and most also agree that a progressively rising CEA titer above an established postoperative baseline generally suggests recurrence. At present there is no accepted standard frequency interval for CEA testing. At Roswell Park Cancer Institute we obtain CEA titers at 6-month intervals for up to 5 years after initial treatment and annually thereafter. However, there is no evidence that survival is improved. In a patient with a single elevated CEA level, a second serum sample should be drawn within 1 month of the initial abnormal CEA before any further aggressive workup. Serum CEA levels are more likely to be elevated when visceral metastases are present than when the recurrence is limited to locoregional areas. Smokers have somewhat higher CEA levels than nonsmokers, and CEA elevations can occur in several benign conditions, such as cirrhosis, inflammatory bowel disease, peptic ulcer disease, pancreatitis, diverticulitis, and renal failure,[25] and after 5-fluorouracil (5-FU) and levamisole adjuvant therapy.[26]

If recurrent or metastatic disease develops, surgical resection offers the only hope of cure. August et al.[4] estimate that approximately 20% of patients with recurrent disease are potentially curable by further surgery and of these only 30% will survive 5 years or more. A number of patients with isolated hepatic metastases from colorectal cancer are amenable to hepatic resection with 5-year survival rates of 20% to 25%.[25,27] In some of these patients metastasis is detected initially on the basis of a serial rise in CEA levels.

Martin et al.[28] published their experience with CEA-directed, second-look laparotomy based on two consecutive elevated CEA levels defined as greater than 7.5 ng/ml. In a prospective study over an 8-year period, 124 asymptomatic patients who had serum CEA levels measured at 4- to 6-week intervals underwent second-look surgery. These patients had surgery if no extraabdominal source was identified on workup to explain an elevated CEA level. The mean time to performance of surgery after the initial elevated CEA was 2.5 months. In the 124 patients undergoing second-look laparotomy, the resectability rate was 60.5%, with a 5-year survival rate of 31%. In this study the long-term cure rate was significantly higher if the second operation was done before the CEA level exceeded 10 ng/ml. These results have not been duplicated in other reports. A possible explanation for this may be the rigorous schedule of CEA monitoring followed by Martin's group.

Kievit et al.[29] have challenged the use of CEA to monitor patients after curative resection of colorectal carcinoma.

Based on a Markov analysis they calculated that the influence of CEA on quality-adjusted life expectancy is minimal. They concluded that CEA monitoring should not be performed because the costs of follow-up, subsequent evaluation, and reoperation based on an elevated CEA level can be quite high, whereas the benefits in terms of days of extended life expectancy may be minimal.

Moertel et al.[26] also evaluated the use of CEA monitoring and concluded that CEA testing was not cost effective. They reanalyzed the results of a study designed to determine the value of adjuvant therapy in patients with stage II and III colon cancer. These patients had postoperative CEA levels measured according to the physician's preference and on no standardized schedule. A CEA value greater than 5 ng/ml was considered abnormal. Eighty-four percent of 1,217 patients had CEA monitoring. Of note was that only 50% of patients had preoperative CEA levels measured. The frequency of CEA monitoring ranged from one assay to as many as 39 assays per patient. Eighty percent of the monitored patients had a CEA level determined at more than half of 14 scheduled evaluations. The false-negative rate (recurrent cancer with a normal CEA level) was 41%. The sensitivity of CEA levels was highest with recurrences in the liver and retroperitoneum (78% and 75%, respectively), whereas it was much lower for lung or peritoneal surface recurrences (42% and 46%, respectively). In this analysis, abdominal explorations performed solely for elevated CEA levels in 29 patients with no other abnormal diagnostic tests (chest x-ray, liver function tests, computed tomography, colonoscopy) were rarely helpful. This is unlike the Ohio State experience, in which resections for cure were performed in four of 29 patients, of whom only one (3.4%) was still alive and disease free after 5 years. Moertel et al.[26] concluded that CEA monitoring infrequently contributed to colorectal cancer cures. However, many have criticized the trial. For example, it is unknown why some patients were monitored for serial CEA levels while others were not, thus weakening the conclusions. Serum CEA levels would be more valuable if efficient treatment of recurrent cancer were available or if long-term follow-up after second-look operations showed improved survival rates. The prospective, randomized, multicenter trial devised by Northover[30] in Great Britain in 1983 under the auspices of the National Institutes of Health and the Cancer Research Campaign promises to address the issue of whether earlier diagnosis of recurrent disease confers any survival benefit.

OTHER TUMOR MARKERS

Many investigators have compared other tumor markers with CEA. Tumor markers such as TAG-72 and carbohydrate antigen CA 19-9 have been evaluated in patients with colorectal cancer.[31-33] TAG-72 is a high-molecular-weight, mucinlike glycoprotein expressed in approximately 40% of patients with malignant colorectal disease at levels considered positive (greater than 6 units per milliliter). Currently there is no approved serological test for TAG-72 antigen in the United States.

In patients with recurrence and normal CEA levels, TAG-72 was increased in 30%, suggesting that TAG-72 could complement CEA monitoring to increase yield.[31] Guadagni et al.[32] monitored TAG-72 and CEA levels in 51 patients after resection. In the 23 patients in whom recurrence developed, the use of TAG-72 plus CEA increased the rate of early detection by 9%. The TAG-72 level is elevated in few patients with benign disease (3%), whereas 10% to 15% of patients with benign disease have an elevated CEA titer. Therefore TAG-72 may prove useful in enhancing the specificity of elevated CEA levels.

The tumor marker CA 19-9 has also been compared with CEA. The evidence is conflicting, but generally CA 19-9 is much less sensitive than CEA (38% versus 84%) and does not provide any more information than monitoring of CEA levels alone.[33]

MONOCLONAL ANTIBODIES

Radiolabeled antibodies have been used to localize colon carcinoma since 1973, when Primus et al.[34] injected a polyclonal antibody into hamsters bearing subcutaneous human colon cancer xenografts. In 1978 the first successful clinical imaging study of anti-CEA antibodies in humans was reported. Mach et al.[35] published the first report of antibody imaging in cancer patients using monoclonal anti-CEA antibodies in 1981. A variety of clinical studies have demonstrated the efficacy of radiolabeled monoclonal antibodies to detect human colorectal carcinoma. Monoclonal antibodies against a variety of tumor-associated antigens can be conjugated to various radionuclides and used to localize tumors in vivo. Promising anti-CEA monoclonal antibodies include ZCE-025, IMMU-4 (NP-4), T84.66, and A5B7. Other non-anti-CEA monoclonal antibodies have been developed that recognize other antigens: 17-1A, 250-30.6, 1A3, and B72.3.

No single antigen is an ideal tumor marker. CEA is the best-characterized tumor-associated antigen. Although most of the colorectal antigens are typically found in 75% to 95% of colon cancer specimens, significant heterogeneity of antigen expression occurs within different sites of tumor in the same patient.[36]

Radioimmunoscintigraphy using radiolabeled monoclonal antibodies against colorectal carcinoma has been employed in tumor localization in patients with rising CEA after curative resection when conventional tests do not reveal a site of recurrence, in preoperative evaluation of patients with hepatic metastases to determine presence of extrahepatic disease, and in intraoperative localization of disease with use of a hand-held gamma detection probe.

Many phase I and II clinical imaging studies have been performed by using radioimmunoscintigraphy to localize both primary and recurrent colorectal cancer. These studies have used anti-CEA and TAG-72 antibodies labeled with various radioisotopes, such as In-111, Tc-99c, and I-131. The overall sensitivity for detection of colorectal cancer has ranged from 60% to 90%.[37,38]

In the initial studies a positive outcome was recorded if any known sites of cancer were imaged. However, it is important to compare the ability of these scans to image tumor sites within the liver and extrahepatic sites individually. For accurate assessment of the sensitivity and specificity of these studies, all suspected lesions must be histologically confirmed.

In-111-labeled antibodies have successfully localized primary (82%) and extrahepatic (44%) tumor sites, regardless of the monoclonal antibody or antigen.[39] Localization of hepatic lesions (18%) is limited because of the marked, nonspecific uptake of the In-111-labeled antigen-antibody complexes in normal liver parenchyma.[39] In-111-labeled antibody also accumulates in the colon, but this can be minimized by the use of laxatives. Technetium-labeled antibodies have successfully localized a high percentage of primary (95%), extrahepatic (80%), and hepatic (71%) tumors.[39]

Beatty et al.[40] evaluated the effect of radioimmunoscintigraphy on patient management in a series of 114 patients with colorectal cancer. This test resulted in a change in management in only 4% of 48 patients with primary tumors. In patients with suspected recurrent colorectal cancer (hepatic metastases, n = 45) or occult recurrences with rising CEA (n = 20), however, the scan led to an additional, previously unplanned surgical procedure in 19 patients (29%). Radioimmunoscintigraphy seems to offer the potential for improvement in the clinical management of a significant number of patients with recurrent colorectal cancer. At present, monoclonal antibody–based tests are still undergoing clinical evaluation. Most patients having this investigation will continue to undergo laparotomy to determine resectability. Radioimmunoguided surgery may be used in these patients. A large, multicenter trial was conducted in patients with primary or suspected recurrent colorectal cancer (rising CEA levels) who underwent surgery in which B72.3 and a hand-held gamma detector were used for intraoperative tumor detection.[41] Tumor labeling was noted in 84% of patients. Occult tumor was identified in 18% of evaluable patients, and changes in operative strategy occurred in 43% of patients. B72.3 appears to be an adequate antibody for use in radioimmunoguided surgery. Other antibodies and fragments are being investigated to improve results.

Moffat et al.[38] conducted a prospective trial comparing radioimmunodetection with IMMU-4 (a murine anti-CEA monoclonal antibody) Tc-99-labeled Fab' fragments against conventional imaging in 35 colorectal cancer patients. Surgical corroboration of findings was obtained in 26 patients. Results were analyzed for each patient and each anatomical site (liver, extrahepatic abdomen, and pelvis). Fifteen patients had evidence of tumor by conventional diagnostic modalities (four with stage IV disease at surgery, five with primary colorectal cancer, and six with disease recurrence), whereas 11 patients had rising CEA levels with no clinical or radiological evidence of recurrence or metastatic disease after curative colorectal resection. Computed tomography was somewhat superior to radioimmunodetection with IMMU-4 in detecting liver metastases (sensitivity of 86.4% versus 72.7%). Radioimmunodetection was far superior in detecting extrahepatic abdominal and pelvic lesions (sensitivities of 90% and 95.2% versus 20% and 40%, respectively). IMMU-4 failed to image pulmonary metastases in five affected patients. IMMU-4 scanning resulted in 10 false-positive scans: six because of late excretion of radioactivity in the colon, two reconstruction artifacts on single photon emission computed tomography, and two with excreted activity accumulating in the bladder. In a prospective study Lechner et al.[42] diagnosed 12 of 12 cases of recurrent colorectal cancer using Tc-99 IMMU-4. In a blinded prospective study by Rodriguez-Bigas et al.[43] comparing computed tomography and radioimmunodetection using Tc-99m-IMMU-4 in 34 patients with primary or metastatic colorectal adenocarcinoma, radioimmunodetection was found to contribute additional information that could have altered treatment in 10 patients.

Doerr et al.[37] studied 18 patients, all with surgical confirmation of disease with In-111 CYT-103 (Oncoscint CR/OV) scanning. All patients had elevated CEA levels. All nine patients with occult disease had surgically confirmed disease at exploration after immunoscintigraphy. Immunoscintigraphy was found to be superior to computed tomography in the detection of pelvic and extrahepatic recurrences (100% versus 43%). Liver metastases were identified equally by both imaging modalities. The In-111 CYT-103 scan findings influenced management in 10 of 18 patients (55%).

Corman et al.[44] reported on a multicenter trial using In-111-Satumomab scans involving 103 patients: 46 with rising CEA and a negative diagnostic evaluation, 29 with known recurrence presumed to be isolated and resectable, and 28 patients with equivocal diagnostic evaluations. The test sensitivity was 73% in patients with confirmed tumor. Results were said to be negative for 35 patients with no evidence of disease, although absence of disease was not confirmed by laparotomy and histopathological analysis. Occult disease was detected in 18 patients. This immunoscintigraphic technique was deemed helpful in the management of 45 patients (44%) and provided information unavailable from other diagnostic modalities.

Intraoperative scanning for localization has generally shown a higher lesion sensitivity than the antibody scan or computed tomography. Martin et al.,[45] using a variety of I-125-labeled antibodies, reported an overall lesion sensitivity of 82% in 37 patients with primary or recurrent colorectal carcinoma. Kuhn et al.[46] found a high lesion sensitivity with In-111-labeled MAb in patients with recurrent colorectal cancer. With the hand-held gamma detection probe 85% of intraabdominal lesions were identified, compared with 80% with abdominal exploration, 30% with computed tomography, and 50% with the preoperative antibody scan. Kuhn et al. reported a change in management in three of 11 patients with recurrent colorectal cancer. Martin et al.[45] found a change in clinical management in 26% of patients with recurrent colon cancer. The intraoperative probe offers the potential for affecting clinical management in a substantial number of patients with primary and recurrent colorectal carcinoma.

Radioimmunoscintigraphy has several drawbacks.[47] The quality and success of imaging depend on the experience and interest of the person interpreting the scans. Some patients with colorectal cancer do not express the antigen to which the diagnostic antibody is directed and thus do not demonstrate tumor localization. A human antimouse antibody (HAMA) response develops in a percentage of patients after initial exposure (50% after the second injection) to murine immunoglobulin. The presence of HAMA may provoke allergic responses, including anaphylaxis, with serial imaging tests. High titers of HAMA may compromise imaging because of the more rapid clearance of the infused radioimmunoconjugate and can interfere with the standard laboratory assay of CEA, causing artifactually increasing or decreasing CEA levels. For accurate determination of CEA level, steps should be taken to remove HAMA from the CEA assay in patients who have been exposed to murine monoclonal antibody. The Fc portion of the intact murine immunoglobulin is particularly immunogenic. The use of murine MAb $F(ab')^2$ and Fab' fragments has reduced the incidence of HAMA.[38] Finally, the outcome of false-positive studies in terms of risk to the patient for additional unnecessary procedures and for the cost of additional diagnostic tests is not well characterized. It is critical to the clinical use of radioimmunodetection that the false-positive rate be low. Urinary catheterization immediately before radioimmunodetection and appropriate bowel preparation with laxatives are essential to minimize the false-positive yield.

Immunoscintigraphy is a disease-specific imaging modality that has become available for use in clinical nuclear medicine facilities. By providing information that complements the findings of standard diagnostic tests, this new technique may help in the design of follow-up strategies.

CONSENSUS STATEMENT IN COLORECTAL CANCER FOLLOW-UP

The American Gastroenterological Association developed a consensus statement dealing with the follow-up of patients with colorectal cancer by reviewing the literature and asking the opinion of several experts.[48] Their analysis suggested that history, physical examination, fecal occult blood test, and liver function tests be performed every 3 to 6 months for 2 years, every 6 to 12 months for the succeeding 2 years, and annually thereafter. They did not recommend varying the intensity of follow-up by TNM stage.

The National Institutes of Health, in a consensus statement in 1981, concluded that the regular and sequential assay of plasma CEA level is the best available noninvasive technique for detecting colorectal cancer relapse in the postoperative surveillance of patients.[49] The Standards Task Force of ASCRS recently published its recommendations for endoscopic follow-up of colorectal cancer patients after curative resection.[50] If the colon was cleared before operation, ASCRS suggested colonoscopy or barium enema at one year postoperatively and then every 3 years. Otherwise, colonoscopy or barium enema was recommended within 6 months of operation and then every 3 years. For the patient with a rectal anastomosis, endoscopic examination of the anastomosis was recommended every 3 months for 2 years, every 6 months in the third year, and annually thereafter. This surveillance strategy is aimed primarily at the detection of metachronous colorectal lesions.

Monitoring Strategies

Colon versus rectum

For colon carcinoma the most common metastatic sites are intraabdominal (hepatic and extrahepatic) sites. Lung and bone metastases occur less commonly. The same patterns of spread also apply to rectal cancer, but in this disease the pelvis represents a common site for recurrence. Locoregional relapse is more common in rectal carcinoma than in colon carcinoma. Adjuvant chemotherapy and radiation have decreased this problem and prolonged survival.[51]

Perineal pain after abdominoperineal resection, other than that arising immediately after surgery, is a symptom of recurrence. Radbruch et al.[52] described an average interval of 7 months between the onset of perineal pain and computed tomography–based diagnosis of recurrence. The delay is mostly due to difficulty in differentiating between postsurgical scar and recurrent tumor, which is an area where monoclonal antibody scans have a potential application.

If local recurrence of rectal cancer can be detected early, 5-year survival rates of 33% may be achieved.[53] This speaks for close follow-up of patients at high risk for local recurrence (rectal tumors with narrow margins, T3 and T4 tumors, and primary tumors with nodal metastases). Patients should be carefully questioned at each office visit regarding symptoms, and physical examination should be directed at the perineal scar or rectal anastomosis, including frequent flexible sigmoidoscopy for 2 to 3 years after resection and less frequent surveillance thereafter. The majority of local recurrences occur within 1 year of the initial surgery. Most local recurrences in rectal cancer are suspected on the basis of symptoms or clinical findings on physical examination. Salvage surgery is rarely feasible for potential cure in patients with severe complaints.

Transrectal ultrasonography (TRUS) and transvaginal endosonography in females after abdominoperineal resection and sphincter-preserving surgery have potential roles in the detection of locoregional disease. TRUS was evaluated by Romano et al.[54] in 42 patients. Eight local recurrences from rectal cancer were detected in follow-up, but there were two false-positive examinations. Beynon et al.[55] showed that endosonography gave valuable information on established recurrence and allowed the detection of recurrent tumors not apparent on routine clinical examination. Charnley et al.[56] found two of 15 local recurrences identified only by endosonography. Biopsy is mandatory for any suspicious area detected using endosonography.

Mascagni et al.[57] evaluated the diagnostic potential of endoluminal (endorectal and endovaginal) ultrasound to detect asymptomatic, resectable, local recurrence after rectal surgery in 120 patients. Seventeen recurrences (14%) were detected. The method showed 97% accuracy, 94% sensitivity, and 98% specificity. The positive predictive value was 85% and the negative predictive value was 99%. Of the 17 patients with recurrences, six were asymptomatic and underwent reoperation. Of the 11 with symptomatic recurrences, only two had reoperation. Two endoluminal ultrasound diagnoses were false-positives, emphasizing the necessity for biopsy in all suspected recurrences.

Data are insufficient to support the routine use of TRUS in all patients after curative radical surgery for rectal cancer. It should be considered for any patient with suspected pelvic recurrence and an accessible lumen for endosonography.

Rectal cancer treated with local excision

Appropriate candidates for local excision of rectal cancer should be at minimal risk for locoregional spread of disease. However, even with careful patient selection, the risk of nodal metastases is 11% to 23%.

Morson et al.[58] studied 119 patients treated with local excision. Ten recurrences were found, five in patients with incomplete local excision. Of the other five patients, three had distant metastases and two underwent salvage surgery, with one dying postoperatively and the other cured by abdominoperineal resection. Bailey et al.[59] treated 63 patients with rectal adenocarcinoma by full-thickness local excision. Four tumors (8%), two of which also had distant disease, recurred locally. Of these, two were successfully treated by repeat resection. The 5-year disease-free survival for the entire group of highly selected patients was 90%.

Transmural rectal cancers have at least a 24% failure rate and are treated more effectively with standard surgery and postoperative radiation therapy.[58] Select patients who undergo local excision with radiation for rectal cancer warrant a follow-up strategy like that for patients who have standard radical surgery. Studies show local failure rates between less than 1% and 50% for local excision. If recurrence develops after local excision and radiation, the patients may be more suitable for salvage surgery than patients with pelvic recurrence after radical surgery for rectal adenocarcinoma. At present a national trial evaluating local excision and chemoradiation for rectal cancer is accruing patients.[60] This trial should help define the risk of recurrence in patients with early rectal cancer.

Modifiers

Individual factors should be considered in any follow-up plan. Elderly patients with associated comorbid conditions, which would preclude acting on information gained from intensive follow-up, should not be subjected to intensive surveillance.

The frequency of follow-up should be based on the prognosis of the patient's primary tumor. The incidence of recurrence depends largely on the stage of the primary tumor (TNM stage I: 0% to 13% risk, stage II: 11% to 61%, stage III: 32% to 88%). Pathological features such as grade, colloid or signet-ring histological findings, venous or lymphatic invasion, perineural invasion, and perforation have been reported to be significant in univariate analysis. However, in multivariate models in which stage is included, many or all of these characteristics lose independent prognostic significance for recurrence or survival.[61] The surveillance strategy after curative resection of colorectal cancer should evaluate the patients most likely to have recurrence (TNM stage III) more intensively than those least likely (TNM stage I). Galandiuk et al.[62] found stage III lesions, the presence of adhesion to or invasion of other organs or both, and perforation to be associated with significantly earlier recurrence.

Patients with elevated serum CEA levels before resection of the primary colorectal cancer have a worse prognosis with a high rate of recurrence in the postoperative period.[63] These patients should be closely monitored. CEA levels may be most helpful in surveillance.

Olson et al.[64] found tumor recurrence to be unrelated to the histological features of the primary colorectal carcinoma. Recurrence occurred in 19% of well-differentiated, 27% of moderately well-differentiated, and 33% of poorly differentiated tumors. The poorly differentiated cancers did seem to have a slightly higher incidence of locoregional-only recurrence, compared with well- and moderately well-differentiated cancers (18.5% versus 4.5% and 9.7%, respectively). The biological behavior of colorectal cancer is diverse, and at present the factors responsible for recurrence are impossible to define precisely.

Adjuvant therapy

By definition, patients receiving adjuvant therapy are at high risk of relapse. These patients generally receive close clinical and biochemical follow-up during the period of adjuvant treatment.

Despite the proven efficacy of adjuvant treatment with 5-FU and levamisole for stage III colon cancer in reducing the incidence of recurrence and improving survival, 40% of patients can still be expected to have a recurrence.[65] Galandiuk et al.[62] found that although 5-FU and levamisole decrease the risk of recurrence in a subset of patients with colon cancer and chemotherapy and radiation reduce the risk of recurrence in a subset of patients with rectal cancer, neither of these regimens affects the relative distribution of recurrences across sites. Time to recurrence was prolonged by adjuvant therapy. The ratio of median times to recurrence among patients with colon cancer receiving adjuvant therapy versus those not receiving such therapy was 1:32. The ratio among patients with rectal cancer receiving chemotherapy and irradiation versus those who did not was 1:17. This suggests that the period of frequent surveillance should be longer, perhaps 3 to 4 years after initial surgery, in patients treated with adjuvant therapy.

Moertel et al.[26] reported falsely elevated CEA levels in 20 patients while they were receiving 5-FU and levamisole. In these patients the CEA level rose because of impaired liver function owing to adjuvant chemotherapy. This is an important finding and must be considered in patients whose CEA levels are elevated during chemotherapy.

METHODS OF SURVEILLANCE

Nonspecific Serology (Excluding Tumor Markers)

Routine serum chemistry and hematological tests have little or no place in the routine follow-up of patients after curative surgery for colorectal cancer, other than to monitor the effects of adjuvant treatment. If the CEA level rises, liver and renal functions must be evaluated to rule out dysfunction of these organ systems as benign causes of CEA elevation. Liver function tests and complete blood count should be performed concurrently with CEA measurement (Table 8-1). Liver function abnormalities may occur with hepatic metastases. Alkaline phosphatase is probably the most sensitive enzyme in detecting these lesions. However, a large volume of metastatic disease may be present in the liver despite normal liver function tests. A combination of CEA greater than 10 ng/ml and alkaline phosphatase greater than 135 U (upper limit of normal: 90 U) has been shown to have an 88% sensitivity rate in diagnosing hepatic metastases but also has a 12% false-positive result.[66] Erythrocyte sedimentation rate and acute-phase reactive proteins have been studied for utility in the follow-up of patients with colorectal cancer.[66,67] Any of these may be nonspecifically elevated in patients with recurrent colorectal cancer, but none add to the information provided by monitoring CEA levels alone.

ENDOSCOPIC SURVEILLANCE

Colonoscopy is an integral part of the routine follow-up of patients with colorectal cancer after potentially curative resection. These patients are at high risk for recurrence of the initial tumor, development of new colon cancers, and formation of colorectal polyps.

All patients undergoing elective colorectal resections for carcinoma should undergo full colonoscopy to the cecum before the initial surgery. In patients with obstructing or perforated lesions, this surveillance examination should be done within 3 to 6 months of primary surgery. Three percent to 7% of patients with colorectal cancer have a synchronous colon cancer that is identified before surgery and should be resected as part of the primary operation.[68] Another 25% have associated polyps that should be removed.

Barium enema is less sensitive than routine endoscopic surveillance in patients after curative colorectal cancer surgery. Nava and Pagana[69] found that barium enema detected only 38% of lesions seen with colonoscopy. Juhl et al.[70] found nine polyps and one asymptomatic anastomotic recurrence in 12 patients with normal barium enemas. The initial approach to examination of the colon and rectum remaining after surgery should be endoscopy. In addition to its superior diagnostic characteristics, colonoscopy allows the resection of significant polyps. Air-contrast barium enema should be used to evaluate patients who cannot undergo colonoscopy or whose colonoscopy did not reach the cecum.

The utility of endoscopic surveillance is twofold: to detect anastomotic recurrence and to detect metachronous colorectal lesions. Anastomotic recurrence seldom occurs as an intraluminal mass. Usually a local or anastomotic tumor recurrence represents seeding of disease in the pericolonic, perimesenteric, or pelvic side wall tissues, with eventual growth into the anastomotic site from outside the intestine.[71] In this situation barium enema may be helpful to identify extramucosal, pericolonic tumor recurrence, although a narrowing on barium enema may represent a benign, anastomotic stricture. Anastomotic recurrences after low anterior resection, which are not unusual, may lend themselves to endoscopic detection. In their series Juhl et al.[70] found that of nine patients with anastomotic recurrence diagnosed between 12 and 30 months after low anterior resection, all had positive findings on sigmoidoscopy. In this series all nine patients were symptomatic and none had disease resectable for cure. Rodriguez-Bigas et al.[43] analyzed the outcome in 50 patients who had anastomotic recurrence after curative colorectal cancer surgery. Forty recurrences (80%) occurred after resection of sigmoid and upper rectal carcinomas. In all 14 patients who were asymptomatic at the time of diagnosis of the anastomotic recurrence, the disease was diagnosed by routine follow-up endoscopy. Seven of these 14 asymptomatic patients had repeat resection, with the anastomosis found to be the only site of recurrence at laparotomy and with appreciable long-term survival. Because of the relatively high recurrence rate at the anastomosis after low anterior resection, consideration should be given to inspecting the anastomosis by rigid or flexible sigmoidoscopy every 6 months for the first 2 to 3 years after surgery for the primary lesion. This would apply primarily to patients with advanced rectal disease. Endoscopic ultrasound is being evaluated for its ability to detect anastomotic recurrences before the patient becomes symptomatic.

Adenoma surveillance reduces the incidence and mortality of colorectal cancer.[72] For up to 6 years after resection of colorectal cancer, routine surveillance endoscopy has an annual interval yield of at least 3% for significant colon polyps and new cancers.[70]

The optimal frequency of colonoscopic studies after colorectal cancer resection has not been defined. At present our follow-up recommendations are as follows. If colonoscopy is not performed before the primary colorectal cancer resection, it should be performed within 3 to 6 months of the surgery. Frequency of subsequent endoscopy depends on the findings at the initial screening. If synchronous polyps are found, the initial follow-up colonoscopy should be done at 6-month intervals until no further metachronous polyps are found in two colonoscopies. If no synchronous polyps are found and patients have a "clean" examination after removal of metachronous polyps, the colonoscopic examination should be done at 3-year intervals. If results of the annual colonoscopy are negative, surveillance every 3 years is probably adequate (Table 8-1).

In the endoscopic surveillance of patients after curative colorectal cancer surgery, selection of subgroups with a higher risk of metachronous cancer may be possible. In Grossman's study[73] patients having one or two first-degree relatives with colorectal cancer tended to have more colorectal lesions found on endoscopic surveillance examinations. Patients with hereditary nonpolyposis colon carcinoma are at particularly high risk for metachronous colorectal lesions and are not spared from metachronous rectal tumors by abdominal colectomy. Svendsen et al.[74] reported that among 396 young patients (less than 40 years of age) with colorectal carcinoma, metachronous cancer developed in 44 at a median of 17 years. Eleven patients (25%) had more than one metachronous cancer or a uterine cancer. These findings support the regular surveillance of young patients with primary colorectal cancer, since they have a long life expectancy and high cumulative risk of new cancer in all remaining colonic segments. Elderly patients with significant comorbid conditions and limited life expectancy can probably have a less rigorous schedule of endoscopic surveillance. Therefore the risks and benefits of endoscopic surveillance must be weighed for each patient and an appropriate, individualized schedule of studies devised.

Radiological Evaluation

Radiological studies in general should not be part of the routine follow-up of patients after curative colorectal cancer surgery. These studies should be prompted by the suspicion of recurrent or metastatic disease based on clinical findings or a serial CEA elevation. To be useful, an imaging study would direct management toward improving the therapeutic outcome, avoiding unnecessary morbidity, or saving money.

Detection of Hepatic Metastases

The most common site of recurrent colorectal carcinoma is the liver. In one third of patients locoregional recurrence occurs, whereas the remainder manifest a more diffuse pattern of metastatic disease.[22]

Several imaging modalities, including radionuclide scintigraphy, ultrasonography, computed tomography, magnetic resonance imaging, and positron emission tomography, have been used to evaluate hepatic metastases from colorectal carcinoma. Radionuclide scintigraphy was widely used in the 1970s and early 1980s because of its low cost and simplicity. Tc-99m sulfur colloid, the agent used, accumulates in the Kupffer cells, which are abundant in the normal liver and absent in the tumor and other hepatic masses. This results in a photopenic (cold) area on the scintigraphic images. The test lacks spatial resolution, sensitivity, and specificity. In general, lesions less than 2 to 2.5 cm in diameter are not detected.[75] Recent advances in single photon emission computed tomography may improve the detectability of liver masses.

Sonography is relatively inexpensive and permits material for cytological examination to be obtained by a guided biopsy. Sonography is operator dependent, and examination may be limited by the presence of intestinal gas. The sensitivity of sonography in detecting liver metastases is low (57%) and falls to 20% with lesions less than 1 cm in diameter.[76]

Computed tomography is the mainstay for the detection of hepatic metastases. Computed tomography should be performed annually except in patients with rectal cancer, who should have baseline abdominal and pelvic computed tomographic scans at 6 months and annually thereafter (Table 8-1). To maximize the yield obtained from computed tomography, the examination and delivery of intravenous contrast agents must be properly performed. Dynamic scanning through the liver should be accomplished within 2 to 3 minutes of the intravenous delivery of contrast material at a rate of 1.5 to 2.5 ml/sec to allow maximal density differentiation between the normal hepatic parenchyma and the metastases. Computed tomography can detect liver metastases in 38% to 91% of patients and is superior to liver scintigraphy and sonography, particularly for lesions smaller than 2 cm.[76] One disadvantage of computed tomography is its nonspecificity, which may create diagnostic problems. For some benign lesions, other tests may be needed to increase the specificity of the diagnosis, such as a radionuclide scan to rule out hemangioma.

Magnetic resonance imaging can be used to detect hepatic metastases. It is more expensive than the other modalities and not as readily available. Magnetic resonance imaging relies on greater tissue contrast between the normal liver and the tumor to improve visualization and detectability. Currently available technology yields a lesion detectability rate of 57% to 82%, which is no better than computed tomography. However, magnetic resonance imaging technology is continuing to improve and may ultimately produce higher detectability rates.

Ward et al.[77] investigated the ability of five hepatic imaging techniques to determine the anatomical location and number of metastases in 19 patients with colorectal cancer. Three computed tomography methods and two magnetic resonance imaging spin-echo pulse sequences (T1- and T2-weighted) were used. The three types of computed tomography scans were EOE–computed tomography (EOE-CT; EOE is an experimental lipid contrast agent), computed tomographic arterial photography (CTAP), and delayed computed tomography (scanning at 4 hours after CTAP). The overall sensitivities were EOE-CT, 83%; CTAP, 78%; delayed computed tomography, 82%; T1-weighted magnetic resonance imaging, 84%; and T2-weighted magnetic resonance imaging, 64%. The false-positive rates were EOE-CT, 16%; CTAP, 31%; delayed computed tomography, 9%; T1-weighted magnetic resonance imaging, 3%; and T2-weighted magnetic resonance imaging, 9%. The authors concluded that T1-weighted magnetic resonance imaging was the most effective hepatic imaging technique.

When hepatic metastases are found and consideration is given to reoperation with curative intent, CTAP or T1-weighted magnetic resonance imaging should be obtained before exploratory laparotomy. In general, patients with four or more liver metastases are not candidates for resection.[27] To prevent unnecessary surgery because of its potential morbidity, the detection of small tumor nodules before laparotomy is to the patient's advantage. When performed properly, CTAP can detect lesions as small as 0.5 cm in diameter.

During exploratory laparotomy for the planned resection of colorectal liver metastases, intraoperative sonographic evaluation of the liver should be mandatory before the resection. In a multiinstitutional Gastrointestinal Tumor Study Group protocol prospectively evaluating the treatment of liver metastases from colorectal cancer, more than 50% of patients said to have resectable disease based on preoperative studies were found at surgery to have unresectable disease.[78] The use of intraoperative ultrasound should therefore diminish the rate of noncurative resections.

Detection of Locoregional Tumor Recurrence

Local recurrence is nonvisceral recurrence of colorectal cancer in sites adjacent to the primary tumor (anastomosis, tumor bed, and regional nodes). A true local recurrence after surgical removal of the primary tumor may offer the possibility of a second operation and hence another chance for cure. Local recurrence occurs in 11% to 30% of patients after potentially curative surgery for colorectal cancer.[19] Approximately one fourth of patients have associated distant metastases.[19] Local recurrences usually occur within 2 years of the initial operation and are more common in rectal and rectosigmoid cancer. Many are symptomatic at diagnosis.

Anastomotic recurrences that involve the mucosa along the suture line can be detected endoscopically, but extraluminal growth in the submucosa or along the serosa and masses in the pericolonic fat may not be recognized. Computed tomography is the best study to define extraluminal masses and the extent of disease.[79] Endoluminal sonography is also being evaluated for this purpose.

Chen et al.[80] found that anastomotic recurrences were better defined by barium enema than by computed tomography scanning (88% versus 61%), which suggests that computed tomography and barium enema are complementary in the detection of local recurrence. This view is not shared by all.

Abdominopelvic computed tomography is accurate and useful in detecting or confirming anastomotic, perianastomotic, or regional nodal recurrence of colorectal carcinoma, particularly in the pelvis. A baseline postoperative computed tomography scan at 6 months in patients with pelvic anastomoses can be used for subsequent comparison (Table 8-1).

Recurrent tumors are sometimes difficult to distinguish from postoperative or postradiation changes on computed tomography, magnetic resonance imaging, and TRUS.[81] Krestin et al.[82] showed that recurrent tumors have a higher signal intensity than fibrotic tissue on T2-weighted imaging, particularly when compared with normal muscle. The accuracy and sensitivity of magnetic resonance imaging in detecting tumor recurrence range from 80% to 88%. Regardless of the imaging modality chosen, a fine-needle aspiration biopsy is needed for definitive differentiation between benign postoperative changes and tumor recurrence. Positron emission tomography has been evaluated for its utility in differentiating between recurrent colorectal cancer and fibrosis. Positron emission tomography performed with ^{18}F-2-fluoro-2-deoxy-D-glucose is an established technique for measuring in vivo tissue metabolism. Ito et al.[83] found that positron emission tomography could distinguish recurrent rectal cancer from fibrosis in 14 of 15 patients with increased uptake of ^{18}F-2-fluoro-2-deoxy-D-glucose seen in the recurrent tumors. Strauss et al.[84] produced similar results in a group of 29 patients, 21 of whom had recurrence. Because of the limited resolution of the positron emission tomography scan, these investigators limited the use of this modality to soft tissue masses greater than 1.5 cm. Positron emission tomography may become particularly useful in patients with equivocal findings using other diagnostic modes. At present it is investigational.

Detection of Extrahepatic Intraabdominal Recurrence

Tumor deposits may be located in retroperitoneal lymph nodes, in remaining intraabdominal organs, or on the peritoneal or serosal surfaces. For detection of nodal metastases and metastases to other viscera such as the ovary, computed tomography is the most useful radiological test.

Peritoneal deposits can be difficult to diagnose without laparotomy. Current imaging modalities generally miss or underestimate peritoneal disease. To be detected, these lesions must be outlined by peritoneal fat and be large enough to be recognized on imaging studies. Computed tomography is the diagnostic modality of choice because of its better spatial resolution, the ability to fill the gastrointestinal tract with contrast material, and limited intestinal motion artifact. However, the sensitivity of computed tomography in detecting these lesions is only 59%.[85] Attempts have been made to improve the detection of peritoneal metastases by instillation of contrast agents into the peritoneal cavity.[86,87] These have not proved to be of much value. Radioimmunoscintigraphy may be useful in the detection of peritoneal metastases.

Detection of Pulmonary Metastases

Chest x-ray examination is part of the routine preoperative evaluation in patients with colorectal carcinoma. No agreement has been reached on the utility of routine chest x-ray evaluations after curative resection. This test identifies isolated pulmonary metastases in approximately 2% of patients with colorectal cancer.[88] Pulmonary metastasectomy may result in 5-year survival rates of 15% to 35%.[89] An abnormal or equivocal chest x-ray should lead to a computed tomography scan of the lung fields to assess the number of pulmonary lesions, unless it is evident from the plain radiograph that multiple tumor nodules are present. A solitary new lesion on chest radiography may represent either a primary lung tumor or a metastatic lesion. Graffner et al.[68] reported that in three of 47 patients the only indicators of recurrent disease were findings on routine chest radiography. These three patients were all asymptomatic. Safi and Beyer[90] studied a population of 1,054 patients after curative colorectal cancer surgery. There were 350 recurrences in this group. In 15 patients the chest x-ray revealed isolated pulmonary metastases. Seven patients underwent resection, and two of these remained free of disease at 5 years. Tornqvist et al.[91] found solitary lung metastases in 13 patients. Seven of these patients underwent pulmonary resection, and four were subsequently free of recurrence. Although yield is small, annual chest radiography should be performed because the lung appears to be a relatively favorable site for salvage surgery (Table 8-1).

Detection of Osseous Metastases

Osseous metastases from colorectal malignancies are rare. Bonheim et al.[92] reported a 4% incidence of bone metastases in a study of 1,046 patients with more than 10 years' follow-up. In the absence of symptoms referable to bone, bone scanning is not required as routine preoperative staging for colorectal cancer patients, nor should it be part of the routine postoperative surveillance. Rectal cancer has a greater propensity than colon cancer to metastasize to bone. The most common sites of osseous metastases are the vertebrae, skull, pelvic bones, and proximal end of the femur and humerus.[93] Bone scanning is the most sensitive study for the detection of bony metastases in symptomatic patients.

PROGNOSIS AFTER RECURRENT COLORECTAL CANCER

Of the 30% to 44% of patients with recurrence after "curative" resection of colorectal cancer, an estimated 20% can be cured by local repeat resection or hepatic or pulmonary metastasectomy.[4] The prognosis of recurrent colorectal cancer depends on the location(s) of recurrence and the extent of disease present at that site. These factors determine re-resectability. Of patients undergoing curative resection, roughly 10% to 40% develop locoregional relapse, 10% to 20% hepatic metastases, 5% to 10% pulmonary metastases, and fewer than 5% bony metastases. In only approximately 15% of these patients is disease recurrence limited to a single site.[19]

In patients with recurrent colorectal cancer, surgical excision offers the only chance for cure. Approximately 20% of patients with locoregional recurrence are cured by aggressive repeat resection. An estimated 10% of patients with recurrent colorectal cancer have resectable liver metastases. Roughly 25% of patients survive 5 years after pulmonary metastasectomy for colorectal cancer. Therefore approximately 16% of patients with recurrent colorectal cancer can be salvaged for cure with aggressive reoperation. Relapse of colorectal cancer in the remaining patients is essentially incurable, with a 5-year survival of less than 5%.

PROGNOSIS OF NEW PRIMARY COLORECTAL CANCER

In 2% to 4% of patients with colorectal cancer a second invasive colorectal adenocarcinoma develops.[94] In most instances, primarily because of endoscopic surveillance programs, these are early-stage lesions amenable to curative resection.

Among 5-year survivors of colorectal adenocarcinoma the risk for a second visceral neoplasm (excluding skin cancer) may be as high as 30%.[95,96] Therefore these patients should have regular health care checks, including breast, gynecological, and prostate examinations, prostate specific antigen monitoring in males, and annual mammography in females.

FUTURE PROSPECTS

In a significant number of patients, high-intensity surveillance after curative surgery for colorectal carcinoma can detect recurrent disease earlier than low-intensity surveillance. Close monitoring has not been conclusively proved to prolong survival. Other issues are the lack of efficacy of time-consuming office visits, the utility and cost of various follow-up studies, and the limited treatment available for relapse, which occurs in the majority of patients with colorectal cancer. Many physicians believe that intensity of surveillance has little impact on patient prognosis.

Multiinstitutional, randomized, prospective trials are needed to evaluate the efficacy of a variety of surveillance programs in the detection and satisfactory treatment of colorectal cancer recurrence. A large number of patients would be necessary to demonstrate a significant improvement in survival when followed in an intensive screening program. The trial should stratify patients based on their recurrence risk, using the primary tumor stage as a variable. Separate surveillance programs should be devised and evaluated for colon and rectal adenocarcinoma, since certain investigations may pertain to one versus the other, based on tumor recurrence patterns.

ROLE OF MOLECULAR BIOLOGY

It is premature to use certain cellular or molecular characteristics as standard determinants of recurrence risk in the follow-up of colorectal cancer patients. Ploidy status and S-phase fraction have not consistently correlated with overall recurrence and survival.[22] In the future these biological features may define in which patients tumors will recur.

The clinical utility of the molecular genetic alterations that characterize colorectal neoplasms has not been established. As the techniques become more refined, however, these markers should improve the management of patients with colorectal cancer. Molecular genetic analysis should also provide prognostic information, which will narrow the spectrum of patients subjected to intensive follow-up regimens.

Mutations in p53, a tumor suppressor gene located on chromosome 17p, are the most common genetic alterations found in human cancers. Hamelin et al.[97] analyzed 85 colorectal cancers, of which 44 (52%) had a p53 mutation. They found a clear association between the detection of p53 mutation and survival. Bell et al.[98] found that the combination of p53 overexpression and c-Ki-*ras* gene mutations predicted a poor prognosis. Recently in a prospective study, investigators reported the correlation between 18q allelic loss and a worse prognosis for patients with stage II colon cancer. Elucidating the relationship between cellular and molecular characteristics and mechanisms of tumor progression and clinical behavior is likely to aid in formulating rational surveillance strategies.

Investigators are studying ways to assess the metastatic potential of tumors. Wielenga et al.[100] have found specific CD 44 variant glycoproteins that are increasingly expressed during colorectal tumor progression, which suggests that they play a role in tumor progression and metastasis.

Further work in identifying patients destined to have tumor progression by examining molecular markers will allow the exclusion of low-risk patients from expensive and time-consuming follow-up. Limited resources can then target the individuals who will benefit from such a program.

REFERENCES

1. Wangensteen OH, Lewis FJ, Tongen LA. The second-look in cancer surgery. Lancet 1951;2:303-7.
2. Gilbersten VA, Wangensteen OH. A summary of thirteen years' experience with the second look program. Surg Gynecol Obstet 1962;114:438-42.
3. Parker SL, Tong T, Bolden S, Wingo PA. Cancer statistics, 1997. CA Cancer J Clin 1997;47:5-27.
4. August DA, Ottow RT, Sugarbaker PH. Clinical perspective of human colorectal cancer metastasis. Cancer Metastasis Rev 1984;3:303-24.
5. Hughes KS, Simon R, Songhorabodi S, et al. Resection of the liver for colorectal carcinoma metastases: a multi-institutional study of patterns of recurrence. Surgery 1986;100:278-84.
6. Finlay IG, McArdle CS. The role of occult hepatic metastases in staging colorectal cancer. Scand J Gastroenterol 1989;150:150-4.
7. Vernava AM, Longo WE, Virgo KS, Coplin MA, Wade TP, Johnson FE. Current follow-up strategies after resection of colon cancer: results of a survey of the American Society of Colon and Rectal Surgeons. Dis Colon Rectum 1994;37:573-83.
8. Foster ME, Hill J, Leaper DJ. Follow-up after colorectal cancer—current practice in Wales and Southwest England. Int J Colorectal Dis 1987;2:118-9.
9. Camunas J, Enriquez JM, Devesa JM, Morales V, Millan I. Value of follow-up in the management of recurrent colorectal cancer. Eur J Surg Oncol 1991;17:530-5.
10. Hulton NR, Hargreaves AW. Is long term follow-up of all colorectal cancer necessary? J R Coll Surg Edinb 1989;34:21-4.
11. Makela J, Haukipauro K, Laitinen S, Kairaluoma MI. Surgical treatment of recurrent colorectal cancer: five-year follow-up. Arch Surg 1989;124:1029-32.
12. Polk HC, Spratt JS. Recurrent colorectal carcinoma: detection, treatment, and other considerations. Surgery 1971;69:9-23.
13. Ovaska J, Jarvinen H, Kujari H, Pertilla I, Mecklin JP. Follow-up of patients operated on for colorectal carcinoma. Am J Surg 1990;159:593-6.
14. Steele G Jr. Follow-up plans after treatment of primary colon and rectum cancer. World J Surg 1991;15:583-8.
15. Gold P, Freedman SO. Demonstration of tumor-specific antigens in colonic carcinomata by immunological tolerance and absorption techniques. J Exp Med 1965;121:439-62.
16. Arnaud JP, Koehl C, Adloff M. Carcinoembryonic antigen (CEA) in the diagnosis and prognosis of colorectal carcinoma. Dis Colon Rectum 1980;23:141-4.
17. Armitage NC, Davidson A, Tsikos D, Wood CB. A study of the reliability of carcinoembryonic antigen blood levels in following the course of colorectal cancer. Clin Oncol 1984;10:141-7.
18. Maglivit GM, Stuckey S. Colorectal carcinoma: evidence for circulating CEA-anti-CEA complexes. Cancer 1983;52:146-9.
19. Sugarbaker PH, Gianola FJ, Dwyer A, Neuman NR. A simplified plan for follow-up of patients with colon and rectal cancer supported by prospective studies of laboratory and radiologic test results. Surgery 1987;102:79-87.
20. Zeng Z, Cohen AM, Urmacher C. Usefulness of carcinoembryonic antigen monitoring despite normal preoperative values in node-positive colon cancer patients. Dis Colon Rectum 1993;36:1063-8.
21. Goslin R, Steele G Jr, Macintyre J, Love SB, Capellaro D. The use of preoperative plasma CEA levels for the stratification of patients after curative resection of colorectal cancers. Ann Surg 1980;192:747-51.
22. Jass JR, Mukawa K, Goh HS, et al. Clinical importance of DNA content in rectal cancer measured by flow cytometry. J Clin Pathol 1989;42:254-9.
23. Rognum TO. CEA, tumour differentiation and DNA ploidy pattern. Scand J Gastroenterol Suppl 1988;149:166-78.
24. Carl J, Bentzen SM, Norgaard-Pedersen B, Kronborg O. Modelling of serial carcinoembryonic antigen changes in colorectal cancer. Scand J Clin Lab Invest 1993;53:751-5.
25. Fuhrman G, Curley S, Hohn D, Roh M. Does improved staging with intraoperative U/S and portal lymph node assessment improve survival following resection of colorectal liver metastases? Scientific Program of the Society of Surgical Oncology, 47th Cancer Symposium, 1994.
26. Moertel CG, Fleming TR, MacDonald JS, Haller DG, Laurie TA, Tangen C. An evaluation of the carcinoembryonic antigen (CEA) test for monitoring patients with resected colon cancer. JAMA 1993;270:943-7.
27. Registry of Hepatic Metastases. Resection of the liver for colorectal carcinoma metastases: a multi-institutional study of indications for resection. Surgery 1988;103:278-88.
28. Martin EW Jr, Minton JP, Carey LC. CEA-Directed second-look surgery in the asymptomatic patient after primary resection of colorectal carcinoma. Ann Surg 1985;202:310-7.
29. Kievit J, Van de Velde CJ. Utility and cost of carcinoembryonic antigen monitoring in colon cancer follow-up evaluation: a Markov analysis. Cancer 1990;65:2580-7.
30. Northover JM. Carcinoembryonic antigen and recurrent colorectal cancer. Br J Surg 1985;72(Suppl):S44-6.
31. Iemura K, Moriya Y. A comparative analysis of the serum levels of NCC-ST-439, CEA and CA 19-9 in patients with colorectal carcinoma. Eur J Surg Oncol 1993;19:439-42.
32. Guadagni F, Roselli M, Cosimelli M, et al. Biologic evaluation of tumor-associated glycoprotein-72 and carcinoembryonic antigen expression in colorectal cancer, Part I. Dis Colon Rectum 1994;37(2 Suppl):S16-S23.
33. Fillela X, Molina R, Pique JM, et al. Use of CA 19-9 in the early detection of recurrences in colorectal cancer: comparison with CEA. Tumour Biol 1994;15:1-6.
34. Primus FJ, Wang FH, Goldenberg DM, Hansen HJ. Localization of human GW-39 tumors in hamsters by radiolabeled heterospecific antibody to carcinoembryonic antigen. Cancer Res 1973;33:2977-82.
35. Mach JP, Buchegger F, Forni M, et al. Use of radiolabeled monoclonal anti-CEA antibodies for the detection of human carcinomas by external photoscanning and tomoscintigraphy. Immunol Today 1981;2:239-49.
36. Toribara NW, Sack TL, Gum JR. Heterogeneity in the induction and expression of carcinoembryonic antigens and related antigens in human colon cancer cell lines. Cancer Res 1989;49:3321-7.
37. Doerr RJ, Herrera L, Abdel-Nabi H. In-111 CYT-103 monoclonal antibody imaging in patients with suspected recurrent colorectal cancer. Cancer 1993;71(12 Suppl):4241-7.
38. Moffat FL, Vargas-Cuba RD, Serafini AN, et al. Radioimmunodetection of colorectal carcinoma using technetium-99m-labeled Fab' fragments of the IMMU-4 anti-carcinoembryonic antigen monoclonal antibody. Cancer 1994;73(3 Suppl):836-45.
39. Kuhn JA, Thomas G. Monoclonal antibodies and colorectal carcinoma: a clinical review of diagnostic applications. Cancer Invest 1994;12:314-23.
40. Beatty JD, Williams LE, Yamauchi D, et al. Presurgical imaging with indium-labeled anti-carcinoembryonic antigen for colon cancer staging. Cancer Res 1990;50 (3 Suppl):922S-6.

41. Martin EW Jr, Cohen AM, Lavery IC, et al. Radioimmunoguided surgery: a preliminary report of a multicenter trial to evaluate the use of the radiolabeled B72.3 monoclonal antibody in colorectal cancer. Scientific Program of the Society of Surgical Oncology, 43rd Cancer Symposium, 1990.
42. Lechner P, Lind P, Binter G, Lesnik H. Anticarcinoembryonic antigen immunoscintigraphy with a 99mTc-Fab' fragment (IMMU-4) in primary and recurrent colorectal cancer: a prospective study. Dis Colon Rectum 1993;36:930-5.
43. Rodriguez-Bigas MA, Stulc JP, Davidson B, Petrelli NJ. Prognostic significance of anastomotic recurrence from colorectal adenocarcinoma. Dis Colon Rectum 1992;35:838-42.
44. Corman ML, Galandiuk S, Block GE, et al. Immunoscintigraphy with 111-In-Satumomab pendetide in patients with colorectal adenocarcinoma: performance and impact on clinical management. Dis Colon Rectum 1994;37:129-37.
45. Martin EW Jr, Tuttle SE, Rousseau M, et al. Radioimmunoguided surgery using monoclonal antibody 17-1A in colorectal cancer. Hybridoma (Suppl) 1986;5:97S-l08S.
46. Kuhn JA, Corbisiero RM, Burns RR, et al. Intraoperative gamma detection probe with presurgical antibody imaging in colon cancer. Arch Surg 1991;126:1398-403.
47. Tempero M. Pitfalls in antibody imaging in colorectal cancer. Cancer 1993;71:4248-51.
48. Fleisher DE, Goldberg SB, Browning TH, et al. Detection and surveillance of colorectal cancer. JAMA 1989;261:580-5.
49. Goldenberg DM, Neville AM, Carter AC, et al. Carcinoembryonic antigen: its role as a marker in the management of cancer: summary of an NIH consensus statement. Br Med J 1981;282:373-5.
50. The American Society of Colon and Rectal Surgeons Standards Task Force. Practice parameters for the detection of colorectal neoplasms. Dis Colon Rectum 1994;35:389-94.
51. Krook JE, Moertel CG, Gunderson LL, et al. Effective surgical adjuvant therapy for high-risk rectal carcinoma. N Engl J Med 1991;324:709-15.
52. Radbruch L, Zech D, Grond S, Meuser T, Lehmann KA. Perianlschmerz und rektumkarzinom-pravalenzbeim lokalrezidiv. Med Klin 1991;86:180-5.
53. Hermanek P, Gall FP, Altendorf A. Lokalrezidive nach rektumkarzinom-entstehung, diagnose, pronose. Langenbecks Arch Chir 1975;338:215-9.
54. Romano G, de Rosa P, Vallone G, Rotondo A, Grassi R, Santangelo ML. Intrarectal ultrasound and computed tomography in the pre- and postoperative assessment of patients with rectal cancer. Br J Surg 1985;72(Suppl):S117-9.
55. Beynon J, Mortensen NJ, McFoy DM, Channer JL, Rigby H, Virjee J. The detection and evaluation of locally recurrent rectal cancer with rectal endosonography. Dis Colon Rectum 1989;32:509-17.
56. Charnley RM, Pyf G, Amar SS, Hardcastle JD. The early detection of recurrent rectal carcinoma by rectal endosonography. SRS Abstracts. Br J Surg 1988;75:1232.
57. Masgagni D, Corbellini L, Urciuoli P, Di Matteo G. Endoluminal ultrasound for early detection of local recurrence of rectal cancer. Br J Surg 1989;76:1176-80.
58. Morson BC, Bussey HJ, Samoorian S. Policy of local excision for early cancer of the colorectum. Gut 1977;18:1045-50.
59. Bailey HR, Huval WV, Max E, Smith RW, Botts DR, Zomora LF. Local excision of carcinoma of the rectum for cure. Surgery 1992;111:555-61.
60. CALGB Protocol 8984. Conservative treatment of adenocarcinoma of the distal rectum: local resection plus adjuvant 5FU/radiation therapy: a phase II study.
61. Deans GT, Parks TG, Rowlands BJ, Spence RA. Prognostic factors in colorectal cancer. Br J Surg 1992;79:608-13.
62. Galandiuk S, Wieand HS, Moertel CG, et al. Patterns of recurrence after curative resection of carcinoma of the colon and rectum. Surg Gynecol Obstet 1992;174:27-32.
63. Wanebo HJ, Bhasker R, Pinsky CM, et al. Preoperative carcinoembryonic antigen level as a prognostic indicator in colorectal cancer. N Engl J Med 1978;299:448-51.
64. Olson RM, Perencevich NP, Malcolm AW, Vanttinen E. Patterns of recurrence following curative resection of adenocarcinoma of the colon and rectum. Cancer 1980;45:2969-74.
65. Moertel CG, Fleming TR, MacDonald JS, et al. Levamisole and fluorouracil for adjuvant therapy of resected colon carcinoma. N Engl J Med 1990;322:352-8.
66. Tartter PI, Slater G, Gelernt I, Aufses A Jr. Screening for liver metastases from colorectal cancer with carcinoembryonic antigen and alkaline phosphatase. Ann Surg 1981;193:357-60.
67. Thynne GS. Plasma carcinoembryonic antigen and erythrocyte sedimentation rate in patients with colorectal carcinoma. Med J Aust 1979;1:592-3.
68. Graffner H, Hultberg B, Johansson B, Moller T, Petersson BG. Detection of recurrent cancer of the colon and rectum. J Surg Oncol 1985;28:156-9.
69. Nava HR, Pagana TJ. Postoperative surveillance of colorectal carcinoma. Cancer 1982;49:1043-7.
70. Juhl G, Larson GM, Mullins R, Bond S, Polk HC Jr. Six-year results of annual colonoscopy after resection of colorectal cancer. World J Surg 1990;14:255-61.
71. Steele G Jr. Standard postoperative monitoring of patients after primary resection of colon and rectum cancer. Cancer 1993;71:4225-35.
72. Winawer SJ, Zauber AG, Ito MN, et al. Prevention of colorectal cancer by colonoscopic polypectomy: the National Polyp Study Workgroup. N Engl J Med 1993;329:1977-81.
73. Grossman S, Milos ML, Tekawa IS, Jewell NP. Colonoscopic screening of persons with suspected risk factors for colon cancer. II. Past history of colorectal neoplasms. Gastroenterology 1989;96:299-306.
74. Svendsen LB, Bulow S, Mellemgaard A. Metachronous colorectal cancer in young patients: expression of the hereditary nonpolyposis colorectal cancer syndrome? Dis Colon Rectum 1991;34:790-3.
75. Castagna J, Benfield JR, Yamada H, Johnson OE. The reliability of liver scans and function tests in detecting metastases. Surg Gynecol Obstet 1972;134:463-6.
76. Schreve RH, Terpstra OT, Ausema L, Lameris JS, van Seijen AJ, Jeekel J. Detection of liver metastases: a prospective study comparing liver enzymes, scintigraphy, ultrasonography and computed tomography. Br J Surg 1984;71:947-9.
77. Ward BA, Miller DL, Frank JA, et al. Prospective evaluation of hepatic imaging studies in the detection of colorectal metastases: correlation with surgical findings. Surgery 1989;105:180-7.
78. Steele G Jr, Bleday R, Mayer RJ, Lindblad A, Petrelli N, Weaver D. A prospective evaluation of hepatic resection for colorectal carcinoma metastases to the liver: Gastrointestinal Tumor Study Group Protocol 6584. J Clin Oncol 1991;9:1105-12.
79. Husband JE, Hodson NJ, Parsons CA. The use of computed tomography in recurrent rectal tumors. Radiology 1988;134:677-82.
80. Chen YM, Ott DJ, Wolfman NT, Gelfand DW, Karsteadt N, Bechtold RE. Recurrent colorectal carcinoma: evaluation with barium enema examination and CT. Radiology 1987;163:307-10.
81. Moss AA. Imaging of colorectal carcinoma. Radiology 1989;170:308-10.
82. Krestin GP, Steinbrich W, Friedmann G. Recurrent rectal cancer: diagnosis with MR imaging versus CT. Radiology 1988;168:307-11.
83. Ito K, Kato T, Tadokoro M, et al. Recurrent rectal cancer and scar: differentiation with PET and MR imaging. Radiology 1992;182:549-52.
84. Strauss LG, Clorius JH, Schlag P, et al. Recurrence of colorectal tumors: PET evaluation. Radiology 1989;170:329-32.
85. Charnsangavej C. New imaging modalities for follow-up of colorectal carcinoma. Cancer 1993;71:4236-40.
86. Halvorsen RA Jr, Panushka C, Oakley QJ, Letourneau JG, Adcock LL. Intraperitoneal contrast material improves the CT detection of peritoneal metastases. AJR Am J Roentgenol 1991;157:37-40.

87. Nelson RC, Chezmar JL, Hoel MJ, Buck DR, Sugarbaker PH. Peritoneal carcinomatosis: preoperative CT with intraperitoneal contrast material. Radiology 1992;182:133-8.
88. Devesa JM, Morales V, Enriquez JM, et al. Colorectal cancer: the bases for a comprehensive follow-up. Dis Colon Rectum 1988;31:636-52.
89. Mountain CF, Khalil KG, Hermes KE, Frozier DH. The contribution of surgery to the management of carcinomatous pulmonary metastases. Cancer 1978;41:833-40.
90. Safi F, Beyer HG. The value of follow-up after curative surgery of colorectal carcinoma. Cancer Detect Prev 1993;17:417-24.
91. Tornqvist A, Ekelund G, Leandoer L. The value of intensive follow-up after curative resection for colorectal carcinoma. Br J Surg 1982;69:725-8.
92. Bonnheim DC, Petrelli NJ, Herrera L, Walsh D, Mittlelman A. Osseous metastases from colorectal carcinoma. Am J Surg 1986;151:457-9.
93. Besbeas S, Stearns, MW Jr. Osseous metastases from carcinomas of the colon and rectum. Dis Colon Rectum 1978;21:266-8.
94. Heald RJ, Lockhart-Mummery HE. The lesion of the second cancer of the large bowel. Br J Surg 1972;59:16-9.
95. Polk HC, Spratt JS, Butcher HR. Frequency of multiple primary malignant neoplasms associated with colorectal carcinoma. Am J Surg 1965;109:71-5.
96. Weir JA. Colorectal cancer: metachronous and other associated neoplasms. Dis Colon Rectum 1975;18:4-5.
97. Hamelin R, Laurent-Puig P, Olschwang S, et al. Association of p53 mutations with short survivals in colorectal cancer. Gastroenterology 1994;106:42-8.
98. Bell S, Scott N, Cross D, et al. Prognostic value of p53 overexpression and c-ki-ras gene mutations in colorectal cancer. Gastroenterology 1993;104:57-64.
99. Jen J, Kim H, Piantadosi S, et al. Allelic loss of chromosome 18q and prognosis in colorectal cancer. N Engl J Med 1994;331:213-21.
100. Wielenga VJ, Heider KH, Offerhaus GJ, et al. Expression of CD 44 variant proteins in human colorectal cancer is related to tumor progression. Cancer Res 1993;53:4754-6.

➢ COUNTERPOINT

Memorial Sloan-Kettering Cancer Center

CAROL J. SWALLOW AND JOSE G. GUILLEM

Numerous recommendations have been set forth for the follow-up of colorectal carcinoma patients after potentially curative primary resection.[1-4] Each schema was developed with the principal goal of detecting disease recurrence early enough to allow for potentially curative repeat resection. Despite this common goal, proposed follow-up schemas vary considerably in the extent and frequency of investigations. This variability is based in part on differences in perception of the ability of various modalities to detect disease recurrence and of efficacy in altering outcome. However, outcome studies estimate that a potentially curative repeat resection is possible in only a minority of patients in whom recurrent colorectal cancer is detected, with an actual cure achieved in at most half of that small group.[5,6] Therefore the ideal follow-up plan should be simple, effective, and economical. Since the risk of a metachronous primary cancer at another site such as breast, ovary, uterine, prostate, or lung may reach 30% in long-term survivors of a colorectal cancer resection,[7-12] appropriate and timely screening for other malignancies may be as rewarding as early detection of recurrence in terms of years of life saved.

PROPOSED FOLLOW-UP SCHEDULE

Rationale

The proposed follow-up schedule includes four components aimed not only at detecting recurrent colorectal cancer but also at preventing other primary cancers or finding them early. Results of this basic evaluation would determine the need for further investigations, via one or more selective evaluations.

Although a program of monthly follow-up examinations is unlikely to translate into increased years of life saved, the follow-up interval should not be so prolonged as to preclude the detection of resectable recurrences. Our follow-up schedule differs from that proposed by Macintosh et al. primarily in the frequency of history, physical examination, sigmoidoscopic examination, and CEA determination during years 3 through 5.

Adjuvant therapy, which is now frequently used, delays recurrence beyond the traditional time points.[13] This suggests that patients should be evaluated at least twice yearly not only during the first 2 years, when most colorectal cancer recurrences are detected,[13] but also during years 3 through 5. We eliminate many of the blood tests and the frequent colonoscopies proposed by Macintosh et al. for reasons to be discussed below. However, we agree that in patients whose general medical condition precludes any further aggressive management, follow-up should be significantly curtailed.

Although Macintosh et al. stress that a follow-up program should be tailored to the patient's risk of recurrence, this concept is not reflected in their follow-up grid (Table 8-1). Averbach and Sugarbaker[6] also alter the recommended follow-up interval according to the perceived level of risk for each patient, distinguishing between low- and high-risk groups. In contrast, we adhere to one basic follow-up regimen for all patients for several reasons.

First, calculation of risk of recurrence remains imprecise, since rates of recurrence vary widely among patients with similarly staged tumors.[14] In addition, despite the initial enthusiasm for precise molecular indicators such as S-phase fraction and allelic loss, these prognostic markers, along with more innovative parameters such as the ratio of matrix metalloproteinase-9 found in tumor versus that in normal mucosa,[15] remain unvalidated.

Furthermore, it may be that patients who are in a low-risk category and yet develop a recurrence are the best candidates for repeat resection. By the same token, patients with biologically aggressive tumors who are at high risk for recurrence may well be those in whom curative repeat resection is not feasible, regardless of how promptly recurrence is detected. Finally, a uniform follow-up regimen based on examinations every few months for all patients is simple and therefore more likely to be adhered to.

Table 8-2 Follow-up of patients with colorectal cancer: Memorial Sloan-Kettering Cancer Center

	YEAR				
	1	2	3	4	5
Office visit	4	4	2	2	2
CEA	4	4	2	2	2
Proctosigmoidoscopy*	4	4	2	2	2
Chest x-ray	1	1	1	1	1
Colonoscopy†	1	0	0	1	0
Transrectal ultrasound	‡	‡	‡	‡	‡
Abdominal computed tomography	‡	‡	‡	‡	‡
Pelvic computed tomography	‡	‡	‡	‡	‡
Chest computed tomography	‡	‡	‡	‡	‡

CEA, Carcinoembryonic antigen.
*Indicated for patients who have undergone sphincter-sparing procedures for rectal cancer.
†If complete colonoscopy was not performed preoperatively, it is performed 3 months postoperatively. Colonoscopy with polypectomy is repeated every 6 months after this initial perioperative colonoscopy until no polyps are detected. If the year 1 colonoscopy is normal, repeat colonoscopy in year 4 and every 3 to 5 years thereafter.
‡Performed as clinically indicated.

Basic Evaluation

Review of symptoms, physical examination, and sigmoidoscopy

Prospective studies have shown that a simple review of symptoms and physical examination provide the first indication of recurrent colorectal cancer in 21% to 48% of cases.[16,17] Symptoms can be reviewed quickly and economically via a questionnaire, followed by a confirmatory interview with a nurse or physician. Included should be inquiries as to general well-being, fatigue, anorexia, weight loss, bowel habits, rectal bleeding, pain, new masses, cough, and neurological symptoms. Physical examination should similarly begin with a general assessment, including evaluation of nutritional status, documentation of weight, and examination for pallor, jaundice, adenopathy, abdominal distention or masses, and hepatosplenomegaly.

In follow-up after resection of rectal cancer, the examination should be tailored to known patterns of recurrence. This should include assessment for groin adenopathy and, if it is detected, fine-needle aspiration. In patients undergoing sphincter-saving procedures, such as a low anterior resection, restorative proctectomy, or local excision, sigmoidoscopy complements the digital rectal examination in detecting and differentiating between anastomotic and the more common perianastomotic pelvic recurrences.[13] A study of recurrent rectal cancer by Rodriguez-Bigas et al.[18] suggests that by detecting asymptomatic (presumably early) recurrences, endoscopy may enhance the chances of curative resection. Any abnormal findings on history or physical examination may prompt use of more selective evaluations, including TRUS and computed tomography of the abdomen, pelvis, or chest. The availability of on-site TRUS and transvaginal ultrasound permits immediate confirmation of certain physical findings. TRUS has proved useful in confirming and further defining suspected local recurrence.[19,20] In some series TRUS has also detected unsuspected recurrences,[21] but its efficacy in this regard has not yet been well defined.

After resection of primary colorectal cancer a follow-up history and physical examination (with sigmoidoscopy after resection of rectal cancer) should be performed every 3 months for the first 2 years and every 6 months for the ensuing 3 years (Table 8-2). At 5 years patients are told that they no longer require specialized follow-up and that they should see their own general physicians for regular health maintenance visits. The rationale for this plan is based on the median time interval for colorectal cancer recurrence; the majority (75%) of recurrences are manifest in the first 2 years, with a decreasing frequency of recurrence up to 5 years.[13,22-26] Approximately 85% of cancers that are destined to recur will do so within 5 years.[27] This temporal pattern may be altered somewhat with more frequent use of adjuvant therapy. Because 20% of cancers that will recur do so during years 3 through 5 and because these later recurrences may in fact become more common in this era of adjuvant therapy, patients are evaluated twice yearly, rather than once yearly, during years 3 through 5.

Although some patients practice primary or secondary tumor prevention techniques without prompting, many do not. Routine follow-up visits after resection provide an opportunity to stress the importance of and confirm compliance with recommendations for yearly breast examination and mammography, gynecological examination with Papanicolaou smear, and prostate examination with prostate-specific antigen determination. The routine review of symptoms and a general physical examination may also raise the suspicion of malignancy in another system. Furthermore, rectal and pelvic examinations involve *en passant* examination of the prostate, uterus, and ovaries. Breast examination may be readily performed if this has not been done in the past year.

Another issue is identification of patients at particularly increased risk for the development of malignancy in any other system, such as patients with familial adenomatous polyposis or hereditary nonpolyposis colon cancer (HNPCC). This risk is routinely assessed by preoperative questionnaire. Follow-up genetic counseling and screening investigations are provided as indicated.

Laboratory tests

Controversy continues to exist around the value of postoperative CEA monitoring. If measured sufficiently frequently and carefully, CEA levels can provide an earlier indication of recurrent disease than does the development of symptoms or physical findings.[17,28-31] The question is whether this lead time enhances resectability and, more important, improves survival rates. Enthusiasm for routine (non-CEA-directed) second-look laparotomy collapsed with the recognition that morbidity in many may outweigh benefit in a few.[32] Some retrospective studies have shown higher rates of resectability and disease-free survival in patients who had frequent postoperative CEA determinations,[26,33,34] whereas others have shown no benefit.[35] Many variables can affect the apparent worth of CEA monitoring in such studies. Among the more significant factors are patient numbers and the rigor with which testing is performed and acted on. Prospective studies addressing this question are rare and include relatively low numbers of subjects.[36,37]

In the multiinstitutional trial in the United Kingdom led by Northover and Slack,[37] all registered patients underwent postoperative CEA determinations. If the CEA level increased (according to strict criteria), patients were randomized to groups in which the attending physician was or was not informed of the rise in CEA. It appears that in the former case, appropriate investigations, explorations, and resections, when feasible, were performed, although this is difficult to confirm. Nevertheless, there was no difference in outcome (resectability or survival) between the two groups (J. Northover, personal communication).

Given the policy at Memorial Sloan-Kettering Cancer Center of aggressive local, liver, and lung resection for patients with recurrent colorectal cancer, physicians are aggressive in detecting such recurrences as early as possible. Although only a small percentage of all patients ultimately undergo curative repeat resection after CEA-directed detection of recurrence, we believe that specialized institutions should continue to pursue cure in this small group of patients.[33,34] Moreover, while acknowledging concerns about the cost effectiveness of the CEA-directed metastatic workup,[33,38] we continue to see patients with resectable liver disease detected solely as a result of a rising CEA level. Averbach and Sugarbaker[6] and others[39-41] have emphasized that liver-only is the pattern of recurrence most reliably detected by CEA measurement and most amenable to curative resection. Postoperative CEA monitoring may also be indicated in institutions testing the effectiveness of new chemotherapeutic agents or biological response modifiers, since early detection of recurrent colorectal cancer at minimal volume may facilitate the antitumor action of such agents.

Blood tests other than CEA are not routinely performed (Table 8-2). There is good evidence that liver function tests do not significantly increase sensitivity to recurrent disease beyond that attained with CEA alone.[42] Routine complete blood counts are not a useful marker of recurrence. Measurement of other tumor markers such as serum NCC-ST 439 and CA 19-9 in conjunction with CEA only minimally enhances the ability to detect recurrent disease.[43-46] Since additional tumor markers would add considerable expense to follow-up and the value of marker-directed early detection is unclear, their routine use is not recommended.

Radiological imaging

After curative resection of a primary colorectal tumor, pulmonary metastases develop in approximately 5% to 10% of patients, with disease confined to the lungs in up to half of these.[6,13,47] Overall, only one fifth of patients with lung metastases are amenable to resection with curative intent, but some authors estimate that at least half of those with lung-only disease can be resected for cure.[47] The 5-year survival rate in patients undergoing resection for cure varies from 20% to 50% in a variety of series, with an average of about 30%.[48-52] Data from Memorial Sloan-Kettering Cancer Center show a 44% 5-year survival rate in 144 patients undergoing lung resection for recurrent colorectal cancer.[52] Although these patients make up a small percentage of those originally undergoing primary resection, a policy of aggressive pulmonary resection mandates optimal surveillance.

Since lung metastases are almost uniformly asymptomatic, radiological imaging is necessary for their detection. Although computed tomography is more sensitive in detecting lung metastases than chest x-ray examination,[53,54] it is also much more expensive. Unless multiple, clearly nonresectable lung metastases are seen on chest x-ray, a confirmatory computed tomography scan of the chest should be done to more precisely define the extent of pulmonary disease. We recommend that plain chest radiography be performed annually up to 5 years postoperatively to cover the period of highest risk for recurrence (Table 8-2).

Colonoscopy

As discussed previously, after removal of a rectal cancer via low anterior resection, restorative proctectomy, or local excision, sigmoidoscopy should be part of each routine physical examination to detect early anastomotic or peri-anastomotic recurrences. Although colonoscopy may detect intraluminal or extraluminal recurrent disease at a colonic anastomotic site, the chief value of colonoscopy is in the detection of metachronous carcinoma and adenomatous polyps, with the potential for endoscopic elimination of the latter. If a complete colonoscopy was not performed preoperatively, it should be performed approximately 3 months postoperatively. This is necessary to rule out a missed carcinoma and to remove polyps.

If the initial perioperative colonoscopy did not reveal metachronous polyps, we agree with the recommendation by Macintosh et al. that complete colonoscopy be repeated 1 year postoperatively (Table 8-2). Recommendations for the frequency of subsequent follow-up colonoscopy depend on the endoscopic findings. Colonoscopy with polypectomy should be repeated every 6 months until no polyps are detected (a clean examination). If the colonoscopy at 1 year is normal, colonoscopy should be performed in another 3 years. If this is normal, a long-term regimen of colonoscopy every 3 to 5 years should then be followed. The National Polyp Study[55] recently showed that colonoscopy every 3 years after an initial colonoscopic polypectomy is as efficacious and safe as an annual colonoscopy in preventing progression of adenomatous polyps to colorectal cancer. In fact, Winawer has stated that after a clean 3-year colonoscopy, the interval can probably be safely extended to 5 years (S. Winawer, personal communication). Our recommendations regarding follow-up colonoscopy after colorectal cancer resection are based on an extrapolation of these data.

Patients with HNPCC represent a special challenge. If this condition is recognized preoperatively, a subtotal colectomy should be performed in otherwise healthy patients who have a colorectal tumor with a potential for cure. The remaining rectum should be examined regularly, since these patients tend to be young with many years at risk for the development of metachronous rectal cancer. The risk of rectal cancer in patients with HNPCC has not been fully defined.

Selective Evaluation

Tests such as TRUS and computed tomography of the abdomen, pelvis, or chest should be undertaken only when the suspicion of recurrence is raised by the modalities already used (Table 8-2). This strategy aims not only to reduce the expense of routine testing but also to limit the investigations that an abnormal test result may elicit. One or more of these ancillary tests is performed first to confirm recurrence at the suspected site. If recurrence proves to be present, a strategic extent-of-disease workup is performed in keeping with individualized therapeutic goals. If curative or palliative repeat resection is deemed feasible and appropriate, a thorough evaluation of extent of disease is required. If repeat resection is not possible or not indicated, some other form of palliative therapy may be selected, which would determine the need if any for further investigation.

REFERENCES

1. Steele G Jr. Follow-up plans after treatment of primary colon and rectum cancer. World J Surg 1991;15:583-8.
2. The American Society of Colon and Rectal Surgeons Standards Task Force. Practice parameters for the detection of colorectal neoplasms. Dis Colon Rectum 1992;35:389-94.
3. Fleisher DE, Goldberg SB, Browning TH, et al. Detection and surveillance of colorectal cancer. JAMA 1989;261:580-5.
4. Goldenberg DM, Neville AM, Carter AC, et al. Carcinoembryonic antigen: its role as a marker in the management of cancer; summary of an NIH consensus statement. Br Med J 1981;282:373-5.
5. August DA, Ottow RT, Sugarbaker PH. Clinical perspective of human colorectal cancer metastasis. Cancer Met Rev 1984;3:303-24.
6. Averbach AM, Sugarbaker PH. Use of tumor markers and radiologic tests in follow-up, In: Cohen AM, Winawer SJ, editors. Cancer of the colon, rectum and anus. New York: McGraw-Hill, 1995:725-51.
7. Weir JA. Colorectal cancer: metachronous and other associated neoplasms. Dis Colon Rectum 1975;18:4-5.
8. Polk HC, Spratt JS, Butcher HR. Frequency of multiple primary malignant neoplasms associated with colorectal carcinoma. Am J Surg 1965;109:71-5.
9. Enblad P, Adami HO, Glimelius B, Krusemo U, Pahlman L. The risk of subsequent primary malignant diseases after cancers of the colon and rectum: a nationwide cohort study. Cancer 1990;65:2091-100.
10. Hoar SK, Wilson J, Blot JW, et al. Second cancer following cancer in the digestive system in Connecticut 1953-82. In: Grenwald P, editor. Multiple cancers in Connecticut and Denmark, National Cancer Institute Monograph 68. Washington, DC: U.S. Government Printing Office, 1993:49-82.
11. Schoenberg BS, Myers MH. Statistical methods for studying multiple primary neoplasms. Cancer 1977;40(4 Suppl):1892-8.
12. Teppo L, Pukkala E, Saxen E. Multiple cancer: an epidemiologic exercise in Finland. J Natl Cancer Inst 1985;75;207-17.
13. Galandiuk S, Wieand HS, Moertel CG, et al. Patterns of recurrence after curative resection of carcinoma of the colon and rectum. Surg Gynecol Obstet 1992;174:27-32.
14. Deans GT, Parks TG, Rowlands BJ, Spence RA. Prognostic factors in colorectal cancer. Br J Surg 1992;79:608-13.
15. Guillem JG, Murray MP, Zeng ZS, Kuranami M, Swallow CJ, Mansilla-Soto J. Matrix metalloproteinases and tissue inhibitor of metalloproteinases in colorectal cancer invasion, metastases, and prognosis. Semin Colon Rectum Surg 1996;7:31-9.
16. Beart RW Jr, O'Connell MJ. Postoperative follow-up of patients with carcinoma of the colon. Mayo Clin Proc 1983;58:361-3.
17. Sugarbaker PH, Gianola FJ, Dwyer A, Neuman NR. A simplified plan for follow-up of patients with colon and rectal cancer supported by prospective studies of laboratory and radiologic test results. Surgery 1987;102:79-87.
18. Rodriguez-Bigas MA, Stulc JP, Davidson B, Petrelli NJ. Prognostic significance of anastomotic recurrence from colorectal adenocarcinoma. Dis Colon Rectum 1992;35:838-42.
19. Beynon J, Mortensen NJ, Foy DM, Channer JL, Rigby H, Virjee J. The detection and evaluation of locally recurrent rectal cancer with rectal endosonography. Dis Colon Rectum 1989;32:509-17.
20. Mascagni D, Corbellini L, Urciuoli P, Di Matteo G. Endoluminal ultrasound for early detection of local recurrence of rectal cancer. Br J Surg 1989;76:1176-80.
21. Charnley RM, Pyf G, Amar SS, Hardcastle JD. The early detection of recurrent rectal carcinoma by rectal endosonography. (SRS Abstracts) Br J Surg 1988;75:1232.
22. McDermott FT, Hughes ES, Pihl E, Johnson WR, Price AB. Local recurrence after potentially curative resection for rectal cancer in a series of 1008 patients. Br J Surg 1985;72:34-7.
23. Michelassi F, Vannucci L, Ayala JJ, Chapel R, Goldberg R, Block GE. Local recurrence after curative resection of colorectal adenocarcinoma. Surgery 1990;108:787-93.
24. Ovaska JT, Jarvinen HJ, Mecklin JP. The value of follow-up programme after radical surgery for colorectal carcinoma. Scand J Gastroenterol 1989;24:416-22.
25. Safi F, Link KH, Beger HG. Is follow-up of colorectal cancer patients worthwhile? Dis Colon Rectum 1993;36:636-44.
26. Schiessel R, Wunderlich M, Herbst F. Local recurrence of colorectal cancer: effect of early detection and aggressive surgery. Br J Surg 1986;73:342-4.
27. Berge I, Ekelund C, Meller B. Carcinoma of the colon and rectum in a defined population. Acta Chir Scand 1973;438(Suppl):1-86.
28. Sugarbaker PH, Zamcheck N, Moore FD. Assessment of serial carcinoembryonic antigen (CEA) assays in postoperative detection of recurrent colorectal cancer. Cancer 1976;38:2310-5.
29. Boey J, Cheung HC, Lai CK, Wong J. A prospective evaluation of serum carcinoembryonic antigen (CEA) levels in the management of colorectal carcinoma. World J Surg 1984;8:279-86.
30. Wanebo HJ, Llaneras M, Martin T, Kaiser D. Prospective monitoring trial for carcinoma of colon and rectum after surgical resection. Surg Gynecol Obstet 1989;169:479-87.
31. Rognum TO. CEA, tumour differentiation and DNA ploidy pattern. Scand J Gastroenterol 1988;149:166-78.
32. Gilbertsen VA, Wangensteen OH. A summary of thirteen years experience with the second look program. Surg Gynecol Obstet 1962;114:438-42.
33. Martin EW Jr, Minton JP, Carey LC. CEA-directed second-look surgery in the asymptomatic patient after primary resection of colorectal cancer. Ann Surg 1985;202:310-7.
34. Minton JP, Hoehn JL, Gerber DM, et al. Results of a 400-patient carcinoembryonic antigen second-look colorectal cancer study. Cancer 1985;55:1284-90.
35. Moertel CG, Fleming TR, Macdonald JS, Haller DG, Laurie JA, Tangen C. An evaluation of the carcinoembryonic antigen (CEA) test for monitoring patients with resected colon cancer. JAMA 1993;270:943-7.
36. Northover JM. Carcinoembryonic antigen and recurrent colorectal cancer. Br J Surg 1985;72(Suppl):S44-6.
37. Northover JM, Slack WW. A randomized controlled trial of CEA-prompted second look surgery in recurrent colorectal cancer: a preliminary report. (abstract) Dis Colon Rectum 1984;27:576.

38. Kievit J, van de Velde CJH. Utility and cost of carcinoembryonic antigen monitoring in colon cancer follow-up evaluation: a Markov analysis. Cancer 1990;65:2580-7.
39. Wanebo JH, Rao B, Pinsky CM, et al. Preoperative carcinoembryonic antigen level as a prognostic indicator in colorectal cancer. N Engl J Med 1978;299:448-51.
40. Sugarbaker PH. Carcinoma of the colon: prognosis and operative choice. Curr Probl Surg 1981;18:753-802.
41. Barillari P, Bolognese A, Chirletti P, Cardi M, Sammartino P, Stipa V. Role of CEA, TPA and CA 19-9 in the early detection of localized and diffuse recurrent cancer. Dis Colon Rectum 1992;35:471-6.
42. Racklin MS, Senagore AJ, Talbott TM. Role of carcinoembryonic antigen and liver function tests in the detection of recurrent colorectal carcinoma. Dis Colon Rectum 1991;34:794-7.
43. Yamaguchi A, Kurosaka Y, Ishida T, et al. Clinical significance of tumor marker NCC-ST 439 large bowel cancers. Dis Colon Rectum 1991;34:921-4.
44. Guadagni F, Roselli M, Cosimelli M, et al. Biologic evaluation of tumor-associated glycoprotein-72 and carcinoembryonic antigen expression in colorectal cancer, Part I. Dis Colon Rectum 1994;37(Suppl 2):S16-23.
45. Iemura K, Moriya Y. A comparative analysis of the serum levels of NCC-ST-439, CEA and CA 19-9 in patients with colorectal carcinoma. Eur J Surg Oncol 1993;19:439-42.
46. Filella X, Molina R, Pique JM, et al. Use of CA 19-9 in the early detection of recurrences in colorectal cancer: comparison with CEA. Tumor Biol 1994;15:1-6.
47. McCormack PM. Surgery for pulmonary metastases. In: Cohen AM, Winawer SJ, editors. Cancer of the colon, rectum and anus. New York: McGraw-Hill, 1995:857-61.
48. Brister SJ, de Varennes B, Gordon PH, Sheiner NM, Pym J. Contemporary operative management of pulmonary metastases of colorectal origin. Dis Colon Rectum 1988;31:786-92.
49. Scheele J, Altendorf-Hofmann A, Stangl R, Gall FP. Pulmonary resection for metastatic colon and upper rectum: is it useful? Dis Colon Rectum 1990;33:745-52.
50. Mori M, Tomoda H, Ishida T, et al. Surgical resection of pulmonary metastases from colorectal adenocarcinoma: special reference to repeated pulmonary resections. Arch Surg 1991;126:1297-302.
51. McAfee MK, Allen MS, Trastek VF, Ilstrup DM, Deschamps C, Pairolero PC. Colorectal lung metastases: results of surgical excision. Ann Thorac Surg 1992;53:780-6.
52. McCormack PM, Ginsberg RB, Bains MS, et al. Accuracy of lung imaging in metastases with implications for the role of thoracoscopy. Ann Thorac Surg 1993;56:863-6.
53. Pass HI, Dwyer A, Makuch R, Roth JA. Detection of pulmonary metastases in patients with osteogenic and soft tissue sarcomas: the superiority of CT scans compared with conventional linear tomograms using dynamic analysis. J Clin Oncol 1985;3:1261-5.
54. Peuchot M, Libshitz HI. Pulmonary metastatic disease: radiologic-surgical correlation. Radiology 1987;164:719-22.
55. Winawer SJ, Zauber AG, O'Brien MJ, et al. Randomized comparison of surveillance intervals after colonoscopic removal of newly diagnosed adenomatous polyps: the National Polyp Study Group. N Engl J Med 1993;328:901-6.

➢ COUNTERPOINT

National Cancer Center Hospital, Japan

YOSHIHIRO MORIYA

The current follow-up strategies for colorectal cancer are aimed at early diagnosis and surgical treatment for recurrence, evaluation and analysis of applied treatment modalities, and detection of metachronous carcinoma at a relatively early stage.

Three main areas of controversy exist. The first is cost. The financial burden of attempting to cure patients with recurrence is considerable. The cost considerations are similar to those raised by mass screening for early detection of primary tumors. The second problem concerns which diagnostic methods to choose. The third is whether any treatment is effective for recurrent disease. Few patients with recurrence are cured.

CURRENT PRACTICE

Some patients are known to have a high risk of recurrent disease. This prognostic information is derived from pathological findings of the primary tumor (such as high T stage and lymph node metastasis). Recurrent tumors in these patients tend to be more difficult to treat than recurrences in patients with low-stage cancer, and the therapies are correspondingly less effective. Ideally all patients should receive follow-up study. In practice, Japanese physicians tend to follow up on high-risk patients most closely, although financial considerations often limit follow-up intensity.

PERIOD OF FOLLOW-UP STUDY

About 75% of recurrences are obvious within 2 years of initial surgery. Programs to detect recurrence should therefore be most intensive during the first 2 years. In this sense I agree with the follow-up program proposed by Macintosh et al. After curative surgery, patients are checked with serum CEA determination, ultrasonography of the liver, chest x-ray examination, and careful physical examination every 3 to 6 months for 2 years, every 6 months for 5 years, and annually thereafter to detect metachronous malignancy (Table 8-3). When surveillance testing detects recurrence, additional examinations (computed tomography scanning, barium enema, colonoscopy, and so forth) are carried out as indicated.

Steele[1] has proposed three possible follow-up plans depending on the practice capabilities of the physician. His analysis supposes that since early detection of recurrent disease does not generally lead to effective therapy, intensive follow-up should be performed only when research trials of new therapy are available.

Data concerning surgery for liver metastases introduce a note of caution. Of 153 patients with hepatic metastasis, 81 (53%) underwent hepatic resection and the 5-year survival rate after hepatectomy was 47%, regardless of the number of hepatic metastases. A similar tendency was observed in patients with pulmonary metastasis. Thirty-nine (37%) of 106 patients with lung metastasis from colorectal cancer underwent metastasectomy, and the 5-year survival rate after pulmonary resection was 32%. Consequently, physicians at the National Cancer Center Hospital in Tokyo continue to emphasize a strict follow-up program leading to early detection and aggressive surgery, if feasible. This clearly can result in successful treatment of recurrent disease.

Table 8-3 Follow-up of patients with colorectal cancer: National Cancer Center Hospital, Japan

	YEAR				
	1	2	3	4	5
Office visit	2-4	2-4	2	2	2
CEA	2-4	2-4	2	2	2
Liver function tests	2-4	2-4	2	2	2
Complete blood count	2-4	2-4	2	2	2
Chest x-ray	2-4	2-4	2	2	2
Abdominal ultrasound	2-4	2-4	2	2	2
Pelvic computed tomography*	3	2	1	1	0
Abdominal computed tomography*	2	2	1	1	0
Colonoscopy or barium enema	1	1	1	1	1

CEA, Carcinoembryonic antigen.
*Performed as part of intensive follow-up when recurrence is suspected.

PATTERNS OF RECURRENCE: COLON VERSUS RECTUM

Patterns of recurrence are different in colon cancer than in rectal cancer. The follow-up regimens should reflect this. For example, the follow-up programs after rectal cancer surgery should emphasize detection of local recurrence and pulmonary metastasis, whereas follow-up after colon cancer surgery should emphasize detection of liver metastasis.

The risk of recurrence depends mainly on the stage of the primary tumor. Rates of recurrence in patients with Dukes A tumor are low for both colonic and rectal cancer. For Dukes C rectal cancer, local recurrence is the most common site (58 of 383 Dukes C cases, 15%), followed by hepatic (46 cases, 12%) and pulmonary sites (40 cases, 10%). On the other hand, local and pulmonary recurrence rates for colonic cancer are low and the most frequently affected site is the liver (40 of 325 Dukes C cases, 12%). Other indicators of high risk are elevated CEA levels before initial surgery, poorly differentiated or signet-ring-cell carcinoma, and venous or lymphatic invasion as revealed by microscopy.

The clinical utility of genetic markers of recurrence risk has not been established. When the mechanism of tumor progression and metastasis at the level of molecular biology has been elucidated, however, more effective follow-up using gene-based markers may be possible.

METHODOLOGY OF FOLLOW-UP STUDY

Office Visits and Physical Examination

Attending physicians should pay careful attention to such symptoms as change in bowel habits and pain, as well as physical findings, particularly digital rectal examination and palpation of the inguinal region in patients after rectal cancer surgery. Digital examination of the rectum is especially important after sphincter-saving procedures to detect locoregional recurrence. CEA measurement, chest radiography, and ultrasound of the liver are generally performed at each visit.

Nonspecific Tests

Liver function tests, kidney function tests, and complete blood count have little value in detecting early recurrence after curative surgery of colorectal cancer. They are often used to monitor side effects of adjuvant chemoradiotherapy, however. Although an elevated alkaline phosphatase level occasionally accompanies hepatic metastasis, this finding is nonspecific. Occasionally a rising level of CEA or other tumor markers may be explained by changes in liver and kidney function, which can be detected by appropriate testing.

Carcinoembryonic Antigen Monitoring

CEA has a 70% to 80% sensitivity in detecting recurrences.[2] The rate of positive CEA and patterns of rising CEA level are different for specific sites of recurrence. Hematogenous metastases are more commonly accompanied by elevated CEA levels than are locoregional recurrences or peritoneal seeding. Steele et al.[3] have shown that CEA monitoring is a poor guide to local recurrence. An early, rapid rise is likely to indicate disseminated disease.[4] However, CEA monitoring and slope analysis can be used to detect hepatic metastasis and to select patients for repeat resection.[4] In general, a slower CEA rise predicts a better chance of a successful salvage procedure.

Calculation of CEA doubling time leads to fewer false-positive results than a single CEA test. Although not yet commonly used, CEA doubling time promises to be an important indicator of recurrent disease.

Other tumor markers such as CA 19-9, TAG-72, and ST-439 have been compared with CEA for clinical usefulness in follow-up programs but have low sensitivity in detecting recurrence.[5] Not surprisingly, use of several tumor markers probably enhances detection of recurrent disease.

Martin et al.[6] reported their experience with CEA-directed second-look laparotomy. They obtained a better cure rate in patients who underwent laparotomy before the CEA level exceeded 10 ng/ml. At present, the need for CEA-directed laparotomy is uncommon because current imaging tests are improving steadily. When recurrent disease predicted by increasing CEA cannot be found, physicians at the National Cancer Center Hospital use frequent imaging studies rather than laparotomy. With this strategy, relatively early detection of recurrent disease is sometimes possible and aggressive salvage surgery for locoregional, hepatic, and pulmonary metastases can be curative.

Chest X-Ray Examination

The 5-year survival rate after pulmonary metastasectomy from colorectal cancer ranges from 15% to 42%.[7] Therefore chest x-ray should be performed every 3 to 6 months for 2 years, every 6 months for the subsequent 3 years, and annually thereafter. Suggestive radiographic findings should prompt computed tomography to judge resectability. Although the incidence of pulmonary metastasis is low in patients with colonic cancer, lung metastases are almost as common as liver metastases in patients with rectal cancer.

Detection of Liver Metastasis

At present, several imaging techniques (ultrasound, computed tomography, and magnetic resonance imaging) are customarily used for early detection of recurrent disease. Ultrasound of the liver is the most frequently used in Japan because it can be performed easily in outpatient clinics by the clinician. Experienced investigators with modern ultrasound equipment can detect very small lesions in the liver.[8] When the CEA level rises or lesions are suspected because of ultrasound abnormalities, more accurate imaging tests, such as contrast-enhanced computed tomography scan, should be used to judge the number and position of the hepatic metastases.[9] In Western countries the sensitivity of ultrasound in detecting liver metastases is lower than has been reported in Japan,[10] perhaps because of the lower incidence of obesity in Japan.

Resection of liver metastases yields better results than does surgery for most other sites of recurrent disease. Physicians at the National Cancer Center Hospital have found that nearly half of patients with liver metastasis from colorectal cancer are candidates for metastasectomy. Therefore early detection of hepatic metastasis is very important in designing rational follow-up strategies.

Colonoscopic Surveillance

Although the primary role of endoscopic surveillance is in diagnosis and treatment of metachronous colorectal lesions, recurrent diseases such as peritoneal seeding and anastomotic and locoregional recurrence in the pelvis are occasionally detected as well. This occurs when the disease causes stenosis, rigidity, or intramucosal invasion of the large bowel. Air-contrast barium enema can yield results similar to colonoscopy in detecting recurrent disease. For detection of locoregional recurrence, endorectal ultrasound (for patients with low anterior resection) and computed tomography (for those with abdominoperineal resection) appear to be more useful than conventional endoscopy. Because recurrent tumors grow primarily in the perimesenteric tissue, mesorectum, or pelvic side wall—that is, extraluminally—they generally are visible from the luminal surface only late in the course of disease.

At present the optimal frequency of colonoscopic surveillance for detecting metachronous colorectal lesions has not been established. Colonoscopic surveillance every 2 or 3 years is recommended for sporadic colorectal cancer. However, patients with higher risk of metachronous cancer (for example, those with first-degree blood relatives who have colorectal cancer, with hereditary nonpolyposis colorectal cancer, or with onset before 40 years old) should receive annual colonoscopic examination.[11]

Radioimmunoscintigraphy Using Radiolabeled Monoclonal Antibodies

Doerr et al.[12] reported that immunoscintigraphy was superior to computed tomography in detecting pelvic and extrahepatic recurrences. Intraoperative scanning using the hand-held gamma detection probe has a higher reported lesion sensitivity than ordinary imaging techniques such as computed tomography.[13] However, radioimmunoguided surgery still presents several problems. The image quality is still poor and depends on the operator's skill. The test lacks sensitivity because some patients with colorectal cancer do not react with the antibody. The learning curve is steep, and the test is expensive. Consequently, radioimmunoscintigraphy for detecting recurrent disease is still thought to be in the research stage.

CONCLUSION

Recurrent colorectal cancers, unlike other gastrointestinal malignancies, can be effectively treated by surgery alone in some cases. In Japan, therefore, early detection of recurrent disease in the liver or lung or at the original primary site is considered important. This policy permits life-prolonging surgery and so improves the survival rate in patients with advanced colorectal cancer. Unfortunately, the effect of chemotherapy on recurrent colorectal cancer is too small to extend life appreciably. Early detection under a strict follow-up program followed by aggressive surgery is in my opinion the only way to improve survival rates in patients with recurrent colorectal cancer.

REFERENCES

1. Steele G Jr. Follow-up plans after treatment of primary cancer of colon and rectum. World J Surg 1991;15:583-8.
2. Armitage NC, Davidson A, Tsikos D, Wood CB. A study of the reliability of carcinoembryonic antigen blood levels in following the course of colorectal cancer. Clin Oncol 1984;10:141-7.
3. Steele G Jr, Ellenberg SE, Ramming K, et al. CEA monitoring among patients in multi-institutional adjuvant GI therapy protocols. Ann Surg 1982;196:162-9.
4. Boey J, Cheung HC, Lai CK, Wong J. A prospective evaluation of serum carcinoembryonic antigen (CEA) levels in the management of colorectal carcinoma. World J Surg 1984;8:279-86.
5. Iemura K, Moriya Y. A comparative analysis of the serum levels of NCC-ST-439, CEA and CA 19-9 in patients with colorectal carcinoma. Eur J Surg Oncol 1993;19:439-42.
6. Martin EW Jr, Minton JP, Carey LC. CEA-directed second-look surgery in the asymptomatic patient after primary resection of colorectal carcinoma. Ann Surg 1985;202:310-7.
7. Goya T, Miyazawa N, Kondo H, Tsuchiya R, Naruke T, Suemasu K. Surgical resection of pulmonary metastases from colorectal cancer: 10-year follow-up. Cancer 1989;64:1418-21.
8. Gunven P, Makuuchi M, Takayasu K, Moriyama N, Yamasaki S, Hasegawa H. Preoperative imaging of liver metastases: comparison of angiography, CT scan, and ultrasonography. Ann Surg 1985; 202:573-9.
9. Nelson RC, Chezmar JL, Sugarbaker PH, Bernardino ME. Hepatic tumors: comparison of CT during arterial portography, delayed CT, and MR imaging for preoperative evaluation. Radiology 1989; 172:27-34.
10. Schreve RH, Terpstra OT, Ausema L. Detection of liver metastases: a prospective study comparing liver enzymes, scintigraphy, ultrasonography and computed tomography. Br J Surg 1994;71:947-9.

11. Svendsen LB, Bulow S, Mellemgaard A. Metachronous colorectal cancer in young patients: expression of the hereditary nonpolyposis colorectal cancer syndrome? Dis Colon Rectum 1991;34:790-3.
12. Doerr RJ, Herrera L, Abdel-Nabi H. In-111 CYT-103 monoclonal antibody imaging in patients with suspected recurrent colorectal cancer. Cancer 1993;71(12 Suppl):4241-7.
13. Martin EW Jr, Tuttle SE, Rousseau M, et al. Radioimmunoguided surgery: intraoperative use of monoclonal antibody 17-1A in colorectal cancer. Hybridoma 1986;5(Suppl 1):S97-108.

➢ COUNTER POINT

Royal Liverpool University Hospital, UK

MICHAEL G. THOMAS AND MICHAEL J. HERSHMAN

Approximately half of patients undergoing potentially curative resection of colorectal cancer die of recurrent disease.[1] The poor prognosis in colorectal cancer stems from its late presentation, and this is unlikely to be altered dramatically unless large bowel neoplasia is detected at an early stage in the dysplasia-adenoma-adenocarcinoma sequence.[1-3] In the future, earlier diagnosis might be achieved by national population screening for gastrointestinal blood loss and a clearer understanding of familial inheritance of this disease.[3-5] Possibly a combination of kindred analysis, population health education, and fecal occult blood testing will have an impact on the stage of presentation of colorectal malignancy. At present, however, recurrence after curative resection appears to reflect mode of presentation, stage and pathology of the tumor, physiology of the patient, and surgeon-related variability. Indeed, only about half of patients with colorectal cancer undergo radical curative resection in regionally based hospitals in the United Kingdom, with an overall 5-year survival of 26.45% for colonic cancer and 28.2% for rectal cancer.[6] Specialist centers can, however, achieve higher rates for potentially curative resection; an 80% rate for rectal cancer has been reported from St. Mark's Hospital.[7-9]

LOCAL RECURRENCE

Reported local recurrence rates after curative resection vary widely (2.6% to 40%),[10,11] and 80% to 90% of such patients die within 5 years.[12,13] Without surgery less than 4% of patients who harbor local recurrence survive 4 years.[14] In addition, only 5% to 20% of patients with local recurrence have resectable disease, and about 90% of these die within the next 3 years.[10] Recurrence of colorectal cancer at the site of an anastomosis can be viewed as a failure of the primary surgical procedure.[15] Winchester and McBride[16] reported a 19% incidence of local recurrence after right-sided colonic resections and a 10% incidence after left-sided colonic resections. Early diagnosis of local recurrence is crucial if repeat resection for cure is contemplated.

Rectal recurrence often occurs in isolation, and although the time taken for local recurrence to appear is variable, it usually occurs within 2 years and most series show a peak at around 6 to 12 months.[10,12,13,17-19] There is also an age-related increase in local recurrence rates.[19] The tumor itself is clearly important; lateral pelvic spread,[20] Dukes stage,[9,12,17,19,21,22] differentiation, and the number of lymph nodes involved all strongly influence recurrence rates.[23,24] Quirke et al.[20] suggest that local recurrence is due to microscopic lateral tumor spread beyond the resection margins. To an extent, this observation might account for the inverse relationship between distance of the tumor from the anal verge and recurrence rates.[12,13,19,25] The limited space in the lower pelvis and rapid spread of tumor may make total pelvic clearance more difficult.[10] The operation itself is, of course, important. Local perforation,[17,26] extension into adjacent organs,[11] inadequate excision of the mesorectum,[27,28] and intraoperative shedding of viable tumor cells may all increase recurrence rates.[29-31] Also, for locally advanced tumors the anterior plane of dissection may limit resectability. Indeed, extension of the dissection to involve the posterior wall of the vagina appears to reduce local recurrence rates in female patients.[11]

Data from the National Cancer Center Hospital in Japan suggest that 36% of patients with Dukes B and C tumors have lateral lymph node involvement.[32] The results of extended radical pelvic lymphadenectomy with 5-year, disease-free survival figures of 69% and symptomatic recurrence rates of 5% are being reported from Japan. Published results on local recurrence after extended dissection do, however, vary.[33] To date the increased morbidity associated with extended lymphatic dissection coupled with a lack of data from randomized trials of radical-versus-nonradical surgery has made radical lymphadenectomy an unattractive addition to curative surgery in Western physicians' eyes.

There is evidence that early detection of local recurrence after radical surgery for rectal cancer leads to better survival.[33] Metaanalysis suggests that intensive follow-up increases the detection of asymptomatic recurrences and metachronous tumors.[34] Also, patients with asymptomatic recurrences are more likely to undergo surgery if the recurrence is detected by a vigorous follow-up protocol.[34] Thus follow-up should be intensive for the first 2 years. Clinical examination alone is not very sensitive and therefore should be supplemented by endoscopy or sigmoidoscopy, radiological imaging, and serology. Computed tomography has been considered the best alternative to simple palpation and sigmoidoscopy, but lesions of 2 cm or greater are required for accurate diagnosis and distinction from fibrosis can be difficult.[35] Imaging techniques such as magnetic resonance imaging might improve sensitivity and specificity in the future.[36]

Debate continues concerning the role of CEA as an early predictor of recurrence. In detecting recurrence in asymptomatic patients, the pattern of CEA level rise is probably more important than single-point elevations.[10,37,38] Caution is required, however, since up to 30% of patients with colorectal cancer recurrence do not show an increase in CEA levels and nonmalignant conditions can cause a rise in levels.[10,38-40] Despite a lack of absolute sensitivity or specificity, CEA appears to be a marker for local recurrence.[38] It has been suggested that intensive follow-up in rectal cancer may have no effect on survival unless combined with measurements of CEA.[34] Clearly this is a controversial claim. In contrast, the preliminary results of the Cancer Research Campaign's CEA second-look trial suggest that knowledge of CEA levels does not affect patient outcome. Therefore, if CEA monitoring does not save lives, should it be undertaken? At present this question remains open. Physicians at the Royal Liverpool University Hospital advocate routine CEA measurements in outpatients as part of follow-up and consider endoluminal magnetic resonance imaging and diagnostic laparoscopy in asymptomatic patients with consistently raised CEA levels.

Endoluminal endosonography performed routinely by use of either a rectal or a vaginal probe can detect local recurrence.[41] In a series of 66 patients who had undergone radical resection for rectal carcinoma, 20% had endosonographic evidence of recurrence. Salvage surgery was possible in four of these 13 cases and in three of these patients recurrence was diagnosed by ultrasound alone.[41] The time interval for scanning is yet to be clearly defined, but a suggested scheme is a baseline scan at 3 months with repeat scanning every 6 months.[41] Although the yield with luminal ultrasound is not high, physicians at our institution advocate its use in selected patients at high risk for local recurrence.[41,42] In addition, our experience with colonoscopic endoluminal ultrasound and intraluminal magnetic resonance imaging is increasing.

Salvage surgery can achieve reasonable results. Vassilopoulos et al.[15] reported a median 5-year survival rate of 49% in patients with complete resection and a survival rate of 12% in patients with microscopic residual disease.[15] Data from St. Mark's Hospital suggest that survival in patients with local recurrence relates to the radical nature of the operation, the absence of severe disease, and a small diameter of the recurrent tumor.[43] Extensive pelvic resection for rectal recurrence involving sacral resection with composite resection of affected viscera and musculoskeletal elements can achieve 4-year survival figures of 33% and disease-free survival in 27% of patients.[14] Such bold surgery is undertaken at a price. Perioperative mortality was 8.5% in the 53 patients of Wanebo et al.,[14] with 50% of the patients requiring an ileal conduit and nearly all having some perioperative morbidity. Tissue diagnosis is obviously essential before extended surgery is planned. Disease-free survival appears to be better in patients with low CEA values and in those in whom the primary procedure was an anterior resection.[14,43] The adequacy of the resection margins, the status of peripelvic lymph nodes, and the presence or absence of bone marrow infiltration can also affect long-term results in salvage surgery.[14] However, a small recurrent tumor diameter might be the most important prognostic indicator.[43]

ADJUVANT THERAPY

Radiation Therapy

The role of radiation therapy in colonic cancer needs to be more clearly defined. Both preoperative and postoperative radiation therapy does, however, appear to be useful in patients with rectal cancer.[10] Radiation therapy can reduce the local recurrence rate but may not alter disease-free survival.[44-46] Low-dose preoperative radiation followed by surgery and postoperative radiation ("sandwich" therapy) does not appear to reduce local recurrence or 5-year survival.[46] When local recurrence follows preoperative radiation therapy, there is no difference in the site and symptoms of the recurrence between irradiated and nonirradiated patients.[47] Controlled trials with high-dose preoperative radiation therapy suggest that patients with rectal carcinoma may have reduced local recurrence rates, but at present no hard evidence suggests a survival benefit.[45,46,48]

Recent trials have shown an increase in survival figures. The first Medical Research Council trial of preoperative radiation therapy suggested a real biological effect of irradiation on the tumor; despite this fact, the trial failed to demonstrate differences in survival or recurrence.[49] The preliminary results of the most recent Medical Research Council trial of preoperative radiation therapy in fixed or partially fixed rectal tumors show a downstaging and downsizing of tumors in the radiation group with a significant reduction in local and distant recurrence rates. There is, however, only a trend toward increased survival, and thus the results are similar to other published trial data.[45,46]

Only one controlled trial has shown a trend toward reduced local recurrence rates with postoperative radiation therapy.[50] The ongoing multicenter trials of both preoperative and postoperative radiation therapy in rectal cancer in the United Kingdom may help define the role of adjuvant radiation in rectal cancer. Palliative radiation therapy in combination with 5-FU does produce significant relief of symptoms and slowing of tumor progression in the treatment of established local recurrence and thus should be considered for patients unsuitable for salvage surgery.[51,52]

Contact radiation is a highly effective local treatment for rectal disease, as eloquently demonstrated in Jean Papillon's monograph on the results of intracavity irradiation at the Centre Leon Berard in Lyon during the past 30 years. Provided that patients are selected carefully and proper treatment schedules are used, excellent control of local disease can be achieved.[53] This modality has allowed a minimal-access approach in patients with early invasive rectal carcinoma or in patients deemed unfit for a laparotomy. Using transanal endoscopic microsurgery (TEM) combined with a modified Papillon technique for intracavity radiation therapy, physicians have achieved encouraging early results.[54]

Chemotherapy

Systemic single-agent chemotherapy in colon cancer has failed to show convincing benefits for disease-free and overall survival in a large number of controlled trials.[10] This, however, may be misleading, since multivariate analysis suggests a possible benefit with 5-FU.[55] When 5-FU was used in combination with levamisole, Moertel et al.[56] were able to demonstrate a 41% reduction in cancer recurrence and an estimated overall reduction in death rate of 33% in patients who had undergone curative resection for Dukes C colonic cancer. The results with B_2 disease were equivocal.[56] Analyzing multiple-agent chemotherapy in colon cancer, the large National Surgical Adjuvant Breast and Bowel Cancer Project indicated that patients given chemotherapy (5-FU with methyl *N*-[2-chloromethyl]-*N*-cyclohexyl *N*-nitrosourea and vincristine) had increased disease-free survival and overall survival compared with control subjects.[50] In addition, the data suggest that postoperative chemotherapy improves disease-free survival in men with rectal cancer under 65 years of age. The Gastrointestinal Tumor Study Group, however, reported a disease-free survival benefit in rectal cancer with combination postoperative chemotherapy and radiation therapy but not chemotherapy alone.[44]

Based on the preceding findings, when adjuvant chemotherapy is used, it should be as a multiple agent regimen with 5-FU and levamisole. All patients who have undergone curative resection for Dukes C colonic carcinoma should be offered 5-FU and levamisole. In addition, combination postoperative radiation therapy with systemic 5-FU-based chemotherapy has been shown to reduce rectal recurrence and improve survival in high-risk patients when compared with postoperative radiation therapy alone.[52] Most chemotherapy regimens last 3 to 6 months, and treatment is resumed on disease progression. The MRC CR-06 trial will attempt to establish whether open-ended chemotherapy has any benefit.

Intrahepatic chemotherapy may be useful in advanced colorectal disease. It produces a slightly increased survival time without an adverse effect on quality of life. Patients with less than 20% of their total liver volume replaced by metastases appear to gain the most benefit.

Immunomodulation, Cytokines, and Photodynamic Therapy

The presence of disseminated epithelial tumor cells can serve as a strong independent predictor of later clinical recurrence.[57] Occult metastases or microfoci of tumor cells are potential targets for monoclonal antibody-mediated, antibody-dependent cellular toxicity, since they lie unshielded in mesenchymal tissues and have low tumor cell bulk.[58] In a randomized trial of postoperative adjuvant monoclonal antibody therapy for Dukes C colorectal cancer, the antibody directed against 17-1A antigen produced a 27% reduction in recurrence rate and a 30% reduction in overall death rate.[58] The immunoglobulin gamma G2a murine monoclonal antibody appeared to have no effect on the disease-free interval. The toxic side effects with the 17-1A antibody were infrequent, and thus monoclonal antibody therapy could be a real alternative to postoperative chemoradiation to treat microscopic residual disease in the future. High-dose interleukin-2 therapies with or without lymphokine-activated killer cells or tumor-infiltrating leukocyte cells have had a disappointing impact on human metastatic colon cancer. In addition, preliminary reports from the MRC CR-04 trial suggest that the addition of interferon to systemic 5-FU regimens does not affect response rate or survival. High-dose cytokine therapy has also been disappointing in colorectal cancer, although future developments may suggest new therapeutic strategies for cytokine use in colon cancer.

No definite statistical evidence has shown that bacillus Calmette-Guérin vaccine can improve disease-free or overall survival from colorectal cancer, although it may protect against death from cardiovascular disease.[10,59] Intraoperative photodynamic therapy is aimed at treating the tumor bed to cause oxidative necrosis of the residual microscopic tumor.[60] This treatment has the benefit of minimal toxicity and side effects.[60,61] Provisional reports have been encouraging.

SYNCHRONOUS AND METACHRONOUS NEOPLASIA

When synchronous adenomas are detected distal to a proven carcinoma, two issues must be addressed. First, susceptibility to neoplastic development is probably increased throughout the colorectum.[62,63] Second, if the adenoma is to be removed endoscopically, the procedure should be delayed until after curative surgery to prevent seeding of colorectal cancer cells in the mucosal defect. In emergency situations when the whole colorectal mucosa has not been evaluated, the presence of synchronous adenoma or early carcinoma must be excluded in the early follow-up period. Colonoscopy is advocated during follow-up in all patients who have urgent or emergency surgery for colorectal cancer.

Meleagros et al.[64] suggest that after temporary fecal diversion performed during curative resection, the stoma should not be closed sooner than 3 months after the operation.[64] Early stoma closure leads to an increase in local recurrence and metastatic disease in rectal carcinoma and higher rates of systemic, metastatic disease in colonic cancer. Probably this is due to the well-documented epithelial hyperplasia seen at the anastomosis after stoma closure.[65,66]

HEPATIC METASTATIC DISEASE

The survival figures for patients with liver metastases that are untreated are, not surprisingly, poor.[67-69] Resection of hepatic metastases can result in long-term survival. Indeed, median survival time is 30 months after hepatectomy for metastatic disease, with 5-year survival rates of 25% to 40% having been reported.[70-72] Hence liver resection is the treatment of choice in patients with favorable disease. Early diagnosis of hepatic metastatic disease is therefore an important aim in follow-up.

The liver is also a frequent site of disease progression after initial hepatic resection for metastatic colorectal cancer. Approximately one third of patients with progressive liver disease have isolated liver metastases, and of these about one third could be candidates for further resection.[73-75] The Mayo Clinic experience in 21 patients demonstrated a median survival of 3.4 years after repeat resection, and these figures are similar to those for initial hepatectomy. Similar results have also been reported in 25 patients from Memorial Sloan-Kettering Cancer Center.[76] Rehepatectomy appears to be achieved with low rates of morbidity and mortality. Thus selected patients with progressive hepatic metastatic disease benefit from resection. As with local rectal recurrence, progressive hepatic disease probably represents disease overlooked at the first hepatectomy.[77] Intraoperative ultrasound improves sensitivity and can therefore be used to reduce hepatic local recurrence after hepatectomy and increase curative hepatectomy rates. Thus intraoperative ultrasound (laparoscopically or at open surgery) is mandatory before hepatic surgery for metastases.

GENETIC IMPLICATIONS IN COLORECTAL NEOPLASIA

Although well-documented familial conditions are easily diagnosed clinically, these account for only approximately 1% of the incidence of large bowel cancer.[78] There is increasing evidence of a hereditary component to the adenomas that occur in familial cancer syndrome patients, as well as many cases of sporadic adenomas.[79-81] Familial clustering of colon cancer is common, with one in five patients with colorectal cancer reporting an affected close relative.[5] Hall et al.[5] studied 83 patients who presented with colorectal cancer below 45 years of age; in the probands of these young patients, the relative risk in close relatives was 5.2, with a high risk in female relatives. The identification of susceptibility serves as a pointer for future metachronous disease and allows for screening of close relatives. There appear to be two broad genetic categories of inherited colon cancers.[82] First are those characterized by defective DNA mismatch repair genes, producing subtle errors in DNA which persist and result in abnormal replication of short nucleotide sequences. These replication errors have been identified by microsatellite probes. Recent studies suggest that five mismatch repair genes are implicated in their development.[83-86] Germline mutations in four of these genes have been observed in families with HNPCC and microsatellite instability is found in most cases of HNPCC.[82,84] In addition, a subset of sporadic colorectal cancers also manifest the mutator phenotype.[87,88] Both HNPCC-related cancers and sporadic cancer with microsatellite instability are associated with predominantly right-sided tumor development.[82,88]

The second genetic category of hereditary colon cancer is associated with mutations in the adenomatous polyposis coli (APC) gene.[89] Mutations in the APC tumor suppressor gene classically cause familial adenomatous polyposis (FAP) or the more recently recognized attenuated FAP (AFAP) phenotype.[89-92] AFAP develops at an earlier age than FAP and is associated with fewer adenomas. Somatic mutations in the APC gene have also been described in sporadic colon cancers.[90]

Mecklin et al.[93,94] and others[95] have shown that large bowel lesions in high-risk families are mainly on the right side. The suggested screening of relatives in families at risk for HNPCC commences at 35 years of age with colonoscopy and continues with screening at 3-year intervals in patients with adenomas and 5-year intervals in those with a "clean" colon until the age of 65. Patients with large adenomas are offered yearly colonoscopy.[5,86,87]

Table 8-4 Follow-up of patients with colorectal cancer (colon cancer): Royal Liverpool University Hospital, UK

	YEAR				
	1	**2**	**3**	**4**	**5**
Office visit*	4	4	3	2	2
Liver function tests	4	4	3	2	2
CEA	4	4	3	2	2
Abdominal ultrasound	2	0	0	0	0
Colonoscopy	2†	0	0	0	0

CEA, Carcinoembryonic antigen.
*Includes genetic evaluation for patients whose cancer is diagnosed before age 50.
†For patients first seen on an emergency basis, colonoscopy is also performed at 3 months to evaluate the rest of the colorectum.

FOLLOW-UP POLICY

Colon Carcinoma

At the Royal Liverpool University Hospital, patients admitted on an elective basis for resection of a colon cancer have had preoperative assessment by colonoscopy or barium enema to exclude synchronous lesions. A baseline CEA measurement and liver function tests are performed along with ultrasonography or computed tomography of the liver. All patients have a preoperative chest x-ray. Tumors are classified according to the criteria of Dukes and Jass staging and are graded for tumor acinar size (as reported from St. Mark's Hospital).[96] After potentially curative resection, patients are seen within 30 days to determine immediate perioperative morbidity and to plan further management. Patients without clear lateral resection margins are entered into the MRC's Adjuvant X-ray and 5-FU Infusion Study trial. Local invasion of the abdominal wall or adjacent structures at operation is marked with titanium surgical clips to allow postoperative radiation therapy to the potential tumor bed. In addition, physicians at the Royal Liverpool University Hospital enter patients into a trial of laparoscopically assisted colectomy that began in June 1996.

Patients are seen postoperatively at 3-month intervals for 2 years, at 4-month intervals for year 3, and at 6-month intervals until discharge at 5 years (Table 8-4). At each outpatient visit, liver function tests are performed and CEA levels are measured. Ultrasonography of the liver is performed at 6 months and 1 year, and follow-up colonoscopy is also performed. In patients who are initially seen on an emergency basis, colonoscopy is performed after 3 months to evaluate the rest of the colorectum. All patients with colon cancer diagnosed before the age of 50 undergo genetic evaluation and are invited to see a clinical geneticist.

Rectal Carcinoma

Patients admitted on an elective basis for resection of rectal cancer have had preoperative assessment by colonoscopy or barium enema and sigmoidoscopy to obtain a tissue diagnosis and exclude synchronous lesions. A baseline CEA measurement, liver function tests, and ultrasonography or computed tomography of the liver are performed. All patients have a preoperative chest x-ray. Endoluminal ultrasound, endoluminal magnetic resonance imaging, or colonoscopic endoluminal ultrasonography and computed tomography are used to evaluate the pelvis in rectal carcinomas, and suitable patients are referred for high-dose preoperative radiation therapy. Their admission date for surgery after preoperative radiation therapy is planned in consultation with the oncology team. Physicians at the Royal Liverpool University Hospital favor a short course of high-dose radiation (2,500 cGy over 5 to 7 days) with surgery within a week of the radiation therapy, with the aim of downgrading and downsizing tumors to allow low anterior resection with total mesorectal excision.[27,28]

Patients with in situ carcinomas (for example, carcinoma within a villous adenoma) within 18 cm of the anal verge are assessed by endoluminal ultrasound or colonoscopic endoluminal ultrasound. If this proves favorable, the patients are treated with 6 weeks of intraluminal contact radiation therapy, followed by transanal endoscopic microsurgery (TEM). Malignant T1 lesions that are less than 3 cm in diameter, within 12 cm of the anal verge, involve less than one third of the lumen, are mobile, and have favorable histological characteristics (well differentiated with no muscularis involvement) have contact radiation therapy for 6 weeks. If residual tumor is present after radiation, it is treated by TEM. Physicians at the Royal Liverpool University Hospital use intrarectal magnetic resonance imaging or ultrasonography for distal rectal tumors and colonoscopic endoluminal ultrasound for proximal rectal and rectosigmoid cancer. Patients with large T1 tumors have preoperative radiation therapy, and lymph node–positive patients are entered in the Quick And Simple And Reliable (QUASAR) trial.

In elderly patients or those unfit for major resection, physicians avoid extensive surgery by combining TEM with postoperative radiation therapy. The use of contact radiation to treat bulky intraluminal disease may cause luminal narrowing because of edema, so that the possibility of laser ablation before radiation therapy should be entertained. Patients with rectal carcinomas who have not received preoperative radiation therapy are offered combination postoperative radiation and multiagent chemotherapy. At present physicians at our institution are evaluating the use of laser photodynamic therapy to treat luminal disease in patients unfit for surgery.

The current policy for the detection of recurrence at the Royal Liverpool University Hospital requires follow-up visits in the outpatient department at 3-month intervals for the first year, 4-month intervals during the second year, and 6-month intervals through year 5 (Table 8-5). When possible, patients are seen at each visit by the surgeon who performed the resection. Clinical examination is combined with rigid sigmoidoscopy, and all patients have serial liver function tests and CEA measurement. Colonoscopy is performed routinely 1 year after surgery. In patients with an isolated elevation of CEA levels, this is repeated. Asymptomatic patients in whom local recurrence is strongly suspected undergo abdominal computed tomography combined with colonoscopic endoluminal ultrasound or intraluminal magnetic resonance imaging. When rectal ultrasound or magnetic resonance imaging indicates malignant disease that cannot be seen or felt on clinical examination, guided biopsy is performed.

Table 8-5 Follow-up of patients with colorectal cancer (rectal cancer): Royal Liverpool University Hospital, UK

	YEAR				
	1	2	3	4	5
Office visit*	4	3	2	2	2
Liver function tests	4	3	2	2	2
CEA	4	3	2	2	2
Sigmoidoscopy	4	3	2	2	2
Colonoscopy	1	1†	1†	1†	1†
Abdominal computed tomography	‡	‡	‡	‡	‡
Colonoscopic endoluminal ultrasound or intraluminal magnetic resonance imaging	‡	‡	‡	‡	‡

CEA, Carcinoembryonic antigen.
*Includes rectal examination.
†Performed for patients with an isolated elevation of CEA levels.
‡Performed for patients with suspected local recurrence.

Physicians at Royal Liverpool University Hospital treat extraluminal local recurrence with a combination of external beam radiation therapy and salvage surgery. Before exploration, patients have abdominal, pelvic, and chest computed tomography performed together with cystoscopy if appropriate. In patients with only intraluminal local recurrence, contact radiation therapy is used to downsize tumor bulk followed by TEM or traditional resection. In a limited number of patients laser ablation is used to reduce bulky intraluminal disease so that intraluminal contact radiation therapy can be performed.

Patients with extensive local recurrence receive palliative radiation therapy with chemotherapy, and those with intraluminal bulky tumor are treated by laser therapy or radiation implants. In patients with extensive pelvic disease that cannot be controlled by radiation therapy, laparoscopic colostomy is offered. Provided the risk of ascitic leakage and port site recurrence is kept in mind, laparoscopic resection or colostomy formation is useful to palliate patients with advanced disease. Laparoscopically assisted palliative resection is useful in a small number of selected cases, and this experience appears to be shared by others.[97]

Family Screening

A family history is obtained for all patients with colorectal cancer. Patients who may have a familial susceptibility to

HNPCC or AFAP are offered screening with colonoscopy and fecal occult blood testing every 3 years beginning at 35 years of age. Microsatellite instability and abnormalities in the DNA mismatch repair and FAP genes are detected by comparing tissue blocks from the index cancer with adjacent apparently normal tissue or DNA from white blood cells. The index case and the kindred are referred to a clinical geneticist so that lifetime risk can be estimated. This allows at-risk individuals to enter a surveillance program.

Hepatic Disease

Physicians at the Royal Liverpool University Hospital aim to detect metastatic liver disease early to allow curative hepatic resection. All patients with radiological evidence of hepatic disease are referred to a surgeon having a special interest in hepatic resection. The current policy at this institution is to repeat the ultrasound and CEA measurement 3 months after initial detection of liver metastases to determine if disease progression has occurred. Patients with disease localized to an anatomical lobe undergo computed tomography of the abdomen, chest, and pelvis to exclude extrahepatic disease. Hepatic resection is then performed if the intraoperative ultrasound findings are favorable. Bilateral hepatic disease and large lesions within the caudate lobe are assessed individually on surgical merit.

After hepatic resection all patients receive at least 3 months of 5-FU chemotherapy. Young patients with an irresectable liver metastasis and no evidence of extrahepatic disease are considered for transplantation. Hepatic cryotherapy is used as an adjuvant to hepatic resection or chemotherapy in advanced hepatic disease. Patients unsuitable for resection, transplantation, or cryotherapy are offered multiagent chemotherapy. Patients with multiple metastases are offered intrahepatic 5-FU as palliative treatment.

Pulmonary Disease

Patients with anatomically localized pulmonary disease and without irresectable extrapulmonary disease are offered resection in combination with chemotherapy. Extensive pulmonary disease is more frequently encountered than localized disease, and these patients are offered palliative chemotherapy.

REFERENCES

1. Rayter Z, Mansi JL, Leicester RJ. Adjuvant chemotherapy for colorectal cancer. Ann R Coll Surg Engl 1995;77:81-4.
2. Gordon N L, Dawson AA, Bennett B, Innes G, Eremin O, Jones PF. Outcome in colorectal adenocarcinoma; two seven-year studies of a population. Br Med J 1993;307:707-10.
3. Hart AR, Wicks AC, Mayberry JF. Colorectal cancer screening in asymptomatic populations. Gut 1995;36:590-8.
4. Hardcastle JD, Thomas WM, Chamberlain J, et al. Randomised, controlled trial of faecal occult blood screening for colorectal cancer: the results of the first 107,349 subjects. Lancet 1989;1:1160-4.
5. Hall NR, Finan PJ, Ward B, Turner G, Bishop DT. Genetic susceptibility to colorectal cancer in patients under 45 years of age. Br J Surg 1994;81:1485-9.
6. Allum WH, Slaney G, McConkey CC, Powel J. Cancer of the colon and rectum in the West Midlands, 1957-1981. Br J Surg 1994;81:1060-3.
7. Karanjia ND, Schache DJ, North WR, Heald RJ. Close shave in anterior resection. Br J Surg 1990;77:510-2.
8. Dixon AR, Maxwell WA, Holmes JT. Carcinoma of the rectum: a 10-year experience. Br J Surg 1991;78:308-11.
9. Lockhart-Mummary HE, Ritchie JK, Hawley PR. The results of surgical treatment for carcinoma of the rectum at St Mark's Hospital from 1948 to 1972. Br J Surg 1976;63:673-7.
10. Abulafi AM, Williams NS. Local recurrence of colorectal cancer: the problem, mechanisms, management and adjuvant therapy. Br J Surg 1994;81:7-19.
11. Buhre LM, Mulder NH, de Ruiter AJ, van Loon AJ, Verschueren RC. Effect of extent of anterior resection and sex on disease-free survival and local recurrence in patients with rectal cancer. Br J Surg 1994; 81:1227-9.
12. Morson BC, Vaughan EG, Bussey HJ. Pelvic recurrence after excision of rectum for cancer. Br Med J 1963;2:13-8.
13. Vandertoll DJ, Beahrs OH. Carcinoma of the rectum and low sigmoid evaluation of anterior resection in 1,766 favorable lesions. Arch Surg 1965;90:793-8.
14. Wanebo HJ, Koness RJ, Vezeridis MP, Cohen SI, Wrobleski DE. Pelvic resection of recurrent rectal cancer. Ann Surg 1994;220:586-97.
15. Vassilopoulos PP, Yoon JM, Ledesma EJ, Mittelman A. Treatment or recurrence of adenocarcinoma of the colon and rectum at the anastomotic site. Surg Gynecol Obstet 1981;152:777-80.
16. Winchester DP, McBride CM. Cancer of the colon: a comparison of survival factors. South Med J 1974;67:1025-30.
17. Phillips RK, Hittinger R, Blesovsky L, Fry JS, Fielding LP. Local recurrence following curative surgery for large bowel cancer: I. The overall picture. Br J Surg 1984;71:12-6.
18. Phillips RK, Hittinger R, Blesovsky L, Fry JS, Fielding LP. Local recurrence following curative surgery for large bowel cancer. II. The rectum and rectosigmoid. Br J Surg 1984;71:17-20.
19. Moossa AR, Ree PC, Marks JE, Levin B, Platz CE, Skinner DB. Factors influencing local recurrence after abdominoperineal resection for cancer of the rectum and rectosigmoid. Br J Surg 1975;62:727-30.
20. Quirke P, Durdey P, Dixon MF, Williams NS. Local recurrence of rectal adenocarcinoma due to inadequate surgical resection: histopathological study of lateral tumour spread and surgical excision. Lancet 1986;2:996-9.
21. Dukes CE, Bussey HJ. The spread of rectal cancer and its effects on prognosis. Br J Cancer 1958;12:309-20.
22. Wood CB, Gillis CR, Hole D, Malcolm AJ, Blumgart LH. Local tumour invasion as a prognostic factor in colorectal cancer. Br J Surg 1981;68:326-8.
23. Grinnel RS. The grading and prognosis of carcinoma of the colon and rectum. Ann Surg 1939;109:500-33.
24. Steinberg SM, Barwick KW, Stablein DM. Importance of tumour pathology and morphology in patients with surgically resected colon cancer: findings from the Gastrointestinal Tumor Study Group. Cancer 1986;58:1340-5.
25. Stearns MW, Binkley GE. The influence of location on the prognosis of operable cancer. Surg Gynecol Obstet 1953;96:368-72.
26. Patel SC, Tovee EB, Langer B. Twenty-five years of experience with radical surgical treatment of carcinoma of the extraperitoneal rectum. Surgery 1977;82:460-5.
27. Heald RJ, Husband EM, Ryall RD. The mesorectum in rectal cancer surgery—the clue to pelvic recurrence? Br J Surg 1982;69:613-6.
28. Heald RJ, Ryall RD. Recurrence and survival after total mesorectal excision for rectal cancer. Lancet 1986;1:1479-82.
29. Umpleby HC, Fermor B, Symes MO, Williamson RC. Viability of exfoliated colorectal carcinoma cells. Br J Surg 1984;71:659-63.
30. Skipper D, Cooper AJ, Marston JE, Taylor I. Exfoliated cells and in vitro growth in colorectal cancer. Br J Surg 1987;74:1049-52.
31. Fermor B, Umpleby HC, Lever JV, Symes MO, Williamson RC. The proliferative and metastatic potential of exfoliate colorectal carcinoma cells. J Natl Cancer Inst 1986;76:347-9.
32. Moriya Y, Hojo K, Sawada T, Koyama Y. Significance of lateral node dissection for advanced rectal carcinoma at or below the peritoneal reflection. Dis Colon Rectum 1989;32:307-15.

33. Moreira LF, Hizuta A, Iwagaki H, Tanaka N, Orita K. Lateral lymph node dissection for rectal carcinoma below the peritoneal reflection. Br J Surg 1994;81:293-6.
34. Bruinvels DJ, Stiggelbout AM, Kievit J, van Houwelingen HC, Habbema JD, van de Velde CJ. Follow-up of patients with colorectal cancer: a meta analysis, Ann Surg 1994;219:174-82.
35. Zaunbauer W, Haertel M, Fuchs WA. Computed tomography in carcinoma of the rectum. Gastrointest Radiol 1981;6:79-84.
36. Balzarini L, Ceglia E, D'Ippolito G, Petrillo R, Tess JD, Musumeci R. Local recurrence of rectosigmoid cancer: what about the choice of MRI for diagnosis? Gastrointest Radiol 1990;15:338-42.
37. Wood CB, Ratcliffe JG, Burt RW, Malcolm AJ, Blumgart LH. The clinical significance of the pattern of elevated serum carcinoembryonic antigen (CEA) levels in recurrent colorectal cancer. Br J Surg 1980;67:46-8.
38. Northover J. Carcinoembryonic antigen and recurrent colorectal cancer. Gut 1986;27:117-22.
39. Ovaska JT, Jarvinen HJ, Mecklin JP. The value of a follow up programme after radical surgery for colorectal carcinoma. Scand J Gastroenterol 1989;24:416-22.
40. Loewenstein MS, Zamcheck N. Carcinoembryonic antigen (CEA) levels in benign gastrointestinal disease states. Cancer 1979;42(3 Suppl):1412-8.
41. Ramirez JM, Mortensen NJ, Takeuchi N, Humphreys MM. Endoluminal ultrasonography in the follow-up of patients with rectal cancer. Br J Surg 1994;81:692-4.
42. Beynon J, Mortensen NJ, Foy DM, Channer JL, Rigby H, Virjee J. The detection and evaluation of locally recurrent rectal cancer with rectal endosonography. Dis Colon Rectum 1989;32:509-17.
43. Gagliardi G, Hawley PR, Hershman MJ, Arnott SJ. Prognostic factors in surgery for local recurrence of rectal cancer. Br J Surg 1995; 82:1401-5.
44. Gastrointestinal Tumor Study Group. Prolongation of the disease-free interval in surgically treated rectal carcinoma. N Engl J Med 1985; 312:1465-72.
45. Gerard A, Buyse M, Nordlinger B, et al. Preoperative radiotherapy as adjuvant treatment in rectal cancer: final results of a randomized study of the European Organization for Research and Treatment of Cancer (EORTC). Ann Surg 1988;208:606-14.
46. Stockholm Rectal Cancer Study Group. Preoperative short-term radiation therapy in operable rectal carcinoma: a prospective randomized trial. Cancer 1990;66:49-55.
47. Sause WT, Pajak TF, Noyes RD. Evaluation of preoperative radiation therapy in operable colorectal cancer. Ann Surg 1994;220:668-75.
48. Holm T, Cedermark B, Rutqvist LE. Local recurrence of rectal adenocarcinoma after curative surgery with and without preoperative radiotherapy. Br J Surg 1994;81:452-5.
49. Second Report of an MRC Working Party. The evaluation of low dose preoperative X-ray therapy in the management of operable rectal cancer; results of a randomly controlled trial. Br J Surg 1984;71:21-5.
50. Fisher B, Wolmark N, Rockette H, et al Postoperative adjuvant chemotherapy or radiation therapy for rectal cancer: results from NSABP protocol R-01. J Natl Cancer Inst 1988;80:21-9.
51. Moertel CG, Childs DS Jr, Reitemeier RJ, Colby MY Jr, Holbrook MA. Combined 5-fluorouracil and supervoltage radiation therapy of locally unresectable gastrointestinal cancer. Lancet 1969;2:865-7.
52. Krook JE, Moertel CG, Gunderson LL, et al. Effective adjuvant therapy for high-risk rectal carcinoma. N Engl J Med 1991;324:709-15.
53. Papillon J. Rectal and anal cancers conservative treatment by irradiation: an alternative to radical surgery. Berlin: Springer-Verlag, 1982.
54. Steel RJ, Hershman MJ, Mortensen NJ, Armitage NC, Schofield JH. Transanal endoscopic microsurgery—initial experience from three centers in the United Kingdom. Br J Surg 1996;83:207-10.
55. Buyse M, Zeleniuch-Jacquotte A, Chalmers TC. Adjuvant therapy of colorectal cancer: why we still don't know. JAMA 1988;259:3571-8.
56. Moertel CG, Fleming TR, Macdonald JS, et al. Levamisole and fluorouracil for adjuvant therapy of resected colon carcinoma. N Engl J Med 1990;322:352-8.
57. Lindemann F, Schlimok G, Dirschedl P, Witte J, Riethmuller G. Prognostic significance of micrometastatic tumour cells in bone marrow of colorectal cancer patients. Lancet 1992;340:685-9.
58. Riethmuller G, Schneider-Gadicke E, Schlimok G, et al. Randomised trial of monoclonal antibody for adjuvant therapy of resected Dukes' C colorectal carcinoma. German Cancer Aid 17-1A Study Group. Lancet 1994;343:1177-83.
59. Wolmark N, Fischer B, Rockette H, et al. Postoperative adjuvant chemotherapy or BCG for colon cancer: results from NSABP protocol C-01. J Natl Cancer Inst 1988;80:30-6.
60. Abulafi AM, Allardice JT, Dean R, Grahn MF, Williams NS. Adjunctive intraoperative photodynamic therapy for colorectal cancer. Gut 1991;32(Suppl 1):2.
61. Allardice JT, Grahn MF, Rowlands AC, et al. Safety studies for intraoperative photodynamic therapy. Lasers Med Sci 1992;7:133-42.
62. Muto T, Bussey HJ, Morson BC. The evolution of cancer of the colon and rectum. Cancer 1974;36:2251-70.
63. Shinya H, Wolff WI. Morphology, anatomic distribution, and cancer potential of colonic polyps. Ann Surg 1979;190:679-83.
64. Meleagros L, Varty PP, Delrio P, Boulos PB. Influence of temporary faecal diversion on long-term survival after curative surgery for colorectal cancer. Br J Surg 1995;82:21-5.
65. Terpstra OT, Dahl EP, Williamson RC, Ross JS, Malt RA. Colostomy closure promotes cell proliferation and dimethylhydrazine-induced carcinogenesis in rat distal colon. Gastroenterology 1981;81:475-80.
66. Umpleby HC, Williamson RC. Anastomotic recurrence in large bowel cancer. Br J Surg 1987;74:873-8.
67. Scheele J, Stangl R, Altendorf-Hoffman A. Hepatic metastases from colorectal carcinoma: impact of surgical resection on the natural history. Br J Surg 1990;77:1241-6.
68. Wood CB, Gillis CR, Blumgart LH. A retrospective study of the natural history of patients with liver metastases from colorectal cancer. Clin Oncol 1976;2:285-8.
69. Jaffe BM, Donegan WL, Watson F, Spratt JS Jr. Factors influencing survival in patients with untreated hepatic metastases. Surg Gynecol Obstet 1968;127:1-11.
70. Hughes KS, Simon R, Songhorabodi S, et al. Resection of the liver for colorectal carcinoma metastases: a multi-institutional study of patterns of recurrence. Surgery 1986;100:278-84.
71. Fortner JG, Silva JS, Golbey RB, Cox EB, Maclean BJ. Multivariate analysis of a personal series of 247 consecutive patients with liver metastases from colorectal cancer. I. Treatment by hepatic resection. Ann Surg 1984;199:306-16.
72. Cady B, McDermot WV. Major hepatic resection for metachronous metastases from colon cancer. Ann Surg 1985;201:204-9.
73. Fortner JG. Recurrence of colorectal cancer after hepatic resection. Am J Surg 1988;155:378-82.
74. Bozetti F, Bignami P, Montalto F, Doci R, Gennari L. Repeated hepatic resection for recurrent metastases from colorectal cancer. Br J Surg 1992;79:146-8.
75. Butler J, Attiyeh FF, Daly JM. Hepatic resection for metastases of the colon and rectum. Surg Gynecol Obstet 1986;162:109-13.
76. Fong Y, Blumgart LH, Cohen A, Fortner J, Brennan MF. Repeat hepatic resection for metastatic colorectal cancer. Ann Surg 1994; 220:657-62.
77. Que FG, Nagorney DM. Resection of recurrent colorectal metastases to the liver. Br J Surg 1994:81;255-8.
78. Jarvinen HJ. Epidemiology of familial adenomatous polyposis in Finland: impact of family screening on the colorectal cancer rate and survival. Gut 1992;33:357-60.
79. Lynch HT, Smyrk T, Lanspa SJ, et al. Flat adenomas in a colon cancer–prone kindred. J Natl Cancer Inst 1988;80:278-82.
80. Burt RW, Bishop DT, Cannon LA, Dowdle MA, Lee RE, Skolnick MH. Dominant inheritance of adenomatous colonic polyps and colorectal cancer. N Engl J Med 1985;312:1540-4.
81. Cannon-Albright LA, Skolnick MH, Bishop T, Lee RG, Burt RW. Common inheritance of susceptibility to colonic adenomatous polyps and associated colorectal cancer. N Engl J Med 1988;319:533-7.

82. Bufill JA. Colorectal cancer genetics: closing the gap between genotype and phenotype. Cancer 1995;76:2389-92.
83. Fishel R, Lescoe MK, Rao MR, et al. The human mutator gene homolog M2H2 and its association with hereditary nonpolyposis colon cancer. Cell 1993;77:167.
84. Lindblom A, Tanndergard P, Werelius B, Nordenskjold M. Genetic mapping of a second locus predisposing to hereditary non-polyposis colon cancer. Nat Genet 1993;5:279-82.
85. Nicolaides NC, Papadopoulos N, Liu B, et al. Mutations of two PMS homologues in hereditary nonpolyposis colon cancer. Nature 1994; 371:75-80.
86. Drummond JT, Li GM, Longley MJ, Modrich P. Isolation of an hMSH2-p160 heterodimer that restores DNA mismatch repair to tumor cells. Science 1995;268:1909-12.
87. Thibodeau SN, Bren G, Schaid D. Microsatellite instability in cancer of the proximal colon. Science 1993;260:816-9.
88. Kim H, Jen J, Vogelstein B, Hamilton SR. Clinical and pathological characteristics of sporadic colorectal carcinomas with DNA replication errors in microsatellite sequences. Am J Pathol 1994;145:148-56.
89. Groden J, Thliveris A, Samowitz W, et al. Identification and characterization of the familial adenomatous polyposis coli gene. Cell 1991; 66:589-600.
90. Nagase M, Nakamura Y. Mutations of the APC (adenomatous polyposis coli) gene. Hum Mutat 1993;2:425-34.
91. Nishisho I, Nakamura Y, Miyoshi Y, et al. Mutations of chromosome 5q21 genes in FAP and colorectal cancer patients. Science 1991; 253:665-9.
92. Kinzler KW, Nilbert MC, Vogestein B, et al. Identification of a gene located at chromosome 5q21 that is mutated in colorectal cancer. Science 1991;251:1366-70.
93. Lynch HT, Kimberling W, Albano WA, et al. Hereditary nonpolyposis colorectal cancer (Lynch syndromes I and II), parts I and II. Cancer 1985;56:934-51.
94. Mecklin JP, Jarvinen HJ, Peltokallio P. Cancer family syndrome: genetic analysis of 22 Finnish kindreds. Gastroenterology 1986; 90:328-33.
95. Mecklin JP, Jarvinen HJ. Clinical features of colorectal carcinoma in cancer family syndrome. Dis Col Rectum 1986;29:160-4.
96. Gagliardi G, Stepniewska KA, Hershman MJ, Hawley PR, Talbot IC. New grade-related prognostic variable for rectal cancer. Br J Surg 1995;82:599-602.
97. Kwok SP, Lau WY, Carey PD, Kelly SB, Leung KL, Li AK. Prospective evaluation of laparoscopically-assisted large-bowel excision for cancer. Ann Surg 1996;223:170-6.

➢ COUNTER POINT

University of Washington Medical Center

MIKA N. SINANAN

In most patients with colorectal carcinoma the disease is detected when it is locally confined and surgically treatable for cure. For about two thirds of patients the initial surgery is indeed curative, and if this group could be accurately defined, the morbidity, uncertainty, and economic cost of follow-up could be avoided. Unfortunately, the best attempts at risk stratification by cancer stage and histological characteristics, as discussed by Macintosh et al., still miss a significant proportion of the patients destined to develop recurrent disease. Thus, until more precise markers for persistent or recurrent colorectal carcinoma are developed, policies for follow-up must be developed for the entire population.

Macintosh et al. describe the goals of a follow-up strategy for patients with colorectal cancer as detection of potentially curable recurrent disease, detection of new (metachronous) cancers, and measurement of the pattern and interval to recurrence to determine the efficacy of the primary cancer treatment. Most diagnostic measures proposed for patients with colorectal cancer are directed toward the first goal. New metachronous colorectal cancers occur at a rate of about 0.35% per year,[1,2] exclusive of defined genetic disorders that increase the risk of new malignancy. Reasonable colonoscopic surveillance policies[3,4] have been established to address this second goal and have been reviewed by Macintosh et al.

The eventual outcome of the primary cancer treatment is the most significant measure of quality and efficacy of care, especially since differences in clinical outcome by institution and practitioner are becoming increasingly important in the managed care of patients. However, simple monitoring of patient status by history is usually sufficient to satisfy the third goal while avoiding invasive and costly investigation. Thus, of the three goals, the detection of potentially curable recurrent disease has the greatest potential impact on a patient's quality of life and survival and remains the subject of considerable controversy.

To develop a program for the detection of recurrent colorectal carcinoma, Macintosh et al. have proposed a series of principles. For ease of reference these are summarized as follows. First, the purpose of surveillance in asymptomatic patients is detection of curable recurrent disease. As is emphasized throughout this book, clinicians should first seek the disease that is most harmful and can be most effectively treated. The stage of the disease and location of the primary cancer (colon versus rectum) are the most important parameters in estimating the likelihood and location of recurrence but are only moderately accurate indicators. Because recurrence can occur with any stage or grade of colorectal carcinoma, no individual patient initially treated for cure should be omitted on the basis of negligible risk. Patients who were not candidates for potentially curative resection of the primary lesion (because of patient or disease factors) should be followed up clinically and treated palliatively.

Recurrence of colorectal carcinoma is a time-limited phenomenon. Most treatable recurrences are detected in the first 2 to 3 years after resection of the primary lesion. Thus surveillance strategies should concentrate resources on that time period. Adjuvant treatment may delay recurrence, so these patients must be followed proportionately longer. Surgery is the only means of potentially curative treatment for recurrent colorectal cancer. There are only three sites where recurrent colorectal cancer may be amenable to repeat resection: the local (anastomotic or resection) site of the initial cancer, the liver, and the lung. Local recurrence is a more significant concern for rectal cancers because wide primary resection is constrained in the pelvis. Distant recurrence in

Table 8-6 Follow-up of patients with colorectal cancer (colon cancer): University of Washington Medical Center

	YEAR				
	1	2	3	4	5
Office visit*	5	4	1	1	1
CEA	5	4	1	1	1
Chest x-ray	2	1	1	0	0
Abdominal computed tomography	2	1	0	0	0
Pelvic computed tomography	2	1	0	0	0
Colonoscopy	1†	0	0	0	0

CEA, Carcinoembryonic antigen.
*Includes genetic (family) screening and counseling performed at baseline for disorders with a suspected or demonstrated genetic transmission (such as familial polyposis or HNPCC syndromes) and for patients who are 50 years of age or less.
†An additional colonoscopy is performed at baseline if complete screening of the colon and rectum is not completed preoperatively. Follow-up after the first year is based on findings from the 12-month study and if indicated is repeated annually for 1 to 3 years.

Table 8-7 Follow-up of patients with colorectal cancer (rectal cancer): University of Washington Medical Center

	YEAR				
	1	2	3	4	5
Office visit*	5	4	1	1	1
CEA	5	4	1	1	1
Chest x-ray	2	1	1	0	0
Abdominal computed tomography	2	1	0	0	0
Pelvic computed tomography	2	1	0	0	0
Sigmoidoscopy	1	2	0	0	0
Colonoscopy	1†	0	0	0	0

CEA, Carcinoembryonic antigen.
*Includes genetic (family) screening and counseling performed at baseline for disorders with a suspected or demonstrated genetic transmission (such as familial polyposis or HNPCC syndromes) and for patients who are 50 years of age or less.
†An additional colonoscopy is performed at baseline if complete screening of the colon and rectum is not completed preoperatively. Follow-up after the first year is based on findings from the 12-month study and if indicated is repeated annually for 1 to 3 years.

the lung and liver can occur after either rectal or colon primary cancers. Most recurrent disease is multifocal. Recurrent cancer that is isolated to one of the three surgically approachable sites is unusual, occurring in only 15% to 20% of patients with recurrent disease. Of this select group, 15% to 30% become long-term survivors after repeat resection.

No single clinical, serological, radiographic, or other examination is optimal for detecting all types of curable recurrent colorectal carcinoma. However, the cost and morbidity of multiple studies mandate a scaled approach, starting with a thorough clinical examination and basic screening studies. Patient education is critical and should emphasize

Table 8-8 Follow-up of patients with colorectal cancer (at increased risk of recurrence)*: University of Washington Medical Center

	YEAR				
	1	2	3	4	5
Office visit†	5	4	2	2	1
CEA	5	4	2	2	1
Chest x-ray	2	1	1	0	0
Abdominal computed tomography	2	1	1	0	0
Pelvic computed tomography‡	2	1	1	0	0
Sigmoidoscopy	1	2	0	0	0
Colonoscopy	1§	0	0	0	0

CEA, Carcinoembryonic antigen.
*Patients at increased risk of recurrence include those with stage T2+N0M0 colorectal cancer with aneuploidy; stage T3N0M0 with angiolymphatic invasion; stage T4N0M0; stage T(any)N1M0; T(any)N(any)M0 with close or positive margins; and any stage cancer treated with adjuvant chemotherapy or chemoradiation.
†Includes genetic (family) screening and counseling performed at baseline for disorders with a suspected or demonstrated genetic transmission (such as familial polyposis or HNPCC syndromes) and for patients who are 50 years of age or less.
‡Performed for patients with rectal cancers.
§An additional colonoscopy is performed at baseline if complete screening of the colon and rectum is not completed preoperatively. Follow-up after the first year is based on findings from the 12-month study and if indicated is repeated annually for 1 to 3 years.

both the purpose of the surveillance program and the importance of early evaluation for subtle symptoms. Regular measurement of the serum CEA level, despite the shortcomings of this test, remains the most cost-effective method of screening for asymptomatic recurrence. It is particularly useful in detecting hepatic and retroperitoneal recurrence.[5] In most clinical situations a confirmed rise in CEA levels should prompt further investigation rather than so-called CEA-directed surgery. Resectability and the potential for cure should first be established by these adjunctive studies.

Although computed tomography portography or T1-weighted magnetic resonance tomography is more accurate at staging the intrahepatic extent of disease, double-spiral computed tomography of the abdomen and chest is emerging as one of the most cost-effective studies for evaluating both the liver and lung when extrapelvic recurrent disease is suspected because of clinical symptoms or rising CEA levels. Pelvic anastomotic recurrence from rectal cancer is best detected by clinical (digital rectal) and endoscopic examination. Endoscopic ultrasound and computed tomography complement these studies. Depending on the clinical assessment of risk after treatment of the primary lesion, baseline endoscopic and radiographic studies should be considered to help distinguish early, subtle recurrence in the pelvic soft tissues from postsurgical and radiation scar.

Since one or more surgical procedures are generally necessary to gain any chance for cure of recurrent colorectal cancer, patients who are not candidates for further surgery (usually because of intercurrent illness) derive no benefit from detection of asymptomatic recurrence and should have only clinical follow-up. Population-wide, there is little proof that identification of presymptomatic recurrence (as compared with symptomatic recurrence) increases the likelihood of resectability, curability, or survival.[6-8] Kievit et al.[9] have provided one of the most suggestive analyses of CEA-driven follow-up that support this argument. Other studies, however, suggest that aggressive screening for recurrent disease does have survival advantage when the screening program is individualized by patient stage, location of disease, and other factors that help stratify risk for recurrence.[10-12]

Although the preceding principles provide an abstract context for designing a follow-up strategy, as a practical matter many clinicians have witnessed successful treatment of recurrent colorectal cancer and been reinforced in their follow-up habits by grateful and often highly functional patients. This experience, as much as any scientific study, commonly drives the follow-up process for individual clinicians and continues to introduce variability in follow-up strategies. Clearly some patients can be cured; however, this can happen only by exposing others to some risk in a process that may require expenditure of significant resources. One characteristic of the current era is that purely financial factors, such as the economic productivity of the survivors versus the cost of saving them, may become preeminent in designing follow-up strategies. It is imperative that clinicians avoid this simplistic approach. Beyond the observations and facts discussed by Macintosh et al. and summarized previously, any surveillance strategy must be guided by a philosophical position regarding the value of those patients who could be saved. Better adjuvant chemotherapy and more effective use of other adjunctive treatment options such as thoracoscopic lung resection, hepatic arterial infusion chemotherapy and cryotherapy, and ethanol injection for liver metastases may in the future increase the value of early detection and lead to even more aggressive follow-up.[13-16]

Given the considerations just discussed, how should physicians proceed? Macintosh et al. provide a schema for follow-up of all comers and modify it with certain caveats provided in the text. I believe, however, that incorporating certain considerations in the algorithm is useful. Specifically, baseline studies and an objective assessment of risk have been incorporated into the follow-up scheme, stratifying patients by location of disease and risk of recurrence. Just as risk stratification is useful in guiding follow-up for recurrent disease, surveillance for metachronous disease should be scaled to the relative significance that such disease holds for the patient. Given the effects of age, intercurrent illness, and the normally greater threat posed by recurrence of the primary tumor (especially for aneuploid or high-stage cancers), colonoscopy to detect rare metachronous lesions (at a cost of at least $1,200 with discomfort and some risk) may not be worthwhile in some patients.

Based on the relative efficacy of individual screening studies detailed by Macintosh et al., Tables 8-6 through 8-8 incorporate modifications in the follow-up of patients with colorectal cancer as performed at the University of Washington Medical Center. The modifications affect baseline studies, highlight differences between colon and rectal cancer, and emphasize the need for genetic screening and counseling in select populations (those 50 years of age or less and with a strong family history, cancer in the setting of familial polyposis, and HNPCC syndromes). Patients at increased risk of recurrence include those with stage T2+N0M0 colorectal cancer with aneuploidy; stage T3N0M0 cancer with angiolymphatic invasion; stage T4N0M0 cancer; stage T(any)N1M0; stage T(any)N(any)M0 with close or positive margins; and any stage cancer treated with adjuvant chemotherapy or chemoradiation. Although individualizing care in this manner would seem to increase the efficiency of follow-up, assessing the true cost effectiveness of such an approach will probably require additional studies.

REFERENCES

1. Kuramoto S, Oohara T. How do colorectal cancers develop? Cancer 1995;75(6 Suppl):1534-8.
2. Cali RL, Pitsch RM, Thorson AG, et al. Cumulative incidence of metachronous colorectal cancer. Dis Colon Rectum 1993;36:388-93.
3. Granqvist S, Karlsson T. Postoperative follow-up of patients with colorectal carcinoma by colonoscopy. Eur J Surg 1992;158:307-12.
4. Chen F, Stuart M. Colonoscopic follow-up of colorectal carcinoma. Dis Colon Rectum 1994;37:568-72.
5. Beart RW Jr, O'Connell MJ. Postoperative follow up of patients with carcinoma of the colon. Mayo Clin Proc 1983;58:361-3.
6. Allen-Mersh TG. Serum CEA in the follow up of colorectal carcinoma: experience in a district general hospital. Ann R Coll Surg Engl 1984;66:14-6.
7. Virgo KS, Vernava AM, Longo WE, McKirgan LW, Johnson FE. Cost of patient follow-up after potentially curative colorectal cancer treatment. JAMA 1995;273:1837-41.
8. Tornqvist A, Ekelund G, Leandoer L. The value of intensive follow up after curative resection for colorectal carcinoma. Br J Surg 1982; 69:725-8.
9. Kievit J, Van de Velde CJ. Utility and cost of carcinoembryonic antigen monitoring in colon cancer follow-up evaluation: a Markov analysis. Cancer 1990;65:2580-7.
10. Bruinvels DJ, Stiggelbout AM, Kievit J, van Houwelingen HC, Habbema JD, van de Velde CJ. Follow-up of patients with colorectal cancer: a meta-analysis. Ann Surg 1994;219:174-82.
11. Ovaska J, Jarvinen H, Kujari H, Perttila I, Mecklin JP. Follow-up of patients operated on for colorectal carcinoma. Am J Surg 1990; 159:593-6.
12. Gerdes H. Surveillance after colon cancer: is it worthwhile? Gastroenterology 1990;99:1849-51.
13. Mori M, Tomoda H, Ishida T, et al. Surgical resection of pulmonary metastases from colorectal adenocarcinoma: special reference to repeated pulmonary resections. Arch Surg 1991;126:1297-301.
14. Scheele J, Altendorf-Hofmann A, Stangl R, Gall FP. Pulmonary resection for metastatic colon and upper rectum cancer: is it useful? Dis Colon Rectum 1990;33:745-52.
15. Preketes AP, Caplehorn JR, King J, Clingan PR, Ross WB, Morris DL. Effect of hepatic artery chemotherapy on survival of patients with hepatic metastases from colorectal carcinoma treated with cryotherapy. World J Surg 1995;19:768-71.
16. Ravikumar TS, Steele G Jr, Kane R, King V. Experimental and clinical observations on hepatic cryosurgery for colorectal metastases. Cancer Res 1991;51:6323-7.

Table 8–9 Follow-up of patients with colorectal cancer by institution

YEAR/PROGRAM	OFFICE VISIT	CBC	LFT	CEA	CXR	COLONO OR BARIUM ENEMA	PELVIC CT
Year 1							
Memorial Sloan-Kettering	4			4	1	1[a]	[b]
Roswell Park	4	2	2	2	1	2[d]	2[e]
Univ Washington I[h]	5[i]			5	2	1[j]	2
Univ Washington II[k]	5[i]			5	2	1[j]	2
Univ Washington III[l]	5[i]			5	2	1[j]	2[m]
Japan: National Cancer Ctr	2-4	2-4	2-4	2-4	2-4	1	3[n]
UK: Royal Liverpool I[h]	4[o]		4	4		2[p]	
UK: Royal Liverpool II[k]	4[q]		4	4		1	
Year 2							
Memorial Sloan-Kettering	4			4	1		[b]
Roswell Park	4	2	2	2	1		1[e]
Univ Washington I[h]	4[i]			4	1		1
Univ Washington II[k]	4[i]			4	1		1
Univ Washington III[l]	4[i]			4	1		1[m]
Japan: National Cancer Ctr	2-4	2-4	2-4	2-4	2-4	1	2[n]
UK: Royal Liverpool I[h]	4[o]		4	4			
UK: Royal Liverpool II[k]	3[q]		3	3		1[s]	
Year 3							
Memorial Sloan-Kettering	2			2	1		[b]
Roswell Park	4	2	2	2	2		1[e]
Univ Washington I[h]	1[i]			1	1		
Univ Washington II[k]	1[i]			1	1		
Univ Washington III[l]	2[i]			2	1		1[m]
Japan: National Cancer Ctr	2	2	2	2	2	1	1[n]
UK: Royal Liverpool I[h]	3[o]		3	3			
UK: Royal Liverpool II[k]	2[q]		2	2		1[s]	

ABD CT abdominal computed tomography
ABD US abdominal ultrasound
ALB albumin
CBC complete blood count
CEA carcinoembryonic antigen
CEUS colonoscopic endoluminal ultrasound
CHEST CT chest computed tomography
COLONO colonoscopy
CXR chest x-ray
LFT liver function tests
MRI magnetic resonance imaging
PROCTO proctosigmoidoscopy
SIG sigmoidoscopy
TRUS transrectal ultrasound
US ultrasound

ABD CT	RECTAL US	PROCTO	CHEST CT	TRUS	ABD US	SIG	COLONOSCOPIC ENDOLUMINAL US OR INTRALUMINAL MRI
[b]		4[c]	[b]	[b]			
1[f,g]	1[e]						
2							
2						1	
2						1	
2[n]					2-4		
					2		
[r]						4	[r]
[b]		4[c]	[b]	[b]			
1	1[e]						
1							
1						2	
1						2	
2[n]					2-4		
[r]						3	[r]
[b]		2[c]	[b]	[b]			
1							
1							
1[n]					2		
[r]						2	[r]

a If complete colonoscopy was not performed preoperatively, it is performed 3 months postoperatively. Colonoscopy with polypectomy is repeated every 6 months after this initial perioperative colonoscopy until no polyps are detected. If the year 1 colonoscopy is normal, repeat colonoscopy in year 4 and every 3 to 5 years thereafter.
b Performed as clinically indicated.
c Indicated for patients who have undergone sphincter-sparing procedures for rectal cancer.
d Performed once preoperatively and once postoperatively. If there is no preoperative colonoscopy, performed at 6 and 12 months.
e Performed for patients with rectal cancer only.
f Performed twice in year 1 for patients with rectal cancer.
g For patients with colon cancer receiving adjuvant therapy, performed at 6 and 12 months.
h Patients with colon cancer.
i Includes genetic (family) screening and counseling performed at baseline for disorders with a suspected or demonstrated genetic transmission (such as familial polyposis or HNPCC syndromes) and for patients who are 50 years of age or less.
j An additional colonoscopy is performed at baseline if complete screening of the colon and rectum is not done preoperatively. Follow-up after the first year is based on findings from the 12-month study, and if indicated is repeated annually for 1 to 3 years.
k Patients with rectal cancer.
l Patients at increased risk of recurrence. Includes those with stage T2+N0M0 colorectal cancer with aneuploidy; stage T3N0M0 with angiolymphatic invasion; stage T4N0M0; stage T(any)N1M0 T(any)N(any)MO with close or positive margins; and any stage cancer treated with adjuvant chemotherapy or chemoradiation.
m Performed for patients with rectal cancers.
n Performed as part of intensive follow-up when recurrence is suspected.
o Includes genetic evaluation for patients whose cancer is diagnosed before age 50.
p For patients first seen on an emergency basis, colonoscopy is also performed at 3 months to evaluate the rest of the colorectum.
q Includes rectal examination.
r Performed for patients with suspected local recurrence.
s Performed for patients with an isolated elevation of CEA levels.

Continued.

Table 8–9 Follow-up of patients with colorectal cancer by institution—cont'd

YEAR/PROGRAM	OFFICE VISIT	CBC	LFT	CEA	CXR	COLONO OR BARIUM ENEMA	PELVIC CT
Year 4							
Memorial Sloan-Kettering	2			2	1	1[a]	[b]
Roswell Park	3	1	1	1	1	1	1[e]
Univ Washington I[h]	1[i]			1			
Univ Washington II[k]	1[i]			1			
Univ Washington III[l]	2[i]			2			
Japan: National Cancer Ctr	2	2	2	2	2	1	1[n]
UK: Royal Liverpool I[h]	2[o]		2	2			
UK: Royal Liverpool II[k]	2[q]		2	2		1[s]	
Year 5							
Memorial Sloan-Kettering	2			2	1		[b]
Roswell Park	3	1	1	1			1[e]
Univ Washington I[h]	1[i]			1			
Univ Washington II[k]	1[i]			1			
Univ Washington III[l]	1[i]			1			
Japan: National Cancer Ctr	2	2	2	2	2	1	
UK: Royal Liverpool I[h]	2[o]		2	2			
UK: Royal Liverpool II[k]	2[q]		2	2		1[s]	

ABD CT	RECTAL US	PROCTO	CHEST CT	TRUS	ABD US	SIG	COLONOSCOPIC ENDOLUMINAL US OR INTRALUMINAL MRI
b		2[c]	b	b			
1							
1[n]					2		
r						2	r
b		2[c]	b	b			
1							
					2		
r						2	r

CHAPTER 9

Anal Carcinoma

University of Washington Medical Center

Mika N. Sinanan, Wui-Jin Koh, and Linda M. Bavisotto

Anal carcinomas are rare lesions, representing 1% to 2% of large bowel cancers and 4% of anorectal malignancies. Several premalignant conditions have been identified. The term "anal carcinoma" encompasses several different types of cancer defined by the cell of origin and location of the lesion.[1] Epidermoid lesions, with or without keratinizing features, make up 80% of anal neoplasms, are derived from the squamous epithelium of the anal skin and anal canal, and are thought to have a viral etiology.[2,3] Basaloid and cloacogenic carcinomas are nonkeratinized, less differentiated forms of epidermoid carcinoma derived from the transitional epithelium of the anal canal proximal to the dentate line. They generally respond to multimodality therapy and have recurrence and survival characteristics similar to those of squamous cell carcinoma of the anus. Adenocarcinoma of the anus, either extending from the rectum or derived from anal glands, makes up an additional 8% to 10% of anal cancers. Melanoma and other rare tumors constitute the remaining lesions. Despite the accessibility of anal cancers to digital palpation and inspection, patient- and physician-related delays in diagnosis are common.[4-6]

Anal cancers are also classified by location based on anatomical landmarks. Those most distal, arising from the squamous epithelium of the anal margin, make up 5% to 10% of all cancers and are defined as occurring from the anal verge out 5 cm on the perianal skin. They are also referred to as perianal carcinomas in the literature. Anal margin cancers occur more frequently in men and are generally detected at an early stage but can metastasize to the inguinal lymph nodes. They tend to be indolent tumors, often permitting curative local resection while preserving the sphincter. Long-term outcome is excellent.[7] Epidermoid cancers of the anal canal form the largest subgroup (85% of all anal carcinomas) and are defined as occurring from the anal columns proximally to the anal verge distally.

The management of anal cancer has evolved over the past 20 years from aggressive primary resection of the anus and rectum (abdominoperineal resection) to a sphincter-sparing, primary radiation or chemoradiation therapeutic approach.[5] Radical surgery is now generally reserved for instances of multimodality therapy failure. Limited surgery with anal preservation and the viral association of these epidermoid tumors potentially increase the risk of recurrence[8,9] and second primary cancers.[10] In patients with a complete response to radiation or chemoradiation and in those who require salvage resection, locoregional nodes are the most common sites of recurrent disease.[11,12] If recurrent disease is confined to the local site and regional nodes, curative resection in an effort to render the patient free of disease still has a survival benefit.

As the primary treatment of anal cancer has evolved toward increased sphincter conservation, careful follow-up has become more important. The goals of a follow-up program are to determine the completeness of response to the primary therapy; to determine the need for further or alternative (primarily surgical salvage) therapy; to detect complications of therapy (radionecrosis, stricture, and the like); to detect recurrent disease; and to define the pattern and extent of recurrent disease, especially disease for which long-term palliative or curative treatment may still be possible.

STAGING OF ANAL CANCER

Several staging techniques have been described for anal cancer and are summarized in Tables 9-1 and 9-2. Boman et al.,[12] following the Dukes model for staging of colorectal carcinoma, described anal canal and anal margin cancers with respect to their depth of penetration, regional nodal involvement, and distant spread. Stage A and stage B disease are localized, with stage A confined to the mucosa and stage B involving the sphincter muscle or pelvic tissues. Stage C involves the regional lymph nodes, and stage D represents distant or unresectable disease.

A more recent staging system (tumor, nodes, metastases [TNM] classification) developed by the American Joint Committee on Cancer and the International Union Against Cancer separates anal canal and margin cancers.[13,14] Both anal margin and canal cancers are staged by size (T), nodal status (N), and presence of distant metastases (M). Like other skin cancers, anal margin cancers are classified as stage I or II if the disease is local, without nodal or adjacent organ involvement (exclusive of the anal sphincter). T1 anal margin cancers are up to 2 cm, T2 lesions between 2 and 5 cm, and T3 lesions over 5 cm in diameter. The T classification does not pertain to depth

Table 9-1 Boman staging method for anal cancer

STAGE	EXTENT OF DISEASE
A	Confined to mucosa, no adenopathy
B	Involving the sphincter, no adenopathy
C	Regional adenopathy
D	Distant or unresectable disease

From Boman BM, Moertel CG, O'Connell MJ, et al. Carcinoma of the anal canal: a clinical and pathologic study of 188 cases. Cancer 1984;54:114-25.

except for T4 lesions that clearly invade deep, extradermal structures such as bone or skeletal muscle. Stage III cancers invade regional organs or have regional nodal involvement. Stage IV denotes distant metastatic disease.

For anal canal cancers, lesions up to 2 cm are classified as T1 and those between 2 and 5 cm are classified as T2. T3 lesions measure over 5 cm, and T4 lesions invade adjacent organs (not including the anal sphincter). Regional nodal involvement may include perirectal nodes (N1), unilateral internal iliac or inguinal nodes (N2), or bilateral internal iliac, inguinal, or perirectal nodes (N3). Stage I and II lesions have no nodal involvement. Stage III indicates regional nodal (N1) disease, regardless of the T size, or T4 disease without adenopathy. Stage IV represents distant disease, usually liver or lung metastases.

CURRENT FOLLOW-UP PRACTICE

Standards of follow-up practice have not been established because of the rare and variable nature of these tumors, the variety of treatment options, and the lack of consensus among gastroenterologists, surgeons, radiation oncologists, and medical oncologists. However, an increasing trend to sphincter-conserving therapy leaves the anus and regional nodal beds present for local examination. Long-term follow-up studies have established with increasing certainty the natural history and patterns of recurrence of this disease and have identified opportunities for meaningful therapeutic intervention in cases of recurrent disease. These are discussed in subsequent sections.

At each follow-up visit, overall patient status, the anal canal and perianal area, the distal rectum, and inguinal lymph nodes should be evaluated. The fact that anal cancer has been associated with an increased incidence of subsequent lung, small intestine, breast, and female genitourinary system cancers (relative risk 2 to 10) should be kept in mind while assessing general health.[9,10] The common occurrence of benign perianal disease (fissures, fistulas, condylomata) in these patients[15,16] and benign scarring from treatment of the primary lesion must be distinguished from recurrent disease. A careful history for new or changing symptoms, a visual, digital, and anoscopic examination of the anus, sigmoidoscopy for the distal rectum, and possibly transrectal ultrasound (TRUS) for submucosal processes[17,18] seem reasonable measures to detect local recurrence. It is important that one physician make sequential examinations so as to distinguish suspicious lesions that require biopsy.[6] In the period

Table 9-2 TNM classification for staging of anal cancer

STAGE	T (SIZE OF TUMOR)	N (NODAL STATUS)	M (PRESENCE OF DISTANT METASTASES)
I	T1	N0	M0
II	T2-3	N0	M0
III	T4	N0	M0
	T1-4	N1-3	M0
IV	T1-4	N0-3	M1

From American Joint Committee on Cancer, Beahrs OH, Henson DE, Hutter RV, Kennedy BJ. Manual for staging of cancer. 4th ed. Philadelphia: JB Lippincott Company, 1992.

after potentially curative multimodality treatment the primary tumor may take up to 4 months to involute.

Regional lymphatic spread from the anus includes the inguinal lymph nodes, internal iliac chain, and lymph nodes of the inferior mesenteric chain. Anal margin tumors spread primarily to the inguinal lymph nodes. In patients treated for these cancers both groins should be carefully examined. Anal canal tumors tend to spread regionally to the groin and to perirectal, internal iliac, and inferior mesenteric lymphatic distribution regions, particularly in patients with a high-grade or advanced-stage lesion. Thus patients with anal canal tumors should be evaluated by clinical examination and, depending on grade and stage of the primary lesion, abdominal and pelvic computed tomographic scans and chest radiographs for detection of more distant disease. Computed tomography has been replaced by pelvic magnetic resonance imaging in some series,[19] although demonstration of a significant benefit from this more expensive technology remains to be shown. If the assay is available, serial changes in the serum level of squamous cell carcinoma antigen (SCCAg; see below) have proved useful in predicting residual or early recurrence and in estimating survival.

The optimal frequency and duration of these examinations have not been established.[18] An initial close observation period with visits every 3 to 4 weeks seems prudent to document the efficacy and toxicity of the sphincter-conserving therapy until the patient's status has stabilized. In addition, new symptoms or complaints must be intensively investigated. The relative ease and safety of access in this area should prompt an early biopsy (preferably under local or regional anesthesia as an outpatient), perhaps repeatedly on any suggestion of residual or recurrent local disease. Once a stable condition is reached after sphincter-conserving therapy, a biopsy of residual scar tissue establishes the 20% to 30% of patients who have persistent microscopic disease and require further therapy, usually resection. A selective, clinically directed biopsy approach has been used at some centers.[20] However, up to 40% of complete clinical responders have viable, persistent tumor cells on deep biopsy, and 55% of those with a residual mass have no viable tumor cells. Thus either persistence or absence of a mass after combination therapy is an unreliable marker for residual disease.[21] Fortunately, analysis of risk factors including stage, immune status, human papillomavirus infection status, response and completeness of therapy, and perhaps SCCAg level helps guide the aggressiveness of follow-up scans and biopsy. The usual interval from initiation of multimodality treatment to biopsy for persistent disease is 12 to 20 weeks.

After the initial period, examinations at 2- to 3-month intervals should be carried out for 24 months,[14,18] then at 6-month to yearly intervals, with the shorter interval for patients at higher risk of local recurrence. Direct inspection and digital palpation of the anus and groins by an experienced clinician are the most important elements of the examination during this follow-up period. Ancillary radiographic procedures are reserved for patients who prompt clinical suspicion of recurrent disease.[22] Most recurrences appear within 2 years of curative treatment.[23] However, recurrence has been documented beyond 15 years,[12,22,24,25] so that individual authors generally agree that these patients must be followed at least that long and perhaps indefinitely.[26,27] A follow-up protocol used at the University of Washington Medical Center, based on studies by Cummings et al.[28] and other national protocols outlined previously, is provided in Table 9-3.

Table 9-3 Follow-up of patients with anal cancer*: University of Washington Medical Center

	YEAR				
	1	2	3	4	5
Office visit†	8	4	1	1	1
Anoscopy	6‡	4	1	1	1
SCCAg	5	2	1	1	1
Transrectal ultrasound	3‡	1	0	0	0
Sigmoidoscopy	2‡	1	0	0	0
Open anal biopsy	1‡	0	0	0	0
Abdominal computed tomography or magnetic resonance imaging	1§	0	0	0	0
Pelvic computed tomography or magnetic resonance imaging	1§	0	0	0	0

SCCAg, Squamous cell carcinoma antigen.
*Follow-up schedule begins on completion of radiation or chemoradiation treatment.
†Includes digital rectal examination.
‡At point of maximal or complete regression of tumor mass. Subsequent follow-up is based on the assumption of a negative biopsy result.
§Performed in high-grade and stages III and IV tumors to document the condition of the internal iliac lymph nodes and presacral space and to provide a basis for later comparison studies.

CURRENT OPTIONS FOR MANAGEMENT OF ANAL CANCER

Cancer of the Anal Margin (Perianal Cancer)

Management of cancer of the anal margin depends on the size of the lesion, the depth and extent of invasion into the anal sphincter, and the status of the inguinal lymph nodes. Options for treatment include both sphincter-conserving and radical (abdominoperineal resection) surgery, primary radiation, combined chemoradiation as described for anal canal cancers, and combinations of these three modalities as have been recently reviewed.[22]

Patients with well- or moderately differentiated, small, superficially invasive perianal cancers (T1 and some T2 lesions) who have no evidence of disease beyond the local area are treated primarily by local excision to clear margins.[16,26,27,29] In most cases resection can be achieved without compromise of anal sphincter function, although partial resection of the sphincter with reconstruction may be necessary. Some authors have recommended the addition of postoperative adjunctive radiation therapy[22] because of the 20% to 30% incidence of locoregional recurrence described for these patients.[27] Radiation treatment seems to be well tolerated.

Patients with deeply invasive perianal cancers (large T2 and all T3 and T4 lesions, as defined by direct examination and TRUS), poorly differentiated cancers, and large tumors usually encompassing over half the circumference of the anus that might otherwise require sphincter (abdominoperineal) resection are candidates for primary radiation[22] or a chemoradiation approach as developed for cancer of the anal canal (see later discussion).[28] The risk of inguinal lymph node and remote metastases, even if they are not clinically detectable at diagnosis, provides a rationale for multimodality, systemic therapy. When treatment is guided by these criteria, results in several series (summarized by Cummings[29]) suggest that sphincter function can be preserved in more than 83% of patients with a 5-year survival rate of 85%.

Cancer of the Anal Canal

Primary surgical therapy

Over the past 20 years, treatment of cancer of the anal canal has undergone an evolution. Until 1974[30] the most common treatment for anal canal cancer was surgery, either local excision or abdominoperineal resection. Only one fourth of anal canal cancers were susceptible to sphincter-conserving local resection,[15] but the results of this treatment, necessarily reserved for the most favorable, early-stage tumors (generally T1 lesions 2 cm or less in diameter) indicated good local control and a 70% to 85% 5-year disease-free survival rate.[12,24,31-33] For more extensive tumors, abdominoperineal resection (including dissection of the internal iliac and inguinal lymph nodes if clinically or pathologically involved[23]) had poorer results. Five-year survival rates averaged 36% to 70%,[11,12,15,23,32] with the lower survival data coming from operative series with more limited resections, a higher incidence of positive surgical margins, and more frequent local recurrence.

Regional lymphadenectomy

The inguinal lymph nodes form the primary lymphatic drainage for tissues of the anal margin and are an important secondary drainage pathway for the anal canal after pararectal, superior hemorrhoidal, and internal iliac groups. As such, primary or delayed involvement of these regional lymphatic pathways has important treatment and survival implications.

Inguinal lymph node involvement at initial presentation has been reported in 4% to 26% of patients with cancer of the anal margin,[6] and without prophylactic nodal treatment it develops metachronously in a further 17%.[16,22,34] Inguinal nodal involvement in these patients is directly related to the grade and depth of invasion of the primary tumor. In the series of anal margin cancers described by Papillon and Chassard,[22] limited lymphadenectomy and external beam radiation (to 4,500 cGy) to the groins resulted in a 67% 5-year survival rate for patients with synchronous groin nodal disease and the salvage of one of four patients with late, isolated groin nodal recurrence. Based on this experience, Papillon and Chassard[22] recommended prophylactic groin nodal radiation for T2N0 and T3N0 lesions of the anal margin and careful evaluation of nodal beds during the follow-up period.

The role of regional lymphadenectomy in the treatment of anal canal carcinoma has been evaluated in a number of series.[34-36] Most studies have shown that prophylactic pararectal and hypogastric lymphatic dissection as part of an extended abdominoperineal resection seems reasonable and can be accomplished with minimal additional morbidity. In contrast, inguinal lymph node dissection is a higher risk procedure. Even under conditions of known groin adenopathy, most authors counsel primary treatment with radiation (with or without chemotherapy) and reserve surgical resection for biopsy-proven residual or recurrent disease.[28] Prophylactic groin radiation is reasonable and should reduce the incidence of late nodal metastases, but prophylactic dissection in the absence of demonstrated inguinal nodal disease has no survival benefit and can result in chronic leg swelling and a poorly healing, painful wound.[23]

Radiation

In the early 1970s, the morbidity of radical resection including the necessity for a colostomy, the disappointing survival results of primary resection for advanced lesions, and new, encouraging survival data from early trials of chemotherapy and radiation treatment prompted the investigation of alternative therapies.[37] Radiation treatment as a sole modality for anal canal carcinoma has been studied most intensively by Papillon et al.[38-40] in Lyon, France. The results of these studies have recently been summarized.[18] Reports by other groups support the findings from Lyon but suggest a wide variation in dosage, technique, and radiation fields.[41,42] Using a two-field technique, Papillon et al.[38-40] administered 4,800 cGy to the perineum and sacrum followed by 2,000 cGy of interstitial ^{192}Ir brachytherapy. Total curative doses up to 6,500 cGy have also been routinely used by other groups,[42,43] although interstitial therapy is less frequently employed.[44] With radiation alone, Papillon et al.[38-40] reported local control in 100% of T1 lesions and more than 80% of all other lesions. The 5-year survival rate for patients with T1 and T2 lesions was 61%, while those with T3 and T4 lesions had a 46% 5-year survival rate. In patients with any involved lymph nodes (N1-3), 5-year survival rate dropped to 27%. Although anal conservation in these series was possible in 67% to 85% of patients, grade III radiation toxicity leading to subsequent surgery was reported in 10%.[18,42] While these results from treatment with radiation alone were encouraging, a trend toward increased toxicity and poorer survival suggests that concomitant chemotherapy, acting as both a radiosensitizer and a systemic agent, might have an important role to play.[45]

Combination therapy (chemoradiation)

Over the past 5 years, combination therapy based on Nigro's original protocol (chemoradiation) has been intensively studied, largely by retrospective case review. The largest reported series of patients undergoing combination therapy for anal canal carcinoma come from several institutions: Detroit (Leichman et al.[46] and Nigro et al.[47-49] at Wayne State), Toronto (Cummings et al.[28,29,45,50] at Princess Margaret Hospital), and New York (Miller et al.[21] and Enker et al.[51] at Memorial Sloan-Kettering Cancer Center). The Radiation Therapy Oncology Group reported on the treatment of 83 patients in a multicenter group trial.[14] Other international studies of combination therapy have also reported their results.[19,52,53] The original protocol described by Leichman et al.[46] included 5-fluorouracil (5-FU) (1 g/m^2 per day, given continuously on days 1 to 4 and 29 to 32), mitomycin C (15 mg/m^2 bolus on day 1), and radiation (3,000 cGy in fractions of 200 cGy using parallel opposing anteroposterior fields to the lesion, true pelvis, and inguinal lymphatic beds, 5 days a week over 3 weeks), followed by deep biopsy at 4 to 6 weeks under anesthesia to assess residual disease. Abdominoperineal resection was reserved for patients with residual disease that could not be locally resected or for recurrent disease.

Several groups have made modifications to the preceding protocol. The influence of radiation dose on survival was evaluated by Myerson et al.,[54] who showed that increasing the radiation dose to 4,000 to 5,000 cGy for stage T2 and T3 patients improved local control and reduced the need for radical surgery.[54] In a parallel study Cummings et al.[28] increased the total radiation dose and split the treatment into two courses to reduce toxicity. John et al.[55] added a second dose of mitomycin C and also boosted the radiation dose with compelling results. Extrapolating from results in esophageal cancer and cancers of the head and neck, some authors have suggested that cisplatin may be as active as mitomycin C in anal cancer yet have a more manageable spectrum of toxicity.[20,35,56] In general, increasing the radiation dose and including mitomycin C or an equivalent agent have been shown to improve survival.

Evaluating the series together shows that combined therapy resulted in local control in 85% to 100% of patients with a 5-year survival rate of 76% to 84%. Anal sphincter function was preserved in 43% to 64% of patients overall, depending on the radiation dose and case mix at presentation. Higher radiation doses in recent reports have apparently improved survival[54] but have also increased the early and late complications of therapy,[14] even with the use of a high-energy linear accelerator. Early skin desquamation and diarrhea, compounded by the hematological effects of mitomycin C, were present in up to 97% of patients.[14] Unfortunately, these problems have made completion of a full course of therapy impossible for a significant proportion of patients. Human immunodeficiency virus (HIV)-positive and other immunosuppressed patients with anal cancer (see later discussion) are an increasingly important group for whom treatment must be individualized[57] and often limited because of unacceptable toxicity with combined therapy.[58] Late complications of combination therapy occur in 16% to 20% of patients[19] and include bowel obstruction, radiation enteritis and cystitis, incontinence, anal stenosis, and chronic diarrhea, with a significant incidence of colostomy in this group.

Prognostic Factors

Identification of patient-related factors or conditions that increase the risk for recurrence or a second primary cancer is helpful in guiding the stringency and interval of follow-up evaluations. Factors that influence the risk of recurrence and prognosis from anal cancer include the stage and histological cell type of the cancer, the grade and DNA ploidy of the tumor, the patient's general health and immune status, the type and completeness of therapy, and the tumor's response to therapy. The molecular characteristics of the tumor and an increasingly recognized association with viral infection or benign anorectal conditions have not as yet been shown to influence prognosis.

Stage, histology, and molecular characteristics

One of the most important characteristics determining the risk for recurrence is the stage of the original tumor.[1] In most studies stage III patients have had a higher likelihood of recurrence than stage I or II patients,[54] although stratification of risk by stage has not been observed by all groups.[28] Another factor bearing on risk of recurrence is the completeness of treatment. In patients treated with combination therapy, those receiving less than the full course of chemotherapy or radiation and those in whom combination therapy failed to eradicate the tumor entirely should also be considered at increased risk.[46] Similarly, for patients treated surgically with either local resection or abdominoperineal resection, close or positive margins establish another high-risk group. Long-term survival has been reported after aggressive treatment of patients with local recurrence or limited distant disease. Thus early detection before bulky or symptomatic recurrence is probably worthwhile.

Anal margin cancers are virtually all of squamous cell origin, and histological variation by grade has not been reported to influence survival. For anal canal cancers, squamous cell histology is associated with a far better response to therapy (see previous discussion) than either adenocarcinoma or melanoma, the two other major types of tumors. In general, nonsquamous cancers of the anorectum are associated with significantly poorer survival despite radical excisional treatment.[59,60] Variation in squamous cell type (basaloid, transitional, or cloacogenic types, each representing a form of nonkeratinizing squamous cell carcinoma of the anal canal) has not been shown to have prognostic significance.[1] For anal canal cancers some studies suggest that histological grade and DNA ploidy may have prognostic value.[61,62] Reports of a high-grade, small cell variant indicate that this marker for poor differentiation is associated with a very poor outcome, regardless of stage.[63]

Intensive characterization of the molecular events occurring around the development of anal squamous neoplasia by Ogunbiyi et al.[64] has shown that aberrant p53 tumor suppressor gene expression is involved in the progression from in situ to invasive squamous cell carcinoma.[64] C-myc[65,66] and E6, an oncoprotein expressed by the DNA-transforming virus human papillomavirus,[67] have both been associated with alteration of p53 in anal squamous cell carcinoma.[64] Overexpression of p53 is associated with malignant potential and prognosis in several types of breast and hematological malignancies,[68] but unfortunately the prognostic significance of p53 in anal cancer is less clear. Immunocytochemical and in situ hybridization studies by Walts et al.[69] have detected p53 in equal proportions of low-grade intraepithelial lesions and invasive anal cancers, suggesting that qualitative detection of p53 alone has little prognostic significance. Measurement of individual tumor p53 content may provide greater prognostic information as these techniques are refined.

High-Risk Groups and Conditions

High-risk groups

The demographics of anal cancer are in evolution. Thirty years ago anal cancer occurred equally in males and females, predominantly during middle age. More recently, anal margin cancers have been found in a higher proportion of men, most less than 60 years of age, while anal canal cancers have occurred at an increasing rate in women over 60.[70-73] These broad epidemiological trends do not, however, establish useful categorizations for surveillance of primary or recurrent disease. Even in one of the highest risk patient demographic groups, male homosexuals practicing anal-receptive intercourse,[74,75] the relative risk of anal cancer compared with the rest of the population is only 33 (4 to 272, 95% confidence limits).[76] Given the rarity of these tumors (an incidence of 0.4 to 1.2 per 100,000 population),[77] the risk to male homosexuals is not sufficient to indicate surveillance for primary anal cancer independent of routine health screening. Even more important in the context of formulating a strategy for patient follow-up, being a member of any group at increased risk for primary anal cancer has not been proved to have independent significance (beyond stage, completeness of treatment, and tumor response) for the risk of recurrent cancer.

Benign anorectal disease

Many common benign anal conditions have been associated with anal cancer. Anal fissure, fistula, perianal abscess, and recurrent bouts of hemorrhoidal inflammation have all been linked temporally (relative risk = 2.4 to 2.6) to the diagnosis of anal cancer. However, careful evaluation of data from Denmark[78] and the U.S. Department of Veterans Affairs[79] suggests that symptoms from a cancer are not infrequently attributed to concomitant benign conditions, artificially increasing their significance. This experience suggests that the clinician should look skeptically at new, unusual, or progressive symptoms from apparently benign, chronic anal conditions. Sporadic cases of anal squamous cell carcinoma arising in chronic hidradenitis suppurativa[80] and perianal Crohn's disease[1,81] suggest that foci of chronic anal inflammation may indeed predispose to anal malignancy but this risk is low.[78] The greater risk is a delay in diagnosis of anal cancer because symptoms are wrongly attributed to a more obvious benign condition. The risk of misdiagnosis also applies to the detection of recurrent disease in patients with chronic, benign anorectal disorders.

Human papillomavirus infection and anal intraepithelial neoplasia

In contrast to the previously discussed benign lesions, a number of other conditions with greater malignant potential have been defined.[26] Genital warts (condyloma acuminatum) caused by infection with human papillomavirus types 6 and 8 have been sporadically associated with invasive anal carcinoma. Although the association between this viral lesion and subsequent malignancy is direct, the risk of malignancy from anal condylomata is still considered low.[82,83] Of greater concern are the conditions of anal intraepithelial neoplasia (AIN) associated with human papillomavirus types 16 and 18[84] and anal Paget's disease (intraepithelial adenocarcinoma). The visible, plaquelike lesion associated with high-grade AIN is termed Bowen's disease (intraepithelial squamous cell carcinoma in situ). Serological studies and measurement of viral DNA have linked both AIN and anal cancer to human papillomavirus type 16,[84,85] suggesting that many if not most squamous cell carcinomas of the anus arise in AIN and that this process is mediated by human papillomavirus.[86] AIN is found in 60% of women with multifocal cervical intraepithelial neoplasia[87] and in an increasing proportion of homosexual males.[88,89] In 4% to 25% of patients with untreated Bowen's disease, invasive squamous cell carcinoma will develop, although this may take up to 15 years.[87,90] Fifty percent of pagetoid lesions are found to have an underlying invasive adenocarcinoma requiring definitive treatment.[1] In the rest, invasive cancer can be expected to develop in up to 40% without treatment.[90] For Bowen's disease and superficial pagetoid lesions, complete excision of the at-risk epithelium is generally curative.[90-93] Patients with AIN lesions associated with human papillomavirus types 16 and 18 may be at increased risk for recurrence and second primary malignancies and thus are subject to close follow-up.[85,90]

Immunodeficiency

The risk associated with HIV infection and, separately, the risk of immunosuppression (therapeutic for transplantation or autoimmune disorders, as a side effect of treatment for other conditions, or after HIV infection) for the development of anal cancer has become an increasingly important issue over the past 10 years. Anal cancer in homosexual, HIV-positive men occurs 84 times more often than in the general population and represents one of the most rapidly growing populations of patients with anal cancer.[94] Indeed, the risk in homosexual, HIV-positive men is appreciably greater than the risk of anal cancer with anal-receptive intercourse alone (relative risk = 33). Although this fact might implicate a specific causal relationship for the HIV virus in anal cancer, most studies suggest that the role of HIV is analogous to other conditions that cause immunosuppression.[95-98] Current reports suggest that homosexual activities predispose to sexual transmission of disease, including human papillomavirus,[99] and that in patients infected with both papillomavirus and HIV, progressive suppression of normal immunity permits proliferation of papillomavirus (especially type 16). Evidence for increased human papillomavirus proliferation in immunocompromised patients has come from direct studies of human papillomavirus prevalence[88] and replication in patients with HIV[100] or other immunodeficiency states,[101] as well as from the clinical observation of human papillomavirus–associated mucosal lesions[89] and refractory anogenital warts in HIV-positive patients.[102] As previously discussed, proliferation of human papillomavirus has been pathogenetically linked to the development of AIN lesions and, subsequently, invasive cancer,[10,103] although the mechanism of malignant transformation remains unclear.[67,95]

Based on analysis of risk categories, Palefsky[100] and other researchers have recommended screening for AIN and anal cancer in three groups: (1) HIV-negative men with a history of anal-receptive intercourse; (2) HIV-positive men or women with CD4 counts less than 500×10^6/L; and (3) women with cervical intraepithelial neoplasia.[100] In these patients, direct and anoscopic inspection should be supplemented by cotton swab cytology, with biopsy reserved for positive cytological results and suspect lesions.[89] Again, whether such high-risk patients deserve any different follow-up after definitive treatment of anal cancer has not been evaluated. As Palefsky[100] pointed out, the intercurrent illness of HIV-positive patients limits life span and usually subjects them to intensive, ongoing evaluation. Close follow-up is probably most beneficial for the first and third groups in terms of overall days of life saved with earlier detection of recurrent disease.

FOLLOW-UP STUDIES

Of patients with a primary anal carcinoma, up to 50% initially complain of rectal bleeding and pain and 25% have a palpable mass. In 25% of patients the anal cancer is diagnosed before symptoms develop,[104] but more often diagnosis is delayed, with up to one third of patients waiting 6 months from the onset of symptoms to diagnosis.[6,105] Although these figures apply to the diagnosis of primary disease rather than recurrence, they suggest the general tendency among patients and physicians to trivialize anorectal symptoms, to ascribe them to benign conditions, and to avoid thorough evaluation of the anorectum for reasons of embarrassment, discomfort, and inconvenience. As with the diagnosis of primary anal cancers, recurrence is usually detected at the time of direct physical examination of the anus. Erroneous or incomplete evaluation has been shown to worsen prognosis.[106]

Physical Examination, Anoscopy, and Biopsy

After curative combination therapy the anus should return to a normal or nearly normal appearance. Tissues may be somewhat less pliable depending on chronic, benign conditions, the effects of radiation, and scarring from biopsies. Mucosal atrophy may predispose to laceration with bowel movements, recurrent fissures, and intermittent bleeding. However, patients should achieve close to a stable condition, a stable degree of continence, and consistent bowel function. During follow-up, physical examinations should be carried out on a schedule as previously described (Table 9-3), with additional visits for any significant change in anorectal function.

Serial digital and anoscopic examinations by a consistent examiner with careful documentation of tissue changes are critical to detection of the subtle changes that might herald local recurrence. Palpation of the anoderm along the entire canal and circumference between the thumb and index finger is important for detecting subtle thickening, masses, or asymmetrical tenderness. More proximally, pararectal adenopathy and rectal tumors are sometimes detected. Anoscopy is useful for evaluation of palpable abnormalities to detect mucosal change (especially dysplastic changes associated with human papillomavirus in at-risk populations[89]) and to visualize regions for biopsy.[5] Sigmoidoscopy serves a similar function in the retroflexed view of the proximal anal canal and provides information about the distal rectum, especially with respect to radiation damage. Colposcopic and cytological examinations of the anus have proved effective for detecting subclinical human papillomavirus infection and the premalignant lesion of anal intraepithelial neoplasia[107] but have not been evaluated after treatment for anal cancer.[89] Depending on patient tolerance, various degrees of anesthesia may be necessary to complete the examination.

Other aspects of the physical examination include bimanual and speculum pelvic examination in women for detection of vaginal lesions and paravaginal adenopathy.[17] Malignant inguinal adenopathy may be distinguished from reactive adenopathy by observing the firm character of the nodes, noting progressive enlargement on serial examinations, and following a policy of early, aggressive biopsy for suspect lymph nodes. In patients treated with abdominoperineal resection, serial inspection of the gluteal cleft is important to distinguish local recurrence from the healing wound. Core needle biopsy is often appropriate for submucosal or deep mass lesions and worrisome lymph nodes, whereas incisional biopsy is usually reserved for superficial masses, suspect ulcers, and intraepithelial mucosal lesions. The vast majority of treatable locoregional recurrences from anal cancer can be detected with careful physical examination and a liberal biopsy policy.

Radiographic Studies

In recent years TRUS and cross-sectional imaging studies of the abdomen and pelvis have proved useful in staging primary cancers of the anus and detecting subtle recurrent lesions. In rare circumstances barium enema may provide additional information about proximal extension of bulky anorectal polypoid lesions.[108]

TRUS, by use of prostatic probes or dedicated endoscopic instruments, is a recent and important innovation in the management of patients with anal cancer. Transducer frequencies of 7.5 to 12 MHz can provide a very high resolution image of the mucosa and underlying muscular elements of the distal rectum and anus.[109] In cancers of the anal canal the ultrasonic image of the lesion and adjacent tissue (including pararectal lymph nodes) has correlated well with the pathological stage. In a study by Roseau et al.,[17] TNM staging of primary lesions and early detection of mural recurrent disease predicted subsequent pathological findings accurately in a group of patients subject to salvage surgery.

Computed tomography or magnetic resonance imaging is most useful in detecting bulky tumor extension for T3 and T4 lesions, deep pelvic (internal iliac and inferior mesenteric artery distribution) adenopathy, and distant metastases in the lung and liver. In a study of 19 posttreatment patients by Cohan et al.,[110] computed tomography correctly identified recurrent disease in 14 (74%). Local tumor recurrence detected by computed tomography had the appearance of ischiorectal or perirectal fat stranding in association with a mass. False positive diagnoses in four patients (21%) included a pelvic abscess, radiation and surgical scar, and radiation necrosis, each verified by tissue biopsy or serial scans. Magnetic resonance imaging has been used successfully in lieu of computed tomography in some studies.[19]

Blood Tests

Two circulating markers for recurrent epidermoid carcinoma of the anus have been described in the literature: SCCAg and CEA. Other routine blood studies such as complete blood count or liver function studies have shown little value in detecting treatable recurrent disease.[111]

SCCAg was first described in association with cancer of the cervix. It has more recently been studied in several cohorts of patients with anal cancer using a radioimmunoassay marketed by Abbott Laboratories. Petrelli et al.[112,113] and others[114] noted that SCCAg had a sensitivity of 59% to 76%, a specificity of 86% to 95%, and a positive predictive value of 62% to 76% for recurrent anal canal cancer. They recommended its use in the long-term follow-up of patients after definitive treatment. Goldman et al.[62] showed that an elevated SCCAg level (SCCAg >2 ng/ml) before treatment of an epidermoid anal cancer predicted residual or recurrent disease in 80% of the patients and a reduction in tumor-specific survival rate from 83% to 45%. Multivariate analysis in the study of Goldman et al.[62] showed that SCCAg elevation was the most significant of all risk factors analyzed for recurrent disease. In contrast, CEA is elevated in only about one fifth of patients before treatment and does not correlate with either prognosis or tumor CEA content, thus limiting its clinical utility.[115]

RECURRENCE AND THE ROLE OF SALVAGE THERAPY

Most recurrences after apparently curative combination treatment of a primary anal cancer occur within 2 years.[23] Late recurrences, some up to 15 years after treatment of a primary lesion, have been documented, with over two thirds isolated to the pelvis.[27,28,51] Late recurrence isolated to the groin lymph nodes is a rare event (4%). Most patients with distant recurrence also have locally recurrent disease. The predominance of locoregional failure suggests that close follow-up, early detection of recurrent disease, and aggressive salvage therapy are critical because unlike the situation with many other malignancies, long-term disease control and cure can still be achieved under these conditions.

Salvage surgical resection is indicated for three groups of patients: (1) those in whom regional treatment has failed; (2) those in whom locally recurrent disease develops after a course of sphincter-sparing treatment; and (3) those with severe radiation injury that prevents sphincter function. Although additional radiation and chemotherapy have been administered for salvage, these modalities are generally reserved for patients with distant metastases. Repeating one or more courses of combination therapy has been effective in less than half of patients with residual or recurrent disease and has introduced considerable morbidity.[19]

Four to 6 weeks after curative sphincter-preserving treatment, 45% of clinical-partial responders and 44% of clinical-complete responders have viable tumor cells at the primary site.[21] Between 15% and 20% of patients with anal canal cancers (usually initially staged as T3 or T4 lesions[19]) have gross residual disease after radiation or combination therapy. Sphincter-sparing local resection is technically feasible and encompasses the entire lesion in a majority of these patients.[21] In the rest, scarring from radiation treatment or bulky residual disease prevents an adequate local resection that will heal.[45] For these patients abdominoperineal resection is necessary; however, deciding which patients will benefit from a more radical resection is often difficult. Both radiographic and clinical examinations including repeated biopsy are often helpful in planning surgical salvage. The incidence of colostomy and salvage abdominoperineal resection for residual disease ranges from 3% to 12%, encompassing both radiation-only and chemoradiation treatment groups.[43,116] Independent of disease stage, survival does not seem to be influenced by the extent of resection (local versus abdominoperineal resection).[51] Unfortunately, surgical salvage is not achieved without risk. Perineal wound healing problems in these patients are common and in some series have been a principal source of morbidity.[54]

Late complications that benefit from surgical treatment have included chronic pain, anal stenosis, anal incontinence, and nonhealing benign ulceration of the anal canal. These occur in 3% to 15% of patients after radiation alone[18,41,44] or combination therapy.[19,45] About half of the patients with such complications eventually require surgical palliation, either a diverting colostomy or abdominoperineal resection. Unfortunately, such patients present particularly complex management problems, with delayed healing and a slow recovery. Recent surgical management of such potentially compromised wounds has benefited from the liberal use of closed suction drains, omental flaps,[117] and, more recently, perineal or transpelvic myocutaneous flaps using nonirradiated tissue.[118] With such techniques, primary wound healing after abdominoperineal resection in the irradiated pelvis is now readily achievable in a majority of patients.

SURVIVAL AFTER RECURRENCE OF ANAL CARCINOMA

Although salvage abdominoperineal resection is important in achieving local control for patients with residual or recurrent pelvic disease, the survival benefit of this procedure has been challenged. Leichman et al.[46] noted a 15% incidence of residual microscopic or gross disease after neoadjuvant treatment, and all of these patients eventually died of distant disease despite salvage abdominoperineal resection. Zelnick et al.[119] have reported a similar bleak experience, with only a 29% 3-year survival rate after salvage abdominoperineal resection. However, Miller et al.[21] reported that 10 of 15 (66%) patients undergoing abdominoperineal resection for biopsy-proven residual disease after a similar protocol were rendered free of disease. In the Radiation Therapy Oncology Group study by Sischy et al.,[14] curative resection to clear margins was possible in five of eight patients (62%) with persistent disease and all of these patients were also rendered disease free. Similar survival benefits have been reported by other groups.[19] Salvage abdominoperineal resection has been shown to increase both local control and survival.

At the time of initial diagnosis, distant metastatic disease is evident in only about 2% of patients.[12] After treatment of an apparently localized primary lesion, unresectable pelvic recurrence and recurrence outside the pelvis are also uncommon events.[22] When detected, they are rarely curable.[28,120] These patients are often candidates for chemotherapy or chemoradiation (e.g., for bony or other regionally accessible metastasis) but tumor response to second or additional rounds of combination therapy is often poor.[121] All patients with distant recurrence will die from their disease. Median survival from detection to death is 1 to 24 months, depending on whether chemotherapy (mitomycin C plus 5-FU or cisplatin plus 5-FU) is administered and how the tumor responds to treatment.[122]

No clear data have shown the effect of a second primary neoplasm versus recurrence of the primary neoplasm on survival. Probably second primaries would be detected at an earlier stage than the original tumor because of the close follow-up and treated just as a recurrence would be treated.

Prior treatment would limit future treatment options for both recurrence and new primary anal cancers.

NONSQUAMOUS CELL CANCERS OF THE ANAL CANAL

Ten percent of anal canal cancers are made up of cell types other than basaloid or squamous. The most common of these, anal adenocarcinoma,[59] makes up 5% to 9% of anorectal neoplasms. Two percent are malignant melanomas, and a variety of sarcomas have also been described.[26] In general, surgery is the primary treatment, but even with radical resection, survival has been poor.

Adenocarcinoma arising from the anus must be distinguished clinically from a distal rectal adenocarcinoma that extends transanally. Primary anal canal adenocarcinomas are thought to arise from anal glands or chronic fistula-in-ano[123] and are often soft, tender masses that tend to bleed. Local excision of small, very superficial lesions is technically feasible in some cases, but most adenocarcinomas require radical resection (abdominoperineal resection). Basik et al.,[59] reporting on the Roswell Park Cancer Institute experience with this disease, treated 10 patients for cure, with long-term disease-free survival in only two patients. The role of combination therapy for adenocarcinoma of the anus has not been systematically evaluated. Follow-up after curative treatment should be no different from that in patients undergoing surgical treatment of anal squamous cell carcinoma, although options for further treatment after recurrence are limited and generally palliative.

The anal canal is the third most common site of melanoma after the skin and eye. These lesions develop near the dentate line in middle-aged patients and may be pigmented or amelanotic.[124] Special stains have been developed to assist in the verification of histologically suspect lesions. Patients with local disease less than 2 mm in depth may be cured, but most patients have a significant mass, regional nodal, or distant disease at the time of diagnosis.[125,126] Abdominoperineal resection seems to improve local control, but 5-year survival is only 10%.[60,125,127,128] Strategies for follow-up of such patients should be indexed to the evaluation of symptomatic recurrence but may change with the availability of better treatment for distant disease.

FUTURE PROSPECTS

The prospects for earlier, more accurate, and more cost-effective detection of recurrent anal cancer must rely on the results of current therapy. Most patients with anal cancer in the United States are treated with local resection or combination therapy, depending on the location and stage of the lesion. Retrospective data show that survival and preservation of the anal sphincter have been remarkably good in these patients. However, prospective validation of these studies is critical and may help identify patients at high risk for complications or tumor recurrence. Once treatment is more standardized, studying the different methods of follow-up (most likely in a multiinstitutional manner) becomes useful. Until treatment is more standardized, however, follow-up protocols are likely to remain linked to the differing treatment protocols used at different institutions. For this reason multiinstitutional trials of follow-up for anal cancer are not advocated at the present time. These studies should also increase understanding of the influence of premalignant lesions or membership in a high-risk group (patients with human papillomavirus infection or AIN) on the type of therapy administered and on the risk of tumor recurrence.

There are prospects for improvements in treatment. These include clarification of the role of radiation and chemoradiation, the types of chemotherapeutic agents employed, and the management of treatment-related toxicity.[45] Employing mitomycin C analogs[14,129] or cisplatin[20] may reduce the toxicity of treatment and allow more patients to achieve a full therapeutic dose without sphincter injury. This especially applies to HIV-positive and other immunosuppressed patients who often cannot tolerate the side effects of current therapy. Adjusting the dosage of radiation under different treatment conditions may have a similar effect. For patients requiring immediate or salvage abdominoperineal resection, technical improvements in the management of the healing, irradiated wound should also reduce morbidity and mortality. Improvements in outcome and survival from primary therapy will further increase the pool of patients subject to follow-up.

Current follow-up schemes for anal cancer await careful cost analysis,[130,131] especially with respect to the benefit of expensive radiographic studies. Whether treatment of such rare tumors should be concentrated in high-volume centers is also an important question.[132] Wider use of serological testing and graduated follow-up schemes, based on a more accurate assessment of recurrence risk, should eventually reduce the cost of follow-up without compromising survival.

REFERENCES

1. Fenger C. Anal neoplasia and its precursors: facts and controversies. Semin Diagn Pathol 1991;8:190-201.
2. Heino P, Goldman S, Lagerstedt U, Dillner J. Molecular and serological studies of human papillomavirus among patients with anal epidermoid carcinoma. Int J Cancer 1993;53:377-81.
3. Aparicio-Duque R, Mittal KR, Chan W, Schinella R. Cloacogenic carcinoma of the anal canal and associated viral lesions: an in situ hybridization study for human papilloma virus. Cancer 1991;68:2422-5.
4. Merlini M, Eckert P. Malignant tumors of the anus: a study of 106 cases. Am J Surg 1985;150:370-2.
5. Tanum G. Diagnosis and treatment of anal carcinoma: an overview. Acta Oncol 1992;31:513-8.
6. Tanum G, Tveit K, Karlsen KO. Diagnosis of anal carcinoma—doctor's finger still the best? Oncology 1991;48:383-6.
7. Deans GT, McAleer JJ, Spence RA. Malignant anal tumours. Br J Surg 1994;81:500-8.
8. Klompje J, Petrelli NJ, Herrera L, Mittelman A. Synchronous and metachronous colon lesions in squamous cell carcinoma of the anal canal. J Surg Oncol 1987;35:86-8.
9. Rabkin CS, Biggar RJ, Melbye M, Curtis RE. Second primary cancers following anal and cervical carcinoma: evidence of shared etiologic factors. Am J Epidemiol 1992;136:54-8.
10. Frisch M, Olsen JH, Melbye M. Malignancies that occur before and after anal cancer: clues to their etiology. Am J Epidemiol 1994;140:12-9.

11. Pyper PC, Parks TG. The results of surgery for epidermoid carcinoma of the anus. Br J Surg 1985;72:712-4.
12. Boman BM, Moertel CG, O'Connell MJ, et al. Carcinoma of the anal canal: a clinical and pathologic study of 188 cases. Cancer 1984;54:114-25.
13. Beahrs OH, Henson DE, Hutter RV, Kennedy BJ, American Joint Committee on Cancer. Manual for staging of cancer. 4th ed. Philadelphia: JB Lippincott Company, 1992.
14. Sischy B, Doggett RL, Krall JM, et al. Definitive irradiation and chemotherapy for radiosensitization in management of anal carcinoma: interim report on Radiation Therapy Oncology Group study No. 8314. J Natl Cancer Inst 1989;81:850-6.
15. Brown DK, Oglesby AB, Scott DH, Dayton MT. Squamous cell carcinoma of the anus: a twenty-five year retrospective. Am Surg 1988;54:337-42.
16. Greenall MJ, Quan SH, Stearns MW, Urmacher C, DeCosse JJ. Epidermoid cancer of the anal margin: pathologic features, treatment, and clinical results. Am J Surg 1985;149:95-101.
17. Roseau G, Palazzo L, Colardelle P, Chaussade S, Couturier D, Paolaggi JA. Endoscopic ultrasonography in the staging and follow-up of epidermoid carcinoma of the anal canal. Gastrointest Endosc 1994;40:447-50.
18. Wagner JP, Mahe MA, Romestaing P, et al. Radiation therapy in the conservative treatment of carcinoma of the anal canal. Int J Radiat Oncol Biol Phys 1994;29:17-23.
19. Tanum G, Tveit KM, Karlsen KO. Chemoradiotherapy of anal carcinoma: tumour response and acute toxicity. Oncology 1993;50:14-7.
20. Rich TA, Ajani JA, Morrison WH, Ota D, Levin B. Chemoradiation therapy for anal cancer: radiation plus continuous infusion of 5-fluorouracil with or without cisplatin. Radiother Oncol 1993;27:209-15.
21. Miller EJ, Quan SH, Thaler HT. Treatment of squamous cell carcinoma of the anal canal. Cancer 1991;67:2038-41.
22. Papillon J, Chassard JL. Respective roles of radiotherapy and surgery in the management of epidermoid carcinoma of the anal margin: series of 57 patients. Dis Colon Rectum 1992;35:422-9.
23. Welch JP, Malt RA. Appraisal of the treatment of carcinoma of the anus and anal canal. Surg Gynecol Obstet 1977;145:837-41.
24. Al-Jurf AS, Turnbull RB, Fazio VW. Local treatment of squamous cell carcinoma of the anus. Surg Gynecol Obstet 1979;148:576-8.
25. Hubens A, Beelaerts W. Late recurrence following treatment of anal canal carcinoma. Acta Chir Belg 1991;91:73-6.
26. Gordon PH. Current status—perianal and anal canal neoplasms. Dis Colon Rectum 1990;33:799-808.
27. Jensen SL, Hagen K, Harling H, Shokouh-Amiri MH, Nielsen OV. Long-term prognosis after radical treatment for squamous-cell carcinoma of the anal canal and anal margin. Dis Colon Rectum 1988; 31:273-8.
28. Cummings BJ, Keane TJ, O'Sullivan B, Wong CS, Catton CN. Epidermoid anal cancer: treatment by radiation alone or by radiation and 5-fluorouracil with and without mitomycin C. Int J Radiat Oncol Biol Phys 1991;21:1115-25.
29. Cummings BJ. Anal cancer. Int J Radiat Oncol Biol Phys 1990;19:1309-15.
30. Nigro ND, Vaitkevicius VK, Considine B Jr. Combined therapy for cancer of the anal canal: a preliminary report. Dis Colon Rectum 1974;17:354-6.
31. Greenall MJ, Quan SH, Urmacher C, DeCosse JJ. Treatment of epidermoid carcinoma of the anal canal. Surg Gynecol Obstet 1985; 161:509-17.
32. Beahrs OH, Wilson SM. Carcinoma of the anus. Ann Surg 1976; 184:422-8.
33. Green JP, Schaupp WC, Cantril ST, Schall G. Anal carcinoma: current therapeutic concepts. Am J Surg 1980;140:151-5.
34. Wolfe HR. The management of metastatic inguinal adenitis in epidermoid cancer of the anus. Proc R Soc Med 1961;61:626-8.
35. Jaiyesimi IA, Pazdur R. Cisplatin and 5-fluorouracil as salvage therapy for recurrent metastatic squamous cell carcinoma of the anal canal [clinical conference]. Am J Clin Oncol 1993;16:536-40.
36. Evans TR, Mansi JL, Glees JP. Response of metastatic anal carcinoma to single agent carboplatin. Clin Oncol (R Coll Radiol) 1993;5:57-8.
37. Moertel CG, Childs DS Jr, Reitmeier RJ, Colby MY Jr, Holbrook MA. Combined 5-fluorouracil and supervoltage radiation therapy of locally unresectable gastrointestinal cancer. Lancet 1969;2:865-7.
38. Papillon J, Montbarbon JF, Gerard JP, Chassard JL, Ardiet JM. Interstitial curietherapy in the conservative treatment of anal and rectal cancers. Int J Radiat Oncol Biol Phys 1989;17:1161-9.
39. Papillon J, Montbaron JF. Epidermoid carcinoma of the anal canal: a series of 276 cases. Dis Colon Rectum 1987;30:324-33.
40. Papillon J. Effectiveness of combined radio-chemotherapy in the management of epidermoid carcinoma of the anal canal. Int J Radiat Oncol Biol Phys 1990;19:1217-8.
41. Touboul E, Schlienger M, Buffat L, et al. Epidermoid carcinoma of the anal canal: results of curative-intent radiation therapy in a series of 270 patients. Cancer 1994;73:1569-79.
42. Salmon RJ, Fenton J, Asselain B, et al. Treatment of epidermoid anal cell cancer. Am J Surg 1984;147:43-8.
43. Martenson JA Jr, Gunderson LL. External radiation therapy without chemotherapy in the management of anal cancer. Cancer 1993; 71:1736-40.
44. Cantril ST, Green JP, Schall GL, Schaupp WC. Primary radiation therapy in the treatment of anal carcinoma. Int J Radiat Oncol Biol Phys 1983;9:1271-8.
45. Cummings B, Keane T, Thomas G, Harwood A, Rider W. Results and toxicity of the treatment of anal canal carcinoma by radiation therapy or radiation therapy and chemotherapy. Cancer 1984; 54:2062-8.
46. Leichman L, Nigro N, Vaitkevicius VK, et al. Cancer of the anal canal: model for preoperative adjuvant combined modality therapy. Am J Med 1985;78:211-5.
47. Nigro ND. The force of change in the management of squamous-cell cancer of the anal canal. Dis Colon Rectum 1991;34:482-6.
48. Nigro ND, Vaitkevicius VK, Considine B Jr. Dynamic management of squamous cell cancer of the anal canal. Invest New Drugs 1989;7:83-9.
49. Nigro ND. Multidisciplinary management of cancer of the anus. World J Surg 1987;11:446-51.
50. Cummings B Jr. Concomitant radiotherapy and chemotherapy for anal cancer. Semin Oncol 1992;19(4 Suppl 11):102-8.
51. Enker WE, Heilwell M, Janov AJ, et al. Improved survival in epidermoid carcinoma of the anus in association with preoperative multidisciplinary therapy. Arch Surg 1986;121:1386-90.
52. Grabenbauer GG, Panzer M, Hultenschmidt B, et al. Prognostische fakkktoren nach simultaner radiochemotherapie des analkanalkarzinoms in einer multizentrischen serie von 139 patienten. Strahlenther Onkol 1994;170:391-9.
53. Goldman S, Ihre T, Seligson U. Squamous-cell carcinoma of the anus: a follow-up study of 65 patients. Dis Colon Rectum 1985; 28:143-6.
54. Myerson RJ, Shapiro SJ, Lacey D, et al. Carcinoma of the anal canal. Am J Clin Oncol 1995;18:32-9.
55. John MJ, Flam M, Lovalvo L, Mowry PA. Feasibility of non-surgical definitive management of anal canal carcinoma. Int J Radiat Oncol Biol Phys 1987;13:299-303.
56. Salem PA, Habboubi N, Anaissie E, et al. Effectiveness of cisplatin in the treatment of anal squamous cell carcinoma. Cancer Treat Rep 1985;69:891-3.
57. Chadha M, Rosenblatt EA, Malamud S, Pisch J, Berson A. Squamous-cell carcinoma of the anus in HIV-positive patients. Dis Colon Rectum 1994;37:861-5.
58. Holland JM, Swift PS. Tolerance of patients with human immunodeficiency virus and anal carcinoma to treatment with combined chemotherapy and radiation therapy. Radiology 1994;193:251-4.
59. Basik M, Rodriguez-Bigas MA, Penetrante R, Petrelli NJ. Prognosis and recurrence patterns of anal adenocarcinoma. Am J Surg 1995;169:233-7.

60. Antoniuk PM, Tjandra JJ, Webb BW, Petras RE, Milsom JW, Fazio VW. Anorectal malignant melanoma has a poor prognosis. Int J Colorectal Dis 1993;8:81-6.
61. Shepherd NA, Scholefield JH, Love SB, England J, Northover JM. Prognostic factors in anal squamous carcinoma:a multivariate analysis of clinical, pathological and flow cytometric parameters in 235 cases. Histopathology 1990;16:545-55.
62. Goldman S, Svensson C, Bronnergard M, Glimelius B, Wallin G. Prognostic significance of serum concentration of squamous cell carcinoma antigen in anal epidermoid carcinoma. Int J Colorectal Dis 1993;8:98-102.
63. Nakahara H, Moriya Y, Shinkai T, Hirota T. Small cell carcinoma of the anus in a human HIV carrier: report of a case. Surg Today 1993;23:85-8.
64. Ogunbiyi OA, Scholefield JH, Smith JH, Polacarz SV, Rogers K, Sharp F. Immunohistochemical analysis of p53 expression in anal squamous neoplasia. J Clin Pathol 1993;46:507-12.
65. Crook T, Wrede D, Tidy J, Scholefield J, Crawford L, Vousden KH. Status of c-myc, p53 and retinoblastoma genes in human papilloma virus positive and negative squamous cell carcinomas of the anus. Oncogene 1991;6:1251-7.
66. Ogunbiyi OA, Scholefield JH, Rogers K, Sharp F, Smith JH, Polacarz SV. C-myc oncogene expression in anal squamous neoplasia. J Clin Pathol 1993;46:23-7.
67. Jakate SM, Saclarides TJ. Immunohistochemical detection of mutant P53 protein and human papillomavirus-related E6 protein in anal cancers. Dis Colon Rectum 1993;36:1026-9.
68. Fung CY, Fisher DE. p53:from molecular mechanisms to prognosis in cancer [editorial]. J Clin Oncol 1995;13:808-11.
69. Walts AE, Koeffler HP, Said JW. Localization of p53 protein and human papillomavirus in anogenital squamous lesions: immunohistochemical and in situ hybridization studies in benign, dysplastic, and malignant epithelia. Hum Pathol 1993;24:1238-42.
70. McConnell EM. Squamous cell carcinoma of the anus—a review of 96 cases. Br J Surg 1970;57:89-92.
71. Grinnell RS. An analysis of forty-nine cases of squamous cell carcinoma of the anus. Surg Gynecol Obstet 1954;98:29-39.
72. Richards JC, Beahrs OH, Woolner LB. Squamous cell carcinoma of the anus, anal canal, and rectum in 109 patients. Surg Gynecol Obstet 1962;114:475-82.
73. Peters RK, Mack TM. Patterns of anal carcinoma by gender and marital status in Los Angeles County. Br J Cancer 1983;48:629-36.
74. Scholefield JH, Thornton Jones H, Cuzick J, Northover JM. Anal cancer and marital status. Br J Cancer 1990;62:286-8.
75. Holly EA, Whittemore AS, Aston DA, Ahn DK, Nickoloff BJ, Kristiansen JJ. Anal cancer incidence: genital warts, anal fissure or fistula, hemorrhoids, and smoking. J Natl Cancer Inst 1989;81:1726-31.
76. Daling JR, Weiss NS, Hislop TG, et al. Sexual practices, sexually transmitted diseases, and the incidence of anal cancer. N Engl J Med 1987;317:973-7.
77. Melbye M, Rabkin C, Frisch M, Biggar RJ. Changing patterns of anal cancer incidence in the United States, 1940-1989. Am J Epidemiol 1994;139:772-80.
78. Frisch M, Olsen JH, Bautz A, Melbye M. Benign anal lesions and the risk of anal cancer. N Engl J Med 1994;331:300-2.
79. Lin AY, Gridley G, Tucker M. Benign anal lesions and anal cancer [letter; comment]. N Engl J Med 1995;332:190-1.
80. Shukla VK, Hughes LE. A case of squamous cell carcinoma complicating hidradenitis suppurativa. Eur J Surg Oncol 1995;21:106-9.
81. Lumley JW, Stitz RW. Crohn's disease and anal carcinoma: an association? A case report and review of the literature. Aust N Z J Surg 1991;61:76-7.
82. Goodman P, Halpert RD. Invasive squamous cell carcinoma of the anus arising in condyloma acuminatum: CT demonstration. Gastrointest Radiol 1991;16:267-70.
83. Butler TW, Gefter J, Kleto D, Shuck EH 3d, Ruffner BW. Squamous-cell carcinoma of the anus in condyloma acuminatum: successful treatment with preoperative chemotherapy and radiation. Dis Colon Rectum 1987;30:293-5.
84. Palmer JG, Shepherd NA, Jass JR, Crawford LV, Northover JM. Human papillomavirus type 16 DNA in anal squamous cell carcinoma [letter]. Lancet 1987;2:42.
85. Palefsky JM, Holly EA, Gonzales J, Berline J, Ahn DK, Greenspan JS. Detection of human papillomavirus DNA in anal intraepithelial neoplasia and anal cancer. Cancer Res 1991;51:1014-9.
86. Palefsky JM. Serologic detection of human papillomavirus-related anogenital disease: new opportunities and challenges [editorial; comment]. J Natl Cancer Inst 1995;87:401-2.
87. Scholefield JH, Hickson WG, Smith JH, Rogers K, Sharp F. Anal intraepithelial neoplasia: part of a multifocal disease process. Lancet 1992;340:1271-3.
88. Law CL, Qassim M, Thompson CH, et al. Factors associated with clinical and sub-clinical anal human papillomavirus infection in homosexual men. Genitourin Med 1991;67:92-8.
89. Surawicz CM, Kirby P, Critchlow C, Sayer J, Dunphy C, Kiviat N. Anal dysplasia in homosexual men: role of anoscopy and biopsy. Gastroenterology 1993;105:658-66.
90. Beck DE, Fazio VW. Premalignant lesions of the anal margin. South Med J 1989;82:470-4.
91. Salmi T, Gronroos M, Nieminen S, Taina E, Maenpaa J. The treatment of perineal and perianal intraepidermal carcinoma with radical extirpation and mesh skin graft: case report. Ann Chir Gynaecol Suppl 1987;202:54-6.
92. Foust RL, Dean PJ, Stoler MH, Moinuddin SM. Intraepithelial neoplasia of the anal canal in hemorrhoidal tissue: a study of 19 cases. Hum Pathol 1991;22:528-34.
93. Rasmussen OO, Christiansen J. Conservative management of Bowen's disease of the anus. Int J Colorectal Dis 1989;4:164-6.
94. Melbye M, Cote TR, Kessler L, Gail M, Biggar RJ. High incidence of anal cancer among AIDS patients: the AIDS/Cancer Working Group. Lancet 1994;343:636-9.
95. Palefsky J. Human papillomavirus infection among HIV-infected individuals: implications for development of malignant tumors. Hematol Oncol Clin North Am 1991;5:357-70.
96. Lipsey LR, Northfelt DW. Anogenital neoplasia in patients with HIV infection. Curr Opin Oncol 1993;5:861-6.
97. Fairley CK, Sheil AG, McNeil JJ, et al. The risk of ano-genital malignancies in dialysis and transplant patients. Clin Nephrol 1994;41:101-5.
98. Penn I. Cancers of the anogenital region in renal transplant recipients:analysis of 65 cases. Cancer 1986;58:611-6.
99. Modesto VL, Gottesman L. Sexually transmitted diseases and anal manifestations of AIDS. Surg Clin North Am 1994;74:1433-64.
100. Palefsky JM. Anal human papillomavirus infection and anal cancer in HIV-positive individuals: an emerging problem [editorial]. AIDS 1994;8:283-95.
101. Sillman FH, Sedlis A. Anogenital papillomavirus infection and neoplasia in immunodeficient women: an update. Dermatol Clin 1991;9:353-69.
102. McMillian A, Bishop PE. Clinical course of anogenital warts in men infected with human immunodeficiency virus. Genitourin Med 1989;65:225-8.
103. Palefsky JM, Gonzales J, Greenblatt RM, Ahn DK, Hollander H. Anal intraepithelial neoplasia and anal papilloma virus infection among homosexual males with group IV HIV disease. JAMA 1990;263:2911-6.
104. Adam YG, Efron G. Current concepts and controversies concerning the etiology, pathogenesis, diagnosis and treatment of malignant tumors of the anus. Surgery 1987;101:253-66.
105. Carter P. Anal cancer: the case for earlier diagnosis [letter; comment]. J R Soc Med 1991;84:695.
106. Jensen SL, Hagen K, Shokouh-Amiri MH, Nielsen OV. Does an erroneous diagnosis of squamous-cell carcinoma of the anal canal and anal margin at first physician visit influence prognosis? Dis Colon Rectum 1987;30:345-51.
107. Sonnex C, Scholefield JH, Kocjan G, et al. Anal human papillomavirus infection: a comparative study of cytology, colposcopy and DNA hybridisation as methods of detection. Genitourin Med 1991;67:21-5.

108. Kahn S, Rubesin SE, Levine MS, Laufer I, Herlinger H. Polypoid lesions at the anorectal junction: barium enema findings. AJR Am J Roentgenol 1993;161:339-42.
109. Roseau G, Palazzo L, Paolaggi JA. Endoscopic ultrasonography in colorectal diseases. Biomed Pharmacother 1992;46:133-8.
110. Cohan RH, Silverman PM, Thompson WM, Halvorsen RA, Baker ME. Computed tomography of epithelial neoplasms of the anal canal. AJR Am J Roentgenol 1985;145:569-73.
111. Tanum G, Hannisdal E, Stenwig B. Prognostic factors in anal carcinoma. Oncology 1994;51:22-4.
112. Petrelli NJ, Palmer M, Herrera L, Bhargava A. The utility of squamous cell carcinoma antigen for the follow-up of patients with squamous cell carcinoma of the anal canal. Cancer 1992;70:35-9.
113. Petrelli NJ, Shaw N, Bhargava A, et al. Squamous cell carcinoma antigen as a marker for squamous cell carcinoma of the anal canal. J Clin Oncol 1988;6:782-5.
114. Fontana X, Lagrange JL, Francois E, et al. Assessment of "squamous cell carcinoma antigen" (SCC) as a marker of epidermoid carcinoma of the anal canal. Dis Colon Rectum 1991;34:126-31.
115. Tanum G, Stenwig AE, Bormer OP, Tveit KM. Carcinoembryonic antigen in anal carcinoma. Acta Oncol 1992;31:333-5.
116. Flam MS, John MJ, Peters MS, et al. Radiation and 5-fluorouracil (5-fluorouracil versus radiation, 5-fluorouracil, mitomycin C [MMC]) in the treatment of anal canal carcinoma: preliminary results of a phase III randomized RTOG/ECOG intergroup trial. Proc Am Soc Clin Oncol 1993;12:192.
117. John H, Buchmann P. Improved perineal wound healing with the omental pedicle graft after rectal excision. Int J Colorectal Dis 1991;6:193-6.
118. McAllister E, Wells K, Chaet M, Norman J, Cruse W. Perineal reconstruction after surgical extirpation of pelvic malignancies using the transpelvic transverse rectus abdominal myocutaneous flap. Ann Surg Oncol 1994;1:164-8.
119. Zelnick RS, Haas PA, Ajlouni M, Szilagyi E, Fox TA Jr. Results of abdominoperineal resections for failures after combination chemotherapy and radiation therapy for anal canal cancers. Dis Colon Rectum 1992;35:574-8.
120. Ellenhorn JD, Enker WE, Quan SH. Salvage abdominoperineal resection following combined chemotherapy and radiotherapy for epidermoid carcinoma of the anus. Ann Surg Oncol 1994;1:105-10.
121. Longo WE, Vernava AM 3d, Wade TP, Coplin MA, Virgo KS, Johnson FE. Recurrent squamous cell carcinoma of the anal canal: predictors of initial treatment failure and results of salvage therapy. Ann Surg 1994;220:40-9.
122. Tanum G. Treatment of relapsing anal carcinoma. Acta Oncol 1993;32:33-5.
123. Morson BC, Sobin LH. Histological typing of intestinal tumors. Geneva: World Health Organization; 1976.
124. Weinstock MA. Epidemiology and prognosis of anorectal melanoma. Gastroenterology 1993;104:174-8.
125. Brady MS, Kavolius JP, Quan SH. Anorectal melanoma: a 64-year experience at Memorial Sloan-Kettering Cancer Center. Dis Colon Rectum 1995;38:146-51.
126. Konstadoulakis MM, Ricaniadis N, Walsh D, Karakousis CP. Malignant melanoma of the anorectal region. J Surg Oncol 1995;58:118-20.
127. Slingluff CL Jr, Seigler HF. Anorectal melanoma: clinical characteristics and the role of abdominoperineal resection. Ann Plast Surg 1992;28:85-8.
128. Frank W, Kurban RS, Hoover HC Jr, Sober AJ. Anorectal melanoma: a case report and brief review of the literature. J Dermatol Surg Oncol 1992;18:333-6.
129. Martenson JA Jr. Sphincter sparing therapy for anal cancer: current status and directions for future research. Hematol Oncol Anals 1994;2:241-7.
130. Virgo KS, Vernava AM, Longo WE, McKirgan LW, Johnson FE. Cost of patient follow-up after potentially curative colorectal cancer treatment. JAMA 1995;273:1837-41.
131. Schulman KA, Yabroff KR. Measuring the cost-effectiveness of cancer care. Oncology 1995;9:523-38.
132. Kimmel SE, Berlin JA, Laskey WK. The relationship between coronary angioplasty procedure volume and major complications. JAMA 1995;274:1137-42.

➢ COUNTER POINT

Memorial Sloan-Kettering Cancer Center

WARREN E. ENKER

I am in overall general agreement with the philosophy of treatment and follow-up of anal epidermoid carcinoma outlined by Sinanan et al. In general, however, my philosophy of long-term follow-up is more selective (based on stage) and less intensive than the follow-up schema adapted from Cummings et al.[1]

INITIAL EVALUATION

Careful evaluation of the patient before treatment is essential, both for the selection of appropriate treatment and for an understanding of the natural history of the disease. Sinanan et al. clearly point out the type of physical examination and imaging studies required for complete evaluation. Emphasis must be placed on evaluating the primary tumor. Staging is composed of objective elements such as size, depth, histological features, and nodal involvement. The primary tumor continues to elude exact measurement. Tumors at such an accessible site should be easily evaluable, but variability in presentation, location, and patient anxiety confound the exact measurement of a primary tumor. The experienced examiner will be able to estimate size within 0.5 cm. Under these circumstances categorizing the patient by appropriate T stage is usually accurate, even if the exact size of the lesion is off by several millimeters. The accurate determination of size is not merely an academic issue. In the Mayo Clinic experience reported by Boman et al.,[2] patients with superficial lesions less than 2 cm in diameter have been successfully treated with excision alone. Survival and local control exceeding 90% are reported.

Adjuncts to exact measurement such as ultrasound, computed tomography, and magnetic resonance imaging all have their own pitfalls. Although a 7.5 MHz ultrasound probe may give ideal resolution of the rectal wall, the focal length of such a probe may require positioning too far from the surface of the primary tumor. In contrast to most primary rectal cancers for which one can adapt to the focal distance of the probe within the rectum, the probe invariably sits right up against the primary tumor in the anal canal. For this reason, estimates of primary tumor size and depth by ultrasound methodology have been less than rewarding. Computed tomography and magnetic resonance imaging are both expensive modalities for evaluating the patient. Although computed tomography provides a more easily interpretable image, magnetic resonance imaging (with or without intrarectal coil) may have the ultimate advantage regarding resolution within layers of the rectal wall. The most critical factor in patient evaluation is a gentle, thorough digital rectal examination by an experienced physician who is capable of performing the examination without discomfort and with constant attention to relieving the patient's anxiety.

INITIAL FOLLOW-UP

Sinanan et al. indicate that the usual interval from initiation of multimodality treatment to biopsy for persistent disease is 12 to 20 weeks. Given the initial 4 to 5 weeks of chemotherapy and radiation and the subsequent round of chemotherapy that some investigators use, the 12- to 20-week period is most appropriate. This period corresponds to an estimated 5 to 13 weeks after the completion of treatment.

Sinanan et al. are wise to select a range of follow-up modalities for observation before biopsy of the primary site for residual disease. A positive biopsy will have many clinical implications. In a recently reported multiinstitutional Eastern Cooperative Oncology Group study, a positive biopsy resulted in abdominoperineal resection of the rectum.[3]

Seasoned observers of patients with anal epidermoid carcinoma are aware of the wide range of rates of primary tumor regression observed. The determinants of the rate of regression are unknown but are undoubtedly influenced by the size and depth of the primary tumor. Thus a primary tumor exceeding 5 cm in diameter might be expected to regress completely by 12 to 16 weeks after the completion of treatment versus 6 to 8 weeks for a lesion that initially measures 2 to 4.9 cm in diameter.

In clinical practice, knowledge that primary tumors may regress at different rates has prompted experienced clinicians to individualize their judgment regarding response to treatment in each patient. This approach differs from the protocol-determined approach, in which patient evaluation is completed at a fixed interval after the completion of initial treatment. In the Eastern Cooperative Oncology Group study cited previously, patients were evaluated 6 to 8 weeks after the completion of treatment,[3] which in my opinion is premature. Thirty-four of 46 patients (74%) had complete regression of the primary tumor. At the same time, 11 of 46 patients (24%) had a partial response to treatment. Because of the dictates of the protocol, these patients went on to abdominoperineal resection. One is led to wonder what would have happened if instead of proceeding to abdominoperineal resection of the rectum, these patients had been allowed another 4 to 6 weeks of observation. Virtually all kinetics of tumor cell death resulting from treatment are cell cycle dependent, requiring an attempt by the tumor cell to replicate. In clinical practice, time to complete regression of the primary tumor must be given wider latitude of observation to avoid the unnecessary morbidity of premature surgical intervention.

The frequency of initial follow-up should be based on the risk of locoregional recurrence. Monthly examinations in the immediate posttreatment period are rarely rewarding. In this respect there is disagreement with the schema proposed by Sinanan et al. (Table 9-3) in which patients undergo monthly examinations for the first 6 months after treatment and bimonthly examinations for the next 6 months. Follow-up can be separated into two categories: patients requiring examination every 2 to 3 months and patients requiring examination every 4 to 6 months initially after treatment (Table 9-4). Patients requiring examination every 2 to 3 months are those at high risk of persistent or locally recurrent disease. This group includes patients whose initial lesions are greater than 5 cm in diameter or have very deep penetration. Patients with lesions between 2 and 5 cm in diameter have a high response rate to treatment with little likelihood of either persistent or locally recurrent disease in the immediate post-treatment period. The likelihood of missing disease that might have been amenable to salvage abdominoperineal resection by examining patients at a 2- to 3-month interval, rather than a 1-month interval, is extremely low.

Table 9-4 Follow-up of patients with anal cancer*: Memorial Sloan-Kettering Cancer Center

	YEAR				
	1	2	3	4	5
Office visit†	2-3‡	2-3‡	2	2	2
Anoscopy	2-3‡	2-3‡	2	2	2
Proctosigmoidoscopy	2§	1	0	0	0
Open anal biopsy	¶	0	0	0	0

*Follow-up schedule begins on completion of the period of evaluation that follows radiation or chemoradiation treatment.
†Includes digital rectal examination.
‡For patients at high risk of persistent or locally recurrent disease, such as those whose initial lesions are greater than 5 cm in diameter or have very deep penetration, bimonthly to quarterly follow-up is indicated.
§Performed at the point of maximal or complete regression of tumor mass. Subsequent follow-up is based on the assumption of a negative biopsy result.
¶Performed as clinically indicated at the point of maximal or complete regression of tumor mass. Subsequent follow-up is based on the assumption of a negative biopsy result.

Patients with superficial lesions under 2 cm in diameter treated by excision alone might also be examined at more frequent intervals because of the absence of multidisciplinary treatment in their management. For patients with lesions 2 to 5 cm in largest single diameter or for all patients 1 year or more after treatment, examination may be conducted at 4- to 6-month intervals based on the clinical and stage-related determination of risks. Most recurrences take place within 2 years, and most deaths within 3 years, after initial diagnosis.

5-YEAR FOLLOW-UP

Based on the follow-up schedule presented by Sinanan et al. in Table 9-3, patients 1 year or more out from treatment are scheduled to undergo examination at 3-month intervals until 24 months and then annually. This program suggests little likelihood of clinical recurrence between the second and third year after treatment. It is my practice to examine patients at 6-month intervals from the end of the second year after treatment through the fifth year of follow-up (Table 9-4). Few patients with recurrence are likely to escape the detection of manageable disease given this time interval.

Despite the reported incidence of recurrence up to 15 years after treatment, the likelihood of such an event is anecdotal, precluding a favorable cost-benefit ratio from annual examination beyond 5 years. Selected patients may be followed for 7 or 8 years, especially if their initial assessment indicated high risk. The key is patient selection based on clinical and stage-related risk factors for recurrence.

The long-term role of TRUS or other imaging studies is debatable. Most locally recurrent lesions can be detected by the sensitive finger of the experienced surgeon. Continuity of care and gentle reassuring examination are much less expensive and of far greater clinical value than any imaging study. TRUS, in particular, is a highly subjective, imager-dependent study. After radiation therapy and possible biopsy, the planes of the rectal wall have fused and it is often impossible to distinguish layers of the rectal wall that might have been observed during preoperative assessment. Furthermore, the majority of lesions that might be observed with TRUS can also be found by digital anorectal examination.

Physical Examination

The accuracy of any anorectal examination is directly related to the patient's ability to relax during examination. Reassurance and the knowledge that the examination will result in absolutely no pain serve the interest of both the physician and the patient. Rarely can the patient's anorectal canal be examined through the thumb and forefinger. In women the thickness of the rectovaginal septum at the level of the anal canal can be evaluated. In the absence of an anterior lesion, thickening of the septum, or anterior abnormalities of any nature, this bidigital examination is unlikely to yield any clinically significant findings.

Flexible Versus Rigid Proctosigmoidoscopy

Flexible proctosigmoidoscopy with a retroflexed view of the upper end of the anal canal is described by Sinanan et al. as a useful procedure in the follow-up of patients with anal cancer. I disagree, emphasizing instead the importance of rigid proctosigmoidoscopy through a well-lit, gently handled scope. Rigid proctosigmoidoscopy provides a direct view of the rectum for the assessment of both the upper anal canal and the rectal mucosa, as in the case of radiation proctitis. It allows a direct view rather than a view through fiberoptic bundles. When gently handled, the rigid proctosigmoidoscope feels no different than the examining finger at this level. The direct view wide channel also permits evaluation of friability in the event of radiation proctitis, direct biopsy, and the like.

ADENOCARCINOMA OF THE ANAL CANAL

Adenocarcinoma of the anus is rare and highly aggressive. Whatever the etiology, these lesions are often locally advanced cancers that are difficult to diagnose clinically. Initially there may be few changes along the anal canal itself because of widespread infiltration of the surrounding tissues. In some cases nodularity can be recognized only at the level of the anorectal junction and biopsy may be difficult. Stricture is common with these locally advanced lesions, interfering with function, causing pain, impeding diagnosis, and particularly making biopsy difficult. On rare occasion, biopsy must be made by interstitial core-needle biopsy rather than superficial biopsy of the anorectal mucosa.

As a rule patients with anal adenocarcinoma have a poor outlook. Treatment should involve preoperative multidisciplinary combined radiation and chemotherapy in virtually all cases. Surgical treatment is almost invariably abdominoperineal resection of the rectum.

Assessing long-term results is difficult. Often these tumors are grouped with other rectal adenocarcinomas and the distinction between the anal and rectal lesions disappears. Nevertheless, anal lesions should be categorized separately. Although the outlook is probably not as dismal as the 30% figure quoted by Sinanan et al., a more accurate estimate of survival is difficult in the absence of clear-cut categories.

MALIGNANT MELANOMA OF THE ANUS

Sinanan et al. accurately summarize the clinical experience of patients with melanoma of the anal canal. The most recent and largest experience recorded has been that of Brady et al.[4] from Memorial Sloan-Kettering Cancer Center in which 85 patients with primary melanoma of the anal canal were treated. The overall 5-year survival rate was approximately 10%. Although the literature is equally divided between patients who survive after wide local excision and those who survive after abdominoperineal resection of the rectum, the Memorial Sloan-Kettering Cancer Center experience is unusual. Of the 10 survivors, nine were women who underwent abdominoperineal resection of the rectum. Although conclusions cannot be drawn from such a small number of patients, these data only fuel the debate between proponents of treatment by abdominoperineal resection and those favoring local excision, particularly in female patients.

REFERENCES

1. Cummings BJ, Keane TJ, O'Sullivan B, Wong CS, Catton CN. Epidermoid anal cancer: treatment by radiation alone or by radiation and 5-fluorouracil with and without mitomycin C. Int J Radiat Oncol Biol Phys 1991;21:1115-25.
2. Boman BM, Moertel CG, O'Connell MJ, et al. Carcinoma of the anal canal: a clinical and pathologic study of 188 cases. Cancer 1984 54: 114-25.
3. Martenson JA, Lipsitz SR, Lefkopoulou M. Results of combined modality therapy for patients with anal cancer (E7283): an Eastern Cooperative Oncology Group study. Cancer 1995;76:1731-6.
4. Brady MS, Kavolius JP, Quan SH. Anorectal melanoma: a 64-year experience at Memorial Sloan-Kettering Cancer Center. Dis Colon Rectum 1995;38:146-51.

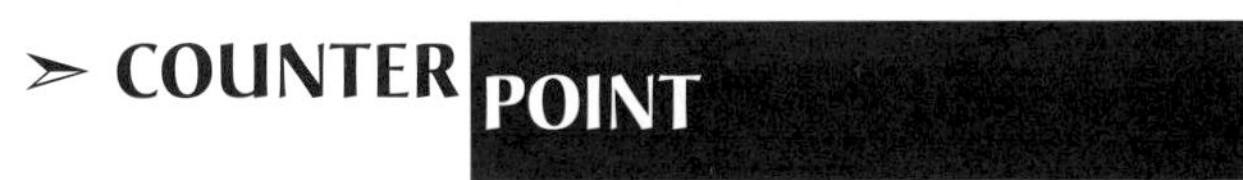

National Cancer Center Hospital, Japan

SHIN FUJITA AND YOSIHIRO MORIYA

Anal carcinomas are rare cancers in Japan. At the National Cancer Center Hospital in Tokyo, only 75 patients with anal

Table 9-5 Follow-up of patients with anal cancer (adenocarcinoma): National Cancer Center Hospital, Japan

	YEAR				
	1	2	3	4	5
Office visit	5*	4	2	2	2
CEA	5*	4	2	2	2
CA 19-9	5*	4	2	2	2
ST439	5*	4	2	2	2
Chest x-ray	2	2	1	1	1
Abdominal ultrasound	2	2	1	1	1
Pelvic computed tomography or magnetic resonance imaging†	1	0	0	0	0

CEA, Carcinoembryonic antigen.
*Includes one evaluation at baseline.
†For patients with advanced cancer only. Magnetic resonance imaging is selected rather than computed tomography if recurrence is suspected.

carcinomas have undergone treatment and follow-up, representing 3% of all patients with large bowel cancer treated nationwide. A major difference between anal carcinomas in Japan and those in the United States is histological type. In the United States epidermoid lesions make up 80% of anal malignancies. In Japan, adenocarcinomas comprise 70% of anal carcinomas and squamous cell carcinomas comprise only 20%.

Adenocarcinomas are usually treated by abdominoperineal resection because radiation therapy and chemotherapy are considered less effective. Squamous cell carcinomas are also treated by radical resection, but some authors have reported that radiation therapy alone or combined with chemotherapy is effective for squamous cell carcinomas of the anal canal.[1-3] Therefore these lesions are usually treated by radiation with or without chemotherapy in Japan. Differences in treatment strategy dictate the need for separate follow-up strategies for adenocarcinomas and squamous cell carcinomas of the anal canal.

CURRENT PRACTICE

Adenocarcinoma of the Anal Canal

The follow-up strategy for patients with adenocarcinoma is the same as that of patients with lower rectal cancer (Table 9-5). Briefly, the follow-up program after baseline measurements are obtained is as follows: at every follow-up visit after curative surgery, careful physical examination of the perineal wound and inguinal lymph nodes is performed and serum levels of CEA and other tumor markers including CA 19-9 and ST439 are measured every 3 months for 2 years. ST439 has been established as a tumor marker for adenocarcinomas of the digestive tract and breast malignancies at the National Cancer Center Research Institute.[4] The sensitivity of ST439 in colorectal cancer patients is 30%.[5] This is lower than the sensitivities of CEA and CA 19-9. However, ST439 can be detected in patients with cancer who have normal levels of CEA and CA 19-9. The CEA level is often increased in some benign diseases such as infection of the upper respiratory tract, hepatitis, and cirrhosis. On the other hand, the false-positive rate of ST439 is relatively low in nonmalignant disease. Therefore the use of ST439 in combination with CEA and CA 19-9 reduces the rate of false-positive results and saves the cost of expensive investigation of a false-positive patient.

Ultrasound of the liver and chest x-rays are evaluated every 6 months for 2 years. In cases of advanced cancer, computed tomography of the pelvis is performed 3 months after surgery for later comparison because the differential diagnosis between inflammatory tissue and recurrence is difficult in some cases. If recurrence is suspected, magnetic resonance imaging of the pelvis is often performed and a surgical biopsy or computed tomography–guided needle biopsy is carried out. When recurrence is confirmed, the areas of recurrent disease and distant metastasis are evaluated for salvage surgery.

Squamous Cell Carcinoma of the Anal Canal

Because of the low incidence of squamous cell carcinoma of the anal canal in Japan, the follow-up strategy for patients with squamous cell carcinoma has not been firmly established. Only five patients have been treated by radiation and chemotherapy at the National Cancer Center Hospital. Residual masses in four of the five patients were resected, and no cancer cells were detected in the specimens.

The remaining case was an example of the successful multimodality treatment described previously. This patient had lymph node metastases in the mesorectum diagnosed by computed tomography scan and TRUS. The tumor was 75 mm in diameter (T3), and there were no distant metastases (M0). This patient was first treated by radiation and chemotherapy according to the regimen proposed by Nigro et al.,[2] with some modification. The patient received 4000 cGy in a total of 20 fractions to the field primary site and pelvis. Mitomycin C (10 mg/m^2 as an intravenous bolus on day 7) and 5-FU (1000 mg/m^2 per 24 hours as a continuous infusion on days 7 through 10) were administered. After treatment the size of the tumor was reduced to 58 mm in diameter and lymph node metastases in the mesorectum were still detected by computed tomography. Thus abdominoperineal resection was performed 1 month after chemoradiation therapy.

During the operation, lymph node metastases around the right obturator artery were detected (N3). Therefore lateral lymph node resection with en bloc excision of internal iliac vessels was performed.[6] Adjuvant chemotherapy of mitomycin C and 5-FU was given 3 weeks after the operation. Pathological examination showed that the tumor was moderately differentiated squamous cell carcinoma and that eight lymph nodes in the mesorectum had metastases. Because this case was far advanced at diagnosis, the patient was followed closely after surgery. Every 3 months computed tomography of the pelvis, ultrasound of the liver, and chest x-ray were performed. This patient had no local recurrence or distant metas-

Table 9-6 Follow-up of patients with anal cancer (squamous cell carcinoma): National Cancer Center Hospital, Japan

	YEAR				
	1	2	3	4	5
Office visit*	5†	4	2	2	2
Anoscopy‡	5†	4	2	2	2
SCCAg	5†	4	2	2	2
Transrectal ultrasound	3†	2	1	1	1
Chest x-ray	2	2	1	1	1
Abdominal ultrasound	2	2	1	1	1
Pelvic computed tomography or magnetic resonance imaging§	1	0	0	0	0

SCCAg, Squamous cell carcinoma antigen.
*Includes digital rectal examination.
†Includes one evaluation at baseline.
‡Performed if recurrence is suspected.
§For patients with advanced cancer only. Magnetic resonance imaging is selected rather than computed tomography if recurrence is suspected.

tases at 3 years after surgery. In other cases, however, this kind of strict follow-up is unnecessary and the follow-up program should be determined by the patient's pathological stage.

Determining whether patients benefit from the follow-up program is of most importance. Because patients with local recurrence can be cured by salvage abdominoperineal resection and patients with distant metastases can be treated by surgery, the purpose of follow-up is early diagnosis of local recurrence and distant metastases. The most effective follow-up program is difficult to determine. The schedule for follow-up of patients with squamous cell carcinoma at the National Cancer Center Hospital is shown in Table 9-6. At each follow-up visit the primary tumor site and inguinal lymph nodes should be evaluated. If recurrence is suspected, anoscopy with biopsy should be performed. Of the routine follow-up tests, digital rectal examination is the most convenient and least expensive method of detecting recurrence. Tanum et al.[7] insist that frequent digital rectal examination is the most important procedure because all local recurrences are diagnosed with such examination and biopsy.

TRUS allows for exact staging and follow-up in irradiated carcinomas.[8] TRUS complements digital rectal examination in the preoperative staging of anal carcinomas. Akasu et al.[9,10] demonstrated that TRUS was more effective in the preoperative assessment of rectal cancer tumor size and lymph node involvement than digital rectal examination, computed tomography, and magnetic resonance imaging. The accuracy rate of TRUS is 69% for tumor size estimation. The accuracy and sensitivity rates of TRUS for assessing lymph node status are 65% and 43%, respectively. This result can also be applied to anal canal cancer. Therefore we recommend that TRUS be performed every 6 months for 2 years.

Computed tomography and magnetic resonance imaging are useful in detecting local recurrence, lateral lymph node metastases, and distant metastases. In tumor size evaluation, accuracy rates of computed tomography and magnetic resonance imaging are lower than that of TRUS. Therefore in the routine follow-up program these modalities are not always necessary. Combined use of the modalities according to tumor stage is considered important because lateral lymph node metastases are not reliably detected by TRUS.

A promising new modality is endorectal surface coil (E-coil) magnetic resonance imaging,[11] which uses a signal receiver inserted into the anus to discern the structure of the pelvic tissues. With this method, tumor extension and perirectal lymph node swelling are more clearly shown than with conventional magnetic resonance imaging. Depth of invasion of rectal cancer was correctly diagnosed by this method in 11 of 12 cases, and lymph node enlargement was also diagnosed in four of seven patients.[11] This evolving technique is promising in the follow-up of patients with anal canal cancer but must still be considered experimental.

FUTURE PROSPECTS

Cost and patient benefits are important considerations in the follow-up program. Both Sinanan et al. and this counterpoint advocate relatively extensive follow-up programs for patients with anal canal cancer. Do these follow-up systems benefit patients or reduce costs? Tanum et al.[7] reported disappointing results of a follow-up program for anal canal cancer. They showed that only three of six locally recurrent cancers were diagnosed while still asymptomatic and that the other three patients had no benefit from the follow-up program, since their local recurrence was diagnosed because of symptoms. The researchers also insisted they did not use computed tomography or magnetic resonance imaging because previous experience showed that no additional information was gained by these procedures. Frequent digital rectal examination is the most important procedure in the follow-up program. Vernava et al.[12] surveyed the follow-up program of all active members of the American Society of Colon and Rectal Surgeons and reported that no standard program of follow-up has been established, even in the follow-up of colorectal cancer patients. Their analysis also showed that the intensity of follow-up of patients did not vary with pathological stage.

These experiences suggest that prospective, randomized, controlled trials for the evaluation of follow-up strategies will be required in the future. In addition, stage-oriented follow-up strategies should be identified because recurrence rates differ among pathological stages. Predicting recurrence by the biological characteristics of the primary tumor using genetic markers will also become increasingly important. If a patient has a tumor that is predicted not to recur, follow-up of that patient will not be necessary. It is hoped that investigations of the mechanisms of invasion and metastases will help to find new markers for early detection and treatment of recurrence and will improve the prognosis of patients with anal canal cancer.

REFERENCES

1. Papillon J. Radiation therapy in the management of epidermoid carcinoma of the anal region. Dis Colon Rectum 1974;17:181-7.
2. Nigro ND, Seydel HG, Considine B, Vaitkevicius VK, Leichman L, Kinzie JJ. Combined preoperative radiation and chemotherapy for squamous cell carcinoma of the anal canal. Cancer 1983;51:1826-9.
3. Doci R, Zucali R, Bombelli L, Montalto F, Lamonica G. Combined chemoradiation therapy for anal cancer: a report of 56 cases. Ann Surg 1992;215:150-6.
4. Sugano K, Ohkura H, Maruyama T, et al. Sandwich radioimmunometric assay with murine monoclonal antibody, NCC-ST-439, for serological diagnosis of human cancers. Jpn J Cancer Res 1988; 79:618-25.
5. Iemura K, Moriya Y. A comparative analysis of the serum levels of NCC-ST-439, CEA and CA 19-9 in patients with colorectal carcinoma. Eur J Surg Oncol 1993;19:439-42.
6. Moriya Y, Hojo K, Sawada T, Koyama Y. Significance of lateral node resection for advanced rectal carcinoma at or below the peritoneal reflection. Dis Colon Rectum 1989;32:307-15.
7. Tanum G, Tveit K, Karlsen KO. Diagnosis of anal carcinoma—doctor's finger still the best? Oncology 1991;48:383-6.
8. Herzog U, Boss M, Spichtin HP. Endoanal ultrasonography in the follow-up of anal carcinoma. Surg Endosc 1994;8:1186-9.
9. Akasu T, Sunouchi K, Sawada T, Tsioulias GJ, Muto T, Morioka Y. Preoperative staging of rectal carcinoma: prospective comparison of transrectal ultrasonography and computed tomography. Gastroenterology 1990;98(5 Part 2):A268.
10. Akasu T, Sugihara K, Moriya Y. Endoscopic ultrasonography of the rectal carcinoma invading the muscularis propria [Japanese]. Stomach Intest 1992;27:1293-1302.
11. Chan TW, Kressel HY, Milestone B, et al. Rectal carcinoma: staging at imaging with endorectal surface coil; work in progress. Radiology 1991;181:461-7.
12. Vernava AM 3d, Longo WE, Virgo KS, Coplin MA, Wade TP, Johnson FE. Current follow-up strategies after resection of colorectal cancer: results of a survey of members of the American Society of Colon and Rectal Surgeons. Dis Colon Rectum 1994;37:573-83.

➢ COUNTERPOINT

Clatterbridge Centre for Oncology, UK

Arthur Sun Myint

Anal carcinoma is not a common malignancy in the United Kingdom. Approximately 300 new cases are diagnosed each year. Following the results of the UKCCCR Phase III Anal Cancer Trial, chemoradiation is now the accepted standard treatment. However, 40% of patients have distant failures and a substantial number of these patients also have locoregional failure. The majority of failures occur within the first 2 years. Therefore proper follow-up is important so that appropriate salvage treatment can be offered in cases of recurrence and so that complications that may require further treatment can be detected.

CURRENT PRACTICE

Initial definitive treatment with chemoradiation allows sphincter-conserving therapy and gives the opportunity for careful locoregional examination during follow-up.[1] Therefore clinical examination alone is important, since both the primary tumor and regional nodes are accessible for inspection and careful palpation. This should be supplemented by endoscopy, radiology, and examination under anesthesia whenever necessary. However, no consensus exists regarding the frequency of follow-up or the types of investigation that should be used. Follow-up also depends on the philosophy and type of treatment that have been offered.

TREATMENT STRATEGY

Anal Margin Tumors

At Clatterbridge Centre for Oncology, patients with well-differentiated, noninfiltrating T1 or small T2 (less than 3 cm in diameter) tumors are treated by local excision.[2] Postoperative radiation therapy is indicated if the resection margins are involved or close (less than 5 mm) to the tumor. A radiation dose of 45 Gy is given in 20 fractions over 28 days. Radical radiation therapy can be given to patients who are not fit for surgery or who refuse it.[3,4] A radiation dose of 54 Gy is given in 20 fractions over 28 days. Patients are treated prone, lying over the rectal board with two wedged radiation portals. One perineal field and a sacral field are used to cover the tumor volume with a 2 cm margin. Prophylactic groin node irradiation is not carried out, provided the patient agrees to close follow-up.

Patients with well- to moderately differentiated larger T2 (greater than 3 cm) and T3 tumors are treated with a radiation dose of 45 cGy in 20 fractions over 4 weeks and are reassessed after 6 weeks. If there is a small residual tumor, a booster dose is given by interstitial implant.[5,6] Patients with poorly differentiated tumors and T4 tumors are treated by chemoradiation as per the schedule for anal canal tumors described in the following discussion. Prophylactic groin node irradiation is also given, since a high risk of nodal involvement exists even if the lymph nodes are not clinically palpable.

Anal Canal Tumors

At Clatterbridge Centre for Oncology, physicians follow the treatment philosophy of Papillon et al.,[5-7] which was adopted in the UKCCCR anal cancer trial. The treatment plan consists of initial chemoradiation with a tumor dose of 45 Gy in 20 fractions over 28 days using the three-field technique with the patient in a prone position. 5-FU (1 g/m^2; days 1 through 4) with mitomycin C (10 mg/m^2; day 1) is given concurrently with radiation during the first week. This is followed by a second cycle using 5-FU (1 g/m^2) alone from day 21 to 24.[8-11] The patient is assessed 6 weeks later, and if there is no response or less than 50% regression of the tumor, surgery is carried out, which usually consists of abdominoperineal resection. If the response is good (greater than 50% regression), a local boost is given with either electrons or, for small residual tumors, interstitial implants using iridium wire with a template.[5,6]

Lymph Nodes

Nodal drainage areas in the groins are not treated prophylactically for well- to moderately differentiated T1 and small T2 (less than 3 cm) tumors. For poorly differentiated and larger tumors, a parallel opposing pair of portals is used. An anterior field to cover the primary and regional lymphatics including both the inguinal regions is used, opposed by a smaller posterior field to cover the primary and adjacent pararectal and pelvic lymph nodes. In patients with palpable lymphadenopathy, if fine-needle aspiration is positive or evokes clinical suspicion, a further local boost to the groin is given using electrons of suitable energy to bring the total tumor dose to 65 cGy. At St. Mark's Hospital, Wolfe[11] found that 49 of 170 patients had inguinal involvement at presentation but only 19 (38.7%) were deemed suitable for block dissection. Five (10.2%) of these were alive and well 5 years later, and only four were alive at 10 years.

For patients in whom prophylactic irradiation is not given initially, close regular follow-up is essential. When metastatic lymphadenopathy is detected, limited or extended lymphadenectomy is carried out depending on the patient's age and general condition. This is followed by postoperative external beam radiation therapy to both groins and local electron boost to each affected side, bringing the total tumor dose to 60 to 65 Gy in 6 weeks.

The prognosis for patients with metachronous nodal metastasis is better than for those with synchronous nodal metastasis at presentation. Wolfe[11] reported that 17 patients in whom late groin nodal metastases developed underwent groin nodal dissection; nine (52%) were alive and well at 5 years. Stearns et al.[12] also found that 15 (75%) of 20 such patients survived 5 years after groin nodal dissection. Golden and Horsley[13] reviewed the literature and found a 20% survival rate at 5 years after groin dissection for synchronous inguinal metastases, versus 59% for metachronous inguinal metastases. In the majority of cases inguinal relapse can be controlled. Treatment failure is usually associated with local or pelvic failure rather than groin metastases.

Distant Metastases

Hematogenous spread is not as common in anal canal cancer as in cancer of the rectum. However, results of the closed phase III UKCCCR anal cancer trial indicated that 40% of the patients died from distant metastatic disease. In their series of 200 cases collected from 31 hospitals in Connecticut, Kluehn et al.[14] reported 13 hepatic and six pulmonary metastases, usually bilateral. Distant metastases are almost exclusively observed in advanced tumors that have invaded the anorectal junction. The proposed new UKCCCR trial will address metastatic disease and evaluate the role of continuing further chemotherapy after initial chemoradiation.

FOLLOW-UP PROTOCOL

Based on the experience at Clatterbridge Oncology Centre, I agree with Sinanan et al. that most recurrences after radical multimodality treatment of primary anal cancer occur within 2 years. Therefore it is important to follow these patients closely during this period, since early detection of recurrent disease will permit aggressive salvage surgical treatment.

Table 9-7 Follow-up of patients with anal cancer: Clatterbridge Centre for Oncology, UK

	YEAR				
	1	2	3	4	5
Office visit*	6	4	2	2	2
Anoscopy	6	4	2	2	2
Proctosigmoidoscopy	4	2	2	2	2

*Includes digital rectal examination.

The follow-up protocol at Clatterbridge Centre for Oncology consists of visits once every 2 months during the first year, every 3 months in the second year, and every 6 months in years 3 through 5 (Table 9-7). Recurrence after 5 years is rare, at which time patients are transferred back to general practitioner care for annual follow-up visits. If patients develop symptoms such as pain, rectal bleeding, or discharge, they are then referred back to the clinic immediately for further assessment.

At each follow-up visit a careful history of new or changing symptoms and thorough physical examination are carried out. Conservative treatment permits careful local examination of the perianal area, anal canal, and lower rectum. Examination of the inguinal region is important, especially if prophylactic irradiation is not carried out at the initial treatment. I find serial digital rectal examination by one observer the most useful assessment, supplemented by anoscopy. Sigmoidoscopy is carried out at 3-month intervals in the first year and 6-month intervals thereafter. Any suspect lesion should be observed and documented carefully. The patient should be reexamined at 4 weeks, and if there is any change, examination under anesthesia should be carried out.

I do not agree with a liberal biopsy policy, which could lead to radionecrosis, especially if the patient had an interstitial implant. Because both the primary tumor and regional lymph nodes can be assessed adequately by clinical examination alone, routine radiological examinations such as intraanal ultrasound,[14] intraanal magnetic resonance imaging, and computed tomography[15] are not carried out. If recurrence is suspected and is proven histologically, further full-stage investigation including computed tomography of the abdomen and pelvis and a chest x-ray are performed before salvage surgery.

Levels of tumor markers such as SCCAg are not checked routinely at Clatterbridge Centre for Oncology. However, SCCAg could be a useful marker[16] and its role in detecting recurrent disease should be evaluated further. I agree with Sinanan et al. regarding the limited role of the tumor marker CEA, and this study also is not carried out routinely.

FUTURE PROSPECTS

Although radiation therapy alone can cure a portion of patients with anal carcinoma, the results from the closed phase III UKCCCR trial indicate that chemotherapy combined with radiation therapy should be standard treatment for patients with this disease. The drug combination used is based on Nigro's original protocol,[9] and its efficiency has been proved by Cummings' series,[10] although this might not be the optimal regimen. Cisplatin-based regimens have shown promising results in other squamous cell carcinomas and have been used synchronously with radiation therapy in small numbers of patients with anal carcinoma. A current UKCCCR phase II trial was established to assess the response to and toxicity of 5-FU and cisplatin in patients with advanced anal carcinoma. Eligible patients are those who relapse after primary treatment or have advanced disease when initially examined and are considered ineligible for primary chemoradiation or radical surgery.

Data from the Radiation Therapy Oncology Group trial showed an improved local control rate for patients receiving mitomycin C in addition to 5-FU and concurrent radiation therapy; therefore mitomycin C warrants consideration in any new treatment regimen. Ideally a three-arm study comparing 5-FU with mitomycin C, 5-FU with cisplatin, and 5-FU with mitomycin C and cisplatin should be carried out. However, since few data are available on three-drug combinations in any squamous cell carcinoma, this arm would need to be piloted in a phase II trial. If found to be acceptable to patients and feasible in the clinic, the study will be introduced into the next UKCCCR trial. Thus it will be possible to determine not only whether cisplatin is a better radiosensitizer than mitomycin C, but also whether the two drugs act synergistically or additively. More important, the study will determine which of the drugs produces fewer side effects.

The next question to address is whether further adjuvant chemotherapy after primary chemoradiation would improve survival and reduce the risk of disseminated disease and death. The dose and fractionation of radiation therapy are also important issues. In the closed UKCCCR trial, initial chemoradiation is followed by boost radiation therapy 6 weeks later. The gap is used to allow the skin reaction to settle and to assess the tumor response before recommending boost treatment or surgery. No data are available to suggest that a shorter gap would be feasible, although some gap or rest period would probably be necessary to allow the acute reactions to settle. Judging from the good initial tumor response rate (92%) in the first trial, boost radiation therapy will be recommended for the majority of patients. Higher doses (for example, 50 Gy in 25 fractions over 5 weeks) with no gap at all may be possible in early tumors (T1) or node-negative cases. Ideally the question of gap should be addressed by a randomized trial.

In any future trials, quality of life should be assessed carefully during the follow-up period so that not only the life years saved but also the quality-of-life years saved can be considered. The question of cost-effective treatment and follow-up should also be addressed so that unnecessary abdominoperineal resection with permanent colostomy and expensive radiological investigations with limited value are not carried out.

REFERENCES

1. Sischy B, Doggett RL, Krall JM, et al. Definitive irradiation and chemotherapy for radiosensitization in management of anal carcinoma: interim report on Radiation Therapy Oncology Group study no. 8314. J Natl Cancer Inst 1989;81:850-6
2. Grenall MJ, Quan SH, Stearns MW, Urmacher C, DeCosse JJ. Epidermoid cancer of the anal margin: pathologic features, treatment, and clinical results. Am J Surg 1985;149:95-101.
3. Martenson JA Jr, Gunderson LL. External radiation therapy without chemotherapy in the management of anal cancer. Cancer 1993; 71:1736-40.
4. Cantril ST, Green JP, Schall GL, Schaupp WC. Primary radiation therapy in the treatment of anal carcinoma. Int J Radiat Oncol Biol Phys 1983;9:1271-8.
5. Papillon J, Montbarbon JF, Gerard JP, Chassard JL, Ardiet JM. Interstitial curietherapy in the conservative treatment of anal and rectal cancers. Int J Radiat Oncol Biol Phys 1989;17:1161-9.
6. Papillon J, Montbaron JF. Epidermoid carcinoma of the anal canal: a series of 276 cases. Dis Colon Rectum 1987;30:324-33.
7. Papillon J. Effectiveness of combined radio-chemotherapy in the management of epidermoid carcinoma of the anal canal. Int J Radiat Oncol Biol Phys 1990;19:1217-8.
8. Moertel CG, Childs DS Jr, Reitmeier RJ, Colby MY Jr, Holbrook MA. Combined 5-fluorouracil and supervoltage radiation therapy for locally unresectable gastrointestinal cancers. Lancet 1969;2:866-7.
9. Nigro ND. The force of change in the management of squamous-cell cancer of the anal canal. Dis Colon Rectum 1991;34:482-6.
10. Cummings BJ. Concomitant radiotherapy and chemotherapy for anal cancer. Semin Oncol 1992;19(4 Suppl 11):102-8.
11. Wolfe HR. The management of metastatic inguinal adenitis in epidermoid cancer of anus. Proc R Soc Med 1961;61:626-8.
12. Stearns MW, Deddish MR, Quan SH. Preoperative roentgen therapy for cancer of the rectum. Surg Gynecol Obstet 1949;109:225-9.
13. Golden CT, Horsley JS 3d. Surgical management of epidermoid carcinoma of the anus. Am J Surg 1976;131:275-80.
14. Kluehn PG, Eisenberg H, Reed JF. Epidermoid carcinoma of the perianal skin and anal canal. Cancer 1968;22:932-8.
15. Roseau G, Palazzo L, Paolaggi JA. Endoscopic ultrasonography in colorectal diseases. Biomed Pharmacother 1992;46:133-8.
16. Cohan RH, Silverman PM, Thompson WM, Halvorsen RA, Baker ME. Computed tomography of epithelial neoplasms of the anal canal. AJR Am J Roentgenol 1985;145:569-73.
17. Petrelli NJ, Shaw N, Bhargava A, et al. Squamous cell carcinoma antigen as a marker for squamous cell carcinoma of the anal canal. J Clin Oncol 1988;6:782-5.

➢ COUNTER POINT

Roswell Park Cancer Institute

MIGUEL A. RODRIGUEZ-BIGAS

Sinanan et al. provide an excellent review of the current management and follow-up of patients with anal carcinoma. They clearly establish the distinction between anal margin carcinomas and anal canal carcinomas and discuss at length the treatment options available for these patients. Physicians treating these patients must clearly define whether the patient has an anal margin or an anal canal squamous cell carcinoma, since the treatment and natural history of these tumors differ.

As mentioned by Sinanan et al., the diagnosis of primary or recurrent anal cancer can be elusive. Therefore serial

Table 9-8 Follow-up of patients with anal cancer*: Roswell Park Cancer Institute

	YEAR				
	1	2	3	4	5
Office visit	7	4	4	2	2
SCCAg	6	4	1	1	1
Transrectal ultrasound	2	1	0	0	0
Chest x-ray	1	1	1	1	1
Pelvic computed tomography	1†	0	0	0	0

SCCAg, Squamous cell carcinoma antigen.
*Follow-up schedule begins on completion of chemoradiation and after findings of full-thickness biopsy are negative.
†Indicated for patients with stage III or IV anal cancer.

examination of the anus, lower rectum, groins, and pelvic organs after treatment, ideally by the same physician, is of utmost importance. Factors that should be considered in planning the follow-up of these patients include stage of the primary tumor, completeness of therapy, and response to therapy. This does not mean that patients with early cancers should be followed differently. Close follow-up of any patient treated for anal canal carcinoma has been the policy at Roswell Park Cancer Institute (Table 9-8).

Patients with squamous cell carcinoma of the anal canal are not at a higher risk of colorectal neoplastic lesions (adenomas or adenocarcinomas) than the general population.[1] Therefore, if asymptomatic patients have no risk factors for colorectal cancer except age, physicians at Roswell Park Cancer Institute follow up with flexible sigmoidoscopy every 3 to 5 years and an annual fecal occult blood test. Computed tomography is performed only to document response to multimodality therapy for patients with involved nodes. A baseline computed tomographic scan is obtained for patients at high risk of recurrence because of their stage. Whether this is cost effective remains to be proved. Several reports have suggested that TRUS can be used to detect recurrence after nonsurgical treatment.[2] Again, the cost effectiveness and benefits in survival have not been established.

At Roswell Park Cancer Institute, SCCAg has been used before and after treatment since 1985.[3] In spite of technological advances, most recurrences are still detected by a careful history and physical examination. In a study at Roswell Park Cancer Institute the most common site of local recurrence after surgical excision of anal canal squamous cell carcinoma was the pelvis or perineum in males, whereas in females it was the posterior vaginal wall.[4] Although the number of patients was small, in female patients who did not undergo posterior vaginectomy at the time of abdominoperineal resection the local recurrence rate was 20% (two of 10 patients); in those who had a posterior vaginectomy the recurrence rate was 9% (two of 22 patients).[4] The present role of surgical excision in squamous cell carcinoma of the anal canal is limited to salvage therapy when multimodality therapy fails or recurrent disease unresponsive to systemic therapy develops.

There is no specific formula for the follow-up of patients with anal cancer. Follow-up must be tailored to take into consideration the aforementioned factors, as well as the fact that the majority of recurrences occur within 2 years of successful treatment.

REFERENCES

1. Klompje J, Petrelli NJ, Herrera L, Mittelman A. Synchronous and metachronous colon lesions in squamous cell carcinoma of the anal canal. J Surg Oncol 1987;35:86-8.
2. Roseau G, Palazzo L, Colardelle P, Chaussade S, Couturier D, Paolaggi JA. Endoscopic ultrasonography in the staging and follow-up of epidermoid carcinoma of the anal canal. Gastrointest Endosc 1994;40:447-50.
3. Petrelli NJ, Palmer M, Herrera L, Bhargava A. The utility of squamous cell carcinoma antigen for the follow-up of patients with squamous cell carcinoma of the anal canal. Cancer 1992;70:35-9.
4. Clark J, Petrelli N, Herrera L, Mittelman A. Epidermoid carcinoma of the anal canal. Cancer 1986;57:400-6.

Table 9-9 Follow-up of patients with anal cancer by institution

YEAR/PROGRAM	OFFICE VISIT	SCCAG	TRUS	CXR	PELVIC CT	ANOSC
Year 1						
Memorial Sloan-Kettering[a]	2-3[b,c]					2-3[b,c]
Roswell Park[f]	7	6	2	1	1[g]	
Univ Washington[h]	8[b]	5	3[i]		1[j,k]	6[i]
Japan: National Cancer Ctr I[l]	5[m]			2	1[j,n]	
Japan: National Cancer Ctr II[o]	5[b,m]	5[m]	3[m]	2	1[j,n]	5[p]
UK: Clatterbridge	6[b]					6
Year 2						
Memorial Sloan-Kettering[a]	2-3[b,c]					2-3[b,c]
Roswell Park[f]	4	4	1	1		
Univ Washington[h]	4[b]	2	1			4
Japan: National Cancer Ctr I[l]	4			2		
Japan: National Cancer Ctr II[o]	4[b]	4	2	2		4[p]
UK: Clatterbridge	4[b]					4
Year 3						
Memorial Sloan-Kettering[a]	2[b]					2
Roswell Park[f]	4	1		1		
Univ Washington[h]	1[b]	1				1
Japan: National Cancer Ctr I[l]	2			1		
Japan: National Cancer Ctr II[o]	2[b]	2	1	1		2[p]
UK: Clatterbridge	2[b]					2
Year 4						
Memorial Sloan-Kettering[a]	2[b]					2
Roswell Park[f]	2	1		1		
Univ Washington[h]	1[b]	1			[j]	1
Japan: National Cancer Ctr I[l]	2			1		
Japan: National Cancer Ctr II[o]	2[b]	2	1	1		2[p]
UK: Clatterbridge	2[b]					2

ABD CT abdominal computed tomography
ABD US abdominal ultrasound
ANOSC anoscopy
CEA carcinoembryonic antigen
CXR chest x-ray
PROCTO proctosigmoidoscopy
SCAAG squamous cell carcinoma antigen
SIG sigmoidoscopy
TRUS transrectal ultrasound

PROCTO	OPEN ANAL BIOPSY	CEA	CA 19-9	ST439	ABD US	SIG	ABD CT
2[d]	[e]						
	1[i]					2[i]	1[j,k]
		5[m]	5[m]	5[m]	2		
					2		
4							
1							
						1	
		4	4	4	2		
					2		
2							
		2	2	2	1		
					1		
2							
		2	2	2	1		
					1		
2							

a Follow-up schedule begins on completion of the period of evaluation that follows radiation or chemoradiation treatment.
b Includes digital rectal examination.
c For patients at high risk of persistent or locally recurrent disease, such as those whose initial lesions are greater than 5 cm in diameter or have very deep penetration, bimonthly to quarterly follow-up is indicated.
d Performed at the point of maximal or complete regression of tumor mass. Subsequent follow-up is based on the assumption of a negative biopsy result.
e Performed as clinically indicated at the point of maximal or complete regression of tumor mass. Subsequent follow-up is based on the assumption of a negative biopsy result.
f Follow-up schedule begins on completion of chemoradiation and a full-thickness biopsy are negative.
g Indicated for patients with stage III or IV anal cancer.
h Follow-up schedule begins on completion of radiation or chemoradiation treatment.
i At point of maximal or complete regression of tumor mass. Subsequent follow-up is based on the assumption of a negative biopsy result.
j Magnetic resonance imaging can be substituted.
k Performed in high-grade and stages III and IV tumors to document the condition of the internal iliac lymph nodes and presacral space and to provide a bssis for later comparison studies.
l Patients with adenocarcinomas.
m Includes one evaluation at baseline.
n For patients with advanced cancer only. Magnetic resonance imaging is selected rather than computed tomography if recurrence is suspected.
o Patients with squamous cell carcinoma.
p Performed if recurrence is suspected.

Continued.

Table 9-9 Follow-up of patients with anal cancer by institution–cont'd

YEAR/PROGRAM	OFFICE VISIT	SCCAG	TRUS	CXR	PELVIC CT	ANOSC
Year 5						
Memorial Sloan-Kettering[a]	2[b]					2
Roswell Park[f]	2	1		1		
Univ Washington[h]	1[b]	1				1
Japan: National Cancer Ctr I[l]	2			1		
Japan: National Cancer Ctr II[o]	2[b]	2	1	1		2[p]
UK: Clatterbridge	2[b]					2

PROCTO	OPEN ANAL BIOPSY	CEA	CA 19-9	ST439	ABD US	SIG	ABD CT
		2	2	2	1		
					1		
2							

CHAPTER 10

Pancreatic Carcinoma

Roswell Park Cancer Institute

JUDY L. SMITH AND NEAL J. MEROPOL

Pancreatic cancer was first described by Morgagni in the 1700s (1682-1771).[1] By 1810 it was already apparent to Baron Alexis Boyer, a professor of practical surgery in Paris, that pancreatic tumors had a uniformly poor prognosis.[2] This remains true despite numerous advances in the surgical and medical care of cancer patients over the past century. In the United States in 1994 pancreatic cancer was newly diagnosed in approximately 27,000 patients and 26,000 patients died of the disease. The population-based death rate has steadily risen over the past 60 years, despite a small but significant gain in overall survival. The 5-year survival rate in 1960 was 1%; currently only 3% to 5% of patients with pancreatic cancer live 5 years.[3] For patients with resectable disease 5-year survival rates of up to 30% have been reported. Ductal adenocarcinoma accounts for approximately 95% of pancreatic cancers, with the remaining 5% mainly nonductal exocrine and endocrine malignancies. This chapter focuses on the follow-up of patients with pancreatic ductal adenocarcinoma after surgical intervention.

POTENTIAL BENEFITS OF SURVEILLANCE

When initially examined by a physician, patients have three patterns of disease: metastatic, locally advanced, or resectable. Between 80% and 90% of patients are found to have unresectable disease at the time of diagnosis, yet the surgeon often has an important role in their care.[4] The usual goals of follow-up and surveillance after treatment of malignancies are to improve survival and quality of life through early detection of recurrence or second primary cancers. In pancreatic adenocarcinoma these goals are often unrealistic. Surgical resection is the backbone of curative treatment, but few patients are cured by resection.[5] Follow-up designed to identify early relapse or recurrence is effective only when treatment that may improve survival or quality of life is available. There is no effective salvage therapy for patients with recurrence of pancreatic cancer. A surveillance program in pancreatic cancer designed to improve survival through early detection of relapse will therefore be ineffective. Because of the overall poor prognosis, detection of second primary cancers is significant only in the extremely small cohort of patients who achieve long-term survival. Surveillance after resection for patients with pancreatic cancer is economically and medically rational only if the primary goal is to improve quality of life.

Centers that are actively pursuing research on the treatment of metastatic or recurrent pancreatic cancer may plan a follow-up regimen with early identification of recurrence as one of its goals. Such programs have little chance of improving patient survival at this time and thus should be economically and emotionally tailored to the patients and their requests. If effective treatment for recurrent disease is identified in the future, recommendations for follow-up must be altered to allow earlier detection.

METHODS OF SURVEILLANCE

History and Physical Examination

History and physical examination are insensitive methods of follow-up but are also inexpensive and noninvasive. A careful interim history and physical examination in patients with pancreatic cancer often guide the physician to potential sites of recurrence. Symptoms and signs such as jaundice, ascites, or pain are ominous and should trigger further investigation. Detection of recurrence before deterioration in performance status probably improves the chance that palliative therapy will enhance quality of life. Physician-patient contact during the appointment also allows the physician to provide emotional support, which is extremely important to the patient's overall well-being.

Radiological Evaluation

Radiological examinations can be helpful in the management and surveillance of patients with pancreatic cancer. Chest roentgenograms can delineate metastasis, but because of the predominance of abdominal recurrences and metastases, computed tomographic scans of the abdomen and pelvis should also be obtained when recurrence is suspected. Computed tomography is useful to evaluate the liver, pancreatic bed, retroperitoneum, and pelvis and to identify peritoneal disease (such as ascites). Although biopsy of lesions identified by these techniques is rarely necessary because of the relentless progression of pancreatic cancer and the accuracy of scanning, some areas are misleading. After resection and adjuvant chemoradiation, thickening of the gastric and duodenal remnant may mimic recurrent cancer. Unopacified loops of bowel in the porta hepatis may also have the appearance of regional recurrence or lymphadenopathy.[6]

Tumor Markers

Numerous tumor markers have been investigated for use in screening and follow-up of pancreatic cancer. These include CA 19-9, carcinoembryonic antigen (CEA), DUPAN-2, and SPAN-1, as well as the enzymes galactosyltransferase II, ribonuclease, and elastase.[7-9] None of these markers is useful for diagnosis or screening for pancreatic cancer because none is sufficiently sensitive or specific. The most extensively studied marker is CA 19-9. It is widely available but is not specific for pancreatic cancer, since levels may be elevated in other gastrointestinal and biliary malignancies. In addition, although up to 96% of patients with pancreatic cancer have an elevated CA 19-9 level at some point during the course of their disease, levels may be normal in the early stages.[8,10] Tumor markers such as CA 19-9 may be more useful for monitoring patients after treatment. Markers that return to normal after resection and subsequently rise often indicate recurrent disease. Care must be taken in interpretation, however, and a careful search for recurrence must be performed before any therapeutic intervention because of the possibility of false-positive results, a separate malignancy, or benign disease.

SURVEILLANCE AND FOLLOW-UP AFTER NONCURATIVE TREATMENT

Noncurative Resections

Between 80% and 90% of patients with pancreatic cancer are found to have metastases or locally unresectable disease at initial diagnosis.[4,11,12] The presentations vary, but jaundice, abdominal and back pain, and profound weight loss are common signs and symptoms.[8,13] Treatment is usually palliative and symptom oriented. Biliary stenting or bypass, nerve blocks and analgesics, gastric bypass, and in some circumstances palliative resection are a few of the options available. Follow-up in these patients may depend on the mode of palliation but must address the inevitable problems.

Biliary-enteric bypass offers a median survival of 4 to 12 months, with an overall survival rate of 14% at 12 months. Endoscopic or transhepatic stenting can be successful in more than 80% of patients, with a mean survival of 4 to 6.5 months.[8,14-17] Symptoms of duodenal obstruction (present in 10% to 16% of patients), recurrent jaundice (17% to 28%), and cholangitis (2%) are not uncommon after these forms of treatment.[8,10,14,18] Duodenal obstruction is an unusual initial symptom of patients with pancreatic adenocarcinoma (less than 5%) but can occur in up to 20% of patients who have not undergone resection.[18,19] When gastric bypass or resection is used for palliation, overall survival and subsequent development of stomach ulcerations (3%) remain the same but poor function or recurrence of the obstruction can occur.[11,20]

Follow-up should include special attention to certain potential problems. Intervention for pain control should be early and aggressive. Because of the unrelenting nature of pancreatic cancer, the policy at Roswell Park Cancer Institute is to minimize testing in these patients unless they are involved in an active clinical protocol. Follow-up should be symptom oriented and minimally invasive. Chest x-ray, computed tomography, and magnetic resonance imaging will not improve quality of life unless indicated by symptoms and will increase costs and stress to this terminally ill group of patients. Symptoms of gastrointestinal obstruction, cholangitis, jaundice, or ulcer disease can be identified through a careful history and physical examination; further testing can be performed if necessary for subsequent treatment.

Patients who do not undergo complete resection should have a monthly office visit for an interim history and physical examination. Blood work and chest radiography should be performed when clinically indicated. Patients receiving experimental therapy should be monitored according to protocol guidelines.

SURVEILLANCE AND FOLLOW-UP AFTER RESECTIONAL THERAPY

Staging

Resection for potential cure is achievable in less than 20% of patients with pancreatic cancer. Factors influencing survival include tumor size, lymph node status, and presence or absence of invasion into parapancreatic structures.[13,21] These factors are delineated in the current American Joint Committee on Cancer staging system (Table 10-1).[22] Pathological staging is essential because even small tumors (T1a) may have up to a 36% incidence of positive nodes. Tsuchiya et al.[23] found that more than 50% of small pancreatic cancers (less than 2 cm) had metastases. It is estimated that less than 4% of patients who undergo resection have early disease (T1aN0M0).[10] Despite the accuracy of the staging systems, almost all patients are at high risk for recurrence and death from their disease and therefore are appropriate candidates for postoperative surveillance.

Patterns of Recurrence

Recurrence after resection occurs locally in 47% to 75% of patients, related to the high rate of invasion into peripancreatic lymphatics, nerves, vessels, and retroperitoneum.[10,24-30] In a review of autopsy material Nagai et al.[31] found that 75% of patients with T1 or T2 tumors had microscopic metastases to lymph nodes not usually resected; Cubilla et al.[32] confirmed this finding. Positive soft tissue margins may occur in up to 38% of patients undergoing resection. Fifty-one percent of 72 patients reviewed by Willett et al.[27] had tumor extension to at least one surgical margin. The residual lymph node and soft tissue disease leads to high local failure rates, which may explain why adjuvant therapy has had limited success.

In addition to locoregional disease, pancreatic cancer recurs in the peritoneum, where seeding can occur in at least 35% of patients.[29] Metastatic and systemic disease occurs in at least 59% to 62% of patients after resection.[29,30]

Table 10-1 Tumor, nodes, metastases (TNM) staging system of pancreatic cancer

PRIMARY TUMOR (T)

TX	Primary tumor cannot be assessed
T0	No evidence of primary tumor
T1	Tumor limited to the pancreas
T1a	Tumor 2 cm or less in greatest dimension
T1b	Tumor more than 2 cm in greatest dimension
T2	Tumor extends directly to any of the following: duodenum, bile duct, or peripancreatic tissues
T3	Tumor extends directly to any of the following: stomach, spleen, colon, or adjacent large vessels

REGIONAL LYMPH NODES (N)

NX	Regional lymph nodes cannot be assessed
N0	No regional lymph node metastasis
N1	Regional lymph node metastasis

DISTANT METASTASIS (M)

MX	Presence of distant metastasis cannot be assessed
M0	No distant metastasis
M1	Distant metastasis

STAGE GROUPING

Stage I	T1	N0	M0
	T2	N0	M0
Stage II	T3	N0	M0
Stage III	Any T	N1	M0
Stage IV	Any T	Any N	M1

From American Joint Committee on Cancer, Beahrs OH, Henson DE, Hutter RVP, Kennedy BJ, editors. Manual for staging of cancer. Philadelphia: JB Lippincott Company, 1992.

Late Complications of Resection

Late complications of surgical resection for pancreatic cancer vary according to the extent and type of resection but nevertheless are closely related (Table 10-2). These problems may be compounded by the anorexia, fatigue, and enteritis that can occur with adjuvant therapy. Tumor recurrence can also occur at any time and mimic these problems. Office visits should include a detailed history of recent problems, with careful attention to symptoms of anorexia, weight loss, nausea, vomiting, bleeding, pain, jaundice, fever, chills, and diarrhea. Caloric intake and evidence of food intolerance should be monitored. Physical examination should emphasize detection of weight loss, lymphadenopathy, hepatomegaly, abdominal or incisional masses, ascites, Blumer's shelf, blood in the stool, and clinical evidence of jaundice. Electrolyte measurements, liver function tests, and complete blood count should be performed if cholangitis, bleeding, or recurrence is suspected.

GUIDELINES FOR FOLLOW-UP

Because no treatment that will improve survival for recurrent or metastatic pancreatic cancer is available, follow-up should emphasize treatment of the complications of surgery, adjuvant therapy, and progressive disease, with focus on maintaining quality of life. Surveillance should be individualized, based on the patient's psychological profile, preference, and symptoms.

Table 10-2 Late complications after surgical resection

Persistent weight loss	Postgastrectomy syndromes
Malnutrition	Dumping
Exocrine insufficiency	Poor gastric emptying
Malabsorption	Marginal ulcerations
Endocrine insufficiency	Peptic ulcer disease
Cholangitis	Diarrhea
Recurrent jaundice	

Table 10-3 Follow-up of patients with pancreatic cancer: Roswell Park Cancer Institute

	YEAR				
	1	2	3	4	5
Office visit	12	4	4	2	2
Complete blood count	6	4	4	2	2
Electrolytes	6	4	4	2	2
Liver function tests	6	4	4	2	2
Chest x-ray	1	*	*	*	*
Abdominal computed tomography	1	*	*	*	*
Pelvic computed tomography	1	*	*	*	*

*Performed if symptoms warrant or if recurrence is suspected.

Little consensus exists among practicing physicians regarding the appropriate follow-up of patients with pancreatic cancer. Surgeons, oncologists, and general practitioners each follow patients according to individual practice patterns.

Postoperative problems and recurrence are so common after resection that follow-up should be conducted on a monthly basis during the first year and a quarterly basis during the second year. If therapy becomes available to treat recurrent or metastatic disease, follow-up will become much more vigorous. The current guidelines for follow-up practiced at Roswell Park Cancer Institute are presented in Table 10-3.

Economic Implications

The original stage of the disease and the use of adjuvant therapy may affect the patient's standard of living and quality of life and may therefore require an alteration in surveillance patterns. Because the overall number of patients available for surveillance after curative resection is small, randomized trials to evaluate the efficacy of surveillance programs are not feasible or necessary. The economic effect of the follow-up guidelines as proposed here is minimal. It is imperative that patients have a personalized approach to follow-up with minimal invasive testing. Considering this, the cost of follow-up is low.

FUTURE PROSPECTS

Much work remains to be done in both diagnosis and treatment of pancreatic cancer. Molecular genetics may provide information about the natural history and biology of the disease and may become useful in the early identification of patients with pancreatic cancer and those patients at risk for the disease. In addition, molecular genetics may play a significant prognostic role and guide physicians in appropriate surveillance and follow-up.

Little is known about the molecular genetics of pancreatic cancer. Numerous studies have shown abnormalities in the c-*erb*B-2 protooncogene and the K-*ras* oncogene.[33-36] K-*ras* mutations are identified in 75% to 90% of patients with pancreatic cancer. C-*erb*B-2 abnormalities are found in approximately 20% of patients. Some early chromosomal abnormalities have also been seen in patients yet have not been completely elucidated.[37] In approximately 43% of patients p53 gene mutations are evident, but to date they have not been associated with extent of tumor, lymph node status, or stage of disease. Early work in this area, however, suggests that survival may be worse in patients with pancreatic cancer with p53 mutations.[38]

There is considerable evidence that transformation to a malignant process is a sequence requiring numerous genetic alterations. Many of these molecular abnormalities are likely to be identified for pancreatic cancer in the future. Intensive research, both in the laboratory and clinically, is needed to advance the knowledge and identification of genetic alterations. This information may further physicians' understanding of the biology of pancreatic cancer and subsequently aid in early identification, treatment, and surveillance of patients.

REFERENCES

1. Brunschwig A. The surgery of pancreatic tumors. New York: The CV Mosby Company, 1942.
2. Sulkowski U, Meyer J, Reers B, Pinger P, Waldner M. The historical development of resection therapy in pancreatic carcinoma. Zentralbl Bl Chir 1991;116:1325-32.
3. Boring CC, Squires TS, Tong T, Montgomery S. Cancer statistics, 1994. CA Cancer J Clin 1994;44:7-26.
4. Connolly MM, Dawson PJ, Michelassi F, Moossa AR, Lowenstein F. Survival in 1001 patients with carcinoma of the pancreas. Ann Surg 1987;206:366-73.
5. van Heerden JA. Pancreatic resection for carcinoma of the pancreas: Whipple versus total pancreatectomy; an institutional perspective. World J Surg 1984;8:880-8.
6. Bluemke DA, Fishman EK, Kuhlman J. CT evaluation following Whipple procedure: potential pitfalls in interpretation. J Comput Assist Tomogr 1992;16:704-8.
7. Satake K, Chung YS, Umeyama K, Takeuchi T, Kim YS. The possibility of diagnosing small pancreatic cancer (less than 4.0 cm) by measuring various serum tumor markers: a retrospective study. Cancer 1991;68:149-52.
8. Warshaw AL, Fernandez-Del Castillo C. Pancreatic carcinoma. N Engl J Med 1992;326:455-65.
9. Livstone EM, Spiro HM. The pancreatic cancer problem. World J Surg 1984;8:803-7.
10. Veronesi U, editor. Surgical oncology: a European handbook. New York: Springer-Verlag, 1989:578-621.
11. Sarr MG, Cameron JL. Surgical palliation of unresectable carcinoma of the pancreas. World J Surg 1994;8:906-13.
12. Crist DW, Sitzmann JV, Cameron JL. Improved hospital morbidity, mortality, and survival after the Whipple procedure. Ann Surg 1987;206:358-65.
13. Douglass HO Jr. Pancreatic cancer. In: Current therapy in hematology/oncology-3. Vol. 3. Brian MC, Carbone PP, editors. New York: BC Decker, Inc., 1988:185-93.
14. Mannell A, van Heerden JA, Weiland LH, Ilstrup DM. Factors influencing survival after resection for ductal adenocarcinoma of the pancreas. Ann Surg 1986;203:403-7.
15. Rooj PD, Rogatko A, Brennan MF. Evaluation of palliative surgical procedures in unresectable pancreatic cancer. Br J Surg 1991; 78:1053-8.
16. Cotton PB. Endoscopic methods for relief of malignant obstructive jaundice. World J Surg 1984;8:854-61.
17. Shepherd HA, Royle G, Ross AP, Diba A, Arthur M, Colin-Jones D. Endoscopic biliary endoprosthesis in the palliation of malignant obstruction of the distal common bile duct: a randomized trial. Br J Surg 1988;75:1166-8.
18. Andersen JR, Sorensen SM, Kruse A, Rokkjaer M, Matzen P. Randomized trial of endoscopic endoprosthesis versus operative bypass in malignant obstructive jaundice. Gut 1989;30:1132-5.
19. Bornman PC, Harries-Jones EP, Tobias R, Van Stiegmann G, Terblanche J. Prospective controlled trial of transhepatic biliary endoprosthesis vs bypass surgery for incurable carcinoma of head of pancreas. Lancet 1986;11:69-71.
20. Lillemoe KD, Sauter PK, Pitt HA, Yeo CJ, Cameron JL. Current status of surgical palliation of periampullary carcinoma. Surg Gynecol Obstet 1993;176:1-10.
21. Cameron JL, Crist DW, Sitzmann JV, et al. Factors influencing survival after pancreaticoduodenectomy for pancreatic cancer. Am J Surg 1991;161:120-5.
22. American Joint Committee on Cancer, Beahrs OH, Henson DE, Robert VP, Kennedy BJ, editors. Manual for staging of cancer. 4th ed. Philadelphia: JB Lippincott Company, 1992.
23. Tsuchiya R, Noda T, Harada N, et al. Collective review of small carcinomas of the pancreas. Ann Surg 1986;203:77-81.
24. Collure DW, Burns GP, Schenk WG Jr. Clinical, pathological and therapeutic aspects of carcinoma of the pancreas. Am J Surg 1994;128:683.
25. Sarr MG, Gladen HF, Beart RW, Jr, van Heckden JA. Role of gastroenterostomy in patients with unresectable pancreatic carcinoma. Surg Gynecol Obstet 1981;152:597.
26. Mannell A, van Heerden JA, Weiland LH, Ilstrup DM. Factors influencing survival after resection for ductal adenocarcinoma of the pancreas. Ann Surg 1986;203:403-7.
27. Willett CG, Lewandrowski K, Warshaw AL, Efird J, Compton CC. Resection margins in carcinoma of the head of the pancreas: implications for radiation therapy. Ann Surg 1993;217:144-8.
28. Bosset JF, Pavy JJ, Gillet M, Mantion G, Pelissier E, Schraub S. Conventional external irradiation alone as adjuvant treatment in resectable pancreatic cancer: results of a prospective study. Radiother Oncol 1992;24:191-4.
29. Johnstone PA, Sindelar WF. Lymph node involvement and pancreatic resection: correlation with prognosis and local disease control in a clinical trial. Pancreas 1993;8:535-9.
30. Johnstone PA, Sindelar WF. Patterns of disease recurrence following definitive therapy of adenocarcinoma of the pancreas using surgery and adjuvant radiotherapy: correlations of a clinical trial. Int J Radiat Oncol Biol Phys 1993;27:831-4.
31. Nagai H, Kuroda A, Morioka Y. Lymphatic and local spread of T1 and T2 pancreatic cancer: a study of autopsy material. Ann Surg 1986;204:65-71.
32. Cubilla AL, Fortner J, Fitzgerald PJ. Lymph node involvement in carcinoma of the head of the pancreas area. Cancer 1978;41:880-7.
33. Sakorafas GH, Lazaris A, Tsiotou AG, Koullias G, Glinatsis MT, Golematis BC. Oncogenes in cancer of the pancreas. Eur J Surg Oncol 1995;21:251-3.

34. Sawabu N, Watanabe H, Yamaguchi Y, Okai T. Mutation of the K-ras oncogene in pancreatic carcinoma, and application of its detection in pancreatic juice to diagnose pancreatic carcinoma. Jpn J Clin Med 1995;53:511-7.
35. Wang ZY, Liu TH, Cui QC. Gene diagnosis of pancreatic adenocarcinoma. Chinese J Pathol 1994;23:270-3.
36. Sakorafas GH, Tsiotou AG. Genetic basis of cancer of the pancreas: diagnostic and therapeutic applications. Eur J Surg 1994;160:529-34.
37. Griffin CA, Hruban RH, Morsberger LA, et al. Consistent chromosome abnormalities in adenocarcinoma of the pancreas. Cancer Res 1995;55:2394-9.
38. Nakamori S, Yashima K, Murakami Y, et al. Association of p53 gene mutations with short survival in pancreatic adenocarcinoma. Jpn J Cancer Res 1995;86:174-81.

➢ COUNTERPOINT

Memorial Sloan-Kettering Cancer Center

KEVIN C. P. CONLON

The prognosis for the majority of patients with pancreatic carcinoma is grim, with an overall long-term survival rate of between 2% and 3%.[1-4] Symptoms are often vague, presentation is delayed, and the majority of patients have advanced disease at diagnosis, which precludes potentially curative therapy.[5]

Between October 1983 and October 1995, 2,228 patients were admitted to Memorial Sloan-Kettering Cancer Center with peripancreatic cancer (Figure 10-1). Ductal adenocarcinoma of the pancreas accounted for 69% of the total number admitted. Only 332 of this group of patients (22%) underwent resection with curative intent. A further 836 (55%) had surgical exploration or bypass. This counterpoint concentrates on the postoperative surveillance of these patients.

At first sight the aims of follow-up for the curative and palliative groups should be inherently different. However, the aggressive nature of pancreatic cancer and lack of effective adjuvant or salvage therapies mean that the general principles of early detection of recurrent disease and identification of second primary malignancies confer minimal benefit on this patient population. In addition, despite some optimistic recent reports that have shown a reduction in the operative mortality and suggested actuarial 5-year survival rates in excess of 20%,[6-8] surgical excision should generally be considered a palliative procedure. Recently physicians at Memorial Sloan-Kettering Cancer Center analyzed the clinicopathological characteristics of 118 patients with ductal adenocarcinoma of the pancreas who underwent resection with curative intent at this institution between 1983 and 1989.[4] The original pathological material from all cases was reviewed. Operative mortality was 3.4%. Median survival was 14.3 months following resection, compared with 4.9 months if no resection was performed (Figure 10-2). Only 12 patients survived 5 years after operation (10.2% overall actual 5-year survival rate). Of these, five patients died of recurrent or metatastic disease between 60 and 64 months. These sobering results are similar to those reported by Nitecki et al.,[9] who reviewed the Mayo Clinic experience between 1981 and 1991 and reported an actuarial 5-year survival rate of 6.8% after resection. Wade et al.,[10] reporting data from the U.S. Department of Veterans

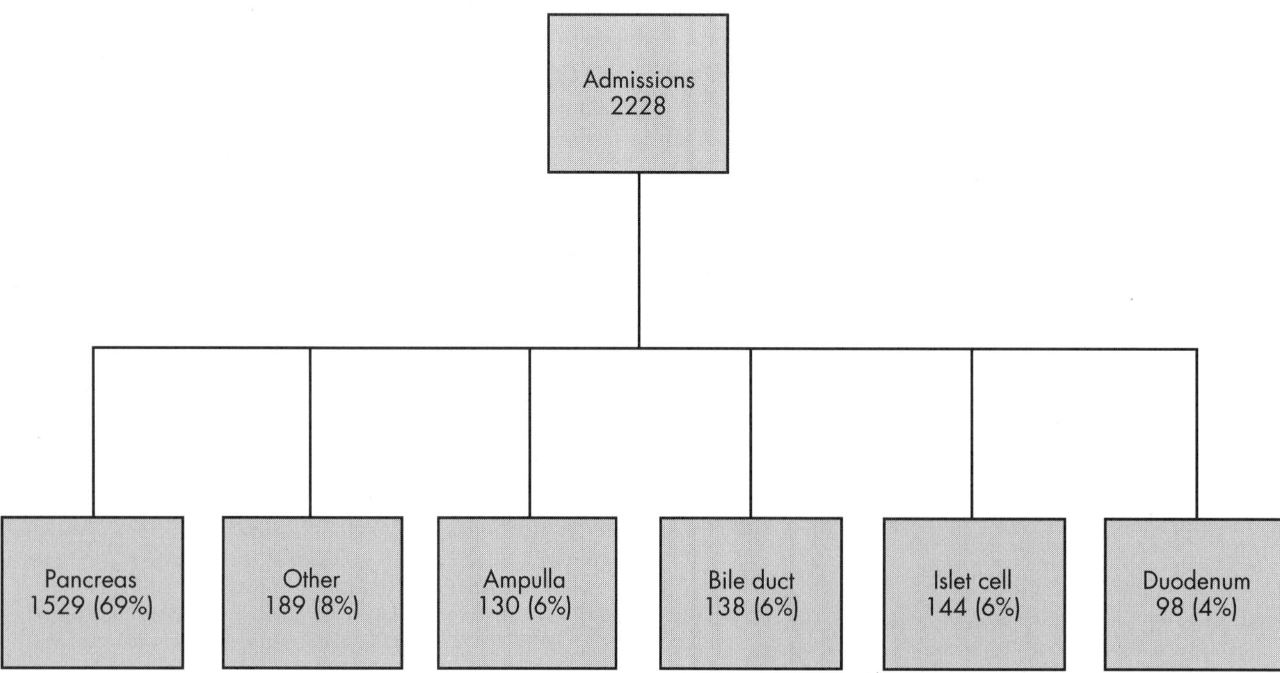

Figure 10-1 Patients admitted to Memorial Sloan-Kettering Cancer Center with a peripancreatic malignancy between October 15, 1983, and October 15, 1995.

Affairs hospital system, concluded that the actuarial 5-year survival after pancreaticoduodenectomy was only 8%.

I strongly believe that for the majority of patients the primary goal of postoperative surveillance should be the maintenance of quality of life. Table 10-4 lists the most common long-term complications after pancreaticoduodenectomy. A follow-up regimen should be tailored to allow appropriate intervention, if required, in each of these areas. In concurrence with Smith and Meropol, surveillance programs tailored primarily to the early detection of recurrent disease should be confined to institutions with active research protocols aimed at the treatment of locally recurrent or metastatic disease. Aggressive surveillance regimens that offer the patient nothing but early identification of recurrent disease confer no benefit and may adversely affect the emotional well-being of the patient and family; thus they should be avoided.

CURRENT PRACTICE

The current regimen at Memorial Sloan-Kettering Cancer Center for the surveillance of patients after pancreatic resection is detailed in Table 10-5. In the early postpancreatectomy period, mild gastrointestinal symptoms such as early satiety, bile reflux gastritis, dumping, or mild gastric outlet obstruction are not infrequent. They can generally be controlled with simple dietary modification. The majority of patients resume their normal diet and maintain weight. Rarely patients with persistent symptoms require prokinetic agents such as erythromycin or metoclopramide. In this group a more frequent schedule of follow-up is needed to assess progress.

Table 10-4 Long-term complications after pancreaticoduodenectomy

POSTGASTRECTOMY SYMPTOMS
Dumping
Diarrhea
Bile-reflux gastritis
Early satiety
Gastric outlet obstruction
Marginal ulceration
NUTRITIONAL AND METABOLIC SEQUELAE
Altered fat and protein absorption
Weight loss
Vitamin and mineral deficiencies
Altered glucose homeostasis
EMOTIONAL SYMPTOMS
Anxiety
Depression
SYMPTOMS CAUSED BY RECURRENT DISEASE
Gastric outlet obstruction
Biliary obstruction
Intestinal obstruction
Ascites
Pain

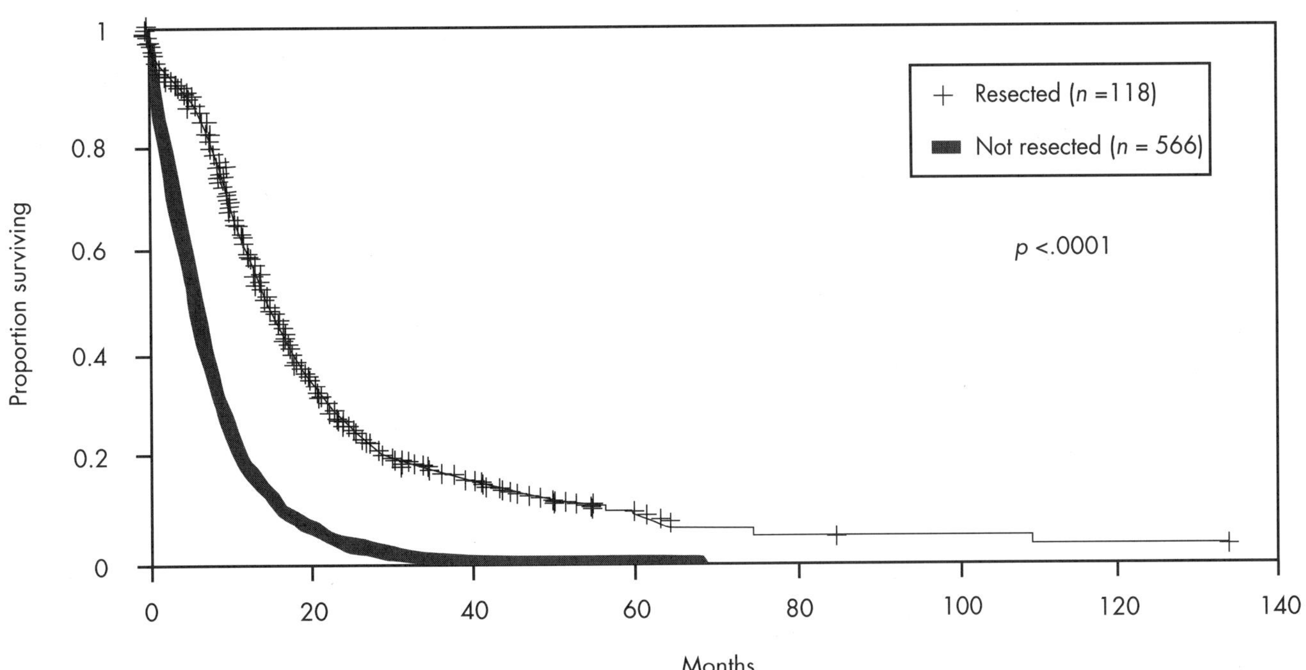

Figure 10-2 Comparison of survival between patients who underwent resection ($n = 118$, median survival = 14.3 months) and patients who did not ($n = 566$, median survival = 4.9 months) ($p < .0001$). (From Conlon KC, Klimstra DS, Brennan MF. Ann Surg 1996;223:273-9.)

Table 10-5 Follow-up of patients with pancreatic cancer: Memorial Sloan-Kettering Cancer Center

	YEAR				
	1	2	3	4	5
Office visit	4	3	3	2	2
Complete blood count	4	3	3	2	2
Multichannel blood tests*	4	3	3	2	2
Chest x-ray	1	0	0	0	0
Abdominal computed tomography	1	0	0	0	0

*Consists of glucose, blood urea nitrogen, creatinine, total bilirubin, uric acid, total protein, albumin, calcium, phosphorus, serum glutamic-oxaloacetic transaminase, lactic dehydrogenase, and alkaline phosphatase.

Pancreatic exocrine insufficiency is not uncommon. The diagnosis can be made clinically (crampy abdominal pains, steatorrhea, and weight loss). Sophisticated metabolic tests are not required. Pancreatic enzyme supplements readily correct the condition and lead to the resumption of normal dietary habits and weight in most cases. Uncontrolled pain and clinically significant depression, although relatively uncommon, have a major impact on a patient's functional state and quality of life. In such patients, if identified, appropriate therapy can control symptoms and improve their quality of life.

Current practice at Memorial Sloan-Kettering Cancer Center is to offer adjuvant therapy to patients after resection. This consists of postoperative radiation therapy with 5-fluorouracil (5-FU). In general, adjuvant radiation involves treatment 5 days a week to a total dose of 5040 cGy. The fractionation is 180 cGy per day to the entire treated volume. Patients receive 5-FU (500 mg/m^2 per day) during the first and last 3 days of their radiation therapy. They also receive weekly 5-FU for 4 months after completion of the radiation therapy. Follow-up includes history and physical examination every 3 months for 1 year after resection, every 4 months during the next 2 years, and every 6 months thereafter (Table 10-5). Because this institution has a number of active protocols dealing with locally recurrent or metastatic disease, physicians obtain a contrast-enhanced, dynamic computed tomographic scan of the abdomen 6 months after resection. Further radiological investigations depend on the clinical situation. Apart from the study at 6 months, computed tomography is not performed routinely on asymptomatic patients.

Follow-up for patients who receive chemoradiation therapy (radiation therapy plus 5-FU plus levamisole) after surgical exploration or bypass for locally advanced disease includes a monthly history, physical examination, and hematological-biochemical profile. Because of the progression of disease these patients are more likely to be symptomatic and thus require more frequent follow-up. Aggressive psychosocial support is given. Radiological investigations are generally not recommended unless symptoms occur (biliary, gastric, or intestinal obstruction) and treatment is indicated. At the time of progression, patients are offered conventional chemotherapy (5-FU or mitomycin C), investigational chemotherapy, or supportive care only.

Patients with metastatic disease are followed in a similar fashion. Treatment options include standard chemotherapy, investigational chemotherapy, or supportive care alone. Follow-up regimens for patients in investigational protocols may differ depending on the requirements of the specific protocol.

SUMMARY

The care of the patient with pancreatic cancer requires a multidisplinary approach, with attention paid to both the physical and emotional needs of the patient. Since physicians currently lack effective adjuvant therapies for this disease, emphasis for the majority of patients should be placed on maintaining quality of life.

REFERENCES

1. Wingo PA, Tong T, Bolden S. Cancer statistics, 1995. CA Cancer J Clin 1995;45:8-30.
2. Gudjonsson B. Cancer of the pancreas: 50 years of surgery. Cancer 1987;60:2284-303.
3. Geer RJ, Brennan MF. Prognostic indicators for survival after resection of pancreatic adenocarcinoma. Am J Surg 1993;165:68-73.
4. Conlon KC, Klimstra DS, Brennan MF. Long-term survival after curative resection for pancreatic ductal adenocarcinoma: clinicopathologic analysis of 5-year survivors. Ann Surg 1996;223:273-9.
5. Conlon KC, Dougherty E, Klimstra DS, Coit DG, Turnbull AD, Brennan MF. The value of minimal access surgery in the staging of patients with potentially resectable peripancreatic malignancy. Ann Surg 1996;223:134-40.
6. Trede M, Schwall G, Saeger HD. Survival after pancreatoduodenectomy: 118 consecutive resections without an operative mortality. Ann Surg 1990;211:447-58.
7. Cameron JL, Crist DW, Sitzmann JV, et al. Factors influencing survival after pancreaticoduodenectomy for pancreatic cancer. Am J Surg 1991;161:120-5.
8. Fernandez-del Castillo C, Rattner DW, Warshaw AL. Standards for pancreatic resection in the 1990s. Arch Surg 1995;130:295-300.
9. Nitecki SS, Sarr MG, Colby TV, van Heerden JA. Long-term survival after resection for ductal adenocarcinoma of the pancreas: is it really improving? Ann Surg 1995;221:59-66.
10. Wade TP, El-Ghazzawy AG, Virgo KS, Johnson FE. The Whipple resection for cancer in U.S. Department of Veterans Affairs hospitals. Ann Surg 1995;221:241-8.

➢ COUNTER POINT

National Kyushu Cancer Center, Japan

YOUSUKE SEO

Pancreatic cancer has increased steadily in incidence over the last four decades and is the fifth leading cause of cancer death in Japan. It was responsible for the death of more than 14,000 Japanese in 1993. Ductal carcinoma comprises 88% of pancreatic cancers in Japan. The resectability rate of duct cell carcinoma of the pancreas has risen recently with the application of extended radical pancreatectomy. Among 852 patients with pancreatic cancer subjected to surgery, 479 (52.6%) underwent resection.[1] The 5-year survival rate was 40% for patients with small (less than 2 cm) lesions undergoing surgery with curative intent.[1]

Therapeutic modalities for resectable cases, however, vary among institutions throughout the country. Either surgery (super-radical pancreatectomy) alone or radical resection with a combination of radiation and chemotherapy (preoperative, intraoperative, or postoperative) is selected in most institutions.[2-5] The most common type of recurrence after super-radical resection is local recurrence, which accounts for 30% to 80% of total recurrent cases. Other areas of recurrence include the liver (66% to 79%), peritoneum (29% to 53%), and lymph nodes (47%). The follow-up of patients with pancreatic ductal adenocarcinoma will be addressed by a review of the Japanese experience.

POTENTIAL BENEFITS OF SURVEILLANCE

Owing to remarkable progress in diagnostic techniques, especially imaging studies, the proportion of pancreatic cancers diagnosed while still small has increased in Japan. Such patients are good candidates for curative surgery. In 1993 tumors less than 2 cm comprised 4.7% of 1,100 cases in Japan.[1] Small pancreatic cancers in the head without jaundice have been reported from several institutions.[6,7] The proportion of unresectable cases in Japan is much smaller than in other countries, as reported by Smith and Meropol. They also state that few patients survive 5 years after curative treatment. However, recent reports show 5-year survival rates to be between 17% and 25%,[8-10] with even better results reported from Japan.[3,4] This has encouraged Japanese physicians to adopt a more intensive follow-up strategy.

I agree with Smith and Meropol about the goals of surveillance after treatment: improvement in quality of life and prolongation of life. An intensive follow-up strategy is supported by reports of curative surgical treatment for recurrent cases and the potentially beneficial effects of chemotherapy and radiation treatments on survival and quality of life.[11,12]

METHODS OF SURVEILLANCE

History and Physical Examination

As pointed out by Smith and Meropol, history and physical examination are not sensitive in detecting tumor recurrence. Nevertheless, the occurrence of new symptoms can prompt the initiation of further diagnostic steps. Major symptoms and signs of pancreatic cancer recurrence after resection are abdominal pain, weight loss, jaundice, and ascites. Therefore Japanese physicians emphasize careful history taking and physical examination.

Radiological Evaluation

Radiological examinations are extremely helpful in the surveillance of patients after therapy for pancreatic cancer. Among the various diagnostic imaging studies, computed tomography is the most useful. Distant metastasis to the liver or lung is detectable with computed tomography, even if the metastatic lesion is less than 2 cm. Thickening of the intestine or a collection of ascites demonstrated by computed tomography is suggestive of peritoneal recurrence. Ultrasonography of the liver is occasionally helpful in diagnosing metastases, so it is commonly performed alternately with computed tomography. Magnetic resonance imaging and celiac angiogram rarely contribute to the detection of recurrent pancreatic cancer.

Tumor Markers

Two commonly used tumor markers of pancreatic cancer in Japan are CEA and CA 19-9. Other markers include DUPAN-2, SPAN-1, CA50, SLX, and elastase I. CA 19-9 is the most sensitive among these markers, with sensitivity and specificity rates of more than 80%.[13,14] Sensitivity rates of other tumor markers in small pancreatic cancer (less than 2 cm) are 50% for elastase I, 22% for CEA, and 13% for CA 19-9.[15] A combination of CA 19-9, DUPAN-2, and SPAN-1 can be a useful marker for the detection of recurrence in more than 80% of patients with pancreatic cancer.[15]

PRIMARY THERAPY

Resectability rates of pancreatic cancer in Japan are much higher than in other countries. According to a report by the Japan Pancreatic Cancer Registry in 1994, the resectability rate was 56.2%.[1]

Most radical operations for pancreatic cancer in Japan are performed by experienced surgeons who specialize in pancreatic surgery at selected hospitals, which is a possible reason for the high resectability and cure rates in Japan. Physicians should suspect early pancreatic cancer when patients have symptoms caused by obstruction of the pancreatic duct, which include mild abdominal pain, back pain, anorexia, and jaundice. Resectable cancers are often difficult to differentiate from nonresectable ones on the basis of symptoms. Abdominal pain and back pain usually represent tumor invasion to an adjacent organ or extrapancreatic nerve plexus.

Treatment modalities for unresectable pancreatic cancer differ among institutions throughout Japan. For locally advanced cases, physicians usually perform staging laparoscopy when routine laboratory and imaging studies are complete, since this is an excellent method for detecting small liver metastases and peritoneal implants, which are difficult to detect by conventional imaging studies. If liver or peritoneal metastases are found on laparoscopy, bypass procedures are often carried out laparoscopically. If the lesion is locally unresectable, chemoradiation therapy is initiated. The beneficial effects of this combination therapy have been reported.[19,20]

Restaging laparoscopy is carried out after chemoradiation to assess resectability, and then either resection or intraoperative radiation therapy for unresectable cases is elected. During intraoperative radiation, gastric or biliary bypass operations and visceral nerve block for pain relief can be performed. Intraoperative radiation therapy affords patients with unresectable but localized cancer a mean survival of approximately 1 year.[16-18] Follow-up of patients with unresectable tumors should focus on relapse of the main tumor and the new appearance of distant metastasis.

Early detection of relapse does not seem to prolong survival or improve the quality of life, since no effective maintenance treatment is available for unresected cases. Attention must be paid to symptoms secondary to the occurrence of gastric ulceration or intestinal obstruction as a complication of radiation therapy, including fever and abdominal pain caused by cholangitis in patients with biliary bypass. Pain is the most important symptom to relieve in patients with advanced pancreatic cancer.

SURVEILLANCE AND FOLLOW-UP AFTER RESECTIONAL THERAPY

Staging

Recent reports from the United States present improvements in the cure rate and survival rate of patients with resectable pancreatic cancer.[8-10] Resection with curative intent is currently undertaken in approximately 50% of patients in Japan.

Besides the factors presented by Smith and Meropol, poor histological differentiation and DNA ploidy have recently been listed as factors influencing survival.[10] The Japanese Pancreas Society has its own staging system for pancreatic cancer, which includes capsular invasion, retroperitoneal invasion, and venous invasion, as well as tumor size and nodal involvement. This staging system reflects prognosis well, but it is complex.[21] Although the resectability rate has risen recently with improvements in survival rate, the recurrence rate remains high in Japan as in other countries.[2,3] Subsequent follow-up plays an important role in the detection of recurrence because curative therapy can occasionally be offered.

Patterns of Recurrence

The pattern of recurrence in patients who undergo super-radical pancreatectomy does not differ much from that described by Smith and Meropol. According to a report from Kanazawa University, a center for super-radical pancreatectomy in Japan, 30 of 45 patients had recurrence after resection. Local retroperitoneal recurrence was found in 80% of 15 patients at autopsy. Liver and peritoneal metastases were noted in 66% and 53%, respectively.[2] Accordingly, the importance of wide retroperitoneal resection including nerve plexuses and lymph node clearance for the prevention of locoregional recurrence deserves emphasis.

LATE COMPLICATIONS OF RESECTION

Late complications of resection depend on the extent of the operative procedure and whether perioperative adjuvant radiation and chemotherapy are used. Malnutrition, for example, can occur because of digestive disturbances or metabolic abnormalities after a complicated reconstruction even without cancer recurrence. Laboratory studies, such as the glucose tolerance test or paraaminobenzoic acid excretion test, can be helpful in differentiating benign from malignant causes of such nutritional problems. Late complications listed by Smith and Meropol are about the same as those seen in Japan.

Table 10-6 Follow-up of patients with pancreatic cancer: National Kyushu Cancer Center, Japan

	YEAR				
	1	2	3	4	5
Office visit	12	4	4	2	2
Complete blood count	12	4	4	2	2
Leucine aminopeptidase	4	4	2	2	2
Multichannel blood tests*	4	4	2	2	2
CEA	4	4	2	2	2
CA 19-9	4	4	2	2	2
DUPAN-2	4	4	2	2	2
SPAN-1	4	4	2	2	2
CA-50	4	4	2	2	2
SLX	4	4	2	2	2
Elastase I	4	4	2	2	2
Chest x-ray	4	4	2	1	1
Chest computed tomography	4	2	2	1	1
Abdominal computed tomography†	2	1	1	1	0
Pelvic computed tomography†	2	1	1	1	0
Abdominal ultrasound†	2	1	1	0	1
Pelvic ultrasound†	2	1	1	0	1

CEA, Carcinoembryonic antigen.
*Includes total protein, glutamate-oxaloacetate transaminase, glutamate-pyruvic transaminase, bilirubin, alkaline phosphatase, cholesterol, blood urea nitrogen, and creatinine.
†Computed tomography and ultrasonography are performed alternately to reduce cost.

GUIDELINES FOR FOLLOW-UP

Because a possibility—albeit small—exists for prolongation of life or improvement in quality of life after detection of recurrence, Japanese physicians advocate vigorous follow-up, using the history, physical examination, measurement of serum tumor marker levels, and imaging studies such as ultrasound, computed tomography, and magnetic resonance imaging. Ultrasound should be performed alternately to reduce costs, even if clinical evidence does not suggest recurrence. Blood chemistries are also used, including total protein, glutamate-oxaloacetate transaminase, glutamate-pyruvic transaminase, bilirubin, alkaline phosphatase, leucine aminopeptidase, cholesterol, blood urea nitrogen, and creatinine.

No protocol of maintenance chemotherapy after curative resection has been established at National Kyushu Cancer Center. Ishikawa et al.[22] advocate perioperative chemotherapy via both the portal vein and hepatic artery for prevention of liver metastasis. I also recommend monthly follow-up during the first year but only every 3 months during the second year. Physicians should continue to follow up patients vigorously, aiming for the early detection of recurrence. The current guidelines for follow-up of patients with pancreatic cancer at National Kyushu Cancer Center are presented in Table 10-6.

REFERENCES

1. Saito Y. Annual report from Japan Pancreas Cancer Registry Committee [Japanese]. Suizo 1994;9:499-527.
2. Kayahara M, Nagakawa T, Ueno K, Ohta T, Takeda T, Miyazaki I. An evaluation of radical resection for pancreatic cancer based on the mode of recurrence as determined by autopsy and diagnostic imaging. Cancer 1993;72:2118-23.
3. Kaneko T, Nakao A, Harada A, et al. A study on recurrence pattern after extended surgery for pancreatic cancer [Japanese]. Jpn J Gastroenterol Surg 1993;26:2423-8.
4. Shibamoto Y, Manabe T, Baba N, et al. High dose, external and intraoperative radiotherapy in the treatment of resectable and unresectable pancreatic cancer. Int J Radiat Oncol Biol Phys 1990;19:605-11.
5. Hiraoka T, Uchino R, Kanemitsu K, et al. Combination of intraoperative radiation with resection of cancer of the pancreas. Int J Pancreatol 1990;7:201-7.
6. Ozaki H. Improvement of pancreatic cancer treatment from the Japanese experience in the 1980s. Int J Pancreatol 1992;12:5-9.
7. Ariyama J. Diagnosis of early pancreatic cancer [Japanese]. Nihon Naikagakkai Zasshi 1992;81:44-7.
8. Grace PA, Pitt HA, Tompkins RK, DenBesten L, Longmire WP Jr. Decreased morbidity and mortality after pancreaticoduodenectomy. Am J Surg 1986;151:141-9.
9. Braasch JW, Deziel DJ, Rossi RL, Watkins E Jr, Winter PF. Pyloric and gastric preserving pancreatic resection: experience with 87 patients. Ann Surg 1986;204:411-8.
10. Cameron JL, Pitt HA, Yeo CJ, Lillemoe KD, Kaufman HS, Coleman J. One hundred and forty-five consecutive pancreaticoduodenectomies without mortality. Ann Surg 1993;217:430-8.
11. Menke-Pluymers MB, Klinkenbijl JH, Tjioe M, Jeekel J. Treatment of locoregional recurrence after intentional curative resection of pancreatic cancer. Hepatogastroenterology 1992;39:429-32.
12. Inoue K, Kosuge T, Shimada K, et al. Repeated radical resection and intraoperative irradiation for recurrent pancreatic ductal adenocarcinoma after pancreatoduodenectomy. Surgery 1995;118:909-11.
13. Masson P, Palsson B, Andren-Sandberg A. Evaluation of CEA, CA 19-9, CA 50, CA-195, and TATI with special reference to pancreatic disorders. Int J Pancreatol 1991;8:333-44.
14. Kawa S, Oguchi H, Tokoo M, et al. Tumor markers for pancreatic cancer. Cancer Research Clin 1992;1:64-70.
15. Ohkura H. Effectiveness of combination assay of tumor marker. Sougou Rinsyo 1990;39:2781.
16. Roldan GE, Gunderson LL, Nagorney DM, et al. External beam versus intraoperative and external beam irradiation for locally advanced pancreatic cancer. Cancer 1988;61:1110-6.
17. Shiply WU, Wood WC, Tepper JE, et al. Intraoperative electron beam irradiation for patients with unresectable pancreatic carcinoma. Ann Surg 1984;200:289-96.
18. Dobelbower RR Jr, Konski AA, Merrick HW 3d, Bronn DG, Schifeling D, Kamen C. Intraoperative electron beam radiation therapy (IOEBRT) for carcinoma of the exocrine pancreas. Int J Radiat Oncol Biol Phys 1991;20:113-9.
19. Jessup JM, Steele G Jr, Mayer RJ, et al. Neoadjuvant therapy for unresectable pancreatic adenocarcinoma. Arch Surg 1993;128:559-64.
20. Hoffman JP, Weese JL, Solin LJ, et al. A pilot study of preoperative chemoradiation for patients with localized adenocarcinoma of the pancreas. Am J Surg 1995;169:71-8.
21. Tsunoda T, Ura K, Eto T, Matsumoto T, Tsuchiya R. UICC and Japanese classifications for carcinoma of the pancreas. Int J Pancreatol 1991;8:205-14.
22. Ishikawa O, Ohigashi H, Sasaki Y, et al. Liver perfusion chemotherapy via both the hepatic artery and portal vein to prevent hepatic metastasis after extended pancreatectomy for adenocarcinoma of the pancreas. Am J Surg 1994;168:361-4.

➢ COUNTERPOINT

Royal Liverpool University Hospital, UK

ANDREW N. KINGSNORTH

Current practice in the treatment of pancreatic cancer has evolved against the background of a steady reduction in operative morbidity and mortality in specialist units in recent years.[1] In a review of 2,172 patients undergoing pancreatic resection in 28 centers, only 150 deaths were reported (6.9%). As a result, the need for postresectional surveillance has increased. Five-year survival rates of 20% to 25% have been reported in some series after curative resection.[2]

Epidemiological data from Great Britain are similar to U.S. data.[3] Since the 1920s, disease frequency has steadily increased, with a slight male preponderance of 1.1 to 1. The incidence reaches a peak in males at 70 to 74 years of age and in females at a somewhat later age. The overall incidence of pancreatic cancer in Great Britain and Wales is 12 per 100,000 people, which translates into about 3,000 new cases per year and represents just over 3% of all malignancies in each sex.[4] Pancreatic cancer ranks sixth for males and eighth for females as a cause of cancer-related death, with an overall 5-year survival of between 2% and 3%. The overall picture therefore is similar to that in the United States.

Treatment of pancreatic cancer has broad economic implications for specialist centers. Expensive, fully equipped diagnostic facilities are made available to a multidisciplinary team consisting of gastroenterologists, surgeons, oncologists, and palliative care specialists. Although its cost effectiveness is unclear, this approach has engendered close cooperation among physicians from different specialties. Multiinstitutional trials are needed to evaluate interventions in two areas: the benefits or hazards of preoperative endoscopic biliary stenting to relieve jaundice and the role of perioperative adjuvant chemoirradiation.

POTENTIAL BENEFITS OF SURVEILLANCE

At Royal Liverpool University Hospital the primary aims are to improve quality of life and to provide support for the patient and family. The methods of surveillance prescribed include history and physical examination, supplemented by routine hematological examinations and serial serum liver enzyme studies. Physicians here do not believe that the routine measurement of tumor markers can detect early recurrence.

Because of resource limitations, computed tomography is used as an adjunct to ultrasonography. If the results of the latter are unsatisfactory or prompt suspicion, a computed tomographic scan is obtained as a subsequent investigation.

Ultrasound, on its own, may detect irrefutable evidence of local recurrence, metastatic liver disease, or ascites.

SURVEILLANCE AND FOLLOW-UP

The follow-up strategies employed at Royal Liverpool University Hospital are similar to those of Roswell Park Cancer Institute, with the exception that palliative care is commonly extended into the community, avoiding hospitalization for terminally ill patients. Improvements in the sensitivity and specificity of tumor markers and refinements in the products of molecular biology research are required before either of these can be translated into clinical practice.

Noncurative Resection

For patients with unfavorable prognostic criteria, such as advanced age, liver metastases, or large tumors, physicians at Royal Liverpool University Hospital favor endoprosthesis placement for palliation of obstructive jaundice.[5] If survival is likely to be less than 6 months, a less rigorous follow-up protocol is used that involves close liaison with primary care physicians, hospice caregivers, or community nurses who work in terminal care. In this way many patients who choose to die at home in their community can be treated humanely. It is then left to the discretion of the patient or the primary caregiver to decide whether a new complication such as vomiting or recurrent jaundice requires immediate further assessment in the surgical unit. Patients expected to survive longer than 6 months are generally offered surgical bypass for obstructive jaundice and, until terminal symptoms intervene, receive monthly office visits with routine history, physical examination, hematology studies, and liver function tests.

Treatment After Resectional Therapy

Because of improvements in functional outcome, a pylorus-preserving Whipple resection for operable lesions is the preferred treatment.[6,7] Survival is not compromised when compared with the conventional Whipple operation.[8] Portal vein resection is occasionally necessary when division of the neck of the pancreas reveals a small area of tumor infiltration along the right lateral border of the superior mesenteric or portal vein. Such patients are at high risk of local recurrence.[9] In addition, lymphatic spread may "skip" tiers of lymph nodes, in which case a lymphatic clearance is recommended, although its efficacy has not yet been proved by randomized trial.[10] Notwithstanding, the main arbiter of local recurrence is extension into peripancreatic soft tissue, which is not effectively encompassed by resection margins.[11] In the experience at Royal Liverpool University Hospital, one third of patients die within the first year, predominantly because of local recurrence, whereas later deaths are predominantly due to liver metastases.

Late Complications of Resection

New-onset diabetes mellitus develops in few patients, but pancreatic exocrine insufficiency is common. Moreover, weight loss occurring more than 1 year after successful resection may not be due to tumor recurrence but to previously borderline exocrine insufficiency becoming a clinically relevant insufficiency. The need for and level of pancreatic exocrine supplements must therefore be constantly monitored.

Although repeat resection for cure or palliation is rarely an option in patients with pancreatic cancer, local recurrence is sometimes limited and amenable to effective surgical palliation. For example, a local recurrence at the biliary-enteric anastomosis or the pancreatic-enteric anastomosis can be explored in appropriate cases with a view to further resection. If a limited volume of disease is discovered, resection can be supplemented by postoperative external beam irradiation. This approach has been taken in a small number of patients at Royal Liverpool University Hospital and has had a relatively rewarding outcome.

Table 10-7 Follow-up of patients with pancreatic cancer: Royal Liverpool University Hospital, UK

	YEAR				
	1	2	3	4	5
Office visit	6	4	4	2	2
Complete blood count	6	4	4	2	2
Liver function tests	6	4	4	2	2
Chest x-ray	3	*	*	*	*
Abdominal ultrasound	3	*	*	*	*
Abdominal computed tomography	*	*	*	*	*

*Performed if symptoms warrant or if recurrence is suspected.

GUIDELINES FOR FOLLOW-UP

Recurrence in patients with pancreatic cancer is almost inevitable. The pattern of recurrence is unpredictable, however, and the differing problems presented by patients require quick action to maintain quality of life. The current guidelines for follow-up at Royal Liverpool University Hospital are presented in Table 10-7.

REFERENCES

1. Johnson CD. Why resect pancreatic cancer? In: Johnson CD, Imrie CW, editors. Pancreatic disease: progress and prospects. London: Springer-Verlag, 1991:97-102.
2. Trede M, Schwall G, Seager HD. Survival after pancreaticoduodenectomy. Ann Surg 1990;211:447-58.
3. Office of population censuses and surveys. Series MBI, No 20, Cancer statistics registrations. England and Wales, London: HMSO, 1987.
4. Glazer G, Coulter C, Crofton ME, et al. Controversial issues in the management of pancreatic cancer: part I. Ann R Coll Surg Engl 1995;77:111-22.
5. van den Bosch RP, van der Schelling GP, Klinkenbijl JH, Mulder PG, van Blenkinstein M, Jeekel J. Guidelines for the application of surgery and endoprostheses in the palliation of obstructive jaundice in advanced cancer of the pancreas. Ann Surg 1994;219:18-24.
6. Kingsnorth AN, Berg JD, Gray MR. A novel reconstructive technique for pylorus-preserving pancreaticoduodenectomy: avoidance of early postoperative gastric stasis. Ann R Coll Surg Engl 1993;75:38-42.

7. Kingsnorth AN, Formela LJ, Chen D, Rehfeld JF. Plasma gastrin and cholecystokinin responses after pylorus-preserving pancreaticoduodenectomy and defunctioned Roux-loop pancreaticojejunostomy. Br J Surg 1994;81:1356-59.
8. Tsao JI, Rossi RL, Lowell JA. Pylorus-preserving pancreaticoduodenectomy: is it an adequate cancer operation? Arch Surg 1994;129:405-12.
9. Allema JH, Reinders ME, van Gullick TM, et al. Portal vein resection in patients undergoing pancreatoduodenectomy for carcinoma of the pancreatic head. Br J Surg 1994;81:1642-6.
10. Nakao A, Harada A, Nonami T, et al. Lymph node metastases in carcinoma of the head of the pancreas region. Br J Surg 1995;82:399-402.
11. Willett CG, Lewandrowski K, Warshaw AL, Efird J, Compton CC. Resection margins in carcinoma of the head of the pancreas: implications for irradiation therapy. Ann Surg 1993;217:144-8.

➢ COUNTER POINT

University of Washington Medical Center

RICHARD H. BELL, JR.

Smith and Meropol correctly emphasize the limited life expectancy of most patients with pancreatic carcinoma and the lack of effective therapy for recurrent disease. For this reason the follow-up of patients with pancreatic cancer is designed to deal with symptoms resulting from progressive or recurrent disease. During follow-up the need for laboratory and radiological testing is guided by the patient's complaints, since therapy is designed to alleviate symptoms rather than to attempt cure of the recurrent cancer.

IMPORTANCE OF TISSUE DIAGNOSIS

Inherent in any rational follow-up of patients with cancer is the necessity for adequate tissue diagnosis. In patients with ductal adenocarcinoma of the pancreas who undergo resection the diagnosis is provided by pathological examination of the operative specimen. In patients with widespread metastatic disease at the time of presentation a diagnosis can and should be based on percutaneous computed tomographic scan– or ultrasound-guided biopsy. Patients with advanced local disease present a problem because their cancer may be declared unresectable on the basis of either computed tomography criteria or exploratory laparotomy but they have no pathological diagnosis. In these circumstances obtaining a tissue diagnosis is critical, since some of these patients may have chronic pancreatitis rather than pancreatic cancer and others may have tumors with a more favorable prognosis, such as lymphoma or islet cell carcinoma.[1] Basing a diagnosis of adenocarcinoma of the pancreas purely on computed tomography findings or operative palpation is inappropriate. The gravity of such a diagnosis for patients and their families demands that tissue confirmation be obtained as often as possible. A definitive histological diagnosis of pancreatic cancer can be achieved 90% of the time by computed tomography–guided fine-needle aspiration of the pancreatic mass in patients who are not candidates for laparotomy[2] or by direct-needle biopsy or by fine-needle aspiration at laparotomy in patients whose cancer is found to be unresectable at operation.[3]

FOLLOW-UP OF PATIENTS WITH UNRESECTABLE DISEASE AT DIAGNOSIS

At diagnosis approximately 90% of patients with pancreatic cancer have tumor extension incompatible with surgical removal.[4] The most common causes of unresectability are hepatic metastases, peritoneal carcinomatosis, nodal involvement outside the bounds of pancreaticoduodenectomy, and invasion of the portal vein, superior mesenteric vein, or superior mesenteric artery. Although operative removal of all tumor is impossible under such conditions, palliative operations to relieve jaundice and gastric outlet obstruction are indicated in patients with reasonable performance status. Currently approximately 50% of patients with pancreatic carcinoma undergo cholecystojejunostomy or choledochojejunostomy with or without gastrojejunostomy as part of their management.[5] Patients with poor performance status or a limited life expectancy usually are treated by endoscopic stent placement for relief of jaundice. The follow-up of patients after palliative surgery or endoscopic stenting focuses on the detection and treatment of three clinical problems: recurrent jaundice, gastric outlet obstruction, and pain.

Recurrent jaundice and cholangitis occur more frequently after endoscopic stent placement than after surgical bypass of the biliary system. In four randomized trials of patients treated by endoscopic stent placement or surgical bypass, the incidence of recurrent jaundice was 19% to 38% after endoscopic stenting, compared with a risk of recurrent jaundice of zero to 16% after operation.[6-9] When endoscopic stents are placed for jaundice caused by pancreatic cancer, the average duration of patency is approximately 4 months. Recurrent jaundice after endoscopic stent placement is treated by stent exchange, which is almost always successful, or by surgical bypass in patients with good performance status. Recurrent jaundice after surgical bypass, although much rarer, is more difficult to treat. An endoscopic approach to the bile duct is not possible after the traditional Roux-en-Y bilioenteric anastomosis. A percutaneous transhepatic approach to the obstructed bile duct may be attempted in patients who otherwise continue to enjoy a reasonable quality of life, but this approach is associated with a significant risk of cholangitis under such circumstances and may be technically impossible if tumor recurrence is extensive. Reoperation is virtually never indicated for recurrent jaundice, since tumor progression in the porta hepatis makes the likelihood of a successful repeat bypass negligible.

In approximately 13% of patients who undergo biliary bypass alone for unresectable pancreatic carcinoma, gastric outlet obstruction requiring surgical correction develops.[10] The diagnosis is based on a history of new onset of vomiting of undigested food and is confirmed by a barium upper gastrointestinal series. When gastric outlet obstruction occurs, computed tomography of the abdomen is appropriate to determine whether the recurrent cancer is relatively localized, suggesting that surgery may add to life expectancy, or whether there is extensive carcinomatosis, in which case gastrojejunostomy is unlikely to add significantly to the quality or length of life.

Most patients with pancreatic cancer have moderate to severe abdominal or back pain before death, presumably from invasion of retroperitoneal neural plexuses. Oral or parenteral narcotics may be administered but frequently have undesirable side effects such as oversedation, nausea, or constipation.[11] A more effective strategy for pain control is percutaneous ablation of the celiac plexus with alcohol, a procedure readily performed in most medical centers. Celiac plexus blockade provides lasting relief of pain in approximately 75% of patients with pancreatic cancer and has a low incidence of complications.[12]

FOLLOW-UP OF PATIENTS AFTER APPARENTLY CURATIVE RESECTION

Medical centers with significant operative experience in pancreatic cancer currently report overall 5-year survival rates after pancreaticoduodenectomy ranging from 7% to 24%,[13-16] although the cure rate in patients with node-negative disease may reach nearly 40%. Smith and Meropol note the traditionally high rate of locoregional recurrence after pancreaticoduodenectomy. Recent modifications in the operative technique of pancreaticoduodenectomy (wider excision of retroperitoneal soft tissue and skeletonization of the superior mesenteric artery during resection of the uncinate process) should decrease the incidence of positive retroperitoneal margins after resection. Similarly, the increasing use of adjuvant radiation therapy for resectable pancreatic cancer should reduce local recurrence, although an increasing percentage of patients will probably have systemic recurrence as the first sign of treatment failure.

Although Smith and Meropol legitimately point out the need to evaluate patients regularly for digestive and other complaints after pancreaticoduodenectomy, most patients enjoy a good quality of life, equivalent in one study to patients undergoing cholecystectomy.[17] Nutrition and weight are usually well maintained. In fact, the onset of digestive complaints or weight loss after a Whipple procedure is often a harbinger of recurrent cancer and should lead to computed tomography of the abdomen.

A study of 14 patients who underwent pancreatectomy for carcinoma indicated that normalization of postoperative CA 19-9 levels to a value of 37 units/ml or less was associated with longer survival than in patients whose CA 19-9 levels failed to normalize.[18] Elevations of CA 19-9 in the postoperative period were also found to precede clinically apparent recurrence by 1 to 7 months. Determination of CA 19-9 in the preoperative and immediate postoperative periods may be justified in terms of providing the patient with some prognostic information. In the absence of effective therapy for recurrent disease, however, obtaining serial values of CA 19-9 in the postoperative period does not seem productive.

Recurrent disease after apparently curative resection usually appears in the liver, on peritoneal surfaces, in the retroperitoneal soft tissue, or in the lungs. It is usually most easily documented by computed tomography.

Overall, about 80% to 85% of patients undergoing apparently curative resection for carcinoma of the pancreas have recurrence. The median time to disease recurrence is approximately 1 year. With the increasing use of adjuvant radiation therapy for carcinoma of the pancreas, a shift from locoregional to distant recurrence is likely to occur. In the absence of effective therapy for recurrent disease, routine radiological or laboratory surveillance in postoperative follow-up is not indicated. The follow-up scheme recom-

Table 10-8 Follow-up of patients with pancreatic cancer: University of Washington Medical Center

	YEAR				
	1	2	3	4	5
Office visit	12	4	4	2	2
Complete blood count	1*	*	*	*	*
Liver function tests	1*	*	*	*	*
Electrolytes	1*	*	*	*	*
Chest x-ray	†	†	†	†	†
Abdominal computed tomography	†	†	†	†	†

*Performed once postoperatively, then only as clinically indicated. May be indicated on a routine basis during adjuvant chemotherapy or radiation therapy.
†Performed only as clinically indicated.

mended by Smith and Meropol is appropriate, although I would eliminate routine postoperative laboratory tests (Table 10-8). The detection of new symptoms in the follow-up period should be pursued with appropriate imaging studies to document recurrence and an attempt should be made to provide palliation of pain and other symptoms.

REFERENCES

1. Benning TL, Silverman JF, Berns LA, Geisinger KR. Fine needle aspiration of metastatic and hematological malignancies clinically mimicking pancreatic carcinoma. Acta Cytol 1992;36:471-6.
2. Edoute Y, Lemberg S, Malberger E. Preoperative and intraoperative fine needle aspiration cytology of pancreatic lesions. Am J Gastroenterol 1991;86:1015-9.
3. Earnhardt RC, McQuone SJ, Minasi JS, Feldman PS, Jones RS, Hanks JB. Intraoperative fine needle aspiration of pancreatic and extrahepatic biliary masses. Surg Gynecol Obstet 1993;177:147-52.
4. Freeny PC, Traverso LW, Ryan JA. Diagnosis and staging of pancreatic adenocarcinoma with dynamic computed tomography. Am J Surg 1993;165:600-6.
5. Wade TP, Radford DM, Virgo KS, Johnson FE. Complications and outcomes in the treatment of pancreatic adenocarcinoma in the United States veteran. J Am Coll Surg 1994;179:38-48.
6. Bornman PC, Harries-Jones EP, Tobias R, Van Stiegmann G, Terblanche J. Prospective controlled trial of transhepatic biliary endoprosthesis versus bypass surgery for incurable carcinoma of head of pancreas. Lancet 1986;1(8472):69-71.
7. Shepherd HA, Royle G, Ross AP, Diba A, Arthur M, Colin-Jones D. Endoscopic biliary endoprosthesis in the palliation of malignant obstruction of the distal common bile duct: a randomized trial. Br J Surg 1988;75:1166-8.
8. Andersen JR, Sorensen SM, Kruse A, Rokkjaer M, Matzen P. Randomized trial of endoscopic endoprosthesis versus operative bypass in malignant obstructive jaundice. Gut 1989;30:1132-5.
9. Dowsett JF, Russell RC, Hatfield AR, et al. Malignant obstructive jaundice: a prospective randomized trial of bypass surgery versus endoscopic stenting [abstract]. Gastroenterology 1989;96:A128.
10. Sarr MG, Cameron JL. Surgical management of unresectable carcinoma of the pancreas. Surgery 1982;91:123-33.
11. Mercadante S. Celiac plexus block versus analgesics in pancreatic cancer pain. Pain 1993;52:187-92.
12. Brown DL, Bulley CK, Quiel EL. Neurolytic celiac plexus block for pancreatic cancer pain. Anesth Analg 1987;66:869-73.
13. Nitecki SS, Sarr MG, Colby TV, van Heerden JA. Long-term survival after resection for ductal adenocarcinoma of the pancreas: is it really improving? Ann Surg 1995;221:59-66.
14. Yeo CJ, Cameron JL, Lillemoe KD, et al. Pancreaticoduodenectomy for cancer of the head of the pancreas: 201 patients. Ann Surg 1995;221:721-31.
15. Geer RJ, Brennan MF. Prognostic indicators for survival after resection of pancreatic adenocarcinoma. Am J Surg 1993;165:68-73.
16. Trede M, Schwall G, Saeger HD. Survival after pancreatoduodenectomy: 118 consecutive resections without an operative mortality. Ann Surg 1990;211:447-58.
17. McLeod RS, Taylor BR, O'Connor BI, et al. Quality of life, nutritional status, and gastrointestinal hormone profile following the Whipple procedure. Am J Surg 1995;169:179-85.
18. Glenn J, Steinberg WM, Kurtzman SH, Steinberg SM, Sindelar WF. Evaluation of the utility of a radioimmunoassay for serum CA19-9 levels in patients before and after treatment of carcinoma of the pancreas. J Clin Oncol 1988;6:462-8.

Table 10-9 Follow-up of patients with pancreatic cancer by institution

YEAR/PROGRAM	OFFICE VISIT	CBC	ELE	LFT	CXR	ABD CT	PELVIC CT	MCBT	LEU
Year 1									
Memorial Sloan-Kettering	4	4			1	1		4[a]	
Roswell Park	12	6	6	6	1	1	1		
Univ Washington	12	1[b]	1[b]	1[b]	[c]	[c]			
Japan: National Kyushu	12	12			4	2[d]	2[d]	4[e]	4
UK: Royal Liverpool	6	6		6	3	[f]			
Year 2									
Memorial Sloan-Kettering	3	3						3[a]	
Roswell Park	4	4	4	4	[f]	[f]	[f]		
Univ Washington	4	[b]	[b]	[b]	[c]	[c]			
Japan: National Kyushu	4	4			4	1[d]	1[d]	4[e]	4
UK: Royal Liverpool	4	4		4	[f]	[f]			
Year 3									
Memorial Sloan-Kettering	3	3						3[a]	
Roswell Park	4	4	4	4	[f]	[f]	[f]		
Univ Washington	4	[b]	[b]	[b]	[c]	[c]			
Japan: National Kyushu	4	4			2	1[d]	1[d]	2[e]	2
UK: Royal Liverpool	4	4		4	[f]	[f]			
Year 4									
Memorial Sloan-Kettering	2	2						2[a]	
Roswell Park	2	2	2	2	[f]	[f]	[f]		
Univ Washington	2	[b]	[b]	[b]	[c]	[c]			
Japan: National Kyushu	2	2			1	1[d]	1[d]	2[e]	2
UK: Royal Liverpool	2	2		2	[f]	[f]			
Year 5									
Memorial Sloan-Kettering	2	2						2[a]	
Roswell Park	2	2	2	2	[f]	[f]	[f]		
Univ Washington	2	[b]	[b]	[b]	[c]	[c]			
Japan: National Kyushu	2	2			1	[d]	[d]	2[e]	2
UK: Royal Liverpool	2	2		2	[f]	[f]			

ABD CT abdominal computed tomography
ABD US abdominal ultrasound
CBC complete blood count
CEA carcinoembryonic antigen
CHEST CT chest computed tomography
CXR chest x-ray
ELAS elastase I
ELE electrolytes
LEU leucine aminopeptidase
LFT liver function test
MCBT multichannel blood tests

CEA	CA 19-9	DUPAN-2	SPAN-1	CA-50	SLX	ELAS	CHEST CT	ABD US	PELVIC US
4	4	4	4	4	4	4	4	2[d]	2[d]
								3	
4	4	4	4	4	4	4	2	1[d]	1[d]
								[f]	
2	2	2	2	2	2	2	2	1[d]	1[d]
								[f]	
2	2	2	2	2	2	2	1	[d]	[d]
								[f]	
2	2	2	2	2	2	2	1	1[d]	1[d]
								[f]	

a Consists of glucose, blood urea nitrogen, creatinine, total bilirubin, uric acid, total protein, albumin, calcium, phosphorus, serum glutamic-oxaloacetic transaminase, lactic dehydrogenase, and alkaline phosphatase.

b Performed once postoperatively, then only as clinically indicated. May be indicated on a routine basis during adjuvant chemotherapy or radiation therapy.

c Performed only as clinically indicated.

d Computed tomography and ultrasonography are performed alternately to reduce cost.

e Includes total protein, glutamate-oxaloacetae transaminase, glutamate-pyruvic transaminase, bilirubin, alkaline phosphatase, cholesterol, blood urea nitrogen, and creatinine.

f Performed if symptoms warrant or if recurrence is suspected.

CHAPTER 11

Hepatobiliary Carcinoma

Memorial Sloan-Kettering Cancer Center

HOWARD M. KARPOFF AND YUMAN FONG

The liver is the most common solid organ site of cancer in the body. Because of its association with viral hepatitis, hepatobiliary carcinoma is a major public health problem, representing 90% of primary liver cancers, and is responsible for more than 1.25 million deaths per year around the world.[1] Other primary cancers of the hepatobiliary tree, including cholangiocarcinoma, gallbladder cancer, and primary sarcomas, occur less frequently but are important clinically because of the essential metabolic and immunological functions of the liver and because the complex anatomical relationships of the biliary tree make even the smallest tumors difficult to treat. For primary cancers of the liver other than lymphoma, surgical excision represents the only potentially curative option. Recurrences resulting either from incomplete resection and the growth of microscopic residual disease or from multicentricity[2] are not uncommon.

Every patient subjected to surgical treatment for a hepatobiliary cancer deserves follow-up. The goals of follow-up, however, vary depending on the type of cancer and stage of disease. These goals may include detection of recurrence, metachronous disease, associated medical problems, or postoperative problems; patient reassurance; and audit of the outcome of therapy. Detection of recurrent and metachronous cancers is important because effective treatment exists. In this chapter the three most common hepatobiliary tumors are discussed: hepatocellular carcinoma, cholangiocarcinoma, and gallbladder cancer. Justification is made for follow-up. There is no consensus regarding follow-up between gastroenterologists and surgeons, and the recommendations given here are those of the Hepatobiliary Surgical Service at Memorial Sloan-Kettering Cancer Center. It is clear from the following discussion that trials of new follow-up modalities are sorely needed, with outcomes determined not only by effectiveness but also by cost.

In terms of etiology, the role of infectious agents other than hepatitis B and C is not discussed because although other infectious agents have been associated with hepatobiliary cancers (such as *Schistosoma japonicum* with hepatobiliary carcinoma and the liver fluke *Opisthorchis viverrini* with cholangiocarcinoma), these agents account for virtually none of the cases seen in the United States. The molecular events leading to hepatobiliary cancers have not been well defined and are not discussed. Research has often focused on how certain etiological agents, such as the hepatitis viruses, cause either specific changes leading to neoplastic transformation or changes predisposing cells to subsequent transformation. Such a discussion is beyond the scope of this chapter. Finally, the chapter does not discuss the follow-up of patients after liver transplantation.

HEPATOCELLULAR CARCINOMA

Current Practice

Hepatocellular carcinoma represents the most common primary solid organ cancer. It is a disease of immense public health significance, causing the deaths of more than 1 million people worldwide each year.[1] The safety of partial hepatectomy for hepatocellular carcinoma has increased over the last three decades to the point that operative mortality rates of less than 5% can routinely be accomplished for noncirrhotic patients. Even for cirrhotic patients, operative mortality rates of approximately 10% can be achieved. Since surgical resection is the only curative therapy for this disease, providing approximately a 30% to 49% 5-year survival rate,[1,3] it represents standard therapy. Close follow-up is justified for patients after resection because effective treatment for recurrence exists. Furthermore, since this malignancy is associated with viral hepatitis and cirrhosis, the risk of metachronous second primary cancers, as well as the development of complications related to portal hypertension and cirrhosis, is significant. These, as well as social and academic reasons, more than justify follow-up.

Patterns of recurrence: effect of staging and histological studies

Distinction must be made between ordinary hepatocellular carcinoma and the fibrolamellar variant, since the clinical picture and outcome of these related diseases are very different[4] and therefore follow-up must also be different. In general, fibrolamellar hepatocellular carcinoma is a disease of the young, with a peak incidence in the late twenties and early thirties. Other characteristics that distinguish ordinary hepatocellular carcinoma from the fibrolamellar form are

Table 11-1 Comparison of hepatocellular carcinoma with fibrolamellar hepatocellular carcinoma*

CHARACTERISTIC	HEPATOCELLULAR CARCINOMA	FIBROLAMELLAR HEPATOCELLULAR CARCINOMA
Male/female	4:1 to 8:1	1:1
Resectability	Less than 25%	50% to 75%
Cirrhosis	60% to 80%	Less than 5%
Alpha-fetoprotein+	80%	Less than 5%
Hepatitis B	65%	Less than 5%

*Based on the authors' review of the literature.

Table 11-2 Results of repeat resection for hepatocellular carcinoma

REFERENCE	TOTAL PRIMARY RESECTIONS	NUMBER UNDER-GOING REPEAT RESECTION	5-YEAR SURVIVAL RATE (%)*
Nagasue, 1990[167]	161	20	26.8
Lin, 1991[86]	188	90	23.5
Matsuda, 1992[88]	100	16	51.2
Zhou, 1993[13]	392	65	41.8
Wu, 1993[31]	Not stated	72	36.1
Kakazu, 1993[26]	268	18	81.5
Imaoka, 1993[14]	275	15	77.0
Nakajima, 1993[168]	149	14	92.0
Shimada, 1994[24]	Not stated	33	40.0
Suenaga, 1994[28]	134	18	36.8
Lo, 1994[10]	277	12	26.0
Bismuth, 1995[169]	222	14	Not stated
Kawasaki, 1995[170]	112	21	Not stated

*Calculated from time of repeat resection.

listed in Table 11-1. The fibrolamellar type generally occurs in noncirrhotic patients, is not associated with viral hepatitis, and is not associated with an increase in circulating alpha-fetoprotein level. This cancer is found more often to be resectable but has a higher propensity to develop nodal metastases.[5] It is much less common than the nonfibrolamellar variety, and in the remainder of the discussion, comments will address the nonfibrolamellar type unless otherwise noted.

Recurrence rates after resection of hepatocellular carcinoma have been reported to be 20% to 80%[6-13] at 5 years, with the liver as a site of recurrence in up to 91% of these patients.[14] Other common sites of metastases include the lung, adrenal glands, other intraabdominal spread, and bone.[15] The incidence of recurrence relates directly to size,[3,16] DNA content,[17,18] nodal involvement, number of lesions resected,[16] vascular involvement by tumor,[3,16,19] and status of the margin of resection.[3,6] One study showed that perioperative blood transfusion was a risk factor for recurrence.[20] However, recurrence is influenced little by the degree of associated parenchymal disease. Cirrhotic patients surviving liver resection appear to have a tumor-free survival rate similar to that of noncirrhotic patients.[6,18,20]

Incidence of new primary cancer

Between 60% and 80% of patients with hepatocellular carcinoma have cirrhosis.[1,21] Clearly, cirrhosis from any cause can lead to malignant transformation of the hepatocyte. Patients with viral hepatitis are especially prone to new neoplasms. Epidemiological studies have determined that the risk for development of hepatocellular carcinoma in the setting of hepatitis B–related cirrhosis is approximately 0.5% per year.[22] Data on the development of hepatocellular carcinoma in the setting of hepatitis C are more preliminary but also more alarming; prevalence rates as high as 5% per year have been reported.[23] The rate of development of second neoplasms certainly is much less than the 60% to 70% chance of developing a recurrence from the first resected cancer. Nevertheless, in patients with cirrhosis, the possibility of development of second neoplasms demands that long-term follow-up be continued even after the chance of recurrence is remote.

Associated medical conditions

Since the patient with hepatocellular carcinoma often has associated cirrhosis, follow-up must have the goal not only of detecting treatable, recurrent cancer, but also of preventing and treating complications of associated parenchymal disease. Patients with alcoholism must be counseled, and patients with hemochromatosis should be followed to determine the need for treatment of iron overload with phlebotomy and iron chelation therapy. Vigilance must be greatest for complications of portal hypertension. It is estimated that up to one fourth of deaths after diagnosis of liver cancer are caused by gastrointestinal bleeding from portal hypertension.[15] Therefore all patients with cirrhosis must be assessed for worsening liver failure and portal hypertension, with constant reevaluation of the need for beta-blockade, diuresis, or portocaval shunting.

Outcome of treatment of recurrence

A major reason for follow-up of patients with hepatocellular carcinoma is that repeat resection is potentially curative for recurrences. A number of reports have shown that although the majority of recurrences after liver resection involve the liver, less than 30% of these are resectable. However, in patients found to have both adequate liver reserve and technically resectable tumors, repeat hepatic resection may be performed safely and result in long-term, disease-free survival.[7] One study comparing repeat liver resections with first-time resections found no difference in blood loss, operative time, and incidence of complications.[24] Not only is surgical excision a relatively safe treatment, aggressive surgical treatment for recurrent disease has been shown to improve outcome and provide long-term survival with a 5-year survival rate between 20% and 80% (Table 11-2).[10,25-30] A study of 72 patients undergoing reoperation for recurrent disease found a

36.1% 5-year survival rate after a second resection and a 36.7% 3-year survival rate after a third resection.[31] A Japanese series of 78 patients undergoing reoperation showed a 54.7% 5-year survival rate after reoperation and a 34.6% 5-year survival rate after a third resection.[30] Comparing palliative treatment, surgery, and transcatheter arterial embolization, patients treated with surgery had the longest survival, with a 48% 5-year survival rate.[27] Surgical resection has also been carried out for selected cases of extrahepatic metastases with long-term survival.[32-34]

Few data exist examining the utility of total hepatectomy and liver transplant in the treatment of recurrent hepatocellular carcinoma.[35] Currently, with the limited number of donors,[35] this approach must be regarded as experimental.

Many ablative techniques have been used for the treatment of hepatocellular carcinoma, including cryoablation,[36,37] transcatheter arterial embolization,[38,39] and percutaneous ethanol injection,[40,41] with varying degrees of effectiveness. Few studies have compared these ablative techniques to repeat resection. The retrospective studies that do exist, however, indicate a significant survival advantage for surgery when compared with transcatheter arterial embolization.[7,42,43] These ablative techniques may provide effective palliation, with specific roles appropriate for each technique. Certainly, in a patient undergoing laparotomy for possible repeat resection, cryoablation should be contemplated if the tumor is found to be unresectable. Percutaneous ethanol injection should be considered for small unresectable recurrences. In a select series of recurrent hepatocellular carcinoma less than 3 cm, treatment with percutaneous ethanol injection had a 5-year survival rate of 46.7%.[44] A combination of transcatheter arterial embolization with percutaneous ethanol injection has also been used with success as palliative therapy for patients with recurrent hepatocellular carcinoma.[45] Ample data are available to suggest that these ablative therapies may provide effective palliation for recurrent disease.[46-48]

Systemic chemotherapy produces partial responses in approximately 20% of patients. The utility of systemic chemotherapy, even in cases of disseminated disease, is debated. For disease localized to the liver, local ablative methods are favored. Some believe that systemic chemotherapy should not be used except in clinical trials because of its low efficacy and high toxicity.[49] Intraarterial chemotherapy has been shown to have consistently higher response rates than systemic treatment.[21] A Japanese study of treatment for recurrent disease compared repeat resection, chemoembolization, and no therapy and demonstrated surgery to be significantly better than chemoembolization, which was better than no treatment.[50] We do not use adjuvant therapy routinely for surgically resectable hepatobiliary disease.

Role of history and physical examination

Histories elicited from patients during follow-up should address symptoms of worsening portal hypertension or liver failure. Symptoms of biliary obstruction, including itching and changes in stool or urine color, should be sought. Any new pain in the right upper quadrant or bone pain should stimulate investigation by appropriate radiological examinations. Physical examination should seek new masses, worsening ascites, and jaundice. Symptomatic tumors, however, usually indicate far advanced recurrence. It is the detection of asymptomatic recurrences by tumor markers or imaging tests that will yield the majority of treatable recurrences.

Table 11-3 Approximate cost of follow-up (in U.S. dollars per test)*

TEST	COST
Alpha-fetoprotein	90
Alkaline phosphatase	15
Alkaline phosphatase isoenzymes	80
Antithrombin III	80
CEA	70
CA 19-9	60
CA-125	100
Gamma-glutamyltransferase	30
Serum glutamic-oxaloacetic transaminase	20
Serum glutamic-pyruvic transaminase	20
Ultrasound	250-400
Computed tomography	500-900
Magnetic resonance imaging	600-1000

CEA, Carcinoembryonic antigen.
*Dollar figures represent average charges for the New York tri-state area.

Role of blood tests and tumor markers

Routine liver function tests are useful for evaluating the status of associated liver diseases. Alterations in liver enzymes such as alkaline phosphatase are seen with recurrences, but no routinely measured liver function test has a high enough predictive value to be considered diagnostic of recurrent cancer. Gamma-glutamyltransferase isoenzymes are being investigated for their utility in following patients after treatment of hepatocellular carcinoma.[51] In this study, gamma-glutamyltransferase-II was positive in 90% of 90 cases and negative in most patients who have only chronic liver disease or extrahepatic tumors. Gamma-glutamyltransferase-II appeared to be more sensitive than alpha-fetoprotein, particularly for smaller tumors and in alpha-fetoprotein-negative tumors. Other variant enzymes of gamma-glutamyltransferase and alkaline phosphatase are also under investigation for their usefulness in diagnosis or follow-up.[52,53] None of these isoenzymes are routinely available, and their use must still be regarded as investigational. A comparison of the costs of the isoenzymes can be found in Table 11-3.

Alpha-fetoprotein remains the standard tumor marker. Approximately 60% to 80% of hepatocellular carcinomas are associated with increased alpha-fetoprotein levels.[54] However, recurrence or progression of a tumor as detected by imaging techniques need not be accompanied by alterations in circulating alpha-fetoprotein levels.[55] Nevertheless, an alpha-fetoprotein level greater than 400 ng/ml is diagnostic of recurrence. During close follow-up, levels are seldom allowed to

Table 11-4 Tumor markers for follow-up of primary liver cancers

MARKER	SENSITIVITY (%)	SPECIFICITY (%)
HEPATOCELLULAR CARCINOMA		
Alpha-fetoprotein[60,62]	44-66	72
Alpha-fetoprotein subspecies[171]	81	85
Alpha-fetoprotein + lentil lectin[58,172,173]	36-73	96-100
Alpha-fetoprotein + DCP[60,66]	78-85	69.4
Alkaline phosphatase[52]	60	*
Antithrombin III	*	*
CA-195[74]	60	22
CA 19-9[73,174]	44	73*
DCP[60,63,66,175]	35-66	Greater than 95
Gamma-glutamyltransferase-II[51-53]	60-90	97
Serum alpha-1-fucosidase[70,71,76]	76-84	91-94
CHOLANGIOCARCINOMA		
CA 19-9[162,177]	*	*
CEA[162,177]	*	*
CA 19-9 + CEA[178]	Accuracy of 86%	
CCA-specific antigen[179]	*	*
DUPAN-2[142,180]	*	*
CA-195[142,180]	*	*
GALLBLADDER CANCER		
CEA[166]	89	88

DCP, Des-gamma-carboxy prothrombin; *CEA,* carcinoembryonic antigen.
*Data not available.

reach such high levels, since the size of the lesion is related to alpha-fetoprotein level. Researchers have begun to examine the utility of isoforms of alpha-fetoprotein as predictors of recurrence. Studies evaluating fucosylated alpha-fetoprotein do not indicate that this form is more effective than alpha-fetoprotein alone.[56] However, an index of fucosylation may be useful in evaluating patients with chronic liver disease when alpha-fetoprotein may be chronically elevated. Additional work has been done evaluating levels of alpha-fetoprotein reactive to lentil lectin, indicating that use of lentil-dependent fractionation of alpha-fetoprotein may be more sensitive and specific than conventional alpha-fetoprotein.[57-59] Tests for these isoforms are cumbersome and are not widely available. At present, conventional alpha-fetoprotein remains the tumor marker of choice. Table 11-4 gives the sensitivity and specificity levels of various tumor markers.

Des-gamma-carboxy prothrombin (DCP), also known as protein induced by vitamin K absence or antagonist II, has been evaluated as a tumor marker for hepatocellular carcinoma and appears to be less sensitive but more specific than alpha-fetoprotein.[60] Even though some researchers have begun to use DCP in monthly screening examinations,[24,26,29] the main utility of this marker may be in combination with alpha-fetoprotein or in the setting of a negative alpha-fetoprotein result. DCP may be elevated in up to 50% of patients who have hepatocellular carcinoma and normal alpha-fetoprotein levels. A study of 165 patients in Japan found that analyzing plasma DCP levels combined with alpha-fetoprotein was useful for both diagnosis and prognosis of hepatocellular carcinoma, as well as for monitoring of postoperative recurrences.[61] Other studies have also supported a role for this marker in combination with alpha-fetoprotein,[11,62-65] these two markers together increasing the sensitivity of detecting recurrent tumors to more than 85%.[66] Few studies have shown DCP to be superior to alpha-fetoprotein, however, and the studies showing little utility for this marker[67,68] have prevented it from gaining wide acceptance.

A number of other serum markers have been suggested as potential diagnostic tools. Markers such as antithrombin III[69] or serum alpha-L-fucosidase[70-72] are being tested, but the data are too preliminary to advocate these as standard markers. CA 19-9[73] and CA-195[74] have not been found useful. Monoclonal antibodies against tumor-specific antigens, such as HG1-219[75] or KM-2,[76] are being investigated, but initial data indicate that the major role for these is in patients with low alpha-fetoprotein levels. None of these tumor markers have surpassed alpha-fetoprotein in usefulness, and the use of any other marker in the follow-up of classic hepatocellular carcinoma must be considered investigational.

The fibrolamellar variant usually does not secrete alpha-fetoprotein; therefore alpha-fetoprotein is usually not used in the follow-up of these patients. Other markers that may be secreted by fibrolamellar hepatocellular carcinoma include neurotensin,[77-79] CEA,[80] and vitamin B_{12}–binding protein capacity.[80-82] Besides CEA, these tests are expensive and not readily available (Table 11-3). The current practice at Memorial Sloan-Kettering Cancer Center is to store serum of any patient with suspected fibrolamellar hepatocellular carcinoma. If final pathological findings on the resected specimen prove the tumor to be fibrolamellar hepatocellular carcinoma, the serum is sent for the various marker studies. Any patient found to have elevated preoperative circulating tumor markers is followed up postoperatively using such markers.

Role of imaging studies

The most likely site of recurrent disease after liver resection is the liver. Ultrasound, computed tomography, and magnetic resonance imaging have been used to monitor for liver and other intraabdominal recurrence. Ultrasound has had the longest record and widest availability and certainly is the least expensive (Table 11-3). However, macroregenerative nodules in the cirrhotic liver may be confused with tumor on ultrasound.[83] Furthermore, certain subtypes of hepatocellular carcinoma, particularly well-differentiated lesions, are isodense with the nonneoplastic liver parenchyma on ultrasound and thus are difficult to distinguish. Techniques such as ultrasound employing microbubbling carbon dioxide may be more sensitive than conventional methods[84] but are not widely used. Nevertheless, a combination of alpha-fetoprotein and abdominal ultrasound is the most common strategy for follow-up.[85,86]

Table 11-5 Follow-up of patients with hepatobiliary cancer (hepatocellular carcinoma): Memorial Sloan-Kettering Cancer Center

	YEAR				
	1	2	3	4	5
Office visit	4	4	4	4	4
Liver function tests*	4	4	4	4	4
Alpha-fetoprotein*,†	4	4	4	4	4
Abdominal ultrasound‡,§	4	4	4	4	4
Abdominal computed tomography§	1	1	1	1	1
Chest x-ray	1	1	1	1	1

*Performed monthly for patients with persistently elevated tumor markers.
†For patients with fibrolamellar hepatocellular carcinoma, substitute neurotensin or other markers found to be elevated in the preresectional blood test.
‡Performed every 6 months for patients with elevated tumor marker levels before surgery.
§Performed every 2 months until recurrence is detected for patients with persistently elevated tumor markers.

Computed tomography and magnetic resonance imaging are more accurate modalities for identification and characterization of new liver lesions. If a potential recurrence is discovered by any modality, further localization studies including computed tomography of the chest, abdomen, and pelvis, magnetic resonance imaging of the liver, or angiography are useful to evaluate the extent of disease and to determine resectability.

Routine follow-up chest x-ray should be performed because of the likelihood of lung metastases. Physicians at Memorial Sloan-Kettering Cancer Center do not routinely perform bone scans except in the case of suspicious symptoms or as part of a preoperative workup for repeat resection when recurrences are found.

Current Recommendations

Many groups have suggested monthly or bimonthly follow-up of patients after resection with blood tests including liver function tests and tumor markers,[24,26,29] and others have suggested an ultrasound examination every 3 months with magnetic resonance imaging[87] or computed tomography scans every 6 to 12 months.[9,24,28,88-90] These schedules are too frequent. Hepatomas are generally slow-growing tumors, with a doubling time of 1 to 19 months (median 4 months).[15] A follow-up schedule of office visits every 3 months is adequate, since it is unlikely that very small recurrences will be identified with certainty, and even less likely that any invasive intervention will be performed for small suspect lesions. When a small lesion is noted, further workup to rule out other sites of recurrence should be performed and the patient followed up more closely.

The routine follow-up of a patient after resection should include an office visit 2 to 3 weeks after hospital discharge. Liver function tests, as well as tumor marker levels, are drawn. For classic hepatocellular carcinoma the tumor marker should usually be alpha-fetoprotein, while for the fibrolamellar variant it should be neurotensin or other markers that have been found to be elevated in the preresectional blood test. For patients found to have elevated tumor marker levels preoperatively a return of tumor marker levels to normal postoperatively should prompt routine follow-up, consisting of office visits every 3 months with physical examination and measurement of liver function tests and tumor marker levels (Table 11-5). Patients should also be followed by an abdominal ultrasound every 6 months and a yearly computed tomography of the abdomen; a chest x-ray is also obtained yearly. The reasons for the diligence in abdominal and particularly liver follow-up are that these are the most common sites of recurrence and that recurrences in the liver can still be treated with good palliation and potential cure. Outcomes of treatment for pulmonary or bony recurrence are never curative, and the outlook is dismal. Therefore follow-up at these sites is undertaken with less diligence.

For patients with no detectable elevations in tumor marker levels before surgery, abdominal ultrasound is used more liberally, usually at intervals of every 3 months. Computed tomographic scans of the abdomen and chest x-rays are still obtained yearly. For patients whose circulating tumor markers do not return to normal levels after surgery the likelihood of persistent disease is high. Patients with persistently elevated tumor marker levels should be seen monthly for repeat liver function tests and tumor marker studies until either the markers return to normal levels or recurrence is detected. Abdominal imaging should be performed every 2 months until the recurrence is detected.

Such close follow-up should be performed for the first 5 years after resection. Even after the first 5 years, patients should be surveyed every 6 months, since the potential for recurrence[10] or new metachronous tumors still exists, particularly in patients with cirrhosis. Complications from cirrhosis and portal hypertension may also arise.

CHOLANGIOCARCINOMA

Current Practice

Cholangiocarcinomas, cancers that arise from the biliary epithelium, are rare, occurring in fewer than 4,500 patients in the United States each year.[91] Although they represent much less of a public health problem than hepatocellular carcinoma, the majority of patients with untreated bile duct cancers die within a year of diagnosis.[92,93] Surgical excision is the treatment of choice; no other therapy offers potential for cure. The most common immediate causes of death are hepatic failure or cholangitis related to tumor growth and inadequate drainage of the biliary tree.[94,95] The objectives of management of cholangiocarcinomas must include not only complete removal of the tumor, but also biliary drainage. It has become clear over the last three decades that curative treatment of tumors involving the upper third of the bile duct depends greatly on aggressive excision, often requiring a major liver resection. Tumors involving the middle or lower third of the bile duct may require a pancreaticoduodenectomy for extirpation. Because such aggressive and radical surgery is needed for resection of disease, resections are usually performed at major referral centers. The radical nature of the procedures required to extirpate disease is reflected in the high morbidity and mortality associated with surgical treatment. Until as recently as 10 years ago, excision of hilar cholangiocarcinomas was associated with a mortality rate as high as 30%[96-100] and excision of distal tumors was associated with a mortality rate as high as 25%.[94,101-105] Recent results indicate a major improvement in safety of these operations, so that resections of hilar tumors can be accomplished with a mortality rate of only approximately 10%,[97,99,106,107] even when liver resections are required. Moreover, pancreaticoduodenectomies may be performed with a perioperative mortality rate of approximately 5%.[108]

Patterns of recurrence and follow-up

For patients with hilar cholangiocarcinoma, complete resection (negative margins) is associated with median survival time on the order of 24 months,[97,99,107,109] which compares favorably with median survival time of 6 to 12 months for patients receiving only palliative bypasses. Surgical resection provides not only improved survival, but also improved quality of survival.[110] The 5-year survival rate after complete resection for both proximal and distal bile duct tumors is approximately 30%.[98,107,111] The greatest risk factors for recurrence are margin-positive resection,[112] node-positive tumor,[113] and vascular involvement by tumor.[114,115] The most likely site of recurrence is local[116] within the bile duct, local lymph nodes, or the liver. The most likely cause of death from recurrent disease is cholangitis or liver failure.[114]

The goals of follow-up after resection are very different from those for hepatocellular carcinoma. Because of the delicate anatomical area within which cholangiocarcinomas occur and the radical procedures required for resection of the primary tumor, a repeat resection with curative intent is unlikely to be possible. Follow-up is therefore directed mainly at diagnosis of symptomatic recurrence to direct palliative therapy, diagnosis of long-term benign complications of surgical treatment (such as biliary stricture and ulcer disease), patient reassurance, and audit of results of treatment. Although cholangiocarcinoma in one site has been associated with second neoplasms in the biliary tree,[117] a major portion of the extrahepatic biliary tree, including the gallbladder, is likely to be resected at the first operation. Therefore surveillance for second neoplasms in the biliary tree is usually not a major goal in the follow-up of patients.

Outcome of treatment of recurrence

Surgical treatment for potential cure has been shown to be effective only in rare recurrent cases.[118] Second local excisions seldom have a curative result. The value of liver transplant for unresectable cholangiocarcinoma is questionable; even more so is the utility of transplant for recurrent disease.[119] The primary aim of treatment of recurrent disease is palliation.

The three main goals of palliation are relief of symptomatic jaundice, relief of cholangitis, and slowing of tumor progression. For biliary drainage to relieve jaundice or cholangitis, either surgical drainage[120] or drainage by percutaneous or endoscopic means can be effective.[121-124] In patients with either previous common bile duct excision or pancreaticoduodenostomy, however, endoscopic drainage has only a limited role, and percutaneous drainage is usually chosen when surgery is to be avoided. Unfortunately, stenting is associated with a high rate of recurrent cholangitis and jaundice.[125,126] Therefore, in patients with limited local recurrence, hepaticojejunostomy may be the most effective palliation.[127] Thus surgical palliation or bypass is our recommendation. However, in patients with very advanced disease and limited life span, percutaneous transhepatic drainage may be preferable.

For primary tumors, intraluminal brachytherapy[120,128] or external beam radiation therapy[129,130] may improve palliation and even survival. If recurrence is clearly very localized, radiation therapy is the best option for control of tumor. In these cases adequate biliary drainage combined with brachytherapy and external beam radiation is favored.

Systemic chemotherapy is a poor alternative, with response rates of 20%.[131] All other therapies must be considered experimental, including intraarterial chemoembolization,[132] regional chemotherapy by infusion,[133,134] somatostatin,[135] or radiation therapy with ^{131}I-anti-CEA.[136] The intent for these treatments of recurrence is palliation.

Role of routine blood tests and tumor markers

A rising alkaline phosphatase or gamma-glutamyltranspeptidase level is a good indicator of evolving biliary obstruction.[137] It does not always indicate tumor recurrence, however, since as many as 10% of patients with biliary surgical reconstruction eventually have a benign anastomotic stricture.[138] Nevertheless, a rising alkaline phosphatase level, particularly in the first few years after resection of tumor, prompts great concern about recurrence.

Patients with a Roux-en-Y biliary reconstruction have a higher chance of peptic ulcer disease.[139] During follow-up, vigilance should be maintained for the development of such complications. Therefore routine blood work used in the follow-up of such patients includes liver function tests, including bilirubin levels and alkaline phosphatase, as well as complete blood count to look for a fall in hematocrit indicative of gastrointestinal bleeding.

A high percentage of biliary malignancies express CEA or other tumor markers such as CA 19-9.[140,141] A new tumor marker, CCA-specific antigen, seen in an animal model and also found in humans, is being evaluated.[141] A study from Czechoslovakia showed higher levels of DUPAN-2 and CA-195 in patients with cholangiocarcinoma than in those with benign common bile duct lesions, but their clinical utilities have yet to be established.[142] The utility of any tumor marker in the follow-up of cholangiocarcinoma, however, is questionable (Table 11-4). Such tests are expensive (Table

Table 11-6 Follow-up of patients with hepatobiliary cancer (cholangiocarcinoma or gallbladder cancer): Memorial Sloan-Kettering Cancer Center

	YEAR				
	1	2	3	4	5
Office visit	4	4	4	4	4
Complete blood count	4	4	4	4	4
Liver function tests	4	4	4	4	4
Chest x-ray	1	1	1	1	1
Abdominal computed tomography*	1	1	1	1	1
CEA	†	†	†	†	†

CEA, Carcinoembryonic antigen.
*Performed twice a year for the first 2 years after cholecystectomy for patients with T1 gallbladder cancer.
†Performed at each office visit after cholecystectomy for patients with T1 gallbladder cancer.

Table 11-7 Risks of spread of gallbladder cancer as related to depth of penetration of primary tumor

DEPTH OF PRIMARY TUMOR		N+ (%)	PERITONEAL DISSEMINATION (%)
T1	Mucosal/muscularis	*	*
T2	Subserosal	29	7
T3	2 cm or less beyond serosa	43	14
T4	More than 2 cm	48	22

Data from Matsumoto Y, Fujii H, Aoyama H, Yamamoto M, Sugahara K, Suda K. Am J Surg 1992;163:239-45.
*No increased risk.

11-3), and recurrence is unlikely to be cured. Moreover, picking up an early recurrence by tumor markers alone is unlikely to change clinical therapy, since palliation of clinical symptoms is the main goal in the treatment of recurrences. Therefore tumor markers should not be routinely used in the follow-up of patients with cholangiocarcinoma. If a patient has jaundice, itching, or sepsis, a workup is performed to determine the cause. It is then that one of the tumor markers may assist in the diagnosis of recurrent malignant disease.

Role of imaging studies

The use of routine imaging studies for follow-up after resection of a cholangiocarcinoma is questionable. These imaging tests are even more expensive than tumor markers. In the absence of symptoms a finding on these imaging studies is unlikely to prompt clinical intervention and is sure to prompt anxiety. There is no clear reason for routinely performing imaging studies on patients after resection, except as a tool to audit outcomes of primary therapy. Clearly, clinical trials on the utility of tumor markers and imaging studies in the follow-up of patients after therapy for cholangiocarcinoma are needed and should be conducted with cost effectiveness as one outcome parameter.

When symptoms of jaundice develop, an abdominal sonogram should be obtained. This can be used to assess intrahepatic ductal dilatation, as well as portal vein patency. The need for further imaging with computed tomography or direct cholangiography is usually dictated by the sonographic findings.

Current Recommendations

The routine follow-up of a patient after resection of cholangiocarcinoma includes an office visit 2 to 3 weeks after hospital discharge. Physical examination, complete blood count, and liver function tests are performed to assess postoperative recovery and complications. Further routine follow-up should consist of office visits every 3 months with physical examination and measurement of liver function tests. A yearly chest x-ray and abdominal computed tomography scan should be obtained (Table 11-6).

GALLBLADDER CANCER

Current Practice

Gallbladder cancer, representing 5,000 cases per year worldwide,[143] is a rare malignancy with a dismal outlook because of its insidious onset, propensity for metastases, and rapid progression.[144] It is associated with cholelithiasis and is found in 1% of gallbladders removed for gallstones. Surgical resection is the treatment of choice and the only potentially curative therapy. However, the 5-year survival rate is less than 20% in all series.[143,145] The extent of surgical resection is controversial, with recommendations ranging from simple cholecystectomy to radical excision that includes extended right hepatectomy and even pancreatectomy. The goal of complete surgical excision can be accomplished only by a procedure that aims to remove the gallbladder, any involved tissue at the cystic duct–common bile duct junction, involved lymphatic tissue, and involved liver tissue. The risk of spread of disease to adjacent tissues and lymphatics can be predicted from the depth of penetration of the tumor through the gallbladder (Table 11-7).[146] For T1 tumors, which are usually discovered by pathological examination after cholecystectomy for cholelithiasis or small polyps, lymphatic metastases are uncommon and no excision beyond a complete cholecystectomy is needed. For T2 to T4 lesions the risk of lymphatic metastases and liver extension is greater. Therefore the common bile duct, periductal nodes, and peripancreatic nodes, as well as the liver tissues adjacent to the gallbladder, should be excised. Even though T4 lesions or lymph node–positive lesions are much more likely to recur, they are by no means incurable.[147] Particularly since alternative therapies have poor outcomes, patients who are otherwise medically fit and have localized disease should undergo radical resection as the only hope for cure.

Patterns of recurrence and follow-up

Clinical data indicate that an aggressive approach is reasonable. In a collected review of the recent Japanese experience

Table 11-8 Staging of gallbladder cancer

TX	Presence of tumor cannot be assessed
T0	No evidence of tumor
Tis	Carcinoma in situ
T1	Mucosal/muscularis
T2	Subserosal
T3	2 cm or less beyond serosa
T4	More than 2 cm
N0	No histological evidence of metastasis to regional lymph nodes
N1	Pericystic and pericholedochal nodes
N2	Retroportal and posterosuperior pancreatic nodes
M0	No (known) distant metastasis
M1	Distant metastasis present

Stage	***Grouping***	***5-Year Survival Rate*** *(%)*[181]
Stage 0	Tis, N0, M0	
Stage I	T1, T2; N0, M0	59
Stage II	T3, T4; N0, M0	40
Stage III	T3, T4; N1, N2; M0	9
Stage IV	T3, T4; N0-N2; M1	7

From American Joint Committee on Cancer, Beahrs OH, Henson DE, Hutter RV, Kennedy BJ, editors. Manual for staging of cancer. Philadelphia: JB Lippincott Company, 1992.

involving 4,567 cases, the 5-year survival rate of patients who did not undergo exploration for resection (n = 765) was zero; for those undergoing exploration but not resection (n = 1342) it was 1.5%; for those subjected to nonradical resections (n = 702) survival was 6.2%; and for those subjected to radical resections it was 50.7%.[147] Median survival for patients with nonresectable disease is on the order of 2 months.[148,149] For tumors with transmural penetration, 5-year survival after simple cholecystectomy is rare, while radical resection offers the potential for long-term survival.[148-152]

Stage of gallbladder cancer (Table 11-8) is a reliable predictor of clinical outcome. Stage I (T1) gallbladder cancers are adequately treated by simple cholecystectomy, while stage I (T2) through stage III gallbladder cancers should be treated by radical resection. Stage IV is incurable and is usually fatal within weeks of diagnosis.[153] Other predictors of recurrence not incorporated into the staging system include spillage of tumor and positive margins.[16,154] Whether gallbladder cancers discovered during laparoscopic cholecystectomy have a poorer prognosis is unknown.[155]

The most common site of recurrence is intraabdominal, presenting as a new liver, periportal, or retropancreatic mass.[156] For these presentations jaundice is not an uncommon sign. Recurrence may also manifest itself as carcinomatosis. Death is likely to be due to biliary sepsis or liver failure.

Gallbladder cancer is usually a rapidly growing tumor that requires a radical surgical resection for eradication. If the surgical resection appropriate for the particular stage of disease is performed, a more extensive resection for recurrence will be difficult to perform. Therefore recurrence is rarely treatable with curative results. The main goal of follow-up after resection of gallbladder cancer is to provide palliation for symptomatic recurrences. The exception is T1 gallbladder cancer treated with a simple cholecystectomy: local recurrence in these patients may be treatable with a more radical resection. Given that the cure rate in T1 or Tis gallbladder cancer is greater than 95%,[153] the cost effectiveness of close follow-up of this group for the few patients who will benefit from early tumor discovery and radical repeat resection begs for investigation. The other goals of follow-up are similar to those of cholangiocarcinomas, which are diagnosis of long-term, benign complications of surgical treatment (biliary stricture, ulcer disease, and so on), patient reassurance, and audit of results of treatment.

Outcome of treatment of recurrence

If recurrent disease is found after resection, prognosis is exceedingly poor. Although anecdotal reports have documented the feasibility of a repeat resection for recurrences,[157] it is the rare case for which a second excision is possible. This is due to a number of factors. The complex reconstruction performed after the primary resection makes early diagnosis of recurrent disease extremely difficult. Although local recurrence is common, it is usually in the context of other intraabdominal spread. Even if the recurrence is locally confined, the previous radical excision makes a second resection technically challenging. Therefore, except for cases of early-stage disease that were treated by cholecystectomy, it is unusual to find a resectable recurrence.

A study from Czechoslovakia demonstrated only a 1% to 5% 5-year survival rate after diagnosis of recurrence.[145] The main goals of treatment are therefore relief of symptomatic jaundice, relief of cholangitis, and a slowing of further tumor progression. Although biliary drainage to relieve jaundice or cholangitis can be accomplished by surgical bypass or by percutaneous or endoscopic means, unlike the situation in cholangiocarcinomas, a nonsurgical approach is usually favored. This stems from the fact that gallbladder cancer is a much more rapid-growing tumor. Patients with stage IV disease usually survive only a few weeks or months. Therefore the long-term patency rates of biliary stents are a secondary issue and the hospitalization and recovery time from a surgical bypass are usually not justified. Most patients with recurrent gallbladder cancer and symptomatic jaundice are treated by percutaneous transhepatic stenting to avoid operative intervention.

Radiation therapy and chemotherapy may play a role in the management of recurrent disease. Few trials have analyzed the effects of radiation therapy and chemotherapy because of the limited numbers of cases per year, but at least one study has shown improvement in survival with adjuvant chemotherapy.[158] Several studies have examined radiation therapy for unresectable gallbladder cancer with good palliation.[159] Intraoperative radiation therapy and high-dose intraluminal brachytherapy[160] have been used for treatment of residual disease, but their palliative uses are unknown.[161] In addition, there have been no large studies reporting the effects of radiation therapy or chemotherapy on recurrent disease. For chemotherapy, numerous case reports exist in the literature of various single agents being employed with effectiveness. In one such case report a retroperitoneal node recurrence after gallbladder cancer was treated with tegafur-uracil and cisplatin-etoposide.[162] Other reports suggest that 5-fluorouracil may improve outcome,[163,164] as may the use of hepatic artery infusion devices.[25,165] Overall, the data do not indicate a definitive role for chemotherapy and radiation therapy in recurrent disease. Therefore the decision to offer such therapy to patients with recurrent disease who have very limited life spans should be carefully considered.

Role of routine blood tests and tumor markers

As in the follow-up of patients after resection of cholangiocarcinomas, liver function tests are used to define the condition of patients with recurrence or benign long-term complications of surgery. CEA is often expressed by gallbladder cancer, and serum CEA levels have been advocated as a tool in the diagnosis of this malignancy (Table 11-4).[166] The use of CEA in follow-up, however, is questionable. It is expensive and unlikely to find a recurrence that will be cured. Detecting an early recurrence by tumor markers alone is unlikely to change clinical therapy, since palliation of clinical symptoms is the main goal in treatment of recurrences. Therefore tumor markers should not be routinely used in the follow-up of patients with gallbladder cancer. If a patient has jaundice, itching, or sepsis, a workup is performed to determine the cause and extent of disease. It is then that CEA may assist in the diagnosis of recurrent malignant disease.

Role of imaging studies

The use of imaging studies to follow gallbladder cancer after resection is not routine. An abnormality on these imaging studies is unlikely to prompt clinical intervention in an asymptomatic patient. The exception to this is the patient with early-stage cancer after simple cholecystectomy. Even though the recurrence rate is low, this is the group for whom repeat resection of recurrences may be possible. Follow-up of these patients by imaging studies in the first 2 years, when the possibility of recurrence is highest, is advocated. Otherwise, except as a tool to audit outcomes of primary therapy, routine imaging studies are unnecessary for patients after resection. As with cholangiocarcinoma, clinical trials on the utility of tumor markers and imaging studies in the follow-up of patients after therapy are needed.

Once jaundice develops, an abdominal sonogram should be obtained. This allows an assessment of intrahepatic ductal dilatation and portal vein patency. The need for further imaging with computed tomography or direct cholangiography is usually dictated by the sonographic findings.

Current Recommendations

The routine follow-up of a patient after resection of gallbladder cancer should include an office visit 2 to 3 weeks after hospital discharge. Physical examination and liver function tests should be performed to assess postoperative recovery and complications. Further routine follow-up should consist of office visits every 3 months with physical examination and measurement of liver function (Table 11-6). A yearly chest x-ray and abdominal computed tomographic scan are obtained. Patients with T1 gallbladder cancer discovered after cholecystectomy have a slightly different follow-up. For these patients biannual computed tomography of the abdomen for the first 2 years and measurement of CEA levels at each office visit are advocated.

REFERENCES

1. Wanebo HJ, Vezeridis MP. Hepatoma. J Surg Oncol Suppl 1993; 3:40-5.
2. Prempracha N, Tengchaisri T, Chawengkirttikul R, et al. Identification and potential use of a soluble tumor antigen for the detection of liver-fluke-associated cholangiocarcinoma induced in a hamster model. Int J Cancer 1994;57:691-5.
3. Sugioka A, Tsuzuki T, Kanai T. Postresection prognosis of patients with hepatocellular carcinoma. Surgery 1993;113:612-8.
4. Craig JR, Peters RL, Edmondson HA, Omata M. Fibrolamellar carcinoma of the liver: a tumor of adolescents and young adults with distinctive clinico-pathologic features. Cancer 1980;46:372-9.
5. Vauthey JN, Klimstra D, Franceschi D, et al. Factors affecting long-term outcome after hepatic resection for hepatocellular carcinoma. Am J Surg 1995;169:28-35.
6. Chen MF, Hwang TL, Jeng LB, Wang CS, Jan YY, Chen SC. Postoperative recurrence of hepatocellular carcinoma: two hundred five consecutive patients who underwent hepatic resection in 15 years. Arch Surg 1994;129:738-42.
7. Dalton RR, Eisenberg BL. Surgical management of recurrent liver tumors. Semin Oncol 1993;20:493-505.
8. Eguchi A, Furuta T, Haraguchi M, Sugimachi K. A valid new approach in treating solitary new lesions after resection of hepatocellular carcinoma. J Surg Oncol 1994;56:263-8.
9. Hashimoto T, Nakayama S, Fukkuhara T, et al. The state of recurrence and the role of hepatectomy in hepatocellular carcinoma. Hepatogastroenterology 1994;41:144-9.
10. Lo CM, Lai EC, Fan ST, Choi TK, Wong J. Resection for extrahepatic recurrence of hepatocellular carcinoma. Br J Surg 1994;81:1019-21.
11. Nakao A, Suzuki Y, Isshiki K, et al. Clinical evaluation of plasma abnormal prothrombin (des-gamma-carboxy prothrombin) in hepatobiliary malignancies and other diseases. Am J Gastroenterol 1991; 86:62-6.
12. Zhou XD, Tang ZY, Yu YQ, et al. Recurrence after resection of alpha-fetoprotein-positive hepatocellular carcinoma. J Cancer Res Clin Oncol 1994;120:369-73.
13. Zhou XD, Yu YQ, Tang ZY, et al. Surgical treatment of recurrent hepatocellular carcinoma. Hepatogastroenterology 1993;40:333-6.
14. Imaoka S, Sasaki Y, Masutani S, et al. Palliative surgical treatment for recurrent and non-resectable hepatocellular carcinoma. Hepatogastroenterology 1993;40:342-6.
15. Okuda K, Ohtsuki T, Obata H, et al. Natural history of hepatocellular carcinoma and prognosis in relation to treatment: study of 850 patients. Cancer 1985;56:918-28.
16. Izumi R, Shimizu K, Ii T, et al. Prognostic factors of hepatocellular carcinoma in patients undergoing hepatic resection. Gastroenterology 1994;106:720-7.

17. Jwo SC, Chiu JH, Chau GY, Loong CC, Lui WY. Risk factors linked to tumor recurrence of human hepatocellular carcinoma after hepatic resection. Hepatology 1992;16:1367-71.
18. Okada S, Shimada K, Yamamoto J, et al. Predictive factors for postoperative recurrence of hepatocellular carcinoma. Gastroenterology 1994;106:1618-24.
19. Yamanaka N, Okamoto E, Toyosaka A, et al. Prognostic factors after hepatectomy for hepatocellular carcinomas: a univariate and multivariate analysis. Cancer 1990;65:1104-10.
20. Yamamoto J, Kosuge T, Takayama T, et al. Perioperative blood transfusion promotes recurrence of hepatocellular carcinoma after hepatectomy. Surgery 1994;115:303-9.
21. Lotze MT, Flickinger JC, Car BI. Hepatobiliary neoplasms. In: Devita VT, Hellman S, Rosenberg SA, editors. Principles of oncology. 4th ed. Philadelphia: JB Lippincott Company, 1993:883-914.
22. Beasley RP. Hepatitis B virus: the major etiology of hepatocellular carcinoma. Cancer 1988;10:1942-56.
23. Di Bisceglie AM. Hepatitis C and hepatocellular carcinoma. Semin Liver Dis 1995;15:64-9, 143.
24. Shimada M, Matsumata T, Taketomi A, Yamamoto K, Itasaka H, Sugimachi K. Repeat hepatectomy for recurrent hepatocellular carcinoma. Surgery 1994;115:703-6.
25. Inoue M, Onda M, Tajiri T, et al. [Two cases of improved quality of life with intra-arterial infusion of CDDP or unresectable gallbladder and pancreatic cancer.] Gan to Kagaku Ryoho [Jpn J Cancer Chemother] 1993;20:1676-8.
26. Kakazu T, Makuuchi M, Kawasaki S, et al. Repeat hepatic resection for recurrent hepatocellular carcinoma. Hepatogastroenterology 1993;40:337-41.
27. Segawa T, Izawa K, Ichinose Y, Tsunoda T, Tsuchiya R, Kanematsu T. [Recurrent hepatocellular carcinoma after hepatic resection.] Nippon Geka Gakkai Zasshi [J Jpn Surg Soc] 1992;93:723-30.
28. Suenaga M, Sugiura H, Kokuba Y, Uehara S, Kurumiya T. Repeated hepatic resection for recurrent hepatocellular carcinoma in eighteen cases. Surgery 1994;115:452-7.
29. Tanikawa K. [Early detection of hepatocellular carcinoma—high risk group and mass survey.] Gan to Kagaku Ryoho [Jpn J Cancer Chemother] 1993;20:864-70.
30. Wu M, Zhang X, Chen H, Yao X, Yang J. Surgical approaches for improving the operating results of primary liver cancer. Gan to Kagaku Ryoho [Jpn J Cancer Chemother] 1992;19Suppl8:1177-81.
31. Wu MC, Chen H, Yan YQ. Rehepatectomy of primary liver cancer. Semin Surg Oncol 1993;9:323-6.
32. Inagaki Y, Unoura M, Urabe T, et al. Distant metastasis of hepatocellular carcinoma after successful treatment of the primary lesion. Hepatogastroenterology 1993;40:316-9.
33. Ueda M, Tsuzuki T. [Aggressive surgery for hepatocellular carcinoma in advanced stage and with recurrence.] Nippon Geka Gakkai Zasshi [J Jpn Surg Soc] 1991;92:1327-9.
34. Une Y, Misawa K, Shimamura T, et al. Treatment of lymph node recurrence in patients with hepatocellular carcinoma. Surg Today 1994;24:606-9.
35. Bismuth H, Chiche L. Comparison of hepatic resection and transplantation in the treatment of liver cancer. Semin Surg Oncol 1993;9:341-5.
36. Onik GM, Atkinson D, Zemel R, Weaver ML. Cryosurgery of liver cancer. Semin Surg Oncol 1993;9:309-17.
37. Zhou XD, Tang ZY, Yu YQ, Ma ZC. Clinical evaluation of cryosurgery in the treatment of primary liver disease. Cancer 1988; 61:1889-92.
38. Nagasue N, Kohno H, Uchida M. Evaluation of preoperative transcatheter arterial embolization in the treatment of resectable primary liver cancer. Semin Surg Oncol 1993;9:327-31.
39. Taniguchi K, Nakata K, Kato Y, et al. Treatment of hepatocellular carcinoma with transcatheter arterial embolization: analysis of prognostic factors. Cancer 1994;73:1341-5.
40. Castells A, Bruix J, Bru C, et al. Treatment of small hepatocellular carcinoma in cirrhotic patients: a cohort study comparing surgical resection and percutaneous ethanol injection. Hepatology 1993; 18:1121-6.
41. Kotoh K, Sakai H, Sakamoto S, et al. The effect of percutaneous ethanol injection therapy on small solitary hepatocellular carcinoma is comparable to that of hepatectomy. Am J Gastroenterol 1994; 89:194-8.
42. Ikeda K, Saitoh S, Tsubota A, et al. Risk factors for tumor recurrence and prognosis after curative resection of hepatocellular carcinoma. Cancer 1993;71:19-25.
43. Segawa T, Izawa K, Tsunoda T, Kanematsu T, Shima M, Matsunaga N. [Evaluation of hepatectomy in small hepatocellular carcinoma—comparison with transcatheter arterial embolization therapy.] Nippon Geka Gakkai Zasshi [J Jpn Surg Soc] 1992;93:1095-9.
44. Tanikawa K, Majima Y. Percutaneous ethanol injection therapy for recurrent hepatocellular carcinoma. Hepatogastroenterology 1993; 40:324-7.
45. Ishii H, Okada S, Nose HK, et al. Survival benefit of percutaneous ethanol injection (PEI) as a combination with transcatheter arterial embolization (TAE) for postoperative recurrence of hepatocellular carcinoma (HCC). Proc Annu Meet Am Soc Clin Oncol 1995; 13:A564.
46. Sasaki Y, Imaoka S, Fujita M, et al. Regional therapy in the management of intrahepatic recurrence after surgery for hepatoma. Ann Surg 1987;206:40-7.
47. Suenaga M, Sugiura H, Kokuba Y, et al. [Strategy for the treatment of hepatocellular carcinoma.] Gan to Kagaku Ryoho [Jpn J Cancer Chemother] 1995;22:45-51.
48. Venook AP, Stagg RJ, Lewis BJ, et al. Chemoembolization for hepatocellular carcinoma. J Clin Oncol 1990;8:1108-14.
49. Ellis LM, Demers ML, Roh MS. Current strategies for the treatment of hepatocellular carcinoma. Curr Opin Oncol 1992;4:741-51.
50. Sasaki Y, Imaoka S, Masutani S, et al. [Regional therapy to prevent recurrence after surgery in hepatocellular carcinoma.] Gan to Kagaku Ryoho [Jpn J Cancer Chemother] 1992;19:1767-70.
51. Xu K, Meng XY, Wu JW, Shen B, Shi YC, Wei Q. Diagnostic value of serum gamma-glutamyl transferase isoenzyme for hepatocellular carcinoma: a 10-year study. Am J Gastroenterol 1992;87:991-5.
52. Ohta H, Watanabe H, Sawabu N. [Isoenzyme as tumor marker.] Nippon Rinsho [Jpn J Clin Med] 1995;53:1124-8.
53. Yamamoto T, Amuro Y, Matsuda Y, et al. Boronate affinity chromatography of gamma-glutamyl transferase in patients with hepatocellular carcinoma. Am J Gastroenterol 1991;86:495-9.
54. Belghiti J, Di Carlo I, Ferreira LL, Bezeaud A, Sauvanet A, Fekete F. [Prognostic value or pre- and postoperative alpha-fetoprotein in the follow-up of patients with surgically-treated hepatocellular carcinoma.] Minerva Chir 1993;48:25-8.
55. Guo Q, Uchida H, Matsuo N, et al. [Study on the evaluation of recurrence of HCC and the effect after transcatheter hepatic arterial embolization—fluctuations in AFP values.] Nippon Igaku Hoshasen Gakkai Zasshi 1993;53:195-203.
56. Yin ZF, Wu MC, Yu ZQ. [The prognostic value of focusylated alpha-fetoprotein measurement in liver cancer patients after surgery.] Chung-Hua Wai Ko Tsa Chih [Chin J Surg] 1994;32:654-6.
57. Hirai H, Taketa K. Lectin affinity electrophoresis of alpha-fetoprotein: increased specificity and sensitivity as a marker of hepatocellular carcinoma. J Chromatogr 1992;604:91-4.
58. Sato Y, Nakata K, Kato Y, et al. Early recognition of hepatocellular carcinoma based on altered profiles of alpha-fetoprotein. N Engl J Med 1993;328:1802-6.
59. Tu Z. [Prospective study on the diagnosis of hepatocellular carcinoma by using alpha-fetoprotein reactive to lentil lectin.] Chung-Hua i Hsueh Tsa Chih [Chin Med J] 1992;72:138-40.
60. Suehiro T, Sugimachi K, Matsumata T, Itasaka H, Taketomi A, Maeda T. Protein induced by vitamin K absence or antagonist II as a prognostic marker in hepatocellular carcinoma: comparison with alpha-fetoprotein. Cancer 1994;73:2464-71.
61. Inoue S, Nakao A, Harada A, Nonami T, Tagaki H. Clinical significance of abnormal prothrombin (DCP) in relation to postoperative survival and prognosis in patients with hepatocellular carcinoma. Am J Gastroenterol 1994;89:2222-6.

62. Brunello F, Marcarino C, Pasquero P, et al. The des-gamma-carboxy prothrombin for the diagnosis of hepatocellular carcinoma. Ital J Gastroenterol 1993;25:9-12.
63. Fujiyama S, Izuno K, Gohshi K, Shibata J, Sato T. Clinical usefulness of des-gamma-carboxy prothrombin assay in early diagnosis of hepatocellular carcinoma. Dig Dis Sci 1991;36:1787-92.
64. Nakao A, Virji A, Iwaki Y, Carr B, Iwatsuki S, Starzl E. Abnormal prothrombin (DES-gamma-carboxy prothrombin) in hepatocellular carcinoma. Hepatogastroenterology 1991;38:450-3.
65. Saitoh S, Ikeda K, Koida I, et al. Serum des-gamma-carboxy prothrombin concentration determined by the avidin-biotin complex method in small hepatocellular carcinomas. Cancer 1994;74:2918-23.
66. Weitz IC, Liebman HA. Des-gamma-carboxy (abnormal) prothrombin and hepatocellular carcinoma: a critical review. Hepatology 1993;18:990-7.
67. Chan CY, Lee SD, Wu JC, et al. The diagnostic value of the assay of des-gamma-carboxy prothrombin in the detection of small hepatocellular carcinoma. J Hepatol 199;13:21-4.
68. Pateron D, Ganne N, Trinchet JC, et al. Prospective study of screening for hepatocellular carcinoma in Caucasian patients with cirrhosis. Hepatology 1994;20:65-71.
69. Grieco A, De Stefano V, Cassano A, et al. Hepatocarcinoma in cirrhosis: is antithrombin III a neoplastic marker? Dig Dis Sci 1991; 36:990-2.
70. Giardina MG, Matarazzo M, Varriale A, Morante R, Napoli A, Martino R. Serum alpha-L-fucosidase: a useful marker in the diagnosis of hepatocellular carcinoma. Cancer 1992;70:1044-8.
71. Marotta F, Chui DH, Safran P, Zhang SC. Serum alpha-L-fucosidase: a more sensitive marker for hepatocellular carcinoma? Dig Dis Sci 1991;36:993-7.
72. Takahashi H, Saibara T, Iwamura S, et al. Serum alpha-L-fucosidase activity and tumor size in hepatocellular carcinoma. Hepatology 1994; 19:1414-7.
73. Fabris C, Basso DA, Leandro G, et al. Serum CA 19-9 and alpha-fetoprotein levels in primary hepatocellular carcinoma and liver cirrhosis. Cancer 1991;68:1795-8.
74. Maharaj B, Pillay S, Padayachi T. Circulating CA-195 in hepatocellular carcinoma and metastatic hepatic carcinoma. Trop Geogr Med 1991;43:329-31.
75. Hada T, Kinoshita Y, Ichimori Y, et al. Establishment of an enzyme immunoassay using monoclonal antibody (HG1-219) and its application for the diagnosis of hepatocellular carcinoma. Jpn J Cancer Res 1992;83:1366-72.
76. Kumagai Y, Chiba J, Sata T, Ohtaki S, Mitamura K. A new tumor-associated antigen useful for serodiagnosis of hepatocellular carcinoma, defined by monoclonal antibody KM-2. Cancer Res 1992; 52:4987-94.
77. Collier NA, Weinbren K, Bloom SR, Lee YC, Hodgson HJ, Blumgart LH. Neurotensin secretion by fibrolamellar carcinoma of the liver. Lancet 1984;1:538-40.
78. Collier NA, Weinbren K, Bloom SR, Lee YC, Hodgson HJ, Blumgart LH. Neurotensin secretion by fibrolamellar carcinoma of the liver. Lancet 1984;1(8376):538-40.
79. Soreide O, Czerniak A, Bradpiece H, Bloom S, Blumgart L. Characteristics of fibrolamellar hepatocellular carcinoma: a study of nine cases and a review of the literature. Am J Surg 1986;151:518-23.
80. Warnes TW, Smith A. Tumor markers in diagnosis and management. Bailleres Clin Gastroenterol 1987;1:63-89.
81. Sheppard KJ, Bradbury DA, Davies JM, Ryrie DR. High serum vitamin B12 binding capacity as a marker of the fibrolamellar variant of hepatocellular carcinoma. [letter] Br Med J Clin Res Ed 1983; 57:286.
82. Wheeler K, Pritchard J, Luck W, Rossiter M. Transcobalamin I as a "marker" for fibrolamellar hepatoma. Med Pediatr Oncol 1986; 14:227-9.
83. Theise ND, Fiel IM, Hytiroglou P, et al. Macroregenerative nodules in cirrhosis are not associated with elevated serum or stainable tissue alpha-fetoprotein. Liver 1995;15:30-4.
84. Hirai T, Ohishi H, Guo Q, et al. [CO_2 US via an implantable port—drug distribution in intraarterial chemotherapy for hepatic tumors and evaluation of effect.] Nippon Igaku Hoshasen Gakkai Zasshi 1993; 53:511-9.
85. Cottone M, Turri M, Caltagirone M, et al. Screening for hepatocellular carcinoma in patients with Child's A cirrhosis: an 8-year prospective study by ultrasound and alphafetoprotein. J Hepatol 1994;21:1029-34.
86. Lin ZY. [Recurrence and treatment of primary liver cancer after radical hepatectomy.] Chung-Hua Wai Ko Tsa Chih [Chin J Surg] 1991; 29:93-6.
87. Huguet C, Bona S, Nordlinger B, et al. Repeat hepatic resection for primary and metastatic carcinoma of the liver. Surg Gynecol Obstet 1990;171:398-402.
88. Matsuda Y, Ito T, Oguchi Y, Nakajima K, Izukura T. Rationale of surgical management for recurrent hepatocellular carcinoma. Ann Surg 1993;217:28-34.
89. Unoura M, Kaneko S, Matsushita E, et al. High-risk groups and screening strategies for early detection of hepatocellular carcinoma in patients with chronic liver disease. Hepatogastroenterology 1993;40:305-10.
90. Xu D, Tang ZY, Yu YQ, et al. Recurrence after resection of alpha-fetoprotein-positive hepatocellular carcinoma. J Cancer Res Clin Oncol 1994;120:369-73.
91. Longmire WP. Tumours of the extrahepatic biliary radicals. In: Hickey RC, ed. Current problems in cancer. Vol. I, No. 2. Chicago: Year Book Medical Publishers, 1976.
92. Kuwayti K, Baggenstoss AH, Stauffer MH, Priestly JI. Carcinoma of the major intrahepatic and extrahepatic bile ducts exclusive of the papilla of Vater. Surg Gynecol Obstet 1957;104:357-66.
93. Okuda K, Kubo Y, Okazaki N, Arishima T, Hashimoto M. Clinical aspects of intrahepatic bile duct carcinoma including hilar carcinoma: a study of 57 autopsy proven cases. Cancer 1977;39:232-46.
94. Ottow RT, August DA, Sugarbaker PH. Treatment of proximal biliary tract carcinoma: an overview of techniques and results. Surgery 1985;97:251-62.
95. Sako S, Seitzinger GL, Garside E. Carcinoma of the extrahepatic ducts: review of the literature and report of six cases. Surgery 1957;41:416-7.
96. Altaee MY, Johnson PJ, Farrant JM, Williams R. Etiologic and clinical characteristics of peripheral and hilar cholangiocarcinoma. Cancer 1991;68:2051-5.
97. Baer HU, Stain SC, Dennison AR, Eggers B, Blumgart LH. Improvements in survival by aggressive resections of hilar cholangiocarcinoma. Ann Surg 1993;217:20-7.
98. Bengmark S, Ekberg H, Evander A, Klofver-Stahl B, Tranberg KG. Major liver resection for hilar cholangiocarcinoma. Ann Surg 1988;207:120-5.
99. Bismuth H, Nakache R, Diamond T. Management strategies in resection for hilar cholangiocarcinoma. Ann Surg 1992 215:31-8.
100. Hadjis NS, Blenkharn JI, Alexander N, Benjamin IS, Blumgart LH. Outcome of radical surgery in hilar cholangiocarcinoma. Surgery 1990;107:597-604.
101. Alexander F, Rossi RL, O'Bryan M, Khettry U, Braasch JW, Watkins E Jr. Biliary carcinoma: a review of 109 cases. Am J Surg 1984;147:503-9.
102. Crile GJ. The advantages of bypass operations over radical pancreaticoduodenectomy in the treatment of pancreatic cancer. Surg Gynecol Obstet 1970;130:1049-53.
103. Herter FP, Cooperman AM, Ahlborn TN, Antinori C. Surgical experience with pancreatic and periampullary cancer. Ann Surg 1982; 195:274-81.
104. Nakase A, Matsumoto Y, Uchida K, Honjo I. Surgical treatment of cancer of the pancreas and the periampullary region: cumulative results in 57 institutions in Japan. Ann Surg 1977;185:52-7.
105. Warren KW, Choe DS, Plaza J, Relihan M. Results of radical resection for periampullary cancer. Ann Surg 1975;181:534-40.

106. Cameron JL, Pitt HA, Zinner MJ, Kaufman SL, Coleman J. Management of proximal cholangiocarcinomas by surgical resection and radiotherapy. Am J Surg 1990;159:91-98.
107. Nagorney DM, Donohue JH, Farnell MB, Schleck CD, Ilstrup DM. Outcomes after curative resections of cholangiocarcinoma. Arch Surg 1993;128:871-9.
108. Geer RJ, Brennan MF. Prognostic indicators for survival after resection of pancreatic adenocarcinoma. Am J Surg 1993;165:68-73.
109. Boerma EJ. Research into the results of resection of hilar bile duct cancer. Surgery 1990;108:572-80.
110. Blumgart LH, Hadjis NS, Benjamin IS, Beazley R. Surgical approaches to cholangiocarcinoma at confluence of hepatic ducts. Lancet 1984;1:66-70.
111. Tompkins RK, Thomas D, Wile A, Longmire WP Jr. Prognostic factors in bile duct carcinoma: analysis of 96 cases. Ann Surg 1981;194:447-57.
112. Yeo CJ, Pitt HA, Cameron JL. Cholangiocarcinoma. Surg Clin North Am 1990;70:1429-47.
113. Reding R, Buard JL, Lebeau G, Launois B. Surgical management of 552 carcinomas of the extrahepatic bile ducts (gallbladder and periampullary tumors excluded): results of the French Surgical Association Survey. Ann Surg 1991;213:236-41.
114. Blumgart LH, Benjamin IS. Cancer of the bile ducts. In: Blumgart LH, editor. Surgery of the liver and biliary tract. 2nd ed. New York: Churchill Livingstone, 1994:967-95.
115. Nakajima T, Kondo Y, Miyazaki M, Okui K. A histopathological study of 102 cases of intrahepatic cholangiocarcinoma. Human Pathol 1988;19:1228-34.
116. Schoenthaler R, Phillips TL, Castro J, Efird JT, Better A, Way LW. Carcinoma of the extrahepatic bile ducts: the University of California at San Francisco experience. Ann Surg 1994;219:267-74.
117. Gertsch P, Thomas P, Baer H, Lerut J, Zimmermann A, Blumgart LH. Multiple tumors of the biliary tract. Am J Surg 1990;159:386-8.
118. Targarona EM, Zografos G, Habib NA. Liver resection for recurrent hilar cholangiocarcinoma. Br J Surg 1993;80:1433.
119. Goldstein RM, Stone M, Tillery GW, et al. Is liver transplantation indicated for cholangiocarcinoma? Am J Surg 1993;166:768-72.
120. Kuvshinoff BW, Armstrong JG, Fong Y, et al. Palliation of irresectable hilar cholangiocarcinoma with biliary drainage and radiotherapy. Br J Surg 1995;82:1522-5.
121. Banerjee B, Teplick SK. Nonsurgical management of primary cholangiocarcinoma: retrospective analysis of 40 cases. Dig Dis Sci 1995;40:701-5.
122. Cheung KL, Lai EC. Endoscopic stenting for malignant biliary obstruction. Arch Surg 1995;130:204-7.
123. Neuhaus H, Hagenmuller F, Griebel M, Claassen M. Percutaneous cholangioscopic or transpapillary insertion of self-expanding biliary metal stents. Gastrointest Endosc 1991;37:31-7.
124. Polydorou AA, Cairns SR, Dowsett JF, et al. Palliation of proximal malignant biliary obstruction by endoscopic endoprosthesis insertion. Gut 1991;32:685-9.
125. Guthrie CM, Haddock G, De Beaux AC, Garden OJ, Carter DC. Changing trends in the management of extrahepatic cholangiocarcinoma. Br J Surg 1993;80:1434-9.
126. Stain SC, Baer HU, Dennison AR, Blumgart LH. Current management of hilar cholangiocarcinoma. Surg Gynecol Obstet 1992;175:579-88.
127. Nordback IH, Pitt HA, Coleman J, et al. Unresectable hilar cholangiocarcinoma: percutaneous versus operative palliation. Surgery 1994;115:597-603.
128. Kurisu K, Hishikawa Y, Miura T, Kanno H, Okamoto E. Radiotherapy of postoperative residual tumor of bile duct carcinoma. Radiat Med 1991;9:82-4.
129. Alfthan H, Haglund C, Roberts P, Stenman UH. Elevation of free beta subunit of human choriogonadotropin and core beta fragment of human choriogonadotropin in the serum and urine of patients with malignant pancreatic and biliary disease. Cancer Res 1992; 52:4628-33.
130. Shiina T, Mikuriya S, Uno T, et al. Radiotherapy of cholangiocarcinoma: the roles for primary and adjuvant therapies. Cancer Chemother Pharmacol 1992;31Suppl:S115-8.
131. Harvey JH, Smith FP, Schein PS. 5-Fluorouracil, mitomycin, and doxorubicin (FAM) in carcinoma of the biliary tract. J Clin Oncol 1984;2:1245-8.
132. Tabara H, Matsuura H, Kohno H, Hayashi T, Nagasue N, Nakamura T. [Intraarterial chemoembolization therapy for unresectable liver cancer using plachitin particles.] Gan to Kagaku Ryoho [Jpn J Cancer Chemother] 1994;21:2225-8.
133. Tsuji Y, Imai M, Katsuki Y, Yasuda T, Nishimura A. [A case of liver metastasis from bile duct cancer effectively treated with hepatic artery infusion chemotherapy.] Gan to Kagaku Ryoho [Jpn J Cancer Chemother] 1994;21:2194-7.
134. Tsushima K, Sakata Y, Shiratori Y, et al. [Cases of advanced cholangiocarcinoma showing partial response by the combination chemotherapy including protracted continuous infusion of 5-FU combined with intravenous administration of low-dose leucovorin and intra-arterial administration of MMC and CQ.] Gan to Kagaku Ryoho [Jpn J Cancer Chemother] 1991;18:2603-5.
135. Tan CK, Podila PV, Taylor JE, et al. Human cholangiocarcinomas express somatostatin receptors and respond to somatostatin with growth inhibition. Gastroenterology 1995;108:1908-16.
136. Stillwagon GB, Order SE, Haulk T, et al. Variable low dose rate irradiation (131I-anti-CEA) and integrated low dose chemotherapy in the treatment of nonresectable primary intrahepatic cholangiocarcinoma. Int J Radiat Oncol Biol Phys 1991;21:1601-5.
137. Vauthey JN, Blumgart LH. Recent advances in the management of cholangiocarcinomas. Semin Liver Dis 1994;14:109-14.
138. Fortner JG, Vitelli CE, Maclean BJ. Proximal extrahepatic bile duct tumors: analysis of a series of 52 consecutive patients treated over a period of 13 years. Arch Surg 1989;124:1275-9.
139. Rieu PN, Jansen JB, Biedmond I, Offerhaus GJ, Joosten HJ, Lamers CB. Short-term results of gastrectomy with Roux-en-Y or Billroth II anastomosis for peptic ulcer: a prospective comparative study. Hepatogastroenterology 1992;39:22-6.
140. Haglund C, Lindgren J, Roberts PJ, Nordling S. Difference in tissue expression of tumor markers CA 19-9 and CA 50 in hepatocellular carcinoma and cholangiocarcinoma. Br J Cancer 1991;63:386-9.
141. Ramage JK, Donaghy A, Farrant JM, Iorns R, Williams R. Serum tumor markers for the diagnosis of cholangiocarcinoma in primary sclerosing cholangitis. Gastroenterology 1995;108:865-9.
142. Roncalli M, Patriarca C, Gambacorta M, Viale G, Coggi G. Expression of new phenotypic markers in cholangiocarcinoma and putative precursor lesions. J Surg Oncol Suppl 1993;3:173-4.
143. Wanebo HJ, Vezeridis MP. Carcinoma of the gallbladder. J Surg Oncol Suppl 1993;3:134-9.
144. Diehl AK. Epidemiology of gallbladder cancer: a synthesis of recent data. J Natl Cancer Inst 1980;65:1209-14.
145. Dvorak J, Smutny S. [Gallbladder carcinoma.] Rozhl Chir 1992;71:76-80.
146. Matsumoto Y, Fujii H, Aoyama H, Yamamoto M, Sugahara K, Suda K. Surgical treatment of primary carcinoma of the gallbladder based on the histologic analysis of 48 surgical specimens. Am J Surg 1992;163:239-45.
147. Ogura Y, Mizumoto R, Isaji S, Kusuda T, Matsuda S, Tabata M. Radical operations for carcinoma of the gallbladder: present status in Japan. World J Surg 1991;15:337-43.
148. Nakamura S, Sakaguchi S, Suzuki S, Muro H. Aggressive surgery for carcinoma of the gallbladder. Surgery 1989;106:467-73.
149. Ouchi K, Owada Y, Matsuno S, Sato T. Prognostic factors in the surgical treatment of gallbladder carcinoma. Surgery 1987;101:731-7.
150. Donohue JH, Nagorney DM, Grant CS, Tsushima K, Ilstrup DM, Adson MA. Carcinoma of the gallbladder: does radical resection improve outcome? Surgery 1990;108:572-80.
151. Shirai Y, Yoshida K, Tsukada K, Muto T, Watanabe H. Radical surgery for gallbladder carcinoma: long-term results. Ann Surg 1992;216:565-8.

152. Wanebo HJ, Castle WN, Fechner RE. Is carcinoma of the gallbladder a curable lesion? Ann Surg 1982;195:624-31.
153. Nevin JE, Moran TJ, Kay S, King R. Carcinoma of the gallbladder: staging, treatment, and prognosis. Cancer 1976;37:141-8.
154. Launoy G, Crenes-Laventure E, Dao T, et al. [Cancer of the gallbladder. Epidemiology, diagnosis and prognostic factors.] Ann Chir 1993;47:18-23.
155. Fong Y, Brennan MF, Turnbull A, Coit DG, Blumgart LH. Gallbladder cancers discovered during laparoscopic surgery: potential for iatrogenic tumor dissemination. Arch Surg 1993;128:1054-6.
156. Oertli D, Herzog U, Tondelli P. Primary carcinoma of the gallbladder: operative experience during a 16 year period. Eur J Surg 1993;159:415-20.
157. Shirai Y, Tsukada K, Ohtani T, Watanabe H, Hatakeyama K. Hepatic metastases from carcinoma of the gallbladder. Cancer 1995; 75:2063-8.
158. Oswalt CE, Cruz AB. Effectiveness of chemotherapy in addition to surgery in treating carcinoma of the gallbladder. Rev Surg 1977;34:436-8.
159. Mahe M, Stampfli C, Romestaing P, Salerno N, Gerard JP. Primary carcinoma of the gallbladder: potential for external radiation therapy. Radiother Oncol 1994;33:204-8.
160. Kurisu K, Hishikawa Y, Taniguchi M, et al. High-dose-rate intraluminal brachytherapy for postoperative residual tumor of gallbladder carcinoma: a case report. Radiat Med 1991;9:241-3.
161. Busse PM, Cady B, Bothe A Jr, et al. Intraoperative radiation therapy for carcinoma of the gallbladder. World J Surg 1991; 15:352-6.
162. Kotoh T, Arima S, Futami K. [A case of retroperitoneal lymph node recurrence with gallbladder cancer responding to UFT and CDDP combination chemotherapy.] Gan to Kagaku Ryoho [Jpn J Cancer Chemother] 1994;21:881-4.
163. Kato K, Koike A, Koide T, et al. [Efficacy of 48-hour infusion of 5-fluorouracil for gallbladder cancer.] Gan to Kagaku Ryoho [Jpn J Cancer Chemother] 1993;20:2341-4.
164. Shibata T, Mishima O, Sato T, et al. [The two cases of examination of chemotherapy in advanced gallbladder carcinoma.] Gan to Kagaku Ryoho [Jpn J Cancer Chemother] 1994;21:1071-5.
165. Hata Y, Morita S, Hisa N, et al. [Evaluation of arterial infusion chemotherapy for advanced gallbladder cancer using implantable port.] Gan to Kagaku Ryoho [Jpn J Cancer Chemother] 1994; 21:2639-43.
166. Roa I, Araya JC, Shiraisch T, et al. [Gallbladder cancer: immunohistochemical expression of CA-19-9, epithelial membrane antigen, dupan-2 and carcinoembryonic antigen.] Rev Med Chil 1992; 120:1218-26.
167. Nagasue N, Uchida M, Makino Y, et al. Incidence and factors associated with intrahepatic recurrence following resection of hepatocellular carcinoma. Gastroenterology 1993;105:488-94.
168. Nakajima Y, Ohmura T, Kimura J, et al. Role of surgical treatment for recurrent hepatocellular carcinoma after hepatic resection. World J Surg 1993;17:792-5.
169. Bismuth H, Chiche L, Castaing D. Surgical treatment of hepatocellular carcinomas in noncirrhotic liver: experience with 68 liver resections. World J Surg 1995;19:35-41.
170. Kawasaki S, Makuuchi M, Miyagawa S, et al. Results of hepatic resection for hepatocellular carcinoma. World J Surg 1995;19:31-4.
171. Burditt LJ, Johnson MM, Johnson PJ, Williams R. Detection of hepatocellular carcinoma-specific alpha-fetoprotein by isoelectric focusing. Cancer 1994;74:25-9.
172. Aoyagi Y, Suzuki Y, Isemura M, et al. The focusylation index of alpha-fetoprotein and its usefulness in the early diagnosis of hepatocellular carcinoma. Cancer 1988;61:769-74.
173. Kuromatsu R, Tanaka M, Tanikawa K. Serum alpha-fetoprotein and lens culinaris agglutinin-reactive fraction of alpha-fetoprotein in patients with hepatocellular carcinoma. Liver 1993;13:177-82.
174. Biermann CW, Lloyd DM, Witte G, Pohlmann G, Klomp HJ, Klapdor R. Chemoembolization of HCC: clinical relevance of AFP, CA 19-9, ferritin and the proliferation marker TPS. [Meeting abstract] J Tumor Mark Oncol 1992;7:56.
175. Suehiro T, Matsumata T, Itasaka H, Taketomi A, Yamamoto K, Sugimachi K. Des-gamma-carboxy prothrombin and proliferative activity of hepatocellular carcinoma. Surgery 1995;117:682-91.
176. Shirai Y, Kawata S, Tamura S, et al. Plasma transforming growth factor-beta 1 in patients with hepatocellular carcinoma: comparison with chronic liver diseases. Cancer 1994;73:2275-9.
177. Meier PN, Manns MP. [Cholangiolar carcinoma.] Leber, Magen, Darm 1994;24:234-8.
178. Adachi E, Maeda T, Matsumata T, et al. Risk factors for intrahepatic recurrence in human small hepatocellular carcinoma. Gastroenterology 1995;108:768-75.
179. Sirisinha S, Prempracha N, Tengchaisri T, Hongsrijinda N, Chinchai T. Identification of tumor markers for cholangiocarcinoma and evaluation of their diagnostic potential. Asian Pac J Allergy Immunol 1994;12:73-81.
180. Dufek V, Petrtyl J, Klener P, Chmel J. [Tumor markers in the diagnosis of tumors in the subhepatic area.] Vnitr Lek 1994;40:350-3.
181. Tashiro S, Konno T, Mochinaga M, Nakakuma K, Murata E, Yokoyama I. Treatment of carcinoma of the gallbladder in Japan. Nippon Shokakibyo Gakkai Zasshi [Jpn J Gastroenterol] 1982; 12:98-104.
182. American Joint Committee on Cancer. Beahrs OH, Henson DE, Hutter RV, Kennedy BJ, editors. Manual for staging of cancer. 4th ed. Philadelphia: JB Lippincott Company, 1992.

➢ COUNTER POINT

National Cancer Center Hospital, Japan

TOMOO KOSUGE, KAZUAKI SHIMADA, JUNJI YAMAMOTO, AND SUSUMU YAMASAKI

A number of factors determine the optimal strategy for postoperative follow-up of patients who have had surgical resection of hepatobiliary neoplasms. An extensive review of the literature and a rational policy of follow-up are provided by Karpoff and Fong. Our recommendations are described here, based on the experience at the National Cancer Center Hospital in Tokyo.

HEPATOCELLULAR CARCINOMA

Background

Hepatocellular carcinoma is common in East Asia and has unique features in its diagnosis and treatment. Hepatitis viral infection is closely related to the development of hepatocellular carcinoma. More than 90% of patients at the National Cancer Center Hospital have chronic liver disease or a history of hepatitis. Karpoff and Fong discuss the predominance of hepatitis B infection in patients with classic hepatocellular carcinoma. However, the proportion of hepatitis B and hepatitis C infections differs considerably from country to country. In Japan more than 70% of patients with hepatocellular carcinoma are positive for hepatitis C viral antibody.[1] The carcinogenic activity of the hepatitis virus persists even after successful treatment and causes metachronous development of hepatocellular carcinoma. Karpoff and Fong refer to two reports[2,3] from the National Cancer Center Hospital as if they showed similar tumor-free postoperative survival between cirrhotic and noncirrhotic patients. In fact, a significantly higher risk of recurrence in cirrhotic patients was described in at least one[2] of the reports. Although a statistically significant difference was not shown in the other study[3] because of the small number of patients included, a potential difference was suggested by the absence of 3-year disease-free survivors among cirrhotic patients and a 42.4% 3-year disease-free survival rate in noncirrhotic patients. The influence of parenchymal disease is more prominent after the third postoperative year. Consequently, permanent follow-up is required in patients with liver dysfunction.

Patterns of Recurrence

Hepatocellular carcinoma has a unique pattern of spread from the primary site. Distribution by way of the portal venous system is common, whereas lymphatic metastases and peritoneal seeding are rare. These features make the liver a predominant site of recurrence after resection. Furthermore, the liver is prone to develop second primary hepatocellular carcinomas. Consequently most recurrent cancers are confined to the remnant liver. A high recurrence rate is also characteristic of hepatocellular carcinoma; 60% to 70% of patients have recurrence within 3 years of initial hepatic resections.[4] Cirrhotic patients also have a considerable risk of recurrence in later years.

Blood Tests and Tumor Markers

Regarding the roles of blood tests and tumor markers, we agree with the tests and frequencies proposed by Karpoff and Fong. Alpha-fetoprotein remains the most useful tumor marker in the follow-up of hepatocellular carcinoma. However, with the development of sensitive imaging modalities, the value of alpha-fetoprotein is decreasing.

Imaging Studies

Using modern imaging modalities such as ultrasound, computed tomography, and magnetic resonance imaging, physicians can find hepatocellular carcinomas as small as 1 cm in diameter. These modalities are complementary in detecting and evaluating intrahepatic lesions. Ultrasound is particularly important in follow-up practice because it is sensitive, noninvasive, and less expensive than other imaging modalities. At the National Cancer Center Hospital, hepatic surgeons are also specialists in ultrasound and perform ultrasound examinations as part of their outpatient activity. The value of ultrasound varies because its reliability depends on the examiner's technique and experience. However, all hepatic surgeons should be familiar with ultrasound, since it is essential for modern hepatic surgery.

Small hyperechoic or hypoechoic lesions are frequently detected with ultrasound. Such lesions include benign regenerative nodules and borderline lesions such as adenomatous hyperplasia; early-stage, well-differentiated hepatocellular carcinoma[5]; and overt hepatocellular carcinoma. In such cases computed tomography with bolus injection of contrast media is useful to distinguish overt hepatocellular carcinoma from other types.[6] The use of helical computed tomography is recommended, if available, because it provides information comparable with a dynamic study. When the mass is hyperdense in the arterial-dominant phase and hypodense in the portal-dominant phase, it is considered to be an overt hepatocellular carcinoma and treatment should be planned. A hypovascular mass smaller than 2 cm in diameter is considered a borderline lesion or early-stage, well-differentiated hepatocellular carcinoma, and its size and shape should be closely followed using ultrasound and computed tomography. Experience with magnetic resonance imaging is increasing rapidly; it appears to be a useful modality.

Treatment

Three effective treatment methods are now available to treat recurrence confined to the liver: repeat hepatic resection,[7] percutaneous ethanol injection,[8] and transcatheter arterial embolization.[9] Our opinion concerning the effectiveness of each treatment is similar to that of Karpoff and Fong. However, it is important to know that each treatment has its unique indications and limitations. Selection of treatment should depend on the location and extent of the recurrent disease and on the patient's hepatic functional reserve (Figure 11-1).

After detection of a hypervascular recurrent nodule, hepatic conventional angiography is carried out, followed by computed tomographic angiography if indicated. Transcatheter arterial embolization or injection of iodized oil is performed partly as treatment and partly as preparation for lipoidal computed tomography, which is performed 1 month later. Evaluation of hepatic function is carried out before angiography to avoid any influence of transcatheter arterial embolization. First the feasibility of repeat hepatectomy is assessed. If surgical resection is not feasible, nonsurgical treatment is selected. Transcatheter arterial embolization is applicable to a wide range of patients. Percutaneous ethanol injection is selected when the number of recurrent nodules is no more than three and the maximal diameter of each nodule is less than 3 cm.

At the National Cancer Center Hospital small hypovascular lesions considered borderline lesions or early-stage, well-differentiated hepatocellular carcinomas are often encountered. Both adenomatous hyperplasia and early-stage hepatocellular carcinoma tend to transform into overt hepatocellular carcinomas.[10] However, surgeons at the National Cancer Center Hospital do not treat small hypovascular lesions until they grow into the overt form because borderline lesions and early-stage hepatocellular carcinoma often remain unchanged for several years and occasionally regress spontaneously. Fine-needle aspiration biopsy is useful to diagnose small hepatic lesions, but it cannot always be fully relied on.[11,12] For example, it is impossible to know whether or not the suspected lesion contains a component of overt hepatocellular carcinoma when the biopsy specimen is composed of

Figure 11-1 Effect of follow-up treatments.

adenomatous hyperplasia or well-differentiated hepatocellular carcinoma. Fortunately, the accuracy of modern imaging modalities in the diagnosis of overt hepatocellular carcinoma is comparable to that of needle biopsy. Consequently, the decision at the National Cancer Center Hospital to start anticancer treatment is based largely on findings of imaging examinations, such as an increase in size, change of internal echo, and appearance of a hypervascular area.

Anticancer treatment should be restricted to overt hepatocellular carcinoma because impairment of hepatic function and progression of cancer are major factors that shorten the patient's life. All effective anticancer treatments impair hepatic function, and excessive treatment should be avoided. Percutaneous ethanol injection for borderline lesions and well-differentiated hepatocellular carcinomas might be advantageous to a patient by preventing transformation into overt hepatocellular carcinoma. However, a new overt hepatocellular carcinoma may then appear, in which case the adverse effect of the prior percutaneous ethanol injection may prevail over any potential advantage.

In contrast to recurrence confined to the liver, no reliable treatment exists for distant metastases. Therefore postoperative surveillance should focus on recurrence in the liver.

Strategy of Follow-Up

A close follow-up strategy is justified considering the patient's high vulnerability to localized recurrence, which can be effectively treated when detected with sensitive diagnostic modalities. Karpoff and Fong advocate less frequent follow-up intervals in patients with a normalized alpha-fetoprotein level. However, it is natural to assume that patients who previously had hepatocellular carcinoma have a higher risk of new hepatocellular carcinomas than would be suggested from prevalence studies of patients with short exposure to the carcinogenic activity of hepatitis virus. Considering that most patients with hepatocellular carcinoma have a history of hepatitis viral infection or liver dysfunction, close follow-up of all such patients is recommended.

Table 11-9 Follow-up of patients with hepatobiliary cancer (hepatocellular carcinoma): National Cancer Center Hospital, Japan

	YEAR				
	1	2	3	4	5
Office visit	6*	4	4	4	4
Complete blood count	6*	4	4	4	4
Liver function tests	6*	4	4	4	4
Electrolytes	6*	4	4	4	4
Alpha-fetoprotein	6*	4	4	4	4
Abdominal ultrasound	6*	4	4	4	4
Abdominal computed tomography	2†	2†	2†	2†	2†

*Includes monthly follow-up for the first 3 months.
†Performed biannually or more frequently as clinically indicated.

Current Practice

Immediately after discharge, patients are seen monthly on an outpatient basis until their general condition becomes stable (Table 11-9). Supportive care is provided to control symptoms caused by impaired hepatic function, such as edema, pleural effusion, and ascites. In this phase, blood samples are examined to assess hepatic function and electrolyte balance. Ultrasound is carried out to evaluate pleural effusion and ascites.

Patients are seen at least every 3 months for 5 years. Complete blood count, liver function tests, electrolytes, and alpha-fetoprotein levels are examined, and ultrasound is carried out. Computed tomography with rapid infusion of contrast media is performed every 6 months. Plain and postcontrast computed tomographic scans with drip infusion are not used because they are less reliable in detecting small hepatocellular carcinomas.[13]

In patients with repeat hepatectomy and percutaneous ethanol injection, tests similar to those after primary resection are indicated. In patients with transcatheter arterial embolization, vascularity of the treated nodules is regularly evaluated using computed tomography at an interval of 3 to 6 months. Transcatheter arterial embolization is repeated when hypervascularity is recognized. Office visits are continued at a prolonged interval, usually every 6 months, even in patients who are doing well after 5 years, because recurrence continues to develop.[2,4]

BILIARY CANCERS

In this section cholangiocarcinoma and gallbladder cancer are discussed together as biliary cancers because factors concerning their follow-up strategies are similar.

Strategy of Follow-Up

Most recurrences of biliary cancers are attributable to remaining cancer cells or incomplete resection. Unlike the situation with hepatocellular carcinoma, development of a second new cancer is exceptional. Consequently the recurrence rate is negligible beyond 5 years after resection. Therefore surveillance for recurrent disease should concentrate on the first 5 years after resection. However, early detection of recurrence is less valuable than in hepatocellular carcinoma because of the scarcity of effective treatment options available for recurrent disease. Repeat resection is rarely possible after a radical primary procedure, and systemic chemotherapy is seldom effective for recurrent disease.[14]

Obstructive jaundice and cholangitis are common consequences of recurrent biliary cancer and frequently bring about a fatal outcome. Similar symptoms can come from benign stricture of the hepatic duct–enteric anastomosis and choledocholithiasis. Control of biliary symptoms contributes to length of survival and quality of life. The types of procedure available for this purpose include percutaneous transhepatic biliary drainage,[15] endoscopic retrograde biliary drainage, and placement of a bilioenteric endoprosthesis,[16] along with several variants of these procedures. Radiation therapy can be combined with drainage procedures for malignant biliary obstruction. Consequently, detection and management of biliary problems are important components of a surveillance program. Ultrasound is feasible for the purpose because of its high sensitivity rate in detecting dilation of the biliary tree.

Table 11-10 Follow-up of patients with hepatobiliary cancer (cholangiocarcinoma or gallbladder cancer): National Cancer Center Hospital, Japan

	YEAR				
	1	2	3	4	5
Office visit	6*	4	4	4	4
Complete blood count	6*	4	4	4	4
Liver function tests	6*	4	4	4	4
Electrolytes	6*	4	4	4	4
CEA	6*	4	4	4	4
CA 19-9	6*	4	4	4	4
Abdominal ultrasound	6*	4	4	4	4
Abdominal computed tomography	1	1	1	1	1

CEA, Carcinoembryonic antigen.
*Includes monthly follow-up for the first 3 months.

Current Practice

Immediately after discharge, monthly office visits are requested for observation and possible treatment of biliary complications (Table 11-10). Complete blood count, liver function tests, and electrolyte studies are performed, and ultrasound is carried out to assess the biliary system. In patients with frequent cholangitis, surveillance focuses on the detection of dilated bile ducts and liver abscesses.

When the patient's condition is stable, blood sampling and ultrasound are carried out every 3 months through year 5. Frequent computed tomography is avoided except when observation with ultrasound is difficult. The frequency of follow-up is reduced to one or two times a year after 5 postoperative years.

SUMMARY

Currently, different follow-up plans are applied to patients with hepatocellular carcinoma and those with biliary cancers. In patients with hepatocellular carcinoma the high probability of recurrence and the existence of effective treatments justify close follow-up focused on intrahepatic recurrence. On the other hand, much attention is paid to biliary complications in patients with biliary cancers.

Optimization of a follow-up plan is valuable. It should reflect the present status of diagnosis and treatment of the disease, which are rapidly developing. For example, modalities to prevent recurrence will be practical in the future and will be included in the follow-up program. Prospective trials to evaluate the cost effectiveness of current follow-up practice may be worthwhile, though advances in practice will not wait for the results of such studies.

REFERENCES

1. The Liver Cancer Study Group of Japan. Primary liver cancer in Japan: clinicopathologic features and results of surgical treatment. Ann Surg 1990;211:277-87.

2. Yamamoto J, Kosuge T, Takayama T, et al. Perioperative blood transfusion promotes recurrence of hepatocellular carcinoma after hepatectomy. Surgery 1994;115:303-9.
3. Okada S, Shimada K, Yamamoto J, et al. Predictive factors for postoperative recurrence of hepatocellular carcinoma. Gastroenterology 1994;106:1618-24.
4. Kosuge T, Makuuchi M, Takayama T, Yamamoto J, Shimada K, Yamazaki S. Long-term results after resection of hepatocellular carcinoma: experience of 480 cases. Hepatogastroenterology 1993;40:328-32.
5. Sakamoto M, Hirohashi S, Shimosato Y. Early stages of multistep hepatocarcinogenesis: adenomatous hyperplasia and early hepatocellular carcinoma. Hum Pathol 1991;22:172-8.
6. Matsui O, Kadoya M, Kameyama T, et al. Benign and malignant nodules in cirrhotic liver: distinction based on blood supply. Radiology 1991;178:493-7.
7. Kakazu T, Makuuchi M, Kawasaki S, et al. Repeat hepatic resection for recurrent hepatocellular carcinoma. Hepatogastroenterology 1993;40:337-41.
8. Sugiura N, Tanaka K, Ohto M, Okuida K, Hirooka N. Treatment of small hepatocellular carcinoma by percutaneous injection of ethanol into tumor with real-time ultrasound monitoring. Acta Hepatol Jpn 1983;24:920.
9. Yamada R, Sato M, Kawabata M, Nakatsuka H, Nakamura K, Takashima S. Hepatic artery embolization in 120 patients with unresectable hepatoma. Radiology 1983;148:397-401.
10. Takayama T, Makuuchi M, Hirohashi S, et al. Malignant transformation of adenomatous hyperplasia to hepatocellular carcinoma. Lancet 1990;336:1150-3.
11. Wee A, Nilsson B, Tan LK, Yap I. Fine needle aspiration biopsy of hepatocellular carcinoma: diagnostic dilemma at the ends of the spectrum. Acta Cytol 1994;38:347-54.
12. Stewart ET. Is a single negative core biopsy, clearly obtained from a suspicious lesion in the cirrhotic liver, sufficient to exclude the diagnosis of hepatocellular carcinoma as the cause of the lesion? AJR Am J Roentgenol 1994;163:1525.
13. Itai Y. Imaging diagnosis with computed tomography. In: Okuda K, Ishak KG, editors. Neoplasms of the liver. Tokyo: Springer-Verlag, 1987:289-300.
14. Falkson G, McIntyre JM, Moertel CG. Eastern Cooperative Oncology Group experience with chemotherapy for inoperable gallbladder and bile duct cancer. Cancer 1984;54:965-9.
15. Makuuchi M, Bandai Y, Ito T, et al. Ultrasonically guided percutaneous transhepatic bile drainage: a single-step procedure without cholangiography. Radiology 1980;135:165-9.
16. Soehendra N, Reynders-Frederix V. Palliative bile duct drainage—a new endoscopic method of introducing a transpapillary drain. Endoscopy 1980;12:8-11.

➢ COUNTERPOINT

Royal Liverpool University Hospital, UK

GRAEME J. POSTON

Primary malignancies of the liver and biliary tract are uncommon in the United Kingdom. The incidence of hepatocellular carcinoma is just under 1,000 new cases each year, and that of cholangiocarcinoma and gallbladder cancer just exceeds 500 new registrations annually for each disease. Because these diseases are uncommon, they are usually managed in specialist tertiary centers. This is in contrast to liver metastases, for which patients frequently are not referred to tertiary level specialists for assessment of resectability or palliative chemotherapy. Currently 11 centers in the United Kingdom undertake one or more liver resections each week and 30-day operative mortalities are uniform among these centers at 2% to 3%. As the indications for hepatectomy increase and physicians become more aware of the therapeutic potential of the procedure, other centers will be established.

I agree with Karpoff and Fong that for patients with primary cancer of the liver and bile ducts, surgical resection is the only treatment modality that offers a potential cure and that the objectives of follow-up management vary among the three primary cancers under consideration.

HEPATOCELLULAR CARCINOMA

In my practice patients fall into three distinct categories of approximately equal size: patients with alcoholic cirrhosis who are largely middle aged or elderly, patients with hepatocellular carcinoma arising spontaneously in the normal liver at any age (including a large proportion—50%—of the fibrolamellar variant), and patients with hepatocellular carcinoma arising after chronic active viral hepatitis, who are often middle aged and often Asian. Operative morbidity and mortality are higher after hepatic resection for hepatocellular carcinoma (8% increase in 30-day mortality) than after hepatectomy for liver metastases (no increase in 30-day mortality). This clearly reflects the nature of the sick livers of the majority of patients with hepatocellular carcinoma compared with patients who have secondary liver tumors. Furthermore, patients with cirrhosis and chronic active hepatitis have, in addition to the risk of metachronous hepatocellular carcinoma, the problems of associated conditions such as portal hypertension, chronic pancreatitis, and diabetes. Because of these additional problems, lifelong follow-up of these patients is inevitable.

Treatment Modalities

Resection with intent to cure should include an adequate resection margin of greater than 1 cm, including satellite micrometastases.[1] Furthermore, perioperative blood transfusion may promote recurrence after hepatectomy for hepatocellular carcinoma.[2] No data supporting the routine use of adjuvant chemotherapy after a potentially curative resection for hepatocellular carcinoma have been reported, and such treatment should not be considered outside the setting of a randomized, controlled clinical trial. Clearly, in the situation of cirrhotic patients with large tumors, clinical compromise must take place between adequacy of resection margins and sufficient volume of the functioning residual liver. In patients with small (less than 5 cm diameter) nonresectable tumors (because of either anatomical location or a general condition precluding major surgical intervention), ablative treatments using alcohol injection, cryosurgery, or interstitial heating with laser are reasonable therapeutic options.[3] However, the use of these techniques should be restricted to specialist centers and ideally they should be offered within the context of ongoing clinical trials and evaluation. Successful cure of hepatobiliary carcinoma has been reported after liver transplantation for hepatic failure in which a small carcinoma was found incidentally within the recipient's own liver.[4-6] However, as stated by Karpoff and Fong, liver transplantation should not be considered a first-line therapy in the management of hepatobiliary carcinoma.

For patients who are not suitable for interventional therapy or who have extrahepatic disease, palliative chemotherapy using adriamycin- or epirubicin-based regimens (given either systemically or regionally) offers some limited improvement in survival for a small percentage (less than 30%) of patients.[7,8] Furthermore, combination therapy (chemotherapy and radiation therapy) may debulk initially unresectable tumors to the point where they become resectable.[9,10] Survival rates after major hepatectomy for large primary liver cancers in European patients with cirrhosis at 1, 2, and 3 years are 66%, 43%, and 37%, respectively.[11]

Objectives of Follow-Up

While agreeing with Karpoff and Fong's objectives of follow-up, I would reprioritize these objectives. The immediate objective after surgery is the detection of postoperative problems. The longer term objectives include detection of treatable recurrence and metachronous primary tumors, management of concurrent medical problems, patient reassurance (where frequency of visits must be balanced with the psychological morbidity associated with such visits), and evaluation of the outcome of therapy.

Patterns of Recurrence and Incidence of New Primary Tumors

The pattern of recurrence and incidence of new primary tumors seen at Royal Liverpool University Hospital is identical to that described at Memorial Sloan-Kettering Cancer Center. The experience of patients with oncologically unstable cirrhotic livers described at Memorial Sloan-Kettering Cancer Center alone justifies lifelong follow-up after successful resection with curative intent. Similarly, the follow-up care of these patients should be shared with the hepatologist and should carefully consider other life-threatening associated disorders, in particular portal hypertension. I have lost one patient from bleeding esophageal varices and encephalopathy during the first 30 days after hepatectomy for hepatocellular carcinoma against the background of alcoholic cirrhosis. No data exist in the United Kingdom on the prevalence of hepatocellular carcinoma in patients with hepatitis C.

Treatment of Recurrence

Karpoff and Fong have outlined the literature on the management of hepatic and extrahepatic recurrent and metachronous hepatocellular carcinoma. Data concerning multiple (2 or more) repeat resections must be viewed carefully, since they come from centers of international excellence.[12-14] In these centers 5-year survival rates exceeding 90% can be achieved after second resection for recurrent hepatocellular carcinoma. It is my experience that repeat hepatectomy, particularly after a major previous procedure on a cirrhotic liver, is not as easy or safe as the first procedure.[14] Limited data are available to support surgical excision of extrahepatic recurrence,[15] but since surgery is the only effective therapeutic modality, this approach should be considered. Alternative forms of ablative therapy for recurrence should be considered only if surgical resection proves impossible, but there are no data that show such treatments to be equal or superior to surgical resection. Going further than Karpoff and Fong, I suggest restricting nonsurgical destructive therapies to tumors less than 5 cm diameter, since above this size the extent of tumor destruction is virtually impossible to assess during treatment. Regional and systemic chemotherapy of recurrent or inoperable hepatocellular carcinoma should be considered only within the context of a clinical trial.

Role of History and Physical Examination in Follow-Up

The primary objective of clinical follow-up is to detect symptoms and signs of recurrent or progressive cancer. Usually, however, by the time recurrent hepatocellular carcinoma becomes symptomatic or clinically detectable, it is incurable and the patient is near death. Patients with hepatocellular carcinoma who have significant weight loss, jaundice, or ascites are virtually certain to have incurable disease. Such patients respond rarely (if at all) to chemotherapy, and treatment should be directed at the symptoms.

Role of Blood Tests and Tumor Markers

With the exception of fibrolamellar hepatocellular carcinoma and the occasional nonfibrolamellar hepatocellular carcinoma that develops in a noncirrhotic liver, these tumors are usually associated with deranged liver function test results. Such patients rarely recover completely after successful hepatectomy, and therefore liver function tests have limited value in predicting or detecting recurrence. Serum alphafetoprotein levels in patients whose tumors secreted alphafetoprotein before resection (90%) remain the mainstay of follow-up in regular practice. The use of gamma-glutamyltransferase isoenzymes, fucosylated alpha-fetoprotein, and other putative serum tumor markers should be confined to clinical studies at present.

The follow-up of fibrolamellar hepatocellular carcinoma is more difficult, since as Karpoff and Fong state, these tumors do not secrete alpha-fetoprotein. Measurements of elevated serum levels of neurotensin and alterations in vitamin B_{12}–binding capacity are not readily available and are not very sensitive or specific. If the serum CEA level was elevated before hepatectomy and reverts to normal after resection, it may prove useful in monitoring progress.

Role of Imaging Studies

The most likely site of further disease is the liver. Hepatocellular carcinoma rarely metastasizes beyond regional lymph nodes before death. Spiral computed tomography and

Table 11-11 Follow-up of patients with hepatobiliary cancer (hepatocellular carcinoma): Royal Liverpool University Hospital, UK

	YEAR				
	1	2	3	4	5
Office visit	3	2	1	1	1
Liver function tests	3	2	1	1	1
Clotting studies*	3	2	1	1	1
Alpha-fetoprotein†	3	2	1	1	1
Abdominal computed tomography	2	2	1	1	1
Chest computed tomography	1‡	0	0	0	0

*Consists of coagulation time and prothrombin time.
†If patient had positive levels preoperatively.
‡Performed at 12 months.

magnetic resonance imaging are the best modalities for monitoring local recurrence, and the two are often complementary. If detectable lung metastases develop, this occurs within a year of resection of the primary tumor, so computed tomography of the lung should be performed once, 1 year after surgery in patients who are otherwise well. Isotope bone scans should be performed only if symptoms indicate the presence of bone metastases, which are rare, before palliative radiation therapy for symptomatic relief.

Current Recommendations

Patients in my practice are seen about 6 weeks after surgery to assess the state of wound healing and general health (Table 11-11). Blood is drawn for liver function tests, including clotting studies (as an indicator of hepatic function) and tumor markers if they were positive preoperatively. If the patients remain well, they are reviewed at 6 months after surgery with a repeat of the tests performed at the 6-week visit as well as computed tomography of the liver. Like Karpoff and Fong, I believe that imaging of otherwise well patients after potentially curative resection of hepatocellular carcinoma should be carried out initially at 6-month intervals. The 12-month visit is a repeat of the 6-month visit with the addition of computed tomography of the lung. Subsequently the patients are seen at 18 and 24 months and annually thereafter at a consultation that follows the protocol of the 6-month visit. The rationale for this approach is that the vast majority of relapses after hepatectomy for hepatocellular carcinoma occur in approximately the first 18 months.[11-15]

Patients with hepatic recurrence are managed by an approach identical to that advocated by Karpoff and Fong. I agree with their management of patients in whom extrahepatic disease develops, as well as patients with persistently elevated tumor marker levels who have no overt clinical or radiological evidence of tumor. Nononcological complications of cirrhosis or chronic active hepatitis should be managed by an appropriate physician.

CHOLANGIOCARCINOMA AND GALLBLADDER CANCER

Cholangiocarcinoma and gallbladder cancer are uncommon in Great Britain. The risk factors for cholangiocarcinoma include ulcerative colitis and sclerosing cholangitis. Gallbladder carcinoma (rare below the age of 70) is never seen in the absence of gallstones. Because they pose similar follow-up management problems, these cancers are considered together.

Both diseases usually present at an advanced stage when they are unresectable and incurable. In the largest U.K. series of cholangiocarcinoma (178 cases collected over a 10-year period from the Hammersmith Hospital), more than 80% were nonresectable at the time of presentation.[16] No one in Britain has an experience similar to that of Nimura et al.[17-19] in Japan who achieved resectability rates greater than 70%. The only treatment modality that offers a chance of cure is radical surgery.[20,21] For tumors that involve the confluence of the hepatic ducts or below, surgery necessitates a biliary drainage procedure and may also include a pancreatoduodenectomy. Radiation therapy (either external beam or intracavity) offers palliation at best and should be combined with endoscopic or percutaneous biliary stenting.[22] There are no data to support systemic chemotherapy, either in the adjuvant setting postsurgery or for palliation outside the setting of a randomized, controlled clinical trial.

Patterns of Recurrence After Surgical Resection

Two factors determine the risk of recurrence after surgical resection of both cholangiocarcinoma and gallbladder cancer: positive resection margins[22] and stage of tumor at presentation.[24-26] Five-year survival rates for British patients after resection with negative resection margins for cholangiocarcinoma and gallbladder cancer are similar to those described by the authors from Memorial Sloan-Kettering Cancer Center.[24-26] Median survival times of patients whose resection margins are involved is 12 months and for patients who undergo palliative stenting or surgical bypass is 6 months.[16,23-26] Additional problems for patients after surgical resection of extrahepatic cholangiocarcinoma and gallbladder cancer include benign fibrotic stricturing at the biliary-enteric anastomosis and an increase in the prevalence of peptic ulcer disease consequent to biliary diversion away from the duodenum.

Objectives of Follow-Up

I agree with Karpoff and Fong in their follow-up objectives for both cholangiocarcinoma and gallbladder cancer, particularly in not setting detection of a second biliary primary tumor as a major aim of follow-up.

Outcome of Treatment of Recurrence

There are little or no data to support a policy of repeat resection of extrahepatic cholangiocarcinoma or recurrent gallbladder cancer for curative intent. In the rare and isolated case of a solitary metachronous intrahepatic primary cholangiocarcinoma arising after a previous hepatectomy for a similar tumor, a repeat hepatectomy could be justified. In this situation the patient should be warned that the overall prognosis is very guarded. Anastomotic recurrence presenting as obstructive jaundice and cholangitis is best managed by percutaneous biliary stenting and palliative external beam radiation therapy.[22]

The goals of palliation of recurrent disease are relief of obstructive jaundice and associated cholangitis and treatment aimed at slowing down tumor progression. Particularly after surgical resection of extrahepatic cholangiocarcinoma the management strategy is complicated by the fact that cholangitis and obstructive jaundice may be due to either local recurrence or benign anastomotic stricture. Obtaining a tissue diagnosis from the site of the biliary enteric anastomosis is often impossible without recourse to a major laparotomy. Other factors may be indicative of recurrent disease, including malignant ascites or peritoneal deposits detected at laparoscopy, hepatic and distant metastases, and rising levels of serum tumor markers such as CA 19-9 and CEA. However, serum tumor markers must be used judiciously in this setting, since they are excreted in bile and may rise as a consequence of obstructive jaundice rather than tumor recurrence. Alternative diagnostic measures include percutaneous transhe-patic cholangiography, which can be combined with an internal or temporary external biliary drainage procedure. Shouldering of a stricture adjacent to the biliary-enteric anastomosis might suggest local recurrence, and bile can be aspirated for cytological examination. Hepatic angiography may be of diagnostic use in detecting recurrence by demonstrating encasement of either the hepatic artery or portal vein by the tumor. Finally, in units with such expertise, fine fiberoptic endoscopy can be attempted via a percutaneous cholangiography catheter.

Stenting of biliary-enteric anastomotic strictures must be performed only if recurrent carcinoma is confirmed. Benign strictures should not be stented. The ideal treatment of a benign anastomotic stricture is surgical revision, preferably to a distant site on the biliary tree (segment 3-4 duct in the recessus of Rex). If surgical revision is not possible, the physician should consider percutaneous balloon cholangioplasty, which may have to be repeated frequently to control episodes of cholangitis.

Role of Routine Blood Tests and Tumor Markers

As Karpoff and Fong state, derangement of liver function tests (particularly rising alkaline phosphatase and bilirubin levels) is indicative of biliary obstruction, which may be due to a benign anastomotic stricture. Frequently the serum alkaline phosphatase level never returns completely to normal after biliary reconstructive surgery. Rising tumor marker levels must be considered with care in the presence of obstructive jaundice.

Role of Imaging Studies

The purpose of further intervention is either to palliate the symptoms of progressive disease or to treat obstructive jaundice and cholangitis resulting from benign anastomotic stricture. Therefore regular imaging of the liver by any radiological modality has little or no point during routine follow-up of an otherwise well patient. If obstructive jaundice develops, ultrasound is the investigation of choice. It will demonstrate the level of obstruction and, if performed by an experienced operator, will show a tumor mass discrete from the surrounding liver parenchyma. Ultrasound may also show vascular encasement, and duplex scanning will demonstrate obstruction to flow in both the hepatic artery and portal vein.

Table 11-12 Follow-up of patients with hepatobiliary cancer (cholangiocarcinoma or gallbladder cancer): Royal Liverpool University Hospital, UK

	YEAR				
	1	2	3	4	5
Office visit	5	2	1	1	1
Liver function tests	5	2	1	1	1
CEA	5	2	1	1	1
CA 19-9	5	2	1	1	1

CEA, Carcinoembryonic antigen.

Current Recommendations

I follow a management strategy similar to that of Karpoff and Fong after surgical resection for either cholangiocarcinoma or gallbladder cancer. Patients are seen at 6 weeks to assess wound healing (Table 11-12). In the rare situation that a percutaneous catheter has been left across a difficult biliary-enteric anastomosis, cholangiography is performed before catheter removal. Blood is drawn for liver function tests, and tumor marker levels, including CEA and CA 19-9, are checked. If patients remain well, they are seen again at 3, 6, 9, and 12 months after surgery and these investigations are repeated. Thereafter patients are seen at 18 and 24 months before proceeding to annual checkups for life. After 5 years the main reason for continued follow-up is the development of late benign stricture of the anastomosis.

REFERENCES

1. Lai EC, You KT, Ng IO, Shek TW. The pathological basis of resection margin for hepatocellular carcinoma. World J Surg 1993;17:786-91.
2. Yamamoto J, Kosuge T, Takayama T, et al. Perioperative blood transfusion promotes recurrence of hepatocellular carcinoma after hepatectomy. Surgery 1994;115:303-9.
3. Livraghi T, Lazzaroni S, Meloni F, et al. Intralesional ethanol in the treatment of unresectable liver cancer. World J Surg 1995;19:801-6.
4. Pichlmayr R, Weimann A, Oldhafer KJ, et al. Role of liver transplantation in the treatment of unresectable liver cancer. World J Surg 1995;19:807-13.
5. McPeake J, Williams R. Liver transplantation for hepatocellular carcinoma. Gut 1995;36:644-6.
6. Tan KC, Rela M, Ryder SD, et al. Experience of orthotopic liver transplantation and hepatic resection for hepatocellular carcinoma of less than 8 cm in patients with cirrhosis. Br J Surg 1995;82:253-6.
7. Ku Y, Fukumoto T, Iwasaki T, et al. Clinical pilot study on high-dose intraarterial chemotherapy with direct hemoperfusion under hepatic venous isolation in patients with advanced hepatocellular carcinoma. Surgery 1995;117:510-9.

8. Yamada R, Kishi K, Sato M, et al. Transcatheter arterial chemoembolization (TACE) in the treatment of unresectable liver cancer. World J Surg 1995;19:795-800.
9. Tang ZY, Yu YQ, Zhou XD, et al. Cytoreduction and sequential reduction for surgically verified unresectable hepatocellular carcinoma: evaluation with analysis of 72 patients. World J Surg 1995; 19:784-9.
10. Sitzmann JV. Conversion of unresectable to resectable liver cancer: an approach and follow-up study. World J Surg 1995;19:790-4.
11. Capussotti L, Borgonovo G, Bouzari H, Smadja C, Grange D, Franco D. Results of major hepatectomy for large primary liver cancer in patients with cirrhosis. Br J Surg 1994;81:427-31.
12. Nakajima Y, Ohmura T, Kimura J, et al. Role of surgical treatment for recurrent hepatocellular carcinoma after hepatic resection. World J Surg 1993;17:792-5.
13. Suenaga M, Sugiura H, Kokuba Y, Uehara S, Kurumiya T. Repeated hepatic resection for recurrent hepatocellular carcinoma in eighteen cases. Surgery 1994;115:452-7.
14. Nagasue N, Kohno H, Hayashi T, et al. Repeat hepatectomy for recurrent hepatocellular carcinoma. Br J Surg 1996;83:127-31.
15. Lo CM, Lai EC, Fan ST, Choi TK, Wong J. Resection for extrahepatic recurrence of hepatocellular carcinoma. Br J Surg 1994;81:1019-21.
16. Blumgart LH, Benjamin IS. Cancer of the bile ducts. In: Blumgart LH, editor. Surgery of the liver and biliary tract, Vol. 2, 2nd ed., Edinburgh: Churchill Livingstone, 1994:967-95.
17. Nimura Y, Hayakawa N, Kamiya J, Kondo S, Shionoya S. Hepatic segmentectomy with caudate lobe resection for bile duct carcinoma of the hepatic hilus. World J Surg 1990;14:535-44.
18. Nimura Y, Hayakawa N, Kamiya J, et al. Combined portal vein and liver resection for carcinoma of the biliary tree. Br J Surg 1991; 78:727-31.
19. Nimura Y, Hayakawa N, Kamiya J, et al. Hepatopancreatoduodenectomy for advanced carcinoma of the biliary tract. Hepatogastroenterology 1991;38:170-5.
20. Sugiura Y, Nakamura S, Iida S, et al. Extensive resection of the bile ducts combined with liver resection for cancer of the main hepatic duct junction: a cooperative study of the Keio Bile Duct Cancer Study Group. Surgery 1994;115:445-51.
21. Miyagawa S, Makuuchi M, Kawasaki S, et al. Outcome of major hepatectomy and pancreatoduodenectomy for advanced biliary malignancies. World J Surg 1996;20:77-80.
22. Kuvshinoff BW, Armstrong JG, Fong Y, et al. Palliation of irresectable hilar cholangiocarcinoma with biliary drainage and radiotherapy. Br J Surg 1995;82:1522-5.
23. Ogura Y, Takahashi K, Tabata M, Mizumoto R. Clinicopathological study on carcinoma of the extrahepatic bile duct with special focus on cancer invasion on the surgical margins. World J Surg 1994;18:778-84.
24. Bhuiya MR, Nimura Y, Kamiya J, Kondo S, Nagino M, Hayakawa N. Clinicopathologic factors influencing survival of patients with bile duct carcinoma: multivariate statistical analysis. World J Surg 1993; 17:653-7.
25. Ouchi K, Suzuki M, Tominaga T, Saijo S, Matsuno S. Survival after surgery for cancer of the gallbladder. Br J Surg 1994;81:1655-7.
26. Chijiiwa K, Tanaka M. Carcinoma of the gallbladder: an appraisal of surgical resection. Surgery 1994;115:751-6.

➢ COUNTERPOINT

Roswell Park Cancer Institute

JUDY L. SMITH

Hepatobiliary cancers are a major health concern worldwide and account for approximately 15,000 deaths each year in the United States.[1] The guidelines for follow-up vary greatly across practices according to the philosophy of the particular institution and the availability of screening modalities.

Table 11-13 Follow-up of patients with hepatobiliary cancer (hepatocellular carcinoma): Roswell Park Cancer Institute

	YEAR				
	1	2	3	4	5
Office visit	12	6	4	4	4
Liver function tests	12	6	4	4	4
Alpha-fetoprotein*	12	6	4	4	4
CEA*	12	6	4	4	4
Chest x-ray	6	6	2	2	2
Abdominal computed tomography	6	6	2	2	2

CEA, Carcinoembryonic antigen.
*Performed if levels were elevated preoperatively.

Hepatocellular carcinoma is a universal health concern. Surgical resection is the standard therapy for and represents the dominant potentially curative modality for the treatment of recurrence. The goal of follow-up is the early detection of primary and recurrent cancers to increase the possibility of curative resection. Secondary aims of follow-up include the treatment of disease (cirrhosis, hepatitis, and hepatic insufficiency) and the palliation of unresectable recurrent disease.

Hepatocellular carcinoma recurs in up to 90% of patients after resection, and intrahepatic recurrence is the major cause of death in these patients.[2-4] Recurrence takes place in the liver alone in 38% to 50% of patients; one third of recurrences may be solitary recurrences or second primary tumors.[4,5] Peritoneum, abdominal wall, and other distant sites are also commonly involved. Most recurrences and deaths occur within the first 18 to 24 months after resection, but recurrence can be seen for 4 or more years. Second primary hepatic malignancies are a lifetime risk for many of these patients.[6,7]

A rigorous follow-up program is expensive and difficult to justify in many solid tumor cases. For patients with hepatocellular carcinoma effective treatment is available for hepatic recurrence if detected early. Resection of recurrence is safe and may improve survival, with 5-year survival rates from 9% to 30%.[2-8] Frequent and intensive surveillance is necessary to provide early diagnosis, since the carcinoma can assume an aggressive pattern of growth.[8] Physicians at Roswell Park Cancer Institute therefore recommend a vigorous program of follow-up for patients with hepatocellular carcinoma after resection as delineated in Table 11-13.

Cholangiocarcinomas and carcinomas of the gallbladder are much less common than hepatocellular carcinoma and much less amenable to treatment after recurrence. Aggressive primary resection is the most effective treatment. Treatment for recurrence invariably fails to provide cure.

Table 11-14 Follow-up of patients with hepatobiliary cancer (cholangiocarcinoma or gallbladder cancer): Roswell Park Cancer Institute

	YEAR				
	1	2	3	4	5
Office visit	4	4	2	2	2
CEA*	5	5	2	2	2
CA 19-9*	5	5	2	2	2
Liver function tests	4	4	2	2	2
Chest x-ray	2	2	1	1	1
Abdominal computed tomography	2	2	1	1	1

CEA, Carcinoembryonic antigen.
*Performed postoperatively and at 3-month intervals if levels were elevated preoperatively.

Follow-up in these patients should be guided by the symptoms and be aimed at the detection of other medical problems, the treatment of surgical complications, and palliation of recurrences. The recommended guidelines for follow-up of these patients at Roswell Park Cancer Institute closely parallel those of Karpoff and Fong and are displayed in Table 11-14.

REFERENCES

1. Parker SL, Tong T, Bolden S, Wingo PA. Cancer statistics, 1996. CA Cancer J Clin 1996;65:5-27.
2. Order SE, Stillwagon GB, Ettinger DS. Primary liver cancers. In: Brain MC, Carbone PC, editors. Current therapy in hematology-oncology, 4th ed. St. Louis: Mosby, 1992:265-9.
3. Ringe B, Pichlmayr R, Wittekind C, Tusch G. Surgical treatment of hepatocellular carcinoma: experience with liver resection and transplantation in 198 patients. World J Surg 1991;15:270-85.
4. Matsuda Y, Ito T, Oguchi Y, Nakajima K, Izukura T. Rationale of surgical management for recurrent hepatocellular carcinoma. Ann Surg 1993;217:28-34.
5. Smalley SR, Moertel CG, Hilton JF, et al. Hepatoma in the noncirrhotic liver. Cancer 1988;62:1414-24.
6. Nagasue N, Yukaya H, Chang YC, et al. Assessment of pattern and treatment of intrahepatic recurrence after resection of hepatocellular carcinoma. Surg Gynecol Obstet 1990;171:217-22.
7. Penn I. Hepatic transplantation for primary and metastatic cancers of the liver. Surgery 1991;110:726-35.
8. Suenaga M, Nakao A, Harada A, et al. Hepatic resection for hepatocellular carcinoma. World J Surg 1992;16:97-105.

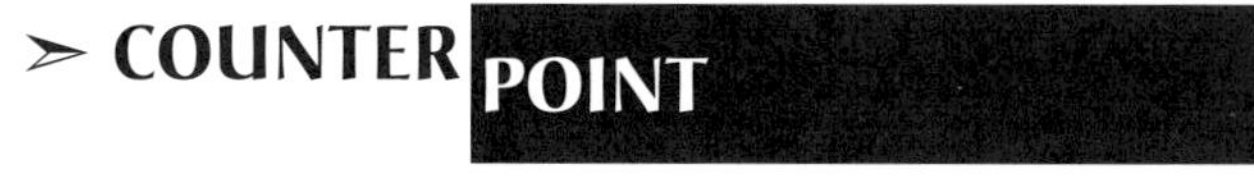

University of Washington Medical Center

W. SCOTT HELTON AND CARLOS A. PELLEGRINI

It is difficult to recommend a simple follow-up regimen that can be applied universally to patients with cancer of the hepatobiliary tree because the natural history, treatment, and prognosis for hepatocellular carcinoma, bile duct cancer, and gallbladder cancer vary considerably. The long-term outcome of patients with these cancers depends on a number of factors in addition to the initial tumor stage and type of treatment. Karpoff and Fong recommend three basic follow-up regimens for patients who have undergone surgical resection of hepatobiliary malignancy, soundly basing their recommendations on a thorough review of current practice, outcome of treatment for recurrent disease, and utility of specific blood tests, tumor markers, and imaging studies. Unfortunately, the majority of patients with hepatocellular carcinoma are not amenable to curative resection and undergo palliative forms of therapy. Therefore, in addition to commenting on Karpoff and Fong's recommendations for follow-up for previously resected patients, follow-up guidelines are provided for patients receiving nonsurgical and noncurative forms of therapy. Furthermore, a number of guidelines are discussed which may be useful in designing highly individualized and cost-effective follow-up strategies for patients with hepatocellular carcinoma.

Karpoff and Fong outline six goals of follow-up for patients with hepatocellular carcinoma. The first two are to detect early, recurrent disease and to treat such disease by repeat surgical resection or nonablative therapy, resulting in improved survival or palliation. Karpoff and Fong correctly point out that the only patients likely to benefit from close postoperative surveillance are those with recurrent hepatocellular carcinoma confined to the liver, since patients with recurrent gallbladder cancer and cholangiocarcinoma are rarely cured. Tumor surveillance should not be performed in asymptomatic patients with any form of incurable hepatobiliary cancer.

Karpoff and Fong's last four goals of follow-up are designed to detect medical and surgical problems, provide patient reassurance, and define outcome. All these goals are important with respect to overall patient care and advancing the therapy for hepatocellular carcinoma. Unfortunately, it is becoming difficult to convince third-party payors and managed care organizations to provide for these services, since meeting these patients' needs has little impact on their survival. Therefore the resources devoted to meeting the last four goals as described by Karpoff and Fong, especially for asymptomatic patients or for patients with incurable disease, should be kept to a minimum.

HEPATOCELLULAR CARCINOMA
General Guidelines for Patient-Specific Follow-Up

Before we comment on Karpoff and Fong's recommendations for follow-up, several issues warrant consideration in an effort to make follow-up patient specific and cost effective (Table 11-15). Patients unwilling to receive additional therapy if recurrent disease is detected should not be monitored for tumor recurrence. Patients receiving palliative therapy should receive follow-up that is specifically designed to monitor and maintain quality of life and symptom relief. Patients with decompensated cirrhosis (for example, Child C) should not be monitored or treated for

Table 11-15 Issues to consider before recommending individualized cost-effective patient follow-up

Patient's willingness to accept and ability to tolerate additional therapy
Palliative versus curative resection
Presence of symptoms
Underlying medical conditions, severity of cirrhosis, and performance status

hepatocellular carcinoma unless liver transplantation is being considered. In patients with unresectable or metastatic cancer, symptoms and progressive disease predominantly dictate the need for office visits, diagnostic tests, therapy, and follow-up. Conversely, asymptomatic patients with known persistent, incurable cancer do not require routine office visits, serial blood tests, or imaging studies. Routine office visits beyond the immediate postoperative period have little role in postoperative tumor surveillance and are not recommended for asymptomatic patients. Frequent office visits are indicated primarily for monitoring and treating patients with advanced liver disease and other medical problems.

Justification for Follow-Up of Patients with Hepatocellular Carcinoma

Karpoff and Fong point out that the only rationale for monitoring patients for recurrent hepatocellular carcinoma is to detect early recurrence confined to the liver that can be treated with the hope of improving survival. We strongly agree with that recommendation, since the evidence is clear that secondary treatment by a variety of means improves survival.[1,2] However, tumor surveillance is recommended for all patients with hepatocellular carcinoma, since additional therapy directed at recurrent disease is justified only when no evidence of extrahepatic disease is present and the patient is able to tolerate additional therapy. Patients with extremely poor prognostic features determined at the time of initial tumor staging (such as patients with expected survival less than 6 months) should not be subjected to postoperative tumor surveillance unless they are enrolled in clinical trials. Further, patients with tumor invasion of the portal vein should not be subjected to routine tumor surveillance or repeated laboratory testing.

Patients with advanced cirrhosis (Child C) and portal vein thrombosis are at significantly increased risk for therapeutic complications. Tumor-specific therapy often accelerates their death.[3,4] Although evidence exists that tamoxifen[5,6] and intraarterial radiation therapy[7] are of some benefit to patients with unresectable hepatocellular carcinoma associated with portal vein thrombosis, the management of patients with such extensive disease should be confined to prospective clinical trials. Patients with limited survival are best served with palliative care only. Under these guidelines only a small group of patients with hepatocellular carcinoma can truly benefit from close tumor surveillance: those with minimal liver disease (such as Child A cirrhosis) treated with curative intent.

We agree with several of Karpoff and Fong's recommendations for follow-up of patients with hepatocellular carcinoma as summarized in their follow-up strategy (Table 11-5). First, patients undergoing resection for cure should be followed up closely with gamma-glutamyltransferase, tumor markers, and imaging studies in an effort to detect treatable recurrent hepatocellular carcinoma of the liver. Second, follow-up should be lifelong for patients with underlying cirrhosis because of the increased risk for a new primary hepatocellular carcinoma. Third, patients without identifiable tumor markers should be followed up more frequently with imaging studies. Chest x-ray should be obtained once a year to detect pulmonary metastases. If pulmonary metastases are detected, treatment may be altered. As stated by Karpoff and Fong, the frequency of monitoring can decrease after 5 years because the risk of recurrence, especially in noncirrhotic patients, decreases over time.

Karpoff and Fong make excellent recommendations for the selective monitoring of patients with fibrolamellar hepatocellular carcinoma based on the unique markers this tumor produces. Although patients with fibrolamellar hepatocellular carcinoma have an overall outcome that is better than patients with standard hepatocellular carcinoma, they still have a significant risk for recurrent intrahepatic tumors, which are usually at the surgical margin. Hence close postoperative tumor surveillance is needed in patients with fibrolamellar hepatocellular carcinoma.

We disagree with several aspects of Karpoff and Fong's recommended surveillance for recurrent hepatocellular carcinoma. They point out that recurrent, treatable hepatocellular carcinoma is unlikely to be detected by physical examination and yet advocate follow-up office visits every 3 months. At the University of Washington Medical Center return office visits to see the surgeon after full recovery from surgery or other ablative therapy are not advocated unless the surgeon is responsible for managing the patient's medical problems related to cirrhosis. Karpoff and Fong point out that gamma-glutamyltransferase and alpha-fetoprotein are the most specific and cost-effective serum markers for detecting recurrent hepatocellular carcinoma, yet they recommend also performing other liver function tests, including bilirubin and alkaline phosphatase, every 3 months. Since standard liver function tests are not specific or sensitive for detecting recurrent hepatocellular carcinoma in the liver, they should not be used for tumor surveillance.

Karpoff and Fong point out that ultrasound is the most common imaging modality used worldwide for monitoring patients for recurrent hepatocellular carcinoma and recommend its routine use. Since both ultrasound and conventional computed tomography miss up to 20% of small hepatocellular carcinomas in the cirrhotic liver,[8] we do not recommend ultrasound for tumor surveillance in patients at risk for recurrent hepatocellular carcinoma. A number of imaging tests with a sensitivity demonstrably better than ultrasound are available for detecting early hepatocellular carcinoma. Prospective trials have demonstrated that com-

Table 11-16 Follow-up of patients with hepatobiliary cancer (recurrent hepatocellular carcinoma after surgical resection for cure): University of Washington Medical Center

	YEAR				
	1	2	3	4	5
Office visit	5	4*	4	4	4
Alpha-fetoprotein	4	4	4	4	4
Gamma-glutamyltransferase	4	4	4	4	4
Helical abdominal computed tomography	3	3	1	1	1
Chest x-ray	1	1	1	1	1

*The frequency of office visits for patients without cirrhosis is once a year beginning in the second year.

Table 11-17 Factors predictive of early intrahepatic recurrence and poor survival

TNM stage and size of primary (T stage)[75,76]
- Portal venous invasion[16]
- Multiple lesions versus single lesion[16]

Intrahepatic metastasis[16]
Presence or absence of a tumor capsule[77]
Chronic liver disease[16]
Inadequate margin at resection (less than 1 cm)[78,79]
Cirrhosis and its severity[16]
- Child A, B survival greater than Child C[16,22,28,56]
- Increased indocyanine green retention[16,80]

Advanced age and decompensated cirrhosis[17]
Macroscopic features: diffuse > encapsulated > fibrolamellar[79]
Nontumorous factors[18,81,82]
- Elevated alanine aminotransferase level (greater than 54 IU)
- Albumin level less than 3.7 mg/dl
- Active hepatic inflammation
- Proliferating cell nuclear antigen labeling index greater than 23%

Serum intercellular adhesion molecule-1[83]
Tumor doubling time[1,84]

puted tomography of the abdomen after intrahepatic arterial lipoidal injection (lipoidal computed tomography) is more sensitive at detecting small carcinomas (less than 2 cm) than ultrasound, conventional magnetic resonance imaging, or angiography combined.[9,10] Although lipoidal computed tomography is considered the most sensitive means of detecting small hepatocellular carcinomas in the cirrhotic liver, this imaging modality still misses a large number of small tumors.[11] Dynamic magnetic resonance imaging and helical computed tomography, also known as spiral computed tomography, can reliably detect hepatocellular carcinoma less than 1 cm in cirrhotic livers[12] and are emerging as the techniques of choice for evaluating liver tumors.[13-15] Lipoidal computed tomography and computed tomography arterial portography are expensive (approximately $3,500 U.S.). Charges for helical computed tomography are approximately $800 U.S. and for dynamic magnetic resonance imaging approximately $1,000 U.S. Therefore, when considering the charges and sensitivities of all imaging studies for detecting small hepatocellular carcinoma, helical computed tomography scan, where available, should be the imaging modality of choice.

Patients should be monitored at 4-month intervals instead of annually by computed tomography, as recommended by Karpoff and Fong. Our recommendation is based on the possibility that recurrent tumors with doubling times of less than 2 months can become detectable within such a time interval. Unless cost constraints limit postoperative monitoring, ultrasound should be used only to monitor for recurrent hepatocellular carcinoma in patients without cirrhosis. Table 11-16 summarizes practices at the University of Washington Medical Center for follow-up of patients with hepatocellular carcinoma previously treated by surgical resection for cure.

Karpoff and Fong recommend more frequent follow-up intervals for patients whose tumor markers do not return to normal postoperatively and for patients with hepatocellular carcinoma without elevated tumor markers. They recommend that these patients have liver function tests, tumor marker studies, and abdominal imaging performed every 2 months until recurrent disease is detected. Patients with persistently elevated tumor markers after curative liver resection have either metastatic disease or additional hepatocellular carcinoma in the liver that has yet to be detected. Efforts should be made to detect these potential sites of recurrence. However, the most cost-effective means of achieving this is to repeat helical computed tomography of the abdomen or perform lipoidal computed tomography no sooner than 2 months postoperatively. If no new lesions are seen in the liver, computed tomography of the chest, if not already performed, is indicated to rule out the presence of pulmonary metastases. No benefit is evident for more frequent office visits and the measurement of serum tumor markers and liver function tests, since these methods of surveillance do not localize recurrent disease. Furthermore, if extrahepatic metastases are detected, additional imaging tests are not indicated. Patients enrolled in clinical trials in whom tumor response to various therapies is being evaluated are exceptions to this rule.

Karpoff and Fong point out that the long-term outcome and risk for developing recurrent hepatocellular carcinoma are dependent on the TNM stage and histology of the primary tumor. There are several other pathological features unique to the tumor and underlying liver pathology in addition to those mentioned that are associated with an increased risk for developing a second hepatocellular carcinoma (Table 11-17). These factors should be taken into account when considering an individual's risk for recurrence and planning the frequency of follow-up. For example, the observation that there is an increased risk for intrahepatic recurrence in patients with hepatic inflammation at the time of initial tumor resection[16-19] suggests that patients with cirrhosis and chronic active hepatitis should be offered close and frequent follow-up.

Follow-Up of Patients with Primary or Recurrent Hepatocellular Carcinoma Treated with Nonresectional Methods

Karpoff and Fong focus on the role of repeat liver resection for recurrent hepatocellular carcinoma, since this results in the best long-term survival when compared with other forms of treatment. However, because of inadequate liver reserve and ability to tolerate further liver resection, only a small percentage of patients with recurrent intrahepatic hepatocellular carcinoma are amenable to repeat liver resection. Thus the majority of patients with recurrent hepatocellular carcinoma confined to the liver are treated by nonresectional techniques[20-25] such as percutaneous ethanol injection,[26-30] transarterial embolization or chemoembolization,[13,31-34] ischemic therapy,[35] cryoablation,[36,37] hormonal therapy,[6] radiation therapy,[38-41] and combination therapy.[20,42-48] Recent experience suggests that survival after some forms of nonresectional therapy for hepatocellular carcinoma is equivalent to that after surgical resection.[36,37,49] Percutaneous ethanol injection alone[28,49-51] or after embolization therapy[52,53] and cryoablation[36,37] can completely eradicate hepatocellular carcinomas. Therefore patients treated with curative intent by nonresectional techniques deserve the same follow-up as patients undergoing surgical resection. In the discussion that follows, current practice patterns are reviewed and our recommendations for the follow-up of patients treated with nonresectional forms of tumor ablation are provided.

Follow-Up of Patients with Hepatocellular Carcinoma Treated by Percutaneous Ethanol Injection

The optimal method and timing of follow-up for patients after percutaneous ethanol injection have not been defined. Encapsulated tumors less than 3 cm in diameter are often completely destroyed with this technique. However, the incidence of residual or locally recurrent disease is approximately 10%.[30] Ultrasound with duplex scanning, computed tomography scan, lipoidal computed tomography, angiographic computed tomography, magnetic resonance imaging,[29] positron emission tomography,[54] serial biopsy,[51] and repeated serum alpha-fetoprotein measurement have all been advocated as methods of assessing residual disease.[55] Areas of high attenuation on computed tomography, increased activity by positron emission tomography, or residual vascularity by duplex scanning or angiography are evidence of residual disease that requires additional ethanol injection into and around the tumor.[28,53] When no residual disease is evident at the site of treatment, follow-up should adhere to the guidelines established for patients undergoing resection for cure.

Clinicians with the largest published experience at treating hepatocellular carcinoma by percutaneous ethanol injection in patients with cirrhosis recommend follow-up with serial abdominal ultrasound and alpha-fetoprotein every 3 months or ultrasound every 3 months alternating with dynamic computed tomography scan every 6 months.[28,51,53,56] Magnetic resonance imaging, although more expensive than helical computed tomography, is also fairly sensitive at detecting persistent carcinoma after percutaneous ethanol injection.[29,57] Lipoidal computed tomography does not accurately assess the presence of persistent tumor after percutaneous ethanol injection and should be performed only in an effort to detect new foci of carcinoma. Total charges for this recommended follow-up strategy, including imaging studies and alpha-fetoprotein, are approximately $3,200 U.S. per year. The ability of such tumor surveillance to improve long-term survival in patients found to have recurrent or secondary hepatocellular carcinoma is not yet established.

Most patients treated with percutaneous ethanol injection have cirrhosis and are at risk for additional lesions. Close follow-up for additional tumors is recommended for patients with compensated Child A or B cirrhosis. Patients with decompensated or Child C cirrhosis should not be monitored or treated for recurrent hepatocellular carcinoma, since the complication rate is high and survival is related to the severity of the underlying liver disease, not to the development of additional tumors. Therefore patients with advanced liver disease should not be subjected to serial imaging studies, liver function tests, or alpha-fetoprotein measurements.

Follow-Up of Patients with Hepatocellular Carcinoma Treated by Cryosurgery

Cryosurgical ablation is being used increasingly to treat patients who have hepatocellular carcinoma with compromised liver function.[36,37,58] Cryosurgery leaves a scar or ghost image in the liver that is indistinguishable from cancer using conventional imaging modalities such as ultrasound, computed tomography, or magnetic resonance imaging, but positron emission tomography with 18-F-fluorodeoxyglucose can readily distinguish cancer from scar tissue.[54] Hence positron emission tomography appears to be an excellent method of detecting residual viable tumors in a lesion previously treated by cryosurgical ablation.[59] Although the utility of positron emission tomography in detecting recurrent hepatocellular carcinoma has not been reported, the potential for this new sensitive imaging modality is great and includes the detection of recurrent disease and the evaluation of response of hepatocellular carcinoma to all forms of nonresectional therapy.[54] Unfortunately, positron emission tomography is relatively expensive (approximately $1,500 U.S.) and not readily available outside of university centers. Therefore the most sensible means of following patients for persistent or recurrent disease is by serial alpha-fetoprotein and computed tomography. Recommendations for the follow-up of patients undergoing percutaneous ethanol injection or cryosurgery are summarized in Table 11-18.

Table 11-18 Follow-up of patients with hepatobiliary cancer (persistent or recurrent hepatocellular carcinoma after nonresectional ablative techniques)*: University of Washington Medical Center

	YEAR				
	1	2	3	4	5
Office visit†	1‡	4	4	4	4
Alpha-fetoprotein	4§	4	4	4	4
Helical abdominal computed tomography	3	3	1	1	1
Abdominal positron emission tomography	1¶	0	0	0	0

*Includes cryosurgery and percutaneous ethanol injection with or without embolic therapy.
†Once alpha-fetoprotein levels return to normal, the frequency of follow-up is every 3 months.
‡First follow-up visit is up to 3 months after treatment.
§Follow-up frequency is every 6 weeks until alpha-fetoprotein levels return to normal, then every 3 months.
¶Persistently elevated alpha-fetoprotein and increased attenuation seen by computed tomography are indicative of incomplete tumor cell killing and should be followed by positron emission tomography or biopsy to detect persistent disease. An alternative to positron emission tomography is to perform additional ethanol injection into and around the area of suspicion.

Follow-Up of Patients Receiving Transplants for Hepatocellular Carcinoma

We agree with Karpoff and Fong that hepatic transplantation should be considered experimental therapy. Although transplantation is relatively commonly used to treat patients with hepatocellular carcinoma, including some with cirrhosis in whom hepatocellular carcinoma was not suspected, no established or consistent guidelines exist for monitoring patients for recurrent hepatocellular carcinoma after orthotopic liver transplantation. Recurrence after orthotopic liver transplantation occurs both in and outside the liver.[60,61] No form of effective treatment currently exists for recurrent disease, and most patients die of metastatic cancer within a year of recurrence.[25] Therefore monitoring patients by computed tomography or alpha-fetoprotein for recurrent disease is not advocated unless the patients are enrolled in a clinical trial in which disease-free survival is being monitored.

Recommended Additional Evaluation When Recurrent Hepatocellular Carcinoma Is Identified by Surveillance

When recurrent hepatocellular carcinoma is detected, patients should be assessed for their willingness to undergo operation, their ability to tolerate additional liver resection, and the risk for nonresectional forms of therapy before further evaluation for extrahepatic metastases. As Karpoff and Fong state, additional studies are needed to exclude extrahepatic hepatocellular carcinoma before initiating additional potentially curative therapy. Karpoff and Fong recommend computed tomography of the chest, abdomen, and pelvis, magnetic resonance imaging, or angiography to exclude extrahepatic disease. In contrast to this approach, we recommend whole-body positron emission tomography as the first additional diagnostic test of choice to exclude the presence of extrahepatic disease. The cumulative charges for computed tomography of the pelvis, abdomen, and chest and bone scans are approximately $3,500 U.S. The charge for positron emission tomography with 18-F-fluorodeoxyglucose is approximately $1,500 U.S., and it is more sensitive than computed tomography for detecting extrahepatic cancer, especially lung and lymph node metastases (unpublished personal observations). When recurrent hepatocellular carcinoma in the liver is identified and extrahepatic cancer is excluded by imaging studies, diagnostic laparoscopy is recommended to exclude peritoneal and surface hepatic metastases not seen by computed tomography before subjecting the patient to laparotomy and repeat liver resection, cryosurgery, or percutaneous ethanol injection. Although no data are available on the cost effectiveness of this approach, several physicians have commented on its utility.[62,63]

Patients with recurrent extrahepatic hepatocellular carcinoma do not obtain survival benefit from any form of therapy directed only at recurrent cancer within the liver. The only potential hope for such patients resides in the development of more effective systemic therapy[41,42] and possibly gene therapy.[64,65] Therefore, unless a patient is enrolled in a clinical trial investigating a novel form of therapy, we do not advocate any form of treatment or additional tumor surveillance once recurrent extrahepatic disease is detected. In contrast, symptomatic patients with intrahepatic or extrahepatic disease may benefit from palliative forms of therapy that may require frequent follow-up.

New and Potentially Better Methods of Tumor Surveillance for Recurrent Hepatocellular Carcinoma

Karpoff and Fong point out that numerous tumor markers for hepatocellular carcinoma are being developed and may become clinically available and affordable in the future. A recently reported sensitive technique worth mentioning is the use of reverse transcriptase polymerase chain reaction for the detection of albumin mRNA, which is expressed on hepatocellular carcinoma cells circulating in the blood.[66] This method has been used to detect early cancer recurrence in patients after liver transplantation.[67]

GALLBLADDER CANCER

Most patients with adenocarcinoma of the gallbladder die within 12 months of their diagnosis. Only patients with early TNM stages of disease have any significant chance of prolonged disease-free survival. Karpoff and Fong recommend that patients with early-stage cancer who previously had a cholecystectomy be followed up with imaging studies for the first 2 years when the risk of recurrence is highest. They justify this by stating that repeat resection of recurrences in this patient population may be possible. We disagree with this opinion for three reasons. First, there are no clinical trial reports of resecting locally recurrent disease that results in prolonged survival. Second, imaging surveillance is expensive. Third, because the threshold of detecting regional recurrence by computed tomography is around 5 mm to 1 cm, by the time metastatic disease is detected by computed tomography the probability of isolated regional recurrence is extremely low because recurrent gallbladder cancer almost always occurs systemically and with diffuse carcinomatosis.

No convincing evidence from any published trial has shown that radical surgical or oncological therapy for advanced stage of gallbladder cancer has any impact on long-term survival. Similarly, few studies have reported substantial benefits of surgery,[68] chemotherapy, or radiation therapy for recurrent disease.[69] Karpoff and Fong point out that in case reports patients with localized recurrent gallbladder cancer have responded to chemotherapy and embolization therapy.[70] Such recurrences are extremely rare, and in our opinion do not justify postoperative tumor surveillance in most patients. Since no substantial improvement in the outcome of patients with recurrent gallbladder cancer has occurred over 40 years, postoperative tumor surveillance should be limited to patients enrolled in neoadjuvant clinical trials.

We agree with the opinion of Karpoff and Fong that imaging surveillance is justified to monitor the outcome of patients enrolled in a clinical trial to assess disease-free survival and in symptomatic patients. Patients outside a clinical trial who remain asymptomatic should not be monitored for tumor recurrence with office visits, tumor markers, liver function tests, chest x-rays, or computed tomography. The lone exception to this recommendation is to offer monitoring for patients who will make significant life-style changes when tumor recurrence is documented.

The recommendation for follow-up of patients with gallbladder cancer at the University of Washington Medical Center is to monitor them for symptomatic recurrence, which is often in the form of jaundice or ascites, by repeated physical examination and serum bilirubin and alkaline phosphatase measurement (Table 11-19). Additional intervention such as percutaneous or endoscopic biliary decompression for obstructive jaundice or a Denver shunt for debilitating malignant ascites may offer some palliation. Since reoperating on patients with recurrent gallbladder cancer, even if it is localized, has no demonstrable survival benefit, any attempt to operate on asymptomatic patients with any form of recurrent disease is strongly discouraged.

Patients with endoscopic or percutaneous biliary stents require close monitoring because of the risk of stent occlusion leading to recurrent jaundice and cholangitis. The median time to occlusion of plastic stents is around 4 months. Hence patients should be monitored every 3 months with alkaline phosphatase and bilirubin for evidence of biliary obstruction. Consideration should be given to elective stent exchange every 3 to 4 months to avoid stent occlusion and cholangitis. On the other hand, patients with advanced stages of gallbladder carcinoma have limited survival and elective stent change may not be cost effective.

Table 11-19 Follow-up of patients with hepatobiliary cancer (cholangiocarcinoma or gallbladder cancer): University of Washington Medical Center

	YEAR				
	1	2	3	4	5
Office visit	4	4	2	2	2
Liver function tests*	4	4	2	2	2
Abdominal ultrasound	†	†	†	†	†

*Includes alkaline phosphatase and bilirubin.
†Recommended for any signs of biliary obstruction.

CHOLANGIOCARCINOMA

Like gallbladder cancer, recurrent cholangiocarcinoma has a dismal prognosis. Intensive postoperative tumor surveillance is therefore unwarranted for patients previously treated for cholangiocarcinoma, since patients rarely benefit from additional therapy for recurrent disease. Therefore follow-up chest x-ray, ultrasound, and abdominal computed tomography are not advocated. Follow-up for asymptomatic patients is restricted to office visits with physical examination for signs of jaundice or ascites. Increasing serum alkaline phosphatase or scleral icterus may herald bile duct obstruction, which can then be stented endoscopically or percutaneously in a timely fashion. Symptomatic patients with recurrent cholangiocarcinoma should have follow-up only as needed for palliation.

CHOLANGIOCELLULAR CARCINOMA

A word should be said about cholangiocellular carcinoma (peripheral cholangiocarcinoma of the liver) since it represents 10% of primary liver cancers.[71,72] Resection is the treatment of choice when there is no evidence of extrahepatic spread.[73,74] Transplantation is not standard therapy.[73] Mean survival time after transplantation is approximately 12 months. Liver resection offers the only chance of survival, and the long-term survival rate is related to initial tumor stage.[73] There are no reports documenting any type of effective therapy for recurrent disease. However, because patients previously undergoing resection for cure are at risk for a second primary cancer in the biliary tree, an argument for surveillance after the original resection can be made. Therefore a follow-up helical computed tomographic scan is recommended once a year for this disease, as well as monitoring of any preoperatively elevated tumor markers such as CEA, CA 19-9, or CA-125. Only prospective trials will determine if such monitoring or treatment will improve patient outcome and prove cost effective.

REFERENCES

1. Okada S, Okazaki N, Nose H, et al. Follow-up examination schedule of postoperative HCC patients based on tumor volume doubling time. Hepatogastroenterology 1993;40:311-5.
2. Kanematsu T, Matsumata T, Takenaka K, Yoshida Y, Higashi H, Sugimachi K. Clinical management of recurrent hepatocellular carcinoma after primary resection. Br J Surg 1988;75:203-6.
3. Okuda K, Ohtsuki T, Obata H, et al. Natural history of hepatocellular cancer and prognosis in relation to treatment: study of 850 patients. Cancer 1985;56:918-28.
4. Chung JW, Park JH, Han JK, Choi BI, Han MC. Hepatocellular carcinoma and portal vein invasion; results of treatment with transcatheter oily chemoembolization. AJR Am J Roentgenol 1995; 165:315-21.
5. Martinez Cerezo FJ, Tomas A, Donoso L, et al. Controlled trial of tamoxifen in patients with advanced hepatocellular carcinoma. J Hepatol 1994;20:702-6.
6. Manesis EK, Giannoulis G, Zoumboulis P, Vafiadou I, Hadziyannis SJ. Treatment of hepatocellular carcinoma with combined suppression and inhibition of sex hormones: a randomized, controlled trial. Hepatology 1995;21:1535-42.
7. Raoul JL, Guyader D, Bretagne J, et al. Randomized controlled trial for hepatocellular carcinoma with portal vein thrombosis: intra-arterial iodine-131-iodized oil versus medical support. J Nucl Med 1994;35:1782-7.
8. Rizzi PM, Kane PA, Ryder SD, et al. Accuracy of radiology in detection of hepatocellular carcinoma before liver transplantation. Gastroenterology 1994;107:1425-9.
9. Bartolozzi C, Lencioni R, Caramella D, Gibilisco G, Cioni R, Vignali C. [Staging of hepatocellular carcinoma. Comparison of ultrasonography, computerized tomography, magnetic resonance, digital angiography, and computerized tomography with lipoidal (in Italian)]. Radiol Med Torino 1994;88:429-36.
10. Gattoni F, Dova S, Volterrani F, Blanc M, Uslenghi C. [Computerized tomography with lipoidal in the assessment of hepatocellular carcinoma (in Italian)]. Radiol Med Torino 1995;89:809-12.
11. Taourel P, Pageaux G, Coste V, et al. Small hepatocellular carcinoma in patients undergoing liver transplantation: detection with CT after injection of iodized oil. Radiology 1995;197:377-80.
12. Oi H, Murakami T, Kim T, Matsushita M, Kishimoto H, Nakamura H. Dynamic MR imaging and early-phase helical CT for detecting small intrahepatic metastasis of hepatocellular carcinoma. AJR Am J Roentgenol 1996;166:369-74.
13. Kawai S, Okamura J, Ogawa M, et al. Prospective and randomized clinical trial for the treatment of hepatocellular carcinoma—a comparison of lipoidal-transcatheter arterial embolization with and without adriamycin (first cooperative study). The Cooperative Study Group for Liver Cancer Treatment from Japan. Cancer Chemother Pharmacol 1992;31(Suppl 1):S1-6.
14. Ferruci JT. Liver tumor imaging: current concepts. Radiol Clin North Am 1994;32:39-54.
15. Bluemke DA, Fishman ER. Spiral CT of the liver. AJR Am J Roentgenol 1993;160:787-92.
16. Kosuge T, Makuuchi M, Takayama T, Yamamoto J, Shimada K, Yamasaki S. Long-term results after resection of hepatocellular carcinoma: experience of 480 cases. Hepatogastroenterology 1993;40:328-32.
17. Fattovich G, Giustina G, Schalm SW, et al. Occurrence of hepatocellular carcinoma and decompensation in Western European patients with cirrhosis type B: the EUROHEP Study Group on Hepatitis B Virus and Cirrhosis. Hepatology 1995;21:77-82.
18. Adachi E, Maeda T, Matsumata T, et al. Risk factors for intrahepatic recurrence in human small hepatocellular carcinoma. Gastroenterology 1995;108:768-75.
19. Tarao K. Shimizu A, Ohkawa S, et al. Development of hepatocellular carcinoma associated with increases in DNA synthesis in the surrounding cirrhosis. Gastroenterology 1992;103:595-600.
20. Tanikawa K. Recent advances in the treatment of hepatocellular carcinoma with reference to the indication of various therapies. Surg Ther 1991;64:172-6.
21. Ravoet C, Blieberg H, Gerard B. Non-surgical treatment of hepatocarcinoma. J Surg Oncol Suppl 1993;3:104-11.
22. Ohto M, Yoshikawa M, Saisho H, Ebara M, Sugiura N. Nonsurgical treatment of hepatocellular carcinoma in cirrhotic patients. World J Surg 1995;19:42-6.
23. Farmer DG, Rosove MH, Shaked A, Busuttil RW. Current treatment modalities for hepatocellular carcinoma. Ann Surg 1994;219:236-47.
24. Venook AP. Treatment of hepatocellular carcinoma: too many options? J Clin Oncol 1994;12:1323-34.
25. Venook A. Liver transplantation for hepatocellular carcinoma. Hepatology 1993;18:218-9.
26. Bastid C, Azar C, Sahel J. Ultrasound guided percutaneous ethanol treatment of hepatic neoplasms: a therapeutic alternative in the nineties. Ultrasound Med Biol 1995;21:129-31.
27. Livraghi T, Vettori C. Percutaneous ethanol injection therapy of hepatoma. Cardiovasc Intervent Radiol 1990;13:146-52.
28. Livraghi T, Giogio A, Marin G, et al. Hepatocellular carcinoma and cirrhosis in 746 patients: long-term results of percutaneous ethanol injection. Radiology 1995;197:101-8.
29. Sironi S, Livraghi T, Del Maschio A. Small hepatocellular carcinoma treated with percutaneous ethanol injection: MR imaging findings. Radiology 1991;180:333-6.
30. Tanikawa K, Majima Y. Percutaneous ethanol injection therapy for recurrent hepatocellular carcinoma. Hepatogastroenterology 1993; 40:324-7.
31. Bismuth H, Morino M, Sherlock D. Primary treatment of hepatocellular carcinoma by arterial chemoembolization. Am J Surg 1992; 163:387-94.
32. Choi BI, Kim HC, Han JK, et al. Therapeutic effect of transcatheter oily chemoembolization therapy for encapsulated nodular hepatocellular carcinoma: CT and pathologic findings. Radiology 1992; 182:709-13.
33. Ngan H, Lai CL, Fan ST, Lai EC, Yuen WK, Tso WK. Treatment of inoperable hepatocellular carcinoma by transcatheter arterial chemoembolization using an emulsion of cisplatin in iodized oil and gelfoam. Clin Radiol 1993;47:315-20.
34. Okamura J, Kawai S, Ogawa M, et al. Prospective and randomized clinical trial for the treatment of hepatocellular carcinoma—a comparison of L-TAE with Farmorubicin and L-TAE with Adriamycin (second cooperative study): the Cooperative Study Group for Liver Cancer Treatment of Japan. Cancer Chemother Pharmacol 1992; 31(Suppl 1):S20-4.
35. Yamada R, Sato M, Kawabata M, Nakatsaka H, Nakamura K, Takashima S. Hepatic artery embolization in 120 with unresectable hepatoma. Radiology 1983;148:397-401.
36. Zhou XD, Tang ZY, Yu YQ, Ma ZC. Clinical evaluation of cryosurgery in the treatment of primary liver cancer: report of 60 cases. Cancer 1988;61:1889-92.
37. Ravikumar TS, Steele GD Jr. Hepatic cryosurgery. Surg Clin North Am 1989;69:433-40.
38. Raoul JI, Bretagne JF, Caucanas JP, et al. Internal radiation therapy for hepatocellular carcinoma: results of a French multicenter phase II trial of transarterial injection of iodine-131-labeled Lipoidal. Cancer 1992;69:346-52.
39. Raoul JL, Guyader D, Bretagne JF, et al. Randomized controlled trial for hepatocellular carcinoma with portal vein thrombosis: intra-arterial iodine-131-iodized oil versus medical support. J Nucl Med 1994;35:1782-7.
40. Novell R, Hilson A, Hobbs K. Ablation of recurrent primary liver cancer using 131I-Lipoidal. Postgrad Med J 1991;67:393-5.
41. Zeng ZC, Tang ZY, Xie H, et al. Radioimmunotherapy for unresectable hepatocellular carcinoma using 131-I-Hepama-1 mAB: preliminary results. J Cancer Res Clin Oncol 1993;119:257-9.

42. Lygidakis NJ, Pothoulakis J, Konstantinidou AE, Spanos H. Hepatocellular carcinoma: surgical resection versus surgical resection combined with pre and post-operative locoregional immunotherapy-chemotherapy: a prospective randomized trial. Anticancer Res 1995;15:543-50.
43. Sitzmann JV, Abrahms R. Improved survival for hepatocellular cancer with combination surgery and multimodality treatment. Ann Surg 1993;217:149-54.
44. Tang ZY, Liu KD, Bao YM, et al. Radioimmunotherapy in the multimodality treatment of hepatocellular carcinoma with reference to second-look resection. Cancer 1990;65:211-5.
45. Tang ZY, Yu YQ, Zhou XD, et al. Treatment of unresectable primary liver cancer: with reference to cytoreduction and sequential resection. World J Surg 1995;19:47-52.
46. Stone MJ, Klintmalm GB, Polter D, et al. Neoadjuvant chemotherapy and liver transplantation for hepatocellular carcinoma: a pilot study in 20 patients. Gastroenterology 1993;104:196-202.
47. Nagasue N, Kohno H, Uchida M. Evaluation of preoperative arterial embolization in the treatment of resectable primary liver cancer. Semin Surg Oncol 1993;9:327-31.
48. Ellis LM, Demers ML, Roh MS. Current strategies for the treatment of hepatocellular carcinoma. Curr Opin Oncol 1992;4:741-51.
49. Livraghi T, Bolondi L, Buscarini L, et al. No treatment resection and ethanol injection in hepatocellular carcinoma: a retrospective analysis of survival in 391 patients with cirrhosis; Italian Cooperative HCC Study Group. J Hepatol 1995;22:522-6.
50. Livraghi T, Bolondi L, Lazzaroni S, et al. Percutaneous ethanol injection in the treatment of hepatocellular carcinoma in cirrhosis: a study on 207 patients. Cancer 1992;69:925-9.
51. Shiina S, Tagawa K, Unuma T, et al. Percutaneous ethanol injection therapy for hepatocellular carcinoma: a histopathologic study. Cancer 1991;68:1524-30.
52. Yamakado K, Hirano T, Kato N, et al. Hepatocellular carcinoma treatment with a combination of transcatheter arterial chemoembolization and transportal ethanol injection. Radiology 1994;193:75-80.
53. Tanaka K, Nakamura S, Numata K, et al. Hepatocellular carcinoma: treatment with percutaneous ethanol injection and transcatheter arterial embolization. Radiology 1992;185:457-60.
54. Torizuka T, Tamaki N, Inokuma T, et al. Value of fluorine-18-FDG-positron emission tomography to monitor hepatocellular carcinoma after interventional therapy. J Nucl Med 1994;35:1965-9.
55. Takayasu K, Moriyama N, Muramatsu Y, et al. The diagnosis of small hepatocellular carcinomas: efficacy of various imaging procedures in 100 patients. AJR Am J Roentgenol 1990;155:49-54.
56. Bolondi L, Gaiani S, Fusconi F, et al. Prognostic factors for survival of small ($\leq$5 cm) untreated hepatocellular carcinoma in the West. Hepatology 1991;14(4 Part 2):171A.
57. DeCobelli F, Castrucci M, Sironi S, et al. [Role of magnetic resonance in the follow-up of hepatocarcinoma treated with percutaneous ethanol injection (PEI) or transarterial chemoembolization (TACE) (in Italian)]. Radiol Med Torino 1994;88:806-17.
58. Zhou XD, Tang ZY, Yu YQ, et al. The role of cryosurgery in the treatment of hepatic cancer: a report of 113 cases. J Cancer Res Clin Oncol 1993;120:100-2.
59. Helton WS, Shields AT, Grahm MM. Technical failures of cryosurgically treated liver tumors demonstrated by FDG-positron emission tomography. Hepatology 1995;22(4 Part 2):107A.
60. Koneru B, Cassavilla A, Bowman J, Iwatsuki S, Starzl TE. Liver transplantation for malignant tumors. Gastroenterol Clin North Am 1988;17:177-93.
61. Yokoyama I, Carr B, Saitsu H, Iwatsuki S, Starzl TE. Accelerated growth rates of recurrent hepatocellular carcinoma after liver transplantation. Cancer 1991;68:2095-100.
62. Greene F, Dorsay D. Laparoscopic evaluation of abdominal malignancy. Cancer Practice 1993;1:29-34.
63. John TG, Greig JD, Crosbie JL, Miles WF, Gorden OJ. Superior staging of liver tumors with laparoscopy and laparoscopic ultrasound. Ann Surg 1994;220:711-9.

64. Huber BE, Richards CA, Kremitsky TA. Retroviral-mediated gene therapy for the treatment of hepatocellular carcinoma: an innovative approach for cancer therapy. Proc Natl Acad Sci U S A 1991; 88:8039-43.
65. Arbuthnot P, Bralet MP, Thomassin H, Danan JL, Brechot C, Ferry N. Hepatoma cell-specific expression of a retrovirally transferred gene is achieved by alpha-fetoprotein but not insulinlike growth factor II regulatory sequences. Hepatology 1995;22:1788-96.
66. Hillaire S, Barbu V, Boucher E, Moukhtar M, Poupon R. Albumin messenger RNA as a marker of circulating hepatocytes in hepatocellular carcinoma. Gastroenterology 1994;106:239-42.
67. Kar S, Carr BI. Detection of liver cells in peripheral blood of patients with advanced-stage hepatocellular carcinoma. Hepatology 1995; 21:403-7.
68. Roa I, Aray J, de Aretxabala X, Wistuba I, Burgos L. [The pathological findings in patients reoperated on for gallbladder cancer (in Spanish)]. Rev Med Chil 1990;118:153-7.
69. Whittington R, Neuberg D, Tester W, et al. Protracted intravenous fluorouracil infusion with radiation therapy in the management of localized pancreaticobiliary carcinoma: a phase I Eastern Cooperative Oncology Group Trial. J Clin Oncol 1995;13:227-32.
70. Kotoh T, Arima S, Futami K. [A case of retroperitoneal lymph node recurrence with gallbladder cancer responding to UFT and CDDP combination chemotherapy (in Japanese)]. Gan To Kagaku Ryoho [Jpn J Cancer Chemother] 1994;21:881-4.
71. Kawarada Y, Mizumoto R. Diagnosis and treatment of cholangiocellular carcinoma of the liver. Hepatogastroenterology 1990;37:176-81.
72. Schlinkert RT, Nagorney DM, Van Heerden JA, Adson MA. Intrahepatic cholangiocarcinoma: clinical aspects, pathology and treatment. HPB Surg 1992;5:95-102.
73. Pichlmayr R, Lamesch P, Weimann A, Tusch G, Ringe B. Surgical treatment of cholangiocellular carcinoma. World J Surg 1995;19:83-8.
74. Chen MF, Jan YY, Wang CS, Jeng LB, Hwang TL. Clinical experience in 20 hepatic resections for peripheral cholangiocarcinoma. Cancer 1989;64:2226-32.
75. Ouchi K, Matsubara S, Fukuhara K, Tominaga T, Matsuno S. Recurrence of hepatocellular carcinoma in the liver remnant after hepatic resection. Am J Surg 1993;166:270-3.
76. Fujio N, Sakai K, Kinoshita H, et al. Results of treatment of patients with hepatocellular carcinoma with severe cirrhosis of the liver. World J Surg 1989;13:211-8.
77. Valls C, Figueras J, Pamies JJ, et al. Preoperative TNM staging of hepatocellular carcinoma in hepatic transplantation: value of lipoidal computed tomography. Transplant Proc 1995;27:2309-10.
78. Chen MF, Hwang TL, Jeng LB, Wang CS, Jan YY, Chen SC. Postoperative recurrence of hepatocellular carcinoma: two hundred five consecutive patients who underwent hepatic resection in 15 years. Arch Surg 1994;129:738-42.
79. Sakon M, Monden M, Umeshita K, et al. The prognostic significance of macroscopic growth pattern of hepatocellular carcinoma. Int Surg 1994;79:38-42.
80. Ohto M, Yoshikawa M, Saisho H, Ebara M, Sugiura N. Nonsurgical treatment of hepatocellular carcinoma in cirrhotic patients. World J Surg 1995;19:42-46.
81. Tarao K, Shimizu A, Harada M, et al. Difference in the in vitro uptake of bromodeoxyuridine between liver cirrhosis with and without hepatocellular carcinoma. Cancer 1989;64:104-9.
82. Chiu JH, Wu LH, Kao HL, et al. Can determination of the proliferating capacity of the nontumor portion predict the risk of tumor recurrence in the liver remnant after resection of human hepatocellular carcinoma? Hepatology 1993;18:96-102.
83. Shimizu Y, Minemura M, Tsukishiro T, et al. Serum concentration of intercellular adhesion molecule-1 in patients with hepatocellular carcinoma is a marker of the disease progression and prognosis. Hepatology 1995;22:525-31.
84. Okada S, Shimada K, Yamamoto J, et al. Predictive factors for postoperative recurrence of hepatocellular carcinoma. Gastroenterology 1994;106:1618-24.

Table 11-20 Follow-up of patients with hepatobiliary cancer by institution

YEAR/PROGRAM	OFFICE VISIT	LFT	AFP	CEA	CXR	ABD CT	CA 19-9
Year 1							
Memorial Sloan-Kettering I[a]	4	4[b]	4[b,c]		1	1[d]	
Memorial Sloan-Kettering II[f]	4	4		[g]	1	1[h]	
Roswell Park I[a]	12	12	12[i]	12[i]	6	6	
Roswell Park II[f]	4	4		5[j]	2	2	5[j]
Univ Washington I[k]	5		4		1		
Univ Washington II[l]	1[m,n]		4[o]				
Univ Washington III[f]	4	4[q]					
Japan: Natl Cancer Ctr I[a]	6[s]	6[s]	6[s]			2[t]	
Japan: Natl Cancer Ctr II[f]	6[s]	6[s]		6[s]		1	6[s]
UK: Royal Liverpool I[a]	3	3	3[u]			2	
UK: Royal Liverpool II[f]	5	5		5			5
Year 2							
Memorial Sloan-Kettering I[a]	4	4[b]	4[b,c]		1	1[d]	
Memorial Sloan-Kettering II[f]	4	4		[g]	1	1[h]	
Roswell Park I[a]	6	6	6[i]	6[i]	6	6	
Roswell Park II[f]	4	4		5[j]	2	2	5[j]
Univ Washington I[k]	4[x]		4		1		
Univ Washington II[l]	4[m]		4				
Univ Washington III[f]	4	4[q]					
Japan: Natl Cancer Ctr I[a]	4	4	4			2[t]	
Japan: Natl Cancer Ctr II[f]	4	4		4		1	4
UK: Royal Liverpool I[a]	2	2	2[u]			2	
UK: Royal Liverpool II[f]	2	2		2			2

ABD CT abdominal computed tomography
ABD PET abdominal positron emission tomography
ABD US abdominal ultrasound
AFP alpha-fetoprotein
CBC complete blood count
CEA carcinoembryonic antigen
CHEST CT chest computed tomography
CLOT clotting studies
CXR chest x-ray
ELE electrolytes
GGT gamma-glutamyltransferase
HEL ABD CT helical abdominal computed tomography
LFT liver function tests

ABD US	CBC	ELE	CLOT	CHEST CT	GGT	HEL ABD CT	ABD PET
4[d,e]							
	4						
					4	3	
						3	1[p]
[r]							
6[s]	6[s]	6[s]					
6[s]	6[s]	6[s]					
			3[v]	1[w]			
4[d,e]							
	4						
					4	3	
						3	
[r]							
4	4	4					
4	4	4					
			2[v]				

a Patients with hepatocellular carcinoma.
b Performed monthly for patients with persistently elevated tumor markers.
c For patients with fibrolamellar hepatocellular carcinoma, substitute neurotensin or other markers found to be elevated in the preresectional blood test.
d Performed every 2 months until recurrence is detected for patients with persistently elevated tumor markers.
e Performed every 6 months for patients with elevated tumor marker levels before surgery.
f Patients with cholangiocarcinoma or gallbladder cancer.
g Performed at each office visit after cholecystectomy for patients with T1 gallbladder cancer.
h Performed twice a year for the first 2 years after cholecystectomy for patients with T1 gallbladder cancer.
i Performed if levels were elevated preoperatively.
j Performed postoperatively and at 3-month intervals if levels were elevated preoperatively.
k Patients with recurrent hepatocellular carcinoma after surgical resection for cure.
l Patients with persistent or recurrent hepatocellular carcinoma after nonresectional ablative techniques; includes cryosurgery and percutaneous ethanol injection with or without embolic therapy.
m Once alpha-fetoprotein levels return to normal, the frequency of follow-up is every 3 months.
n First follow-up visit is up to 3 months after treatment.
o Follow-up frequency is every 6 weeks until alpha-fetoprotein levels return to normal, then every 3 months.
p Persistently elevated alpha-fetoprotein and increased attenuation seen by computed tomography are indicative of incomplete tumor cell killing and should be followed by positron emission tomography or biopsy to detect persistent disease. An alternative to positron emission tomography is to perform additional ethanol injection into and around the area of suspicion.
q Includes alkaline phosphatase and bilirubin.
r Recommended for any signs of biliary obstruction.
s Includes monthly follow-up for the first 3 months.
t Performed biannually or more frequently as clinically indicated.
u If patient had positive levels preoperatively.
v Consists of coagulation time and prothrombin time.
w Performed at 12 months.
x The frequency of office visits for patients without cirrhosis is once a year beginning in the second year.

Continued.

Table 11-20 Follow-up of patients with hepatobiliary cancer by institution—cont'd

YEAR/PROGRAM	OFFICE VISIT	LFT	AFP	CEA	CXR	ABD CT	CA 19-9
Year 3							
Memorial Sloan-Kettering I[a]	4	4[b]	4[b,c]		1	1[d]	
Memorial Sloan-Kettering II[f]	4	4		[g]	1	1[h]	
Roswell Park I[a]	4	4	4[i]	4[i]	2	2	
Roswell Park II[f]	2	2		2[j]	1	1	2[j]
Univ Washington I[k]	4		4		1		
Univ Washington II[l]	4[m]		4				
Univ Washington III[f]	2	2[q]					
Japan: Natl Cancer Ctr I[a]	4	4	4			2[t]	
Japan: Natl Cancer Ctr II[f]	4	4		4		1	4
UK: Royal Liverpool I[a]	1	1	1[u]			1	
UK: Royal Liverpool II[f]	1	1		1			1
Year 4							
Memorial Sloan-Kettering I[a]	4	4[b]	4[b,c]		1	1[d]	
Memorial Sloan-Kettering II[f]	4	4		[g]	1	1[h]	
Roswell Park I[a]	4	4	4[i]	4[i]	2	2	
Roswell Park II[f]	2	2		2[j]	1	1	2[j]
Univ Washington I[k]	4		4		1		
Univ Washington II[l]	4[m]		4				
Univ Washington III[f]	2	2[q]					
Japan: Natl Cancer Ctr I[a]	4	4	4			2[t]	
Japan: Natl Cancer Ctr II[f]	4	4		4		1	4
UK: Royal Liverpool I[a]	1	1	1[u]			1	
UK: Royal Liverpool II[f]	1	1		1			1
Year 5							
Memorial Sloan-Kettering I[a]	4	4[b]	4[b,c]		1	1[d]	
Memorial Sloan-Kettering II[f]	4	4		[g]	1	1[h]	
Roswell Park I[a]	4	4	4[i]	4[i]	2	2	
Roswell Park II[f]	2	2		2[j]	1	1	2[j]
Univ Washington I[k]	4		4		1		
Univ Washington II[l]	4[m]		4				
Univ Washington III[f]	2	2[q]					
Japan: Natl Cancer Ctr I[a]	4	4	4			2[t]	
Japan: Natl Cancer Ctr II[f]	4	4		4		1	4
UK: Royal Liverpool I[a]	1	1	1[u]			1	
UK: Royal Liverpool II[f]	1	1		1			1

ABD US	CBC	ELE	CLOT	CHEST CT	GGT	HEL ABD CT	ABD PET
4[d,e]							
	4						
					4	1	
						1	
[r]							
4	4	4					
4	4	4					
			1[v]				
4[d,e]							
	4						
					4	1	
						1	
[r]							
4	4	4					
4	4	4					
			1[v]				
4[d,e]							
	4						
					4	1	
						1	
[r]							
4	4	4					
4	4	4					
			1[v]				

CHAPTER 12

Bronchogenic Carcinoma

Memorial Sloan-Kettering Cancer Center

ROBERT J. DOWNEY, NAEL MARTINI, AND ROBERT J. GINSBERG

Complete resection is the treatment of choice for localized non–small cell lung cancer (NSCLC). However, after an apparently complete resection, tumors recur at rates estimated at 20% to 30% for stage I tumors (Table 12-1), 50% for stage II, and 70% to 80% for stage III tumors at 5 years.[1] Recurrences may be either locoregional or distant. Once lung cancer recurs, prognosis is limited, with 2-year survival rates of 37%, 20%, and 14% for stages I, II, and III, respectively.[2] Small cell bronchogenic carcinoma, which accounts for approximately 20% of patients, is rarely curable. Follow-up for patients with small cell carcinoma of the lung is beyond the scope of this chapter and is not discussed.

Some local and distant recurrences may be treated by surgical resection or palliative modalities such as external beam radiation or brachytherapy. Therefore, after surgical resection for lung cancer, close supervision of the patient is important to identify and treat recurrent or new primary disease as early as possible. First, patterns of recurrence after resection of NSCLC are reviewed, including sites and survival statistics. Methods of surveillance for recurrent disease are then discussed, as well as the results of surgical treatment for recurrent disease.

TYPES OF RECURRENCE

Local recurrence is defined as clinically manifest disease within the same hemithorax or at the bronchial stump. Regional recurrence is disease in the lymphatic drainage basins, including the mediastinum and neck. Distant recurrence is defined as histologically identical disease in the contralateral lung or elsewhere outside the hemithorax.

Local Recurrence and Metachronous Primaries

A resection is considered complete and potentially curative when no gross residual tumor remains at the conclusion of the operation and all resection margins are histologically free of tumor. The extent of pulmonary resection necessary to achieve a complete resection is determined by the size and location of the tumor. Lobectomy is preferred for peripheral tumors.[3] For centrally located tumors, bilobectomy, sleeve lobectomy, or pneumonectomy may be necessary to encompass all disease. The rate of isolated local recurrence for stage I tumors treated with a complete resection and limited mediastinal lymph node dissection is 10% to 30% over 3 to 5 years.[4-6] For stage II disease the rate is 30%, and for stage III, 40%.[7]

Table 12-1 Recurrence estimates after pulmonary resection

	YEARS AFTER RESECTION OF STAGE I LUNG CANCER					
	0-1	1-2	2-3	3-4	4-5	5-6
Recurrences (No.)	48	35	21	11	10	10
Rate/100 patient-years	15.0	12.8	8.7	5.2	5.2	2.7

When the tumor is small and peripheral, a lesser resection—such as a segmentectomy or wedge excision—may be acceptable, particularly for patients with limited pulmonary reserve. Although long-term survival may follow lesser resections, the risks of local recurrence for stage I tumors are increased threefold for wedge excision and 2.4-fold for segmental excision compared with lobectomy.[8,9]

Patients with incomplete resection of their primary tumor do poorly, even when the residual disease is only microscopically evident at the bronchial margin.[10] Recurrence at the bronchial stump, in the chest wall, or in the remaining portion of a lobe when a lesser resection than lobectomy has been performed must be considered to be due to an inadequate initial excision. In other words, local recurrence and regional lymph node metastasis after resection represent persistent disease, not second primary carcinomas. The remainder of this discussion does not address such patients.

Distant Recurrence

No matter the initial stage, approximately two thirds of patients have the first evidence of recurrence in distant organs.[9] In descending order of frequency the sites of distant recurrence are the brain, bone, liver, and adrenal glands.[5]

In a small subgroup of patients (7%) solitary sites of metastatic disease develop after completely resected lung cancer.[11] Occasionally these sites can be effectively treated, allowing the patient the possibility of long-term survival.

For example, patients with solitary brain metastases treated by surgical excision, combined with resection of primary locoregional disease and systemic chemotherapy, may achieve a 15% to 20% 5-year survival rate (median survival time: 21 months).[12] No large series are available regarding other solitary sites of metastasis treated in this aggressive fashion, but isolated instances of long-term survival have been cited in the literature. For this reason, in follow-up after complete resection the history and physical examination should be directed toward metastatic sites potentially amenable to treatment.

Second Primary Malignancies

When a complete resection of a primary lung carcinoma has been performed, any new lesion—even if in the same lung—may represent a new primary tumor. The risk of a second primary malignancy remains relatively stable over time, whereas the risk of recurrent disease after resection of a primary tumor is greatest in the first 2 years after resection. The rate of diagnosis of new lung cancers in patients with prior resections ranges from 0.016 to 0.026 occurrences per patient per year for the first 5 years.[10,13] We have reviewed 118 patients from the Memorial Sloan-Kettering Cancer Center tumor registry who were alive 10 years from their initial diagnosis and treatment of their primary lung cancers.[14] New cancers of the lung developed in 19 of 118 patients (16%) 6 to 22 years after treatment of their first lung cancer. The diagnosis of a metachronous primary is most convincing when the new lesion is in the contralateral lung and of a different histological type. Attempts have been made to use DNA ploidy patterns and p53 gene structure analyses to distinguish recurrent from second primary disease.[15] In evaluating new lesions in the postresection patient, the physician must remember that benign pulmonary lesions may also develop. Tissue diagnosis is therefore essential whenever a new lesion appears after an apparently adequate resection of a primary lung cancer.

METHODS OF FOLLOW-UP

History and Physical Examination

After the immediate recovery period a status check visit is recommended every 3 months for the first year, every 4 months for the second year, and once to twice a year thereafter (Table 12-2). Most physicians recommend only a yearly checkup after 5 years. Between 5% and 15% of recurrences occur beyond 5 years. The risk of a new primary cancer persists at a rate of 1% to 3% per year. Late recurrences are reported to occur sporadically after 10 years (1% to 3% per year); therefore a yearly checkup thereafter is also recommended.

At each follow-up visit the patient's general condition is assessed and physical examination performed. A careful history is essential; symptoms are the first manifestation of recurrent or metastatic disease in at least 50% of patients. Even if the patient is asymptomatic, physical examination should include the supraclavicular region to detect any

Table 12-2 Follow-up of patients with bronchogenic carcinoma (non–small cell lung cancer): Memorial Sloan-Kettering Cancer Center

	YEAR				
	1	2	3	4	5
Office visit	4	3	1-2	1-2	1-2
Chest x-ray	3-4	3-4	2	2	2
CEA	*	*	*	*	*
Chest computed tomography	*	*	*	*	*

CEA, Carcinoembryonic antigen.
*Performed only when clinically indicated.

adenopathy, the upper abdomen to assess liver size, and the incision to detect any wound-related complications. If present, symptoms guide the examination. Locoregional recurrence often produces recurrent or new chest pain, persistent cough, hoarseness caused by recurrent laryngeal nerve palsy, or symptoms of superior vena caval obstruction. Nonspecific signs, such as continued weight loss or anorexia, may herald liver metastases. Intracranial metastatic disease is usually associated with neurological signs such as visual disturbances, mental change, and speech or gait disturbances. New and unremitting skeletal pain suggests bone metastases.

Biochemical Studies

Elevated serum calcium, alkaline phosphatase, serum glutamic oxalate transaminase, and lactic dehydrogenase levels are nonspecific markers of recurrent cancer. Whether biochemical determinations should be included in routine follow-up examinations of postsurgical patients is a matter of judgment. Physicians at Memorial Sloan-Kettering Cancer Center do not use these tests routinely but advise patients to remain under the care of their internist or family practitioner for comprehensive screening of nonneoplastic disorders, which usually includes an electrocardiogram and hematological and biochemical studies.

Measurement of carcinoembryonic antigen (CEA) is valuable as a follow-up test only in patients whose level was abnormal before surgery. An elevated CEA level generally returns to normal after resection. If this occurs, serial CEA assessment becomes worthwhile. Thus far no other specific tumor marker for NSCLC has been detected. Neuron-specific enolase and thymidine kinase are being investigated as potential markers for recurrent small cell lung cancer.[16] It is hoped that markers for both small cell cancer and NSCLC will become available, allowing the detection not only of early primary lung cancer, but also of treatable recurrences after resection.

Chest Radiographs and Computed Tomography

The most useful examination to detect locoregional recurrence or a second primary tumor is the chest x-ray. The clinical practice at Memorial Sloan-Kettering Cancer Center is to recommend a posteroanterior and lateral chest x-ray

2 weeks after surgery as a baseline after stabilization of surgical changes. Plain films are then obtained at 3- to 4-month intervals for 2 years, at 6-month intervals for 3 years, and yearly thereafter. Chest x-rays are always compared with previous films. If no interval change is identified and no pulmonary pathological condition is suspected, no further testing is usually necessary. Additional tests (usually computed tomography of the chest) are generally prompted by symptoms, signs, or new chest x-ray findings.

Routine computed tomography of the asymptomatic patient does not appear to be helpful. Scanning is currently performed only when clinical features suggest that recurrent disease is likely. However, no prospective study of its usefulness and cost effectiveness in follow-up has been conducted.

Locoregional recurrence is often difficult to detect in patients, especially after pneumonectomy, because of the failure of x-rays to penetrate the hemithorax or mediastinum. Computed tomography of the chest has proved impressive in detecting recurrence in patients with suggestive symptoms and unrevealing chest x-rays. Patients frequently have recurrent ipsilateral chest pain or a dry hacking cough, suggesting recurrent disease. Before computed tomography was available, such symptoms often remained enigmatic for months. Recurrent disease in the ipsilateral hemithorax or mediastinum is now more easily detected. Other modalities of thoracic imaging such as magnetic resonance imaging[17] and scintigraphy,[18] which may assist in distinguishing postoperative scarring from recurrent malignancies, are being evaluated but as yet have no proven advantages over computed tomography.

Sputum Cytology

From 1974 to 1984, mass screening with sputum cytology was performed in an effort to detect lung cancer at a presymptomatic and presumably resectable stage. Unfortunately, these efforts demonstrated that although higher resectability rates were achieved, improved survival could not be demonstrated for the screened population. The subsequent development of two monoclonal antibodies developed against small cell cancer and NSCLC has led to a multicenter trial to determine the efficacy of sputum cytological examination in detecting second primary lung cancers.[19] Accrual of patients by the Lung Cancer Early Detection Working Group is currently approximately 50% complete.

After resection of a lung cancer, patients often quit smoking of their own accord. If no complications occur and no recurrence ensues, such patients usually have no cough. Routine sputum examinations are then unrewarding. Exceptions to this rule may include patients whose initial symptom was hemoptysis, who had a histological finding of squamous cell carcinoma on bronchoscopic specimens, or who had a radiographically occult lung cancer.[19] The value of sputum cytology in detecting second aerodigestive tumors in this patient population is as yet unproved, however.

Bronchoscopy

Serial bronchoscopy is not generally indicated. However, this examination should be considered in special circumstances, including patients in whom tumor is very near or at the bronchial resection margin, patients with severe dysplasia or in situ changes at the resection margin, or patients with known multiple bronchial epithelial tumors. A new, unexplained cough or hemoptysis necessitates consideration of diagnostic bronchoscopy, even if chest x-rays remain negative. The introduction of fiberoptic bronchoscopy has made examination simple and extremely well tolerated without general anesthesia. It should be advised when symptoms, signs, or radiological or cytological findings suggest locally recurrent disease.

RESULTS OF TREATMENT OF RECURRENT DISEASE AND SECOND PRIMARY CANCERS

Results of Salvage Therapy for Locoregional Recurrences

Two potentially curative options exist for locally recurrent NSCLC: resection or radiation. In 1954, Beattie et al.[20] performed the first surgical attempt at cure of a recurrence by a carinal resection after a right pneumonectomy. In the years since this demonstration of technical feasibility, only scant information has appeared regarding the effectiveness of repeat resection. Recent series include those of Dartevelle and Khalife[21] and Kulka et al.,[22] each reporting a median survival of only 12 months in a total of 46 patients undergoing a diverse group of repeat resections for recurrent lung cancer. External beam therapy offers another therapeutic option that has been reported in limited series; median survival times do not exceed 12 to 14 months.[23,24] These poor results again emphasize the need for definitive resection with attention to margins and lymph node resection at the time of initial surgery.

Surgical Resection of Second Primaries

The risk and extent of resection of a second primary lung cancer depend in part on the extent of the prior operation. Repeat resection within a previous surgical field probably increases the operative risk. A completion pneumonectomy (removal of all residual lung parenchyma after an ipsilateral wedge resection, segmentectomy, or lobectomy) carries a mortality of 10% to 20%.[25,26] Resections that leave a patient with less than two lobes (for example, a left upper lobectomy combined with a right pneumonectomy) severely compromise pulmonary reserve and are not generally advisable. However, a contralateral wedge resection after a pneumonectomy can often be tolerated.[27] In the few patients who have second primary lung cancers that can be encompassed by surgical resection and who would not become respiratory cripples, survival after resection may be expected to be 33% at 5 years and 20% at 10 years.[28]

RISK REDUCTION BY BEHAVIOR MODIFICATION AND CHEMOPREVENTION

The causal relationship between cigarette smoking and lung cancer is well established, but few studies have addressed the effect of continued smoking on the risk of a second primary lung cancer. The diagnosis of lung cancer leads some patients to quit smoking: at 1 year and 2 years after diagnosis, 53% and 40% of smokers are reported to have quit completely.[29] Smoking cessation appears to translate into a decreased susceptibility to a second primary lung cancer. Patients who were able to stop after small cell lung cancer was diagnosed had a four-fold reduction in risk of having a second primary lung cancer.[30] The most important aspect of follow-up surveillance to limit morbidity and mortality from a second primary lung cancer may be to actively encourage smoking cessation.

Attempts are under way to determine whether dietary supplements may reduce the risk of second primary lung cancers.[31] Previous studies suggested that diets low in beta-carotene and vitamin A are associated with an increased risk of lung cancer.[32,33] Unfortunately, the initial results of the Alpha-Tocopherol Beta-Carotene Cancer Prevention Study (a prospective, randomized, double-blind, placebo-controlled, primary prevention trial undertaken to determine whether supplementation or "chemoprevention" would reduce the risk of primary lung cancer in smokers) not only failed to show a reduction in the incidence, but also demonstrated an 8% higher mortality rate among recipients of supplements.[34] A national trial of chemoprevention to prevent second malignancies of the aerodigestive tract is under way.

FUTURE PROSPECTS

After apparently curative resection of a primary lung carcinoma, patients are at risk for locoregional recurrence, distant metastases, or the development of a second primary lung carcinoma. Careful surveillance of these patients is favored, emphasizing a careful history focused on the development of new symptoms, a physical examination directed primarily to the most probable sites of recurrent disease, and chest x-rays. The most useful additional study for the asymptomatic patient may be serial computed tomographic scans, although the benefit is unproven.

Given the current cost containment climate in medicine, scrutiny of all measures of surveillance for cost effectiveness is to be expected.[35,36] A recent study from the M.D. Anderson Cancer Center[37] found that routine follow-up and surveillance of all patients who had undergone a complete resection for lung cancer altered treatment strategy in less than 3%. We believe that surveillance, as outlined in this chapter, of the patient who has undergone resection of a primary lung cancer is still justified by the benefit to patients with treatable recurrences and new primary lung cancers.

REFERENCES

1. Martini N. Surgical treatment of non–small lung cancer by stage. Semin Surg Oncol 1990;6:248-54.
2. Ichinose Y, Yano T, Yokoyama H, et al. Postrecurrent survival of patients with non-small-cell lung cancer undergoing a complete resection. J Thorac Cardiovasc Surg 1994;108:158-61.
3. Martini N, McCaughan BC, McCormack PM, Bains MS. The extent of resection for localized lung cancer: lobectomy. In: Kittle CF, editor. Current controversies in thoracic surgery. Philadelphia: WB Saunders Company, 1986:171-4.
4. Martini N, Bains MS, Burt ME, et al. Incidence of local recurrence and second primary tumors in resected stage I lung cancer. J Thorac Cardiovasc Surg 1995;109:120-9.
5. Feld R, Rubinstein LV, Weisenberger TH, The Lung Cancer Study Group. Sites of recurrence in resected stage I non-small-cell lung cancer: a guide for future studies. J Clin Oncol 1984;2:1352-8.
6. The Ludwig Lung Cancer Study Group. Patterns of failure in patients with resected stage I and II non-small-carcinoma of the lung. Ann Surg 1987;205:67-71.
7. The Lung Cancer Study Group. Effects of postoperative mediastinal radiation on completely resected stage II and stage III epidermoid cancer of the lung. N Engl J Med 1986;315:1377-81.
8. Martini N, Ghosh P, Melamed MR. Local recurrence and new primary carcinoma after resection. In: Delarue NC, Eschapasse H, editors. International trends in general thoracic surgery. Vol 1. Philadelphia: WB Saunders Company, 1985:164-9.
9. Ginsberg RJ, Rubinstein L. Randomized trial of lobectomy versus limited resection for T1N0 non-small cell lung cancer. Ann Thorac Surg 1995;60:615-23.
10. Pairolero PC, Williams DE, Bergstralh EJ, Piehler JM, Bernatz PE, Payne WS. Postsurgical stage I bronchogenic carcinoma: morbid implications of recurrent disease. Ann Thorac Surg 1984;38:331-8.
11. Albain KS, Crowley JJ, Le Blanc M, Livingston RB. Survival determinants in extensive-stage non-small-cell lung cancer: the Southwest Oncology Group experience. J Clin Oncol 1991;9:1618-26.
12. Burt M, Wronski M, Arbit E, Balicich JH, The Memorial Sloan-Kettering Cancer Center Thoracic Surgical Staff. Resection of brain metastases from non-small-cell lung carcinoma: results of therapy. J Thorac Cardiovasc Surg 1992;103:399-410.
13. Thomas P, Rubinstein L, The Lung Cancer Study Group. Cancer recurrence after resection: T1N0 non–small cell lung cancer. Ann Thorac Surg 1990;49:242-7.
14. Temeck BK, Flehinger BJ, Martini N. A retrospective analysis of 10-year survivors from carcinoma of the lung. Cancer 1984;53:1405-8.
15. Ichinose Y, Hara N, Ohta M, Kuda T, Asoh H, Chikama H. DNA ploidy patterns of tumors diagnosed as metachronous or recurrent lung cancers. Ann Thorac Surg 1991;52:469-73.
16. Fischbach W, Schwarz-Wallrauch C, Jany B. Neuron-specific enolase and thymidine kinase as an aid to the diagnosis and treatment monitoring of small cell lung cancer. Cancer 1989;63:1143-9.
17. Kono M, Adachi S, Kusumoto M, Sakai E. Clinical utility of Gd-DTPA-enhanced magnetic imaging in lung cancer. J Thorac Imaging 1993;8:18-26.
18. Hatfield MK, MacMahon H, Ryan JW, et al. Postoperative recurrence of lung cancer: detection by whole-body gallium scintigraphy. AJR Am J Roentgenol 1986;147:911-5.
19. Tockman MS, Erozan YS, Gupta P, Piantadosi S, Mulshine JL, Ruckdeschel JC. The early detection of second primary lung cancers by sputum immunostaining. Chest 1994;106:385S-90S.
20. Beattie EJ Jr, Davis C Jr, O'Kane C, Friedberg SA. Surgical intervention in recurrent bronchogenic carcinoma. JAMA 1954;155:835-7.
21. Dartevelle P, Khalife J. Surgical approach to local recurrence and the secondary primary lesion. In: Delarue NC, Eschapasse H, editors. International trends in general thoracic surgery. Vol 1, Philadelphia: WB Saunders Company, 1985:156-63.
22. Kulka F, Kostic S. Surgical alternatives in ipsilateral recurrence of bronchogenic carcinoma. Eur J Cardiothorac Surg 1988;2:430-2.
23. Kopelson G, Choi NC. Radiation therapy for postoperative local-regionally recurrent lung cancer. Int J Radiat Oncol Biol Phys 1980;6:1503-6.
24. Curran WJ Jr, Herbert SH, Stafford PM, et al. Should patients with post-resection locoregional recurrence of lung cancer receive aggressive therapy? Int J Radiat Oncol Biol Phys 1992;24:25-30.
25. McGovern EM, Trastek VF, Pairolero PC, Payne WS. Completion pneumonectomy: indications, complications, and results. Ann Thorac Surg 1988;46:141-6.
26. Gregoire J, Deslauriers J, Guojin L, Rouleau J. Indications, risks, and results of completion pneumonectomy. J Thorac Cardiovasc Surg 1993;105:918-24.
27. Levasseur P, Regnard JF, Icard P, Dartevelle P. Cancer surgery on a single residual lung. Eur J Cardiothorac Surg 1992;6:639-40.

28. Faber LP. Resection for second and third primary lung cancer. Semin Surg Oncol 1993;9:135-41.
29. Gritz E, Nisenbaum R, Elashoff, Holmes EC. Smoking behavior following diagnosis in patients with stage I non–small lung cancer. Cancer Causes Control 1991;2:105-12.
30. Richardson GE, Tucker MA, Venzon DJ, et al. Smoking cessation after successful treatment of small-cell lung cancer is associated with fewer smoking-related second primary cancers. Ann Intern Med 1993;119:383-90.
31. Kellof GJ, Boone CW, Steele VK, Perloff M, Crowell J, Doody LA. Development of chemopreventative agents for lung and upper aerodigestive tract cancers. J Cell Biochem Suppl 1993;17F:2-17.
32. Peto R, Doll R, Buckely JD, Sporn MB. Can dietary beta-carotene materially reduce human cancer rates? Nature 1981;290:201-8.
33. Menkes MS, Comstock GW, Vuilleumier JP, Helsing KJ, Rider AA, Brookmeyer R. Serum beta-carotene, vitamins A and E, selenium, and the risk of lung cancer. N Engl J Med 1986;315:1250-4.
34. The Alpha-Tocopherol, Beta-Carotene Cancer Prevention Study Group. The effect of vitamin E and beta-carotene on the incidence of lung cancer and other cancers in male smokers. N Engl J Med 1994; 330:1029-35.
35. Virgo KS, McKirgan LW, Caputo MCA. Posttreatment management options for patients with lung cancer. Ann Surg 1995;222:700-10.
36. Naunheim KS, Virgo KS, Coplin MA, Johnson FE. Clinical surveillance testing after lung cancer operations. Ann Thorac Surg 1995; 60:1612-16.
37. Walsh GL, O'Connor M, Willis KM, et al. Is follow-up of lung cancer patients following resection medically indicated and cost effective? Ann Thorac Surg 1996;60:1563-72.

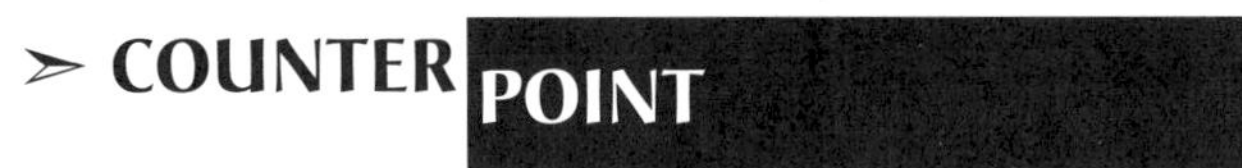

National Kyushu Cancer Center, Japan

YUKITO ICHINOSE

To clarify the precise recurrence pattern of completely resected lung cancer and to investigate whether intensive treatment for recurrence influences survival, physicians at National Kyushu Cancer Center have performed a prospective trial of the intensive follow-up care of patients with completely resected lung cancer since January 1993. As of November 1995, 35 of 129 registered patients have had recurrences. The National Kyushu Cancer Center surveillance strategy to detect recurrence within the first 24 months after operation, when the majority of recurrences are known to occur, is based on an analysis of this trial.

PATIENTS AND METHODS

From January 1993 to May 1995, 129 patients with completely resected lung cancer were entered into the trial. The follow-up schedule is presented in Table 12-3. When an abnormality in the general examination (including symptoms, physical examination, complete blood count, blood chemistry, and tumor markers) was found, computed tomography, magnetic resonance imaging, or bone scanning was performed. The recurrent disease was then confirmed by a biopsy whenever clinically feasible. The median follow-up time was 19 months and ranged from 5 to 35 months. Of 129 patients, 35 demonstrated recurrence. The characteristics of the registered patients and those with recurrence are shown in Table 12-4.

Table 12-3 Follow-up of patients with bronchogenic carcinoma (intensive follow-up)*: National Kyushu Cancer Center, Japan

	YEAR				
	1	2	3	4	5
Office visit	6	6	3	3	3
Complete blood count	6	6	3	3	3
Blood chemistry†	6	6	3	3	3
CEA	6	6	3	3	3
Sialyl Lewis X	6	6	3	3	3
SCCAg	6	6	3	3	3
Chest x-ray	4	4	2	2	2
Sputum cytology‡	3	3	3	3	3
Brain computed tomography	2	2	1	1	1
Chest computed tomography	2	2	1	1	1
Upper abdominal computed tomography	2	2	1	1	1
Bone scintigraphy	2	2	1	1	1

CEA, Carcinoembryonic antigen; *SCCAg,* squamous cell carcinoma antigen.
*Strategy tested in an ongoing National Kyushu Cancer Center trial.
†Includes serum calcium, alkaline phosphatase, glutamic oxalate transaminase, and lactic dehydrogenase levels.
‡Performed in patients with resected squamous cell carcinoma and for either current or former smokers.

MODE AND TIME OF RECURRENCE

As shown in Table 12-5, among the 35 patients with recurrent disease, local recurrence alone occurred in 5 (14%) patients, distant recurrence alone in 25 (71%) patients, and combined recurrence in five (14%) patients. The most frequent organ with distant metastasis was lung (35%, 10 of 31), followed by bone (29%, 9 of 31), and brain (19%, 6 of 31). The median time to recurrence was 6 months and ranged from 2 to 24 months. Recurrence took place in 29 (83%) and 33 (94%) patients within 12 and 18 months after the operation, respectively.

EXAMINATIONS LEADING TO THE DIAGNOSIS OF RECURRENCE

Table 12-6 summarizes the examinations leading to the diagnosis of recurrence. Of the 35 patients with recurrence, 13 (37%) had symptoms related to the recurrent disease and one (3%) had cervical lymph node swelling that was detected by physical examination. Seven of nine patients (78%) with bone metastases and three of six patients (50%) with brain metastases had symptoms such as skeletal pain and neurological abnormalities, respectively.

High levels of serum tumor markers were the initial evidence of recurrence in 13 of the 35 patients (37%) with

Table 12-4 Characteristics of registered patients and patients with recurrence

	REGISTERED PATIENTS (n = 129)	PATIENTS WITH RECURRENCE (n = 35)
Gender		
Female/male	41/88	10/25
Age		
Mean ± standard deviation (range)	63.7 ± 9.2 (41-81)	65.0 ± 9.6 (41-77)
Pathological stage		
I	73	11
II	12	2
IIIA	32	16
IIIB	3	3
IV*	9	3
Histology		
Adenocarcinoma	81	21
Squamous cell carcinoma	29	9
Others	19	5

Data from National Kyushu Cancer Center trial.
*Nine patients in stage IV had ipsilateral pulmonary metastasis that was completely removed by either a wedge resection or a segmentectomy.

Table 12-5 Mode of recurrence

SITE OF RECURRENCE	NUMBER OF PATIENTS
Local recurrence	5
Lymph node*	2
Pleura	1
Pleura + lymph node	1
Bronchial stump	1
Distant recurrence	25
Lung	8
Brain	5
Bone	8
Liver	1
Liver + bone	1
Others	2
Combined (local + distant)	5
Lymph node + lung	1
Lymph node + liver	2
Lymph node + brain	1
Bronchial stump + lung	1

Data from National Kyushu Cancer Center trial.
*Hilar or mediastinal lymph node.

Table 12-6 Examinations leading to the diagnosis of recurrence

EXAMINATION	NUMBER OF PATIENTS	SITE OF RECURRENCE*						TOTAL RECURRENCES
		LOCAL	LUNG	BONE	BRAIN	LIVER	OTHERS	
Symptoms + physical examination	14	2	1	7	3	1	2	16
Tumor marker	13	6	5	2		3		16
Chest x-ray	4	1	3					4
Chest computed tomography	1	1	1					2
Brain computed tomography	3				3			3
Abdominal computed tomography	0							0
Bone scintigraphy	0							0
Sputum cytology	0							0
Total	35	10	10	9	6	4	2	41

Data from National Kyushu Cancer Center trial.
*When recurrence was simultaneously diagnosed based on more than one examination, the most convenient and least expensive positive test leading to the diagnosis was recorded. Symptoms plus physical examination was considered most convenient and least costly, followed by tumor marker, chest x-ray, and computed tomography scan.

recurrent disease. In addition, two patients with recurrence-related symptoms had high levels of tumor markers. Fifteen patients (43%) showed abnormal tumor marker levels. CEA and sialyl Lewis X abnormalities were observed in 12 and five patients, respectively. It is also noteworthy that nine (75%) of 12 patients with high levels of CEA at the time of recurrence had a normal serum level before the operation.

In asymptomatic patients with recurrence, three brain recurrences, one local recurrence, and one lung recurrence were detected by computed tomography. However, no recurrent disease was detected by an upper abdominal computed tomographic scan. No instances of recurrent disease were detected by bone scintigraphy, sputum cytology, complete blood count, or blood chemistry.

CONCLUSION

Although definitive conclusions cannot be drawn from the present analysis, some lessons for the design of follow-up surveillance strategies are clear. As Downey et al. point out, a careful history focusing on the development of new symptoms is the most important factor in detecting recurrence. Tumor markers, especially CEA, seem to be useful in follow-up examinations, even in patients with normal preoperative serum CEA levels. A computed tomographic scan does not

Table 12-7 Follow-up of patients with bronchogenic carcinoma (non–small cell lung cancer): National Kyushu Cancer Center, Japan

	YEAR				
	1	2	3	4	5
Office visit	4-6	3-4	2	2	2
Chest x-ray	4-6	3-4	2	2	2
CEA	4-6	3-4	2	2	2

CEA, Carcinoembryonic antigen.

Table 12-8 Follow-up of patients with bronchogenic carcinoma (non–small cell lung cancer): Roswell Park Cancer Institute

	YEAR				
	1	2	3	4	5
Office visit	3	3	3	2	1
Chest x-ray	3	3	3	2	1

provide meaningful information for most asymptomatic patients. Bone scintigraphy, sputum cytology, complete blood count, and blood chemistry excluding tumor markers are generally not useful in detecting recurrence. A combination of symptoms, physical examination, tumor markers (especially CEA), and chest x-ray led to the diagnosis of recurrence in 31 (89%) of 35 patients with recurrence. Based on these observations the follow-up schedule employed at National Kyushu Cancer Center (Table 12-7) is recommended. However, whether a follow-up strategy can favorably affect a patient's survival remains unclear.

➢ COUNTER POINT

Roswell Park Cancer Institute

JOHN D. URSCHEL

Downey et al. have outlined a sensible and fairly standard approach to the follow-up of patients after resection of non–small cell lung cancer. The purpose of follow-up is to detect cancer recurrences and second primary lung cancers.[1] Although most patients with lung cancer recurrence are not candidates for curative treatment, timely initiation of palliative treatment strategies may improve quality of life. Patients with second primary lung cancers detected during routine follow-up often have early-stage disease that is curable by surgical resection.

The schedule of follow-up recommended by Downey et al. is followed, with minor variations, by many North American thoracic surgeons,[2] including physicians at Roswell Park Cancer Institute (Table 12-8). The essential elements of follow-up visits are history, physical examination, and chest x-ray. Symptoms, signs, and abnormal chest x-ray findings warrant other investigations, such as laboratory studies, computed tomography, and bronchoscopy. However, as Downey et al. point out, there is no evidence to support the use of these additional investigations in routine lung cancer follow-up.

The cost effectiveness of basic lung cancer follow-up programs, such as that recommended by Downey et al., has been questioned.[3-5] To control costs in a managed care environment, there is a temptation to shift the responsibility for follow-up of patients with lung cancer from the operating surgeon to the primary care physician. This could offer cost savings, but experience in both academic and community settings has caused me to doubt the wisdom of this strategy of cost containment. Primary care physicians who lack expertise in lung cancer may order more investigations for possible cancer recurrence than their more experienced specialist colleagues. No matter who is responsible for lung cancer follow-up, evidence-based guidelines are needed.

Outcomes research in cancer follow-up is an area of current interest. Follow-up programs for breast and colon cancer have been extensively studied,[6-9] and this research is reviewed elsewhere in the text. For these malignancies intensive follow-up protocols are difficult to justify. Lung cancer follow-up has not received as much research attention, but retrospective studies suggest that intensive lung cancer follow-up gives little survival benefit.[4,5] It is hoped that in the future, lung cancer follow-up protocols will be based on evidence rather than on surgical tradition and clinical intuition. Until that time the guidelines provided by Downey et al. are sensible and worth following.

REFERENCES

1. Rocco PM, Antkowiak JG, Takita H, Urschel JD. Long-term outcome after pneumonectomy for nonsmall cell lung cancer. J Surg Oncol 1996;61:278-80.
2. Naunheim KS, Virgo KS, Coplin MA, Johnson FE. Routine clinical surveillance testing following lung cancer surgery: current practice and attitudes. Ann Thorac Surg 1995;60:1612-6.
3. Heibert CA. The "cured" lung cancer patient: is follow-up by the surgeon worthwhile? Ann Thorac Surg 1995;60:1557-8.
4. Walsh GL, O'Connor M, Willis KM, et al. Is follow-up of lung cancer patients following resection medically indicated and cost effective? Ann Thorac Surg 1996;60:1563-72.
5. Virgo KS, McKirgan LW, Caputo MC, et al. Post-treatment management options for patients with lung cancer. Ann Surg 1995;222:700-10.
6. The GIVIO Investigators. Impact of follow-up testing on survival and health-related quality of life in breast cancer patients: a multicenter randomized controlled trial. JAMA 1994;271:1587-92.
7. Rosselli Del Turco M, Palli D, Cariddi A, Ciatto S, Pacini P, Distante V. Intensive diagnostic follow-up after treatment of primary breast cancer: a randomized trial; National Research Council Project on Breast Cancer Follow-Up. JAMA 1994;271:1593-7.
8. Bruinvels DJ, Stiggelbout AM, Kievit J, van Houwelingen HC, Habbema JD, van de Velde CJ. Follow-up of patients with colorectal cancer: a meta-analysis. Ann Surg 1994;219:174-82.
9. Virgo KS, Vernava AM, Longo WE, McKirgan LW, Johnson FE. Cost of patient follow-up after potentially curative colon cancer treatment. JAMA 1995;273:1837-41.

➣ COUNTER POINT

University of Washington Medical Center

JOHN A. JOHNKOSKI AND DOUGLAS E. WOOD

Lung cancer is now the most common cause of death from malignancy in both men and women and is responsible for nearly 170,000 deaths annually in the United States.[1] Although the largest group at risk, tobacco users, is easily identified, routine screening for lung cancer has been demonstrated not to be cost effective.[2] Once NSCLC is diagnosed, however, the treatment of choice for patients is complete resection. Unfortunately, after a potentially curative resection, tumors recur at a significant rate, depending on the stage of tumor and the adequacy of resection.[3] Of the tumors that do recur, 50% of recurrences appear in the first 2 years postoperatively and 90% by 5 years, with second primary lung cancers occurring at a rate of 1% to 3% per year.[4]

Follow-up of patients after curative resection is important for a number of reasons. The most obvious is for early recognition of recurrent or new primary disease, with the goal of discovering a recurrence when it is still resectable and potentially curable. Follow-up of these patients is also important because they are at an increased risk for other malignancies, usually of the aerodigestive tract. Another, less apparent reason for follow-up of these patients is so that the treatment of their malignancy may be evaluated. Only through these observations can any judgment be made regarding the efficacy of the treatment. It has been suggested that because routine follow-up only alters the course for a minority of patients, it is not cost effective.[5] Although it is certainly true that some means of follow-up are less cost effective than others, the lack of a standard means of evaluating the management of these patients will ultimately lead to less efficacious and certainly less cost-effective care.

Several controversies exist concerning follow-up after potentially curative resection, including the frequency of follow-up visits, which tests are most effective at detecting recurrent or new disease, and who should be responsible for the follow-up of these patients. In this era of cost awareness it is increasingly important to eliminate unnecessary office visits, limit the use of expensive diagnostic technology, and minimize redundancy between the primary care physician and thoracic surgeon.

Downey et al. review patterns of recurrence after curative resection of NSCLC, methods of surveillance for recurrent and new primary disease, and results of surgical resection for recurrent disease. In this counterpoint several points regarding the frequency and modality of follow-up in these patients are addressed. The cost effectiveness of different modalities used in follow-up and the issue of which member of the health care team is best suited to follow up these patients postoperatively are also discussed.

Table 12-9 Follow-up of patients with bronchogenic carcinoma (non–small cell lung cancer): University of Washington Medical Center

	YEAR				
	1	2	3	4	5
Office visit	3	3	2	2	1
Chest x-ray	3	3	2	2	1

FREQUENCY OF FOLLOW-UP

Nearly half of recurrences are evident within 2 years of potentially curative resection, with the rate of recurrence dependent on the initial stage. Approximately two thirds of these are distant metastases, rather than locoregional recurrence.[6,7] By 5 years postoperatively, 90% of the recurrences will have occurred, with the remaining 10% occurring over the next 5 years. Any regimen of time intervals selected for routine follow-up visits will be inherently somewhat arbitrary but should take into consideration the timing of curable recurrences.

Downey et al. advocate an initial visit 2 weeks postoperatively, followed by visits every 3 to 4 months for the first 2 years, every 6 to 12 months up to 5 years, and annually thereafter. This is a reasonable regimen, accounting for the fact that most recurrences are evident within the first 2 years and representing the general practice. A similar regimen is followed at the University of Washington Medical Center, with visits every 4 months for 2 years, every 6 months for the next 2 years, and annually thereafter. Most patients with NSCLC are in an age group in which they should be examined by their primary physician on an annual basis. This should suffice for follow-up after 4 to 5 years as long as the primary physician is familiar with the modalities and importance of lung cancer follow-up.

MODALITIES OF FOLLOW-UP

History and Physical Examination

A postoperative visit should include a careful history and directed physical examination (Table 12-9). Approximately 75% of patients have symptoms of their recurrence, making a thorough history one of the most valuable "tests" that exists for recurrent lung cancer. Symptoms may be the result of locoregional recurrence, such as new chest pain, persistent cough, new hoarseness, or symptoms of superior vena cava syndrome. Distant metastases represent two thirds of recurrences and may be heralded by site-specific symptoms. Changes in mental status or new neurological symptoms are among the most common findings and are associated with intracranial metastases, whereas continuing weight loss and anorexia are very poor prognostic signs and are often indicative of spread of disease to the liver. New bone or joint pain is usually the first symptom of bony metastases. After resection of NSCLC, all patients should have a directed physical examination at each follow-up visit. In addition to examining the incision, the physician should look for signs of metastatic disease, including supraclavicular adenopathy, hepatomegaly, new neurological deficits, bone pain, and weight loss. Furthermore, any new symptoms should prompt a more detailed examination and diagnostic studies.

A recent study has questioned the utility of routine follow-up after potentially curative resection of NSCLC.[5] The researchers maintain that routine follow-up may not be necessary because 76% of patients with recurrent disease have symptoms and half of those with symptoms sought medical attention before their scheduled appointment. This is an interesting and somewhat provocative conclusion to draw from these data. Given the same information, we would argue that the high rate of symptoms makes the history an efficient way of detecting recurrent disease. In addition, the fact that half of the patients with symptoms sought treatment early means that half of the patients did not seek medical attention for their symptoms, which emphasizes the value of routine appointments. This same group found that only two of 135 recurrences were evident on physical examination. This may indicate that the examination is far less effective in detecting recurrent disease. However, it can be performed in less than 5 minutes and is an inexpensive adjunct to the history.

Radiological Studies

Chest x-ray has been good in detecting locoregional recurrence of lung cancer, with nearly an 80% sensitivity rate in two studies.[5,8] The added benefit is that chest radiography is relatively inexpensive, available at even a small hospital or clinic, and probably more reliably interpreted than other radiological studies that might be used in this setting. Chest x-rays should be obtained at each postoperative visit and should become part of the annual examination after 5 years (Table 12-9). All studies should be compared with prior films, since new changes may be subtle.

Symptoms of recurrence or changes on the chest x-ray should prompt the physician to obtain a computed tomographic scan of the chest. The computed tomographic scan is superior to chest x-ray in identifying mediastinal spread of disease and can be useful in guiding further diagnostic studies of the mediastinum, such as cervical mediastinoscopy or anterior mediastinotomy (Chamberlain procedure). The computed tomographic scan of the chest obtained for workup of a new pulmonary nodule has the benefit of further defining the location and characteristics of the nodule as well as the presence of other pulmonary nodules not detected by chest x-ray. This is important, since local recurrence at a previous surgical staple line clearly has different implications than multiple bilateral pulmonary nodules suggestive of metastatic disease. A computed tomographic scan should extend through the liver and adrenal glands to evaluate these organs for evidence of metastatic disease. Computed tomography may also be helpful in the routine follow-up of patients who have undergone pneumonectomy. The loss of all lung tissue makes the mediastinum ipsilateral to the resection difficult to evaluate, and the area at highest risk after this type of resection. However, mediastinal recurrence after pneumonectomy is almost always unresectable and usually represents metastatic nodal disease with a low likelihood of cure. There is no prospective study to attest to the value of a computed tomographic scan after pneumonectomy, and obtaining one in this patient population is not currently part of the practice at the University of Washington Medical Center.

A relatively small study by Gorich et al.[8] demonstrated an advantage of computed tomography over chest x-ray in detecting both local recurrence and new lymph node involvement. The researchers advocate the routine use of computed tomography in the postoperative period to detect recurrent or new primary disease at an earlier and possibly more resectable stage. This is an interesting finding but should be confirmed by a larger trial, since the routine use of computed tomography would be expensive and might well result in needless anxiety for the patient and unnecessary biopsies or resections because of false-positive results. The use of magnetic resonance imaging to differentiate scarring from recurrent carcinoma is currently being evaluated and may at some point play a role in postoperative surveillance.[9] At present the only radiological study that can be recommended for routine use after resection of NSCLC is chest x-ray.

Biochemical Studies

At present the only biochemical study that is of value in the follow-up of patients after resection of NSCLC is measurement of CEA,[10] which is helpful only when the level is elevated preoperatively and falls to normal levels after resection. We have not found CEA useful at the University of Washington Medical Center, and it is not clear how widely CEA is used. Other nonspecific tests for metastatic disease such as serum calcium, alkaline phosphatase, serum glutamic-oxaloacetic transaminase, and lactic dehydrogenase levels may be helpful for evaluating the extent of known metastatic disease or as a guide to the response to subsequent therapy. However, they have no proven role in routine follow-up after curative resection. A biochemical marker for NSCLC would be useful for the follow-up of patients after resection, as well as for screening populations at high risk for lung cancer. This is under investigation at the University of Washington.

Sputum Cytology

Sputum cytology has not been proved useful either for screening for primary lung cancer or for detecting recurrent disease.[11,12] We agree with Downey et al. that this test should not be part of the routine follow-up of these patients. The use of monoclonal antibodies directed at both small cell and non–small cell cancers of the lung in the examination of sputum samples is under evaluation and may yield a useful test for the detection of recurrent disease. At this time, however, the routine use of sputum cytology cannot be recommended.

Bronchoscopy

Bronchoscopy has evolved into a procedure that can be easily performed in the outpatient setting and is tolerated well by awake patients. It is not indicated for routine follow-up but should be reserved for patients who have symptoms of recurrence. Bronchoscopy is in the second tier of diagnostic studies, along with computed tomography. In addition, bronchoscopy may be useful for patients with known bronchial epithelial tumors or in situations in which the line of resection was close to tumor. Bronchoscopy also enables the physician to obtain a tissue diagnosis and more accurately determine whether further resection will be possible. Furthermore, in instances of unresectable endobronchial disease, it allows the surgeon to determine the need for and usefulness of palliative procedures, such as rigid bronchoscopy with coring out of tumor, laser ablation of tumor, and stenting of extensive endobronchial disease that threatens the airway.

COST EFFECTIVENESS OF FOLLOW-UP

In this era of increased concern about the costs of medical care, it is crucial to consider the cost effectiveness of follow-up after potentially curative resection of NSCLC. A recent report by Walsh et al.[5] raised the provocative question of whether follow-up of these patients is cost effective on a routine basis. The authors were able to document that only 3% of their patients received further therapy directed at cure. If further curative therapy were the only benefit of follow-up, it might be tempting to agree with this position. However, these figures ignore the patients who received palliative care with subsequent improvement in the quality of life and survived longer because recurrent disease was detected at follow-up. Walsh et al. also stated that survival for patients with recurrent disease detected in the asymptomatic stage was 34 months, compared with 19 months for patients who had symptomatic recurrence. It is difficult to know whether this represents a difference in tumor biology or is the result of earlier institution of palliative measures. Most likely it is a combination of both factors. However, to exclude these patients from routine follow-up would be to deprive them of palliative care in many cases. Furthermore, what these results underscore is the importance of obtaining a curative resection at the first operation. Clearly, recurrent NSCLC has a dismal prognosis and is amenable to further surgical resection in only a fraction of cases.

Assuming that follow-up of patients after curative resection of NSCLC is worthwhile, physicians must make every effort to make it as efficient and cost effective as possible. The frequency of follow-up outlined previously is appropriately tailored to the rate of recurrence and probably represents the minimum with which most practitioners would feel comfortable. The other major variables in determining the cost of follow-up are the modalities used. A postoperative return visit to the clinic or office is one of the least expensive charges in medicine today, and the history and physical examination have been shown to be very sensitive in detecting recurrent disease. Of all the other studies or tests that may be routinely obtained in the postoperative setting, the only one with proven value is the chest x-ray. Fortunately, it is also one of the least expensive and most easily obtained studies. In light of this, it is clear that a thorough history and directed physical examination, along with standard posteroanterior and lateral chest x-rays, are cost effective and should constitute the basis for routine follow-up. Except in selected instances discussed previously, they should guide the use of all other, more expensive studies in the detection of recurrent disease.

RESPONSIBILITY OF THE SURGEON IN FOLLOW-UP

The increased attention to cost containment in the practice of medicine raises the issue of who is responsible for postoperative follow-up of patients. Ideally the member of the health care team who knows the most about lung cancer, its therapy, and the indications for further resection or palliative care should be the one to oversee care of the patient after resection for lung cancer. In most instances this person is the thoracic surgeon. In settings in which this would require an inordinate amount of travel for the patient, the necessary information may be communicated by letter or telephone between the primary physician and surgeon. This should not, however, affect the frequency or modalities of follow-up. The other situation in which the surgeon will most likely not be the primary caregiver involves the patient with metastatic disease. The treatment of patients with extensive recurrent or widely metastatic disease should ideally be managed by a medical oncologist, often with additional consultations with a radiation oncologist and thoracic surgeon. The operating surgeon plays a vital role in these discussions, since he or she is uniquely acquainted with the patient's anatomy and best suited to make recommendations regarding further resection or palliation of the airway.

SUMMARY

Most practitioners are convinced of the value of routine follow-up for patients who have had curative resection for lung cancer. The treatment of metastatic disease is limited to palliation and is not significantly affected by recognition of asymptomatic disease. However, patients with locoregional recurrence or a new primary tumor in the lung may be considered for curative resection if the cancer is discovered at an early stage. With the ever-increasing importance of cost containment in medical care, and given the proliferation of expensive technologies that may be applied in the evaluation of these patients, the challenge is to develop and adhere to a plan of follow-up care that is both cost effective and efficient at detecting recurrent disease. Follow-up consisting of a history, directed physical examination, and standard posteroanterior and lateral chest x-rays every 4 months for 2 years, every 6 months for the next 2 years, and annually thereafter should meet both of these objectives and should be readily attained in the majority of practice settings (Table 12-9).

REFERENCES

1. Wingo PA, Tong T, Bolden S. Cancer statistics, 1995. CA Cancer J Clin 1995;45:8-30.
2. Fontana RS, Sanderson DR, Woolner LB, et al. Screening for lung cancer: a critique of the Mayo Lung Project. Cancer 1991;67:1155-64.
3. Martini N, Ginsberg RJ. Non-small cell lung cancer/postresection follow-up. In: Pearson FG, editor. Thoracic surgery. New York: Churchill Livingstone, 1995:759-63.
4. Martini N. Surgical treatment of non-small cell lung cancer by stage. Semin Surg Oncol 1990;6:248-54.
5. Walsh GL, O'Connor M, Willis KM, et al. Is follow-up of lung cancer patients following resection medically indicated and cost effective? Ann Thorac Surg 1996;60:1563-72.
6. Mountain C. Therapy of stage I and II non-small cell lung cancer. Semin Oncol 1983;10:71-80.
7. Feld R, Rubinstein L, Weisemberger T, Lung Cancer Study Group. Sites of recurrence in resected stage I non-small cell lung cancer: a guide for future studies. J Clin Oncol 1984;2:1352-8.

Table 12-10 Follow-up of patients with bronchogenic carcinoma (non–small cell lung cancer) by institution

YEAR/PROGRAM	OFFICE VISIT	CXR	CEA	CHEST CT	CBC
Year 1					
Memorial Sloan-Kettering	4	3-4	a	a	
Roswell Park	3	3			
Univ Washington	3	3			
Japan: National Kyushu[b]	6	4	6	2	6
Japan: National Kyushu	4-6	4-6	4-6		
Year 2					
Memorial Sloan-Kettering	3	3-4	a	a	
Roswell Park	3	3			
Univ Washington	3	3			
Japan: National Kyushu[b]	6	4	6	2	6
Japan: National Kyushu	3-4	3-4	3-4		
Year 3					
Memorial Sloan-Kettering	1-2	2	a	a	
Roswell Park	3	3			
Univ Washington	2	2			
Japan: National Kyushu[b]	3	2	3	1	3
Japan: National Kyushu	2	2	2		
Year 4					
Memorial Sloan-Kettering	1-2	2	a	a	
Roswell Park	2	2			
Univ Washington	2	2			
Japan: National Kyushu[b]	3	2	3	1	3
Japan: National Kyushu	2	2	2		
Year 5					
Memorial Sloan-Kettering	1-2	2	a	a	
Roswell Park	1	1			
Univ Washington	1	1			
Japan: National Kyushu[b]	3	2	3	1	3
Japan: National Kyushu	2	2	2		

BRAIN CT brain computed tomography
CBC complete blood count
CEA carcinoembryonic antigen
CHEST CT chest computed tomography
CXR chest x-ray
SCCAG squamous cell carcinoma antigen
SPUTUM sputum cytology
UPPER ABD CT upper abdominal computed tomography

8. Gorich J, Beyer-Enke SA, Flentje M, Zuna I, Vogt-Moykopf I, Van Kaick G. Evaluation of recurrent bronchogenic carcinoma by computed tomography. Clin Imaging 1990;14:131-7.
9. Kono M, Adachi S, Kusumoto M, Sakai E. Clinical utility of Gd-DTPA-enhanced magnetic imaging in lung cancer. J Thorac Imaging 1993;8:18-26.
10. Macchia V, Mariano A, Cavalcanti M. Tumor markers and lung cancer: correlation between serum and bronchial secretion levels of CEA, TPA, CanAg CA-50, NSE and ferritin. Int J Biol Markers 1987;2:151-6.
11. Fontana RS, Sanderson DR, Taylor WF, et al. Early lung cancer detection: results of the initial (prevalence) radiologic and cytologic screening in the Mayo Clinic Study. Am Rev Respir Dis 1984; 130:561-5.
12. Frost JK, Ball WC Jr, Levin ML, et. al. Early lung cancer detection: results of the initial (prevalence) radiologic and cytologic screening in the John Hopkins study. Am Rev Respir Dis 1984;130:549-54.

BLOOD	SIALYL LEWIS X	SCCAG	SPUTUM	BRAIN CT	UPPPER ABD CT	BONE SCAN
6[c]	6	6	3[d]	2	2	2
6[c]	6	6	3[d]	2	2	2
3[c]	3	3	3[d]	1	1	1
3[c]	3	3	3[d]	1	1	1
3[c]	3	3	3[d]	1	1	1

a Performed only when clinically indicated.
b Strategy tested in an ongoing National Kyushu Cancer Center trial.
c Includes serum calcium, alkaline phosphatase, glutamic oxalate transaminase, and lactic dehydrogenase levels.
d Performed in patients with resected squamous cell carcinoma and for either current or former smokers.

CHAPTER 13

Soft Tissue Sarcoma

University of Washington Medical Center

Richard J. O'Donnell, James D. Bruckner, and Ernest U. Conrad III

Soft tissue sarcomas are a relatively rare and histologically diverse set of malignancies that arise principally from connective tissues throughout the body. In Sweden the annual incidence is 18 per million.[1] A slightly higher rate has been calculated in the United States, with estimates ranging from 6,000 to 11,400 new cases per year.[2,3] Historically, 5-year survival for this group as a whole has been less than 50%,[4] but more recent applications of multimodality therapy have improved the outlook considerably. For patients with nonmetastatic disease at diagnosis, 5-year disease-free survival rates are on the order of 70% to 80%.[5-8]

Although the last decade has seen a plethora of texts, monographs, and articles heralding these advances in diagnosis, treatment, and prognosis, little has been codified regarding the appropriate follow-up of patients with soft tissue sarcoma. As treatment protocols become more complex and as more patients survive for longer time periods, monitoring their progress will become increasingly important. Doing so in a safe but cost-effective manner will be necessitated by constraints on health care resources. Unfortunately, because of the low incidence of soft tissue sarcoma, little if anything about the overall economic impact of this disease exists in the published literature.

Because surveillance begins early in the care of patients treated with neoadjuvant strategies, this chapter begins with a brief overview of the current status of the initial treatment of soft tissue sarcomas. Since surveillance varies according to a given patient's perceived risk factors, prognosis and patterns of recurrence are considered. The discussion then focuses on the follow-up of patients with localized disease treated with curative intent. Adult extremity lesions, which occur most frequently, are emphasized, but information about head and neck, thoracic, abdominal, and pediatric tumors is included where appropriate. A matrix for monitoring patient health and for surveillance of local, regional, and distant recurrences is presented. Treatment and prognosis of recurrent disease are also discussed, as are prospects for improving follow-up care of patients with soft tissue sarcoma.

CURRENT MANAGEMENT OF SOFT TISSUE SARCOMA

Diagnosis and Staging

As in any area of medical practice, evaluation of the patient with a soft tissue mass begins with a comprehensive history and physical examination. It then proceeds with appropriate laboratory and radiographic studies en route to determining the tissue diagnosis and tumor stage.

History

Soft tissue sarcomas arise throughout the body in the following distributions: extremities (60%), trunk (30%), and head and neck (10%).[9] Lower extremity lesions are three times more common than those of the upper extremity, and 75% occur at or above the knee.[9] Retroperitoneal tumors account for 40% of truncal soft tissue sarcomas, and tumors of the abdominal and chest walls, mediastinum, pelvis, and breast account for the remainder.[9]

A painless mass is the most common presentation. It is necessary to determine when the mass was first noted and how rapidly it has grown. Acute pain is thought to occur from hemorrhage within the tumor, whereas chronic pain results from extensive tumor necrosis.[10] Pain, paresthesias, and weakness can all be consequences of nerve irritation or involvement. Peripheral edema may result from venous compression. Limitation of function may follow from muscular or juxtaarticular extension. Visceral organ dysfunction can occur from thoracic, retroperitoneal, abdominal, or pelvic sarcomas. A review of systems should concentrate on pulmonary and gastrointestinal symptoms, as well as constitutional findings such as fever, fatigue, anorexia, and weight loss.

Elements of a patient's past medical history may also be of relevance. Prototypical conditions associated with the development of sarcomas include neurofibromatosis type I (neurofibrosarcoma),[11] Stewart-Treves syndrome (lymphangiosarcoma),[12] and the acquired immunodeficiency syndrome (Kaposi's sarcoma),[13] among others.[14-17] Sarcomas are known to arise after radiation exposure,[18-20] but associations with chemical agents,[21] foreign bodies,[22] and prior trauma are less well established.

Table 13-1 Laboratory examination of bone and soft tissue malignancy

ROUTINE TESTS
Blood urea nitrogen
Creatinine
Urinalysis
Aspartate aminotransferase
Alkaline phosphatase
Glucose
Thyroid function tests
Complete blood count with differential
Erythrocyte sedimentation rate
Calcium
Phosphorus
SPECIALIZED TESTS
Serum immunoelectrophoresis
Peripheral blood smear
Bone marrow smear
Parathyroid hormone
Vitamin D
Carcinoembyronic antigen
Acid phosphatase
Prostate specific antigen
CA-127 level

Table 13-2 Radiological examination of soft tissue sarcoma

ROUTINE TESTS
Plain radiographs
Site
Chest
Computed tomography
Site
Chest
Abdomen
Magnetic resonance imaging of site
Technetium-99m bone scintigraphy
Positron emission tomography
SPECIALIZED TESTS
Angiography
Lymphangiography
Ultrasound
Gallium scintigraphy
Indium-labeled white blood cell
Scintigraphy

Physical examination

Soft tissue masses should be examined to determine size, consistency, and relationship to surrounding structures. Tenderness, warmth, erythema, and surrounding edema should be noted. Any soft tissue mass larger than 5 cm and denser than muscle, even if nontender, should be evaluated further.

The neurovascular status of the extremities must be documented. Lymphadenopathy must be considered. Abdominal, rectal, and pelvic examinations should focus on masses and organomegaly. Pulmonary findings such as pleural effusion, although unusual at initial presentation, should not be overlooked.

Laboratory examination

Patients with suspected bone or soft tissue malignancy necessarily undergo a number of routine blood screens to evaluate their general health, with more specialized tests added as the differential diagnosis warrants (Table 13-1). Hypoglycemia is seen as a paraneoplastic phenomenon with some soft tissue sarcomas.[23] Hypophosphatemia and hypercalcemia have also been reported.[24,25] Unfortunately, no laboratory test exists that is either sensitive or specific for the diagnosis of soft tissue sarcoma.

Radiological examination

To further assist in staging and preoperative planning, a number of routine and specialized radiological studies are performed (Table 13-2). The site of the primary tumor should be evaluated with plain radiographs (x-rays), computed tomography (for trunk and extremity primary lesions), or magnetic resonance imaging (for extremity primary lesions). Though magnetic resonance imaging is generally considered superior to computed tomography for extremity soft tissue sarcomas,[26-28] a preoperative computed tomography scan is also helpful in assessing intralesional calcification and the relationship of the tumor to cortical bone.[29] Magnetic resonance imaging and computed tomography together are also recommended for pelvic and spinal sarcomas, and computed tomography alone is generally used for thoracic and intraabdominal tumors.

Metastatic disease should be investigated with a computed tomographic scan of the chest and abdomen as well as bone scintigraphy.[30-32] We have also gained considerable experience with positron emission tomography[33-36] as a guide to the grade of the primary tumor, as a screen for metastatic disease, and for the assessment of response to neoadjuvant therapy. Since the advent of these tests, other means of analysis such as arteriography,[37] lymphangiography,[38] ultrasound,[39] and gallium scintigraphy[40] have fallen into disuse.

Pathological examination

To complete the staging evaluation of a soft tissue tumor before definitive treatment, a biopsy must be performed according to strict surgical principles. This can be accomplished in one of several ways.

Closed or needle biopsy, with or without radiological (computed tomography–guided) control, is minimally invasive and is the most commonly used technique in some centers.[41,42] It is preferred for lesions to which access is problematic (abdominal, pelvic, or spinal primary tumors). The disadvantage of this method is that the quantity of tissue obtained may be insufficient for diagnosis and grading.

An incisional procedure is the standard means of biopsy of a soft tissue neoplasm. The use of proper technique in per-

Table 13-3 American Joint Committee on Cancer stage grouping for soft tissue sarcoma

HISTOPATHOLOGICAL GRADING (G)

GX	Grade cannot be assessed
G1	Well-differentiated
G2	Moderately differentiated
G3	Poorly differentiated
G4	Undifferentiated

DEFINITION OF TNM

Primary Tumor (T)

TX	Primary tumor cannot be assessed
T0	No evidence of primary tumor
T1	Tumor 5 cm or less in greatest dimension
T2	Tumor more than 5 cm in greatest dimension

Regional Lymph Nodes (N)

NX	Regional lymph nodes cannot be assessed
N0	No regional lymph node metastasis
N1	Regional lymph node metastasis

Distant Metastasis (M)

MX	Presence of distant metastasis cannot be assessed
M0	No distant metastasis
M1	Distant metastasis

STAGE GROUPING

Stage 1A	G1	T1	N0	M0
Stage 1B	G1	T2	N0	M0
Stage IIA	G2	T1	N0	M0
Stage IIB	G2	T2	N0	M0
Stage IIIA	G3,4	T1	N0	M0
Stage IIIB	G3,4	T2	N0	M0
Stage IVA	Any G	Any T	N1	M0
Stage IV	Any G	Any T	Any N	M1

Modified from American Joint Committee on Cancer: Beahrs OH, Henson DE, Hutter RV, Kennedy BJ, editors. Manual for staging of cancer. Philadelphia: JB Lippincott Company, 1992.

forming incisional biopsies is essential to avoid compromising definitive surgery, especially when limb salvage is planned.[43-46] Excisional biopsy is advised only for small lesions (less than 3 to 4 cm) that can be easily excised with a wide margin without undue functional compromise, or when an incisional biopsy would contaminate tissue that would be difficult to resect at a later date, such as pelvic lesions.[29]

The pathological specimen is first examined to determine histological type and whether malignancy is present. Routine histological staining is performed, followed by specialized studies (immunohistochemistry, electron microscopy, and cytogenetics, including flow cytometry).[47] Cytogenic analysis of chromosomal aberrations is particularly helpful in the diagnosis of pediatric soft tissue tumors.[48,49]

Soft tissue sarcomas are further classified as well differentiated (grade 1), moderately well-differentiated (grade 2), poorly differentiated (grade 3), or, less commonly, undifferentiated (grade 4), according to criteria such as cellularity, pleomorphism, and mitotic activity. Grading depends in part on histological type, since some exhibit a narrow range of biological behavior, while others have a spectrum of aggressiveness.[50,51]

Staging

The most widely accepted staging system for soft tissue sarcomas is that of the American Joint Committee on Cancer (Table 13-3).[50] It is based on the tumor, nodes, metastases (TNM) method. An alternative means of classifying both bone and soft tissue sarcomas, based on grade, tumor extent, and the presence or absence of metastases, has been advocated by the Musculoskeletal Tumor Society.[52-54]

Treatment

Surgery remains the mainstay of therapy for soft tissue sarcoma. Nonoperative therapy, consisting principally of high-dose radiation therapy, is generally reserved for large, inaccessible tumors for which surgical extirpation is not possible. Although an inverse relationship exists between tumor size and ability to attain local control,[55] some success has been reported with aggressive radiation therapy for unresectable lesions.[56,57]

Surgery alone

Historically the management of soft tissue sarcomas has been surgical, without the use of adjuvant therapies. As noted by Yang et al.,[9] the use of surgery alone for extremity tumors regardless of stage resulted in acceptable local control only with a high rate of amputation.[58-62] Limb-sparing and other conservative surgical techniques have come into vogue as the addition of adjuvant and neoadjuvant strategies has improved local control rates without jeopardizing survival.[63,64]

Currently, surgery is accepted as the sole method of treatment for small (less than 7 cm in diameter), extremity soft tissue sarcomas without evidence of regional or distant metastases. A local recurrence rate of 10% with a 5-year survival rate greater than 90% has been reported.[65]

Surgery plus radiation therapy

As noted previously, surgery alone for extremity sarcomas achieves a local control rate of greater than 80% only at the expense of a high percentage of extensive ablative procedures.[9] Furthermore, surgery alone provides local control in only 50% to 75% of truncal and 30% to 40% of retroperitoneal lesions.[66] Radiation therapy has therefore been advocated as a means to improve local control, combined where appropriate with more conservative surgical measures.

Postoperative external beam radiation therapy to a total dose of approximately 66 Gy has achieved good local control while maintaining survival.[7,67-72] Currently this method applied to extremity, as well as head and neck, sarcomas results in 92% local control and 76% long-term disease-free survival rates.[7] Less success with more gastrointestinal morbidity has been described for this approach to retroperitoneal sarcomas.[73,74]

The combination of preoperative and postoperative radiation therapy has been advocated because the former provides the practical advantages of a smaller field exposure, lower risk of contamination from operative spillage of a mass that is at least partially necrotic, and the potential to resect shrunken tumors that were previously unresectable. Disadvantages include difficulties with histological evaluation of the resected specimen and wound complications.[66] To date, 97% local control and 65% 5-year disease-free survival rates have been reported.[7]

The inclusion of brachytherapy (iridium-192 afterloaded catheters) in the treatment plan has attracted considerable interest. Advantages include reduced treatment length and optimal dose distribution. Local control rates on the order of 95% have been recorded.[75,76] Newer techniques awaiting further investigation include intraoperative external beam,[74] proton beam,[77] and fast neutron beam[78] therapies.

Surgery plus radiation therapy plus chemotherapy

Despite the advances made in radiation oncology, the realization that local recurrence of soft tissue sarcoma may not be causally related to distant recurrence and hence overall patient survival[1,79-81] and the encouraging results found with chemotherapy of pediatric rhabdomyosarcoma,[82] osteosarcoma,[83] and Ewing's sarcoma[84] have prompted investigation into the potential applicability of adjuvant and neoadjuvant chemotherapy protocols for soft tissue sarcoma.

Of five randomized trials of adjuvant doxorubicin versus control,[5,8,85-87] only that from Bologna[8] demonstrated a significant disease-free and overall survival benefit for the chemotherapy arm. This study, however, has been criticized on statistical grounds.[88,89] Of five randomized trials of adjuvant combination chemotherapy versus control,[6,89-92] almost all have shown a significant benefit in terms of local control. Although one study with relatively few patients has shown statistically significant improvement in metastatic rate and overall survival in the chemotherapy arm,[92] the remainder, including the largest study to date,[89] have not confirmed these findings.

Interest has thus turned to neoadjuvant chemotherapy, which has the theoretical advantage of being able to treat both the primary tumor and micrometastatic disease immediately after diagnosis and staging are complete. As with preoperative radiation therapy, tumor response can improve the ease and safety of surgical resection while assisting the clinical and pathological assessment of prognosis. Soft tissue sarcomas often respond dramatically to chemotherapy, with flow cytometric estimates of cell proliferation being predictive of short-term effects.[93]

Several centers are investigating neoadjuvant regimens for high-grade soft tissue sarcomas.[94-102] At M.D. Anderson Cancer Center, for example, patients receive preoperative cyclophosphamide, doxorubicin, and dacarbazine, with or without vincristine, followed by definitive local therapy (surgery with or without radiation therapy).[94] Patients with evidence of tumor progression despite chemotherapy undergo immediate local therapy (preoperative radiation plus surgery).[94] Postoperative chemotherapy is given to responders.[94] At the University of California, Los Angeles, patients receive intravenous doxorubicin, cisplatin, and ifosfamide, followed by 28 Gy radiation before surgery.[100] The European Organization for Research and Treatment of Cancer is currently conducting a prospective study of high-risk patients randomly selected to receive three courses of neoadjuvant doxorubicin, ifosfamide, or no chemotherapy before proceeding to surgery with or without radiation therapy.[89]

Our Protocol

At the University of Washington Medical Center, treatment of patients with soft tissue sarcoma is individualized according to the estimated risk of local and distant recurrence.

Low-risk patients

All low-grade and small (less than 7 cm) intermediate-grade tumors are treated initially with wide surgical resection. Postoperative radiation therapy is added in cases of marginal or intralesional surgical margins. Follow-up is based on a low-risk surveillance matrix.

High-risk patients

Patients with high-grade or large (7 cm or greater) intermediate-grade tumors are entered into a phase II study involving neoadjuvant chemotherapy, surgery, and adjuvant chemotherapy and radiation therapy.[103] Preoperatively, three cycles of doxorubicin and cisplatin or ifosfamide are administered every 28 days. Surgical resection is undertaken with a goal of achieving at least a marginal or wide surgical excision, and limb-sparing techniques are used when feasible. Patients then receive an additional five cycles of adjuvant chemotherapy, beginning within 1 month of surgery. Patients who are to receive radiation therapy have three cycles of adjuvant chemotherapy before radiation, followed by the final two cycles of chemotherapy. Surveillance, which begins during neoadjuvant treatment and continues indefinitely, is discussed later.

Prognosis

The literature about prognostic factors that relate to soft tissue sarcomas is extensive and often confusing. In general, patients with extremity neoplasms enjoy a more favorable survival prognosis than patients with tumors in other locations.[104,105] When multivariate analyses of extremity tumors are reviewed, the most generally accepted adverse prognostic factors are higher grade,[62,104,106-112] larger size,[108,109,111,113] and histological evidence of necrosis.[1,51,106,113] Other studies have identified other adverse survival prognosticators, including positive margins,[62,108,109] need for extensive ablative surgery,[108-110] and older age.[62,108-110,112] Adverse prognostic indicators for local recurrence include positive margins,[1,62,108-110,112,115] limb-sparing surgery,[108,109,115] and older age.[108-110]

SURVEILLANCE OF PATIENTS WITH SOFT TISSUE SARCOMA

Appropriate follow-up encompasses both monitoring of general health and surveillance for locally, regionally, or distantly recurrent disease. The former requires an understanding of the potential side effects of multimodality therapy, while the latter necessitates knowledge of the likely patterns and risk of tumor recurrence and appropriate diagnostic measures. Treatment and prognosis for local and metastatic recurrence are briefly considered before the presentation of a suggested surveillance matrix.

General Medical, Surgical, and Mental Health

Before treatment begins, the patient with a soft tissue mass undergoes the aforementioned laboratory and radiological diagnostic screening procedures. Before open biopsy the appropriate tests for preoperative medical clearance, such as electrocardiography, are conducted. Performance status[50] should be assessed and clinical photographs taken.

Patients with low-risk lesions who undergo wide excisional biopsy are entered into the postsurgical surveillance protocol described below. Patients with high-risk lesions who undergo incisional biopsy (or computed tomography–guided biopsy) must begin a presurgical neoadjuvant surveillance protocol immediately.

For patients receiving neoadjuvant chemotherapy, necessary pretreatment tests include a complete blood count (including absolute neutrophil and platelet counts); electrolyte levels (including magnesium), blood urea nitrogen and creatinine (including creatinine clearance), and liver function tests. Since almost all soft tissue sarcoma regimens involve doxorubicin, which is cardiotoxic,[116] radionuclide angiography to determine left ventricular ejection fraction must be performed. For protocols that include cisplatin a baseline audiogram is needed. Once chemotherapy (whether neoadjuvant or adjuvant) has commenced, interim history, physical, laboratory, and radiographic examinations should continue as outlined below.

For patients receiving radiation therapy, pretreatment musculoskeletal function must be assessed. Special attention should be directed toward joints and major neuromuscular units involved in the radiation field.

Once surgery is complete, the wound and surgical site must be carefully monitored for swelling, erythema, warmth, or drainage, which could herald the development of a seroma, hematoma, or infection. Wound healing is altered by irradiation and chemotherapy.[117] Complications are avoided by scrupulous attention to closed suction drainage of the wound, sterile dressings, and activity limitation until healing is well under way. Thereafter close cooperation with physical and occupational therapists, orthotists, and prosthetists maximizes functional recovery.[118]

Throughout the treatment course the psychosocial well-being of the patient with soft tissue sarcoma must be remembered. This is best addressed by a multidisciplinary team, including psychiatrists, social workers, and an oncology nursing staff.[119-121]

Local Recurrence

Patterns

As general health returns to baseline once neoadjuvant, surgical, and adjuvant treatments are complete, surveillance must be directed toward the possibility of recurrence of the primary lesion. Potter et al.[122] reported a series of 307 patients with fully resectable, high-grade soft tissue sarcomas treated at the National Cancer Institute with surgery alone or in combination with chemotherapy or radiation therapy or both. In all, 25 of 307 patients (8%) had an initial recurrence that was local. Of the recurrences, 21 (7%) were isolated and four (1%) occurred in combination with other areas of recurrence. Thus local recurrence accounted for 25 of 107 (23%) initial recurrences and regional and distant sites accounted for the remaining 77%.[122] The average time to all initial recurrences was 18 months (range, 0.5 to 72.0 months),[122] which is in accord with the estimation that 80% of local recurrences occur within 2 years of surgery.[123,124]

Diagnosis

The clinician should remain alert for a history of recurrent pain; extremity recurrences might be evidenced by paresthesias, head and neck recurrences with dysphonia or dysphagia, and abdominal tumors with gastrointestinal distress. Physical examination should focus on the delineation of warmth, swelling, or a frank mass within the surgical field. Laboratory studies are not particularly helpful for diagnosing a local recurrence.

Radiological surveillance of locally recurrent disease should start with routine plain x-rays of the primary site. Altered soft tissue shadows, periosteal reaction of underlying bones, or abnormal bowel gas patterns should be studied. Bone scintigraphy can document perturbation of nearby bone, as well as search out more widely metastatic disease.

The mainstay of monitoring for local recurrence is magnetic resonance imaging. The ability to alter pulse sequences and to add gadolinium enhancement allows distinctions to be made among recurrent tumor, normal structures, and postoperative changes such as edema, seroma, hematoma, and posttreatment scarring.[125-127] Obtaining magnetic resonance imaging at 6 months after surgery allows for the resolution of postoperative edema and provides a baseline for comparison with subsequent abnormalities. Although magnetic resonance imaging has proved more sensitive than computed tomography for the detection of locally recurrent disease,[128] the latter technique is still useful in certain circumstances, such as the surveillance of chest and abdominal primary lesions.

Treatment

Whenever possible in cases of isolated local recurrence, repeat wide or radical surgical excision should be under-

Table 13-4 Results of reoperation for completely resected isolated locally recurrent soft tissue sarcoma

STUDY	PATIENTS (*n*)	EXTREMITY LESIONS (%)	5-YEAR SURVIVAL RATE (%)
Jaques et al., 1990[130]	39	0	35
Potter et al., 1985[122]	20	31	35
Sauter et al., 1993[124]	30	45	49
Singer et al., 1992[131]	21	62	67
Giuliano et al., 1982[129]	33	66	87

Modified from Sauter ER, Hoffman JP, Eisenberg BL. Semin Oncol 1993;20:451-5.

Table 13-5 Patterns of initial recurrence of high-grade soft tissue sarcomas

	POTTER ET AL., 1985[122] (%, n = 107)	HUTH AND EILBER 1988[137] (%, n = 85)
Lung ± other sites	59	64
Isolated lung	52	40
Local ± other sites	23	22
Isolated local	20	15
Lymph ± other sites	5	2
Bone ± other sites	7	11
Liver ± other sites	4	4
Any other site	14	12

taken.[124] The importance of careful documentation of surgical margins cannot be overemphasized. Negative surgical margins can be obtained in approximately 90% of patients in whom surgery is attempted.[122,124,129] Additional treatment with radiation or chemotherapy should be considered where appropriate.

For local disease in a patient with regional or distant recurrences, aggressive resection with curative intent is contemplated infrequently. In the series reported by Potter et al.,[122] only one of 15 (7%) patients with multiple sites of initial recurrence became disease free. Nonetheless, palliative resection of locally recurrent disease in this circumstance may be necessary.

Prognosis

Sauter et al.[124] have summarized the literature showing favorable outcomes, especially for patients with extremity lesions, in whom complete resection of isolated locally recurrent disease can be accomplished (Table 13-4).

Although there has long been concern that local recurrence is causally related to metastatic disease,[62,110,123,132-136] increasing evidence from multivariate analyses of population-based studies supports the view that local recurrence is a marker for, rather than a cause of, distant disease.[1,79,80] Most recently the size and timing of local recurrence were found to be more predictive of metastasis than the presence of local recurrence per se.[81] However, as pointed out by Gustafson,[1] the fact that local recurrence is not the common source of metastasis should not discourage appropriate aggressive treatment of isolated local disease that is potentially curable.

Regional and Distant Recurrence

Patterns

As far as surveillance is concerned, the pattern of initial regional and distant recurrence is of paramount importance. The most common mode of spread of soft tissue sarcoma in the study of Potter et al.[122] was that of isolated pulmonary metastases, accounting for 56 of 107 (52%) of all initial recurrences. Bone and liver metastases were present in only seven of 107 (7%) and four of 107 (4%) patients with initial recurrences, respectively.[122] Regional lymph node spread was relatively rare as an initial presentation, occurring alone or in combination with other sites in only five of 107 (5%) cases.[122] The average time to any recurrence was 18 months (range, 0.5 months to 72 months).[122] These data are in accord with those of Huth and Eilber[137] (Table 13-5).

The pattern of initial recurrence is mostly a function of primary site, since 70% of extremity lesions recur initially as isolated lung metastases, while truncal tumors tend to exhibit local recurrences initially and retroperitoneal tumors appear first as diffuse abdominal sarcomatosis.[122] Much less is known about the predictability of initial recurrence according to the histological type of tumor.[138]

Diagnosis

Unfortunately, pulmonary and other distant metastases are typically asymptomatic until quite advanced. A history of cough, pleuritic chest pain, dyspnea, or hemoptysis is occasionally elicited.[139] Regional lymph node metastases sometimes occur as a painful swelling. Physical examination should concentrate on auscultation and percussion of the lungs, as well as inspection of any masses. Routine laboratory examination is most often nonspecific and may point to a decline in general health (such as anemia or hypoalbuminemia), to iatrogenic complications (such as nephrotoxicity from chemotherapeutic agents), or, in the case of abnormal liver function tests, to hepatic metastases.

Radiological studies form the basis for surveillance of distant disease. Numerous reports have demonstrated the superior sensitivity of computed tomography scans of the chest compared with conventional radiography for the detection of pulmonary metastases.[140,141] Nonetheless, plain chest x-ray is considered more specific than computed tomography and so is still recommended as part of routine follow-up every 1 to 3 months.[139] Technetium-99m bone scanning is recommended on a less frequent basis, and computed tomography of the liver only in cases of positive laboratory values.[129] Lymphangiography is seldom useful in the diagnosis of lymphatic metastatic deposits.[10]

Table 13-6 Surveillance matrix during neoadjuvant and adjuvant chemotherapy

STRATEGY	DURING EACH CYCLE	AFTER EACH CYCLE	AFTER SECOND AND THIRD CYCLES	BEFORE DOXORUBICIN AND AFTER 450 mg/m²
Physical examination	X	X		
Complete blood count, neutrophil, platelets, electrolytes, blood urea nitrogen/creatinine	X			
Liver function tests		X		
Plain chest x-ray		X		
Chest computed tomography			X	
Magnetic resonance imaging of primary site			X	
Cardiac radionuclide angiography				X

Treatment

Since pulmonary metastases are generally asymptomatic, resection is considered only for cure and not for palliation. For metastases to be considered for surgical resection, several basic requirements need to be met: (1) the primary tumor should be controlled or controllable; (2) there should be no extrapulmonary metastases; (3) the pulmonary metastases should be fully resectable; and (4) the patient must have adequate pulmonary reserve to survive the resection.[139,142] In addition, pulmonary metastases that progress despite chemotherapy should probably not be considered for resection. Technically, the procedure can be carried out via thoracotomy, median sternotomy, or thoracoscopy. Complete resection is possible in more than 90% of patients selected for surgery, with perioperative mortality of approximately 1%.[143] Resection of second (recurrent) pulmonary metastases is also possible.

Resection of metastases to bone or lymph nodes is occasionally necessary for palliative reasons such as painful inguinal lymphadenopathy that threatens limb neurovascularity. Hepatectomy for soft tissue sarcoma metastases is very rarely indicated.[144]

Prognosis

Numerous reports highlight the potential benefits of pulmonary resection for soft tissue sarcoma metastases.[142,143,145-148] The overall 5-year survival rate is 25%.[143] For secondarily recurrent pulmonary metastases that are fully resected, the median survival time is approximately 2 years.[149-150]

Occurrence of a Second Primary Cancer

Patients with soft tissue sarcoma are subject to the development of a second primary neoplasm of the same histological type, either synchronously or metachronously, as has been documented, for example, in neurofibromatosis type I[151] or malignant fibrous histiocytoma.[152] More frequent, however, is the metachronous occurrence of a second primary of different histology, either related or unrelated to prior treatment. In a review of 8,815 patients with sarcoma from the National Cancer Institute's Surveillance, Epidemiology and End Results Program registered between 1973 and 1986, 240 (3%) developed a metachronous second primary sarcoma.[153] Of these 240, 74 (31%) were thought to be radiation induced, while the remainder arose de novo.[153] The 5-year survival rate for patients with a single sarcoma was 53% compared with 26% for those with a second primary lesion, a statistically significant difference.[153] Recognition of this phenomenon might reduce delays in diagnosis of these often advanced secondary lesions.

Surveillance Matrix Recommendations

At the University of Washington Sarcoma Clinic, surveillance of soft tissue sarcoma patients begins on entry into the phase II neoadjuvant study protocol. Routine phlebotomy is performed during each course of chemotherapy, and interim history, physical examination, and chest x-rays are performed at monthly intervals. Computed tomography of the chest and magnetic resonance imaging of the primary site are performed after the second chemotherapy cycle. If the tumor has progressed, the patient proceeds directly to surgery. If the tumor is stable or shows evidence of shrinkage or necrosis, the third preoperative cycle is completed and repeat computed tomographic scans and magnetic resonance images are obtained just before surgery. Once surgery is complete, adjuvant chemotherapy begins within 1 month, with the same laboratory and chest x-ray routine. However, radionuclide angiography is now performed when the cumulative doxorubicin dosage reaches 450 mg/m² and thereafter before each dose of doxorubicin (Table 13-6).

Once treatment is complete, high-risk patients are reexamined every 2 months for the first year, every 3 months for the second year, and every 6 months thereafter. Chest x-rays alternate with computed tomographic scans of the chest. After a baseline plain film and magnetic resonance images obtained at 2 months, these site-directed tests are performed on a yearly basis (Table 13-7).

These matrices are meant to serve as guidelines only. For instance, when clinical suspicion is high, magnetic resonance imaging of the site can be performed more frequently. On the other hand, for patients with low-risk tumors who do not receive adjuvant therapy, surveillance intervals can be

Table 13-7 Follow-up of patients with soft tissue sarcoma (high-risk patients): University of Washington Medical Center

	YEAR				
	1	2	3	4	5
Office visit	7*	4	2	2	2
Urinalysis	4*	4	2	2	2
Complete blood count	4*	4	2	2	2
Erythrocyte sedimentation rate	4*	4	2	2	2
Multichannel blood tests†	4*	4	2	2	2
Chest computed tomography	4*	2	1	1	1
Chest x-ray	3	2	1	1	1
Site film	2*	1	1	1	1
Site magnetic resonance imaging	2	1	1	1	1
Bone scan	1	1	1	1	1

*Includes one test performed at baseline.
†Consists of blood urea nitrogen, creatinine, aspartate aminotransferase, alkaline phosphatase, glucose, calcium, and phosphorus.

Table 13-8 Follow-up of patients with soft tissue sarcoma (low-risk patients): University of Washington Medical Center

	YEAR				
	1	2	3	4	5
Office visit	5*	4	1	1	1
Chest x-ray	3*	2	1	1	1
Urinalysis	2	2	0	0	0
Complete blood count	2	2	0	0	0
Erythrocyte sedimentation rate	2	2	0	0	0
Multichannel blood tests†	2	2	0	0	0
Chest computed tomography	2	2	0	0	0
Site film	2*	1	0	0	0
Site magnetic resonance imaging	2	1	1	1	1
Bone scan	1	1	1	1	1

*Includes one test performed at baseline.
†Consists of blood urea nitrogen, creatinine, aspartate aminotransferase, alkaline phosphatase, glucose, calcium, and phosphorus.

increased. In general, these patients are examined every 3 months for the first 2 years and yearly thereafter (Table 13-8). Adherence to such a schedule requires diligence on the part of both the patient and the clinician, especially since patients sometimes live far from the tertiary care facility and are often part of managed care plans in which the emphasis is on cost containment and avoidance of "unnecessary" tests.

FUTURE PROSPECTS

Improved delineation of prognostic factors for local or systemic soft tissue sarcoma recurrence could ultimately assist in patient follow-up. Promising advances have been reported in immunocytochemistry (detection of bone marrow metastases in neuroblastoma),[154] molecular biology (altered expression of the retinoblastoma gene product),[155] biochemistry (proliferating cell nuclear antigen in malignant fibrous histiocytoma),[156] cytogenetics (flow cytometric analysis of DNA content),[105] and nuclear medicine (technetium-99m hexamethyl-propyleneamineoxime assessment of tumor vascularity).[157]

New surveillance methods are also under development. Hoefnagel et al.[158] have described radioimmunoscintigraphy techniques helpful in the follow-up of patients with rhabdomyosarcoma. Pino et al.[159] have found ultrasound to be an effective means of detection of local soft tissue sarcoma recurrence, even at sizes between 0.5 cm and 5 cm. Nadel[160] has demonstrated that thallium-201 scintigraphy and single photon emission computed tomography are helpful in imaging of metastases in pediatric sarcomas. Finally, Conrad et al.[36] have shown positron emission tomography to predict histological grade and response to neoadjuvant treatment, while Tse et al.[34] have shown positron emission tomography to be useful in the imaging of pulmonary metastases in osteosarcoma.

REFERENCES

1. Gustafson P. Soft tissue sarcoma: epidemiology and prognosis in 508 patients. Acta Orthop Scandinavica 1994;65 Suppl 259:1-31.
2. Ross JA, Severson RK, Davis S, Brooks JJ. Trends in the incidence of soft tissue sarcomas in the United States from 1973 through 1987. Cancer 1993;72:486-90.
3. Wingo PA, Tong T, Bolden S. Cancer statistics, 1995. CA Cancer J Clin 1995;45:8-30.
4. Axtell LM, Asire AJ, Myers MH. Cancer patient survival, 1960-1973. NIH Publication no. 77-992. Bethesda, Md: National Cancer Institute, 1976.
5. Wilson RE, Wood WC, Lerner HL, et al. Doxorubicin chemotherapy in the treatment of soft-tissue sarcoma: combined results of two randomized trials. Arch Surg 1986;121:1354-9.
6. Chang AE, Kinsella T, Glatstein E, et al. Adjuvant chemotherapy for patients with high-grade soft-tissue sarcomas of the extremity. J Clin Oncol 1988;6:1491-500.
7. Suit HD, Mankin HJ, Wood WC, et al. Treatment of the patient with stage M0 soft tissue sarcoma. J Clin Oncol 1988;6:854-62.
8. Gherlinzoni F, Pignatti G, Fontana M, Giunti A. Soft tissue sarcomas: the experience at the Istituto Ortopedico Rizzoli. Chir Organi Mov 1990;75 Suppl 1:150-4.
9. Yang JC, Glatstein EJ, Rosenberg SA, Antman KH. Sarcomas of soft tissues. In: DeVita VT, Hellman S, Rosenberg SA, editors. Cancer: principles & practice of oncology. 4th ed. Philadelphia: JB Lippincott Company, 1993:1435-88.
10. Shiu MH, Brennan MF. Clinical features and diagnosis of soft tissue sarcoma. In: Shiu MH, Brennan MF, editors. Surgical management of soft tissue sarcoma. Philadelphia: Lea & Febiger, 1989:23-38.
11. Heard G. Malignant disease in von Recklinghausen's neurofibromatosis. Proc Royal Soc Med 1963;56:502-3.
12. Stewart FW, Treves N. Lymphangiosarcoma in postmastectomy lymphedema: a report of six cases in elephantiasis chirurgica. Cancer 1948;1:64-81.

13. Safai B, Diaz B, Schwartz J. Malignant neoplasms associated with human immunodeficiency virus infection. CA Cancer J Clin 1992; 42:74-95.
14. Reed WB, Nickel WR, Campion G. Internal manifestations of tuberous sclerosis. Arch Dermatol 1963;87:715-28.
15. Fraumeni JF Jr, Vogel CL, Easton JM. Sarcomas and multiple polyposis in a kindred: a genetic variety of hereditary polyposis? Arch Intern Med 1968;121:57-61.
16. Schweisguth O, Gerard-Marchant R, Lemerle J. Nævomatose basocellulaire association a un rhabdomyosarcome congenital. Arch Franç Péd 1968;25:1083-93.
17. Usui M, Ishii S, Yamawaki S, Hirayama T. The occurrence of soft tissue sarcomas in three siblings with Werner's syndrome. Cancer 1984;54:2580-6.
18. O'Neil MB Jr, Cocke W, Mason D, Hurley EJ. Radiation-induced soft-tissue fibrosarcoma: surgical therapy and salvage. Ann Thorac Surg 1982;33:624-8.
19. Halperin EC, Greenberg MS, Suit HD. Sarcoma of bone and soft tissue following treatment of Hodgkin's disease. Cancer 1984; 53:232-6.
20. Souba WW, McKenna RJ Jr, Meis J, Benjamin R, Raymond AK, Mountain CF. Radiation-induced sarcomas of the chest wall. Cancer 1986;57:610-5.
21. Kang H, Enzinger FM, Breslin P, et al. Soft tissue sarcoma and military service in Vietnam: a case-control study. J Natl Cancer Inst 1987;79:693-9.
22. Brand KG. Foreign body induced sarcomas. In: Becker FF, editor. Cancer. New York: Plenum, 1975:485-511.
23. Weiss SW, Enzinger FM. Malignant fibrous histiocytoma: an analysis of 200 cases. Cancer 1978;41:2250-66.
24. Renton P, Shaw DG. Hypophosphatemic osteomalacia secondary to vascular tumors of bone and soft tissue. Skeletal Radiol 1976;1:21-4.
25. Bertelsen CA, Eilber FR. Paraneoplastic syndromes with soft-tissue sarcoma: a report of two unusual cases. J Surg Oncol 1983;24:170-2.
26. Aisen AM, Martel W, Braunstein EM, McMillin KI, Phillips WA, Kling TF. MRI and CT evaluation of primary bone and soft-tissue tumors. AJR Am J Roentgenol 1986;146:749-56.
27. Bland KI, McCoy DM, Kinard RE, Copeland EM 3d. Application of magnetic resonance imaging and computerized tomography as an adjunct to the surgical management of soft tissue sarcomas. Ann Surg 1987;205:473-81.
28. Chang AE, Matory YL, Dwyer AJ, et al. Magnetic resonance imaging versus computed tomography in the evaluation of soft tissue tumors of the extremities. Ann Surg 1987;205:340-8.
29. Springfield DS. Evaluation of bone and soft tissue tumors. In: Lewis ML, editor. Musculoskeletal oncology: a multidisciplinary approach. Philadelphia: WB Saunders Company, 1992:1-11.
30. McNeil BJ. Rationale for the use of bone scans in selected metastatic and primary bone tumors. Semin Nucl Med 1978;8:336-45.
31. Enneking WF, Chew FS, Springfield DS, Hudson TM, Spanier SS. The role of radionuclide bone-scanning in determining the resectability of soft-tissue sarcomas. J Bone Joint Surg Am 1981;63:249-57.
32. Kirchner PT, Simon MA. The clinical value of bone and gallium scintigraphy for soft-tissue sarcomas of the extremities. J Bone Joint Surg Am 1984;66:319-27.
33. Nieweg OE, Pruim J, Hoekstra HJ, et al. Positron emission tomography with fluorine-18-fluorodeoxyglucose for the evaluation of therapeutic isolated regional limb perfusion in a patient with soft-tissue sarcoma. J Nucl Med 1994;35:90-2.
34. Tse N, Hoh C, Hawkins R, Phelps M, Glaspy J. Positron emission tomography diagnosis of pulmonary metastases in osteogenic sarcoma. Am J Clin Oncol 1994;17:22-5.
35. Shulkin BL, Mitchell DS, Ungar DR, et al. Neoplasms in a pediatric population: 2-[F-18]-fluoro-2-deoxy-D-glucose PET studies. Radiology 1995;194:495-500.
36. Conrad EU 3d, Eary JF, Bavisotto L, Mankoff D. Quantitative [F-18] FDG PET imaging in sarcoma. In: Abstracts of the 8th annual meeting of the International Symposium on Limb Salvage; 1995 May 10-12; Florence, Italy. Florence: ISOLS, 1995:177.
37. Levin DC, Watson RC, Baltaxe HA. Arteriography in diagnosis and management of acquired peripheral soft-tissue masses. Radiology 1972;103:53-8.
38. Weingrad DN, Rosenberg SA. Early lymphatic spread of osteogenic and soft-tissue sarcomas. Surgery 1978;84:231-40.
39. Lange TA, Austin CW, Seibert JJ, Angtuaco TL, Yandow DR. Ultrasound imaging as a screening study for malignant soft tissue tumors. J Bone Joint Surg Am 1987;69:100-5.
40. Finn HA, Simon MA, Martin WB, Darakjian H. Scintigraphy with gallium-67 citrate in staging of soft-tissue sarcomas of the extremity. J Bone Joint Surg Am 1987;69:886-91.
41. Åkerman M, Rydholm A, Persson BM. Aspiration cytology of soft-tissue tumors: the 10-year experience at an orthopedic oncology center. Acta Orthop Scand 1985;56:407-12.
42. Ball AB, Fisher C, Pittam M, Watkins RM, Westbury G. Diagnosis of soft tissue tumours by Tru-Cut biopsy. Br J Surg 1990;77:756-8.
43. Enneking WF. The issue of the biopsy. J Bone Joint Surg Am 1982; 64:1119-20.
44. Mankin HJ, Lange TA, Spanier SS. The hazards of biopsy in patients with malignant bone and soft-tissue tumors. J Bone Joint Surg Am 1982;64:1121-7.
45. Simon MA. Biopsy of musculoskeletal tumors. J Bone Joint Surg Am 1982;64:1253-7.
46. Simon MA, Bierman JS. Biopsy of bone and soft-tissue lesions. In: Schafer M, editor. Instructional course lectures. Vol. 43. Chicago: AAOS, 1994:521-6.
47. Kreicbergs A. DNA cytometry of musculoskeletal tumors: a review. Acta Orthop Scand 1990;61:282-97.
48. Fletcher JA, Kozakewich HP, Hoffer FA, et al. Diagnostic relevance of clonal cytogenetic aberrations in malignant soft-tissue tumors. N Engl J Med 1991;324:436-42.
49. Barr FG, Chatten J, D'Cruz CM, et al. Molecular assays for chromosomal translocations in the diagnosis of pediatric soft tissue sarcomas. JAMA 1995;273:553-7.
50. American Joint Committee on Cancer. Soft tissues. In: Beahrs OH, Henson DE, Hutter RV, Kennedy BJ, editors. Manual for staging of cancer. 4th ed. Philadelphia: JB Lippincott Company, 1992:127-33.
51. Costa J, Wesley RA, Glatstein E, Rosenberg SA. The grading of soft tissue sarcomas: results of a clinicohistopathologic correlation in a series of 163 cases. Cancer 1984;53:530-41.
52. Enneking WF, Spanier SS, Goodman MA. Current concepts review: the surgical staging of musculoskeletal sarcoma. J Bone Joint Surg Am 1980;62:1027-30.
53. Springfield DS. Staging systems for musculoskeletal neoplasia. In: Schafer M, editor. Instructional course lectures. Vol. 43. Chicago: AAOS, 1994:537-42.
54. Nelson TE, Enneking WF. Staging of bone and soft-tissue sarcomas revisited. In: Stauffer RN, Ehrlich MG, Fu FH, Kostuik JP, Manske PR, Sim FH, editors. Advances in operative orthopaedics. Vol. 2. St. Louis: Mosby, 1994:379-91.
55. Tepper JE, Suit HD. Radiation therapy of soft tissue sarcomas. Cancer 1985;55:2273-7.
56. Cade S. Soft tissue tumors: their natural history and treatment. Proc Royal Soc Med 1951;19:19-36.
57. Windeyer B, Dische S, Mansfield CM. The place of radiotherapy in the management of fibrosarcoma of the soft tissues. Clin Radiol 1966;17:32-40.
58. Shiu MH, Castro EB, Hajdu SI, Fortner JG. Surgical treatment of 297 soft tissue sarcomas of the lower extremity. Ann Surg 1975;182:597-602.
59. Gerner RE, Moore GE, Pickern JW. Soft tissue sarcomas. Ann Surg 1975;181:803-8.
60. Simon MA, Enneking WF. The management of soft-tissue sarcomas of the extremities. J Bone Joint Surg Am 1976;58:317-27.

61. Simon MA, Spanier SS, Enneking WF. Management of adult soft-tissue sarcomas of the extremities. Surg Annu 1979;11:363-402.
62. Markhede G, Angervall L, Stener B. A multivariate analysis of the prognosis after surgical treatment of malignant soft-tissue tumors. Cancer 1982;49:1721-33.
63. National Institutes of Health consensus development panel on limb-sparing treatment of adult soft tissue sarcomas and osteosarcomas: introduction and conclusions. Cancer Treat Symp 1985;3:1-5.
64. Williard WC, Hajdu SI, Casper ES, Brennan MF. Comparison of amputation with limb-sparing operations for adult soft tissue sarcoma of the extremity. Ann Surg 1992;215:269-75.
65. Geer RJ, Woodruff J, Casper ES, Brennan MF. Management of small soft-tissue sarcoma of the extremity in adults. Arch Surg 1992;127: 1285-9.
66. Mazanet R, Antman KH. Adjuvant therapy for sarcomas. Semin Oncol 1991;18:603-12.
67. Lindberg RD, Martin RG, Romsdahl MM. Surgery and postoperative radiotherapy in the treatment of soft tissue sarcomas in adults. AJR Am J Roentgenol 1975;123:123-9.
68. Suit HD, Russell WO, Martin RG. Sarcoma of soft tissue: clinical and histopathologic parameters and response to treatment. Cancer 1975;35:1478-83.
69. Lindberg RD, Martin RG, Romsdahl MM, Barkley HT Jr. Conservative surgery and postoperative radiotherapy in 300 adults with soft-tissue sarcomas. Cancer 1981;47:2391-7.
70. Leibel SA, Tranbaugh RF, Wara WM, Beckstead JH, Bovill EG, Phillips TL. Soft tissue sarcomas of the extremities: survival and patterns of failure with conservative surgery and postoperative irradiation compared to surgery alone. Cancer 1982;50:1076-83.
71. Suit HD, Mankin HJ, Wood WC, Proppe KH. Preoperative, intraoperative, and postoperative radiation in the treatment of primary soft tissue sarcoma. Cancer 1985;55:2659-67.
72. Suit HD, Mankin HJ, Willett CG, Gebhardt MC, Wood WC, Skates S. Limited surgery and external radiation in soft tissue sarcomas. In: Ryan JR, Baker LO, editors. Recent concepts in sarcoma treatment. Dordrecht: Kluwer, 1988:94-103.
73. Glenn J, Sindelar WF, Kinsella T, et al. Results of multimodality therapy of resectable soft-tissue sarcomas of the retroperitoneum. Surgery 1985;97:316-25.
74. Kinsella TJ, Sindelar WF, Lack E, Glatstein E, Rosenberg SA. Preliminary results in a randomized study of adjuvant radiation therapy in resectable adult retroperitoneal soft tissue sarcomas. J Clin Oncol 1988;6:18-25.
75. Brennan MF, Hilaris B, Shiu MH, et al. Local recurrence in adult soft-tissue sarcoma: a randomized trial of brachytherapy. Arch Surg 1987;122:1289-93.
76. Schray MF, Gunderson LL, Sim FH, Pritchard DJ, Shives TC, Yeakel PD. Soft tissue sarcoma: integration of brachytherapy, resection, and external irradiation. Cancer 1990;66:451-6.
77. Suit HD, Willett CG. Radiation therapy of sarcomas of the soft tissues. In: Pinedo HM, Verweij J, Suit HD, editors. Soft tissue sarcomas: new developments in the multidisciplinary approach to treatment. Boston: Kluwer, 1991:61-74.
78. Laramore GE, Griffith JT, Boespflug M, et al. Fast neutron therapy for sarcomas of soft tissue, bone, and cartilage. Am J Clin Oncol 1989;12:320-6.
79. Rööser B, Gustafson P, Rydholm A. Is there no influence of local control on the rate of metastases in high-grade soft-tissue sarcoma? Cancer 1990;65:1727-9.
80. Gustafson P, Rööser B, Rydholm A. Is local recurrence of minor importance for metastases in soft tissue sarcoma? Cancer 1991;67:2083-6.
81. Choong PF, Gustafson P, Rydholm A. Size and timing of local recurrence predicts metastasis in soft tissue sarcoma: growth rate index analyzed retrospectively in 134 patients. Acta Orthop Scand 1995;66:147-52.
82. Maurer HM, Gehan E, Crist W, et al. Intergroup rhabdomyosarcoma study (IRS)-III: a preliminary report of overall outcome. Proc Am Soc Clin Oncol 1989;6:296.
83. Rosen G, Caparros B, Huvos AG, et al. Preoperative chemotherapy for osteogenic sarcoma: selection of postoperative adjuvant chemotherapy based on the response of the primary tumor to preoperative chemotherapy. Cancer 1982;49:1221-30.
84. Burgert EO Jr, Nesbit ME, Garnsey LA, et al. Multimodal therapy for the management of nonpelvic, localized Ewing's sarcoma of bone: intergroup study IESS-II. J Clin Oncol 1990;8:1514-24.
85. Antman K, Ryan L, Broden E, et al. Pooled results from three randomized adjuvant studies of doxorubicin versus observation in soft tissue sarcoma: 10 year results and review of the literature. In: Salmon SE, editor. Adjuvant therapy of cancer. Vol. 6. Philadelphia: WB Saunders Company, 1990:529-43.
86. Alvegård TA, Sigurdsson H, Mouridsen H, et al. Adjuvant chemotherapy with doxorubicin in high-grade soft tissue sarcoma: a randomized trial of the Scandinavian Sarcoma Group. J Clin Oncol 1989;7:1504-13.
87. Eilber FR, Giuliano AE, Huth JF, Morton DL. A randomized prospective trial using postoperative adjuvant chemotherapy (adriamycin) in high-grade extremity soft-tissue sarcoma. Am J Clin Oncol 1988;11:39-45.
88. Mertens WC, Bramwell VH. Adjuvant chemotherapy of soft tissue sarcomas. In: Verweij J, Pinedo HM, Suit HD, editors. Multidisciplinary treatment of soft tissue sarcomas. Boston: Kluwer, 1993:117-33.
89. Bramwell V, Rouesse J, Steward W, et al. Adjuvant CYVADIC chemotherapy for adult soft tissue sarcoma–reduced local recurrence but no improvement in survival: a study of the European Organization for Research and Treatment of Cancer Soft Tissue and Bone Sarcoma Group. J Clin Oncol 1994;12:1137-49.
90. Benjamin RS, Terjanian TO, Fenoglio CJ. The importance of combination chemotherapy for adjuvant treatment of high-risk patients with soft-tissue sarcomas of the extremities. In: Salmon SE, editor. Adjuvant therapy of cancer. Vol. 5. Orlando: Grune & Stratton, 1987:735-44.
91. Edmonson JH, Fleming TR, Ivins JC, et al. Randomized study of systemic chemotherapy following complete excision of nonosseous sarcomas. J Clin Oncol 1984;2:1390-6.
92. Ravaud A, Bui NB, Coindre JM, et al. Adjuvant chemotherapy with CYVADIC in high risk soft tissue sarcoma: a randomized prospective trial. In: Salmon SE, editor. Adjuvant therapy of cancer. Vol. 6. Philadelphia: WB Saunders Company, 1990:556-66.
93. Schmidt RA, Conrad EU 3d, Collins C, Rabinovitch P, Finney A. Measurement and prediction of the short-term response of soft tissue sarcomas to chemotherapy. Cancer 1993;72:2593-601.
94. Pezzi CM, Pollock RE, Evans HL, et al. Preoperative chemotherapy for soft-tissue sarcomas of the extremities. Ann Surg 1990;211:476-81.
95. Soulen MC, Weissmann JR, Sullivan KL, et al. Intraarterial chemotherapy with limb-sparing resection of large soft-tissue sarcomas of the extremities. J Vasc Interv Radiol 1992;3:659-63.
96. Cany L, Bui NB, Stöckle E, Coindre JM, Kantor G, Ravaud A. Chimiothérapie d'induction et tratement combiné conservateur des sarcomes des tissus mous de l'adulte. Bull Cancer 1992;79:1077-85.
97. Kónya A, Vigváry A. Neoadjuvant intraarterial chemotherapy of soft tissue sarcomas. Ann Oncol 1992;3 Suppl 2:S127-9.
98. Priebat DA, Trehan RS, Malawar MM, Schulof RS. Induction chemotherapy for sarcomas of the extremities. In: Sugarbaker PH, Malawar MM, editors. Musculoskeletal surgery for cancer: principles and techniques. New York: Thieme, 1992:96-120.
99. Rahóty P, Kónya A. Results of preoperative neoadjuvant chemotherapy and surgery in the management of patients with soft tissue sarcoma. Eur J Surg Oncol 1993;19:641-5.
100. Engel CJ, Eilber FR, Rosen G, Selch MT, Fu YS. Pre-operative chemotherapy for soft-tissue sarcomas of the extremities: the experience at the University of California, Los Angeles. In: Pinedo HM, Verweij J, Suit HD, editors. Multidisciplinary treatment of soft tissue sarcomas. Boston: Kluwer, 1993:135-41.
101. Casper ES, Gaynor JJ, Harrison LB, Panicek DM, Hajdu SI, Brennan MF. Preoperative and postoperative adjuvant combination chemotherapy for adults with high grade soft tissue sarcoma. Cancer 1994;73:1644-51.

102. Rossi CR, Vecchiato A, Foletto M, et al. Phase II study on neoadjuvant hyperthermic-antiblastic perfusion with doxorubicin in patients with intermediate or high grade limb sarcomas. Cancer 1994;73:2140-6.
103. Collins C, Conrad EU 3d, Schmidt RA, et al. Neoadjuvant chemotherapy of soft tissue sarcoma: clinical and pathologic correlates of response. Proc Am Soc Clin Oncol 1993;12:469.
104. Torosian MH, Friedrich C, Godbold J, Hajdu SI, Brennan MF. Soft-tissue sarcoma: initial characteristics and prognostic factors in patients with and without metastatic disease. Semin Surg Oncol 1988;4:13-9.
105. Budach W, Budach V, Socha B, Stuschke M, Streffer C, Sack H. DNA content as a predictor of clinical outcome in soft tissue sarcoma patients. Eur J Cancer 1994;30A:1815-21.
106. Trojani M, Contesso G, Coindre JM, et al. Soft-tissue sarcomas of adults: study of pathological prognostic variables and definition of a histopathological grading system. J Cancer 1987;33:37-42.
107. Ueda T, Aozasa K, Tsujimoto M, et al. Multivariate analysis for clinical prognostic factors in 163 patients with soft tissue sarcoma. Cancer 1988;62:1444-50.
108. Collin CF, Friedrich C, Godbold J, Hajdu S, Brennan MF. Prognostic factors for local recurrence and survival in patients with localized extremity soft-tissue sarcoma. Semin Surg Oncol 1988; 4:30-7.
109. Brennan MF, Shiu MH. Presentation, demographics, and prognostic factors of soft tissue sarcoma. In: Shiu MH, Brennan MF, editors. Surgical management of soft tissue sarcoma. Philadelphia: Lea & Febiger, 1989:45-57.
110. Berlinö, Stener B, Angervall L, Kindbloom LG, Markhede G, Odén A. Surgery for soft tissue sarcoma in the extremities: a multivariate analysis of the 6-26-year prognosis in 137 patients. Acta Orthop Scand 1990;61:475-86.
111. Gaynor JJ, Tan CC, Casper ES, et al. Refinement of clinicopathologic staging for localized soft tissue sarcoma of the extremity: a study of 423 adults. J Clin Oncol 1992;10:1317-29.
112. Singer S, Corson JM, Gonin R, Labow B, Eberlein TJ. Prognostic factors predictive of survival and local recurrence for extremity soft tissue sarcoma. Ann Surg 1994;219:165-73.
113. van Unnik JAM, Coindre JM, Contesso C, et al. Grading of soft tissue sarcomas: experience of the EORTC Soft Tissue and Bone Sarcoma Group. Eur J Cancer 1993;29A:2089-93.
114. Peabody TD, Monson D, Montag A, Schell MJ, Finn H, Simon MA. A comparison of the prognoses for deep and subcutaneous sarcomas of the extremities. J Bone Joint Surg Am 1994;76:1167-73.
115. Collin C, Hajdu SI, Godbold J, Friedrich C, Brennan MF. Localized operable soft tissue sarcoma of the upper extremity: presentation, management, and factors affecting local recurrence in 108 patients. Ann Surg 1987;205:331-9.
116. Dresdale A, Bonow RO, Wesley R, et al. Prospective evaluation of doxorubicin-induced cardiomyopathy resulting from postsurgical adjuvant treatment of patients with soft tissue sarcomas. Cancer 1983;52:51-60.
117. Springfield DS. Surgical wound healing. In: Verweij J, Pinedo HM, Suit HD, editors. Multidisciplinary treatment of soft tissue sarcomas. Boston: Kluwer, 1993:81-98.
118. Ragnarsson KT. Rehabilitation of patients with physical disabilities caused by tumors of the musculoskeletal system. In: Lewis ML, editor. Musculoskeletal oncology: a multidisciplinary approach. Philadelphia: WB Saunders Company, 1992:429-48.
119. Snow BR, Gusmorino P, Pinter I. Behavioral medicine and cancer: a clinical guide. In: Lewis ML, editor. Musculoskeletal oncology: a multidisciplinary approach. Philadelphia: WB Saunders Company, 1992:449-63.
120. Rosenberg G, Gropper M. Psychosocial dimensions of bone cancer: social work services and human resources. In: Lewis ML, editor. Musculoskeletal oncology: a multidisciplinary approach. Philadelphia: WB Saunders Company, 1992:465-76.
121. Ryniker DM, Freudman LS, Weiner DM, Cord C, Castoria HA, McLean K. Nursing considerations. In: Lewis ML, editor. Musculoskeletal oncology: a multidisciplinary approach. Philadelphia: WB Saunders Company, 1992:501-48.
122. Potter DA, Glenn J, Kinsella T, et al. Patterns of recurrence in patients with high-grade soft-tissue sarcomas. J Clin Oncol 1985; 3:353-66.
123. Cantin J, McNeer GP, Chu FC, Booher RJ. The problem of local recurrence after treatment of soft tissue sarcoma. Ann Surg 1968; 168:47-53.
124. Sauter ER, Hoffman JP, Eisenberg BL. Diagnosis and surgical management of locally recurrent soft-tissue sarcomas of the extremity. Semin Oncol 1993;20:451-5.
125. Biondetti PR, Ehman RL. Soft-tissue sarcomas: use of textural patterns in skeletal muscle as a diagnostic feature in postoperative MR imaging. Radiology 1992;183:845-8.
126. Vanel D, Shapeero LG, De Baere T, et al. MR imaging in the follow-up of malignant soft-tissue tumors: results of 511 examinations. Radiology 1994;190:263-8.
127. Munk PL, Poon PY, Chhem RK, Janzen DL. Imaging of soft-tissue sarcomas. Canad Assoc Radiol J 1994;45:438-46.
128. Reuther G, Mutschler W. Detection of local recurrent disease in musculoskeletal tumors: magnetic resonance imaging versus computed tomography. Skeletal Radiol 1990;19:85-90.
129. Giuliano AE, Eilber FR, Morton DL. The management of locally recurrent soft-tissue sarcoma. Ann Surg 1982;196:87-91.
130. Jaques DP, Coit DG, Hajdu SI, Brennan MF. Management of primary and recurrent soft-tissue sarcoma of the retroperitoneum. Ann Surg 1990;212:51-9.
131. Singer S, Antman K, Corson JM, Eberlein TJ. Long-term salvageability for patients with locally recurrent soft-tissue sarcomas. Arch Surg 1992;127:548-54.
132. Suit HD, Tepper JE. Impact of improved local control on survival in patients with soft tissue sarcoma. Int J Radiat Oncol Biol Phys 1986;12:699-700.
133. Emrich LJ, Ruka W, Driscoll DL, Karakousis CP. The effect of local recurrence on survival time in adult high-grade soft tissue sarcomas. J Clin Epidemiol 1989;42:105-10.
134. Stotter AT, A'Hern RP, Fisher C, Mott AF, Fallowfield ME, Westbury G. The influence of local recurrence of extremity soft tissue sarcoma on metastasis and survival. Cancer 1990;65:1119-29.
135. Barr LC, Stotter AT, A'Hern RP. Influence of local recurrence on survival: a controversy reviewed from the perspective of soft tissue sarcoma. Br J Surg 1991;78:648-50.
136. Suit HD. Local control and patient survival. Int J Radiat Oncol Biol Phys 1992;23:653-60.
137. Huth JF, Eilber FR. Patterns of metastatic spread following resection of extremity soft-tissue sarcomas and strategies for treatment. Semin Surg Oncol 1988;4:20-6.
138. Vezeridis MP, Moore R, Karakousis CP. Metastatic patterns in soft-tissue sarcomas. Arch Surg 1983;118:915-8.
139. Gardner TE, Daly JM. Diagnosis and management of distant recurrence in soft-tissue sarcomas. Semin Oncol 1993;20:456-61.
140. Chang AE, Schaner EG, Conkle DM, Flye MW, Doppman JL, Rosenberg SA. Evaluation of computed tomography in the detection of pulmonary metastases: a prospective study. Cancer 1979;43:913-6.
141. Pass HI, Dwyer A, Makuch R, Roth JA. Detection of pulmonary metastases in patients with osteogenic and soft-tissue sarcomas: the superiority of CT scans compared with conventional linear tomograms using dynamic analysis. J Clin Oncol 1985;3:1261-5.
142. Martini N, McCormack PM, Bains MS, Beattie EJ. Surgery for solitary and multiple pulmonary metastases. NY State J Med 1978; 78:1711-4.
143. Martini N, McCormack PM. Pulmonary resection in sarcoma metastases. In: Ryan JR, Baker LO, editors. Recent concepts in sarcoma treatment. Dordrecht: Kluwer, 1988:197-200.
144. Jaques DP, Coit DG, Casper ES, Brennan MF. Hepatic metastases from soft-tissue sarcoma. Ann Surg 1995;221:392-7.

145. Huth JF, Holmes E, Vernon SE, Callery CD, Ramming KP, Morton DL. Pulmonary resection for metastatic sarcoma. Am J Surg 1980; 140:9-16.
146. Roth JA, Pass HI, Wesley MN, White D, Putnam JB, Seipp C. Comparison of median sternotomy and thoracotomy for resection of pulmonary metastases in patients with adult soft-tissue sarcomas. Ann Thorac Surg 1986;42:134-8.
147. Calkins ER, Ramming KP. Therapy of pulmonary metastases from sarcoma. In: Eilber FR, Morton DL, Sondak VL, Economou JS, editors. The soft tissue sarcomas. Orlando: Grune & Stratton, 1987: 267-77.
148. McCormack PE, Bains MS, Martini N. Surgical resection of pulmonary metastases from soft tissue sarcoma. In: Shiu MH, Brennan MF, editors. Surgical management of soft tissue sarcoma. Philadelphia: Lea & Febiger, 1989:263-73.
149. Casson AG, Putnam JE, Natarajan G, et al. Efficacy of pulmonary metastasectomy for recurrent soft tissue sarcoma. J Surg Oncol 1991;47:1-4.
150. Pogrebniak HW, Roth JA, Steinberg SM, Rosenberg SA, Pass HI. Reoperative pulmonary resection in patients with metastatic soft tissue sarcoma. Ann Thorac Surg 1991;52:197-203.
151. Krumerman MS, Stingle W. Synchronous malignant glandular schwannomas in congenital neurofibromatosis. Cancer 1978;41: 2444-51.
152. Nathanson SD, Zarbo RJ, Sarantou T. Metachronous second primary malignant fibrous histiocytoma in two skeletal muscles. J Surg Oncol 1992;49:259-65.
153. Robinson E, Bar-Deroma R, Rennert G, Neugut AI. A comparison of the clinical characteristics of second primary and single primary sarcoma: a population based study. J Surg Oncol 1992;50:263-6.
154. Moss TJ, Reynolds CP, Sather HN, Romansky SG, Hammond GD, Seeger RC. Prognostic value of immunocytologic detection of bone marrow metastases in neuroblastoma. N Engl J Med 1991;324:219-26.
155. Cance WG, Brennan MF, Dudas ME, Huang CM, Cordon-Cardo C. Altered expression of the retinoblastoma gene product in human sarcomas. N Engl J Med 1990;323:1457-62.
156. Dreinhöfer KE, Åkerman M, WillJé H, Anderson C, Gustafson P, Rydholm A. Proliferating cell nuclear antigen (PCNA) in high-grade malignant fibrous histiocytoma: prognostic value in 48 patients. Int J Cancer 1994;59:379-82.
157. Hill S, Heary T, Flower MA, Cronin B, McCready VR, Thomas JM. Blood flow measurement in extremity soft tissue sarcoma with technetium-99m hexamethyl-propyleneamineoxime and single photon emission computed tomography. Br J Surg 1994;81:1609-11.
158. Hoefnagel CA, Kapucuö, de Kraker J, van Dongen A, Voûte PA. Radioimmunoscintigraphy using In-111 antimyosin Fab fragments for the diagnosis and follow-up of rhabdomyosarcoma. Eur J Cancer 1993;29A:2096-100.
159. Pino G, Conzi GF, Murolo C, et al. Sonographic evaluation of local recurrences of soft tissue sarcomas. J Ultrasound Med 1993;12:23-6.
160. Nadel HR. Thallium-201 for oncological imaging in children. Semin Nucl Med 1993;23:243-54.

➢ COUNTERPOINT

Memorial Sloan-Kettering Cancer Center

JONATHAN J. LEWIS

Soft tissue sarcomas are rare and unusual neoplasms. They comprise a diverse group of tumors that share a common embryological origin from mesoderm, except for neurosarcomas, which are neuroectodermal. They also tend to behave alike. Treatment principles are therefore similar for all these tumors. Approximately 50% of patients with sarcomas die of their disease. Although sarcomas may develop in any anatomical site, approximately 50% occur in the extremities. This counterpoint focuses on the biology, evaluation, and management of soft tissue sarcomas in adults (greater than 16 years of age).

Table 13-9 Memorial Sloan-Kettering Cancer Center staging system

PROGNOSTIC FACTORS	*Favorable Factors*	*Adverse Factors*
Size	Less than 5 cm	Greater than or equal to 5 cm
Site	Superficial	Deep
Histological grade	Low	High

MEMORIAL SLOAN-KETTERING CANCER CENTER STAGING

Number of Adverse Factors	*Stage*
0	0
1	I
2	II
3	III
Metastasis	IV

Modified from Lewis JJ, Brennan MF: Soft tissue sarcomas. In: Current problems in surgery. St. Louis: Mosby, 1996.

EVALUATION AND STAGING OF PRIMARY TUMORS

At Memorial Sloan-Kettering Cancer Center physicians use a staging system (Table 13-9) based on the histological grade, site, and size of the primary tumor and the presence or absence of metastases.[1] A retrospective review of 1,215 patients from 13 institutions found histological grade to be a critical determinant of outcome.[2] Histological grade is based on degree of mitosis, cellularity, presence of necrosis, differentiation, and stromal content. Various grading systems exist, but for planning therapy the broad categories of low grade or high grade suffice. Clearly such arbitrary and subjective decisions may be difficult, but they facilitate practical management of the patient. Low-grade lesions have a low (less than 15%) risk of subsequent metastasis, and high-grade lesions have a high (greater than 50%) risk.

Size has historically been considered a less important determinant of biological behavior, but large lesions tend to be associated with late recurrence. High-grade lesions less than 5 cm in maximum diameter have limited risk for metastatic disease if treated appropriately at the first encounter. Reevaluations of current staging systems tend to emphasize combinations of grade and size.[3] It is important to recognize that prognostic factors for outcome, such as grade and size, may have variable importance with time. For example, in early metastases (less than 2 years), grade is the dominant predictive variable. In contrast, for late metastases (greater than 5 years), size and initial microscopic margins are important variables.[4]

Table 13-10 Prognostic factors for extremity soft tissue sarcoma[1,19]

OUTCOME VARIABLE	FACTORS PROGNOSTIC BY MULTIVARIATE ANALYSIS
Local recurrence	Presentation with recurrent disease
	Gross or microscopically positive surgical margin
Distant metastasis	High histological grade
	Deep location
	Size 5 cm or greater
Postmetastasis survival	Age 60 years or greater
	Time from presentation to metastasis
	Metastasis to sites other than single lung
Disease specific mortality	High histological grade
	Deep location
	Size 5 cm or greater

Modified from Lewis JJ, Brennan MF: Soft tissue sarcomas. In: Current problems in surgery. St. Louis: Mosby, 1996.

Lymph node metastases occur in less than 3% of soft tissue sarcomas in adults.[5] Therefore physicians at Memorial Sloan-Kettering Cancer Center do not perform lymphangiography for staging. For extremity lesions the lung is the principal site for metastases of high-grade lesions[6]; for visceral lesions the liver is the principal site.[7] Thus, for initial staging, patients with low-grade extremity lesions require a chest x-ray and those with high-grade lesions a computed tomographic scan of the chest. Patients with visceral lesions should have their liver imaged as part of the initial abdominal computed tomography or magnetic resonance imaging. Physicians at Memorial Sloan-Kettering Cancer Center do not generally perform angiography, since it adds little data that will change the management strategy.

PROGNOSTIC FACTORS FOR OUTCOME

Several multivariate analyses of prognostic factors for patients with soft tissue sarcoma have been reported.[1,8-19] The two largest single-institution analyses of extremity lesions[1,19] are from Memorial Sloan-Kettering Cancer Center and analyze 423 and 1,041 patients, respectively. Both emphasize the importance of careful selection of outcome variables for analysis of the impact of prognostic factors. The most recent analysis[19] prospectively collected data from a population of 1,041 adult patients with localized extremity soft tissue sarcoma. The patients were treated between 1982 and 1994. Patient, tumor, and pathological factors were analyzed by univariate and multivariate techniques to identify prognostic factors for the end points of local recurrence, metastatic recurrence, disease-specific survival, and postmetastasis survival (Table 13-10). The 5-year survival rate for this cohort of patients was 76%, with a median follow-up duration of 3.95 years.

It should be emphasized that these prognostic factors have been derived from studies of patients with localized extremity sarcoma. Although extremity sarcomas make up approximately 50% of cases, these results should not be generalized to the greater population of patients with soft tissue sarcoma. Indeed, site itself is a determinant of prognosis and survival. Separate analyses of prognostic factors for retroperitoneal, head and neck, and visceral sarcomas have recently been published.[20-25]

PRINCIPLES OF MANAGEMENT OF THE PRIMARY TUMOR

Management algorithms used at Memorial Sloan-Kettering Cancer Center are shown in Figures 13-1 and 13-2. In contrast to the University of Washington Sarcoma Clinic, the definition of a small tumor here is less than 5 cm (compared with less than 7 cm). Surgery remains the dominant modality of curative therapy for all soft tissue sarcomas.[26] Although surgery is the central thrust of treatment, the development of effective local adjuvant therapies has facilitated less aggressive surgical procedures. Whenever practical, function- and limb-sparing procedures should be performed. Provided that the entire tumor is removed, less radical procedures have not been demonstrated to adversely affect local recurrence rates or outcomes.[27,28]

The only potentially curative treatment for patients with retroperitoneal or visceral sarcoma is surgical resection with negative microscopic margins. Resectability rates for patients with primary and recurrent lesions range from 53% to 59%.[29-31] Resection often involves en bloc multiorgan resection to achieve negative margins. The most common reason for unresectability is the presence of major vascular involvement (aorta or vena cava), peritoneal metastases, or distant metastases.[31] Resection of adjacent organs including the kidney, colon, pancreas, and spleen is necessary in 50% to 80% of cases to enable complete resection.[29,30,32] There is no evidence that partial resection or debulking improves survival.[29] Deliberate partial resection should be confined to palliative surgery.

Radiation Therapy

Combined surgical resection and adjuvant external beam radiation therapy have been used by several investigators.[33-36] The data from these investigations reveal that adjuvant radiation therapy improves local control over surgery alone. In these series local recurrence rates for extremity sarcomas range from 8% to 20%. The results also confirm recurrence data reported from the National Cancer Institute randomized prospective study comparing limb-sparing surgery with postoperative radiation to amputation.[27]

Adjuvant radiation may also be given using the brachytherapy technique.[37-41] The role of adjuvant radiation brachytherapy was addressed in a randomized prospective trial at Memorial Sloan-Kettering Cancer Center in which 126 patients with completely resected extremity and superficial trunk sarcomas were randomly selected to receive either adjuvant brachytherapy or no further therapy.[40,41] With a median follow-up of 67 months, the local recur-

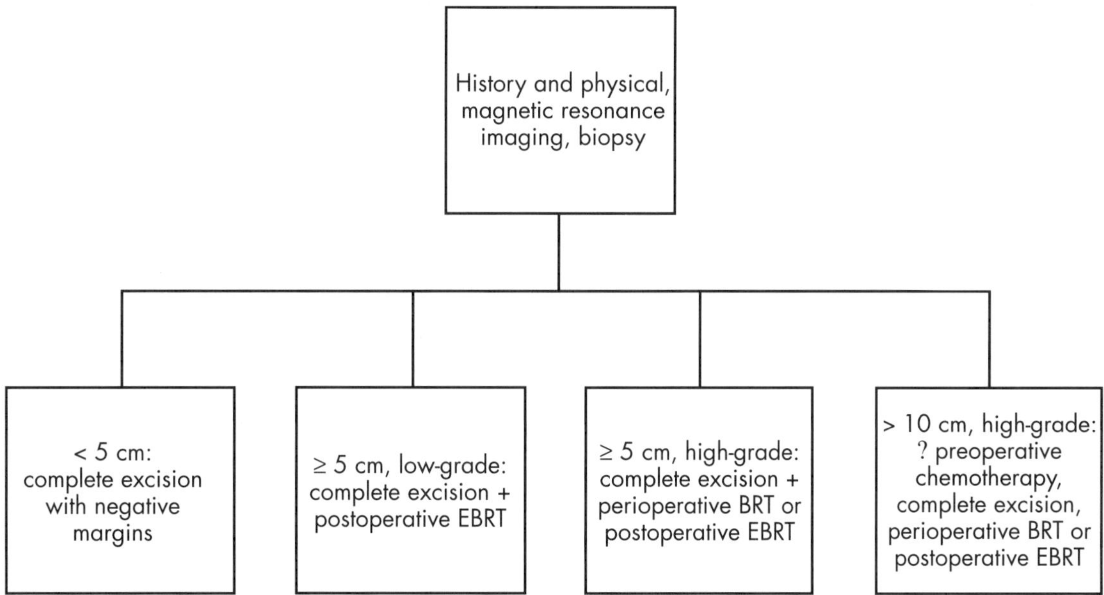

Figure 13-1 Algorithm for the management of primary extremity soft tissue sarcoma using a biological rationale (size and grade of tumor). *BRT,* Brachytherapy; *EBRT,* external beam radiation therapy. (Modified from Lewis JJ, Brennan MF: Soft tissue sarcomas. Current Problems in Surgery. St. Louis: Mosby, 1996.)

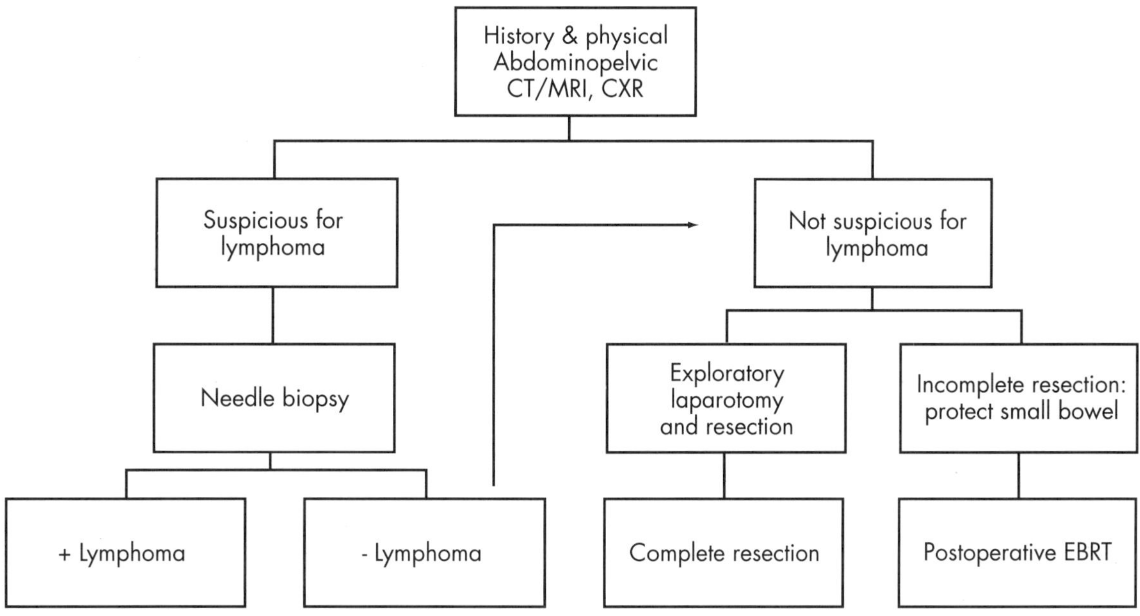

Figure 13-2 Algorithm for the management of primary retroperitoneal or visceral soft tissue sarcoma. Fine-needle aspiration biopsy is not routinely used. *CT,* Computed tomography; *MRI,* magnetic resonance imaging; *CXR,* chest x-ray; *EBRT,* external beam radiation therapy. (Modified from Lewis JJ, Brennan MF: Soft tissue sarcomas. Current Problems in Surgery. St. Louis: Mosby, 1996.)

rence rate in the group receiving adjuvant brachytherapy was 18%, versus 33% in the group receiving no further therapy. Subset analysis revealed that improvement in local control was in the group of patients with high-grade lesions. At this institution brachytherapy is the adjuvant therapy of choice for patients with completely resected, high-grade extremity sarcomas of 5 cm or greater. It provides the same efficacy of local control as other techniques, with the advantage of permitting the completion of treatment within 10 to 14 days.

Chemotherapy

Adjuvant chemotherapy has not been proved to be efficacious, although a preoperative regimen may provide some benefit in patients with large, high-grade lesions.[42] Adjuvant chemotherapy for soft tissue sarcoma should be regarded as investigational and is rarely indicated except in a clinical trial.[42,43] Adjuvant chemotherapy has a potential role in patients who are at high risk for metastatic disease. Most physicians would agree that adjuvant chemotherapy should not be given to patients with low-grade or small (less than 5 cm) primary sarcomas in an extremity. Because of the inherent good prognosis and overall survival of these patients, they are not appropriate candidates for clinical trials evaluating the efficacy of adjuvant systemic therapy.[3]

Multiple nonrandomized studies of adjuvant chemotherapy for soft tissue sarcoma have been described.[27,44-47] These nonrandomized studies are subject to inherent selection bias and are therefore difficult to interpret. Some retrospective results suggest that disease-free survival rates may be better in patients treated with adjuvant chemotherapy, compared with historical control patients who were treated by resection alone. Multiple prospective randomized trials evaluating adjuvant chemotherapy have been published.[48-51] Only two of 12 studies have demonstrated a significant improvement in disease-free and overall survival for patients receiving adjuvant chemotherapy.[49,50] The diversity of sarcoma types, together with the low incidence, makes it difficult to accrue enough patients for randomization balanced by size, grade, and subtype. Thus, the randomized trials performed to date often lack sufficient statistical power to detect clinically meaningful differences in survival. Adjuvant chemotherapy for soft tissue sarcoma should be regarded as investigational and should not be administered to patients outside the confines of an investigational protocol trial.

Table 13-11 Follow-up of patients with soft tissue sarcoma (extremity sarcomas of any grade less than 5 cm in diameter plus low-grade extremity sarcomas at least 5 cm in diameter): Memorial Sloan-Kettering Cancer Center

	YEAR				
	1	2	3	4	5
Office visit	2	2	2	2	2
Chest x-ray	1	1	1	1	1
Complete blood count	1	1	1	1	1
Liver function tests	1	1	1	1	1
Chest computed tomography	*	*	*	*	*
Abdominal computed tomography	*	*	*	*	*
Pelvic computed tomography	*	*	*	*	*

*Performed only when metastatic recurrence is suspected.

Table 13-12 Follow-up of patients with soft tissue sarcoma (high-grade extremity sarcomas at least 5 cm in diameter): Memorial Sloan-Kettering Cancer Center

	YEAR				
	1	2	3	4	5
Office visit	4	4	4	2*	2*
Chest x-ray	2*	2*	2*	2*	2*
Complete blood count	1	1	1	1	1
Liver function tests	1	1	1	1	1
Chest computed tomography	†	†	†	†	†
Abdominal computed tomography	†	†	†	†	†
Pelvic computed tomography	†	†	†	†	†

*Performed at quarterly intervals for patients with extremity lesions greater than 10 cm in diameter.
†Performed only when metastatic recurrence is suspected.

POSTTREATMENT FOLLOW-UP AND MANAGEMENT OF RECURRENT DISEASE

Extremity Sarcomas

Despite optimal multimodality therapy, recurrent disease develops in at least one third of patients with a median disease-free interval of 18 months.[52] Local extremity recurrence appears as a nodular mass or series of nodules arising in the surgical scar. Physicians at Memorial Sloan-Kettering Cancer Center do not use routine radiological surveillance for local recurrence in the extremity. The mainstay of monitoring for local recurrence is physical examination (Tables 13-11 and 13-12). If local recurrence is suspected, computed tomography or magnetic resonance imaging and possibly a fine-needle aspiration biopsy may be performed. In contrast, patients with local recurrence of retroperitoneal or visceral sarcoma usually have nonspecific symptoms, often only after recurrence has reached a substantial size. Therefore these patients are routinely followed up with computed tomography of the abdomen and pelvis (Tables 13-11 and 13-13). After a workup to determine the extent of disease, patients with isolated local recurrence should undergo repeat resection. The results of second resection are good, and two thirds of these patients have long-term survival. Adjuvant radiation therapy should be used after surgery. The approach depends on the method and extent of previous radiation.

The site of distant metastasis is a function of the site of the primary tumor. For extremity lesions the most common site of metastasis is the lung. It is the only site of recurrence in approximately half of patients.[6] Chest x-ray is therefore a crucial component in the follow-up of these patients. Computed tomography of the chest is usually performed only when indicated by an abnormal or new finding on chest x-ray. Extrapulmonary metastases are uncommon and occur as a late manifestation of widely disseminated disease. Physi-

Table 13-13 Follow-up of patients with soft tissue sarcoma (retroperitoneal, gastrointestinal, or visceral sarcomas): Memorial Sloan-Kettering Cancer Center

	YEAR				
	1	2	3	4	5
Office visit	4	4	4	2	2
Complete blood count	4	4	4	2	2
Liver function tests	4	4	4	2	2
Abdominal computed tomography	4	4	4	2	2
Pelvic computed tomography	4	4	4	2	2
Chest x-ray	*	*	*	*	*
Chest computed tomography	*	*	*	*	*

*Performed only when metastatic recurrence is suspected.

cians at Memorial Sloan-Kettering Cancer Center do not routinely use technetium-99m bone scanning or liver imaging and do not perform a metastatic survey unless indicated. Excision is recommended for patients whose primary tumors are controlled or controllable, who have no extrathoracic disease, and who are medically fit, if complete resection of all lung disease appears possible.[6,53] Patients with unresectable pulmonary metastases or extrapulmonary metastatic sarcoma have a uniformly poor prognosis and are best treated with systemic chemotherapy. Recently the combination of mesna, ifosfamide, doxorubicin, and dacarbazine has been shown to have a 47% response rate and a 10% complete response rate.[54] Trials evaluating this combination and other ifosfamide-doxorubicin combinations with cytokine support are under way.

Retroperitoneal Sarcomas

In patients with completely resected tumors the 5-year actuarial survival rate ranges between 54% and 64%.[29,30,55] Survival rates for patients who have incomplete resection range from 10% to 36%. Local recurrence occurs in the majority of these patients, with rates between 53% and 68% reported.[30,56] The median time to recurrence is 16 months. Based on these data, patients should be examined postoperatively every 3 months for the first 3 years (Table 13-13). Computed tomography is commonly performed at 3- to 6-month intervals. Complete resection of locally recurrent disease is possible in about 44% of patients and may be associated with a prolonged 5-year survival rate of up to 50%.[29] The issue of follow-up and treatment of recurrence depends on the philosophy of the physician responsible for follow-up. How often to offer repeat resection to asymptomatic patients with recurrent retroperitoneal sarcoma is a difficult decision. What is clear is that, as with primary retroperitoneal sarcoma, resection should be offered only for palliation or if the potential for complete resection exists.

Gastrointestinal and Visceral Sarcomas

Despite complete resection, recurrence rates are still high, ranging from 42% to 90%, with a median time to recurrence of 18 to 24 months.[22,57] The liver is the most common site of recurrence (50% to 65%), although intraperitoneal recurrence develops in about 30% of patients and 8% have other sites of distant metastases.[57] If the intraabdominal recurrence is completely resected, survival is improved; this should be attempted in patients who have low operative risk.[7,57,58] The extent of disease may limit the application of resection, and certainly when hepatic resection is contemplated, anything less than complete resection is not indicated.[7]

SUMMARY AND SURVEILLANCE RECOMMENDATIONS

At Memorial Sloan-Kettering Cancer Center the follow-up of patients with soft tissue sarcoma is based on their risk of recurrence. This is predicated on the site, size, and grade of the primary tumor (Tables 13-11 to 13-13). Physicians at this institution differ from those at the University of Washington Sarcoma Clinic in that less frequent follow-up intervals (3- versus 2-month intervals) are used early on. In addition, plain films and magnetic resonance imaging of the primary site are not generally used for routine follow-up but rather as indicated based on physical examination. Urinalysis, thyroid function tests, and erythrocyte sedimentation rate are not considered as part of the routine follow-up. Patients with primary extremity tumors that are less than 5 cm and completely excised receive clinical follow-up every 6 months for 5 years and every 12 months thereafter (Table 13-11). These patients also undergo chest x-ray examination every 12 months. Patients with low-grade primary extremity tumors 5 cm or greater in diameter receive the same follow-up as those with small lesions of all grades (Table 13-11).

Large, high-grade primary tumors in an extremity mandate closer follow-up. Patients with high-grade tumors 5 to 10 cm in diameter receive clinical follow-up every 3 months for 3 years and every 6 months thereafter (Table 13-12). In addition, they undergo chest x-ray every 6 months. Patients with high-grade tumors greater than 10 cm in diameter are examined clinically and by chest x-ray every 3 months indefinitely (Table 13-12). Physicians at Memorial Sloan-Kettering Cancer Center do not routinely perform computed tomography of the chest to survey for lung metastases. In patients receiving postoperative radiation therapy or chemotherapy, routine follow-up is combined with the follow-up required for radiation therapy or chemotherapy.

Patients with retroperitoneal, gastrointestinal, or visceral sarcomas are examined clinically every 3 months for the first 3 years (Table 13-13). In addition, these patients undergo computed tomography of the abdomen and pelvis every 3 months. After 3 years patients are followed up clinically and by computed tomography every 6 months. As previously noted, how often to offer repeat resection to asymptomatic patients with recurrent retroperitoneal sarcoma is difficult to determine.

ACKNOWLEDGMENTS

This work is supported by the National Institutes of Health Grant CA 47179. The significant support and contribution of Murray F. Brennan, M.D., is sincerely appreciated.

REFERENCES

1. Gaynor JJ, Tan CC, Casper ES, et al. Refinement of clinicopathologic staging for localized soft tissue sarcoma of the extremity: a study of 423 adults. J Clin Oncol 1992;10:1317-29.
2. Russel WO, Cohen J, Enzinger F, et al. A clinical and pathological staging system for soft tissue sarcomas. Cancer 1977;4:1562-70.
3. Geer RJ, Woodruff J, Casper ES, Brennan MF. Management of small soft-tissue sarcoma of the extremity in adults. Arch Surg 1992;127: 1285-9.
4. Lewis JJ, Leung D, Casper ES, Woodruff JM, Brennan MF. Multifactorial analysis of long-term (>5 year) survival in primary extremity sarcoma. Proc Soc Surg Oncol 1995.
5. Fong Y, Coit J, Woodruff JM, Brennan MF. Lymph node metastasis from soft tissue sarcoma in adults: analysis of data from a prospective database of 1772 sarcoma patients. Ann Surg 1993;217:72-7.
6. Gadd MA, Casper ES, Woodruff JM, McCormack PM, Brennan MF. Development and treatment of pulmonary metastases in adult patients with extremity soft tissue sarcoma. Ann Surg 1993;218:705-12.
7. Jaques DP, Coit DG, Casper ES, Brennan MF. Hepatic metastases from soft tissue sarcoma. Ann Surg 1995;221:392-7.
8. Markhede G, Angervall L, Stener B. A multivariate analysis of the prognosis after surgical treatment of malignant soft-tissue tumors. Cancer 1982;49:1721-33.
9. Sears HF, Hopson R, Inouye W, et al. Analysis of staging and management of patient with sarcoma: a ten-year experience. Ann Surg 1980;191:488-93.
10. Trojani M, Contesso G, Coindre JM, Rizzo T, Grotzinger PJ. Soft-tissue sarcomas of adults: study of pathological prognostic variables and definition of a histopathological grading system. Int J Cancer 1984;33:37-42.
11. Rydholm A, Berg NO, Gullberg B, Persson BM, Thorngren KG, et al. Prognosis for soft-tissue sarcoma in the locomotor system: a retrospective population-based follow-up study of 237 patients. Acta Pathol Microbiol Scand 1984;92:375-86.
12. Heise HW, Myers MH, Russell WO, et al. Recurrence-free survival time for surgically treated soft tissue sarcoma patients: multivariate analysis of five prognostic factors. Cancer 1986;57:172-7.
13. Tsujimoto M, Aozasa K, Ueda T, Morimura Y, Komatsubara Y, Doi T. Multivariate analysis for histologic prognostic factors in soft tissue sarcomas. Cancer 1988;62:994-8.
14. Rooser B, Attewell R, Berg NO, Rydholm A. Prognostication in soft tissue sarcoma: a model with four risk factors. Cancer 1988;61:817-23.
15. Mandard AM, Petiot JF, Marnay J, et al. Prognostic factors in soft tissue sarcomas: a multivariate analysis of 109 cases. Cancer 1989; 63:1437-51.
16. Emrich LJ, Ruka W, Driscoll DL, Karakousis CP. The effect of local recurrence on survival time in adult high-grade soft tissue sarcomas. J Clin Epidemiol 1989;42:105-10.
17. Stotter AT, A'hern RP, Fisher C, Mott AF, Fallowfield ME, Westbury G. The influence of local recurrence of extremity soft tissue sarcoma on metastasis and survival. Cancer 1990;65:1119-29.
18. Alvegard TA, Berg NO, Baldetorp B, et al. Cellular DNA content and prognosis of high-grade soft tissue sarcoma: the Scandinavian Sarcoma Group experience. J Clin Oncol 1990;8:538-47.
19. Pisters PW, Leung DH, Woodruff J, Shi W, Brennan MF. Analysis of prognostic factors in 1,041 patients with localized soft tissue sarcomas of the extremities. J Clin Oncol 1996. In press.
20. Bevilacqua RG, Rogatko A, Hajdu SI, Brennan MF. Prognostic factors in primary retroperitoneal soft-tissue sarcomas. Arch Surg 1991; 126:328-34.
21. Kraus DH, Dubner S, Harrison LB, et al. Prognostic factors for recurrence and survival in head and neck soft tissue sarcomas. Cancer 1994;74:697-702.
22. McGrath PC, Neifeld JP, Lawrence W Jr, Kay S, Horsley JS 3d, Parker GA. Gastrointestinal sarcomas: analysis of prognostic factors. Ann Surg 1987;206:706-10.
23. Ng EH, Pollock RE, Munsell MF, Atkinson EN, Romsdahl MM. Prognostic factors influencing survival in gastrointestinal leiomyosarcomas: implications for surgical management and staging. Ann Surg 1992;215:68-77.
24. Meijer S, Peretz T, Gaynor JJ, Tan C, Hajdu SI, Brennan MF. Primary colorectal sarcoma: a retrospective review and prognostic factor study of 50 consecutive patients. Arch Surg 1990;125:1163-8.
25. Olah KS, Dunn JA, Gee H. Leiomyosarcoma have a poorer prognosis than mixed mesodermal tumours when adjusting for known prognostic factors: the result of a retrospective study of 423 cases of uterine sarcoma. Br J Obstet Gynaecol 1992;99:590-4.
26. Brennan MF. Management of extremity soft-tissue sarcoma. Am J Surg 1989;158:71-8.
27. Rosenberg SA, Tepper J, Glatstein E, et al. The treatment of soft-tissue sarcomas of the extremities: prospective randomized evaluations of (1) limb-sparing surgery plus radiation therapy compared with amputation and (2) the role of adjuvant chemotherapy. Ann Surg 1982;196:305-15.
28. Sondak VK, Economou JS, Eilber FR. Soft tissue sarcomas of the extremity and retroperitoneum: advances in management. Adv Surg 1991;24:333-59.
29. Jaques DP, Coit DG, Hajdu SI, Brennan MF. Management of primary and recurrent soft-tissue sarcoma of the retroperitoneum. Ann Surg 1990;212:51-9.
30. Dalton RR, Donohue JH, Mucha P Jr, van Heerden JA, Reiman HM, Chen SP. Management of retroperitoneal sarcomas. Surgery 1989; 106:725-33.
31. Storm FK, Mahvi DM. Diagnosis and management of retroperitoneal soft-tissue sarcoma. Ann Surg 1991;214:2-10.
32. Alvarenga JC, Ball AB, Fisher C, Fryatt I, Jones L, Thomas JM. Limitations of surgery in the treatment of retroperitoneal sarcoma. Br J Surg 1991;78:912-6.
33. Lindberg RD, Martin RG, Romsdahl MM, Barkley HT Jr. Conservation surgery and postoperative radiotherapy in 300 adults with soft-tissue sarcomas. Cancer 1981;47:2391-7.
34. Potter DA, Glenn J, Kinsella T, et al. Patterns of recurrence in patients with high-grade soft-tissue sarcomas. J Clin Oncol 1985; 3:353-66.
35. Leibel SA, Tranbaugh RF, Wara WM, Beckstead JH, Bovill EG, Phillips TL. Soft tissue sarcomas of the extremities: survival and patterns of failure with conservative surgery and postoperative irradiation compared to surgery alone. Cancer 1982;50:1076-83.
36. Suit HD, Mankin HJ, Wood WC, Proppe KH. Preoperative, intraoperative, and postoperative radiation in the treatment of primary soft tissue sarcoma. Cancer 1985;55:2659-67.
37. Hilaris B, Shiu M, Nori D. Limb sparing therapy for locally advanced soft tissue sarcomas. Endocu Therapy/Hypothermia Oncol 1985;1:17-24.
38. Schray MF, Gunderson LL, Sim FH, Pritchard DJ, Shives TC, Yeakel PD. Soft tissue sarcoma: integration of brachytherapy, resection, and external irradiation. Cancer 1990;66:451-6.
39. Habrand JL, Gerbaulet A, Pejovic MH, et al. Twenty years experience of interstitial iridium brachytherapy in the management of soft tissue sarcomas. Int J Radiat Oncol Biol Phys 1991;20:405-11.
40. Brennan MF, Hilaris B, Shiu MH, et al. Local recurrence in adult soft tissue sarcoma: a randomized trial of brachytherapy. Arch Surg 1987;122:1289-93.
41. Harrison LB, Franzese F, Gaynor JJ, Brennan MF. Long-term results of a prospective randomized trial of adjuvant brachytherapy in the management of completely resected soft tissue sarcomas of the extremity and superficial trunk. Int J Radiat Oncol Biol Phys 1993; 27:259-65.

42. Casper ES, Gaynor JJ, Harrison LB, Panicek DM, Hajdu SI, Brennan MF. Preoperative and postoperative adjuvant combination chemotherapy for adults with high grade soft tissue sarcoma. Cancer 1994; 73:1644-51.
43. Mazanet R, Antman KH. Adjuvant therapy for sarcomas. Semin Oncol 1991;18:603-12.
44. Sordillo PP, Magill GB, Shiu MH, Lesser M, Hajdu WI, Golbey RB. Adjuvant chemotherapy of soft part sarcomas with ALOMAD (S4). J Surg Oncol 1981;18:345-53.
45. Das Gupta TK, Patel MK, Chaudhuri PK, Briele HA. The role of chemotherapy as an adjuvant to surgery in the initial treatment of primary soft tissue sarcomas in adults. J Surg Oncol 1982;19:139-44.
46. Rosenberg SA, Kent H, Costa J, et al. Prospective randomized evaluation of the role of limb-sparing surgery, radiation therapy, and adjuvant chemoimmunotherapy in the treatment of adult soft-tissue sarcomas. Surgery 1978;84:62-9.
47. Mills EE. Adjuvant chemotherapy of adult high-grade soft tissue sarcomas. J Surg Oncol 1982;21:170-5.
48. Ravaud A, Bui NB, Coindre JM, et al. Adjuvant chemotherapy with CYVADIC in high risk soft tissue sarcoma: a randomized prospective trial. In: Salmon SE, editor. Adjuvant therapy of cancer VI. Philadelphia: WB Saunders Company, 1990:556-66.
49. Bui NB, Maree D, Coindre JM, et al. First results of a prospective randomized study of CYVADIC adjuvant chemotherapy in adults with operable high risk soft tissue sarcoma. Proc Am Soc Clin Oncol 1989;8:318.
50. Picci P, Bacci G, Gherlinzoni F, et al. Results of randomized trial for the treatment of localized soft tissue tumors (STS) of the extremities in adult patients. In: Ryan JR, Baker LO, editors. Recent concepts in sarcoma treatment. The Netherlands: Kluwer Academic, 1988:144-8.
51. Gherlinzoni F, Bacci G, Picci P, et al. A randomized trial for the treatment of high-grade soft-tissue sarcomas of the extremities: preliminary observations. J Clin Oncol 1986;4:552-8.
52. Brennan MF, Casper ES, Harrison LB, Shiu MH, Gaynor J, Hajdu SI. The role of multimodality therapy in soft tissue sarcoma. Ann Surg 1991;214:328-38.
53. Roth JA, Putnam JB Jr, Wesley MN, Rosenberg SA. Differing determinants of prognosis following resection of pulmonary metastases from osteogenic and soft tissue sarcoma patients. Cancer 1985; 55:1361-6.
54. Elias A, Ryan L, Aisner J, Antman KH. Mesna, doxorubicin, ifosfamide, dacarbazine (MAID) regimen for adults with advanced sarcoma. Semin Oncol 1990;17:41-9.
55. Farhood AI, Hajdu SI, Shiu MH, Strong EW. Soft tissue sarcomas of the head and neck in adults. Am J Surg 1990;160:365-9.
56. Westbury G. Amputations for soft tissue sarcoma. Ann R Coll Surg Engl 1991;73:163-4.
57. Ng EH, Pollock RE, Romsdahl MM. Prognostic implications of patterns of failure for gastrointestinal leiomyosarcomas. Cancer 1992; 69:1334-41.
58. Demers ML, Roh MS, Ellis LM. Liver resection improves survival for metastatic sarcoma. Proc Soc Surg Oncol 1995;181.

➢ COUNTERPOINT

National Kyushu Cancer Center, Japan

HIROKAZU CHUMAN

There are many histological subtypes of soft tissue sarcoma and several grading systems, making discussion of the natural history and prognosis complicated. Although this is a relatively rare disease, efforts have been made to improve treatment results by assessing prognosis. In the last several years multivariate analyses of prognostic factors have revealed risk factors for lesions localized in the extremities. Histopathological grade, depth of location, and tumor size are considered independent unfavorable characteristics for distant metastasis and mortality.[1-16] Because no nationwide tumor registration system exists in Japan, the exact incidence of the disease is not clear. Generally the incidence of malignant soft tissue sarcoma is 2 per 100,000 persons, suggesting that about 3,000 cases per year occur in Japan. Japanese surgeons usually conduct the follow-up of patients on whom they operate and even administer chemotherapy for advanced cases. The follow-up strategies vary somewhat among centers.

Table 13-14 Surgical staging of soft tissue sarcoma by the Musculoskeletal Tumor Society

STAGE	GRADE	RESECTION	METASTASIS
IA	Low grade	Intracompartmental	No distant metastasis
IB	Low grade	Extracompartmental	No distant metastasis
IIA	High grade	Intracompartmental	No distant metastasis
IIB	High grade	Extracompartmental	No distant metastasis
III	Any	Any	Distant metastasis

Data from Enneking WF, Spanier SS, Goodman MA. J Bone Joint Surg Am 1980;62:1027-30.

This counterpoint focuses on soft tissue sarcoma arising in the extremities. The optimal management of this disease has not been established. Clinicians classify patients by known risk factors, observe the clinical course, and tailor treatment accordingly. Existing treatments for primary lesions and current trials of preoperative therapy for patients with locally advanced disease or distant metastases warrant mention.

In Japan surgery is performed according to a modified sarcoma staging system based on the concept of compartmentalization (Table 13-14) proposed by Enneking et al.[18] The local recurrence rate after limb salvage surgery is now less than 10%, as low as that after amputation, which has increased the survival rate of patients with low-grade soft tissue sarcomas. The 5-year disease-free survival rate of those with high-grade soft tissue sarcomas is nearly 70%. The prognosis of patients who have high-grade soft tissue sarcoma with distant metastasis remains poor.[18-28] Although chemotherapy often has severe side effects, adjuvant regimens have been used. Unfortunately, most randomized studies of adjuvant chemotherapy with doxorubicin[29-36] or combination regimens[37-44] have shown no benefit.

DIAGNOSIS AND TREATMENT

The first complaint of most patients is a painless mass. Computed tomography and magnetic resonance imaging are usually conducted in such instances (Table 13-15). If a sarcoma is suspected, chest x-ray and computed tomography are valuable staging tools. Angiography is useful only if vascular reconstruction is contemplated. Biopsy is the next step.

In planning surgery, careful evaluation of the anatomical setting of the tumor is essential to maximize local control

Table 13-15 Evaluation of primary soft tissue sarcomas before treatment

Primary lesions
Physical findings
Plain radiographs
Computed tomography
Magnetic resonance imaging for tumors in the extremities or pelvis
Special tests (in patients in whom complex reconstruction is anticipated)
Angiography
Ultrasound
Distant metastasis
Plain chest x-ray
Computed tomography of the lung or abdomen
Histological diagnosis and grading
Open biopsy
Excisional biopsy

Table 13-16 Surgical procedures conducted in Japan

Marginal resection	Resection through the reactive zone
Wide resection	Resection in the normal tissues around the reactive zone
Curative wide resection	Resection with a 5 cm margin of grossly normal tissue around the reactive zone
Radical resection	Resection of the compartment including the tumor

(Tables 13-16 and 13-17). To preserve limb function, reconstruction of excised major blood vessels, bone, and joints may be required. Table 13-17 outlines current strategies of treatment according to stage. Preoperative induction therapy using radiation,[45-50] arterial infusion chemotherapy (cisplatin or doxorubicin based[51]), and systemic chemotherapy with ifosfamide, cisplatin, or derivatives of doxorubicin is being evaluated at Japanese centers. These adjuvant therapies are not regarded as standard, and further studies are necessary.

The treatment for patients in whom distant metastasis is detected at the time of diagnosis generally includes radical resection of the primary lesion. This usually improves quality of life by preventing the primary lesion from growing into a huge mass. Chemotherapy is typically started after resection of the primary lesion.

Recurrence at the primary site is treated with further surgery, which has had encouraging outcomes, making surveillance after primary therapy quite justifiable. Many reports have described the results of salvage surgery as being comparable to those of primary surgery.

FOLLOW-UP MANAGEMENT AFTER TREATMENT OF A PRIMARY LESION

The initial evidence of recurrence is usually local disease in low-grade tumors and distant metastasis in high-grade tumors. A rational follow-up scheme should take this into account. Recent multivariate analyses of prognostic factors based on the TNM staging system[52] proposed by the American Joint Committee on Cancer are important for prognostication. This staging system emphasizes tumor grade, and thus Japanese physicians tend to divide patients with sarcoma into two groups—high grade and low grade—for follow-up management.

Table 13-17 Typical therapies for primary soft tissue sarcoma in Japan

STAGE*	PRIMARY TREATMENT
IA	Surgery (wide or curative wide resection)
IB	Surgery (wide or curative wide resection with vascular or skeletal reconstruction)
IIA	Surgery (curative wide or radical resection)
IIB	Surgery and adjuvant therapy such as preoperative radiation therapy, arterial infusion of doxorubicin or neoadjuvant chemotherapy with CYVADIC or MAID
III	Palliative therapy after surgery or trials of chemotherapy (CYVADIC, MAID, doxorubicin derivatives, or carboplatin)

CYVADIC, Cyclophosphamide, vincristine, doxorubicin, and dacarbazine; *MAID,* mesna, doxorubicin, ifosfamide, and dacarbazine.
*Musculoskeletal Tumor Society staging system.

Low-Grade Sarcoma

Recurrence of low-grade (G1 or G2) soft tissue sarcoma, particularly G1 cases, may take more than 10 years. Some reports have indicated that the risk of recurrence does not decrease with the passage of time.[16] One report stated that recurrences often appear within about 6 months of marginal resection or intratumoral resection, which suggests that follow-up consultation should be performed at intervals of approximately 6 months. Local recurrence is apt to develop in the subcutaneous tissue or near the resection scar of the primary lesion, and cases with superficial primary lesions often recur superficially. It is important that patients be instructed in self-examination, since the patient often finds the abnormality between visits.

Many local recurrences of deeply seated extremity and truncal sarcomas are asymptomatic and impalpable. Thus regular examinations by computed tomography or magnetic resonance imaging are required. Even for low-grade sarcomas such examinations should be performed every 6 to 12 months (Tables 13-18 and 13-19). Deeply seated and huge tumors tend to recur, and surveillance should be more intensive in such patients.

Most low-grade soft tissue sarcomas do not respond to chemotherapy or radiation therapy. The standard treatment for locally recurrent low-grade sarcoma is radical repeat resection or amputation, which can often be curative.

High-Grade Sarcoma

Although the local recurrence rate after radical resection of high-grade lesions is as low as 10%, distant metastasis often

Table 13-18 Follow-up of patients with soft tissue sarcoma (low-grade sarcoma with superficial or small lesions): National Kyushu Cancer Center, Japan

	YEAR				
	1	2	3	4	5
Office visit	2	1	1	1	1
Chest x-ray	2	1	1	1	1
Site ultrasound	2	1	1	1	1
Site x-ray	2	1	1	1	1

Table 13-19 Follow-up of patients with soft tissue sarcoma (low-grade sarcoma with deeply seated or large primary lesions): National Kyushu Cancer Center, Japan

	YEAR				
	1	2	3	4	5
Office visit	3	2	2	1	1
Chest x-ray	3	2	2	1	1
Site ultrasound	3	2	2	1	1
Site x-ray	3	2	2	1	1
Site magnetic resonance imaging	2	1	1	1	1
Chest computed tomography	1	1	1	1	1
Abdominal computed tomography	1	1	1	1	1

occurs.[1-16] Again, tumor size and deep location are risk factors for distant metastasis.

Regular chest x-rays should be obtained every 2 to 3 months for about 3 years (Table 13-20). After 3 years the metastasis rate in high-grade soft tissue sarcoma is as low as that in low-grade cases.[16] Many Japanese surgeons perform follow-up consultation at intervals of 2 or 3 months for the first 3 years after treatment and then every 4 to 6 months for another 5 years. Computed tomographic scans of the chest and abdomen are useful in detecting small metastatic lesions but have not been evaluated yet in Japan for sensitivity, specificity, and cost-benefit aspects. In Japan, standard follow-up management usually involves chest x-ray and computed tomography or magnetic resonance imaging at intervals of about 6 months.

If unresectable metastases are detected, medical treatment should start immediately. Chemotherapy is still imperfect; only 20% to 30% of patients respond to doxorubicin or ifosfamide,[18-28] which are the most effective agents currently available. Japanese physicians do not agree about the benefit of thoracotomy or hepatectomy for resectable metastases. Lung metastases from low-grade tumors can be successfully treated by resection in some cases, but all forms of therapy for distant metastases from high-grade tumors are usually noncurative.

Table 13-20 Follow-up of patients with soft tissue sarcoma (high-grade sarcoma): National Kyushu Cancer Center, Japan

	YEAR				
	1	2	3	4	5
Office visit	5	4	2	2	2
Chest x-ray	5	4	2	2	2
Site ultrasound	5	4	2	2	2
Chest computed tomography	2	2	2	2	2
Abdominal computed tomography	2	2	2	2	2
Site x-ray	2	2	2	2	2
Site magnetic resonance imaging	2	2	2	2	2

PREOPERATIVE AND POSTOPERATIVE ADJUVANT TREATMENT

Limb salvage surgery can be performed on many patients, who often retain good postoperative function of the affected limb. Many reports have described the utility of adjuvant radiation therapy.[45-50] The local recurrence rate is about 10% for low-grade lesions and 10% to 30% for high-grade lesions. Computed tomography and magnetic resonance imaging facilitate treatment planning. In Japan, several trials of adjuvant chemotherapy before limited surgery have shown encouraging results (Table 13-17) but no consensus exists as to the optimum regimen.

Postoperative chemotherapy (doxorubicin; doxorubicin plus dacarbazine; and cyclophosphamide, vincristine, doxorubicin, and dacarbazine [CYVADIC] therapy) has been disappointingly ineffective.[29-44] Most of these studies have been based on historical control subjects, and few randomized studies have been performed in Japan.

FUTURE PROSPECTS

Histological tumor grading is currently so subjective as to be decidedly different among institutions. Many studies of grading and prognostic factors have given slightly different conclusions. Immunostaining for substances such as proliferating cell nuclear antigen and quantification of cell-cycle parameters by flow cytometry may supplement or replace grading systems. There are currently no useful serum tumor markers for soft tissue sarcoma in adults, nor any practical screening method to detect this disorder in high-risk, asymptomatic patients, but DNA-based tests for lesions in the Rb and other relevant genes hold promise.

Study of the clinical behavior of soft tissue sarcoma is hindered by the many subtypes that have been described. It is now possible to collect many cases of each subtype using computer-based registries, which will facilitate clinical research. Effective and less toxic therapy for distant metastasis is urgently required. Promising drugs must be evaluated by randomized, comparative studies. The optimal follow-up management strategy remains to be determined and should be studied in clinical trials. Cost-benefit analyses of all phases of management of patients with sarcoma will become increasingly important.

REFERENCES

1. Markhede G, Angervall L, Stener B. A multivariate analysis of the prognosis after surgical treatment of malignant soft-tissue tumors. Cancer 1982;49:1721-33.
2. Trojani M, Contesso G, Coindre JM, et al. Soft-tissue sarcomas of adults: study of pathological prognostic variables and definition of a histopathological grading system. Int J Cancer 1984;33:37-42.
3. Tsujimoto M, Aozasa K, Ueda T, Morimura Y, Komatsubara Y, Doi T. Multivariate analysis for clinical prognostic factors in soft tissue sarcomas. Cancer 1988;62:994-8.
4. Ueda T, Aozasa K, Tsujimoto M, et al. Multivariate analysis for clinical prognostic factors in 163 patients with soft tissue sarcoma. Cancer 1988;62:1444-50.
5. Mandard AM, Petiot JF, Marnay J, et al. Prognostic factors in soft tissue sarcomas: a multivariate analysis of 109 cases. Cancer 1989;63:1437-51.
6. Rydholm A, Berg NO, Gullberg B, Persson BM, Thorngren KG. Prognosis for soft tissue sarcoma in the locomotor system: a retrospective population-based follow-up study of 237 patients. Acta Pathol Microbiol Immunol Scand 1984;92:375-86.
7. Collin C, Godbold J, Hajdu S, Brennan M. Localized extremity soft tissue sarcoma: an analysis of factors affecting survival. J Clin Oncol 1987;5:601-12.
8. Sears HF, Hopson R, Inouye W, Rizzo T, Grotzinger PJ. Analysis of staging and management of patients with sarcoma: a ten year experience. Ann Surg 1980;191:488-93.
9. Heise HW, Myers MH, Russell WO, et al. Recurrence-free survival time for surgically treated soft tissue patients: multivariate analysis of five prognostic factors. Cancer 1986;57:172-7.
10. Alvegard TA, Berg NO, Baldetorp B, et al. Cellular DNA content and prognosis of high-grade soft tissue sarcoma: the Scandinavian Sarcoma Group Experience. J Clin Oncol 1990;8:538-47.
11. Rooser B, Attewell R, Berg NO, Rydholm A. Prognostication in soft tissue sarcoma: a model with four risk factors. Cancer 1988;61;817-23.
12. Bell RS, O'Sullivan B, Liu FF, et al. The surgical margin in soft tissue sarcoma. J Bone Joint Surg Am 1989;71:370-5.
13. Stotter AT, A'Hern RP, Fisher C, Mott AF, Fallowfield ME, Westbury G. The influence of local recurrence of extremity soft tissue sarcoma on metastasis and survival. Cancer 1990;65:1119-29.
14. Rooser B, Attewell R, Berg NO, Rydholm A. Survival in soft tissue sarcoma: prognostic variables identified by multivariate analysis. Acta Orthop Scand 1987;58:516-22.
15. Emrich LJ, Ruka W, Driscoll DL, Karakousis CP. The effect of local recurrence on survival time in adults with high-grade soft tissue sarcomas. J Clin Epidemiol 1989;42:105-10.
16. Gaynor JJ, Tan CC, Casper ES, et al. Refinement of clinicopathologic staging for localized soft tissue sarcoma of the extremity: a study of 423 adults. J Clin Oncol 1992;10:1317-29.
17. American Joint Committee on Cancer, Beahrs OH, Henson DE, Hutter RVP, Kennedy BJ, editors. Manual for staging of cancer, 4th edition, Philadelphia: JB Lippincott Company, 1992:131-3.
18. Enneking WF, Spanier SS, Goodman MA. Current concepts review: the surgical staging of musculoskeletal sarcoma. J Bone Joint Surg Am 1980;62:1027-30.
19. Wilson RE, Wood WC, Lerner HL, et al. Doxorubicin chemotherapy in the treatment of soft tissue sarcoma: combined results of two randomized trials. Arch Surg 1986;121:1354-9.
20. Antman K, Ryan L, Borden E, et al. Pooled results from three randomized adjuvant studies of doxorubicin versus observation in soft tissue sarcoma: 10 year results and review of literature. In: Salmon SE, editor. Adjuvant therapy of cancer VI. Philadelphia: WB Saunders Company, 1990:529-43.
21. Baker LH. Adjuvant chemotherapy for soft tissue sarcomas. In: Ryan JR, Baker LO, editors. Recent concepts in sarcoma treatment. Dordecht, the Netherlands: Kluwer Academic, 1988:131-8.
22. Alvegard TA, Sigurdsson H, Mouridsen H, et al. Adjuvant chemotherapy with doxorubicin in high-grade soft tissue sarcoma: a randomized trial of the Scandinavian Sarcoma Group. J Clin Oncol 1989;7:1504-13.
23. Eilber FR, Guiliano AE, Huth JF, Morton DL. A randomized prospective trail using postoperative adjuvant chemotherapy (adriamycin) in high-grade extremity soft-tissue sarcoma. Am J Clin Oncol 1988;11:39-45.
24. Gherlinzoni F, Bacci G, Picci P, et al. A randomized trial for the treatment of high-grade soft tissue sarcomas of the extremities: preliminary observations. J Clin Oncol 1986;4:552-8.
25. Gherlizoni F, Pignatti G, Fontana M, Giunti A. Soft tissue sarcomas: the experience at the Istituto Ortopedico Rizzoli. Chir Organi Mov 1990;75:150-4.
26. Picci P, Bacci G, Gherlizoni F, et al. Results of a randomized trial for a treatment of localized soft tissue tumors of the extremities in adult patients. In: Ryan JR, Baker LO, editors. Recent concepts in sarcoma treatment. Dordecht, the Netherlands: Kluwer Academic, 1988:144-55.
27. Benjamin RS, Terjanian TO, Genoglio CJ, et al. The importance of combination chemotherapy for adjuvant treatment of high risk patients with soft tissue sarcomas of the extremities. In: Salmon SE, editor. Adjuvant therapy of cancer V. New York: Grune & Stratton, 1987:735-44.
28. Edmonson JH, Fleming TR, Ivins JC, et al. Randomized study of systemic chemotherapy following complete excision of nonosseous sarcoma. J Clin Oncol 1984;2:1390-6.
29. Baker AR, Chang AE, Glastein E, et al. National Cancer Institute experience in the management of high grade extremity soft tissue sarcoma. In: Ryan JR, Baker LO, editors. Recent concepts in sarcoma treatment. Dordecht, the Netherlands: Kluwer Academic, 1988:123-9.
30. Rosenberg SA, Tepper J, Glatstein E, et al. The treatment of soft-tissue sarcomas of the extremities: prospective randomized evaluations of (1) limb-sparing surgery plus radiation therapy compared with amputation and (2) the role of adjuvant chemotherapy. Ann Surg 1982;196:305-15.
31. Rosenberg SA. Adjuvant chemotherapy of adult patients with soft tissue sarcoma. In: DeVita V, Hellman S, Rosenberg SA, editors. Important advances in oncology. Philadelphia: JB Lippincott Company, 1985:273-94.
32. Bui NB, Maree D, Coindre JM, et al. First results of a prospective randomized study of CYVADIC adjuvant chemotherapy in adults with operable high risk soft tissue sarcoma. Proc Am Soc Clin Oncol 1989;8:318.
33. Ravaud A, Bui NB, Coindre JM, et al. Adjuvant chemotherapy with CYVADIC in high risk soft tissue sarcoma: a randomized prospective trial. In: Salmon SE, editor. Adjuvant therapy of cancer VI. New York: Grune & Stratton, 1990:556-66.
34. Bramwell V, Rouesse J, Steward W, et al. Adjuvant CYVADIC chemotherapy for adult soft tissue sarcoma—reduced local recurrence but no improvement in survival: a study of the European Organization for Research and Treatment of Cancer Soft Tissue and Bone Sarcoma Group. J Clin Oncol 1994;12:1137-49.
35. Antman K, Crowley J, Balcerzak SP, et al. An intergroup phase III randomized study of doxorubicin and dacarbazine with or without ifosfamide and mesna in advanced soft tissue and bone sarcomas. J Clin Oncol 1993;11:1276-85.
36. Bramwell V, Mouridsen HT, Santoro A, et al. Cyclophosphamide vs ifosfamide and mensa: final report of a randomized phase II trial in adult soft tissue sarcoma. Eur J Cancer Clin Oncol 1987;23:311-21.
37. Edmonson JH, Ryan LM, Blum RH, et al. Randomized comparison of doxorubicin alone versus ifosfamide plus doxorubicin or mitomycin, doxorubicin, and cisplatin against advanced soft tissue sarcomas. J Clin Oncol 1993;11:1269-75.
38. Santoro J, Mouridsen HT, Steward W. A randomized EORTC study in advanced soft tissue sarcomas: ADM vs ADM + IFOS vs CYVADIC. Proc Am Soc Clin Oncol 1990;9:309.

39. Baker L, Benjamin R, Fine G, et al. Combination chemotherapy in management of disseminated soft tissue sarcomas. Proc Am Soc Clin Oncol 1979;20:378.
40. Borden EC, Amato DA, Rosenbaum C, et al. Randomized comparison of three adriamycin regimens for treatment of metastatic soft tissue sarcomas. J Clin Oncol 1987;5:840-50.
41. Gottlieb JA, Baker LH, Quagliana JM, et al. Chemotherapy of sarcomas with a combination of adriamycin and dimethyl triazeno imidazole carboxamine. Cancer 1972;30:1632-8.
42. Omura GA, Major FJ, Blessing JA, et al. A randomized study of adriamycin with and without dimethyl triazoenoimidazole carboxamine in advanced uterine sarcomas. Cancer 1983;52:626-32.
43. Pinedo HM, Bramwell VH, Mouridsen HT, et al. CYVADIC in advanced soft tissue sarcoma: a randomized study comparing two schedules; a study of the EORTC Soft Tissue and Bone Sarcoma Group. Cancer 1984;53:1825-32.
44. Schoenfeld DA, Rosenbaum C, Horton J, et al. A comparison of adriamycin versus vincristine and adriamycin, and cyclophosphamide versus vincristine, actinomycin-D, and cyclophosphamide for advanced sarcoma. Cancer 1982;50:2757-62.
45. Abbatucci JS, Boulier N, de Ranieri J, et al. Local control and survival in soft tissue sarcomas of the limbs, trunk walls and head and neck: a study of 113 cases. Int J Radiat Oncol Biol Phys 1986;12: 579-86.
46. Denton JW, Dunham WK, Salter M, Urist MM, Balch CM. Preoperative regional chemotherapy and rapid-fraction irradiation for sarcomas of the soft tissue and bone. Surg Gynecol Obstet 1984;158: 545-51.
47. Eilber FR, Mirra J, Eckart J, et al. Intraarterial adriamycin, radiation therapy, and surgical excision for extremity skeletal and soft tissue sarcomas. Dev Oncol 1984;26:141-52.
48. Hoekstra HJ, Schraffordt Koops H, Molenaar WM, et al. A combination of intraarterial chemotherapy, preoperative and postoperative radiotherapy, and surgery as limb-saving treatment of primarily unresectable high-grade soft tissue sarcomas of the extremities. Cancer 1989;63:59-62.
49. Tsuchiya H, Tomita K, et al. Intraarterial cisplatin and caffeine with/without doxorubicin for musculoskeletal high-grade spindle cell sarcoma. Oncol Reports 1994;1:27-36.
50. Goodnight JE Jr, Bargar WL, Voegeli T, Blaisdel FW. Limb-sparing surgery for extremity sarcomas after preoperative intraarterial doxorubicin and radiation therapy. Am J Surg 1985;150:109-13.
51. Karakousis CP, Emrich LJ, Rao U, Krishnamsetty RM. Feasibility of limb salvage and survival in soft tissue sarcomas. Cancer 1986;57: 484-91.
52. Mantravadi RV, Trippon MJ, Patel MK, Walker MJ, Das Gupta TK. Limb salvage in extremity soft-tissue sarcoma: combined modality therapy. Radiology 1984;152:523-6.
53. Brennan MF, Hilaris B, Shiu MH, et al. Local recurrence in adult soft-tissue sarcoma: a randomized trial of brachytherapy. Arch Surg 1987;122:1289-93.
54. Pisters PW, Harrison LB, Woodruff JM, Gaynor JJ, Brennan MF. A prospective randomized trial of adjuvant brachytherapy in the management of low-grade soft tissue sarcomas of the extremity and superficial trunk. J Clin Oncol 1994;12:1150-5.

➢ COUNTER POINT

Royal Liverpool University Hospital, UK

Sam J. Leinster

The concept of evidence-based medicine is becoming increasingly accepted,[1] and new treatment schedules are subjected to assessment in clinical trials before being accepted into routine practice. Less attention has been paid to assessing the value of follow-up protocols, many of which are based on best guess and consensus rather than objective evidence of benefit. To show benefit, an evaluation must demonstrate that not only can recurrence be detected earlier if the patient is in a follow-up program rather than being brought to medical attention when symptoms appear, but also that such earlier presentation actually affects the long-term outcome. To be cost effective, a follow-up program must lead significantly often to an intervention that prolongs the survival of the patient. When interventions are likely to be purely palliative, diagnosing recurrence before symptoms develop has no advantage. Surveillance during the treatment period is not, strictly speaking, follow-up and should be regarded as treatment monitoring to which different considerations pertain.

As shown by O'Donnell et al. in Table 13-4, aggressive treatment of isolated local recurrence can result in long-term control in a useful proportion of patients.[2] Attempts to detect local recurrence therefore have face validity. Whether regular magnetic resonance imaging provides any survival advantage over regular physical examination is yet to be demonstrated. There is in any case little advantage in performing magnetic resonance imaging twice in the first year after therapy as indicated in the follow-up recommendations by O'Donnell et al. (Tables 13-7 and 13-8), since the post-operative changes render interpretation impossible. Baseline magnetic resonance imaging early in the second year after treatment seems much more satisfactory, although even at that point acute changes may persist. When financial constraints exist, it may be better to use magnetic resonance imaging as a diagnostic tool thereafter, applying it only if recurrence is suspected on clinical grounds rather than as a routine annual study (Table 13-21). Clearly a study of the different strategies is needed to determine whether outcomes differ.

Since 80% of local recurrences occur within 2 years of treatment,[2,3] continuing close surveillance with expensive imaging after this point seems to have little value. Patients may well be as effective in detecting treatable recurrences as physicians. This has been demonstrated for malignant melanoma[4-6] but has not been reported for sarcoma. It may be more effective in sarcomas of the extremities than in retroperitoneal or other sarcomas of the trunk.

The other site of recurrence where early intervention may result in cure is the lung. Since curative resection is likely to be possible only when the metastases are asymptomatic, follow-up by imaging is essential but argument remains as to the best screening modality for chest metastases. Although computed tomography is more sensitive than a plain chest x-ray, there is no evidence that this extra sensitivity is reflected in an improved cure rate. The role of computed tomographic scanning in the follow-up period should be in the exclusion of undetected multiple metastases in a patient whose chest x-ray shows a solitary metastasis that

Table 13-21 Follow-up of patients with soft tissue sarcoma: Royal Liverpool University Hospital, UK

	YEAR				
	1	2	3	4	5
Office visit	4	4	2	2	2
Urinalysis	4	4	2	2	2
Complete blood count	4	4	2	2	2
Multichannel blood tests*	4	4	2	2	2
Chest x-ray	2	2	1	1	1
Chest computed tomography	†	†	†	†	†
Site magnetic resonance imaging	‡	1§	‡	‡	‡

*Consists of blood urea nitrogen, creatinine, aspartate aminotransferase, alkaline phosphatase, glucose, calcium, and phosphorus.
†Performed only if clinically indicated or if the chest x-ray prompts suspicion.
‡Performed only if recurrence is suspected on the basis of clinical findings.
§Performed to provide a baseline for future studies. If magnetic resonance imaging is performed earlier, changes that are due to the operative trauma and are difficult to differentiate from recurrence may still be present, leading to unnecessary further investigations.

appears to be suitable for resection (Table 13-21). The frequency of routine chest x-ray also needs to be defined in a proper study.

Routine isotope bone scanning or liver examinations are not indicated during follow-up, since no curative procedure can be undertaken and there is no point in treating the asymptomatic stages of recurrences. These investigations have a role, of course, in the evaluation of the patient on first presentation when the treatment strategy is being planned.

Regular physical examination and chest x-ray are justified for the first 2 years, since recurrence is common within this period and early intervention may result in long-term cure. Thereafter the argument for regular follow-up is less clear and should be the subject of specific studies (Table 13-21).

REFERENCES

1. Rosenberg W, Donald A. Evidence based medicine: an approach to clinical problem-solving. Br Med J 1995;310:1122-6.
2. Sauter ER, Hoffman JP, Eisenberg BL. Diagnosis and surgical management of locally recurrent soft-tissue sarcomas of the extremity. Semin Oncol 1993;20:451-5.
3. Cantin J, McNeer GP, Chu FC, Booher RJ. The problem of local recurrence after treatment of soft tissue sarcoma. Ann Surg 1968; 168:47-53.
4. Jillela A, Mani S, Nair B, et al. The role of close follow-up of melanoma patients with AJCC stages I-III: a preliminary analysis. Proc Am Soc Clin Oncol 1995;14:413.
5. Shumate CR, Urist MM, Maddox WA. Melanoma recurrence surveillance: patient or physician based? Ann Surg 1995;221:566-71.
6. Ruark DS, Shaw HM, Ingvar C, Thompson JF, McCarthy WH. Who detects the first recurrence in stage I cutaneous malignant melanoma: patient or doctor? 46th Ann Symp Soc Surg Oncol 1993;149.

➢ COUNTER POINT

Roswell Park Cancer Institute

JAMES E. SPELLMAN, JR.

O'Donnell et al. present a concise overview of the current issues of management and follow-up of the patient with soft tissue sarcoma. The recommendations delivered herein are presented in light of current practices at Roswell Park Cancer Institute, with particular reference to extremity lesions. Emphasis is placed on lesions considered to put the patient at high risk for recurrence, thus deserving of entrance onto neoadjuvant or adjuvant protocols. O'Donnell et al. present a thorough regimen for the follow-up of patients treated on protocol, designed to identify recurrences at both clinical and preclinical stages. Identifying recurrent disease in patients who had initially been rendered disease free is extremely important because most recurrences are treatable with resultant prolongation of survival. Patients must therefore undergo stringent staging evaluations before entrance into a neoadjuvant trial to avoid group bias caused by understaging. Some questions remain as to which patients should be placed onto protocols. The evaluation and follow-up of many patients outside the constraints of protocols may not necessarily be as extensive as that proposed by O'Donnell et al. Today's medical environment is forcing the physician to be cost conscious yet still maintain high standards of care. Follow-up evaluations therefore should be focused according to the risk of recurrence.

The risk of local recurrence for extremity soft tissue sarcomas should ideally be no more than 10% with current treatment modalities. Tumor size, grade, and location all play a role in defining the risk of local recurrence. Tumor size and grade also influence the risk of distant spread, although it is less certain that local recurrence alters that risk.[1] The modalities used in specific clinical situations to effect good local control have been under some debate.[2-7] Adjuvant chemotherapy has not improved overall survival in most studies.[8-11] Distant recurrence clearly affects survival. As stated, the lungs are the most common site of distant recurrence for extremity soft tissue sarcomas. Attention to this site in the follow-up of the patient is extremely important because lung recurrences may be resected for cure.[12]

The follow-up of patients with extremity soft tissue sarcoma at Roswell Park Cancer Institute is similar to that proposed by O'Donnell et al. (Table 13-22). Patients undergoing postoperative surveillance are evaluated every 3 months for 2 years and every 6 months for the next 3 years. Lifetime yearly evaluations are recommended after the fifth year. A thorough physical examination and chest x-ray are obtained at each visit. Complete blood count and liver function tests are also performed at each visit to aid in the assessment of patient general welfare, particularly for those undergoing or having undergone adjuvant treatment. A computed tomo-

Table 13-22 Follow-up of patients with soft tissue sarcoma (extremity): Roswell Park Cancer Institute

	YEAR				
	1	2	3	4	5
Office visit	4	4	2	2	2
Complete blood count	4	4	2	2	2
Liver function tests	4	4	2	2	2
Chest x-ray	4	4	2	2	2
Site magnetic resonance imaging	1	1	1	1	1
Chest computed tomography	*	*	*	*	*

*Indicated for patients with a minor abnormality in the initial preoperative study requiring follow-up for interval changes.

graphic scan of the chest is not routinely obtained unless an initial preoperative study in a high-risk patient discloses a minor abnormality that must be followed for interval changes. Magnetic resonance imaging of the operative site is performed yearly. Bone scanning has not proved useful, although it has been recommended by others.[13] While the efficacy of this follow-up regimen has not yet been formally evaluated at Roswell Park Cancer Institute, physicians at this institution believe that the vast majority of recurrences are detected while still in a treatable state.

One issue that deserves some mention is the patient with a retroperitoneal or intraabdominal sarcoma. Although a detailed description of the treatment of these tumors is beyond the scope of this discussion, recommendations for follow-up may be pertinent to both sites. Retroperitoneal sarcomas represent approximately 15% of soft tissue sarcomas. Of retroperitoneal tumors, 82% are malignant and 55% are sarcomas.[14] Retroperitoneal tumors have gained a reputation for regional invasion and local recurrence. Tumor size, grade, and invasion of adjacent organs are features important in the staging of these tumors. Completeness of resection and grade of the tumor are important prognostic factors.[15] Patients undergoing a complete resection have an overall 5-year survival rate of 64%.[16] In patients who receive complete resection, tumor grade is a significant prognostic factor.[15] However, local recurrence may occur in as many as 90% of patients.[14] In a series of 114 patients reported by Jaques et al.,[17] 49% of completely resected tumors recurred. Fifty-four percent of completely resected high-grade tumors recurred at a median time of 15 months. Forty-four percent of completely resected low-grade tumors recurred at a median time of 42 months. Thus vigilance is imperative, even for completely resected low-grade tumors. Pulmonary metastases occurred in 6%, and hepatic metastases occurred in 9%. Complete resection of recurrent nonmetastatic disease in this series was possible in 44% of patients. These patients enjoy a significant prolongation in overall survival. Neither adjuvant chemotherapy nor radiation therapy has shown benefit in this disease.[15-17]

Smooth muscle tumors of the gastrointestinal tract represent 1% or less of primary tumors at these sites and account for 2% of sarcomas in adults.[18-20] Tumor grade, size, and invasion of adjacent structures are important prognostic features. When complete resection is possible, tumor grade represents a major prognostic factor, with 5-year survival rates of 18% for high-grade tumors and 72% for low-grade tumors.[20] Recurrence after complete resection occurs in 44% of patients. Hepatic metastases (42%) and local recurrences (42%) are the major patterns of recurrence for patients undergoing complete resection. Mean time to recurrence is about 9 months. As with retroperitoneal tumors, neither chemotherapy nor radiation therapy as adjuvant treatment has shown a survival benefit. Maintaining frequent follow-up on these patients is important because complete resection of recurrent disease confers a survival advantage.

Depending on referral patterns, diffuse intraabdominal spread or sarcomatosis develops in a number of patients with retroperitoneal or intraabdominal sarcoma. These patients may also benefit from surgical extirpation of their disease, similar to patients with less extensive recurrence. A series of 72 patients with disseminated intraabdominal soft tissue sarcoma was evaluated by Karakousis et al.[21] to determine the benefit of a surgical debulking program. The tumor was completely resected grossly in 64% of patients. The median survival for patients with completely resected disease was 23 months, versus 9 months for patients whose disease was not resected completely. After complete resection, patients with high-grade tumors survived longer by a median of 6 months, while patients with low-grade tumors survived longer by a median of 28 months ($p \leq .001$).

Although the duration of disease-free status is limited in these patients, many are eligible for reexploration and resection of recurrences and are able to enjoy quality time with their families that they would miss with other modalities of treatment. When the disease can no longer be completely resected, the surgeon should consider ceasing exploration of the patient. Hepatic metastases are frequent in these patients, and the issue of resection in such cases is often met with trepidation. Jaques et al.[22] reviewed 65 patients with sarcoma metastatic to the liver. Fourteen patients underwent resection with a median survival of 33 months. This compares with a median survival of 12 months for patients who did not undergo resection. The difference was not statistically significant. A good-quality magnetic resonance image can be useful in determining potential resectability and in the follow-up of these patients.

The follow-up of patients with retroperitoneal, intraabdominal, or diffuse intraabdominal sarcoma must be frequent and detailed. At Roswell Park Cancer Institute this entails a physical examination, chest x-ray, complete blood count, and liver function tests for the first 2 years and every 6 months thereafter (Table 13-23). In addition, computed tomographic scans of the abdomen and pelvis are obtained at least every 3 months for the first 2 years and every 6 months thereafter, depending on the clinical situation. For patients with resected

Table 13-23 Follow-up of patients with soft tissue sarcoma (intraabdominal and retroperitoneal): Roswell Park Cancer Institute

	YEAR				
	1	2	3	4	5
Office visit	4	4	2	2	2
Complete blood count	4	4	2	2	2
Liver function tests	4	4	2	2	2
Chest x-ray	4	4	2	2	2
Abdominal computed tomography	4	4	2	2	2
Pelvic computed tomography	4	4	2	2	2
Chest computed tomography	*	*	*	*	*
Liver magnetic resonance imaging	†	†	†	†	†

*Indicated for patients with a minor abnormality in the initial preoperative study or who require follow-up for interval changes on chest x-ray.
†Indicated for patients with resected liver lesions or a possible new lesion in the liver.

liver lesions or a possible new lesion in the liver, magnetic resonance imaging is performed. For patients with primary disease who remain well after resection, the visits are extended to every 6 months after 2 years. This continues for another 3 years, after which the visits are placed on a yearly basis. Adherence to a stringent follow-up routine is necessary to detect recurrences while they are still resectable.

REFERENCES

1. Gustafson P, Rooser B, Rydholm A. Is local recurrence of minor importance for metastases in soft tissue sarcoma? Cancer 1991; 67:2083-6.
2. Karakousis CP, Emrich LJ, Rao U, Khalil M. Limb salvage in soft tissue sarcomas with selective combination of modalities. Eur J Surg Oncol 1991;17:71-80.
3. Rydholm A, Gustafson P, Rooser B, et al. Limb-sparing surgery without radiotherapy based on anatomic location of soft tissue sarcoma. J Clin Oncol 1991;9:1757-65.
4. Geer RJ, Woodruff J, Casper ES, Brennan MF. Management of small soft-tissue sarcoma of the extremity in adults. Arch Surg 1992;127: 1285-9.
5. Harrison LB, Franzese F, Gaynor JJ, Brennan MF. Long-term results of a prospective trial of adjuvant brachytherapy in the management of completely resected soft tissue sarcomas of the extremity and superficial trunk. Int J Radiat Oncol Biol Phys 1993;27:259-65.

Table 13-24 Follow-up of patients with soft tissue sarcoma by institution

YEAR/PROGRAM	OFFICE VISIT	CBC	LFT	CXR	SITE MRI	CHEST CT	ABD CT
Year 1							
Memorial Sloan-Kettering I[a]	2	1	1	1		[b]	[b]
Memorial Sloan-Kettering II[c]	4	1	1	2[d]		[b]	[b]
Memorial Sloan-Kettering III[e]	4	4	4	[b]		[b]	4
Roswell Park I[f]	4	4	4	4	1	[g]	
Roswell Park II[h]	4	4	4	4		[i]	4
Univ Washington I[k]	7[l]	4[l]		3	2	4[l]	
Univ Washington II[n]	5[l]	2		3[l]	2	2	
Japan: National Kyushu I[o]	2			2			
Japan: National Kyushu II[p]	3			3	2	1	1
Japan: National Kyushu III[q]	5			5	2	2	2
UK: Royal Liverpool	4	4		2	[r]	[s]	

ABD CT abdominal computed tomography
CBC complete blood count
CHEST CT chest computed tomography
CXR chest x-ray
ESR erythrocyte sedimentation rate
LFT liver function test
LIVER MRI liver magnetic resonance imaging
MCBT multichannel blood tests
SITE US site ultrasound
SITE MRI site magnetic resonance imaging
URIN urinalysis

6. Fein DA, Lee WR, Lanciano RM, et al. Management of extremity soft tissue sarcomas with limb-sparing surgery and postoperative irradiation: do total dose, overall treatment time, and the surgery-radiotherapy interval impact on local control? Int J Radiat Oncol Biol Phys 1995;32:969-76.
7. Edmonson JH. Chemotherapeutic approaches to soft tissue sarcomas. Semin Surg Oncol 1994;10:357-63.
8. Antman K, Ryan L, Borden E, et al. Pooled results from three randomized adjuvant studies of doxorubicin versus observation in soft tissue sarcoma: 10 year results and review of the literature. In: Salmon SE, editor. Adjuvant therapy of cancer. Vol VI. Philadelphia: WB Saunders Company, 1990:529-43.
9. Antman K, Suit H, Amato D, et al. Preliminary results of a randomized trial of adjuvant doxorubicin for sarcomas: lack of apparent difference between treatment groups. J Clin Oncol 1984;2:601-8.
10. Chang AE, Kinsella T, Glatstein E, et al. Adjuvant chemotherapy for patients with high-grade soft-tissue sarcomas of the extremity. J Clin Oncol 1988;6:1491-500.
11. Pisters PW, Harrison LB, Woodruff JM, Gaynor JJ, Brennan MF. A prospective randomized trial of adjuvant brachytherapy in the management of low-grade soft tissue sarcomas of the extremity and superficial trunk. J Clin Oncol 1994;12:1150-5.
12. Gadd MA, Casper ES, Woodruff JM, McCormack PM, Brennan MF. Development and treatment of pulmonary metastases in adult patients with extremity soft tissue sarcoma. Ann Surg 1993;218:705-12.
13. Finn HA, Simon MA, Martin WB, Darakjian H. Scintigraphy with gallium-67 citrate in staging of soft tissue sarcomas of the extremity. J Bone Joint Surg Am 1987;69:886-91.
14. Storm FK, Mahvi DM. Diagnosis and management of retroperitoneal soft-tissue sarcoma. Ann Surg 1991;214:2-10.
15. Bevilacqua RG, Rogatko A, Hajdu SI, Brennan MF. Prognostic factors in primary retroperitoneal soft-tissue sarcomas. Arch Surg 1991; 126:328-34.
16. Karakousis CP, Velez AF, Emrich LJ. Management of retroperitoneal sarcomas and patient survival. Am J Surg 1985;150:376-80.
17. Jaques DP, Coit DG, Hajdu SI, Brennan MF. Management of primary and recurrent soft-tissue sarcoma of the retroperitoneum. Ann Surg 1990;212:51-9.
18. Shiu MH, Farr GH, Papachristou DN, Hajdu SI. Myosarcomas of the stomach: natural history, prognostic factors and management. Cancer 1982;49:177-87.
19. Shiu MH, Farr GH, Egeli RA, Quan SH, Hajdu SI. Myosarcomas of the small and large intestine: a clinicopathologic study. J Surg Oncol 1983;24:67-72.
20. Conlon KC, Casper ES, Brennan MF. Primary gastrointestinal sarcomas: analysis of prognostic variables. Ann Surg Oncol 1995;2:26-31.
21. Karakousis CP, Blumenson LE, Canavese G, Rao U. Surgery for disseminated abdominal sarcoma. Am J Surg 1992;163:560-4.
22. Jaques DP, Coit DG, Casper ES, Brennan MF. Hepatic metastases from soft-tissue sarcoma. Ann Surg 1995;221:392-7.

PELVIC CT	LIVER MRI	SITE US	SITE X-RAY	URIN	MCBT	ESR	BONE SCAN
b							
b							
4							
4	j						
			2[l]	4[l]	4[l,m]	4[l]	1
			2[l]	2	2[m]	2	1
		2	2				
		3	3				
		5	2				
				4	4[t]		

a Patients with extremity sarcomas of any grade less than 5 cm in diameter plus low-grade extremity sarcomas greater than 5 cm in diameter.
b Performed only when metastatic recurrence is suspected.
c Patients with high-grade extremity sarcomas at least 5 cm in diameter.
d Performed at quarterly intervals for patients with extremity lesions greater than 10 cm in diameter.
e Patients with retroperitoneal, gastrointestinal, or visceral sarcomas.
f Extremity soft tissue sarcoma patients.
g Indicated for patients with a minor abnormality in the initial preoperative study requiring follow-up for interval changes.
h Patients with intraabdominal and retroperitoneal soft tissue sarcoma.
i Indicated for patients with a minor abnormality in the initial preoperative study or who require follow-up for interval changes on chest x-ray.
j Indicated for patients with resected liver lesions or a possible new lesion in the liver.
k For high-risk patients.
l Includes one test performed at baseline.
m Consists of blood urea nitrogen, creatinine, aspartate aminotransferase, alkaline phosphatase, glucose, calcium, and phosphorus.
n For low-risk patients.
o Low-grade sarcoma patients with superficial or small lesions.
p Low-grade sarcoma patients with deeply seated or large primary lesions.
q High-grade sarcoma patients.
r Performed only if recurrence is suspected on the basis of clinical findings.
s Performed only if clinically indicated or if the chest x-ray prompts suspicion.
t Consists of blood urea nitrogen, creatinine, aspartate aminotransferase, alkaline phosphatase, glucose, calcium, and phosphorus.
u Performed to provide a baseline for future studies. If magnetic resonance imaging is performed earlier, changes that are due to the operative trauma and are difficult to differentiate from recurrence may still be present, leading to unnecessary further investigations.

Continued.

Table 13-24 Follow-up of patients with soft tissue sarcoma by institution–cont'd

YEAR/PROGRAM	OFFICE VISIT	CBC	LFT	CXR	SITE MRI	CHEST CT	ABD CT
Year 2							
Memorial Sloan-Kettering I[a]	2	1	1	1		[b]	[b]
Memorial Sloan-Kettering II[c]	4	1	1	2[d]		[b]	[b]
Memorial Sloan-Kettering III[e]	4	4	4	[b]		[b]	4
Roswell Park I[f]	4	4	4	4	1	[g]	
Roswell Park II[h]	4	4	4	4		[i]	4
Univ Washington I[k]	4	4		2	1	2	
Univ Washington II[n]	4	2		2	1	2	
Japan: National Kyushu I[o]	1			1			
Japan: National Kyushu II[p]	2			2	1	1	1
Japan: National Kyushu III[q]	4			4	2	2	2
UK: Royal Liverpool	4	4		2	1[u]	[s]	
Year 3							
Memorial Sloan-Kettering I[a]	2	1	1	1		[b]	[b]
Memorial Sloan-Kettering II[c]	4	1	1	2[d]		[b]	[b]
Memorial Sloan-Kettering III[e]	4	4	4	[b]		[b]	4
Roswell Park I[f]	2	2	2	2	1	[g]	
Roswell Park II[h]	2	2	2	2		[i]	2
Univ Washington I[k]	2	2		1	1	1	
Univ Washington II[n]	1			1	1		
Japan: National Kyushu I[o]	1			1			
Japan: National Kyushu II[n]	2			2	1	1	1
Japan: National Kyushu III[q]	2			2	2	2	2
UK: Royal Liverpool	2	2		1	[r]	[s]	
Year 4							
Memorial Sloan-Kettering I[a]	2	1	1	1		[b]	[b]
Memorial Sloan-Kettering II[c]	2[d]	1	1	2[d]		[b]	[b]
Memorial Sloan-Kettering III[e]	2	2	2	[b]		[b]	2
Roswell Park I[f]	2	2	2	2	1	[g]	
Roswell Park II[h]	2	2	2	2		[i]	2
Univ Washington I[k]	2	2		1	1	1	
Univ Washington II[n]	1			1	1		
Japan: National Kyushu I[o]	1			1			
Japan: National Kyushu II[n]	1			1	1	1	1
Japan: National Kyushu III[q]	2			2	2	2	2
UK: Royal Liverpool	2	2		1	[r]	[s]	

PELVIC CT	LIVER MRI	SITE US	SITE X-RAY	URIN	BLOOD	ESR	BONE SCAN
[b]							
[b]							
4							
4	[j]						
			1	4	4[m]	4	1
			1	2	2[m]	2	1
		1	1				
		2	2				
		4	2				
				4	4[t]		
[b]							
[b]							
4							
2	[j]						
			1	2	2[m]	2	1
							1
		1	1				
		2	2				
		2	2				
				2	2[t]		
[b]							
[b]							
2							
2	[j]						
			1	2	2[m]	2	1
							1
		1	1				
		1	1				
		2	2				
				2	2[t]		

Continued.

Table 13-24 Follow-up of patients with soft tissue sarcoma by institution–cont'd

YEAR/PROGRAM	OFFICE VISIT	CBC	LFT	CXR	SITE MRI	CHEST CT	ABD CT
Year 5							
Memorial Sloan-Kettering I[a]	2	1	1	1		[b]	[b]
Memorial Sloan-Kettering II[c]	2[d]	1	1	2[d]		[b]	[b]
Memorial Sloan-Kettering III[e]	2	2	2	[b]		[b]	2
Roswell Park I[f]	2	2	2	2	1	[g]	
Roswell Park II[h]	2	2	2	2		[i]	2
Univ Washington I[k]	2	2		1	1	1	
Univ Washington II[n]	1			1	1		
Japan: National Kyushu I[o]	1			1			
Japan: National Kyushu II[n]	1			1	1	1	1
Japan: National Kyushu III[q]	2			2	2	2	2
UK: Royal Liverpool	2	2		1	[r]	[s]	

PELVIC CT	LIVER MRI	SITE US	SITE X-RAY	URIN	BLOOD	ESR	BONE SCAN
b							
b							
2							
2	j						
			1	2	2m	2	1
							1
		1	1				
		1	1				
		2	2				
				2	2t		

CHAPTER 14

Cutaneous Melanoma

Memorial Sloan-Kettering Cancer Center

DANIEL G. COIT

Although the yearly incidence of melanoma, estimated at 34,000 new cases in the United States in 1995,[1] is not nearly that of the more common tumors such as those of breast, lung, prostate, and colon, the trend in incidence is striking. Melanoma is increasing in incidence more rapidly than any other human malignancy. Furthermore, not all of these tumors are early, since the death rate from melanoma is increasing more rapidly than all human tumors with the exception of lung cancer. If the current trend continues as expected, it is estimated that someone born in the year 2000 will have approximately a one in 90 chance of developing melanoma at some point during his or her lifetime. With the incidence of this disease doubling every 13 years in the United States, melanoma is projected to become the most common human malignancy within the next century. The potential for this to become a major public health issue, not only for diagnosis and treatment, but also for follow up after treatment, is very real.

The economic implications alone are enormous. Melanoma is primarily a disease of young people, with the median age at diagnosis around 45 years. In addition, the majority of patients treated with melanoma are cured of their disease. It is imperative that physicians define an acceptable follow-up program, since the financial burden on the health care system imposed by unnecessarily intense follow-up will be substantial. On the other hand, follow-up must be of adequate intensity to detect treatable, potentially curable recurrences in this young cohort, since many patient-years are at stake.

RATIONALE FOR FOLLOW-UP

The rationale for follow-up of cancer patients in general has been stated elsewhere in this volume. These are worth reiterating with specific reference to melanoma.

Detection of Recurrence

The basic assumption in the follow-up of patients with cancer is that early detection of recurrence will affect long-term outcome. Recurrence is not always treatable and, if treatable, is not always curable. As described below, the relationship between the intensity of follow-up of the patient with melanoma and the prognosis is difficult to define. There are a number of other reasons for an organized follow-up program of melanoma patients.

Detection of a Second Primary Melanoma

Patients who have had a primary cutaneous melanoma treated are at increased risk for a second primary melanoma.[2-5] This lifetime risk is estimated at 4% to 6% and is higher in patients with atypical or dysplastic nevi or a strong family history of melanoma.[6-8] Thus ongoing dermatological surveillance is an essential component of follow-up after treatment for melanoma. Under surveillance, subsequent primary melanomas tend to be much thinner and to have a better prognosis. In patients with multiple primary melanomas, prognosis tends to be governed by the thickest lesion as an independent factor. Dermatological surveillance is also important in detecting other nonmelanoma skin cancers in this group of patients, who frequently give a history of significant prior sun exposure.

Patient Education

An integral part of the follow-up of patients with melanoma is education. This includes the teaching of self-examination, not only for primary cutaneous lesions, but also for regional nodal areas. Patients should be taught to recognize the classic characteristics of cutaneous melanoma in friends and family. In addition, the importance of and methods for avoidance of excess sun exposure, perhaps the only melanoma risk factor over which patients have significant control, should be a routine part of the follow-up visit. These methods include using sunblock, wearing protective clothing, and avoiding the midday sun.

Screening for Other Primary Malignancies

Patients with melanoma may be at slightly increased risk for other invasive noncutaneous malignancies.[9] In addition, many patients with melanoma have no other physician, being otherwise young and healthy. In the absence of other medical care, routine surveillance strategies are appropriate. Although a description of strategies is beyond the scope of this chapter, they include breast examination with routine screening mammography on a schedule as recommended by the American Cancer Society and a digital rectal examination with stool guaiac and prostate examination in men over the age of 50. Reminding women of the importance of routine pelvic examinations with a Papanicolaou (Pap) smear is appropriate. Follow-up visits afford the opportunity for a brief review of systems, with evaluation of any significant intercurrent symptoms. Finally, in patients with known risk factors for specific malignancies, ensuring that appropriate surveillance strategies are employed is most important, particularly in the absence of any other treating physician. Examples of the latter strategies are a screening colonoscopy in patients with a family history of colon cancer or a periodic chest x-ray in patients with a history of heavy smoking.

Identification of Family Kindreds

Approximately 5% to 11% of patients with melanoma have a family history of the disease or will have affected relatives in the future.[8,10] Longitudinal follow-up of these patients facilitates the identification of families at risk for melanoma, affording the opportunity to bring them under the umbrella of dermatological surveillance. This is important not only for early detection of new lesions, but also for genetic screening and counseling.

Psychosocial Support

One of the most important aspects of ongoing follow-up in patients with melanoma is the sense of reassurance patients have after a negative examination. The diagnosis of melanoma in this otherwise healthy population, unaccustomed to chronic disease, is accompanied by enormous anxiety about the future. With every normal checkup this anxiety lessens. The clinician, aided by algorithms to be described later in the chapter, can estimate for patients the degree of risk of recurrence at any point in time after initial treatment, as well as the likelihood of future recurrence. In addition to reassurance on an individual basis, the organization and supervision of patient support groups have proved enormously rewarding. Most patients with melanoma have never met anyone else with the disease. Sitting face to face with other patients of similar disease stage, particularly if they are doing well years after the diagnosis, can be reassuring in a way that no amount of individual counseling can provide. Furthermore, at least one study has suggested that psychosocial counseling may favorably affect the prognosis of patients with melanoma.[11]

Documentation of End Results

Clinicians must record and document the end results of patient treatment. This provides internal quality control. For example, if the regional nodal recurrence rate exceeds that seen in the literature, the surgical technique may be inadequate. Furthermore, keeping a record is important for refining physicians' understanding of the natural history of the disease and for defining prognostic factors and high-risk groups. Only through the careful documentation of end results can physicians make observations, either retrospectively or prospectively, that assist in refining management decision algorithms.

CURRENT PRACTICE

A rational program of follow-up for patients treated definitively for their primary cancer should be based on a thorough understanding of the natural history of the disease. Specifically, since the objective of follow-up is to detect recurrence, an understanding of the patterns of recurrence should aid the physician in selecting a specific panel of examinations and investigations. An understanding of the time to recurrence should help the physician determine the frequency with which examinations and investigations should be performed. A great deal is known about the natural history of patients with malignant melanoma with respect to these two parameters.

Pattern of Recurrence

Approximately 25% of patients with clinical stage I and II melanoma will have recurrence.[12-15] The pattern of recurrence after definitive treatment of clinical stage I melanoma has been well described.

With prolonged follow-up, in retrospective series, local recurrence has been documented in up to 13% to 17% of patients. In a more recent prospective, randomized trial reported by Balch et al.,[16] local recurrence was observed in only 2% to 4% of patients after a median follow-up of 4 years. In-transit metastases are seen as the initial site in less than 10% of patients who have recurrences.

The most common site of recurrent disease after definitive management of primary clinical stage I melanoma is the regional nodal basin, occurring in 40% to 60% of patients.[12,17] The incidence of regional nodal recurrence as the initial site of failure is highly dependent on whether elective lymph node dissection was a component of the original treatment. McCarthy et al.[15] found that the first site of recurrence was in the regional nodes in 50% to 60% of patients with recurrence who did not have antecedent elective lymph node dissection as a part of their initial treatment, compared with less than 10% in those who had undergone elective lymph node dissection. Systemic metastases are seen in 23% to 38% of patients, with the majority of these visceral and the remainder distant subcutaneous or remote nodal disease.

In a comprehensive review of the subject by Gadd and Coit[19] the majority of clinical recurrences after lymph node dissection were solitary and of those the majority were accessible on physical examination, being locoregional, remote soft tissue, or nodal. In that series more than two thirds of initial recurrences of melanoma were detectable by physical examination. Isolated visceral recurrences were less common as the initial site of relapse, with the lung the most common site. Thus, as physicians develop a strategy for where and how to look for recurrence, clearly physical examination is the cornerstone.

In addition to detecting recurrence of the primary tumor, close follow-up will result in the discovery of a second primary melanoma in approximately 2% to 4% of patients.[2-5] In the setting of an ongoing follow-up program, second primary melanomas tend to be thinner with an excellent prognosis.

Based on the preceding data, the follow-up of patients after definitive treatment for clinical stage I melanoma should involve a diligent physical examination, with attention focused on a complete dermatological examination and on the locoregional area, as well as remote nodes. Periodic chest x-rays are useful in detecting asymptomatic pulmonary recurrence. The yield of routine blood work in detecting occult visceral disease is quite low, since these tests are not sensitive indicators of recurrent disease.

Time to Recurrence

Of recurrences, 55% to 67% become apparent by 2 years and 65% to 81% by 3 years after definitive treatment of the primary tumor. Logically, therefore, patients should be examined at more frequent intervals during that period and at increasing intervals thereafter.

In patients treated for melanoma metastatic to regional nodes at initial diagnosis (pathological stage III), the time to recurrence is earlier than that for patients without regional nodal metastases. In the series from Memorial Sloan-Kettering Cancer Center, 80% of recurrences after lymph node dissection with positive nodes became apparent within the first 2 years. In addition, although isolated regional nodal recurrence after lymph node dissection occurs with a finite frequency,[19-21] the majority of recurrences are systemic.

A significant incidence of late recurrence, more than 10 years after initial treatment, occurs in patients with malignant melanoma.[22-30] These patients tend to have thinner primary lesions than patients with earlier recurrence and almost always initially have negative nodes. The pattern of recurrence that appears after 10 years is similar to that of early recurrence. In general, the prognosis after late recurrence is similar to that of patients with early recurrence.[31]

What Is Known About Current Practice

The National Cancer Institute has published a consensus statement on the diagnosis and treatment of early melanoma.[32] Recommendations for follow-up office visits after surgical therapy include an interval of 6 months in patients without atypical moles and without a family history of melanoma for the first 2 years. If the patient is disease free for 2 years, yearly visits thereafter are advised. For patients with atypical moles or a positive family history, shorter intervals between examination, such as 3 to 6 months, are recommended. The decision to extend the interval after 2 years should be based on the stability and characteristics of the atypical moles. Follow-up should consist of a rigorous physical examination. Screening for occult visceral metastases is believed to be unnecessary. For patients with melanoma in situ, serial skin examinations at regular intervals are advised. Furthermore, screening of first-degree family members is thought to be important.

A number of reviews have described the current practice in the follow-up of patients after treatment for their melanoma, both from individual centers and as consensus statements. Kelly et al.[14] analyzed the risk of recurrence of melanoma tabulated by year and stratified by intervals of tumor thickness and from this derived a follow-up schedule. Patients with melanomas less than 0.76 mm thick were seen every 6 months for the first year, then yearly. Patients with tumors 0.76 to 1.49 mm thick were seen every 6 months. Patients with tumors measuring 1.5 to 4.0 mm were seen every 3 months for the first year, every 4 months for the second through fourth years, and twice yearly thereafter. Patients with melanomas thicker than 4.0 mm were seen every 2 to 3 months for the first year, every 3 months for years 2 through 4, and every 6 months thereafter. This study, however, was based on a relatively small number of patients in each individual group.

McCarthy et al.[15] reported on a larger series of patients from the Sydney Melanoma Unit in Australia, looking at 3,171 patients followed up for 2.5 to 36.2 years. During the course of that study 886 (28%) had recurrence. As with the previous study these researchers looked at the interval to first recurrence stratified by primary tumor thickness. They described a suggested follow-up interval of once yearly for patients with melanomas less than or equal to 0.7 mm. Patients with melanomas measuring 0.8 to 1.5 mm were seen every 6 months for 3 years, then yearly thereafter, while those with melanomas measuring 1.6 to 3.0 mm were seen every 2 months for the first year, every 4 months for the second year, every 6 months for the third year, every 9 months for years 4 and 5, and yearly thereafter. For melanomas over 3.0 mm in thickness, follow-up was recommended every 1½ months for the first year, every 2 months for the second year, every 4 months for years 3 through 5, and yearly thereafter.

In addition to describing the time to and incidence of recurrence, McCarthy et al.[15] described the patterns of initial recurrence in patients, stratified by whether elective lymph node dissection was performed as a part of initial treatment. Although they did not specify a suggested regimen of investigations at each follow-up visit, the data showed clearly that nodal recurrence was by far the most common initial site of recurrent disease in patients without elective lymph node dissection, while visceral metastases were much more common as the first site of failure when elective lymph node dissection was a part of the primary treatment.

Romero et al.[18] polled 11 physicians who are experts in the care of patients with melanoma and collated their recommendations for follow-up. As with the prior two studies, the recommended frequency of follow-up was related to tumor thickness. Based on a general consensus with minor variation, the majority of experts agreed that patients with melanomas 0.75 mm in thickness or less should be seen every 6 months for years 1 and 2 and yearly thereafter. Patients with melanomas 0.76 to 1.5 mm are seen every 3 months for years 1 and 2, every 6 months for years 3 through 5, and yearly thereafter, while patients with melanomas greater than 1.5 mm in thickness are seen every 3 months for years 1 through 3, every 6 months for years 4 and 5, and yearly thereafter. Again, this study focused more on interval to recurrence than on pattern of recurrence, and no specific recommendations were made as to investigations beyond a physical examination at the time of follow-up.

The follow-up strategy in patients with clinical stage I melanoma should be modified by a number of parameters. The consensus is that because thicker melanomas tend to recur more often and earlier,[22] these patients should be seen more frequently, particularly in the initial years. Balch et al.[33] have also reported that tumor ulceration and anatomical location influence the likelihood of recurrence and have suggested that these factors should play a role in the design of the follow-up schedule.[34]

Furthermore, as shown by McCarthy et al.,[15] although elective lymph node dissection as a component of initial treatment may or may not affect the likelihood of subsequent recurrence, it certainly affects the pattern of subsequent recurrence. Patients undergoing elective lymph node dissection are less likely to have nodal recurrence as a component of their initial recurrence, with systemic visceral recurrences predominating in this group. Patients not undergoing elective lymph node dissection are more likely to have regional nodes as their initial site of recurrence. This is important because patients with regional nodal recurrence have a better prognosis than those with systemic recurrence. Thus close follow-up of patients who have not undergone regional nodal resection may have a greater impact on prognosis than close follow-up of patients who have already had their nodes removed.

The impact of adjuvant therapy as a component of initial treatment on the pattern of recurrent disease is unknown. No statement can be made as to any modification of the proposed follow-up schedules based on this variable.

The frequency of follow-up should be modified according to the treatment options available if recurrence is detected. Local and nodal recurrences may be treated by surgical resection in almost any setting. Regional in-transit recurrence suitable for isolation limb perfusion should be treated in a center where there is sufficient experience with the technical details and the management of complications of this procedure. Options for treatment of visceral recurrence are limited. Offering more intensive follow-up at centers where more options are available for treatment if recurrence is detected seems reasonable. Specifically, more intensive follow-up of patients may be appropriate in an academic center specializing in the multimodality treatment of melanoma. Patients whose follow-up takes place in a local community, where investigational treatment strategies will not be pursued in the event of systemic recurrence, might be followed up less rigorously, looking more for surgically treatable second primary cancers or locoregional recurrences.

Role of Physical Examination

As can be inferred from these data, a comprehensive physical examination is the cornerstone of follow-up of patients with melanoma. With a 5% lifetime risk of a second primary melanoma, a periodic complete dermatological examination is vital. This is especially true in patients with known multiple primary melanomas, multiple atypical moles, or a strong family history.[6-8] In addition, a comprehensive locoregional examination is mandatory, since with the early detection of locoregional recurrence, early surgical intervention may alter the natural history of the recurrence. A careful examination for local recurrence, satellitosis, and visible or palpable in-transit disease is important. In addition, examination of regional nodes, particularly in patients who did not undergo regional lymph node dissection at the time of initial definitive treatment, is mandatory. Up to 30% of patients with locoregional recurrence can be saved with aggressive surgical treatment.

In patients with recurrence in remote nodes or soft tissue metastases, physical examination is the optimal method of detection. Detecting these is particularly important because the survival rate after surgical resection in this group of patients is 20% to 25%.[35] Visceral metastases are much less frequently detected by physical examination. Pulmonary metastases are almost always asymptomatic and detected radiologically, whereas brain and gastrointestinal metastases are usually symptomatic, often in the absence of significant physical findings.

Role of Laboratory Tests

Since the majority of recurrences are detectable by physical examination, the laboratory plays a relatively limited role in the follow-up of melanoma patients. Periodic hemoglobin determinations can pick up subclinical gastrointestinal tract metastases. Periodic liver function tests may detect early evidence of hepatic metastases. However, in the absence of symptoms, it is not clear that early detection of these lesions affects the natural history of the disease.

Recently the development of serum markers to help detect recurrence has attracted attention. Reintgen et al.[36] have been interested in defining the role of LASA-P. Of 270 patients with melanoma who had determinations of LASA-P and NSE, 30% had a recurrence at some point within their clinical course. The sensitivity and specificity of NSE were 27% and 77%, respectively. The sensitivity and specificity of LASA-P were 65% and 76%, respectively. The authors suggested that LASA-P may be a useful marker in follow-up of patients with melanoma. Work is ongoing in this regard.

Mani et al.[37] observed that an elevated serum S-100 level is often seen in patients with high tumor burden (largest lesion more than 6 cm in diameter or greater than five sites of metastases). However, neither S-100 nor NSE was useful in detecting a low or medium tumor burden. Mani et al.[37] found that NSE could not distinguish between patients with low tumor burden and normal volunteers. Reintgen et al.[36] found that S-100 alone had a sensitivity and specificity in detecting recurrent melanoma of 43% and 94%, respectively. They found the highest sensitivity, 71%, when combining LASA-P with S-100. However, the specificity of this combination was only 55%.

Wong et al.[39] reported on a cohort of 270 patients prospectively followed with serial determinations of serum antigen-specific immune complex (ASIC). At a median follow-up time of 25 months, 77 patients (30%) had recurrence. The authors found the level of ASIC to be highly correlated with stage at presentation. Although cancer recurred in only 25 of 135 (16%) of ASIC-negative patients, 55 of 118 (47%) of ASIC-positive patients had recurrences in the follow-up period. Thus the positive predictive value of ASIC was 47% and the negative predictive value was 84%. The investigators believed that this was a preliminary but promising methodology for follow-up of patients at risk for melanoma recurrence.

Horikoshi et al.[40] noted an elevation in urinary or serum 5-S-cysteinyldopa in seven of nine patients with recurrent melanoma 3 to 36 months before these recurrences were clinically apparent. Studies are ongoing to define the sensitivity, specificity, and positive and negative predictive values of this technique.

Radiology

Periodic chest x-rays seem reasonable in patients at risk for systemic metastases. Of all solitary sites of visceral recurrence, the lungs are the most frequent. Furthermore, in patients undergoing complete resection of a solitary site of visceral metastatic disease, the long-term survival rate is maximized after pulmonary resection.[35] Since these patients are usually asymptomatic, almost all of these lesions are detected by periodic chest x-ray.

Routine computed tomographic scanning, on the other hand, has an extremely low yield in the absence of clinical symptoms, physical findings, or abnormal laboratory values.[41] The same can be said about nuclear medicine scans. In general, these examinations should not be used in routine follow-up of patients with melanoma.

Treatment of Recurrence

While the treatment of recurrent melanoma is beyond the scope of this review, the frequency and intensity with which the physician looks for recurrence should be in part related to the treatment options available. Treatment of recurrence can be divided into that with curative intent, that with palliative intent, and that involving investigational therapy. Recurrences treated with curative intent involve second primary melanomas, locoregional recurrences, and solitary remote nodal or soft tissue recurrences.[35] In addition, pulmonary recurrences, particularly those that have remained solitary over a period of observation, can often be resected with the expectation of long-term cure in up to 20%.[42-44] In all patients treated for recurrent melanoma with curative intent, a comprehensive extent of disease evaluation is appropriate before treatment of all but second primary cancers.

Patients treated with palliative intent, that is, those with brain metastases, gastrointestinal tract metastases, or multiple remote nodal or soft tissue metastases, need a less comprehensive extent of disease evaluation. Patients offered surgery should have a reasonable life expectancy and be able to tolerate the proposed procedure with minimal morbidity.

Physician- Versus Patient-Detected Recurrence

A number of legitimate concerns have arisen recently with regard to who detects recurrences and whether this has any prognostic implications. Brandt et al.[45] reported on a cohort of 206 patients with melanomas less than 1.5 mm thick. With a short follow-up of 3 months to 24 years (median not specified), melanomas recurred in 11 patients, only five of whom were alive after treatment of their recurrence. The authors concluded that the yield of intensive follow-up with respect to improving prognosis of the entire group did not justify the effort or expense in patients with thin melanomas.

Jillella et al.[46] reported on a cohort of 279 patients, AJCC stages I through III, who were followed up prospectively. With a median follow-up time of 4.5 years, cancer recurred in 49 (17.6%) of the patients. Of 196 patients who were AJCC stages I and II at presentation, 32 (16%) had recurrence; all of those recurrences were detected by the patients. Of 83 patients who were AJCC stage III at presentation, 17 (20%) had recurrence; only three of these were detected by physicians, and the remainder were detected by the patient. In all, 46 of 49 recurrences (94%) were patient detected.

Shumate et al.[47] reported on 195 evaluable cases of melanoma recurrence and found that symptoms were present in 90% of patients, accurately predicting the site of recurrence. In their review 128 of 195 patients (66%) had their recurrence diagnosed at a previously scheduled visit, while 67 of 195 patients (34%) had a return before a scheduled visit. There was no difference in outcome between patient- and physician-detected recurrences.

Ruark et al.[48] reported on 257 patients with recurrent melanoma in whom both the site of recurrence and the individual detecting the recurrence were clearly identified. In 72% of cases the patient detected the recurrence, whereas the physician detected recurrence in the remaining 28%. The overall 5-year survival rate after recurrence was identical whether the patient or physician detected the initial recurrence.

Baughan et al.[49] reported on an audit of a melanoma follow-up clinic involving 331 patients seen over a 10-year period, of whom 65 (20%) had recurrence. Of the recurrences, 41 (63%) were patient detected and 20 (37%) were physician detected. There was no difference in survival between the two groups once recurrence was detected. Despite this and significant reported patient anxiety before scheduled clinic appointments, 95% of the patients were highly satisfied with the structured follow-up program, preferring scheduled visits to a policy of coming back when necessary. All five of these studies indicate that patient education may be a much more important component of post-treatment management than intensive physical follow-up, as assessed by the impact on prognosis once recurrence is detected.

FUTURE PROSPECTS

The optimal follow-up program for patients with melanoma is not likely ever to be defined by a prospective, randomized study. If such a program could be defined and carried out, it would be an important study, given the burgeoning number of young patients with this disease. The optimal trial design would compare outcomes in patients randomly assigned to intensive follow-up, combined with patient education, frequent physical examinations, and diagnostic testing, to another group randomly selected for education alone without intensive physician contact. Although the expectation is that the outcomes in both groups would be similar, this type of trial is probably not feasible given the current medicolegal climate.

A molecular biological technique being investigated for identification of patients at high risk for recurrence is flow cytometry, looking at both ploidy and S-phase fraction of the primary tumor.[50,51] In addition, a great deal of effort has been expended recently on trying to define a melanoma gene, with particular attention focused on nonrandom alterations in chromosomes 9 and 10 seen in patients with dysplastic nevi and primary melanoma.[10]

A number of investigators have used polymerase chain reaction methodology to detect melanoma cells in blood or bone marrow. This technique appears to be extremely sensitive, although its clinical utility has yet to be defined.[52]

A number of other techniques are in preclinical development and may well assist in the follow-up of patients with melanoma. A number of groups[53-55] have suggested that 2-fluorine-^{18}F-2-deoxy-d-glucose positron emission tomography scans may be more accurate than computed tomographic scanning in the detection of metastatic melanoma. This technique, however, does not appear to be sensitive in picking up small pulmonary metastases.

Technetium 99m–labeled monoclonal antibodies have also been evaluated in an attempt to detect clinically occult metastatic melanoma. The sensitivity of this technique has been variously reported at 45% to 90%.[56] It has the drawback of sensitizing the patient to mouse protein, precluding subsequent therapeutic administration of cytotoxic murine monoclonal antibodies. Furthermore, at present it does not appear to be sensitive enough to warrant routine clinical application.

FINAL RECOMMENDATIONS

There is no optimal formula for the follow-up of patients with melanoma. The schedules described in Tables 14-1 through 14-3 serve as guidelines or points of departure that should be modified in both frequency and number of investigations performed according to a range of parameters.

Table 14-1 Follow-up of patients with cutaneous melanoma (primary tumors less than 1 mm thick, negative nodes): Memorial Sloan-Kettering Cancer Center

	YEAR				
	1	2	3	4	5
Office visit	2	2	1	1	1
Chest x-ray	1	1	1	1	1
Complete blood count	1	1	1	1	1
Liver function tests	1	1	1	1	1

Table 14-2 Follow-up of patients with cutaneous melanoma (primary tumors at least 1 mm thick, negative nodes): Memorial Sloan-Kettering Cancer Center

	YEAR				
	1	2	3	4	5
Office visit	3-4	3-4	3	2	2
Complete blood count	1-2	1-2	1-2	1	1
Liver function tests	1-2	1-2	1-2	1	1
Chest x-ray*	1	1	1	1	1

*Performed twice a year during years 1 and 2 for patients with primary tumors greater than 4 mm thick.

Table 14-3 Follow-up of patients with cutaneous melanoma (positive nodes): Memorial Sloan-Kettering Cancer Center

	YEAR				
	1	2	3	4	5
Office visit	4	4	3	2	2
Chest x-ray	2	2	1	1	1
Complete blood count	2	2	1	1	1
Liver function tests	2	2	1	1	1

From a cost-benefit point of view, more resources should be focused on detecting treatable locoregional recurrences, although even with those, it is difficult to document improved outcome after treatment of physician-detected as opposed to patient-detected relapse. Clearly the intensity of dermatological surveillance for a second primary melanoma depends on such factors as family history and the presence, number, and degree of atypia of other nevi. Patients also differ in their need for emotional support and reassurance, an important component of a scheduled follow-up program.

The optimal duration of follow-up is unknown. Late recurrences more than 10 years after treatment of localized melanoma are well recognized, and the risk of a second primary melanoma continues for life. Patients enrolled in specific programs evaluating new treatment approaches must be followed up closely to define the impact of those programs on patterns of relapse and survival.

REFERENCES

1. Wingo PA, Tong T, Bolden S. Cancer statistics, 1995. CA Cancer J Clin 1995;45:8-30.
2. Kang S, Barnhill RL, Mihm MC Jr, Sober AJ. Multiple primary cutaneous melanomas. Cancer 1992;70:1911-6.
3. Austin PF, Stankard CS, Cruse CW, Schroer K, Glass F, Reintgen DS. Multiple primary melanomas: evidence for the efficacy of screening and evidence against the minimalistic philosophies of cancer follow-up care. 46th Annual Cancer Symp Soc Surg Oncol 1993;150.
4. Gupta BK, Piedmonte MR, Karakousis CP. Attributes and survival patterns of multiple primary cutaneous malignant melanoma. Cancer 1991;67:1984-9.
5. Slingluff CL Jr, Vollmer RT, Seigler HF. Multiple primary melanoma: incidence and risk factors in 283 patients. Surgery 1993;113: 330-9.
6. Rivers JK, Kopf AW, Vinokur AF, et al. Clinical characteristics of malignant melanoma developing in persons with dysplastic nevi. Cancer 1990;65:1232-6.
7. Rigel DS, Rivers JK, Kopf AW, et al. Dysplastic nevi: markers for increased risk for melanoma. Cancer 1989;63:386-9.
8. Carey WP Jr, Thompson CJ, Synnestvedt M, et al. Dysplastic nevi as a melanoma risk factor in patients with familial melanoma. Cancer 1994;74:3118-25.
9. Gutman M, Cnaan A, Inbar M, et al. Are malignant melanoma patients at higher risk for a second cancer? Cancer 1991;68:660-5.
10. Kraehn GM, Schartl M, Peter RU. Human malignant melanoma: a genetic disease? Cancer 1995;75:1228-37.
11. Fawzy FI, Fawzy NW, Hyun CS, et al. Malignant melanoma. Effects of an early structured psychiatric intervention, coping, and affective state on recurrence and survival 6 years later. Arch Gen Psychiatry 1993;50:681-9.
12. Fusi S, Ariyan S, Sternlicht A. Data on first recurrence after treatment for malignant melanoma in a large patient population. Plast Reconstr Surg 1993;91:94-8.
13. Slingluff CL Jr, Dodge RK, Stanley WE, Seigler HF. The annual risk of melanoma progression. Implications for the concept of cure. Cancer 1992;70:1917-27.
14. Kelly JW, Blois MS, Sagebiel RW. Frequency and duration of patient follow-up after treatment of a primary malignant melanoma. J Am Acad Derm 1985;13:756-60.
15. McCarthy WH, Shaw HM, Thompson JF, Milton GW. Time and frequency of recurrence of cutaneous stage I malignant melanoma with guidelines for follow-up study. Surg Gynecol Obstet 1988;166:497-502.
16. Balch CM, Urist MM, Karakousis CP, et al. Efficacy of 2-cm surgical margins for intermediate-thickness melanomas (1 to 4 mm): results of a multi-institutional randomized surgical trial. Ann Surg 1993;218:262-9.
17. Reintgen DS, Vollmer R, Tso CY, Seigler HF. Prognosis for recurrent stage I malignant melanoma. Arch Surg 1987;122:1338-42.
18. Romero JB, Stefanato CM, Kopf AW, Bart RS. Follow-up recommendations for patients with stage I malignant melanoma. J Dermatol Surg Oncol 1994;20:175-8.
19. Gadd MA, Coit DG. Recurrence patterns and outcome in 1019 patients undergoing axillary or inguinal lymphadenectomy for melanoma. Arch Surg 1992;127:1412-6.
20. Warso MA, Das Gupta TK. Melanoma recurrence in a previously dissected lymph node basin. Arch Surg 1994;129:252-5.
21. Monsour PD, Sause WT, Avent JM, Noyes RD. Local control following therapeutic nodal dissection for melanoma. J Surg Oncol 1993;54:18-22.
22. Schultz S, Kane M, Roush R, et al. Time to recurrence varies inversely with thickness in clinical stage 1 cutaneous melanoma. Surg Gynecol Obstet 1990;171:393-7.
23. Briele HA, Beattie CW, Ronan SG, Chaudhuri PK, Das Gupta TK. Late recurrence of cutaneous melanoma. Arch Surg 1983;118:800-3.
24. Callaway MP, Briggs JC. The incidence of late recurrence (greater than 10 years); an analysis of 536 consecutive cases of cutaneous melanoma. Br J Plast Surg 1989;42:46-9.
25. Crowley NJ, Seigler HF. Late recurrence of malignant melanoma: analysis of 168 patients. Ann Surg 1990;212:173-7.
26. Shaw HM, Beattie CW, McCarthy WH, Milton GW. Late relapse from cutaneous stage I malignant melanoma. Arch Surg 1985;120: 1155-9.
27. Pearlman NW, Takach TJ, Robinson WA, Ferguson J, Cohen AL. A case-control study of late recurrence of malignant melanoma. Am J Surg 1992;164:458-61.
28. Koh HK, Sober AJ, Fitzpatrick TB. Late recurrence (beyond ten years) of cutaneous malignant melanoma: report of two cases and a review of the literature. JAMA 1984;251:1859-62.
29. Raderman D, Giler S, Rothem A, Ben-Bassat M. Late metastases (beyond ten years) of cutaneous malignant melanoma: literature review and case report. J Am Acad Dermatol 1986;15:374-8.
30. Day CL, Mihm MC Jr, Sober AJ, et al. Predictors of late deaths among patients with clinical stage I melanoma who have not had bony or visceral metastases within the first 5 years after diagnosis. J Am Acad Derm 1983;8:864-8.
31. Crowley NJ, Seigler HF. Relationship between disease-free interval and survival in patients with recurrent melanoma. Arch Surg 1992; 127:1303-8.
32. National Cancer Institute. After treatment of early melanoma, should patients and family members be followed? Why and how? NIH Consens Dev Conf Cons Statement 1992;10:1-26.
33. Balch CM, Soong SJ, Murad TM, Ingalls AL, Maddox WA. A multifactorial analysis of melanoma. II. Prognostic factors in patients with stage I (localized) melanoma. Surgery 1979;86:343-51.
34. Soong SJ, Shaw HM, Balch CM, McCarthy WH, Urist MM, Lee JY. Predicting survival and recurrence in localized melanoma: a multivariate approach. World J Surg 1992;16:191-5.
35. Coit DG. Role of surgery for metastatic malignant melanoma: a review. Semin Surg Oncol 1993;9:239-45.
36. Reintgen DS, Cruse CW, Wells KE, Saba HI, Fabri PJ. The evaluation of putative tumor markers for malignant melanoma. Ann Plast Surg 1992;28:55-9.
37. Mani S, Poo WJ, Cuny C. S100 as a potential serum marker in metastatic melanoma. Proc Am Soc Clin Oncol 1994;13:398.
38. Miliotis G, Cruse W, Puleo C, et al. The evaluation of new putative tumor markers for melanoma. 47th Annual Cancer Symp Soc Surg Oncol 1994;169.
39. Wong JH, Xu SH, Skinner K, Foshag LJ, Morton DL. Prospective evaluation of the use of antigen-specific immune complexes in predicting the development of recurrent melanoma. Arch Surg 1991; 126:1450-4.
40. Horikoshi T, Ito S, Wakamatsu K, Onodera H, Eguchi H. Evaluation of melanin-related metabolites as markers of melanoma progression. Cancer 1994;73:629-36.
41. Buzaid AC, Sandler AB, Mani S, et al. Role of computed tomography in the staging of primary melanoma. J Clin Oncol 1993;11: 638-43.
42. Harpole DH Jr, Johnson CM, Wolfe WG, George SL, Siegler HF. Analysis of 945 cases of pulmonary metastatic melanoma. J Thorac Cardiovasc Surg 1992;103:743-50.
43. Wong JH, Euhus DM, Morton DL. Surgical resection for metastatic melanoma to the lung. Arch Surg 1988;123:1091-5.
44. Gorenstein LA, Putnam JB, Natarajan G, Balch CA, Roth JA. Improved survival after resection of pulmonary metastases from malignant melanoma. Ann Thorac Surg 1991;52:204-10.
45. Brandt SE, Welvaart K, Hermans J. Is long-term follow-up justified after excision of a thin melanoma (less than or equal to 1.5 mm)? A retrospective analysis of 206 patients. J Surg Oncol 1990;43:157-60.
46. Jillela A, Mani S, Nair B, et al. The role of close follow-up of melanoma patients with AJCC stages I-III: a preliminary analysis. Proc Am Soc Clin Oncol 1995;14:413.

47. Shumate CR, Urist MM, Maddox WA. Melanoma recurrence surveillance: patient or physician based? Ann Surg 1995;221:566-71.
48. Ruark DS, Shaw HM, Ingvar C, Thompson JF, McCarthy WH. Who detects the first recurrence in stage I cutaneous malignant melanoma: patient or doctor? 46th Annual Symp Soc Surg Oncol 1993;149.
49. Baughan CA, Hall VL, Leppard BJ, Perkins PJ. Follow-up in stage I cutaneous malignant melanoma: an audit. Clin Oncol (R Coll Radiol) 1993;5:174-80.
50. Heaton KM, Rippon MB, el-Naggar A, Tucker SL, Ross MI, Balch CM. Prognostic implications of DNA index in patients with stage III cutaneous melanoma. Am J Surg 1993;166:648-53.
51. Karlsson M, Boeryd B, Carstensen J, Kagedal B, Bratel AT, Wingren S. DNA ploidy and S-phase fraction in primary malignant melanoma as prognostic factors for stage III disease. Br J Cancer 1993;67:134-8.
52. Dale PS, Wang Y, Conrad A, et al. Multiple marker polymerase chain reaction assay for evaluating circulating melanoma cells. Proc Am Soc Clin Oncol 1995;14:413.
53. Kirgan D, Guenther J, Bhattatiry M, et al. The importance of whole body PET scans on the management of metastatic malignant melanoma [abstract]. Proc Am Soc Clin Oncol 1994;13:396.
54. Pounds TR, Valk PE, Spitler L, Haseman MK, Myers RW, Lutrin CL. Metabolic PET imaging in detection of metastatic melanoma: comparison to CT imaging. Proc Am Soc Clin Oncol 1995;14:416.
55. Gritters LS, Francis IR, Zasadny KR, Wahl RL. Initial assessment of positron emission tomography using 2-fluorine-18-fluoro-2-deoxy-d-glucose in the imaging of malignant melanoma. J Nucl Med 1993; 34:1420-7.
56. Blend MJ, Ronan SG, Salk DJ, Gupta TK. Role of technetium 99m-labelled monoclonal antibody in the management of melanoma patients. J Clin Oncol 1992;10:1330-7.

➢ COUNTERPOINT

National Cancer Center Hospital, Japan

AKIFUMI YAMAMOTO

The yearly incidence of melanoma in Japan is estimated at 1,500 to 2,000 new cases,[1,2] and in recent years this level has been maintained or slightly increased. The incidence of melanoma in Japan is much lower than in the United States and has shown no trend toward marked increase. Because of the low incidence the public lacks sufficient medical knowledge about the disease, so that most patients are at advanced stages when they visit hospitals, leading to poor treatment outcomes. A large-scale educational campaign through the mass media must therefore be performed. It is important to make patients and their families understand the disease and the need for follow-up after treatment.

In Japan few nationwide studies on large numbers of patients with melanoma have been reported and there is almost no literature discussing follow-up of the disease. In this counterpoint the discussion of follow-up for patients with melanoma is based on an analysis of 494 patients treated through 1995 at the National Cancer Center Hospital, which has the most experience in treating patients with melanoma in Japan.

DETECTION OF RECURRENCE

The basic purpose of the follow-up of patients with cancer is early detection of recurrence. Although recurrent cancer is not always treatable and curable, early detection permits a better chance of cure. Close follow-up is therefore of great importance. However, it also involves a substantial financial burden and the need for frequent visits, which may create mental stress for patients or decrease their quality of life. An acceptable follow-up program with appointments at adequate intervals is required.

Detection of a Second Primary Melanoma

It has been well documented that patients who have had a primary cutaneous melanoma treated are at risk for a second primary melanoma.[3-6] This lifetime risk is estimated at 4% to 6%, but in Japanese patients the risk is very low. Second primary melanomas are rare, affecting only one of the 494 patients (0.2%) at the National Cancer Center Hospital. Therefore follow-up for the detection of a second primary melanoma is not considered as important in Japan, although follow-up clearly contributes to early detection of second primary melanomas or nonmelanoma skin cancers.

Patient Education

An integral part of the follow-up of patients with melanoma is education. Education is of great significance for self-examination by patients and for patients' family and friends to understand the disease. Patients should be taught to avoid excessive sun exposure to prevent the development of both melanoma and nonmelanoma skin cancer.

Screening for Other Primary Malignancies

In Japan no report has been made that patients with melanoma are at increased risk for other invasive noncutaneous malignancies. Screening systems are being organized in Japan, in which patients with high-incidence malignancies, such as gastric, lung, breast, uterine, and colorectal cancers, are screened in groups in the physician's office or local community hospital. As a routine part of follow-up of patients with melanoma to screen for the presence of metastases, physicians in Japan perform blood tests, chest x-rays, ultrasound of the abdomen, gallium tumor scintigraphy, and other examinations that permit the adventitious detection of other invasive noncutaneous malignancies, although with low frequency. For example, measurement of tumor markers such as alpha-fetoprotein and carcinoembryonic antigen as part of a blood examination may lead to the detection of primary hepatic or colorectal cancer.

Identification of Family Kindreds

In Japan the risk of melanoma in family members of patients with melanoma is extremely low and estimated at less than 1%. Therefore the identification of family kindreds appears to be less important in Japan.

Psychosocial Support

An important aspect of follow-up in patients with melanoma is the sense of reassurance that they have after a negative examination. At follow-up visits clinicians can give psychological support to patients anxious about the future.

Documentation of End Results

It is imperative that clinicians record and document the end results of patient treatment. This can improve the management of melanoma.

CURRENT PRACTICE

A rational program of follow-up for patients treated definitively for their primary cancer should be based on a thorough understanding of the natural history of the disease. An understanding of patterns of recurrence and time to recurrence should be used to design panels of follow-up examinations and to determine the frequency with which those examinations and investigations should be performed.

Pattern of Recurrence

In the aforementioned series recurrence took place in 18.2% of patients with clinical stage I to II melanoma. Of the patients with clinical stage I melanoma, 8.3% had recurrence, with 80% of these regional nodal recurrence and the remainder regional skin recurrence and in-transit metastasis. Of the patients with clinical stage II melanoma, 26.4% had recurrence, with 64.8% of these regional nodal recurrence and most of the remainder visceral metastases involving the lung, bone, brain, and other organs. In patients with advanced disease at diagnosis, the initial sites of extranodal metastasis were the cutaneous-subcutaneous (53%), lung (26%), liver (9%), bone (9%), and brain (3%).[7]

Based on the preceding data the follow-up of patients with clinical stage I melanoma should involve a complete dermatological examination and a diligent physical examination with special attention to the locoregional lymph nodes. Although the follow-up of patients with clinical stage II melanoma depends greatly on whether patients undergo elective lymph node dissection, a diligent physical examination should be performed similar to that performed for patients with clinical stage I melanoma. Periodic chest x-rays, ultrasound of the abdomen, nuclear medicine scans, and other examinations are also necessary.

Time Course to Recurrence

Retrospective analysis of patients at the National Cancer Center Hospital in Japan showed that recurrences in patients with clinical stage I melanoma became apparent at a minimum of 1 year and 7 months to a maximum of 9 years (median 6 years) after definitive treatment of the primary cancer, with a tendency for relatively late recurrence. This suggests that follow-up once or twice a year is sufficient. Recurrences in patients with clinical stage II melanoma were found at a minimum of 2 months to a maximum of 12 years (median 1.5 years) after definitive treatment of the primary tumor, with 57.9% of these becoming apparent within the first 2 years and 94.7% within the first 5 years. Within the first 2 years, therefore, follow-up should be performed every 3 months. Recurrences in patients with clinical stage III melanoma were recognized at a minimum of 1 month to a maximum of 5 years and 11 months (median 1 year) after definitive treatment of the primary tumor, with 61.7% of these becoming apparent within the first year, 79.0% within the first 2 years, and 96.3% within the first 5 years. This suggests that it is necessary to perform follow-up every 3 months within the first 2 years and to continue strict observation within the first 5 years. These data indicate that short intervals between examinations are necessary in patients with clinical stage II to III melanoma, particularly during the first 2 years after definitive treatment of the primary tumor, with increasing intervals after 5 years.

What Is Known About Current Practice

With regard to the follow-up of patients with melanoma, few organized studies have been reported in Japan. Physicians at the National Cancer Center Hospital classify patients with melanoma according to the TNM classification defined by the International Union Against Cancer for follow-up. As a rule, physicians consider it advisable to tailor follow-up based on the thickness of tumor. Patients with melanomas 0.75 mm or less in thickness and those with tumors 0.76 to 1.5 mm in thickness were not markedly different in prognosis,[8] and it is reasonable to group these patients together as 1.5 mm or less for follow-up. The 5-year survival was 89.3% in patients with tumors 1.51 to 3.0 mm in thickness, 62.6% in those with tumors measuring 3.01 to 4.0 mm, and 52.3% in those with tumors measuring 4.01 mm or more, showing that prognosis is poorer with tumors thicker than 3.0 mm.[8] Elective lymph node dissection is generally performed for patients with melanomas thicker than 3.0 mm. Therefore a reasonable follow-up schedule would divide patients into those with tumors 1.51 to 3.0 mm in thickness and those with tumors thicker than 3.01 mm. The 5-year survival of patients with clinical stage III melanoma who had no regional lymph node metastasis was 81.2%, but that of patients having regional nodal metastasis was 51.0%, showing an apparent difference in prognosis.[8] It is reasonable to make specific follow-up schedules for patients with regional nodal metastasis and for those without such metastasis.

Role of Physical Examination

Physical examination is the most important procedure in the follow-up of patients with melanoma. A careful visual observation and palpation can detect local recurrence, satellitosis, in-transit metastasis, and regional nodal metastasis and can also reveal metastases to remote nodes or soft tissue. Prognosis may be improved by surgical resection of these lesions. There is, however, almost no likelihood that visceral metastases will be detected by physical examination.

Role of Laboratory Tests

The laboratory plays a relatively limited role in the follow-up of patients with melanoma. In Japan the measurement of serum 5-S-cysteinyldopa level is considered useful in confirming the condition of patients with melanoma and in detecting recurrence.[9,10] Studies about this methodology are ongoing at a limited number of medical institutions,

Table 14-4 Follow-up of patients with cutaneous melanoma (primary tumors less than or equal to 1.5 mm thick, negative nodes): National Cancer Center Hospital, Japan

	YEAR				
	1	2	3	4	5
Office visit	2	2	1	1	1
5-S-cysteinyldopa	2	2	1	1	1
Lactate dehydrogenase	2	2	1	1	1
CEA	2	2	1	1	1
Alpha-fetoprotein	2	2	1	1	1
Chest x-ray	1	1	1	1	1

CEA, Carcinoembryonic antigen.

Table 14-5 Follow-up of patients with cutaneous melanoma (primary tumors 1.51 to 3 mm thick, negative nodes): National Cancer Center Hospital, Japan

	YEAR				
	1	2	3	4	5
Office visit	4	4	3	2	2
5-S-cysteinyldopa	2	2	1	1	1
Lactate dehydrogenase	2	2	1	1	1
CEA	2	2	1	1	1
Alpha-fetoprotein	2	2	1	1	1
Chest x-ray	1	1	1	1	1

CEA, Carcinoembryonic antigen.

including the National Cancer Center Hospital, and this technique may prove useful in follow-up care. The measurement of serum lactic dehydrogenase levels in patients with melanoma may also be useful to detect recurrence. Blood examination is easy to perform and permits measurement of tumor markers such as alpha-fetoprotein and carcinoembryonic antigen for other cancers. Currently it is recommended that laboratory tests be performed at relatively short intervals.

Radiology

In the follow-up of patients with melanoma at risk for systemic metastases, periodic chest x-rays are of the greatest importance because lung metastasis is most frequent and some patients with solitary lung metastasis can be saved by surgical treatment. Ultrasound of the abdomen can reveal liver or intraperitoneal lymph node metastases and should be a part of the follow-up strategy. Nuclear medicine scans are useful in detecting bone or brain metastasis, although they are not as sensitive as other examinations. Computed tomographic scanning is valuable to confirm lesions suspected on the basis of screening.

Treatment of Recurrence

Follow-up can permit early detection of recurrence and treatment with curative intent, resulting in a better prognosis. Even in patients who cannot tolerate operation and should receive other treatments, detecting metastasis in early stages when the tumor is as small in volume as possible and has not yet spread to multiple organs will increase response to treatment and improve life expectancy.

Physician- Versus Patient-Detected Recurrence

In the follow-up of patients with melanoma in the Japanese series, 36 (58.1%) of the 62 regional nodal and cutaneous-subcutaneous recurrences were patient detected and the remaining 26 (41.9%) were physician detected. Since the survival rate was 15.4% in the former cases and 19.4% in the latter, it is evident that patient education is important. Most visceral metastases are asymptomatic and detected by physicians, but the prognosis for these patients is dismal.

Table 14-6 Follow-up of patients with cutaneous melanoma (primary tumors greater than 3 mm thick, negative nodes): National Cancer Center Hospital, Japan

	YEAR				
	1	2	3	4	5
Office visit	4	4	3	2	2
5-S-cysteinyldopa	2	2	2	2	2
Lactate dehydrogenase	2	2	2	2	2
CEA	2	2	2	2	2
Alpha-fetoprotein	2	2	2	2	2
Chest x-ray	2	2	1	1	1
Abdominal ultrasound	2	2	1	1	1

CEA, Carcinoembryonic antigen.

FUTURE PROSPECTS

In Japan the optimal follow-up program for patients with melanoma is not likely to be defined by a prospective, randomized study, and this type of study appears not to be feasible. I suggest that ongoing follow-up should be performed according to the program currently regarded as optimal, with modification from time to time when new findings or useful examinations are discovered.

FINAL RECOMMENDATIONS

No optimal formula has been defined for the follow-up of patients with melanoma in Japan. Physicians at the National Cancer Center Hospital consider it necessary to perform ongoing follow-up based on the schedules described in Tables 14-4 through 14-7, so that they will be able to evaluate new treatment approaches and to make the pathophysiology of melanoma clearer. Because the incidence of second primary melanoma or familial melanoma is extremely low in Japan, follow-up for the detection of these has little significance. The most important purpose is to detect treatable local recurrence, since visceral metastases can rarely be treated successfully. Clinicians should not only make every

Table 14-7 Follow-up of patients with cutaneous melanoma (positive nodes): National Cancer Center Hospital, Japan

	YEAR				
	1	2	3	4	5
Office visit	4	4	3	2	2
5-S-cysteinyldopa	4	4	2	2	2
Lactate dehydrogenase	4	4	2	2	2
CEA	4	4	2	2	2
Alpha-fetoprotein	4	4	2	2	2
Chest x-ray	3	2	2	2	2
Abdominal ultrasound	2	2	1	1	1
Nuclear medicine scan	1	1	1	1	1

CEA, Carcinoembryonic antigen.

effort to improve the prognosis of patients with melanoma through follow-up, but also modify it into a better program when new findings or useful examinations are discovered.

REFERENCES

1. Ishihara K, Ikeda S, Mori S. Diagnosis, treatment and statistics of cutaneous malignant tumors in Japan. Skin Cancer 1994;9:7-17.
2. Ishihara K, Ikeda S, Hirone T, et al. Prognostic factors of malignant melanoma. Skin Cancer 1989;4:349-61.
3. Kang S, Barnhill RL, Mihm MC Jr, Sober AJ. Multiple primary cutaneous melanoma. Cancer 1992;70:1911-6.
4. Austin PF, Stankard CS, Cruse CW, Schroer K, Glass F, Reintgen DS. Multiple primary melanoma: evidence for the efficacy of screening and evidence against the minimalistic philosophies of cancer follow-up care. 46th Ann Cancer Symp Soc Surg Oncol 1993;150.
5. Gupta BK, Piedmonte MR, Karakousis CP. Attributes and survival patterns of multiple primary cutaneous malignant melanoma. Cancer 1991;67:1984-9.
6. Slingluff CL Jr, Vollmer RT, Seigler HF. Multiple primary melanoma: incidence and risk factors in 283 patients. Surgery 1993;113: 330-9.
7. Yamamoto A, Ishihara K. A statistical study of 242 cases of malignant melanoma. Acta Sch Med Univ Gifu 1987;35:207-37.
8. Ishihara K. Malignant melanoma statistics in Japan. Skin Cancer 1994;9:52-68.
9. Horikoshi T, Ito S, Wakamatsu K, Onodera H, Eguchi H. Evaluation of melanin-related metabolites as markers of melanoma progression. Cancer 1994;73:629-36.
10. Yamazaki N, Ishihara K, Wakamatsu K, Ito S. Evaluation of serum 5-S-cysteinyldopa as a biochemical marker of progression of malignant melanoma. Eur J Dermatol 1994;4:329-32.

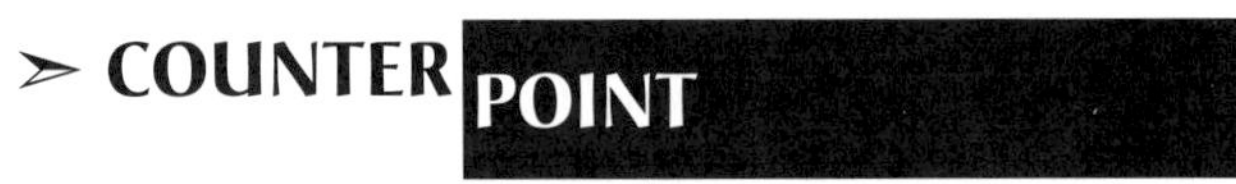

Royal Liverpool University Hospital, UK

SAM J. LEINSTER

Coit has thoroughly reviewed the evidence with regard to melanoma follow-up, and there is nothing to add to it. The translation of that evidence into recommendations for follow-up is, however, open to question. The pattern of follow-up suggested by Coit is based on acceptance of the rationale the author sets out. A critical appraisal of the rationale is therefore essential.

RATIONALE FOR FOLLOW-UP

Detection of Recurrence

No one would disagree that the fundamental assumption in cancer follow-up is that early detection of recurrence will improve long-term survival. There is, however, an unspoken assumption that follow-up by a physician will result in earlier detection than would occur if the patient were asked to report back at the first sign of any problems. This is based on the belief that the earlier treatment commences, the better will be the outcome. All of these assumptions must be tested before a treatment strategy can be formulated. A functional strategy must also take into account the fact that late recurrence can be seen.[1]

The evidence presented by Coit shows clearly that the majority of recurrences (63% to 94%) are detected by patients themselves rather than physicians.[2-5] Patients whose recurrences are detected by physicians do not have a better prognosis than those who detect their own recurrence.[3-5] I cannot find any evidence to the contrary. Based on this evidence, an intensive program of follow-up for the purpose of detecting recurrence is difficult to justify.

Detection of a Second Primary Cancer

The increased risk of a second primary melanoma is real but seems to be confined to particular groups of patients, particularly those with atypical nevi and a family history.[6] Surveillance may be effective in this group, but teaching all patients (including those at high risk) to maintain effective surveillance on themselves may also be possible. Population studies show that public education can result in the de novo presentation of thinner melanomas.[7] If this effect can be achieved in populations that are notoriously resistant to health education programs, similar results should be obtainable in patients who are already motivated as a result of having had a melanoma treated. Once again, there is a lack of evidence that physician surveillance will be more effective than patient education. A similar argument applies to the detection of other skin cancers in this group.

Patient Education

Patients should be encouraged to take active responsibility for their own follow-up and a program of patient education is essential. There are no studies of how frequently this education should be reinforced (if it should be reinforced at all), and better ways to reinforce education than through discussion at a follow-up visit may exist. Reiteration of information the patient does rapidly come to regard as routine will not necessarily encourage behavior modification.

Screening for Other Primary Malignancies

The effectiveness of screening in reducing mortality from other primary malignancies is the subject of considerable debate. Where screening is shown to be effective, it should be part of a structured program and not be conducted on an ad hoc basis. Within the United Kingdom the overall health maintenance of patients is the responsibility of their registered general practitioners, who arrange for screening not only for cancer, but also for other serious health problems such as hypertension or diabetes mellitus. Using melanoma follow-up as a focus for general health maintenance is not justified. Major screening programs such as those for breast or cervical cancer are funded and monitored by the Department of Health.

Identification of Family Kindreds

For many patients with familial melanoma the family history is elicited at the initial visit. When there is no family history of melanoma, the patient can be asked to report if a case subsequently occurs within the family. The patient does not need to visit the physician regularly to ensure that this information is recorded. Once the possibility of a familial link is apparent, other family members can be informed and advised to consult a physician. Since they will probably not all be within the same geographical area, they may have to seek help in their own locality.

Psychosocial Support

Psychosocial support for patients with cancer is paramount because up to 40% of patients may have significant psychological morbidity.[8] The psychological symptoms must be specifically sought. Patients expect the oncologist to be interested in their physical symptoms and may not disclose their psychological problems without specific enquiry being made.[9] If the patient has major psychological problems, the relief experienced at being told there is no recurrence will be temporary. Studies in the follow-up of other cancers show that the review visit is anxiety provoking in itself. Patients forget concerns about tumors until the time for review approaches, when all their worries come flooding back. The sense of reassurance after a negative examination is thus relieving an anxiety that was generated by waiting for that examination. The lessening of anxiety is more likely to be a function of the passage of time than the accumulation of negative examinations. The argument that psychosocial counseling may improve prognosis is an argument for establishing effective psychotherapeutic programs, not for instituting follow-up.

Documentation of End Results

The only noncontroversial reason for regular follow-up of patients with melanoma is the documentation of the end results of treatment. Good information is necessary if treatment programs are to be properly evaluated. In a health care system where every patient has a personal registered general practitioner, such information may be derived indirectly by requesting data from that physician. Patients with recurrence will be referred back in any case, and an annual verification of the well-being of the remainder can be carried out by mail.

Table 14-8 Follow-up of patients with cutaneous melanoma (primary tumors less than 0.76 mm thick, negative nodes): Royal Liverpool University Hospital, UK

	YEAR				
	1	2	3	4	5
Office visit	1	0	0	0	0

FOLLOW-UP SCHEDULE

The follow-up schedule should be determined by the patient's best interests. It does not seem reasonable to determine follow-up on the basis of what intervention the center conducting the follow-up is able to offer in the event that recurrence is detected. The patient should be offered the best follow-up possible, and if disease that cannot be treated by the supervising physician is detected, the patient should be offered the chance of referral to a center where the appropriate treatment can be offered. What then is the best follow-up schedule?

The major weakness of all the follow-up schedules discussed, including the National Cancer Institute consensus statement,[10] is that they appear to assume that follow-up will influence survival. As shown previously, for the majority of patients detection of recurrence by a physician at routine follow-up does not improve survival over detection by the patient. Follow-up visits seem pointless for unselected patients. Clearly a prospective, randomized study of close follow-up versus a policy of trusting the patient to return when recurrence is detected is needed. Alternatives to the suggested schedules are set out in the following sections.

Patients with Tumors Less Than 0.76 mm in Thickness

The chance of recurrence in this group of patients is low. Obviously, a postoperative visit is needed so that the histology and prognosis can be discussed with the patient (Table 14-8). At this visit the patient can be instructed about the need to be vigilant for new primary melanomas and to report any family members in whom melanoma develops. Patients do not need to be seen again, and physicians at Royal Liverpool University Hospital have adopted the policy of discharging them after the first postoperative visit. This is clearly different from the strategy at Memorial Sloan-Kettering Cancer Center, but annual review is illogical, since the gap between follow-up visits is so long that diagnosis could be delayed rather than expedited.

Patients with Tumors Greater Than 0.76 mm in Thickness

The risk of recurrence increases with increasing thickness of the tumor and with other factors such as the presence of ulceration. This group of patients warrants follow-up, and Coit's suggested schedule for physical examination in the

Table 14-9 Follow-up of patients with cutaneous melanoma (primary tumors at least 0.76 mm thick, negative nodes): Royal Liverpool University Hospital, UK

	YEAR				
	1	2	3	4	5
Office visit	3-4	3-4	3	0	0
Complete blood count*	1-2	1-2	1-2	0	0
Liver function tests*	1-2	1-2	1-2	0	0
Chest x-ray*	1	1	1	0	0

*The need for these tests and their appropriate frequency should form part of a comparative study of the effectiveness of follow-up in this group of patients.

first 3 years seems appropriate (Table 14-9). There is no evidence that chest x-rays and blood tests contribute to overall outcome, but the arguments for them are strong enough to indicate the need for a comparative study to include radiography and blood tests in the comparison.

Between 65% and 81% of recurrences take place during the first 3 years of follow-up. Thereafter the number of recurrences that will be detected at follow-up is low. Therefore it is more efficient and probably more effective to give responsibility to the patient and cease regular follow-up. This differs from Coit's recommendation of continued annual follow-up. A potential problem is that patients who have become accustomed to follow-up may be reluctant to stop attending. To avoid this the patient should be told from the beginning what will occur.

Patients with Positive Nodes

The follow-up of patients with positive nodes is more intensive; prolonged follow-up is indicated. Follow-up should continue for at least 5 years; the follow-up strategy recommended by Coit is reasonable (Table 14-10). Although this schedule is followed at Royal Liverpool University Hospital, the value of the various tests is open to challenge and is based on consensus rather than evidence of effectiveness.

Patients with Atypical Moles or a Family History

The National Cancer Institute recommendation for 3-month interval follow-up for a minimum of 2 years seems reasonable for patients who have atypical moles or a family history of melanoma.

SUMMARY

If the era of evidence-based medicine is to become a reality, courage will be needed to act in accordance with the evidence rather than with the consensus view. In the follow-up of melanoma, there is little evidence to support organized follow-up programs despite the consensus viewpoint. Large, long-term, prospective studies are needed to clarify the best practice in follow-up as well as primary treatment.

Table 14-10 Follow-up of patients with cutaneous melanoma (positive nodes)*: Royal Liverpool University Hospital, UK

	YEAR				
	1	2	3	4	5
Office visit	4	4	3	2	2
Chest x-ray	2	2	1	1	1
Complete blood count	2	2	1	1	1
Liver function tests	2	2	1	1	1

*The follow-up strategy I recommend is identical to the strategy recommended by Coit of Memorial Sloan-Kettering Cancer Center.

REFERENCES

1. McEwan L, Smith JG, Matthews JP. Late recurrence of localized cutaneous melanoma: its influence on follow-up policy. Plast Reconstr Surg 1990;86:527-34.
2. Brandt SE, Welvaart K, Hermans J. Is long-term follow-up justified after excision of a thin melanoma (less than or equal to 1.5 mm)? A retrospective analysis of 206 patients. J Surg Oncol 1990;43:157-60.
3. Jillela A, Mani S, Nair B, et al. The role of close follow-up of melanoma patients with AJCC stages I-III: a preliminary analysis. Proc ASCO 1995;14:413.
4. Shumate CR, Urist MM, Maddox WA. Melanoma recurrence surveillance: physician or patient based? Ann Surg 1995;221:566-71.
5. Ruark DS, Shaw HM, Ingvar C, Thompson JF, McCarthy WH. Who detects the first recurrence in stage I cutaneous malignant melanoma: patient or doctor? 46th Ann Symp Soc Surg Oncol 1993;149.
6. Mackie RM, McHenry P, Hole D. Accelerated detection with prospective surveillance for cutaneous malignant melanoma in high-risk groups. Lancet 1993;341:1618-20.
7. Herd RM, Cooper EJ, Hunter JA, et al. Cutaneous malignant melanoma: publicity, screening clinics and survival—the Edinburgh experience 1982-90. Br J Dermatol 1995;132:563-70.
8. Greer S, Moorey S, Baruch JD, et al. Adjuvant psychological therapy for patients with cancer: a prospective randomised trial. Br Med J 1992;304:675-80.
9. Maguire P, Faulkner A, Regnard C. Eliciting the current problems of the patient with cancer—a flow diagram. Palliat Med 1993;7:151-6.
10. National Institutes of Health Consensus Conference. After treatment of early melanoma, should patients and family members be followed? Why and how? NIH Consens Dev Conf Cons Statement 1992;10:1-26.

➢ COUNTERPOINT

Roswell Park Cancer Institute

James E. Spellman, Jr.

Coit presents an in-depth assessment of the important issues surrounding the follow-up of patients with melanoma, insightfully blending issues of risk and tests and offering prospects for the future with real concerns regarding cost containment. As pointed out, melanoma is a growing health concern. Recommendations for follow-up are currently based on the risk of recurrence. This risk has in part been defined by factors of prognostic importance that enable physicians to stratify patients into groups of greater or lesser risk for recurrence. These recommendations are guidelines and will certainly be modified as physicians develop ways to lessen a patient's risk of recurrence. As mentioned in Coit's synopsis, future prospects might depend on the development of molecular techniques to identify not only patients at high risk for recurrence, but also patients whose recurrence is undetectable through current technology.

One area where little effort has been expended in the United States to date is patient education. Here, the family practitioner may greatly reduce risk and costs. Cristofolini et al.[1] demonstrated that significant savings in the treatment of melanoma could be realized through the use of educational health campaigns directed at raising public awareness of risk reduction and early diagnosis. In today's environment of dwindling resources, reducing the cost of treatment and follow-up by lowering the number of patients with advanced disease or high risk may lessen the burden on an already financially stressed health care system.

The recommendations for follow-up of patients with melanoma proposed by Coit are similar in content and frequency to those currently used by the Melanoma Division at Roswell Park Cancer Institute (Tables 14-11 and 14-12). If at the end of 5 years of follow-up patients are well, annual visits are instituted. These recommendations are based on time to recurrence, as well as patterns and frequency of recurrence. Factors influencing the risk of recurrence for node-negative and node-positive patients have previously been elucidated.[2,3] The frequency of follow-up visits and the testing performed at these visits are designed to ensure that the risk of missing a clinical recurrence is less than 1%.[4] Requiring such a stringent detection rate may seem excessive. However, the majority of recurrences are treatable and demonstrate a survival benefit as a result of early intervention.

Despite the vigilant follow-up described by Coit, melanoma is a capricious disease. Recurrences beyond 10 years after treatment of the primary tumor do occur.[5] Even within the lowest risk group (patients with lesions of Breslow thickness 0.75 mm or less), there are those with lesions of Clark's levels IV and V who may be considered high risk.[6] Physicians must be cognizant of these unusual circumstances and not become complacent in the follow-up of patients.

Two new areas in the treatment of melanoma may present the physician with further information on which to base decisions for risk assessment and follow-up. A multiinstitutional trial is under way evaluating the efficacy of treating microscopic nodal disease based on the identification of the sentinel node.[7] In addition, recently published results of the Eastern Cooperative Oncology Group trial EST 1684 have demonstrated a benefit of the adjuvant use of interferon alpha-2b in patients with deep primary (T4) or regionally metastatic (N1) melanoma.[8] If proven beneficial, these treatments may dramatically alter future follow-up patterns for a significant proportion of the melanoma population.

Table 14-11 Follow-up of patients with cutaneous melanoma (primary tumors less than 1 mm thick, negative nodes): Roswell Park Cancer Institute

	YEAR				
	1	2	3	4	5
Office visit	2	2	1	1	1
Chest x-ray	2	2	1	1	1
Complete blood count	2	2	1	1	1
Liver function tests	2	2	1	1	1

Table 14-12 Follow-up of patients with cutaneous melanoma (primary tumors at least 1 mm thick, negative nodes or primary tumors of any thickness, positive nodes): Roswell Park Cancer Institute

	YEAR				
	1	2	3	4	5
Office visit	4	4	2	2	2
Chest x-ray	4	4	2	2	2
Complete blood count	4	4	2	2	2
Liver function tests	4	4	2	2	2

The follow-up of patients with melanoma has been well presented by Coit. The recommendations given are similar to those espoused by Roswell Park Cancer Institute and should be followed by all who undertake the care of patients with melanoma. Important issues regarding follow-up lie on the horizon. The institution of new therapies and the development of more sensitive detection techniques are certain to color decisions. In addition, dwindling resources may influence the way physicians are able to care for their patients while attempting to maintain the highest standards of care possible.

REFERENCES

1. Cristofolini M, Bianchi R, Boi S, et al. Analysis of the cost-effectiveness ratio of the health campaign for the early diagnosis of cutaneous melanoma in Trentino, Italy. Cancer 1993;71:370-4.
2. Balch CM, Soong SJ, Milton GW, et al. A comparison of prognostic factors and surgical results in 1,786 patients with localized (stage I) melanoma treated in Alabama, USA, and New South Wales, Australia. Ann Surg 1982;196:677-84.
3. Balch CM, Soong SJ, Murad TM, Ingalls AL, Maddox WA. A multifactorial analysis of melanoma. III. Prognostic factors in melanoma patients with lymph node metastases (stage II). Ann Surg 1981;193:377-88.
4. McCarthy WH, Thompson JF, Milton GW. Time and frequency of recurrence of cutaneous stage I malignant melanoma with guidelines for follow-up study. Surg Gynecol Obstet 1988;166:497-502.
5. Briele HA, Beattie CW, Ronan SG, Chaudhuri PK, Das Gupta TK. Late recurrences of cutaneous melanoma. Arch Surg 1983;118:800-3.
6. Morton DL, Davtyan DG, Wanek LA, Foshag LJ, Cochran AJ. Multivariate analysis of the relationship between survival and the microstage of primary melanoma by Clark level and Breslow thickness. Cancer 1993;71:3737-43.

7. Morton DL, Wen DR, Cochran AJ. Management of early-stage melanoma by intraoperative mapping and selective lymphadenectomy. Surg Oncol Clin North Am 1992; 1:247-59.
8. Kirkwood JM, Strawderman MH, Ernstoff MS, Smith TJ, Borden EC, Blum RH. Interferon alpha-2b adjuvant therapy of high-risk resected cutaneous melanoma: the Eastern Cooperative Oncology Group trial EST 1684. J Clin Oncol 1996;14:7-17.

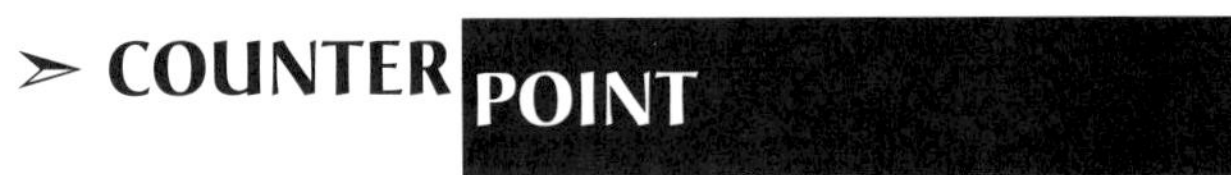

University of Washington Medical Center

DAVID R. BYRD

Critical challenges to traditional strategies for the follow-up of patients with cancer are long overdue. Cutaneous melanoma is a cancer with unpredictable clinical behavior for which follow-up planning often has been based on patient and physician anxiety rather than a critical analysis of the goals of follow-up. Coit has clearly and thoughtfully described the essential components and rationale for a modern approach to follow-up. Modifications to his suggestions are offered in Tables 14-13 and 14-14, which include recent information challenging the utility of laboratory testing and chest x-ray in asymptomatic patients.

FOLLOW-UP AFTER TREATMENT WITH CURATIVE INTENT

Coit has clearly stated the reasons for follow-up in the melanoma population, such as identification of recurrent disease amenable to additional treatment with curative intent, surveillance for new primary cutaneous melanomas, ongoing patient education to prevent and identify other health problems, and surveillance for nonmelanoma malignancies. Other factors include identification of familial melanoma or cancer family syndromes, alleviation of patient anxiety, and documentation of disease outcomes.

In Tables 14-1 through 14-3 Coit provides general guidelines for the frequency of follow-up examination and laboratory and radiological testing for patients with primary melanoma. Each table represents suggested follow-up for a different stage at diagnosis and appropriately reflects the wealth of retrospective information that is known about the time to recurrence and the patterns of failure for each stage. The cornerstone of follow-up is patient history and physical examination, and the suggested intervals reflect an accurate distillation of several articles that have critically examined the role of the physician and patient in the recognition of recurrence. Modification of these guidelines is appropriate for many patients based on differences in patient anxiety and concomitant risk factors. Although many patients are relieved by regular, frequent examinations, others have several days or weeks of escalating anxiety before each visit that may cause other somatic complaints.[1]

A recent article has legitimately challenged the role of blood tests and chest x-rays in the follow-up of patients with melanoma.[2] This study retrospectively analyzed 261 patients with high-risk melanoma who were enrolled in a prospective, randomized adjuvant trial through the North Central Cancer Treatment Group (NCCTG) from 1984 to 1990. Follow-up was intensive and included patient history, physical examination, complete blood count, blood chemistry panel, and chest x-ray. Of the 145 evaluable patients who had recurrence, 94% of recurrences were identified by patient history (68%) or physical examination (26%). Nine patients (6%) had an abnormal chest x-ray. In no instance was an abnormal laboratory test the sole indicator of recurrence.

In an asymptomatic patient it is reasonable to eliminate any routine blood testing during follow-up. In addition to the preceding study, no conclusive or even compelling evidence has appeared showing that laboratory testing is better than evaluation by history and physical examination in detecting early recurrences that are treatable with curative intent. An increasingly common scenario is the pursuit of subtle elevations of liver function tests found on routine blood testing. High-resolution computed tomography is then frequently performed and may identify subtle but indeterminate hepatic densities (which are often completely unrelated to the abnormal blood findings for which the scan was ordered). Patients are then subjected to invasive attempts at tissue diagnosis that are often inconclusive or are told that an interval scan in 2 to 3 months will discriminate between benign and malignant lesions. This not only markedly increases the costs of follow-up, but also adds considerable unnecessary anxiety for the patient. There is some optimism that newer sensitive whole blood or serum testing can identify viable circulating melanoma cells or cell products, but correlation with clinical outcome is lacking. At present, no

Table 14-13 Follow-up of patients with cutaneous melanoma (primary tumors less than 1 mm thick, negative nodes): University of Washington Medical Center

	YEAR				
	1	2	3	4	5
Office visit	2	2	1	1	1
Chest x-ray	1	1	1	1	1

Table 14-14 Follow-up of patients with cutaneous melanoma (primary tumors at least 1 mm thick, negative nodes or primary tumors of any thickness, positive nodes): University of Washington Medical Center

	YEAR				
	1	2	3	4	5
Office visit	3-4	3-4	2	2	2
Chest x-ray	1	1	1	1	1

effective treatment is available for metastatic melanoma that has spread beyond regional lymph nodes.

The role of interval chest x-rays in the follow-up of patients with melanoma is less clear. Although long-term survival may be achieved in a small subgroup of patients undergoing lung resection for isolated pulmonary metastases, the majority of patients with pulmonary metastases have multiple lesions or other distant metastatic sites and are not candidates for resection. Identifying the earliest sign of a pulmonary metastasis may be less important than identifying the subgroup of patients with indolent metastatic disease with solitary lesions. Since an isolated pulmonary metastasis may occur with equal frequency before and after 2 years of follow-up,[2] yearly chest x-rays would seem to yield an appropriate cost-effective balance during the first 5 years of follow-up.

Tables 14-13 and 14-14 provide a simplified hybrid of the suggested follow-up by Coit and the conclusions of the NCCTG as performed at the University of Washington Medical Center. New NCCTG protocol guidelines do not require routine laboratory tests and limit chest x-rays to once a year. Other cooperative oncology groups will likely follow similar guidelines. Future modifications will undoubtedly reflect the pressures of cost containment in the current health care environment.

RESIDUAL OR PROGRESSIVE DISEASE

In patients with residual or progressive disease after treatment, the major goal of follow-up should be to maintain or enhance the quality of life and performance status of the patient, since the chance of cure is negligible with current treatments. These patients face abandonment by those to whom they have entrusted their personal health, a fear that for some is nearly as intense as fear of their disease. This is often the most difficult clinical situation for cancer clinicians, since their extensive medical training and use of modern medical technology have failed to cure the patient. These patients benefit from personal contact with a caring physician, health care provider, medical social worker, and a patient care support group, since each of these offers complementary problem recognition and treatment skills.

The interval of scheduled clinic visits should reflect the anticipated rapidity of change in symptoms, the patient's anxiety, sense of well-being, and need to participate with the provider in assessing and determining subsequent treatment or direction of care, and identification of clinically silent toxic results of treatment and determination of tumor response in patients receiving systemic treatment. Patients with progressive melanoma often expect access to a caring professional on demand. This can be provided by visit, phone, or even electronic mail. No rigid schedule is clinically relevant to an individual patient. A careful history and examination during each scheduled and unscheduled visit may uncover subtle or underestimated symptoms that are treatable.

The compassionate and most appropriate follow-up of patients with advanced melanoma will remain one of the greatest challenges to the treating clinician. Physicians skilled enough to meet the medical and psychosocial needs of their patients will carry the additional challenge of teaching these skills to students of oncology and of communicating the legitimate needs of these patients to insurance companies and other health care payors.

REFERENCES

1. Loprinzi CL. Follow-up testing for curatively treated cancer survivors: what to do? JAMA 1995;273:1877-8.
2. Weiss M, Loprinzi CL, Creagan ET, Dalton RJ, Novotny P, O'Fallon JR. Utility of follow-up tests for detecting recurrent disease in patients with malignant melanomas. JAMA 1995;274:1703-5.

Table 14-15 Follow-up of patients with cutaneous melanoma by institution

YEAR/PROGRAM	OFFICE VISIT	CXR	CBC	LFT
Year 1				
Memorial Sloan-Kettering I[a]	2	1	1	1
Memorial Sloan-Kettering II[b]	3-4	1[c]	1-2	1-2
Memorial Sloan-Kettering III[d]	4	2	2	2
Roswell Park I[a]	2	2	2	2
Roswell Park II[e]	4	4	4	4
Univ Washington I[a]	2	1		
Univ Washington II[e]	3-4	1		
Japan: Natl Cancer Ctr I[f]	2	1		
Japan: Natl Cancer Ctr II[g]	4	1		
Japan: Natl Cancer Ctr III[h]	4	2		
Japan: Natl Cancer Ctr IV[d]	4	3		
UK: Royal Liverpool I[i]	1			
UK: Royal Liverpool II[j]	3-4	1[k]	1-2[k]	1-2[k]
UK: Royal Liverpool III[a,l]	4	2	2	2
Year 2				
Memorial Sloan-Kettering I[a]	2	1	1	1
Memorial Sloan-Kettering II[b]	3-4	1[c]	1-2	1-2
Memorial Sloan-Kettering III[d]	4	2	2	2
Roswell Park I[a]	2	2	2	2
Roswell Park II[e]	4	4	4	4
Univ Washington I[a]	2	1		
Univ Washington II[e]	3-4	1		
Japan: Natl Cancer Ctr I[f]	2	1		
Japan: Natl Cancer Ctr II[g]	4	1		
Japan: Natl Cancer Ctr III[h]	4	2		
Japan: Natl Cancer Ctr IV[d]	4	2		
UK: Royal Liverpool I[i]				
UK: Royal Liverpool II[j]	3-4	1[k]	1-2[k]	1-2[k]
UK: Royal Liverpool III[a,l]	4	2	2	2

ABD US abdominal ultrasound
AFP alpha-fetoprotein
CBC complete blood count
CEA carcinoembryonic antigen
CXR chest x-ray
LDH lactic dehydrogenase
LFT liver function tests
5-S-CYST 5-S-cysteinyldopa

5-S-CYST	LDH	CEA	AFP	ABD US	TUMOR SCAM
2	2	2	2		
2	2	2	2		
2	2	2	2	2	
4	4	4	4	2	1
2	2	2	2		
2	2	2	2		
2	2	2	2	2	
4	4	4	4	2	1

a Patients with primary tumors less than 1 mm thick, negative nodes.
b Patients with primary tumors at least 1 mm thick, negative nodes.
c Performed twice a year during years 1 and 2 for patients with primary tumors greater than 4 mm thick.
d Patients with positive nodes.
e Patients with primary tumors at least 1 mm thick, negative nodes or primary tumors of any size, positive nodes.
f Patients with primary tumors less than or equal to 1.5 mm thick, negative nodes.
g Patients with primary tumors 1.51 to 3 mm thick, negative nodes.
h Patients with primary tumors greater than 3 mm thick, negative nodes.
i Patients with primary tumors less than 0.76 mm thick, negative nodes.
j Patients with primary tumors at least 0.76 mm thick, negative nodes.
k The need for these tests and their appropriate frequency should form part of a comparative study of the effectiveness of follow-up in this group of patients.
l The follow-up strategy this author recommends is identical to the strategy recommended by Coit of Memorial Sloan-Kettering Cancer Center.

Continued.

Table 14-15 Follow-up of patients with cutaneous melanoma by institution–cont'd

YEAR/PROGRAM	OFFICE VISIT	CXR	CBC	LFT
Year 3				
Memorial Sloan-Kettering I[a]	1	1	1	1
Memorial Sloan-Kettering II[b]	3	1	1-2	1-2
Memorial Sloan-Kettering III[d]	3	1	1	1
Roswell Park I[a]	1	1	1	1
Roswell Park II[e]	2	2	2	2
Univ Washington I[a]	1	1		
Univ Washington II[e]	2	1		
Japan: Natl Cancer Ctr I[f]	1	1		
Japan: Natl Cancer Ctr II[g]	3	1		
Japan: Natl Cancer Ctr III[h]	3	1		
Japan: Natl Cancer Ctr IV[d]	3	2		
UK: Royal Liverpool I[i]				
UK: Royal Liverpool II[j]	3	1[k]	1-2[k]	1-2[k]
UK: Royal Liverpool III[a,l]	3	1	1	1
Year 4				
Memorial Sloan-Kettering I[a]	1	1	1	1
Memorial Sloan-Kettering II[b]	2	1	1	1
Memorial Sloan-Kettering III[d]	2	1	1	1
Roswell Park I[a]	1	1	1	1
Roswell Park II[e]	2	2	2	2
Univ Washington I[a]	1	1		
Univ Washington II[e]	2	1		
Japan: Natl Cancer Ctr I[f]	1	1		
Japan: Natl Cancer Ctr II[g]	2	1		
Japan: Natl Cancer Ctr III[h]	2	1		
Japan: Natl Cancer Ctr IV[d]	2	2		
UK: Royal Liverpool I[i]				
UK: Royal Liverpool II[j]				
UK: Royal Liverpool III[a,l]	2	1	1	1

5-S-CYST	LDH	CEA	AFP	ABD US	TUMOR SCAN
1	1	1	1		
1	1	1	1		
2	2	2	2	1	
2	2	2	2	1	1
1	1	1	1		
1	1	1	1		
2	2	2	2	1	
2	2	2	2	1	1

Continued.

Table 14-15 Follow-up of patients with cutaneous melanoma by institution—cont'd

YEAR/PROGRAM	OFFICE VISIT	CXR	CBC	LFT
Year 5				
Memorial Sloan-Kettering I[a]	1	1	1	1
Memorial Sloan-Kettering II[b]	2	1	1	1
Memorial Sloan-Kettering III[d]	2	1	1	1
Roswell Park I[a]	1	1	1	1
Roswell Park II[e]	2	2	2	2
Univ Washington I[a]	1	1		
Univ Washington II[e]	2	1		
Japan: Natl Cancer Ctr I[f]	1	1		
Japan: Natl Cancer Ctr II[g]	2	1		
Japan: Natl Cancer Ctr III[h]	2	1		
Japan: Natl Cancer Ctr IV[d]	2	2		
UK: Royal Liverpool I[i]				
UK: Royal Liverpool II[j]				
UK: Royal Liverpool III[a,l]	2	1	1	1

5-S-CYST	LDH	CEA	AFP	ABD US	TUMOR SCAN
1	1	1	1		
1	1	1	1		
2	2	2	2	1	
2	2	2	2	1	1

CHAPTER 15

Breast Carcinoma

Roswell Park Cancer Institute

STEPHEN B. EDGE, ELLIS G. LEVINE, MARK A. ARREDONDO, AND HALUK TEZCAN

Breast cancer is the most common cancer in women requiring follow-up in modern oncology practice. Although lung cancer recently eclipsed breast cancer as the leading cause of cancer death in women, a much higher proportion of women survive breast cancer. In the United States annually, breast cancer develops in 182,000 women and 46,000 die of the disease.[1] Thus more than 1 million women in the United States at any one time are under surveillance for recurrence within 10 years of treatment.

Not only is breast cancer common, but surveillance must extend into the second decade of follow-up. Because of the large proportion of women surviving breast cancer, strategies for follow-up must also account for the risk of new primary breast cancer as well as other cancers. Follow-up must allow for the impact of primary therapy on recurrence risk and time to recurrence. For example, breast-sparing surgery changes the nature of local disease follow-up and adjuvant systemic therapy may delay recurrence.

Cancer recurrence surveillance strategies hinge on whether detection of recurrence before appearance of symptoms increases the odds of favorable outcome measured by length or quality of life. The clinical practice after primary therapy has been follow-up with various imaging and laboratory studies to detect recurrences at an earlier asymptomatic stage. The intent is to treat these recurrences earlier and to improve the length and quality of life of affected women. Despite intensive surveillance more than two thirds of patients still present with symptomatic metastases.[2] Furthermore, no highly effective systemic therapy has been developed for metastatic breast cancer. Treatment for recurrence is curative in only a few circumstances, such as local recurrence after breast-sparing therapy. Treatment for bony or visceral metastases is not curative except in isolated cases and in a small percentage of the few who undergo high-intensity chemotherapy. Few data indicate that treatment of subclinical metastatic disease improves outcome. There is hope that in the future—possibly the near future—new, more effective therapies will be developed. However, until more effective therapy is available, follow-up strategies should be consistent with the uncertainty about whether early detection of metastatic disease offers longer or higher quality of life.

Because of the large number of women involved, determination of the most appropriate surveillance strategy has an important impact in human and economic terms. Withholding effective tests affects thousands of lives, but blind application of tests is inappropriately expensive if it offers no medical or emotional benefit. Because of the numbers involved, breast cancer surveillance has been studied extensively by the academic community. In addition, health care payors are seeking objective data on effectiveness of follow-up testing to determine what insurance benefits should be provided.[3]

Surveillance practice in the United States varies widely.[4-6] Many factors influence practice. Among these are the expectations of patients that physicians should be able to screen for and treat recurrence. With increased networking among patients, individuals not receiving aggressive follow-up hear about additional blood and imaging tests from women receiving intensive surveillance. Appropriately, such patients ask their own physicians about these tests and may have them performed. Furthermore, patients seeing several physicians may have different tests performed by each one. A recent example of this is a primary physician ordering quarterly CA 15-3 tests for a woman with ductal carcinoma in situ.

Cold facts must be tempered by sensitivity to the concerns of women facing breast cancer follow-up. Breast cancer is a lifelong diagnosis that irreversibly changes the lives of affected women and their families. Providers must remain cognizant of emotional issues. Follow-up visits which the physician considers routine are stress-laden events for the woman whose life hangs in the balance. Understanding, individual and group support, and ongoing education are vital to helping women maintain physical and mental well-being.

GENERAL MEDICAL SURVEILLANCE

General Considerations

Breast cancer follow-up must include attention to general medical care. Most women survive breast cancer. It is important that general medical care not slip between the cracks of specialty care. In the changing environment of health care organization, responsibility for follow-up may fall on a wide variety of professionals. Whoever provides care should determine that the woman's overall medical needs are met.

Most women continue follow-up with specialty physicians (oncologists and surgeons). Many curtail primary care visits under a potentially erroneous assumption that the specialist oversees all care. The specialist must either provide the care or ensure that the woman continues with her primary care providers. A trend within some health maintenance organizations is for primary care specialists to provide all cancer follow-up care. Primary care physicians performing cancer follow-up must be aware of oncological issues and provide necessary examinations, screening tests, and emotional support services.

Risk and Genetic Counseling

Approximately 15% of breast cancers occur in identifiable inherited patterns. An important element of breast cancer follow-up is addressing concerns about family risk for cancer. As understanding of breast cancer biology and genetics expands, more accurate testing and risk prediction will be available. Those providing breast cancer follow-up should be aware of the facts and should make available to patients and families the resources in their community for genetic counseling and testing.[7]

ESTROGEN REPLACEMENT THERAPY

Postmenopausal estrogen replacement therapy reduces the risk of early death from cardiovascular disease and osteoporosis. Estrogens are generally withheld from women with breast cancer out of concern that recurrence not be promoted.[8-10] Unfortunately, there are essentially no data on the use of estrogen in women with breast cancer. Because of the real benefits of estrogen and the high proportion of women with early-stage breast cancer who will never have a recurrence, this question is under reexamination. The Eastern Cooperative Oncology Group breast committee reviewed this issue and is considering a clinical trial that will examine the question.[11] One single-institution study is under way.[12] At this time routine estrogen replacement is not recommended for women after treatment of breast cancer.

SCREENING FOR NONBREAST SECOND MALIGNANCIES

Women with breast cancer are at slightly increased risk for colon, ovarian, and endometrial cancers. Some women may have breast cancer as part of a known inherited syndrome. Appropriate screening for these cancers is an important element of breast cancer follow-up. Minimum follow-up should include colon cancer screening by the American Cancer Society guidelines and a yearly pelvic examination and Papanicolaou (Pap) smear. Any new screening strategies developed for these cancers should be considered for inclusion in breast cancer follow-up.

SECOND PRIMARY BREAST CANCER

In women with breast cancer a new primary cancer may develop in the opposite breast or, after breast-conserving therapy, in the same breast. After 10 years the risk of a new breast cancer is equal to or even greater than the risk of recurrence of the index cancer. In the Memorial Sloan-Kettering Cancer Center series of node-negative breast cancer, a new primary malignancy was detected in the contralateral breast in 9% of patients at 10 years and in 13.9% at 20 years.[13] Tamoxifen adjuvant therapy reduces the risk of contralateral breast cancer by about 40%.[14] All women with breast cancer should undergo lifelong screening for a new breast cancer with monthly self-examination, yearly professional examination, and yearly mammography (Table 15-1).

Table 15-1 Follow-up of patients with breast cancer: Roswell Park Cancer Institute

	YEAR				
	1	2	3	4	5
Office visit	4	2	2	2	2
Liver function tests*	4	2	2	2	2
Mammography†	2	1	1	1	1
Pelvic examination	1	1	1	1	1
Papanicolaou test	1	1	1	1	1
Chest x-ray	1	1	1	1	1
Bone scan	‡	‡	‡	‡	‡
Abdominal computed tomography	‡	‡	‡	‡	‡
Abdominal ultrasound	‡	‡	‡	‡	‡
Chest computed tomography	‡	‡	‡	‡	‡
Pelvic ultrasound	‡	‡	‡	‡	‡
Endometrial biopsy	‡	‡	‡	‡	‡
CEA	§	§	§	§	§
CA 15-3	§	§	§	§	§

CEA, Carcinoembryonic antigen.
*Consists of alkaline phosphatase and lactic dehydrogenase.
†Mammography should begin at 6 months after radiation for breast-conserving therapy.
‡Performed if clinically indicated.
§If recurrence is documented, it may be useful for assessing treatment response.

IMPACT OF CANCER THERAPY: TOXICITY AND TREATMENT-INDUCED CANCER

Adjuvant systemic therapy reduces the risk of recurrence and prolongs survival.[15] Recurrences may also be delayed, prolonging the period of recurrence risk. Adjuvant tamoxifen, cytotoxic chemotherapy, and radiation also carry some long-term risks, including increased risk of other cancers.

Tamoxifen

The use of tamoxifen as adjuvant therapy for early-stage breast cancer increased steadily through the 1980s. It has few immediate side effects, especially in postmenopausal women.[14] However, in addition to its antiestrogenic effects, tamoxifen has weak estrogen agonist activity. It may therefore have an effect on the endometrium similar to that of unopposed estrogen, leading to an increased risk of endometrial cancer and possibly other uterine tumors. The estrogenic effect of tamoxifen also increases the rate of thromboembolic disease. Evidence has been reported of a slight increased risk of gastrointestinal cancers with tamoxifen, but concerns about liver cancer with tamoxifen appear unfounded.[16]

Multiple studies demonstrate an elevated risk of endometrial cancer with tamoxifen.[17-20] The Swedish Adjuvant Tamoxifen Trial was the first controlled trial to document this risk.[20,21] This study compared tamoxifen at 40 mg per day for 2 and 5 years versus a placebo. The risk of endometrial cancer in the tamoxifen group was six times that of the placebo. There was a nonsignificant trend to higher risk with longer term therapy.

The level of risk at the current standard tamoxifen dose (20 mg per day) is best estimated from the National Surgical Adjuvant Breast and Bowel Project (NSABP) B-14 placebo-controlled trial of tamoxifen in women with estrogen receptor–positive, node-negative cancer.[19] Tamoxifen decreased the annual rate of breast cancer relapse from 45 out of 1,000 women to 25 out of 1,000 and increased the annual rate of endometrial cancer from zero to 1.2 per 1,000 for women taking tamoxifen (relative risk 7.5). However, with only two cases of endometrial cancer in the control group, a more appropriate comparison may be found in Surveillance, Epidemiology, and End Results (SEER) data, which would predict seven endometrial cancers in the control group, yielding a relative risk of 2.2.

Tamoxifen-associated endometrial cancer probably has no more or less aggressive behavior than endometrial cancer in women not treated with tamoxifen. One group reported that tamoxifen-associated endometrial cancer is more aggressive.[22] However, in virtually every other series the majority of cancers are early stage and low grade, with stage and expected cure rates that do not differ from endometrial cancer in women not treated with tamoxifen.[17,19,20,23] Postmenopausal women appear to be at most risk for endometrial cancer with tamoxifen,[17-19] but it has developed in premenopausal women. A recent metaanalysis of this issue concluded that tamoxifen increases the annual risk of endometrial cancer from one in 1,000 to two in 1,000. Moreover, the analysis concludes that there is no strong association with duration of therapy, that endometrial cancer in tamoxifen-treated women does not carry an unusually poor prognosis, and that the benefit of tamoxifen outweighs the risk in terms of lives saved.[24]

Endometrial cancer screening should be included in the follow-up of all women taking tamoxifen. All women taking tamoxifen should be questioned at each visit about symptoms suggestive of gynecological disorders and should undergo a pelvic examination and Pap smear annually. The majority of women with tamoxifen-associated endometrial cancer have postmenopausal bleeding. Therefore this symptom should prompt full evaluation, including sampling of the endometrium. If results are negative, appropriate hormonal therapy for the bleeding is reasonable. If bleeding persists, hysteroscopy, dilation and curettage, and possibly hysterectomy are indicated.

The roles of routine uterine ultrasound and endometrial biopsy are controversial. Many women taking tamoxifen have demonstrable endometrial abnormalities. Endometrial thickness, uterine size, and uterine blood flow measured by transvaginal ultrasound are significantly greater in tamoxifen-treated women.[25-29] Between 80% and 90% of postmenopausal women taking tamoxifen have endometrial thickness greater than the normal 5 mm. Endometrial biopsy reveals a significantly higher incidence of proliferative changes in women taking tamoxifen compared with control groups.[25-28] In 111 postmenopausal women randomly assigned in a tamoxifen breast cancer prevention trial, the placebo group and tamoxifen groups had, respectively, 90% and 61% atrophic endometrium, 6% and 13% proliferative endometrium, zero and 16% atypical hyperplasia, and 2% and 8% polyps.[28] None had endometrial cancer. There was a significant correlation between endometrial thickness and histological abnormalities. All women with atypical hyperplasia or polyps had endometrial thickness greater than 8 mm.

The role of routine endometrial screening for women taking tamoxifen remains unresolved. The risk of endometrial cancer death from a cancer not detected until an advanced stage is very low. The result of such screening may be withdrawal of tamoxifen in a high proportion of women, denying them the benefit of tamoxifen. Strategies such as periodic progesterone therapy for all women taking tamoxifen, or selectively for those who demonstrate endometrial abnormalities, require clinical investigation. There is no evidence to support the use of routine screening endometrial biopsy or uterine ultrasound.[30,31]

Chemotherapy

Long-term toxicity from standard adjuvant breast cancer chemotherapy is rare. Symptomatic cardiac toxicity of anthracyclines is rare at the cumulative doses used in breast cancer treatment.

Chemotherapy does not appear to increase the risk of other solid tumors. The only malignancy consistently associated with the use of chemotherapy after a diagnosis of breast cancer has been myelodysplastic syndrome/acute leukemia (MDS/AL). These diagnoses represent a continuum. Fortunately, the adjuvant chemotherapy regimens that are currently applied—cyclophosphamide, methotrexate, and 5-fluorouracil (5-FU); cyclophosphamide and adriamycin; and cyclophosphamide, adriamycin, and 5-FU—appear to be associated with no or minimal added risk of this greatly feared complication.[32-36] Although high rates of MDS/AL have been reported after the adjuvant therapy of breast cancer, their association has been with agents both no longer typically used (chlorambucil and prednimustine) and continued at a duration much longer than currently recommended.[37]

Despite the assurances provided by the preceding data, the momentum toward the use of more dose-intensive regimens has caused the issue of MDS/AL to resurface. The report of six leukemias (typically of the M4/M5 subtype and with 11q23 chromosomal abnormalities) over an alarmingly short follow-up period in the NSABP B-25 trial has raised concerns. In NSABP B-25, women are randomly assigned to receive cyclophosphamide at 1200 mg/m^2 × 4 versus 2400 mg/m^2 × 2 versus 2400 mg/m^2 × 4 along with doxorubicin at 60 mg/m^2.[38] Although the cumulative incidence of MDS/AL reported is less than 1%, more cases are anticipated. Ultimately, if an increase in MDS/AL rates proves to be an unwelcome accompaniment of dose-intensive therapies, this risk will need to be weighed against the additional benefits provided by these therapies. No specific monitoring for chemotherapy-induced neoplasms is necessary.

Surgery and Radiation

Long-term risks of surgery in women with breast cancer include lymphedema and surgical deformity. Physicians should understand that recovery of body image is an important element of breast cancer treatment. When a mastectomy is necessary for cancer treatment, women should be informed of reconstruction and cosmetic options. In most cases reconstruction can be performed at the time of the mastectomy. For those who choose not to do this, those who were not offered this option, or those for whom it was deemed inappropriate, delayed reconstruction should be made available.

Lymphedema is a permanent swelling of the arm after surgery or irradiation of the axilla in breast cancer. With less radical surgery in recent decades, the incidence of lymphedema has dropped. At least mild lymphedema develops in 5% to 20% of women.[39,40] Lymphedema may not develop for many months or years after treatment. The combination of radiation and axillary dissection for women with more extensive nodal involvement increases the risk of lymphedema.[41,42] All women should be warned of the risk and signs of lymphedema and cellulitis. Surveillance history and examination of patients should include evaluation for lymphedema.

Long-term effects of radiation are relatively uncommon. Brachial plexus symptoms develop in less than 2%, are usually self-limiting, and are related to the extent of nodal radiation and use of chemotherapy.[43] Rib fracture is rare. Pneumonitis develops in 1% of patients or less.[44] Radiation to the left chest wall with a mastectomy or breast-conserving therapy slightly increases the risk of death from ischemic heart disease.[45,46]

Radiation also conveys a slight risk of second malignancy. Sarcomas of the breast, angiosarcoma of the skin, and osteosarcoma may occur in as many as 0.2% with a mean latency period of more than 10 years.[47-49] Lung cancer risk is increased on the side treated. The relative risk of lung cancer determined by a study of SEER data and the Connecticut State Tumor Registry is 2.0 and 1.8 or an estimated nine cases per 10,000 treated patients at 10 years.[50,51] Risk is markedly increased in smokers after 10 years (a relative risk of 32).[52] However, because the data derive from women treated before 1980 when the volume of lung treated was much greater than now, these figures probably overstate the risk.[51,52] Adjuvant radiotherapy does not seem to increase the risk of contralateral breast cancer.[53]

PATTERNS OF RECURRENCE AND SURVEILLANCE FOR RECURRENCE

Patterns of Recurrence: An Overview

It is necessary to understand the patterns of breast cancer recurrence, the time frame of recurrence, and the impact of adjuvant therapy to develop surveillance strategies. In the majority of women with breast cancer, recurrence never develops. However, the risk of recurrence extends over many years. It is possible that all women with invasive breast cancer have microscopic metastases at diagnosis. Some believe that recurrence simply reflects the rate of proliferation of a given cancer.[54] The risk of recurrence for invasive breast cancer varies from less than 5% to greater than 80% depending on factors including tumor size, grade, and lymph node status. Other prognostic indicators and a combination of factors under investigation may allow more accurate outcome prediction.[55,56] When such prediction is a reality, adjuvant treatment and follow-up surveillance strategies may require reconsideration.

Breast cancer may recur in the local tumor bed (breast or mastectomy scar), in regional lymph nodes, and at distant sites. The most common site of distant metastases is bone, followed by lung and pleura, liver, soft tissue, and brain.[57,58] Recurrence risk is highest in the first 2 to 5 years after diagnosis[58-60] and decreases with time.[61] However, as many as 10% of recurrences occur beyond 10 years.[13,54,61,62] Therefore, although surveillance for recurrence is best focused on the early years, it must extend into the second decade of follow-up.

Most series report that both local and distant recurrence risks peak in the early years of follow-up and then decrease. However, Veronesi et al.[63] reported that local recurrence after breast-conserving therapy remained stable at about 1% per year over the first 10 years, compared with the early high rate and late low rate of distant failure (Figure 15-1).

Adjuvant therapy alters the patterns of recurrence. Local recurrence risk is reduced by cytotoxic chemotherapy and by tamoxifen.[16,64,65] Distant recurrence risk is reduced by adjuvant therapy, but even for those with eventual recurrence, adjuvant therapy may have delayed the time to first recurrence. Adjuvant chemotherapy may affect distant site risks differently, having a greater impact on soft tissue and less impact on bony and visceral metastases.[64]

The data supporting follow-up testing for various local and distant sites are reviewed below, followed by concrete recommendations for each site. The follow-up tests performed at Roswell Park Cancer Institute are presented in Table 15-1. In general terms, breast cancer follow-up relies on clinical history and examination plus mammography and chest x-ray. Except for women with intraductal cancer, recommendations do not differ by disease stage. Although it is

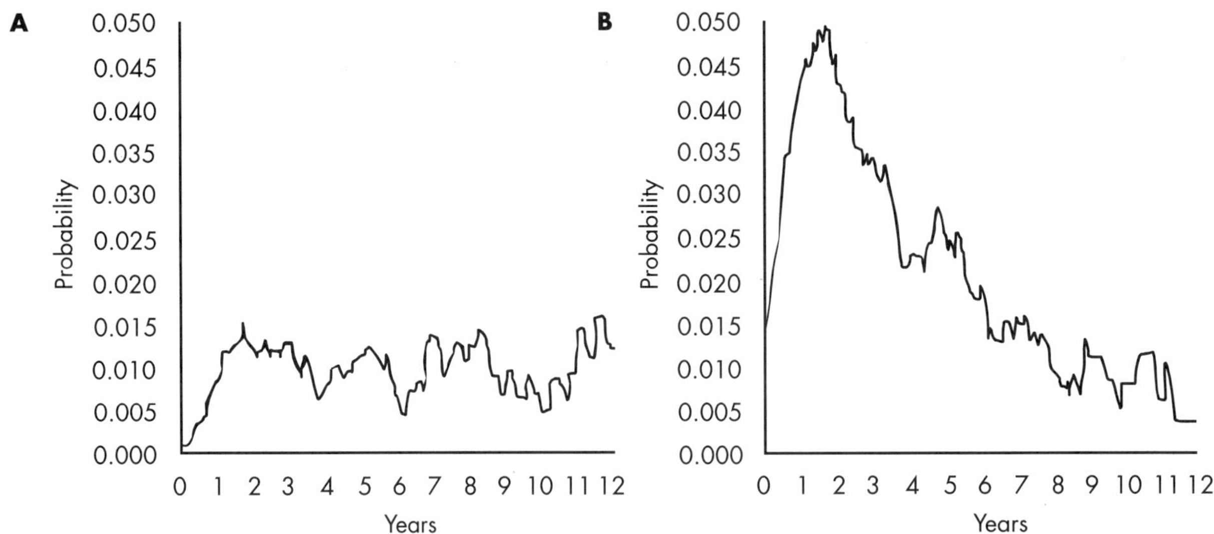

Figure 15-1 Time course of, **A**, local and, **B**, distant recurrence after breast cancer diagnosis for 1,124 women treated by breast-conserving surgery, radiation, and appropriate systemic adjuvant therapy (yearly event probability). (Data from Veronesi U, Marubini E, Del Vecchio M, et al. J Natl Cancer Inst 1995;87:19-27.)

tempting to perform more intensive testing on women with more advanced disease, the data do not support this practice.

Locoregional Recurrence

Isolated locoregional recurrence accounts for 15% to 30% of first recurrences. Supraclavicular nodal recurrence is considered metastatic (M1) disease according to the rules of the International Union Against Cancer and the American Joint Committee on Cancer. Unfortunately, many reports combine local and regional recurrence in the same figure and include supraclavicular recurrence as regional recurrence.

In a recent series locoregional recurrence after mastectomy occurred by 5 years in 8.4% of patients (164 of 1,243), of whom half were node negative,[66] 11% (245 of 2,240) by 10 years at Guy's Hospital,[57] and 8% (37 of 430) by 8 years (66% node negative) in a Norwegian series.[59] Local relapse risk after mastectomy is related to tumor size and nodal status. After radical mastectomy in 716 women, rates of locoregional failure, identified as the site of first recurrence after 10 years, were 6% of node-negative and 18% of node-positive women.[60] When women with simultaneous distant and locoregional recurrences are included, the locoregional recurrence rates were 8% for node-negative and 27% for node-positive women. Two recent series confirm this high rate of locoregional recurrence after mastectomy in node-positive disease, even among women who received adjuvant systemic therapy. The Ludwig Group reported locoregional failure in 13% of 491 women with one to three positive nodes and 18% of 327 women with more than three positive nodes.[67] The North Central Cancer Treatment Group reported an isolated locoregional recurrence rate of 20% and total locoregional recurrence of 36% for 564 women who received adjuvant chemotherapy in controlled trials at 8 years after mastectomy.[68]

Although most reports do not distinguish between chest wall (local) and nodal (regional) recurrence, those that do show that one half to two thirds of locoregional recurrences are found in the chest wall. The Ludwig Group reported combined chest wall and contralateral breast cancer recurrence rates of 7% local versus 12% total locoregional recurrence in women with one to three positive nodes and 8.6% local versus 18% total locoregional recurrence in women with more than three positive nodes.[67] In the Norwegian series two thirds (22 of 37) of locoregional recurrences occurred in the chest wall only and one third (15 of 37) included supraclavicular and axillary nodal recurrence.[59] Radiation therapy after mastectomy reduces the incidence of local recurrence but does not improve survival.[69]

Breast-conserving therapy provides an ultimate outcome equivalent to total mastectomy.[70] In most circumstances breast-conserving therapy consists of wide local excision (lumpectomy), axillary lymph node dissection, and whole breast radiation therapy (with or without a radiation boost to the site of the primary tumor). In the United States breast-conserving therapy is being used in an increasing proportion of patients with early-stage breast cancer. In addition, it is appropriate in some circumstances after cytoreductive chemotherapy for larger cancers.

The average risk of local recurrence in T1 and T2 breast cancer after breast-conserving therapy is about 10%.[70] Factors influencing the local failure risk include tumor size, lymph node status, and histological features including grade, peritumoral lymphatic permeation, surgical margins, and the extent of intraductal cancer associated with an invasive cancer.[63] Radiation after surgical excision is an integral part of breast-conserving therapy. Local failure risk is 20% to 40% if whole breast radiation is omitted.[65,71] Systemic adjuvant therapy influences the rate of local recurrence.[16,65] In the NSABP B-14 study of tamoxifen in node-negative, estrogen receptor–positive breast cancer, only 2% of women receiving tamoxifen after breast-conserving therapy had local recurrence.

Most ipsilateral breast cancer events after breast-conserving therapy are true recurrences of the primary tumor. However, the treated breast is also at risk of a new primary cancer. Distinguishing between a new primary and a recurrence may be difficult. Between 5% and 30% of ipsilateral events are in a site in the breast distant from the original tumor, and these events tend to occur later than those in the original quadrant, presumably signifying a new primary tumor.[72,73]

Although local recurrence after breast-conserving therapy is generally an isolated event, women who have local recurrence are at greater risk for distant metastases than those who do not.[63,74] Most series report that about two thirds of women with local recurrences will be successfully treated and not subsequently have distant metastases.[72,74] One group reported that women who have recurrence of invasive disease are at a greater than 50% risk of distant recurrence.[75] Local recurrence may simply be an indicator of more aggressive disease and not a source of the metastases itself.[63] This view is shared by the NSABP, which documented that after treatment with breast-conserving therapy without radiation compared with treatment with radiation, a similar number (but smaller proportion) of women who had local recurrence did not have metastatic disease.[72] Treatment for local recurrence after breast-conserving therapy in most circumstances is total mastectomy. Select cases may be treated by reexcision of the tumor without mastectomy or with lumpectomy and radiation if radiation was originally withheld (ductal carcinoma in situ or select patients with invasive cancer in clinical trials).

Distant disease recurrence risk is the same for women treated by breast-conserving therapy and mastectomy. Local recurrence risk is a major issue in selecting initial treatment and in planning follow-up care. In selection of the mode of local therapy the risks of local recurrence after breast-conserving therapy must be balanced against the real risk of local recurrence after mastectomy. The Royal Marsden Hospital reported total locoregional failure in 15% of women treated with wide excision and radiation, compared with 13% of women treated by mastectomy.[76]

Ductal carcinoma in situ may also be treated by breast-conserving therapy.[77] Ductal carcinoma in situ carries virtually no risk of systemic recurrence. Breast recurrence after this disease is invasive in about 50% of cases. Factors that influence local recurrence risk include tumor size, adequacy of resection, use of radiation therapy, and the histological subtype of ductal carcinoma in situ. Noncomedo (papillary, solid, and cribriform) carcinoma and low-grade ductal carcinoma in situ confer a lower risk of local failure than the comedo form. The risk of local recurrence with lumpectomy plus radiation in ductal carcinoma in situ is also approximately 10%. Controversy continues over the use of radiation therapy. The only controlled trial of radiation in ductal carcinoma in situ showed that radiation reduced the local failure rate by two thirds.[78] However, many authorities believe that small lesions, particularly of the noncomedo, low-grade subtypes, have a low recurrence risk and that radiation should not be administered to these women.[79]

The risk of local failure after lobular carcinoma in situ is included for completeness. Lobular carcinoma in situ is not truly a cancer. The diagnosis of lobular carcinoma in situ increases a woman's risk of future breast cancer at any location in either breast. This risk is about 0.5% to 1% per year after diagnosis of lobular carcinoma in situ.[80,81] Women with lobular carcinoma in situ should be followed up with periodic examinations and an annual mammography and be counseled regarding breast cancer risk like any woman with increased breast cancer risk. No other intervention is warranted.[82]

Surveillance for Locoregional Recurrence

Local recurrence after mastectomy

Regular screening for local recurrence after mastectomy is important because intervention controls disease in a significant proportion of women.[83] Where possible, excision of the recurrent disease, followed by chest wall radiation, permanently controls local disease in approximately 50% of women. Many of these women will not have recurrence at distant sites.[69,84,85]

The only effective screening test for local recurrence is regular physical examination. Women should be encouraged to perform self-examination on the mastectomy scar. Suspect findings include a change in the thickness or width of the scar, skin nodules, fixation of the skin to chest wall structures, or erythema similar to that of inflammatory breast cancer.

Local recurrences generally occur as palpable cutaneous lesions. Mammography of the chest wall scar or axilla after mastectomy is technically possible, but periodic mastectomy site mammography detected no local recurrences that were not suspected clinically in a series of 827 women.[86] In another study, mastectomy site mammography was found to be inferior to clinical examination and ultrasound.[87] Surveillance with mastectomy site mammography is therefore not indicated in breast cancer follow-up.

Local recurrence after breast-conserving therapy

Monitoring for local recurrence after breast-conserving therapy includes the triad of self-examination, professional examination, and mammography. After completion of radiation the breast undergoes predictable changes in physical and mammographic appearance.[88] Change is the most rapid in the first 6 months, but some changes take longer to stabilize (Figure 15-2). Any remaining seroma and mass in the lumpectomy site generally disappear by 6 months. Skin dis-

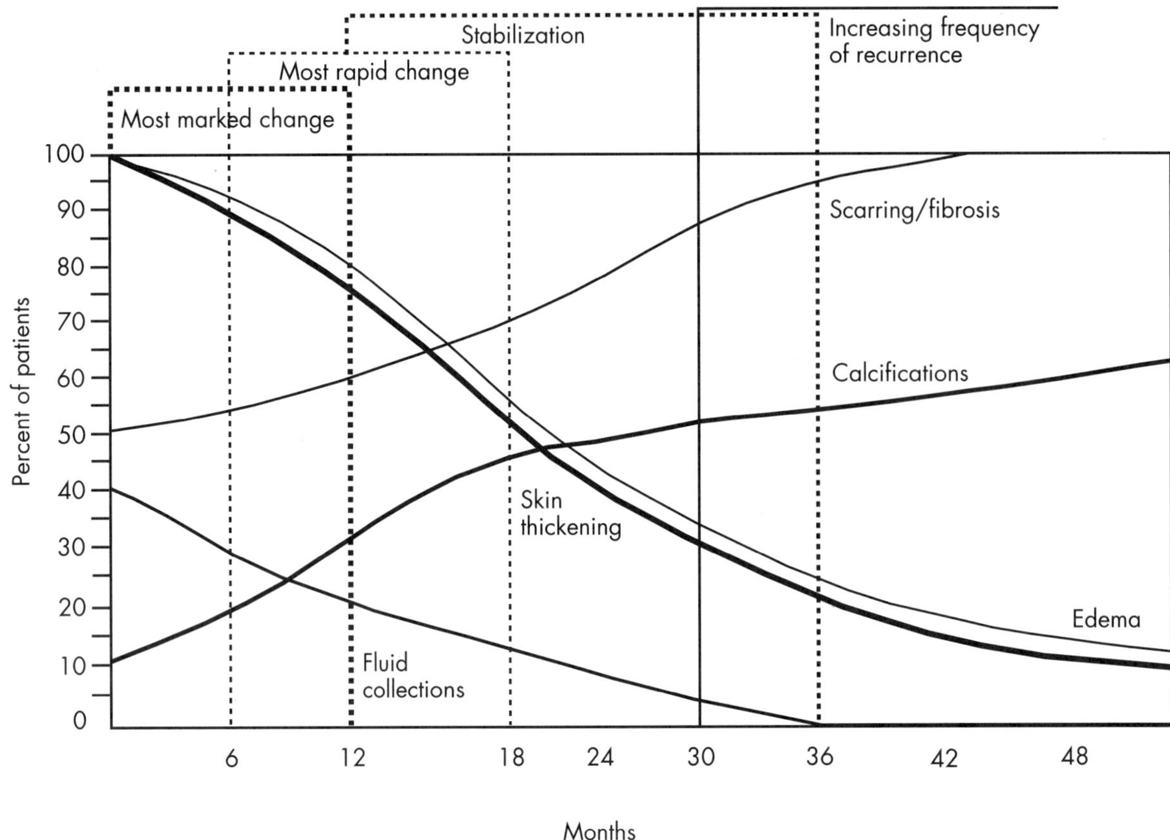

Figure 15-2 Time course of changes in the conservatively treated breast. (Modified from Mendelson EB. Radiol Clin North Am 1992;30:107–38.)

coloration from radiation generally peaks and subsides by 6 months. The degree of change is mostly stabilized by 12 months after radiation, with further slow improvement subsequently. Skin retraction over the biopsy site develops in a small fraction of women and is permanent. A seroma or scar felt as a mass may be a permanent finding in some cases. Enlargement of a mass in the biopsy site or skin changes after this time should prompt suspicion of recurrence and careful evaluation. The woman should be encouraged to perform self-examination and to alert her physician of any changes. The breast and regional nodes should be examined at every follow-up visit.

Mammography should be performed before radiation to ensure completeness of resection.[88] The first postradiation mammography should be performed 6 months after radiation, although some physicians believe it should be delayed until 9 to 12 months.[89] Earlier mammography is of no value because of the edema and skin changes. Thus a mammogram obtained before 6 months does not serve as a useful baseline. The risk of recurrence in this time-frame is low.

The second postradiation mammogram should be obtained 6 months later to demonstrate stability of the breast parenchyma.[88,90] If the breast is mammographically stable and there are no suspect findings, mammography should be performed annually. If substantial nodularity or stable calcification is present, mammography can be repeated earlier. To avoid confusion between the radiologist and clinician over which mammogram is the annual film, all mammograms should include the contralateral breast.

Mammography should be supplemented by ultrasound according to standard clinical guidelines. Other ancillary imaging tests may prove useful in the future. Gadolinium-enhanced magnetic resonance imaging may aid in determining if clinical or mammographic findings represent recurrent cancer, but its role as a surveillance test is as yet undefined.[91]

Many clinicians perform mammography at 6-month intervals for 2, 3, or more years after radiation.[88,92] The only harm of increased frequency of mammography is the added expense and worry for the patient. Taking all these factors into account, a recent multispecialty society task force published guidelines for mammography after breast-conserving therapy, recommending studies at 6 and 12 months after radiation, followed by annual screening (Table 15-1).[70]

Local recurrence after breast reconstruction

For women who need mastectomy, reconstruction of a breast mound is an excellent alternative for cosmetic and psychological benefits. Options include subpectoral implants (including tissue expanders) and autogenous tissue transfer. Reconstruction can be performed in most cases at the time of mastectomy without compromising cancer care. The risk of local recurrence after reconstruction is the same as after mastectomy without reconstruction. In a series of 306 women treated by immediate reconstruction (95% were implants), 16 (5%) had chest wall recurrence and 11 (3%) had regional node recurrence.[93]

Treatment for local recurrence is the same as after mastectomy without reconstruction: resection of known disease and radiation. If the implant is not removed with the recurrence, radiation leads to capsular contracture, which is often painful, in about half of patients.[93] With treatment, local recurrence after reconstruction has the same implications for ultimate outcome as discussed previously. A concern is that reconstruction will delay the detection of locoregional recurrence. This appears to be unfounded, since the outcome for these women is no different than for those without reconstruction.[84,93]

Physical examination and history are the most important tests for recurrence. Imaging studies have generally not been used for the reconstructed mound.[94] An x-ray is performed on tissue that lacks all the architectural characteristics of the breast, and therefore the hallmarks of cancer on breast mammography may not apply to the reconstructed breast. Surgical changes in the muscle, fat, and skin of the mound may appear suspect compared with breast mammography. These include calcifications, masses of fat necrosis, and foreign body reactions.[95] Mammography of the mound might detect recurrence in the skin or subcutaneous tissue. Lesions on the chest wall, a common site of local recurrence, are as likely to be missed as they are in breast mammography. On the other hand, isolated cases of local recurrence in the reconstructed breast mound have been described.[94] One group recommends mammography every 6 months.[96] However, the weight of evidence at this time is that the yield of mammography of the simulated breast is low and is not valuable in follow-up.[88]

Regional recurrence after mastectomy and breast-conserving therapy

Axillary nodal recurrence occurs in a small fraction of women after mastectomy. Physical examination is the most sensitive screening test for axillary recurrence and should be performed at every follow-up visit. Local recurrence in the axilla may produce pain. Neurological changes in the arm or increasing stiffness of the shoulder may herald recurrence in or around the brachial plexus. Careful physical examination of the axilla and the supraclavicular region identifies the majority of such recurrences. Lateral mammographic views of the axilla after mastectomy performed in two large practices discovered no additional lesions in comparison with physical examination.[88,97] Imaging with computed tomography or magnetic resonance imaging supplements physical examination in this situation and may help distinguish between postsurgery radiation scarring and recurrent cancer.[98,99]

The International Union Against Cancer and the American Joint Committee on Cancer classify supraclavicular nodal disease as distant metastatic disease. However, supraclavicular nodal recurrence may be successfully controlled by radiation alone or in combination with systemic therapy. A significant proportion of women with isolated supraclavicular recurrence have prolonged disease-free life after radiation therapy. Examination of the supraclavicular and cervical node chains on both sides is an integral part of every breast cancer follow-up examination (Table 15-1).

Surveillance for locoregional recurrence should include history, self-examination, and periodic physical examination (Table 15-1). Mammography of the mastectomy site or reconstructed breast is not necessary. Mammography of the conserved breast should be performed at 6 and 12 months after completion of radiation (or after surgery if radiation is not performed) and annually thereafter, including the contralateral breast.

Distant Metastases: An Overview

After curative surgery with or without adjuvant therapy, 5% to 80% of women with varied prognostic factors are expected to have recurrence within 5 years of their primary therapy. More than half of these recurrences are distant metastases involving bone, lung or pleura, liver, central nervous system, or other organs.[2,66,100]

Many investigators have tried to identify prognostic factors (tumor or treatment characteristics) that may predict recurrence in distant organs. Estrogen receptor–negative tumors tend to recur in visceral sites (lung, pleura, liver, or central nervous system) more often than those that are estrogen receptor positive.[101,102] Estrogen receptor status does not predict the time to relapse or incidence of distant metastases.[101] In a retrospective study the mean S-phase fraction of the primary tumor was higher in patients with recurrence in the liver or brain than in patients whose relapse was locoregional.[103] Kamby et al.[104] reviewed the effects of adjuvant systemic therapy on the pattern of metastases in the Danish Breast Cancer Cooperative Group protocol-77 experience. Although systemic chemotherapy (cyclophosphamide alone or cyclophosphamide, methotrexate, and 5-FU) in premenopausal or perimenopausal women reduced the total number of metastatic sites, the incidence of liver disease was increased compared with the untreated control subjects. In this study the tamoxifen-treated patients had an increased incidence of lung metastases without a change in the overall incidence of distant metastases. Miura et al.[105] studied the ethnic differences in the patterns of relapse of breast cancer patients from Japan and the United Kingdom. The Japanese patients had a significantly higher incidence of metastases in the supraclavicular fossa (22 of 36 local recurrences) and the lung (12 of 52 distant recurrences) compared with patients from the United Kingdom (12 of 37 local recurrences and 5 of 78 distant recurrences, respectively). Currently, none of these factors are compelling enough to cause a change in the overall practice of breast cancer follow-up.

The detection of asymptomatic metastases depends on the screening study used and its sensitivity and specificity. The incidence, presentation, and methods of detection of common sites of distant metastases are described below.

Bone Metastases

The skeletal system is the most common site for distant metastases after treatment for primary breast cancer. Between 8% and 21% of all women treated for primary breast cancer have recurrence first and only in the bone when followed up with yearly or more frequent radionuclide bone scans.[2,66,106] Bone metastases represent 26% to 38% of all recurrences and 41% to 51% of distant metastases.[2,58,66,106] In an additional 10% to 20% of women the bone is involved in conjunction with another site, most commonly the lung or liver. The risk of recurrence is highest in the first 3 years after treatment of primary breast cancer.[2,107] Almost 80% of the bone metastases that are found as an initial recurrence occur during this interval.

The most common site for bone metastases is the pelvis, followed by the spine, skull, and ribs. Bone metastases usually cause pain or neurological symptoms because of nerve root or cord compression. The radionuclide bone scan is the most sensitive imaging study to detect bone metastases from recurrent breast cancer. Sensitivity has been estimated to be 98% or better.[108] Specificity of the bone scan, however, depends heavily on the experience of the interpreter and clinical and x-ray correlation of the hot spots. In a retrospective study by Jacobson et al.[109] of the 239 new bone scan abnormalities detected during the follow-up of 242 breast cancer patients, only 54 (23%) were actual metastases. Various criteria have been proposed to improve the specificity of an abnormal study: the number of lesions, site of the lesion, type (lytic or blastic) of lesions on the plain radiographs, and normal-appearing plain radiographs in a patient with abnormal uptake on bone scan. Jacobson et al.[109] have demonstrated that with increasing numbers of new lesions on bone scan, the likelihood of metastases increases. All patients with five or more new lesions were eventually found to have metastatic disease. The involvement of the axial skeleton is more likely to represent metastases than rib involvement. Plain radiographs of the abnormal lesions are helpful, since lytic or blastic lesions correlate more with malignancy than sclerotic lesions. In addition, the finding of a normal radiograph in the area of an abnormal bone scan is highly suggestive of early metastases. Despite these adjunctive criteria, specificity of the bone scan remains radiologist dependent and ranges between 12% and 66%.

The initial enthusiasm for posttreatment surveillance using bone scans was generated in part by the report by Gerber et al.[110] in 1977. They showed that bone scan was a sensitive test to detect early recurrences in patients with breast cancer. Of 47 patients with breast cancer with follow-up bone scans, 12 had bone metastases detected by a bone scan, and in 11 of these patients the bone was the first site of recurrence. Based on their observation they suggested that routine follow-up bone scans may detect early recurrences in the bone and the subsequent initiation of early chemotherapy or immunotherapy may change the outcome. Hence bone scans (every 6 months to annually) became a routine follow-up test until the mid-1980s, at which time various investigators questioned the role of this test.

In retrospective analyses of the data collected during cooperative group studies in which routine bone scans for follow-up were undertaken (at yearly or shorter intervals), the majority of patients with breast cancer (more than 75%) who had bone metastases had bone pain, pathological fracture, or abnormal serum chemistry findings, prompting unscheduled studies.[59,106,111] Alternatively, only 18% to 35% of patients with bone metastases were asymptomatic and the metastases were detected with a routine scheduled bone scan.[106,111] In the NSABP B-09 study in which a follow-up bone scan was performed every 6 months for 3 years and annually thereafter, 250 bone scans were performed to detect each asymptomatic patient with bone metastasis.[106] Two recent surveys of U.S. oncologists have demonstrated a change in trend; only 20% to 25% of physicians routinely order annual or more frequent bone scans after curative breast surgery and adjuvant therapy.[4,5]

Two recent prospective, randomized studies from Italy add further support to the inability of routine bone scans to prolong survival. The Italian investigators in the Gruppo Interdisciplinare Valutazione Interventi in Oncologia (GIVIO) compared intensive follow-up with nonintensive follow-up.[2] For the former cohort, bone scans were performed annually for 2 years, then every other year. Among the latter, bone scans were performed only when clinically indicated. The number of bone metastases detected in the first 5 years was the same in both groups. Rosselli Del Turco et al.[66] compared intensive follow-up—bone scans every 6 months for the first 5 years—with nonintensive follow-up. The intensive follow-up group had more distant metastases detected, including in the bone, than the clinical follow-up group. However, both studies showed no difference between the two groups in overall survival at 5 years.

Plain radiographs of the skeletal system are not sensitive (approximately 40%) for the detection of early metastases and therefore are not recommended for follow-up. Computed tomography offers three-dimensional information and high-quality images but is impractical for imaging more than a defined area and is prohibitively expensive. Magnetic resonance imaging produces excellent images of the bone marrow and allows differentiation between benign and malignant disease processes within the marrow cavity. However, as with computed tomography, magnetic resonance imaging is unlikely to become a routine test because of its expense and limited availability.

Osteoblasts are rich in alkaline phosphatase. Since release of this enzyme into the circulation gives some indication of osteoblastic activity, it has been used as a marker of bone metastases in various malignancies. Pedrazinni et al.[112] reviewed the utility of elevated serum alkaline phosphatase in detecting bone metastases. In this retrospective study 1,371 patients were followed up with yearly bone scans and alkaline phosphatase. The sensitivity of the alkaline phosphatase was 50%, which is somewhat higher than other studies.[113] In another retrospective study Hannisdal et al.[59] showed that an alkaline phosphatase level that was elevated 10% above each individual's baseline had a sensitivity of 35% in detecting distant metastases. In a smaller study by Hayward et al.[114] alkaline phosphatase and serum lactic dehydrogenase were shown to be good negative predictors. In 105 patients with normal levels of alkaline phosphatase and lactic dehydrogenase, only one (0.95%) had a positive bone scan. Although alkaline phosphatase measurement is not sensitive (20% to 35%) enough to be used for early detection of bone metastasis, elevated levels of either alkaline phosphatase or lactic dehydrogenase may prompt the physician to obtain a bone scan or liver imaging in an otherwise asymptomatic patient.[113,114]

Surveillance for bony metastases should include periodic directed history and physical examination (Table 15-1). Alkaline phosphatase and lactic dehydrogenase determination is included twice a year at Roswell Park Cancer Institute. Bone scan, x-rays, and magnetic resonance imaging should be reserved for evaluation of clinically suspect symptoms or signs.

Intrathoracic Recurrence

The lung and pleura combined are the second most common site for distant metastases after primary surgical treatment for breast cancer with or without adjuvant therapy.[2,59,66,102,107,115-119] The recurrence rate of breast cancer in the lung and pleura as the initial site of disease is 5% and ranges from 2% to 10% in various studies that had a median follow-up of 5 or more years.[2,59,66,102,107,115-119] This site constitutes about 18% (range 12% to 29%) of all distant metastases at the time of breast cancer recurrence. As with all metastases, the risk of recurrence is highest in the first 3 years after diagnosis and decreases gradually with each following year.[2]

Parenchymal lung metastases (fewer than six metastases) are usually asymptomatic.[116] Only 5% of patients with a single nodule and 35% with multiple pulmonary nodules are symptomatic at presentation.[118] These patients have nonspecific complaints of cough and decreased exercise tolerance. In contrast to parenchymal lesions, pleural lesions are usually symptomatic (89%), producing cough, shortness of breath, or pain.[118]

Chest x-ray has been the screening test of choice for recurrences in the lung and pleura. Chest x-ray is a sensitive imaging modality for pleural effusions as small as 150 ml. Its ability to resolve parenchymal lesions begins at around 1 to 2 centimeters. The sensitivity of chest x-ray in detecting breast cancer metastases to the chest has been estimated to be 86%.[118] Although multiple pulmonary nodules are highly suggestive of metastatic breast disease, pleural effusion, solitary nodules, or pulmonary infiltrates are nonspecific findings. A single nodule raises the possibility of a primary lung cancer.

The availability and relatively low cost of chest x-ray have been reasons for its use in routine screening of patients with breast cancer after primary therapy. Despite its ability to detect asymptomatic metastases in the chest a median of 13 months earlier than among patients presenting with symptoms, the long-term survival has not differed between the groups.[120] Ciatto et al.[118] reviewed the impact of chest x-ray in the follow-up of 1,697 patients with breast cancer. During the follow-up period, 523 patients had relapse, 67 patients had isolated lung and pleural metastases, and another 71 patients had metastases in multiple sites, including the lung and pleura. Of the 67 patients (58%) with isolated lung and pleura metastases, 39 were asymptomatic. In this study 11,543 chest x-ray examinations were performed to detect these 39 asymptomatic chest recurrences. No difference in survival was measured from the time of therapy for metastatic disease between the asymptomatic group (39 patients) with isolated metastases and the group with symptoms (28 patients). The failure of routine chest x-ray examination to improve survival has been observed in many other retrospective studies.[116,121-123]

Two randomized studies from Italy support the conclusion obtained from retrospective studies that routine follow-up chest x-ray has no benefit in improving survival or quality of life. The GIVIO investigators compared intensive follow-up with nonintensive follow-up.[2] The former group had chest x-rays every 6 months, whereas the latter had chest x-ray performed only when clinically indicated. There was no difference in the incidence of lung and pleural metastases, overall survival, and quality of life between the two groups in the first 5 years. Rosselli Del Turco et al.[66] compared intensive follow-up—chest x-ray every 6 months—with nonintensive follow-up. The number of lung and pleural metastases detected was higher in the group receiving intensive follow-up (28 of 622) than that with nonintensive follow-up (18 of 621). However, the overall 5-year survival for both groups was identical. Quality-of-life parameters were not assessed in this study.

Computerized axial scanning has better resolution than chest x-ray, resulting in greater sensitivity. At present the lack of evidence of improved survival after earlier detection of distant metastases and the institution of current treatment modalities do not warrant the routine use of more expensive imaging modalities for follow-up of asymptomatic patients. The diagnostic use of computed tomography should be limited to cases in which chest x-ray is inadequate for the diagnosis of a symptomatic patient. Surveillance for intrathoracic recurrence should consist of periodic history and physical examination and annual chest x-ray (Table 15-1).

Liver Metastases

The liver is the third most common site for metastatic recurrence after primary therapy for breast cancer. Isolated liver metastases constitute approximately 3% to 9% of recurrences and 5% to 11% of distant metastases.[2,100,115,119] The majority of recurrences in the liver are associated with concurrent locoregional or other distant metastasis (in the bone or lung).[119,124] As with all recurrences, the risk of liver metastases is highest in the first 2 to 3 years (yearly incidence of 1% to 2%) and then gradually declines.[107,124]

Two thirds of patients with liver metastases have either new complaints or an enlarged liver on routine physical examination. The most frequent complaint is a dull ache in the right upper quadrant of the abdomen. Patients may also have nonspecific complaints such as nausea, vomiting, malaise, and weight loss. Jaundice is not a common presenting symptom.[124] On physical examination, typical findings include an enlarged liver with an irregular edge that is usually hard and nodular, ascites, and jaundice. About one third of patients with liver metastases are asymptomatic.

Radionuclide scanning, ultrasound, computed tomography, or magnetic resonance imaging can be used to image the liver for the detection of hepatic lesions. Several studies have evaluated the sensitivity and specificity of each of these modalities in detecting hepatic metastases.[125,126] When compared with computed tomography or ultrasound in the detection of metastatic disease of the liver, magnetic resonance imaging has the same or better sensitivity and superior specificity. The availability and expense of the three imaging studies should determine the initial choice of imaging modality. If the ultrasound or computed tomography results are not conclusive, the physician may consider magnetic resonance imaging to confirm the diagnosis.

Alkaline phosphatase, aspartate aminotransferase, and total bilirubin are relatively inexpensive studies that may aid in the diagnosis of liver metastases. About 90% of the patients with liver metastases have elevated alkaline phosphatase. Aspartate aminotransferase elevation can be seen in 70% of patients. Total bilirubin elevation is less common in early disease.

Screening for liver metastases using imaging studies has not been popular because of the low incidence of isolated liver recurrences and expense of these studies. Kauczor et al.[127] retrospectively reviewed 2,657 abdominal ultrasound examinations of 414 patients with breast cancer over a 5-year follow-up period.[127] Only 26 of 2,657 examinations (less than 1%) demonstrated liver metastases.

The GIVIO investigators compared an intensive follow-up group (yearly ultrasound studies) with a control group (imaging studies performed only when clinically indicated) in a randomized manner.[2] The disease-free and overall survival rates of both groups were identical in the first 5 years. Imaging studies (ultrasound, computed tomography, or magnetic resonance imaging) therefore should be reserved for confirmation of clinical or laboratory suspicion of liver involvement. Surveillance for liver metastases should consist of periodic history and physical examination and biannual alkaline phosphatase measurement (Table 15-1).

Central Nervous System Metastases

The incidence of central nervous system metastases as a site of first recurrence is relatively low (2% to 7%).[100,119] Since routine imaging of the brain is not performed, almost all patients have central nervous system symptoms or positive physical examination findings. The most common complaint is new onset of headache. Nearly half of patients with central nervous system symptoms have metastases visible on computed tomography with contrast enhancement.

Magnetic resonance imaging is a more sensitive test than computed tomography and is rapidly becoming the preferred choice, but it may be reserved for patients with new central nervous system symptoms when clinical suspicion of metastases is high and computed tomography fails to identify a lesion. The role of positron emission tomography in evaluating central nervous system disease in the breast cancer patient is unknown.

The low incidence of central nervous system disease as the first site of recurrence after primary therapy and the expense of computed tomography and magnetic resonance imaging are reasons not to perform routine imaging of the brain (Table 15-1). Recurrence in the brain is associated with a poorer survival than recurrence in other distant sites.[58,102]

TUMOR MARKERS

Breast malignancies can produce biological molecules that can be detected in the tumor itself or in serum. An association between a circulating tumor-related antigen and the presence of breast cancer must exist to allow the serum test to be useful in cancer surveillance. Since an absolute tumor marker that can accurately diagnose a specific malignancy is not available, it is the quantitative difference between a value considered normal (within methodological limits of detection) and that measured in the presence of cancer that qualifies a molecule as a tumor marker.[128] The most widely studied serum-circulating tumor markers in breast cancer follow-up are tumor-associated antigens such as CEA and CA 15-3, although the science of tumor marker biology is expanding and many other tumor markers are being investigated.

CEA is a family of closely related but highly variable, strongly immunogenic glycoproteins identified in virtually any mucin-producing epithelial cancer[129] and can be shed into the bloodstream. CEA is detected in cancerous breast tissue in 32% to 56% of cases[130,131] and in the serum of 7% to 26% of patients with breast cancer overall.[132,133] The CEA level is elevated in 10%, 15%, 35%, and 60% of patients, respectively, with stages I, II, III, and IV breast cancer.[134] Although elevation of initial CEA can reflect a greater risk of recurrence (16% versus 5%),[135,136] 20% to 40% of patients with advanced disease do not have elevated levels during follow-up[137,138] and 10% of patients with progressive disease show a decline in serial CEA measurements.[135,137-139]

Despite limitations, many groups have studied the predictive value of CEA serial determinations in breast cancer surveillance to detect recurrence. In follow-up of 1,626 patients an elevated or rising CEA level preceded documentable breast cancer recurrence in 34% of 312 patients with recurrence (true-positive rate), but with a false-positive rate of 9% (elevated or rising CEA concentration in the absence of recurrence).[134] In another tabulated review, Hayes[140] found that the time from clinically occult to clinically apparent metastatic disease ranged from 3 to 18 months, but with median lead times ranging from only 4.8 to 6.9 months.[140] Rather than a single, postoperative measurement, a serial rise in CEA levels during follow-up (especially values significantly greater than 10 ng/ml) is a better predictor of relapse. However, serial determinations to verify increasing levels will narrow the lead time and diminish any theoretical advantage of identifying clinically occult recurrence.[141] Most studies have described serial measurements at 3-month intervals.

CA 15-3 is a highly glycosylated, heterogeneous glycoprotein, initially identified by monoclonal antibodies prepared against human milk fat globule antigen.[142] It is representative of a family of mucin-associated antigens such as mucinlike carcinoma-associated antigen, CAM26 and CAM29, and CA549,[143-146] which appear to be similar in sensitivity and specificity to CA 15-3.[137,147-150] CA 15-3 can be found in 78% of breast carcinomas by immunochemistry[151] and in serum in 31% of patients with primary breast cancer[133] and 73% of those with metastatic breast cancer.[142] As tabulated by Hayes,[152] an increasing or elevated CA 15-3 level can predict breast cancer relapse with a sensitivity of 45% to 77% (the percentage of patients with metastasis and elevated CA 15-3), a specificity of 94% to 98% (the percentage of patients without metastasis and nonelevated CA 15-3), and a positive predictive value of 41% to 92% (the percentage of patients with elevated CA 15-3 subsequently documented with metastatic disease) at median lead times ranging from 4 to 7 months. In one study of women with metastases the incidence of an elevated CA 15-3 level was significantly greater than that for CEA (63% compared with 41%), with preferential CA 15-3 increase in patients with bone metastases or local recurrences but not liver metastases.[142] This preferential increase based on site of metastases was not confirmed in another study of 129 patients.[153] In this cohort of women with initial locoregional recurrence only who ultimately proved to have metastatic disease, an elevated CA 15-3 concentration did predict a shorter time to distant disease (10 months) than in those with nonelevated CA 15-3 (21 months).

To enhance the predictive value of serial serum tumor marker measurements, many groups have studied the combined detection of CEA and CA 15-3. When optimized cutoff levels (to 97.5% specificity) are used, CEA is 10% to 15% lower in sensitivity than CA 15-3 in detecting clinically occult recurrence, but the combined measurement of CEA and CA 15-3 may increase sensitivity by 5% to 10%.[137,154] However, the clinical utility is still not defined. In one study, although an elevated CA 15-3 level was the first sign of recurrence in 46% of women (elevated CEA in 7%), the lead time to systemic disease was only 2.7 ± 2.6 months (mean ± standard deviation).[155] While a CA 15-3 level above 50 U/ml had a positive predictive value of 100% in 16 patients with recurrence (9% of 168 patients followed with initial stage I breast cancer), the positive predictive value was only 56% when any elevation above normal (30 U/ml) was considered.[156] In addition, approximately 6,000 serial serum measurements of CEA and CA 15-3 (at 1-month intervals) were obtained in 196 patients with lymph node–positive breast cancer before elevated values emerged to predict recurrence.[157] In this study the sensitivity of an elevated serum marker as the first sign of recurrence happened to be better for CEA (54%) than for CA 15-3 (39%), but more clinically relevant was that the lead time was less than 6 months for 77% of patients in whom an elevated tumor marker represented clinically occult recurrence. As stated, this detection of clinically occult recurrence was based on serial measurements obtained at 1-month intervals, since a prior study by the same group had found that when tumor markers were measured at 3-month intervals, 50% of patients with elevated levels already had clinically identifiable metastases.[158] As with routine CEA measurements, most studies have described serial CA 15-3 determinations at 3-month intervals.

An additional concern that may limit the utility of serial postoperative serum tumor markers is the recognized inherent variance in laboratory measurements, which influences the sensitivity and specificity of testing.[159] Serial measurements at short intervals can result in variation up to 105% for CEA and 90% for CA 15-3. Multiplicative measurements on individual samples can show a variance in values of up to 40% for CEA and 20% to 23% for CA 15-3. Circadian variability (at 4-hour intervals) in serum CEA measurements has also been described.[157,159-161] Both tumor markers can be elevated in benign conditions.[162] To minimize this inherent variability, submitting serum samples to a single laboratory (rather than many laboratories) may be advisable and elevated values should be confirmed by repeated measurements at 1-month intervals to identify a significant increase (20% to 25%).[157,163] Testing is otherwise best performed at 3-month intervals.[137] It is also important to recognize that basal levels in otherwise normal women increase with age. The mean levels of CEA increase from 1.75 mg/L at an age under 50 years to 2.5 mg/L at ages 70 to 75 years. The mean levels of CA 15-3 increase with age from 15 kU/L at an age under 50 years to 25 kU/L at ages 75 to 80 years.[137]

It is apparent that despite a generally low positive predictive value, elevated levels of serum tumor markers (CEA and CA 15-3) will identify a percentage of patients with clinically occult recurrence with an average lead time of 6 months or less. The small clinical worth of a relatively short lead time in the absence of defined plans for intervention should dissuade clinicians from routinely measuring serum tumor markers in patients with early-stage breast cancer (stages I and II) until large, multiinstitutional studies can better define the value of such practices. One such study is being conducted by the Cancer and Leukemia Group B. The utility of a serial tumor marker measurement to monitor neoadjuvant treatments or therapy for advanced or metastatic disease is also under investigation.[164,165] Pending these data, determination of tumor markers is not warranted in breast cancer follow-up (Table 15-1).

IMPACT OF SURVEILLANCE AS A BASIS FOR FOLLOW-UP GUIDELINES

The merits of individual components of the follow-up schedule to detect recurrent breast cancer are addressed previously. However, is the combination of these components more relevant and effective? If not, are physicians placing too much emphasis on detection of recurrent disease in the follow-up routine? Are there other compelling reasons to see patients regularly?

Aims of breast cancer follow-up programs include the early detection and treatment of recurrence, which is the overwhelming emphasis of most programs; the early detection of new primaries in the contralateral breast or of recurrent or new primaries in a previously irradiated breast; and the evaluation of neoadjuvant and adjuvant treatments among patients enrolled in clinical trials. Follow-up programs also involve monitoring long-term complications of treatment, patient rehabilitation and psychological support, and family and patient risk counseling.[166,167] Issues related to the early detection of new primary malignancies have already been addressed and are not reiterated here. Monitoring of patients on clinical protocols that may use investigational drugs, doses, or schedules is a special case for which close and routine follow-up is justifiable, not only to determine the validity of the hypothesis, but also to determine the incidence of unanticipated and anticipated toxicities. Nonetheless, because only a small percentage of women are entered in such studies, the relevance of the debate—to follow closely or not—is little influenced.

The effectiveness of surveillance is predicated on two assumptions: that most recurrences are detected at surveillance visits and that treatment of recurrences discovered prematurely and presumably earlier in their development offers a better chance of cure or long-term survival.[168] A multitude of studies have proved the first assumption wrong. Only 20% to 30% of recurrences are discovered at routine follow-up visits; in other instances symptoms or signs noted by the patient have resulted in an interval appointment.[2,107,119,166,169-171] When all clinic visits are considered, only approximately 1% result in the discovery of an asymptomatic recurrence.[172] Furthermore, the overwhelming majority of recurrences represent metastatic, incurable disease; that is, they are discovered late.[173]

Are sufficient recurrences detected on routine visits to influence the long-term survival of all patients so followed? Retrospective and nonrandomized studies have provided conflicting results. Some studies suggest that patients with asymptomatic recurrences live longer,[107,119,170] whereas other studies do not.[122,171] However, the positive studies have been appropriately criticized for their inherent inability to eliminate either lead-time bias (patients with disease detected by early diagnosis survive longer than those whose disease is detected at the occurrence of new signs or symptoms, even when treatment is worthless) or length-time bias (slow-growing tumors are preferentially detected by the early diagnosis process, since they are detectable longer). The lack of trend among these studies suggests that nothing short of a randomized, controlled trial would be able to clarify the situation.

Two randomized, controlled trials have been published. The study by the GIVIO group involved the follow-up of 1,320 women younger than 70 years of age with stages I, II, and III unilateral primary breast cancer at 20 general hospitals in Italy.[2] Patients were assigned to intensive surveillance (office visits every 3 months, then every 6 months; liver function tests at the same interval; chest x-ray every 6 months; bone scan every 12 months; and liver echography every 12 months) or a control regimen, in which patients were seen with the same frequency but had only clinically indicated tests performed. Both groups received yearly mammography aimed at detecting contralateral breast cancer. Although metastases were found among 31% of asymptomatic patients in the intensive regimen compared with 21% of asymptomatic patients in the control group, overall survival was no different between the two groups after a median follow-up of 71 months (Figure 15-3). The investigators reasonably concluded that follow-up based on routine execution of a battery of diagnostic tests is not superior to clinical follow-up.

In the other multicenter study, also conducted in Italy, 1,243 consecutive patients surgically treated for unilateral invasive breast carcinoma with no evidence of metastases were randomly assigned to intensive versus nonintensive follow-up.[66] For both groups physical examination was performed every 3 months in the first 2 years and every 6 months in the following 3 years and mammography was performed annually. The intensively followed group also had chest x-rays and bone scans performed every 6 months. Not unexpectedly, the 5-year disease-free survival rate was lower ($p < .05$) among patients followed up more intensively (Figure 15-4). However, no difference was found in 5-year overall mortality (18.5% versus 19.5%) between the two follow-up groups (Figure 15-5). The investigators reasonably concluded that periodic chest x-rays and bone scans allowed the earlier detection of distant metastases but had no impact on prognosis.

Although the prospective and retrospective studies reviewed previously do not support the contention that treatment of intensively followed patients prolongs survival longer than treatment of those followed clinically, such studies have used conventional treatment strategies only. Is it possible that more aggressive strategies employed at the time of detection of asymptomatic disease would influence progression-free survival and overall survival to a degree heretofore unrealized? Could high-dose therapy followed by autologous bone marrow or peripheral stem cell support improve results in patients whose breast cancer is considered incurable? Should physicians rethink the notion that rigorous follow-up does not provide a better clinical outcome?

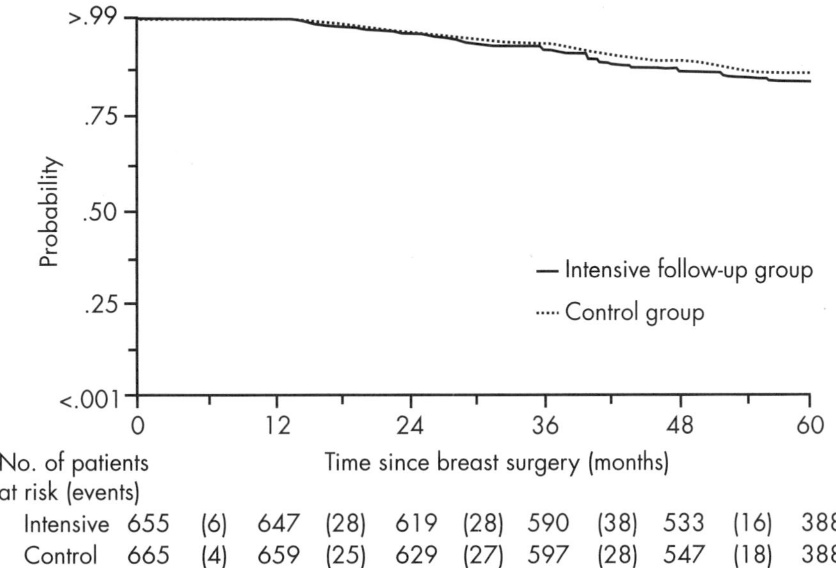

Figure 15-3 Overall survival in the GIVIO randomized comparison of intensive surveillance versus follow-up consisting of clinically indicated tests only. Data are based on 655 patients in the intensive follow-up group who experienced 132 events of disease and 665 patients in the control group who experienced 122 events of disease (log rank test = 0.656; $p = .42$). (Modified from GIVIO Investigators. JAMA 1994;271:1587-92.)

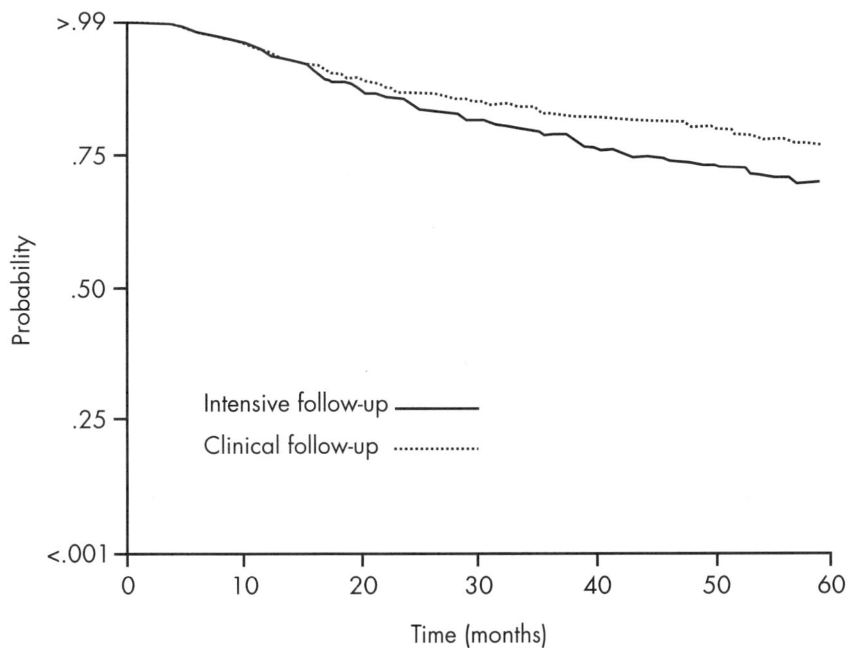

Figure 15-4 Comparison of intensive versus clinically indicated follow-up: disease-free survival. (Significant at $p < .05$.) (Modified from Rosselli Del Turco M, Palli D, Cariddi A, Ciatto S, Pacini P, Distante V. JAMA 1994;271:1593-7.)

High-dose chemotherapy attended by transplantation has been the subject of intense interest because its ability to improve common outcome variables among patients with breast cancer has been repeatedly shown. Specifically, complete responses have been seen among two thirds of selected patients with locally advanced or metastatic disease and unmaintained progression-free intervals continue among 15% to 30% of all patients at median lengths of follow-up of 3 years and greater.[174-176] Moreover, partial responses induced by conventional therapy have been converted to

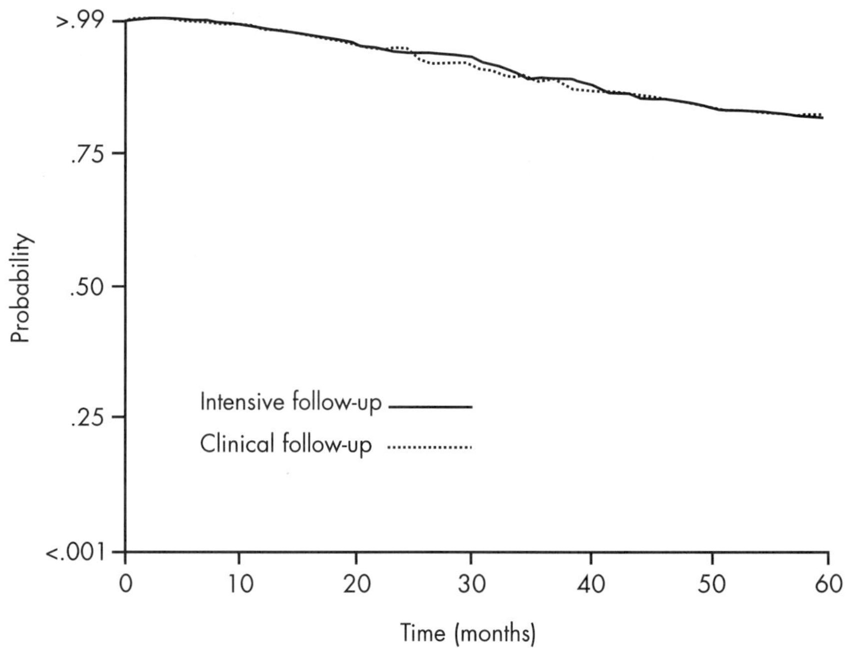

Figure 15-5 Comparison of intensive versus clinically indicated follow-up: overall mortality at 5 years. (Modified from Rosselli Del Turco M, Palli D, Cariddi A, Ciatto S, Pacini P, Distante V. JAMA 1994;271:1593-7.)

complete responses after high-dose chemotherapy.[176] Peters et al.[177] have demonstrated a 72% event-free survival rate at a median follow-up time of 3.3 years among women with greater than 10 positive nodes and no evident metastatic disease after the use of high-dose cyclophosphamide, cisplatin, and carmustine as consolidation after standard-dose adjuvant chemotherapy. The overwhelming majority of these women have micrometastatic disease.[177] All of these results are better, considerably so in some instances, than would be anticipated with standard therapy.

On the other hand, among patients with metastatic disease treated with transplantation protocols, median survivals have not been clearly different from those for standard therapy.[176,178] Moreover, quality-of-life issues have not been routinely addressed.

In a comprehensive review comparing high-dose chemotherapy and autologous bone marrow transplantation with conventional doses of chemotherapy, Eddy[179] examined the effectiveness, benefits, and risks of both procedures (Table 15-2).[179] Gross comparisons suggested that transplantation protocols were associated with higher complete and overall response rates but that median response times, median survival times, and overall survival times were similar between the two approaches. In addition, transplantation protocols were associated with higher treatment-related mortality rates, high rates of nonmortal toxicity, and a high rate of side effects.

Simply stated, survival and median response times do not differ enough between the two approaches either to allow unguarded acceptance of high-dose chemotherapy followed by autologous bone marrow transplantation outside of the context of a randomized clinical trial or to alter follow-up approaches after the treatment of primary breast cancer. Fortunately, such a randomized trial is under way. A multicenter study led by the Philadelphia Bone Marrow Transplant Group is conducting a comparison between conventional maintenance with cyclophosphamide, methotrexate, and 5-FU and high-dose chemotherapy with cyclophosphamide, thiotepa, and carboplatin plus autologous bone marrow and peripheral stem cell rescue in women with metastatic breast cancer responding to conventional induction therapy.

If life cannot be prolonged, can the quality of that life be improved by regular radiographically and laboratory-based follow-up? Although this idea has many proponents, objective evidence is underdeveloped or nonexistent. Regular chest x-rays are espoused in part because treatment of pleural effusions, pericardial metastases, and mediastinal disease is probably more effective when treatment is given earlier.[180] However, this impression has never been substantiated and it appears likely that the treatment of these conditions in asymptomatic or minimally symptomatic patients, many of whom may never require intervention, may generally cause more, rather than less, debility.

Similarly, the performance of bone scanning or skeletal surveys for the early detection of bone metastases and the subsequent prophylaxis of pathological fractures, a laudable goal, has not been the subject of prospective studies.[181] However, radiographical detection of asymptomatic metastases with the potential to cause immobility seems likely to be an infrequent event and cost ineffective for several rea-

Table 15-2 Summary of studies of high-dose chemotherapy with autologous bone marrow transplantation

	BEST GUESS OF PROBABILITY OR MAGNITUDE OF OUTCOME*		
HEALTH OUTCOMES	REGULAR-DOSE CHEMOTHERAPY	HDC WITH ABMT	DIFFERENCE
BENEFITS			
Relief of symptoms	?	?	?
Complete response rate	8%	36%	+28%
Overall response rate	39%	70%	+31%
Median response time	9.6 mo	8 mo	-1.6 mo
Median survival time	16.6 mo	16 mo	-0.6 mo
2-year survival rate	39%	43%	+4%
RISKS (RATE)			
Mortality due to bone marrow toxicity	1%	12%	+11%
Extramedullary toxicity	0%	30%	+30%
Secondary effects of bone marrow suppression; infection	3%	75%	+72%
Side effects of chemotherapy			
Alopecia	75%	100%	+25%
Nausea	50%	100%	+50%
Vomiting	40%	100%	+60%
Stomatitis	20%	75%	+50%
Diarrhea	10%	75%	+65%

Modified from Eddy DM. J Clin Oncol 1992;10:657-70.
HDC, High-dose chemotherapy; *ABMT,* autologous bone marrow transplantation.
*Estimates are rounded. Note that a wide range of uncertainty surrounds every estimate.

sons. First, bone metastases typically become evident with localized pain that is gradual in onset, progressive over weeks or months, and more severe at night. Painful lesions are also more likely to fracture than asymptomatic ones. Moreover, up to 8% of patients with pure lytic lesions, the type most predisposed to fracture, have false-negative bone scans and the criteria for selecting patients for treatments and procedures that potentially avert pathological fracture are not even agreed on.[182,183]

The argument against routine studies for the early detection of spinal cord compression is similar. Fully 93% of patients have back pain preceding or early in the development of spinal cord compression because of bone or nervous system compromise.[184] Although bone scans are positive in 100% of patients with breast cancer in whom spinal cord compression develops, the positive predictive value of this study in the absence of back pain or other symptoms is probably less than 1%. Therefore with few exceptions the patient, rather than any follow-up study, will alert the physician to the possibility of spinal cord compromise. In sum, the ability of intensive follow-up studies to have even a minor impact on the breast cancer patient's quality of life appears limited, but the area is fertile for additional research.

Do psychological benefits accrue to patients followed up regularly? The study by Morris et al.[172] investigating the attitudes of 285 women followed up after potentially curative treatment of primary breast cancer would suggest so. In the survey 85% preferred regular follow-up in a breast clinic to an attendance-only-when-symptomatic approach and 70% preferred regular breast clinic visits to those with their general practitioner for this purpose. Furthermore, 80% said they felt reassured and less anxious after attending the breast clinic.

The preceding findings are not universal. Patients have criticized the lack of psychological support provided by physicians.[185] This result is not unexpected, since physicians often lack formal training in this aspect of the patient-physician interaction. Furthermore, the study of Muss et al.[186] infers that the comfort derived by women on follow-up visits is based on misunderstandings. More than 90% of women believed that early detection improved long-term outlook, their chance for cure, or their chance to respond to therapy. Few patients were aware of the limitations of follow-up visits. Rosselli Del Turco et al.[66] reasonably object to the lack of attention paid to the psychological distress that may affect women who receive routine follow-up. Presumably women waiting for test results or risking additional diagnostic procedures because of false-positive results would be distressed, being reminded that recurrence or an adverse effect of treatment is an ever-present hazard.

In the randomized study by the GIVIO investigators[2] in which women were followed up intensively with diagnostic tests versus clinically indicated follow-up alone, a prospective examination of quality of life was conducted. A standardized assessment was performed on all patients free of disease using self-administered questionnaires at 6, 12, 24, and 60 months after randomization. When the questionnaires were assembled, an extensive review of cancer-specific and general quality-of-life instruments used in research with cancer patients until 1985 was performed. These instruments included the Functional Living Index-Cancer Scale, the Sickness Impact Profile, the Profile of Mood States, and the Cancer Inventory of Problem Situation. Although 70% of respondents at each of four assessments preferred to be seen frequently by a physician and undergo diagnostic tests even if free of symptoms, results showed that type of follow-up did not affect various dimensions of health-related quality of life. Mean scores referring to overall health and quality-of-life perception, emotional well-being, body image, social functioning, symptoms, and satisfaction with care were similar and not significantly different.

In sum, women's preferences for routine and aggressive follow-up may be related to a misunderstanding of its ultimate ability to alter the course of their disease. Psychological benefits derived, then, may represent only a house of cards. Moreover, no evidence has been presented that women suffer adverse psychological effects when routine diagnostic testing is withheld.

Can other arguments be made for regular follow-up? There are several, including the assurance of rehabilitation and full return of function; monitoring of late effects of treatment-accelerated bone loss, cardiovascular sequelae, secondary malignancies, and sexual dysfunction; and screening for other high-risk tumors in the breast cancer population, such as ovarian and endometrial cancer. Regular follow-up also allows an opportunity to help the family adjust to the patient's disease and to educate family members about the hereditary consequences of some forms of breast cancer.[167] However, relatively few visits could accomplish many of these tasks. Furthermore, additional studies looking for other malignancies or complications of treatment are likely to evoke protests regarding cost-effectiveness because of either the relative rarity of a positive finding or physicians' present inability to intervene meaningfully once a problem is identified.

FUTURE PROSPECTS AND CONCLUSION

Follow-up strategies are based on the uncertainty of disease outcome. Major advances in follow-up depend on the development of improved therapies and will come from either improved prediction of recurrences or the discovery of specific breast cancer tests. Application of molecular biology to breast cancer staging may allow a more accurate outcome prediction. Techniques under investigation include screening of bone marrow at the time of diagnosis for micrometastases using probes for epithelial cell markers or breast cancer–specific markers and similar molecular screening of lymph nodes for micrometastases that cannot be detected by histological examinations. Unfortunately, no serum tumor marker specific for breast cancer is on the horizon.

For women today, what can be concluded? Perhaps all tasks can be accomplished by a minimum of one and a maximum of two or three visits a year (Table 15-1). History, physical examination, and attention to the woman's psychological status are the important elements of these visits. Except for mammography on a yearly basis, the utility of diagnostic tests is poor and their use should be discouraged.

REFERENCES

1. Wingo PA, Tong T, Bolden S. Cancer statistics, 1995. CA Cancer J Clin 1995;45:8-30.
2. The GIVIO Investigators. Impact of follow-up testing on survival and health-related quality of life in breast cancer patients: a multicenter randomized controlled trial. JAMA 1994;271:1587-92.
3. Kattlove H, Liberati A, Keeler E, Brook RH. Benefits and costs of screening and treatment for early breast cancer: development of a basic benefit package. JAMA 1995;273:142-8.
4. Loomer L, Brockschmidt JK, Muss HB, Saylor G. Postoperative follow-up of patients with early breast cancer: patterns of care among clinical oncologists and a review of the literature. Cancer 1991;67:55-60.
5. Simon MS, Hoff M, Hussein M, Martino S, Walt A. An evaluation of clinical follow-up in women with early stage breast cancer among physician members of the American Society of Clinical Oncology. Breast Cancer Res Treat 1993;27:211-9.
6. Richert-Boe KE. Heterogeneity of cancer surveillance practices among medical oncologists in Washington and Oregon. Cancer 1995;75:2605-12.
7. Hoskins KF, Stopfer JE, Calzone KA, et al. Assessment and counseling for women with a family history of breast cancer: a guide for clinicians. JAMA 1995;273:577-85.
8. Theriault RL, Sellin RV. Estrogen-replacement therapy in younger women with breast cancer. Monogr Natl Cancer Inst 1994;16:149-52.
9. Hutchinson-Williams KA, Gutmann JN. Estrogen replacement therapy (ERT) in high-risk cancer patients. Yale J Biol Med 1991; 64:607-26.
10. Pritchard KI, Sawka CA. Menopausal estrogen replacement therapy in women with breast cancer. Cancer 1995;75:1-3.
11. Cobleigh MA, Berris RF, Bush T, et al. Estrogen replacement therapy in breast cancer survivors: a time for change; Breast Cancer Committees of the Eastern Cooperative Oncology Group. JAMA 1994;272: 540-5.
12. Vassilopoulou-Sellin R, Theriault RL. Randomized prospective trial of estrogen-replacement therapy in women with a history of breast cancer. Monogr Natl Cancer Inst 1994;16:153-9.
13. Rosen PP, Groshen S, Kinne DW, Norton L. Factors influencing prognosis in node-negative breast carcinoma: analysis of 767 T1N0M0/T2N0M0 patients with long-term follow-up. J Clin Oncol 1993;11:2090-100.
14. Jaiyesimi IA, Buzdar AU, Decker DA, Hortobagyi GN. Use of tamoxifen for breast cancer: twenty-eight years later. J Clin Oncol 1995;13:513-29.
15. Hortobagyi GN, Buzdar AU. Current status of adjuvant systemic therapy for primary breast cancer: progress and controversy. CA Cancer J Clin 1995;45:199-226.
16. Rutqvist LE, Johansson H, Signomklao T, Johansson U, Fornander T, Wilking N. Adjuvant tamoxifen therapy for early stage breast cancer and second primary malignancies: Stockholm Breast Cancer Study Group. J Natl Cancer Inst 1995;87:645-51.
17. Seoud MA, Johnson J, Weed JC Jr. Gynecologic tumors in tamoxifen-treated women with breast cancer. Obstet Gynecol 1993;82:165-9.
18. van Leeuwen FE, Benraadt J, Coebergh JW, et al. Risk of endometrial cancer after tamoxifen treatment of breast cancer. Lancet 1994;343:448-52.
19. Fisher B, Costantino JP, Redmond CK, Fisher ER, Wickerham DL, Cronin WM. Endometrial cancer in tamoxifen-treated breast cancer patients: findings from the National Surgical Adjuvant Breast and Bowel Project (NSABP) B-14. J Natl Cancer Inst 1994;86:527-37.

20. Fornander T, Hellstrom AC, Moberger B. Descriptive clinicopathologic study of 17 patients with endometrial cancer during or after adjuvant tamoxifen in early breast cancer. J Natl Cancer Inst 1993;85:1850-5.
21. Fornander T, Rutqvist LE, Cedermark B, et al. Adjuvant tamoxifen in early breast cancer: occurrence of new primary cancer. Lancet 1989;1:117-20.
22. Magriples U, Naftolin F, Schwartz PE, Carcangiu ML. High-grade endometrial carcinoma in tamoxifen-treated breast cancer patients. J Clin Oncol 1993;11:485-90.
23. Barakat RR, Wong G, Curtin JP, Vlamis V, Hoskins WJ. Tamoxifen use in breast cancer patients who subsequently develop corpus cancer is not associated with a higher incidence of adverse histologic features. Gynecol Oncol 1994;55:164-8.
24. Jordan VC, Assikis VJ. Endometrial carcinoma and tamoxifen: clearing up a controversy. Clin Cancer Res 1995;1:467-74.
25. Lahti E, Blanco G, Kauppila A, Apaja-Sarkkinen M, Taskinen PJ, Laatikainen T. Endometrial changes in postmenopausal breast cancer patients receiving tamoxifen. Obstet Gynecol 1993;81:660-4.
26. Cohen I, Rosen DJ, Shapira J, et al. Endometrial changes with tamoxifen: comparison between tamoxifen-treated and nontreated asymptomatic, postmenopausal breast cancer patients. Gynecol Oncol 1994;52:185-90.
27. Uziely B, Lewin A, Brufman G, Dorembus D, Mor-Yosef S. The effect of tamoxifen on the endometrium. Breast Cancer Res Treat 1993;26:101-5.
28. Kedar RP, Bourne TH, Powles TJ, et al. Effects of tamoxifen on uterus and ovaries of postmenopausal women in a randomized breast cancer prevention trial. Lancet 1994;343:1318-21.
29. Tepper R, Cohen I, Altaras M. Doppler flow evaluation of pathologic endometrial conditions in postmenopausal breast cancer patients treated with tamoxifen. J Ultrasound Med 1994;13:635-40.
30. Henderson IC. Should tamoxifen use be curtailed because of the risk of endometrial cancer? Breast Diseases: A Year Book Quarterly 1994;5:18-23.
31. Hindle WH. Tamoxifen therapy and the endometrium: gynecologic considerations. Breast Diseases: A Year Book Quarterly 1994;5:24-6.
32. Valagussa P, Moliterni A, Terenziani M, Zambetti M, Bonadonna G. Second malignancies following CMF-based adjuvant chemotherapy in resectable breast cancer. Ann Oncol 1994;5:803-8.
33. Curtis RE, Boice JD Jr, Stovall M, et al. Risk of leukemia after chemotherapy and radiation treatment for breast cancer. N Engl J Med 1992;326:1745-51.
34. Fisher B, Brown AM, Dimitrov NV, et al. Two months of doxorubicin-cyclophosphamide with and without interval reinduction therapy compared with 6 months of cyclophosphamide, methotrexate, and fluorouracil in positive-node breast cancer patients with tamoxifen-nonresponsive tumors: results from the National Surgical Adjuvant Breast and Bowel Project B-15. J Clin Oncol 1990;8:1483-96.
35. Buzdar A, Hortobagyi GN, Kau S, et al. Long-term efficacy and toxicities of doxorubicin-containing adjuvant therapy in breast cancer—MD Anderson Cancer Center studies; Fourth International Congress on Anti-Cancer Chemotherapy. 1993 Feb 2-5; Paris, 1993:59.
36. Ragaz J, Yun J, Spinelli J. Analysis of incidence of secondary acute myelogenous leukemias (2nd AML) in breast cancer patients (BCP) treated with adjuvant therapy (AT)—association with therapeutic regimens [abstract]. Proc Am Soc Clin Oncol 1995;14:112.
37. Levine EG, Bloomfield CD. Leukemias and myelodysplastic syndromes secondary to drug, radiation, and environmental exposure. Semin Oncol 1992;19:47-84.
38. DeCillis A, Anderson S, Wickerham DL, et al. Acute myeloid leukemia (AML) in NSABP B-25. Proc Am Soc Clin Oncol 1995; 14:98.
39. Kissin MW, Querci della Rovere G, Easton D, Westbury G. Risk of lymphoedema following the treatment of breast cancer. Br J Surg 1986;73:580-4.
40. Hoe AL, Iven D, Royle GT, Taylor I. Incidence of arm swelling following axillary clearance for breast cancer. Br J Surg 1992;79:261-2.
41. Ryttov N, Holm NV, Qvist N, Blichert-Toft M. Influence of adjuvant irradiation on the development of late arm lymphedema and impaired shoulder mobility after mastectomy for carcinoma of the breast. Acta Oncol 1988;27:667-70.
42. Larson D, Weinstein M, Goldberg I, et al. Edema of the arm as a function of the extent of axillary surgery in patients with stage I-II carcinoma of the breast treated with primary radiotherapy. Int J Radiat Oncol Biol Phys 1986;12:1575-82.
43. Pierce SM, Recht A, Lingos TI, et al. Long-term radiation complications following conservative surgery (CS) and radiation therapy (RT) in patients with early stage breast cancer. Int J Radiat Oncol Biol Phys 1992;23:915-23.
44. Levitt SH, Fletcher GH. Trials and tribulations: do clinical trials prove that irradiation increases cardiac and secondary cancer mortality in the breast cancer patient? Int J Radiat Oncol Biol Phys 1991;21:523-7.
45. Rutqvist LE, Lax I, Fornander T, Johansson H. Cardiovascular mortality in a randomized trial of adjuvant radiation therapy versus surgery alone in primary breast cancer. Int J Radiat Oncol Biol Phys 1992;22:887-96.
46. Gyenes G, Fornander T, Carlens P, Rutqvist LE. Morbidity of ischemic heart disease in early breast cancer 15-20 years after adjuvant radiotherapy. Int J Radiat Oncol Biol Phys 1994;28:1235-41.
47. Taghian A, de Vathaire F, Terrier P, et al. Long-term risk of sarcoma following radiation treatment for breast cancer. Int J Radiat Oncol Biol Phys 1991;21:361-7.
48. Brady MS, Garfein CF, Petrek JA, Brennan MF. Post-treatment sarcoma in breast cancer patients. Ann Surg Oncol 1994;1:66-72.
49. Pendlebury SC, Bilous M, Langlands AO. Sarcomas following radiation therapy for breast cancer: a report of three cases and a review of the literature. Int J Radiat Oncol Biol Phys 1995;31:405-10.
50. Inskip PD, Stovall M, Flannery JT. Lung cancer risk and radiation dose among women treated for breast cancer. J Natl Cancer Inst 1994;86:983-8.
51. Neugut AI, Robinson E, Lee WC, Murray T, Karwoski K, Kutcher GJ. Lung cancer after radiation therapy for breast cancer. Cancer 1993;71:3054-7.
52. Neugut AI, Murray T, Santos J, et al. Increased risk of lung cancer after breast cancer radiation therapy in cigarette smokers. Cancer 1994;73:1615-20.
53. Storm HH, Andersson M, Boice JD Jr, et al. Adjuvant radiotherapy and risk of contralateral breast cancer. J Natl Cancer Inst 1992;84: 1245-50.
54. Quiet CA, Ferguson DJ, Weichselbaum RR, Hellman S. Natural history of node-negative breast cancer: a study of 826 patients with long term follow-up. J Clin Oncol 1995;13:1144-51.
55. Mansour EG, Ravdin PM, Dressler L. Prognostic factors in early breast carcinoma. Cancer 1994;74:381-400.
56. Ravdin PM. A practical view of prognostic factors for staging, adjuvant treatment planning, and as baseline studies for possible future therapy. Hematol Oncol Clin North Am 1994;8:197-211.
57. Coleman RE, Rubens RD. The clinical course of bone metastases from breast cancer. Br J Cancer 1987;55:61-6.
58. Kamby C, Rose C, Ejlertsen B, et al. Stage and pattern of metastases in patients with breast cancer. Eur J Cancer Clin Oncol 1987;23: 1925-34.
59. Hannisdal E, Gundersen S, Kvaloy S, et al. Follow-up of breast cancer patients stage I-II: a baseline strategy. Eur J Cancer 1993; 29A:992-7.
60. Valagussa P, Bonadonna G, Veronesi U. Patterns of relapse and survival following radical mastectomy: analysis of 716 consecutive patients. Cancer 1978;41:1170-8.
61. Rosen PP, Groshen S, Saigo PE, Kinne DW, Hellman S. A long-term study of survival in stage I (T1N0M0) and stage II (T1N1M0) breast carcinoma. J Clin Oncol 1989;7:355-66.
62. Rosen PP, Groshen S, Kinne DW. Prognosis in T2N0M0 stage I breast carcinoma: a 20 year follow-up study. J Clin Oncol 1991; 9:1650-61.

63. Veronesi U, Marubini E, Del Vecchio M, et al. Local recurrences and distant metastases after conservative breast cancer treatments: partly independent events. J Natl Cancer Inst 1995;87:19-27.
64. Goldhirsch A, Gelber RD, Price KN, et al. Effect of systemic adjuvant treatment on first sites of breast cancer relapse. Lancet 1994; 343:377-81.
65. Fisher B, Anderson S. Conservative surgery for the management of invasive and noninvasive carcinoma of the breast: NSABP trials; National Surgical Adjuvant Breast and Bowel Project. World J Surg 1994;18:63-9.
66. Rosselli Del Turco M, Palli D, Cariddi A, Ciatto S, Pacini P, Distante V. Intensive diagnostic follow-up after treatment of primary breast cancer: a randomized trial; National Research Council Project on Breast Cancer Follow-up. JAMA 1994;271:1593-7.
67. Goldhirsch A, Gelber RD, Castiglione M. Relapse of breast cancer after adjuvant treatment in premenopausal and perimenopausal women: patterns and prognoses. J Clin Oncol 1988;6:89-97.
68. Pisansky TM, Ingle JN, Schaid DJ, et al. Patterns of tumor relapse following mastectomy and adjuvant systemic therapy in patients with axillary lymph node–positive breast cancer: impact of clinical, histopathologic, and flow cytometric factors. Cancer 1993;72:1247-60.
69. Houghton J, Baum M, Haybittle JL. Role of radiotherapy following total mastectomy in patients with early breast cancer: The Closed Trials Working Party of the CRC Breast Cancer Trials Group. World J Surg 1994;18:117-22.
70. Winchester DP, Cox JD. Standards for breast-conservation treatment. CA Cancer J Clin 1992;42:134-62.
71. Cajucom CC, Tsangaris TN, Nemoto T, Driscoll D, Penetrante RB, Holyoke ED. Results of salvage mastectomy for local recurrence after breast-conserving surgery without radiation therapy. Cancer 1993;71:1774-9.
72. Fisher ER, Anderson S, Redmond C, Fisher B. Ipsilateral breast tumor recurrence and survival following lumpectomy and irradiation: pathological findings from NSABP protocol B-06. Semin Surg Oncol 1992;8:161-6.
73. Dershaw DD, McCormick B, Osborne MP. Detection of local recurrence after conservative therapy for breast carcinoma. Cancer 1992; 70:493-6.
74. Haffty BG, Fischer D, Beinfield M, McKhann C. Prognosis following local recurrence in the conservatively treated breast cancer patient. Int J Radiat Oncol Biol Phys 1991;21:293-98.
75. Abner AL, Recht A, Eberlein T, et al. Prognosis following salvage mastectomy for recurrence in the breast after conservative surgery and radiation therapy for early-stage breast cancer. J Clin Oncol 1993;11:44-8.
76. Rayter Z, Gazet JC, Ford HT, Easton DF, Coombes RC. Comparison of conservative surgery and radiotherapy with mastectomy in the treatment of early breast cancer. Eur J Surg Oncol 1990;16:486-92.
77. Hetelekidis S, Schnitt SJ, Morrow M, Harris JR. Management of ductal carcinoma in situ. CA Cancer J Clin 1995;45:244-53.
78. Fisher B, Costantino J, Redmond C, et al. Lumpectomy compared with lumpectomy and radiation therapy for the treatment of intraductal breast cancer. N Engl J Med 1993;328:1581-6.
79. Schwartz GF, Finkel GC, Garcia JC, Patchefsky AS. Subclinical ductal carcinoma in situ of the breast: treatment by local excision and surveillance alone. Cancer 1992;70:2468-74.
80. Gump FE. Lobular carcinoma in situ (LCIS): pathology and treatment. J Cell Biochem Suppl 1993;17G:53-8.
81. Osborne MP, Hoda SA. Current management of lobular carcinoma in situ of the breast. Oncology 1994;8:45-9.
82. Carson W, Sanchez-Forgach E, Stomper P, Penetrante R, Tsangaris TN, Edge SB. Lobular carcinoma in situ: observation without surgery as an appropriate therapy. Ann Surg Oncol 1994;1:141-6.
83. Jardines L, Callans LS, Torosian MH. Recurrent breast cancer: presentation, diagnosis, and treatment. Semin Oncol 1993;20:538-47.
84. Salvadori B, Rovini D, Squicciarini P, Conti R, Cusumano F, Grassi M. Surgery for local recurrences following deficient radical mastectomy for breast cancer: a selected series of 39 cases. Eur J Surg Oncol 1992;18:438-41.
85. Tennvall-Nittby L, Tengrup I, Landberg T. The total incidence of loco-regional recurrence in a randomized trial of breast cancer TNM stage II: The South Sweden Breast Cancer Trial. Acta Oncol 1993;32:641-6.
86. Fajardo LL, Roberts CC, Hunt KR. Mammographic surveillance of breast cancer patients: should the mastectomy site be imaged? AJR Am J Roentgenol 1993;161:953-5.
87. Rissanen TJ, Makarainen HP, Mattila SI, Lindholm EL, Heikkinen MI, Kiviniemi HO. Breast cancer recurrence after mastectomy: diagnosis with mammography and US. Radiology 1993;188:463-7.
88. Mendelson EB. Evaluation of the postoperative breast. Radiol Clin North Am 1992;30:107-38.
89. Orel SG, Troupin RH, Patterson EA, Fowble BL. Breast cancer recurrence after lumpectomy and irradiation: role of mammography in detection. Radiology 1992;183:201-6.
90. Sardi A, Eckholdt G, McKinnon WM, Bolton JS. The significance of mammographic findings after breast-conserving therapy for carcinoma of the breast. Surg Gynecol Obstet 1991;173:309-12.
91. Gilles R, Guinebretiere JM, Shapeero LG, et al. Assessment of breast cancer recurrence with contrast-enhanced subtraction MR imaging: preliminary results in 26 patients. Radiology 1993;188:473-78.
92. Hassell PR, Olivotto IA, Mueller HA, Kingston GW, Basco VE. Early breast cancer: detection of recurrence after conservative surgery and radiation therapy. Radiology 1990;176:731-5.
93. Noone RB, Frazier TG, Noone GC, Blanchet NP, Murphy JB, Rose D. Recurrence of breast carcinoma following immediate reconstruction: a 13-year review. Plast Reconstr Surg 1994;93:96-106.
94. Mund DF, Wolfson P, Gorczyca DP, Fu YS, Love SM, Bassett LW. Mammographically detected recurrent nonpalpable carcinoma developing in a transverse rectus abdominus myocutaneous flap: a case report. Cancer 1994;74:2804-7.
95. Schiller VL, Bos C, Brenner RJ, Turner RR. Foreign body reaction to suture material mimicking malignant microcalcifications in the breast. AJR Am J Roentgenol 1994;162:729.
96. Strax P. Imaging: follow-up of breast cancer reconstruction cases. Cancer 1991;68:1157-8.
97. Propeck PA, Scanlan KA. Utility of axillary views in postmastectomy patients. Radiology 1993;187:769-71.
98. Moskovic E, Curtis S, A'Hern RP, Harmer CL, Parsons C. The role of diagnostic CT scanning of the brachial plexus and axilla in the follow-up of patients with breast cancer. Clin Oncol (R Coll Radiol) 1992;4:74-7.
99. Dixon AK, Wheeler TK, Lomas DJ, Mackenzie R. Computed tomography or magnetic resonance imaging for axillary symptoms following treatment of breast carcinoma? A randomized trial. Clin Radiol 1993;48:371-6.
100. Chaudary MA. Patterns of recurrence in Western and Japanese women with breast cancer. Breast Cancer Res Treat 1991;18(Suppl 1):S115-8.
101. Campbell FC, Blamey RW, Elston CW, Nicholson RI, Griffiths K, Haybittle JL. Oestrogen-receptor status and sites of metastasis in breast cancer. Br J Cancer 1981;44:456-9.
102. Clark GM, Sledge GW Jr, Osborne CK, McGuire WL. Survival from first recurrence: relative importance of prognostic factors in 1,015 breast cancer patients. J Clin Oncol 1987;5:55-61.
103. Hatschek T, Carstensen J, Fagerberg G, Stal O, Grontoft O, Nordenskjold B. Influence of S-phase fraction on metastatic pattern and post-recurrence survival in a randomized mammography screening trial. Breast Cancer Res Treat 1989;14:321-7.
104. Kamby C, Rose C, Ejlertsen B, et al. Adjuvant systemic treatment and the pattern of recurrences in patients with breast cancer. Eur J Cancer Clin Oncol 1988;24:439-47.
105. Miura S, Yoshida M, Murai H, Hayward JL, Chaudary MA. Patterns of recurrence and relapse—Anglo-Japanese comparative study. Breast Cancer Res Treat 1991;18(Suppl 1):127-30.
106. Wickerham L, Fisher B, Cronin W. The efficacy of bone scanning in the follow-up of patients with operable breast cancer. Breast Cancer Res Treat 1984;4:303-7.

107. Tomin R, Donegan WL. Screening for recurrent breast cancer—its effectiveness and prognostic value. J Clin Oncol 1987;5:62-7.
108. Khandekar JD, Burkett FE, Scanlon EF. Sensitivity (S), specificity (SP), and predictive value (PV) of bone scans (BS) in breast cancer (BC) [abstract]. Proc Am Assoc Cancer Res/Am Soc Clin Oncol 1978;19:379.
109. Jacobson AF, Stomper PC, Jochelson MS, Ascoli DM, Henderson IC, Kaplan WD. Association between number and sites of new bone scan abnormalities and presence of skeletal metastases in patients with breast cancer. J Nucl Med 1990;31:387-92.
110. Gerber FH, Goodreau JJ, Kirchner PT, Fouty WJ. Efficacy of preoperative and postoperative bone scanning in the management of breast carcinoma. N Engl J Med 1977;297:300-3.
111. Pandya KJ, McFadden ET, Kalish LA, Tormey DC, Taylor SG 4th, Falkson G. A retrospective study of earliest indicators of recurrence in patients on Eastern Cooperative Oncology Group adjuvant chemotherapy trials for breast cancer: a preliminary report. Cancer 1985;55:202-5.
112. Pedrazzini A, Gelber R, Isley M, Castiglione M, Goldhirsch A. First repeated bone scan in the observation of patients with operable breast cancer. J Clin Oncol 1986;4:389-94.
113. Mayne PD, Thakrar S, Rosalki SB, Foo AY, Parbhoo S. Identification of bone and liver metastases from breast cancer by measurement of plasma alkaline phosphatase isoenzyme activity. J Clin Pathol 1987;40:398-403.
114. Hayward RB, Frazier TG. A reevaluation of bone scans in breast cancer. J Surg Oncol 1985;28:111-3.
115. Ojeda MB, Alonso MC, Bastus R, Alba E, Piera JM, Lopez Lopez JJ. Follow-up of breast cancer stages I and II: an analysis of some common methods. Eur J Cancer Clin Oncol 1987;23:419-23.
116. Hietanen P. Chest radiography in the follow-up of breast cancer. Acta Radiol Oncol 1986;25:15-8.
117. Valagussa P, Tess JD, Rossi A, Tancini G, Banfi A, Bonadonna G. Adjuvant CMF effect on site of first recurrence, and appropriate follow-up intervals, in operable breast cancer with positive axillary nodes. Breast Cancer Res Treat 1981;1:349-56.
118. Ciatto S, Herd-Smith A. The role of chest x-ray in the follow-up of primary breast cancer. Tumori 1983;69:151-4.
119. Rutgers EJ, van Slooten EA, Kluck HM. Follow-up after treatment of primary breast cancer. Br J Surg 1989;76:187-90.
120. Andreoli C, Buranelli F, Campa T, et al. Chest x-ray survey in breast cancer follow-up: a contrary view. Tumori 1987;73:463-5.
121. Logager VB, Vetergaard A, Herrstedt J, Thomsen HS, Zedeler K, Dombernowsky P. The limited value of routine chest x-ray in the follow-up of stage II breast cancer. Eur J Cancer 1990;26:553-5.
122. Stierer M, Rosen HR. Influence of early diagnosis on prognosis of recurrent breast cancer. Cancer 1989;64:1128-31.
123. Umbach GE, Holzki C, Bender HG. Postoperative follow-up and clinical outcome in patients treated for breast cancer [abstract]. Proc Am Soc Clin Oncol 1987;6:56.
124. Hoe AL, Royle GT, Taylor I. Breast liver metastases—incidence, diagnosis and outcome. J R Soc Med 1991;84:714-6.
125. Viachos L, Trakadas S, Gouliamos A, et al. Comparative study between ultrasound, computed tomography, intra-arterial digital subtraction angiography, and magnetic resonance imaging in the differentiation of tumors of the liver. Gastrointest Radiol 1990;15:102-6.
126. Curati WL, Halevy A, Gibson RN, Carr DH, Blumgart LH, Steiner RE. Ultrasound, CT and MRI comparison in primary and secondary tumors of the liver. Gastrointest Radiol 1988;13:123-8.
127. Kauczor HU, Voges EM, Wieland-Schneider C, Mitze M, Thelen M. Value of routine abdominal and lymph node sonography in the follow-up of breast cancer patients. Eur J Radiol 1994;18:104-8.
128. Chu TM. Biochemical markers for human cancer. In: Seifert G, editor. Morphological tumor markers, general aspects and diagnostic relevance. New York: Springer-Verlag, 1987:19-46.
129. Kloppel G, Caselitz J. Epithelial tumor markers: oncofetal antigens (carcinoembryonic antigen, alpha fetoprotein) and epithelial membrane antigen. In: Seifert G, editor. Morphological tumor markers, general aspects and diagnostic relevance. New York: Springer-Verlag, 1987:103-32.
130. Haga S, Watanabe O, Shimizu T, et al. The clinical value of tissue carcinoembryonic antigen in breast cancer. Japan J Surg 1991;21: 278-83.
131. Esteban JM, Felder B, Ahn C, Simpson JF, Battifora H, Shively JE. Prognostic relevance of carcinoembryonic antigen and estrogen receptor status in breast cancer patients. Cancer 1994;74:1575-83.
132. Wang DY, Bulbrook RD, Hayward JL, Hendrick JC, Franchiomont P. Relationship between plasma carcinoembryonic antigen and prognosis in women with breast cancer. Eur J Cancer 1975;11:615-8.
133. Safi F, Kohler I, Rottinger E, Beger H. The value of the tumor marker CA 15-3 in diagnosing and monitoring breast cancer: a comparative study with carcinoembryonic antigen. Cancer 1991;68:574-82.
134. Beard DB, Haskell CM. Carcinoembryonic antigen in breast cancer: clinical review. Am J Med 1986;80:241-5.
135. Myers RE, Sutherland DJ, Meakin JW, Kellen JA, Malkin DG, Malkin A. Carcinoembryonic antigen in breast cancer. Cancer 1978;42:1520-6.
136. Ballesta AM, Molina R, Filella X, Jo J, Gimenez N. Carcinoembryonic antigen in staging and follow-up of patients with solid tumors. Tumour Biol 1995;16:32-41.
137. Stenman UH, Heikkinen R. Serum markers for breast cancer. Scand J Clin Lab Invest Suppl 1991;206:52-9.
138. Lamerz R, Leonhardt A, Ehrhart H, von Lieven H. Serial carcinoembryonic antigen (CEA) determinations in the management of metastatic breast cancer. Oncodevell Biol Med 1980;1:123-35.
139. Krieger G, Wander HE, Prangen M, Bandlow G, Beyer JH, Nagel GA. [Determination of the carcinoembryonic antigen (CEA) for predicting the success of therapy in metastatic breast cancer]. [German] Dtsch Med Wochensch 1983;108:610-4.
140. Hayes DF, Kaplan W. Evaluation of patients after primary therapy. In: Harris JR, Lippman ME, Morrow M, Hellman S, editors. Diseases of the breast. Philadelphia: Lippincott-Raven, 1996:629-48.
141. Falkson HC, Falkson G, Portugal MA, van der Watt JJ, Schoeman HS. Carcinoembryonic antigen as a marker in patients with breast cancer receiving postsurgical adjuvant chemotherapy. Cancer 1982; 49:1859-65.
142. Hayes DF, Zurawski VR Jr, Kufe DW. Comparison of circulating CA15-3 and carcinoembryonic antigen levels in patients with breast cancer. J Clin Oncol 1986;4:1542-50.
143. Seregni E, Crippa F, Botti C, et al. Mucin-like carcinoma-associated antigen (MCA) in breast cancer: clinical experience at the National Cancer Institute of Milan. Int J Biol Markers 1993;8:124-9.
144. Dnistrian AM, Schwartz MK, Greenberg EJ, Smith CA, Dorsa R, Schwartz DC. CA 549 as a marker in breast cancer. Int J Biol Markers 1991;6:139-43.
145. Boccardo F, Bombardieri E, Zanardi S, et al. Preliminary study on serum levels of mucinous like cancer antigen (MCA) in patients with breast disease: comparison with CEA. Int J Biol Markers 1991;6:12-20.
146. Yasasever V, Karologlu D, Erturk N, Dalay N. Diagnostic value of the tumor markers in breast cancer. Eur J Gynaecol Oncol 1994; 15:33-6.
147. Nicolini A, Ferdeghini M, Colombini C, Carpi A. Evaluation of serum CA549, CA M26 and CA M29 levels in the post-operative follow-up of breast cancer patients. J Nucl Med Allied Sci 1990;34:309-13.
148. Clocchiatti L, De Biasi F, Cartei G, et al. Evaluation of the circulating glycoprotein CA549 in mammary cancer and other malignancies. Tumori 1991;77:395-8.
149. Bieglmayer C, Szepesi T, Kopp B, et al. CA15.3, MCA, CAM26, CAM29 are members of a polymorphic family of mucin-like glycoproteins. Tumour Biol 1991;12:138-48.
150. Jotti GS, Bombardieri E. Circulating tumor markers in breast cancer. Anticancer Res 1990;10:253-8.
151. Kufe D, Inghirami G, Abe M, Hayes D, Justi-Wheeler H, Schlom J. Differential reactivity of a novel monoclonal antibody (DF3) with human malignant versus benign breast tumors. Hybridoma 1984; 3:223-32.
152. Hayes DF. Tumor markers for breast cancer: current utilities and future prospects. Hematol Oncol Clin North Am 1994;8:485-506.

153. Geraghty JG, Coveney EC, Sherry F, O'Higgins NJ, Duffy MJ. CA 15-3 in patients with locoregional and metastatic breast carcinoma. Cancer 1992;70:2831-4.
154. al-Jarallah MA, Behbehani AE, el-Nass SA, et al. Serum CA-15.3 and CEA patterns in postsurgical follow-up, and in monitoring clinical course of metastatic cancer in patients with breast carcinoma. Eur J Surg Oncol 1993;19:74-9.
155. Nicolini A, Colombini C, Luciani L, Carpi A, Giuliani L. Evaluation of serum CA15-3 determination with CEA and TPA in the postoperative follow-up of breast cancer patients. Br J Cancer 1991;64: 154-8.
156. O'Hanlon DM, Kerin MJ, Kent PJ, et al. A prospective evaluation of CA15-3 in stage I carcinoma of the breast. J Am Coll Surg 1995;180:210-2.
157. Jager W. The early detection of disseminated (metastasized) breast cancer by serial tumour marker measurements. Eur J Cancer Prev 1993;2(Suppl 3):133-9.
158. Jager W, Cilaci S, Merkle E, Palapelas V, Lang N. Analysis of the first signs of metastases in breast cancer patients. Tumordiagn Ther 1991;12:60-4.
159. Gion M, Cappelli G, Mione R, et al. Evaluation of critical differences of CEA and CA 15.3 levels in serial samples from patients operated for breast cancer. Int J Biol Markers 1994;9:135-9.
160. Gion M, Cappelli G, Mione R, et al. Variability of tumor markers in the follow-up of patients radically resected for breast cancer. Tumor Biol 1993;14:325-33.
161. Touitou Y, Levi F, Bogdan A, Benavides M, Bailleul F, Misset JL. Rhythm alteration in patients with metastatic breast cancer and poor prognostic factors. J Cancer Res Clin Oncol 1995;121:181-8.
162. Jacobs EL, Haskell CM. Clinical use of tumor markers in oncology. Curr Probl Cancer 1991;15:299-360.
163. van Dalen A, van der Linde DL, Heering KJ, van Oudalblas AB. How can treatment response be measured in breast cancer patients? Anticancer Res 1993;13:1901-4.
164. Dixon AR, Jackson L, Chan SY, Badley RA, Blamey RW. Continuous chemotherapy in responsive metastatic breast cancer: a role for tumour markers? Br J Cancer 1993;68:181-5.
165. Kiang DT, Greenberg LJ, Kennedy BJ. Tumor marker kinetics in the monitoring of breast cancer. Cancer 1990;65:193-9.
166. Tomiak EM, Piccart MJ. Routine follow-up of patients following primary therapy for early breast cancer: what is useful? Acta Clin Belg 1993;15:38-42.
167. Wertheimer MD. Against minimalism in breast cancer follow-up. JAMA 1991;265:396-7.
168. Schapira DV. Breast cancer surveillance—a cost-effective strategy. Breast Cancer Res Treat 1993;25:107-11.
169. Marrazzo A, Solina G, Puccia V, Fiorentino E, Bazan P. Evaluation of routine follow-up after surgery for breast carcinoma. J Surg Oncol 1986;32:179-81.
170. Dewar JA, Kerr GR. Value of routine follow-up of women treated for early carcinoma of the breast. Br Med J 1985;291:1464-7.
171. Zwaveling A, Albers GH, Felthuis W, Hermans J. An evaluation of routine follow-up for detection of breast cancer recurrences. J Surg Oncol 1987;34:194-7.
172. Morris S, Corder AP, Taylor I. What are the benefits of routine breast cancer follow-up? Postgrad Med J 1992;68:904-7.
173. Tomiak E, Piccart M. Routine follow-up of patients after primary therapy for early breast cancer: changing concepts and challenges for the future. Ann Oncol 1993;4:199-204.
174. Ayash LJ. High dose chemotherapy with autologous stem cell support for the treatment of metastatic breast cancer. Cancer 1994;74: 532-5.
175. Shpall EJ, Jones RB, Bearman S. High-dose therapy with autologous bone marrow transplantation for the treatment of solid tumors. Curr Opin Oncol 1994;6:135-8.
176. Triozzi PL. Autologous bone marrow and peripheral blood progenitor transplant for breast cancer. Lancet 1994;344:418-9.
177. Peters WP, Ross M, Vredenburgh JJ, et al. High-dose chemotherapy and autologous bone marrow support as consolidation after standard-dose adjuvant therapy for high-risk primary breast cancer. J Clin Oncol 1993;11:1132-43.
178. Mulder NH, Mulder PO, Sleijfer DT, et al. Induction chemotherapy and intensification with autologous bone marrow reinfusion in patients with locally advanced and disseminated breast cancer. Eur J Cancer 1993;29A:668-71.
179. Eddy DM. High-dose chemotherapy with autologous bone marrow transplantation for the treatment of metastatic breast cancer. J Clin Oncol 1992;10:657-70.
180. Horton J. Follow-up of breast cancer patients. Cancer 1984;53:790-7.
181. Theriault RL, Hortobagyi GN. Bone metastasis in breast cancer. Anticancer Drugs 1992;3:455-62.
182. Pritchard DJ, Burch PA. Orthopedic complications. In: Holland JF, Freii E III, Bast RC Jr , Kufe DW, Morton DL, Weichselbaum RR, editors. Cancer medicine. 3rd ed. Philadelphia: Lea & Febiger, 1993:2290-3.
183. Glover DJ, Grabelsky S, Glick JH. Oncological emergencies and special complications. In: Calabresi P, Schein PS, Bast Jr RC, Kufe DW, Morton DL, Weichselbaum RR, editors. Medical oncology: basic principles and clinical management of cancer. 2nd ed. New York: McGraw-Hill, Inc., 1993:1021-72.
184. Harrison KM, Muss HB, Ball MR, McWhorter M, Case D. Spinal cord compression in breast cancer. Cancer 1985;55:2839-44.
185. Heitanen P. Response to follow-up of breast cancer. Strahlenther Onkol 1985;161:678-80.
186. Muss HB, Tell GS, Case LD, Robertson P, Atwell BM. Perceptions of follow-up care in women with breast cancer. Am J Clin Oncol 1991;14:55-9.

➢ COUNTERPOINT

Memorial Sloan-Kettering Cancer Center

BRIAN J. O'HEA AND PATRICK I. BORGEN

As Edge et al. have appropriately pointed out, breast cancer is an enormous public health concern. Despite the alarming statistics presented, however, the 5-year survival rate for breast cancer increased for the first time ever during the interval from 1983 to 1990.[1] As the incidence of breast cancer rises and if mortality rates continue to fall, the cohort of breast cancer survivors with special follow-up needs will continue to grow.

Posttreatment surveillance programs traditionally focus on the early detection of cancer recurrence. Follow-up visits are frequently dominated by questions concerning visit frequency, extent-of-disease testing, diet, genetic testing, hormone replacement therapy, and subsequent pregnancy. This counterpoint addresses some of these difficult questions and outlines the breast cancer follow-up program at Memorial Sloan-Kettering Cancer Center.

GENERAL MEDICAL SURVEILLANCE

Primary Care

Current speculation postulates an association between dietary fat intake and outcome in patients with breast cancer.[2] Sakamoto et al.[3] found that for postmenopausal patients with localized breast cancer the 10-year survival rate in Japan was nearly twice that in the United States. There was no appreciable difference, however, among premenopausal patients. A more recent Canadian study showed that a diet high in saturated fats before the development of breast cancer was associated with an increased risk of dying from the disease.[4] Although the results of these and other studies do not establish a causal relationship between fat intake and breast cancer survival, the survival differences identified could not be explained by differences in any other currently accepted prognostic factor.

Memorial Sloan-Kettering Cancer Center is participating in the ongoing Women's Intervention Nutrition Study.[5] In this study postmenopausal patients are randomly assigned to either a dietary intervention group (15% calories from fat) or a dietary control group, with cancer relapse and survival as end points. In the future, dietary manipulation and other life-style modifications may become important to patients with breast cancer. To this end we agree with Edge et al. that the primary care physician should remain an active participant in the general health as well as the breast health of breast cancer survivors.

Genetic Counseling

The cloning of the breast cancer predisposition gene *BRCA1* in 1994 ushered in a new era of breast cancer research.[6] A *BRCA1* mutation carries with it a 73% risk of breast cancer by age 50, which becomes an 87% risk by age 70.[7] In addition, *BRCA1* mutation carriers have a 44% risk of ovarian cancer by age 70. Significantly increased risks for colon cancer (relative risk 4.11) and prostate cancer (relative risk 3.33) are also found in susceptible probands.[7] These risks, however, are much lower than the breast and ovarian risks, translating into absolute risks by age 70 of 8% and 6%, respectively.[7] With the widespread clinical availability of *BRCA1* testing on the near horizon, physicians can expect that a subset of patients may want to be tested. The results of this testing will have enormous implications in terms of family planning, increased surveillance in other family members, and even consideration of prophylactic surgery. In addition, genetic testing may expose the patient to the risk of employment- and insurance-related discrimination. At Memorial Sloan-Kettering Cancer Center physicians have developed an integrated program with the clinical genetics department that will provide *BRCA1* and eventually *BRCA2* testing for selected patients and their families within the framework of comprehensive pre-test and post-test counseling. Physicians must brace for the increased number of patients who will request genetic testing as these analyses become commercially available. Certainly, genetic counseling and ultimately genetic testing should be available at any institution offering comprehensive follow-up care of patients with breast cancer.

Hormone Replacement Therapy

One of the most controversial topics facing breast cancer survivors today is the safety of hormone replacement therapy.[8] In an attempt to answer this question more completely, a prospective clinical trial of hormone replacement in breast cancer survivors is under way at M.D. Anderson Cancer Center, as alluded to by Edge et al.[9] Breast cancer survivors are given hormones after a disease-free interval of 2 years in the case of estrogen receptor–negative tumors and a disease-free interval of 10 years if the receptor status of the original tumor is unknown. Unfortunately, it will take years to learn even the preliminary results of this study, which is designed to detect a difference in recurrence rate of 10% or more. Moreover, the safety of hormone replacement therapy in patients known to have estrogen receptor–positive tumors will not be determined because these patients are not included in the study.

Recently there has been interest in alternatives to the commonly prescribed estrogens for hormone replacement therapy. Clonidine has been used to ameliorate hot flashes.[10] Calcium and fluoride supplements have been used to reduce the demineralization of bone. However, whether these supplements alone can reduce osteoporosis in postmenopausal patients deprived of estrogen is unclear. Etidronate also appears to reduce osteoporosis and fractures in postmenopausal patients.[11]

Phytoestrogens are nonsteroidal substances of plant origin, particularly abundant in soy products. These naturally occurring substances are thought to exert both estrogen agonist and antagonist-like effects. The abundance of soy products in the Japanese diet has been postulated to explain the extremely low incidence of hot flashes in the Japanese population.[12] Phytoestrogens may ameliorate menopausal symptoms in patients for whom hormone replacement presents an unacceptable risk.

Perhaps the greatest benefit of hormone replacement therapy for postmenopausal patients is the reduction in the risk of cardiovascular disease. However, a low-fat diet, cholesterol-lowering medication, regular exercise, and smoking cessation can also reduce the risk of cardiovascular disease for patients in whom estrogen therapy is thought to be risky. We agree with Edge et al. that until more definitive evidence is available, hormone replacement therapy should not routinely be recommended after breast cancer. We encourage patients to use other nonhormonal remedies that may diminish disabling menopausal symptoms without potentially adding to the risk of breast cancer recurrence.

Second Primary Malignancies

The most common second primary malignancy in patients with breast cancer is carcinoma of the opposite breast. In a report from Memorial Sloan-Kettering Cancer Center, Rosen et al.[13] found that in 9% of patients a subsequent contralateral cancer developed after 18 years. The average annual hazard rate per person at risk was calculated to be 0.8% per year. Most breast cancer survivors are also at slightly increased risk for the development of other nonbreast malignancies. In the Connecticut Tumor Registry, 41,109 breast cancer cases were identified between 1935 and 1982.[14] Of 2,661 women monitored for more than 20 years, 340 (12.8%, relative risk 1.6) subsequently had a second primary malignant tumor, a rate that was statistically significant. Of these second primary tumors, 34% were in the contralateral breast, 22% in the colon or rectum, 9% in the lung, 6% in the uterus, and 4% in the ovary. The elevated incidence of each of these second primary cancers was statistically significant, with relative risks in the 1.5 to 2 range.[14]

Pregnancy After Breast Cancer

Young patients with breast cancer often ask about the safety of subsequent pregnancies, particularly with regard to tumor recurrence and survival. Some breast cancer survivors interested in subsequent pregnancies express a desire for a sense of "normalcy" and a way to "reconnect."[15] Others say that being pregnant would make them feel complete and help them to get well again. These feelings are tempered by concerns about tumor recurrence and mortality.

Currently available data on this subject come only from retrospective studies, most of which show a relatively favorable 5-year survival rate of 50% to 75% in patients with a pregnancy after breast cancer.[16,17] Other studies have actually reported a survival advantage imparted by pregnancy after breast cancer.[18,19] Despite various attempts to find matched control subjects in these studies, significant selection bias probably exists because only patients who showed no evidence of disease became pregnant. Sankila et al.[19] have referred to this inescapable selection bias as the "healthy mother effect."

Unfortunately, in addition to selection bias, these reports are apt to suffer recollection bias, since only patients who are alive and doing well are likely to be included in retrospective studies. In fact, Petrek[20] estimates that the 41 patients reported in the Memorial Sloan-Kettering Cancer Center study[21] represent only 10% of patients with breast cancer treated during that time interval who have subsequently become pregnant. Clearly it is possible to identify a cohort of patients with pregnancies after breast cancer that does as well as retrospectively matched control subjects. It remains unclear, however, how the cohort of patients does as a whole and whether limited information on a small subset of the entire cohort can be used legitimately to make treatment decisions for individual patients.

More complete data will require the creation of a prospective database including all patients with breast cancer who subsequently become pregnant. Until more definitive data support the safety of pregnancy after breast cancer, we do not encourage patients to become pregnant.

THERAPY-INDUCED CANCER

Tamoxifen

The beneficial effects of tamoxifen are impressive. In the Early Breast Cancer Trialists' Collaborative Group metaanalysis, adjuvant tamoxifen therapy was found to reduce the annual odds of tumor recurrence by 25%, while the annual odds of death were reduced by 17%.[22] In a second metaanalysis of eight trials of adjuvant hormonal therapy, tamoxifen reduced the risk of contralateral breast carcinoma by 35%.[23]

Although tamoxifen has increased the incidence of endometrial carcinoma when used as adjuvant treatment for breast cancer, the influence is thought to be small.[24] Recently a report from Memorial Sloan-Kettering Cancer Center looked at 20 cases of endometrial carcinoma in 232 patients with breast cancer undergoing dilation and curettage.[25] All 20 cases of endometrial carcinoma occurred in patients with abnormal bleeding. Not a single case of endometrial carcinoma was found in 23 tamoxifen users who were asymptomatic. Clearly patients taking tamoxifen should undergo yearly pelvic examinations and Pap smears, with endometrial sampling for any abnormal vaginal bleeding. We agree with Edge et al. that endometrial biopsy and endometrial ultrasound are not routinely recommended for otherwise asymptomatic patients taking tamoxifen.

It is worth mentioning that routine yearly endometrial sampling is a requirement for patients currently being entered into the NSABP P-1 tamoxifen chemoprevention trial. Patient accrual for this trial came to a halt after an increased risk of endometrial carcinoma was found among tamoxifen users in the NSABP B-14 trial. This otherwise aggressive surveillance for endometrial carcinoma is understandable, however, within the context of a chemoprevention trial in otherwise healthy individuals.

SURVEILLANCE FOR BREAST CANCER RECURRENCE

Locoregional Recurrence

The incidence of locoregional recurrence after mastectomy varies greatly in the literature. At 10 years of follow-up in the NSABP B-04 study the locoregional recurrence rate after total mastectomy was approximately 7%.[26] Recurrence after mastectomy has traditionally been associated with an ominous prognosis. Gilliand et al.[27] retrospectively reviewed 60 patients with chest wall recurrence after mastectomy, all of whom eventually died of breast cancer up to 232 months after treatment. In a review of 204 patients by Bedwinek et al.[28] the 5-year disease-free survival for patients with isolated locoregional recurrence was a mere 13%. A solitary recurrence, largest tumor recurrence less than 1 cm, and a disease-free interval greater than 24 months were all factors predictive of a better outcome. If any two of these factors were present, 5-year survival was 52%.

Axillary recurrence tends to have an even worse prognosis. Deckers[29] reviewed the results of patients in the NSABP B-04 study who were randomly assigned to receive no axillary treatment at all. Clinically apparent axillary disease subsequently developed in 68 patients, 58 (81%) of whom have failed systemically at a median time of 17 months after recurrence.

The treatment of locoregional recurrence after mastectomy usually involves a combination of local excision and radiation therapy. The 5-year local control rate was reported as 57% in one series.[30] Solitary chest wall recurrences, small isolated recurrences, and recurrences that were totally excised had the best local control rates at lower radiation therapy doses. Bedwinek et al.[31] reported that 62% of patients with uncontrollable locoregional disease had symptoms that impaired their quality of life. A program of surveillance for early detection of locoregional recurrence after mastectomy is unlikely to result in breast cancer cures. However, recurrences that are detected earlier may be smaller, isolated, more easily treatable, and associated with longer disease-free survival. More convincingly, early detection of locoregional recurrence may improve local control and impart a quality-of-life benefit in doing so.

Ipsilateral Breast Failure After Breast Conservation

Breast conservation appears to provide survival rates equivalent to mastectomy in most patients with early breast cancer. Recently the 12-year results of the NSABP B-06 study were published.[32] The ipsilateral in-breast failure rate at 10 years was 10%. The failure rate for node-negative patients was 12%, as compared with 5% in the node-positive group, suggesting that adjuvant chemotherapy plays a role in reducing local recurrence.

Although the use of mammography after breast conservation at Memorial Sloan-Kettering Cancer Center is similar to that described by Edge et al., the following should be noted. When a new breast cancer develops as microcalcifications, postexcision mammography is recommended to exclude the possibility of residual calcifications. This postexcision mammogram also serves as a new baseline.

At the time of breast conservation, physicians at Memorial Sloan-Kettering Cancer Center routinely place six hemoclips around the periphery and the base of the wide-excision cavity, not only to assist in the accurate delivery of the radiation boost, but also to guide them in searching for recurrent disease on subsequent mammograms. Posttreatment scarring is often seen as a mammographically dense mass located within the area marked by the hemoclips. Recurrent carcinoma, however, often extends well beyond the perimeter of the old excision site as defined by the clips.

Edge et al. are correct in their assessment that a sizeable percentage of patients with local recurrence after breast conservation ultimately do well after salvage mastectomy. In 1991 physicians at Memorial Sloan-Kettering Cancer Center published the results of salvage mastectomy in 46 patients.[33] The data on results of 45 evaluable patients with a median follow-up of 80 months after salvage have been reviewed. Results show an actuarial 5-year overall survival rate of 74% and disease-free survival rate of 72%. Actuarial 10-year survival rates are 62% (overall) and 56% (disease free). A disease-free interval of greater than 24 months was associated with a significantly improved 10-year survival rate (87% versus 40%, p = .0052), as was early tumor stage at initial diagnosis (87% versus 31%, p = .03). In a recent review of ipsilateral breast recurrence in Milan, Veronesi et al.[34] reported a 5-year survival rate of 69% in 151 patients with isolated in-breast recurrence, results similar to those at Memorial Sloan-Kettering Cancer Center.

Detection of ipsilateral recurrence after breast conservation requires mammography and physical examination only. In the conserved irradiated breast, edema, scarring, and fibrosis can contribute to the difficulty of subsequent physical examinations. We use fine-needle aspiration to evaluate the less suspect, ill-defined thickening often detected at the treatment site. Excisional biopsy can be reserved for instances in which fine-needle aspiration is equivocal or for more clinically suspect lesions.

Metastatic Disease

In the follow-up of patients with breast cancer, metastatic disease is the finding physicians fear most. Although metastatic disease is as yet incurable, a recent metaanalysis of 50 randomized trials suggested that effective chemotherapy may prolong survival by as long as 6 months.[35] The crux of the issue concerning breast cancer follow-up is how aggressive physicians should be in pursuit of asymptomatic metastases.

Two recent prospective randomized trials could not demonstrate a survival advantage imparted by intensive follow-up of breast cancer patients.[36,37] The study from the Italian GIVIO group gives detailed data on the method of detecting recurrent disease. This study was designed to detect a 20% relative reduction in mortality with 80% power for patients undergoing intensive surveillance.[37] In both the intensive and nonintensive follow-up groups the physical examination schedule was the same. The presentation, evaluation, and treatment of symptomatic patients were also the same in both groups. Therefore intensive follow-up affected only the detection of metastases in asymptomatic patients undergoing laboratory or imaging studies.

In the intensive follow-up group, asymptomatic metastatic disease was identified in 39 patients. Five of the 39 patients in whom metastatic disease was found by physical examination can be excluded because their metastatic disease would have also been detected by physical examination in the nonintensive follow-up group. Thus 34 patients remain in the intensive follow-up group in whom metastatic disease was identified by methods other than history (symptoms) and physical examination. In the nonintensive follow-up group 26 asymptomatic patients with metastatic disease were identified. Therefore the intensive follow-up schedule resulted in earlier detection of metastatic disease in only eight of 655 patients (1.2%).

The GIVIO study does not establish conclusively that early detection of metastatic disease is useless. With such a marginally increased rate of detection it is not surprising that the intensive follow-up group had no survival advantage. Rather, the intensive follow-up program as offered in this trial seems to have failed primarily in its ability to detect preclinical metastatic disease.

In addition, the report from the GIVIO investigators indicates that conventional laboratory and imaging modalities do not effectively detect asymptomatic metastatic disease. The basic principles of tumor biology hold that systemic treatment of micrometastatic disease is likely to be most effective when the tumor burden is small.[38] Early detection and prompt treatment of metastatic disease are consistent with these principles and at least in theory should enhance the utility of systemic therapy.

Early detection of subclinical metastatic disease is particularly exciting when coupled with newer, more promising therapeutic modalities. In a recent randomized trial in South Africa, high-dose chemotherapy was compared with a conventional dosage schedule in patients with metastatic breast cancer.[39] High-dose chemotherapy was associated with a significantly higher response rate and median survival time (90 weeks versus 45 weeks) when compared with the conventional schedule. Two pilot studies under way at Memorial Sloan-Kettering Cancer Center are evaluating the potential role of tumor vaccine in the treatment of breast cancer. Patients with rising levels of tumor markers without identifiable disease are eligible to be immunized with either MUC-1-KLH conjugate or sTn cluster-KLH conjugate. The study end point is the induction of an immune response as evidenced by either a helper T cell or a cytotoxic T cell response.

Edge et al. make a good case against the routine monitoring of tumor markers in otherwise asymptomatic patients. In general, 40% to 50% of patients have a rise in either CEA or CA 15-3 levels before the development of metastases, with lead times ranging from 3 to 18 months.[40] The ability of tumor markers to predict tumor recurrence and progression of disease is under further investigation at Memorial Sloan-Kettering Cancer Center. We remain optimistic about the ability of tumor markers to identify preclinical systemic disease, particularly within the context of ongoing trials employing aggressive, innovative therapeutic modalities.

SUMMARY

Appropriate follow-up of breast cancer survivors will become increasingly important given the intense scrutiny of financial resource allocation and utilization. The focus and goal of follow-up programs are the early detection of recurrent disease. The efficacy of these efforts, however, is contingent upon the notion that routine surveillance in otherwise asymptomatic patients is beneficial. Whether newer, more effective chemotherapeutic modalities will convincingly substantiate the theoretical advantage of vigilant screening for asymptomatic metastatic disease remains to be seen.

At Memorial Sloan-Kettering Cancer Center physicians aggressively pursue local control in patients who otherwise show no sign of systemic disease. In the same way physicians are realistic but vigilant in the search for preclinical metastatic disease. It is in the latter patients, whose tumor burdens may be small, that the newer therapeutic modalities may be most effective.

In reaction to the current climate of cost containment, managed care, and capitation, disease management algorithms have evolved as an attempt to standardize care and maximize cost effectiveness. Table 15-3 gives an example of a breast cancer surveillance schedule that may soon be part of a more complex breast cancer treatment pathway at Memorial Sloan-Kettering Cancer Center. Although cost will continue to be a major factor in health care reform and will definitely influence any breast cancer follow-up algorithm, physicians must strive to do what is ultimately best for patients.

Table 15-3 Follow-up of patients with breast cancer: Memorial Sloan-Kettering Cancer Center

	YEAR				
	1	2	3	4	5
Office visit*	3	3	3	2	2
Liver function tests	3	3	3	2	2
CEA†	3	3	3	2	2
CA 15-3†	3	3	3	2	2
Pelvic examination	1	1	1	1	1
Papanicolaou test	1	1	1	1	1
Mammography‡	1	1	1	1	1
Chest x-ray	1	1	1	1	1

CEA, Carcinoembryonic antigen.
*Clinical follow-up examinations are alternated among the surgeon, radiation oncologist, medical oncologist, and occasionally the primary care physician.
†Although routine monitoring of CA 15-3 and CEA is not performed on all patients, medical oncologists remain optimistic about the potential impact of therapeutic intervention based solely on rising tumor markers.
‡Yearly mammography is recommended after an initial posttreatment mammogram in the conserved breast.

REFERENCES

1. Wingo PA, Tong T, Bolden S. Cancer statistics, 1995. CA Cancer J Clin 1995;45:8-30.
2. Morrison AS, Lowe CR, MacMahon B, Ravnihar B, Yuasa S. Some international differences in treatment and survival in breast cancer. Int J Cancer 1976;18:269-73.
3. Sakamoto G, Sugano H, Hartman WH. [Comparative clinicopathological study of breast cancer among Japanese and American women.] [in Japanese] Gan No Rinsho 1979;25:161-70.
4. Wynder EL, Kajitani T, Kuno J, et al. A comparison of survival rates between American and Japanese patients with breast cancer. Gynecol Obstet 1963;111:196-200.
5. Chlebowski RT, Blackburn GL, Buzzard IM, et al. Adherence to a dietary fat intake reduction program in postmenopausal women receiving therapy for early breast cancer: the Women's Intervention Nutrition Study. J Clin Oncol 1993;11:2072-80.
6. Miki Y, Swensen J, Shattuck-Eidens D, et al. A strong candidate for the breast and ovarian cancer susceptibility gene BRCA1. Science 1994;266:66-71.
7. Ford D, Easton DF, Bishop DT, Narod SA, Goldgar DE. Risks of cancer in BRCA1-mutation carriers. Breast Cancer Linkage Consortium. Lancet 1994;343:692-5.
8. DiSaia PJ, Grosen EA, Odicino F, et al. Replacement therapy for breast cancer survivors. Cancer 1995;76(Suppl 1):2075-8.
9. Vassilopoulou-Sellin R, Theriault RL. Randomized prospective trial of estrogen-replacement therapy in women with a history of breast cancer. Monogr Natl Cancer Inst 1994;16:153-9.
10. Nagamani M, Kelver ME, Smith ER. Treatment of menopausal hot flashes with transdermal administration of clonidine. Am J Obstet Gynecol 1987;156:561-5.
11. Strom T, Thamsborg G, Steiniche T, Genant HK, Sorensen OH. Effect of intermittent cyclical etidronate therapy on bone mass and fracture rate in women with postmenopausal osteoporosis. N Engl J Med 1990;322:1265-71.
12. Adlercreutz H, Hamalainen E, Gorbach S, Goldin B. Dietary phytooestrogens and the menopause in Japan. Lancet 1992;339:1233.

13. Rosen PP, Groshen S, Kinne DW, Hellman S. Contralateral breast carcinoma: an assessment of risk and prognosis in stage I (T1N0M0) and stage II (T1N1M0) patients with 20-year follow-up. Surgery 1989;106:904-10.
14. Harvey EB, Brinton LA. Second cancer following cancer of the breast in Connecticut, 1935-82. Monogr Natl Cancer Inst 1885;68:99-112.
15. Dow KH. Having children after breast cancer. Cancer Practice 1994;2:407-13.
16. Cheek JH. Cancer of the breast in pregnancy and lactation. Am J Surg 1973;126:729-31.
17. Cooper DR, Butterfield J. Pregnancy subsequent to mastectomy for cancer of the breast. Ann Surg 1970;171:429-33.
18. von Schoultz E, Johansson H, Wilking N, Rutqvist LE. Influence of prior and subsequent pregnancy on breast cancer prognosis. J Clin Oncol 1995;13:430-4.
19. Sankila R, Heinavaara S, Hakulinen T. Survival of breast cancer patients after subsequent term pregnancy: "healthy mother effect." Am J Obstet Gynecol 1994;170:818-23.
20. Petrek JA. Pregnancy safety after breast cancer. Cancer 1994;74:528-31.
21. Harvey JC, Rosen PP, Ashikari P, Robbins GF, Kinne DW. The effect of pregnancy on the prognosis of carcinoma of the breast following radical mastectomy. Surg Gynecol Obstet 1981;153:723-5.
22. Early Breast Cancer Trialists' Collaborative Group. Systemic treatment of early breast cancer by hormonal, cytotoxic, or immune therapy: 133 randomised trials involving 31,000 recurrences and 24,000 deaths among 75,000 women. Lancet 1992;339:71-85.
23. Nayfield SG, Karp JE, Ford LG, Dorr FA, Kramer BS. Potential role of tamoxifen in prevention of breast cancer. J Natl Cancer Inst 1991;83:1450-9.
24. Jordan VC, Assikis VJ. Endometrial carcinoma and tamoxifen: clearing up a controversy. Clin Cancer Res 1995;1:467-74.
25. Gibson LE, Barakat RR, Venkatraman ES, et al. Endometrial pathology at dilatation and curettage in breast cancer patients: comparison of tamoxifen users and nonusers. Proc Am Soc Clin Oncol 1994;863.
26. Fisher B, Redmond C, Fisher ER, et al. Ten-year results of a randomized clinical trial comparing radical mastectomy and total mastectomy with or without irradiation. N Engl J Med 1985;312:674-81.
27. Gilliland MD, Barton RM, Copeland EM 3d. The implications of local recurrence of breast cancer as the first site of therapeutic failure. Ann Surg 1983;197:284-7.
28. Bedwinek JM, Lee J, Fineberg B, Ocwieza M. Prognostic indicators in patients with isolated local-regional recurrence of breast cancer. Cancer 1981;47:2232-5.
29. Deckers PJ. Axillary dissection in breast cancer: when, why, how much, and for how long? Another operation soon to be extinct? J Surg Oncol 1991;48:217-9.
30. Halverson KJ, Perez CA, Kuske RR, Garcia DM, Simpson JR, Fineberg B. Isolated local-regional recurrence of breast cancer following mastectomy: radiotherapeutic management. Int J Radiat Oncol Biol Phys 1990;19:851-8.
31. Bedwinek JM, Fineberg B, Lee J, Ocwieza M. Analysis of failures following local treatment of isolated local-regional recurrence of breast cancer. Int J Radiat Oncol Biol Phys 1981;7:581-5.
32. Fisher B, Anderson S, Redmond CK, Wolmark N, Wickerham DL, Cronin WM. Reanalysis and results after 12 years of follow-up in a randomized clinical trial comparing total mastectomy with lumpectomy with or without irradiation in the treatment of breast cancer. N Engl J Med 1995;333:1456-61.
33. Osborne MP, Borgen PI, Wong GY, Rosen PP, McCormick B. Salvage mastectomy for local and regional recurrence after breast-conserving operation and radiation therapy. Surg Gynecol Obstet 1992;174:189-94.
34. Veronesi U, Marubini E, Del Vecchio M, et al. Local recurrences and distant metastases after conservative breast cancer treatments: partly independent events. J Natl Cancer Inst 1995;87:19-27.
35. A'Hern RP, Ebbs SR, Baum MB. Does chemotherapy improve survival in advanced breast cancer? A statistical overview. Br J Cancer 1988;57:615.
36. Rosselli Del Turco M, Palli D, Cariddi A, Ciatto S, Pacini P, Distante V. Intensive diagnostic follow-up after treatment of primary breast cancer: National Research Council Project on breast cancer follow-up. JAMA 1994;271:1593-7.
37. The GIVIO Investigators. Impact of follow-up testing on survival and health-related quality of life in breast cancer patients: a multicenter randomized controlled trial. JAMA 1994;271:1587-92.
38. Davidson NE, Lippman ME. Adjuvant therapy for breast cancer. In: Lippman ME, Lichter AS, Danforth DN, editors. Diagnosis and management of breast cancer. Philadelphia: WB Saunders, 1980:348-74.
39. Bezwoda WR, Seymour L, Dansey RD. High-dose chemotherapy with hematopoietic rescue as primary treatment for metastatic breast cancer: a randomized trial. J Clin Oncol 1995;13:2483-9.
40. Hayes DF. Tumor markers for breast cancer: current utilities and future prospects. Hematol Oncol Clin North Am 1994;8:485-506.

➢ COUNTER POINT

National Cancer Center Hospital

TAKASHI FUKUTOMI

Although excellent results have been achieved in the treatment of breast cancer, recurrence is seen in approximately 25% to 30% of Japanese patients who undergo surgery. In this counterpoint the clinical application of prognostic factors and methods for postoperative surveillance are discussed, with emphasis on the direction that the National Cancer Center Hospital is taking.

PROGNOSTIC FACTORS

It would be clinically useful if physicians could determine prospectively the biological aggressiveness of breast cancer and predict whether metastasis or local recurrence is likely to occur. However, even today, histopathologically confirmed axillary lymph node metastasis is the most important prognostic factor. Figure 15-6 shows the survival curves after mastectomy depending on whether the axillary lymph nodes were involved. Japanese patients with breast cancer show approximately a 5% to 15% 10-year survival advantage, ignoring prognostic variables, when compared with their Caucasian counterparts.[1] It is difficult to analyze prognostic factors and to evaluate the efficacy of postoperative adjuvant therapy because of better overall treatment results in Japanese patients. In addition to lymph node involvement a number of prognostic factors have been investigated at the National Cancer Center Hospital, including menopausal status, tumor size, histological grade, hormone receptor status, c-*erb*B-2 expression, p53 expression, and cathepsin D in breast cancer cells.

Histological grade is a useful prognostic factor, particularly in node-negative cases (Table 15-4). The prognosis of node-negative patients with a tumor having p53 expression is also significantly poorer than of those without p53 expression (Figure 15-7).[2] In contrast, c-*erb*B-2 expression is positive in 35% of intraductal and predominantly intraductal carcinomas.[3] Physicians at the National Cancer Center Hos-

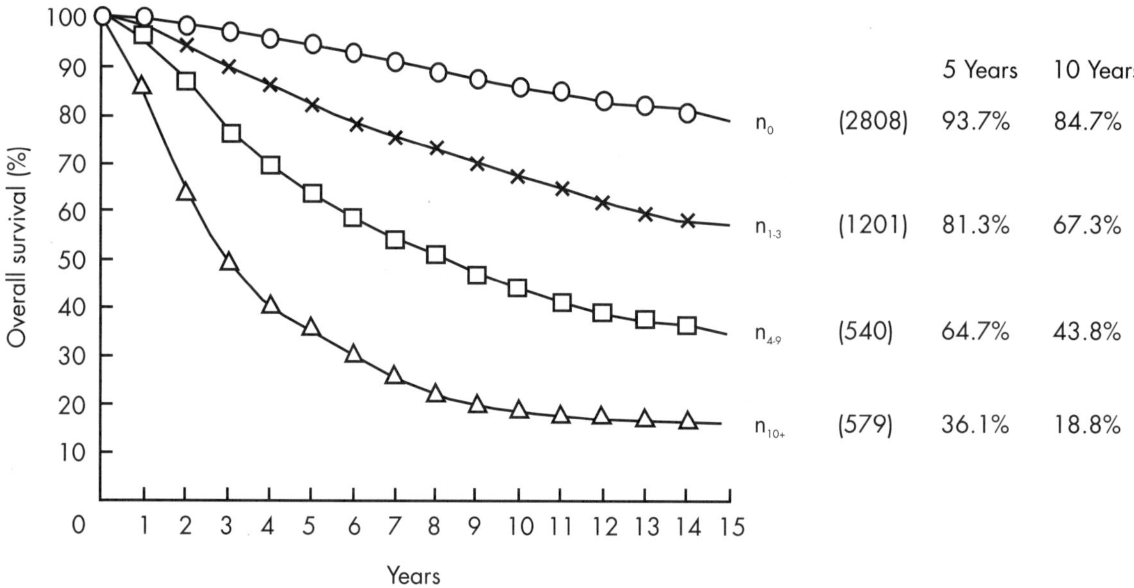

Figure 15-6 Overall survival by lymph node status. (Data from the National Cancer Center Hospital.)

Table 15-4 Risk factors in univariate analysis with respect to recurrence within 2 years*

	TOTAL NUMBER OF PATIENTS (n = 154)	NUMBER WITH RECURRENCE (%) (n = 32)	RISK RATIO (95% CONFIDENCE INTERVAL)
p53			
–	121	19 (15.7)	1.00
+	33	13 (39.4)	3.28 (1.43-7.53)
c-*erb*B-2			
–	120	25 (20.8)	1.00
+	15	1 (6.7)	0.24 (0.03-2.00)
++	19	6 (31.6)	1.75 (0.58-5.26)
+ and ++	34	7 (20.6)	0.95 (0.36-2.54)
Cathepsin D			
–	62	20 (32.3)	1.00
+	70	7 (10.0)	0.22 (0.08-0.59)
++	22	5 (22.7)	0.45 (0.12-1.67)
+ and ++	92	12 (13.4)	0.26 (0.10-0.64)
Histological grade			
Grade 1	26	1 (3.8)	1.00
Grade 2	87	12 (13.8)	5.07 (0.6-41.7)
Grade 3	41	19 (46.3)	42.6 (4.35-417)
Histological type			
Noninvasive	26	3 (11.5)	1.00
Invasive	128	29 (22.7)	2.29 (0.6-8.3)
ID or IL	114	29 (25.4)	
SP	14	0 (0)	

Data from Iwaya K, Tsuda H, Fukutomi T, et al.[6]
–, Negative; +, weakly positive; ++, strongly positive; *ID*, invasive ductal carcinoma; *IL*, invasive lobular carcinoma; *SP*, "special types" of invasive carcinoma.

pital suggest that node-negative patients with histological grade 3 tumor or positive p53 expression should receive intensive follow-up and postoperative adjuvant therapy.

The prognosis of node-positive patients with positive c-*erb*B-2 expression is significantly poorer than the prognosis of those with negative c-*erb*B-2 (Figure 15-8).[3,4] Mutations of p53 and expression of c-*erb*B-2 occur mostly in patients with grade 3 tumors but are not associated with lymph node status.[3,5] Hormone receptor status is inversely correlated with these genetic alterations.[3] Cathepsin D was

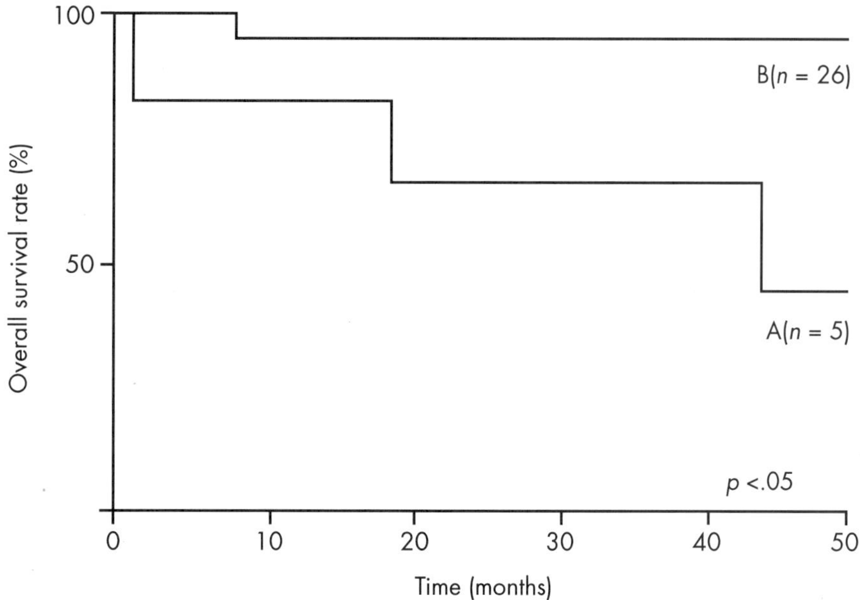

Figure 15-7 Kaplan-Meier overall survival curves for patients with breast carcinoma with regard to immunoreaction with PAb-1801. *A*, Positive cases. *B*, Negative cases. (Modified from Iwaya K, Tsuda H, Hiraide H, et al. Jpn J Cancer Res 1991;82:835-40.)

not found to be useful. Alterations in the two genes can be used as indicators of disease prognosis independent of lymph node status. It seems that these gene alterations occur in breast cancers showing a high proliferation rate irrespective of any invasion. Therefore physicians at the National Cancer Center Hospital routinely evaluate all cases of breast cancer after mastectomy by using several parameters, including histological grade, lymph node involvement, hormone receptor status, and expression of c-*erb*B-2 and p53 determined by immunohistochemistry. Histological grade is used as an indicator of follow-up surveillance for all stages of breast cancer to select cases with a poorer prognosis, while c-*erb*B-2 and p53 are used clinically as prestratification factors before carrying out the chemoendocrine therapy protocol for node-positive disease.

PATTERNS OF RECURRENCE

Tables 15-5 and 15-6 show the first site of recurrence, the incidence of recurrence as assessed histologically by lymph node involvement, and the disease-free period found in 779 recurrent breast cancer cases at the National Cancer Center Hospital. Based on the analysis of these cases the patterns of recurrence after mastectomy can be summarized in the following ways. First, the most important prognostic factor in patients with breast cancer is the number of lymph nodes involved. Second, patients with higher stage disease tend to have a shorter disease-free interval.

The initial sites of recurrence are local lesions (28%), bone (26%), lung and pleura (33%), and liver (8%), these sites comprising 95% of recurrent sites. The lower incidence of liver metastasis as the first site of recurrence may be because of poorer ability to diagnose liver metastasis than lung or bone metastases. Comparative studies in patients with breast cancer in Japan and Great Britain have shown that Japanese patients with breast cancer have a slightly higher incidence of supraclavicular lymph node and lung metastases than their English counterparts, whereas a higher incidence of bone metastases was found in the English patients.[7]

The peak incidence of recurrence is within 2 to 3 years of the mastectomy, with a median disease-free interval of 24 months and a mean disease-free interval of 35 months. Approximately 85% of recurrences occurred within 5 years. Classification according to the metastatic site showed that the median disease-free period was 17 months for skin and chest wall metastases, 20 months for liver metastases, and approximately 24 to 28 months for lung, bone, and regional lymph node metastases.

PRACTICAL PROCEDURES FOR FOLLOW-UP SURVEILLANCE

In the outpatient clinic at the National Cancer Center Hospital, postoperative follow-up surveillance includes a history and physical examination, which are thought to be the most important modalities. Inspection and palpation of the local region (ipsilateral chest wall, axillary region, supraclavicular region, and contralateral breast), as well as blood tests (liver function tests and tumor markers ST 439, CEA, and CA 15-3), are performed once every 6 months in node-negative patients for 5 years. Patients who are node-negative with histological grade 3 tumors or whose tumors exhibit positive p53 expression are followed up in the same way as node-positive patients. History and physical examinations as well as blood tests are performed once every 3 months for 2 years. Patients are then seen biannually, similar to node-

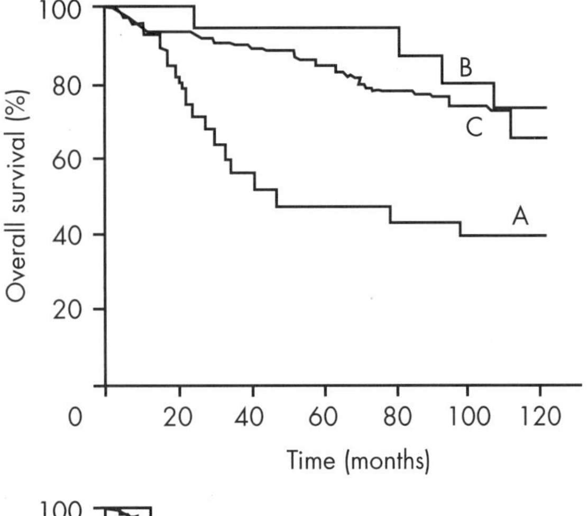

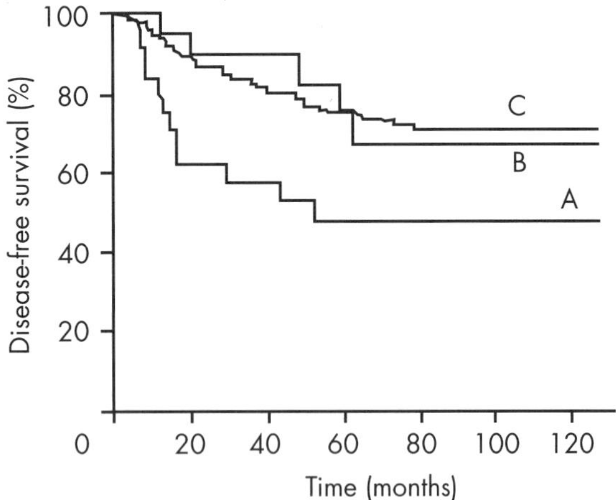

Figure 15-8 Survival curves of patients with breast carcinoma. Overall survival curves *(upper)* and disease-free survival curves *(lower)* for, *A*, the group with strong staining (++) of c-*erb*B-2 protein; *B*, the group with weak staining (+) of c-*erb*B-2 protein; and, *C*, the group with no staining (–) of c-*erb*B-2 protein. (Modified from Tsuda H, Hirohashi S, Shimosato Y, et al. Jpn J Cancer Res 1990;81:327-32.)

negative patients, after 2 years. Chest x-ray, ultrasound examinations of the abdomen, and bone scintigram scans are performed annually in all cases (both node-positive and node-negative) for up to 5 years after surgery.

If the number of metastatic lymph nodes is at least 10, or at least four with c-*erb*B-2 positive expression or histological grade 3, a higher rate of recurrence can be predicted and the disease-free interval tends to be shorter. The diagnostic tests previously mentioned are performed every 6 months for 2 years after surgery. History, physical examination, and blood tests are performed every 6 months in all patients between 5 and 10 years after surgery. Examinations are performed once a year after 10 years. In recent years computed tomography has often been used to confirm the presence of metastases, particularly in the liver. Liver scintigraphy, however, is rarely performed. When bone metastases are suspected, magnetic resonance imaging can be helpful because it improves the detection rate of bone metastases to approximately 95%. Various tumor markers have been useful in predicting the recurrence of breast cancer and assessing disease progression, as well as the efficacy of treatment. Three tumor markers—CEA, CA 15-3, and ST 439—are used at the National Cancer Center Hospital.

Table 15-5 Rates of first site of recurrence and disease-free interval in 779 recurrent breast cancer cases at the National Cancer Center Hospital, Tokyo

SITE OF RECURRENCE	NUMBER OF CASES (%)	DISEASE-FREE MONTHS MEDIAN (RANGE)
Skin	128 (19%)	17 (2-194)
Lymph nodes	62 (9%)	27 (2-157)
Bone	176 (26%)	24 (3-160)
Lung	185 (27%)	26 (3-216)
Pleura	40 (6%)	28 (5-121)
Liver	53 (8%)	20 (2-153)
Brain	19 (3%)	24 (3-132)
Other*	16 (2%)	——

*Includes the thyroid, ovary, peritoneum, and choroid.

Table 15-6 Relationship between lymph node metastasis and disease-free interval in 779 cases of recurrent breast cancer at the National Cancer Center Hospital, Tokyo

LYMPH NODE METASTASIS	NUMBER OF CASES (%)	DISEASE-FREE MONTHS MEDIAN (RANGE)*
Negative (56%)	138 (20)	43 (3-183)
Positive (44%)	558 (80)	22 (3-216)

*$p < .01$.

Local recurrence rates in the treated breast after breast conservation therapy have been reported to be between 5% and 20%.[8] The probability of occurrence of contralateral breast carcinoma is approximately 5%. In patients with cancer recurrence in the ipsilateral breast or on the contralateral side, early detection will obviously improve the prognosis. Therefore physicians at the National Cancer Center Hospital routinely perform inspection and palpation of both breasts at least once every 6 months, as well as performing mammography annually.

Questions have been raised about performing routine checkups in asymptomatic patients. Rosselli Del Turco et al.[9] reported that intensive surveillance by the use of diagnostic tests did not improve prognosis in patients with breast cancer in a randomized trial in Italy. The investigators also reported that frequent laboratory tests and roentgenography after primary treatment of breast cancer did not improve survival or influence health-related quality of life.[10] They reported that chest x-ray examination and mammography need only be performed annually. Bone scintigrams, abdominal ultrasonography, and tumor markers were not thought to be valuable in follow-up surveillance.

Table 15-7 Minimal requirements for follow-up after treatment of primary breast cancer with curative intent recommended by the European Organization for Research and Treatment of Cancer

Follow-up starts after the completion of surgery, radiation therapy, or adjuvant chemotherapy. Routine adjuvant tamoxifen treatment requires no special follow-up investigations.

MINIMAL TIME SCHEDULE

First year: 3-month interval between follow-up visits
Second to fifth year: biannual follow-up visits
After 5 years: annual follow-up visits for life

MINIMAL FOLLOW-UP INVESTIGATIONS

History
Physical examination with emphasis on the treated site of the breast, the contralateral breast, and regional lymph node areas
Annual mammography
All other investigations performed only when indicated

Data from EORTC Breast Cancer Cooperative Group. Manual for clinical research in breast cancer. Leuven, Belgium: 5th EORTC Breast Cancer Working Conference, 1991:61.

Table 15-8 Follow-up of patients with breast cancer (node-negative patients*): National Cancer Center Hospital, Japan

	YEAR				
	1	2	3	4	5
Office visit	2	2	2	2	2
Liver function tests	2	2	2	2	2
CEA	2	2	2	2	2
CA 15-3	2	2	2	2	2
ST 439	2	2	2	2	2
Mammography	1	1	1	1	1
Chest x-ray	1	1	1	1	1
Bone scan	1	1	1	1	1
Abdominal ultrasound	1	1	1	1	1

CEA, Carcinoembryonic antigen.
*Excluding patients with histological grade 3 tumor or positive p53 expression. Such patients are followed up in the same way as node-positive patients.

In addition, such unnecessary procedures have financial implications. In Japan 70% to 90% of medical costs are reimbursed by the health insurance system supported by the government. The European Organization for Research and Treatment of Cancer recommended minimal time schedules and follow-up investigations as listed in Table 15-7.[10]

Overall I support the belief that intensive follow-up has little impact on patient prognosis. However, because evaluation of therapeutic outcomes in each research protocol requires rather intensive surveillance, physicians at the National Cancer Center Hospital conduct follow-up as previously described (Tables 15-8 and 15-9).

Table 15-9 Follow-up of patients with breast cancer (node-positive and select node-negative patients*): National Cancer Center Hospital, Japan

	YEAR				
	1	2	3	4	5
Office visit	4	4	2	2	2
Liver function tests	4	4	2	2	2
CEA	4	4	2	2	2
CA 15-3	4	4	2	2	2
ST 439	4	4	2	2	2
Mammography	1	1	1	1	1
Chest x-ray	1†	1†	1	1	1
Bone scan	1†	1†	1	1	1
Abdominal ultrasound	1†	1†	1	1	1

CEA, Carcinoembryonic antigen.
*Includes node-negative patients with histological grade 3 tumor or positive p53 expression.
†Performed twice a year for patients whose number of metastatic lymph nodes is at least 10, irrespective of histological grade and c-*erb*B-2 expression, and for patients whose number of metastatic lymph nodes is at least four with c-*erb*B-2 positive expression or histological grade 3 tumor.

REFERENCES

1. Allen DS, Bulbrook MA, Hayward JL, et al. Recurrence and survival rates in British and Japanese women with breast cancer. Breast Cancer Res Treat 1991;18(Suppl 1):S131-4.
2. Iwaya K, Tsuda H, Hiraide H, et al. Nuclear p53 immunoreaction associated with poor prognosis of breast cancer. Jpn J Cancer Res 1991;82:835-40.
3. Tsuda H, Iwaya K, Fukutomi T, Hirohashi S. p53 mutations and c-*erb*B-2 amplification in intraductal and invasive breast carcinomas of high histological grade. Jpn J Cancer Res 1993;84:394-401.
4. Tsuda H, Hirohashi S, Shimosato Y, et al. Immunohistochemical study on overexpression of c-*erb*B-2 protein in human breast cancer: its correlation with gene amplification and long-term survival of patients. Jpn J Cancer Res 1990;81:327-32.
5. Tsuda H, Hirohashi S, Shimosato Y, et al. Correlation between histologic grade of malignancy and copy number of c-*erb*B-2 gene in breast carcinoma: a retrospective analysis of 175 cases. Cancer 1990;65:1794-800.
6. Iwaya K, Tsuda H, Fukutomi T, Tsugane S, Suzuki M, Hirohashi S. Histologic grade and p53 immunoreaction as indicators of early recurrence of node-negative breast cancer. Jpn J Clin Oncol 1997;27:6-12.
7. Chaudary MA. Patterns of recurrence in Western and Japanese women with breast cancer. Breast Cancer Res Treat 1991;18(Suppl 1):S115-8.
8. Haffty BG, Fisher D, Rose M, Beinfield M, McKhann C. Prognostic factors for local recurrence in the conservatively treated breast cancer patient: a cautious interpretation of the data. J Clin Oncol 1991;9:997-1003.
9. Rosselli Del Turco M, Palli D, Cariddi A, Ciatto S, Pacini P, Distante V. Intensive diagnostic follow-up after treatment of primary breast cancer: National Research Council Program on breast cancer follow-up. JAMA 1994;271:1593-7.
10. The GIVIO Investigators. Impact of follow-up testing on survival and health-related quality of life in breast cancer patients: a multicenter randomized controlled trial. JAMA 1994;271:1587-92.
11. EORTC Breast Cancer Cooperative Group. Manual for clinical research in breast cancer. Leuven, Belgium: 5th EORTC Breast Cancer Working Conference, 1991:61.

➢ COUNTER POINT

Royal Liverpool University Hospital, UK

JOHN WINSTANLEY

The approach to the follow-up of breast cancer taken by Edge et al. leaves one with the strong sense that the special relationship between the United Kingdom and the United States is not only political but medical as well, for there are few differences in the strategy of breast cancer follow-up between the two countries (Table 15-10). Those differences that do exist arise for the most part because of the logistical organization and manpower provision within the health care system in the United Kingdom.

Table 15-10 Follow-up of patients with breast cancer: Royal Liverpool University Hospital, UK

	YEAR				
	1	2	3	4	5
Office visit	2	2	2	1	1
Mammography*	1	1	1	1	1
Bone scan	†	†	†	†	†
Abdominal computed tomography	†	†	†	†	†
Abdominal ultrasound	†	†	†	†	†
Chest computed tomography	†	†	†	†	†
Pelvic ultrasound	†	†	†	†	†
Endometrial biopsy	†	†	†	†	†
CEA	‡	‡	‡	‡	‡
CA 15-3	‡	‡	‡	‡	‡

CEA, Carcinoembryonic antigen.
*Mammography should begin at 6 months after radiation for breast-conserving therapy.
†Performed if clinically indicated.
‡If recurrence is documented, it may be useful for assessing treatment response.

GENERAL MEDICAL SURVEILLANCE AND SCREENING FOR OTHER CANCERS

Although vigilance for malignancies in other organs is something that would be supported in principle, it is nonetheless perceived as a counsel of perfection. Manpower restrictions mean that routine screening for colorectal cancer in patients with breast cancer would normally be undertaken only in those with a strong family history of colon cancer or who also had breast cancer. No routine screening exists for colon cancer in the United Kingdom other than that provided by private health insurers. The same applies to endometrial carcinoma. Although it is accepted as a risk after prolonged tamoxifen use, the manpower to screen for this does not exist within the National Health Service. Moreover, since the prognosis, even if it does occur, is good, no pressure exists as yet to fund this service. Cervical carcinoma is covered by a national screening program; however, this is organized by the primary health care team and not the surgical oncologist. The surgeon caring for a patient with breast cancer is therefore concerned primarily with that cancer and its sequelae rather than the general oncological health of the patient.

SURVEILLANCE FOR RECURRENT TUMORS IN THE BREAST

In the United Kingdom the Royal College of Radiologists recently produced a report on the radiological follow-up of breast cancer, in which the consensus was that some form of regular mammography is mandatory for both the normal unaffected breast and the remaining breast in cases of conservation, although the optimal interval between screening tests is not clear. The current practice at Royal Liverpool University Hospital is to screen at annual intervals until a patient reaches an age at which she would not be considered fit for surgical intervention should a small impalpable recurrence or new tumor be found. This is by necessity a pragmatic approach. For instance, intensive screening of a patient of 65 with severe cardiac or pulmonary disease for recurrent carcinoma in a conserved irradiated breast seems inappropriate when there is little prospect of surgical intervention and the only other option is perhaps a change in hormonal therapy. Conversely, physicians would see much merit in screening a very fit 70-year old in whom the options for further surgical procedures, or even chemotherapy, remain open.

Physicians at Royal Liverpool University Hospital omit a mammogram at 6 months. All patients with palpable disease have mammography performed at diagnosis so that other occult tumors in the breast should be apparent. In the event that separate tumors or extensive ductal carcinoma in situ is present, physicians at this institution normally recommend mastectomy, making mammography for residual disease at 6 months redundant. In the case of impalpable screening-detected disease the United Kingdom National Breast Screening Programme has strict quality assurance standards requiring that all specimens excised be radiographed and discussed at a joint disciplinary meeting to ensure that all disease has been excised and appropriately treated. Furthermore, only designated pathologists, radiologists, and surgeons are allowed to treat such cancers. This process makes mammography at 6 months redundant.

Although it may be true, as Edge et al. point out, that in some instances unstable breast parenchyma may be identified, the general view in the United Kingdom and at Royal Liverpool University Hospital in particular is that the identification and treatment of such disease are unlikely to affect overall outcome and therefore the increased workload is not justified. The role of magnetic resonance imaging is as yet undefined. However, reports from the United Kingdom and Europe indicate that it has significant potential for identifying recurrent disease in the conserved breast[1] and in that respect may prove a useful tool in conjunction with mammography. With sufficient resources, magnetic resonance imaging could become the first-line screening tool for recurrent and primary disease and for screening the young breast at risk.

Controversy over the management of ductal carcinoma in situ exists in the United Kingdom as in the United States. This is the subject of a four-arm trial that is linked with a European trial comparing radiation therapy and tamoxifen. A similar trial exists for invasive ductal carcinomas of either special type or Bloom and Richardson grade 1. Accrual to these trials is slow, and no interim results are available. The policy with regard to the follow-up of lobular carcinoma in situ at Royal Liverpool University Hospital is the same as that outlined by Edge et al. (Table 15-1).

BREAST RECONSTRUCTION AND SURVEILLANCE

Attitudes toward reconstruction are becoming more liberal in the United Kingdom. At Royal Liverpool University Hospital approximately 50% of patients undergoing mastectomy choose reconstruction. Traditionally this has been performed with implants, but the use of live tissue reconstruction is becoming more popular. I have never seen the delayed detection of local recurrence as a problem and feel the psychological benefits of improved body image far outweigh any theoretical risk of delay in diagnosing recurrent disease.

SCREENING FOR DISTANT METASTASES

Screening for distant metastases is not the current policy at Royal Liverpool University Hospital. Although chest x-ray and liver function tests are relatively inexpensive and simple to perform, it is generally perceived that distant disease carries a poor prognosis and that little would be achieved by aggressive investigation. Indeed, it can be argued that there are positive disadvantages to alerting patients to recurrent disease that is likely to prove difficult to control. A similar attitude exists with regard to tumor markers in that they are not used in routine follow-up. Nevertheless, in some centers in Europe and the United Kingdom interest has been shown in using combinations of tumor markers to monitor progress and therapeutic response in proven recurrent disease. As a consequence, a European tumor marker collaborative group is being established to investigate this aspect of tumor marker use via a clinical trial.

REFERENCES

1. Lewis-Jones HG, Whitehouse GH, Leinster SJ. The role of magnetic resonance imaging in the assessment of local recurrent breast carcinoma. Clin Radiol 1991;43:197-204.

➢ COUNTERPOINT

University of Washington Medical Center ▪ Fred Hutchinson Cancer Research Center

JULIE R. GRALOW AND BENJAMIN O. ANDERSON

Breast cancer follow-up has three major goals: surveillance for cancer recurrence, monitoring for toxicities related to therapy, and maximizing overall health and quality of life for the cancer survivor. Most studies have found that intensive surveillance for early detection of distant metastases does not improve survival. With this information, managed health care systems push for reduced specialist involvement. Breast cancer survivors have complicated needs that require long-term follow-up by an oncology specialist. Third-party payors' data sets often fail to address quality-of-life issues such as body image and sexuality, menopausal symptoms, issues of survivorship, and the need to improve physical, work, and social functioning.

The strategy for breast cancer patient follow-up at the University of Washington Breast Cancer Specialty Center is to reduce the risk of cancer recurrence through careful risk assessment and evaluation of prognostic factors at initial treatment, followed by appropriate adjuvant therapy aimed at preventing recurrence. Patients are monitored for locoregional and distant recurrence based on prognostic factors at diagnosis, along with active surveillance for second breast cancers and potential treatment complications. Routine follow-up must address quality of life, general health, and emotional issues related to the diagnosis of breast cancer.

GENERAL MEDICAL SURVEILLANCE

General medical surveillance of patients with breast cancer should focus on routine health maintenance, as well as issues more specific to breast cancer. Factors affecting quality of life in these patients include menopause and reproduction, sexuality and body image, and fear of recurrence and survivorship. Because the majority of women with breast cancer ultimately survive their cancer, a critical component of breast cancer follow-up is to assure patients that routine health surveillance and risk reduction are not omitted.

Menopause and Reproductive Issues

Hormone replacement therapy after breast cancer

Managing menopausal symptoms and their sequelae in patients with breast cancer is challenging. Whether estrogen actually increases breast cancer risk in the general population is unknown.[1-4] However, women with a personal history of breast cancer may have increased susceptibility to the tumor-promoting effects of estrogen. Thus estrogen replacement therapy in breast cancer survivors is controversial and generally not recommended.

Although we share the concerns of Edge et al. regarding estrogen in patients with a history of breast cancer, all mortality causes must be considered when making decisions about estrogen for these patients. In the limited available reports of estrogen use in breast cancer survivors, no adverse sequelae have been demonstrated.[5,6] The prohibition of estrogen for low-risk patients with breast cancer may diminish both quality of life (because of vasomotor and urogenital symptoms, for instance) and overall survival by increasing the risk of coronary artery disease and osteoporotic fracture.[7] Death from nonneoplastic conditions is common among node-negative patients with breast cancer, and cardiovascular disease is the most common nonneoplastic cause of death.[8]

Until randomized clinical trials addressing the issue are completed, physicians at the University of Washington Breast Cancer Specialty Center generally avoid exogenous administration of estrogen to patients with breast cancer. However, a past history of breast cancer is not viewed as an absolute contraindication for supplemental estrogen use. In selected patients at very low risk of recurrence and more than 5 years from diagnosis, the potential benefits of estrogen may outweigh the theoretical risks. In this group estrogen can be prescribed with close follow-up.

Alternatives to hormone replacement therapy in patients with breast cancer

Since current medical practice recommends avoiding estrogen replacement therapy for most women with breast cancer, alternative recommendations must be made. Non-estrogen approaches for the prevention and treatment of osteoporosis include maintaining skeletal integrity with weight-bearing exercise, walking, and avoidance of trauma, a diet rich in calcium and limited in caffeine, alcohol, and protein, and avoidance of smoking. For patients at high risk of osteoporotic fracture, vitamin D metabolites, antiresorptive agents, and tamoxifen may be helpful. Cardiovascular risk may be improved by controlling hyperlipidemia and hypertension, discontinuing smoking, increasing exercise, and losing weight. Estrogen remains the most effective treatment for vasomotor symptoms associated with estrogen depletion, including hot flashes, night sweats, and insomnia, although Bellergal (phenobarbital, belladonna, and ergotamine tartrate) is effective in some patients.[9] Other drugs that can be used include sedatives and tranquilizers, nonsteroidal antiinflammatory drugs, alpha-adrenergics such as clonidine, and antidopaminergics. Such alternative therapies as vitamins, biofeedback, stress management, and exercise are occasionally effective.[10,11] Symptoms of urogenital atrophy including urinary incontinence, dyspareunia, and vaginal discharge and irritation are known sequelae of estrogen loss. Non-estrogen-containing lubricants and moisturizers, such as those with a polycarbophil base, can assist in sexual comfort and improve vaginal symptoms. Women who remain sexually active usually have less vaginal atrophy than those who are abstinent.[12] Kegel exercises and vaginal dilators may be beneficial to improve urogenital tone. Low-dose, intermittent estrogen vaginal cream can probably be given safely with concurrent tamoxifen, since systemic estrogen levels are relatively low and are unlikely to compete with tamoxifen by this route.[13]

Caution must be taken when using naturopathic treatments for menopausal symptoms because the active ingredients of some herbal remedies are natural estrogen-like compounds.[14,15] The effect of these agents on the risk of breast cancer recurrence is unknown. We are also cautious about recommending the routine administration of progestins and androgens to patients with breast cancer for the treatment of menopausal symptoms. The role of progesterone and androgen receptors in the regulation and differentiation of breast cancer cells is not well understood.[16-19] Education and counseling regarding menopausal changes, especially in young women with chemotherapy-induced ovarian dysfunction, can reduce fear and improve perception of symptoms.

Pregnancy after a diagnosis of breast cancer

Pregnancy after a diagnosis of breast cancer has not been shown to affect overall survival, disease recurrence, or metastasis.[20-22] Physicians at the University of Washington Breast Cancer Specialty Center generally support patients who wish to become pregnant after breast cancer treatment but recommend waiting 2 years after diagnosis and treatment.

Emotional Issues and Quality of Life

Breast cancer is a lifelong diagnosis that irreversibly changes the lives of affected women and their families. Approximately one third of breast cancer survivors experience significant psychiatric morbidity during the first 3 years of treatment. Anxiety and depression occur in one fourth to one third of patients with breast cancer. Self-esteem and body image problems are common.[23-26] The potential psychological, sexual, and physical dysfunction caused by both the diagnosis and treatment of breast cancer can decrease the quality of a woman's life. If these problems can be identified early, counseling and intervention may be helpful.[27-30]

Many options are available to help patients cope with breast cancer diagnosis and treatment. Support groups, psychological counseling programs, community-based programs, and volunteer programs such as the American Cancer Society's Reach to Recovery program can be effective. The availability of education and support programs should be stressed. Regular assessment of quality-of-life issues should be part of routine follow-up visits, questioning the patient about physical and sexual functioning, pain, nutrition, sleep, psychological well-being, social functioning, energy, and fatigue, as well as general health.

Breast Cancer Risk Reduction

A personal history of breast cancer is a strong risk factor for development of subsequent primary breast cancers.[31] De novo breast cancer is the most frequent second cancer in patients with breast cancer, with an annual risk of 0.3% to 1.0%.[32] The risk of contralateral breast cancer is two to four times higher with invasive or in situ lobular carcinoma. Any patient with breast cancer needs close surveillance of both breasts, including imaging, physical examination, and reinforcement concerning the importance of self-examination.

A correlation between nutrition, exercise, weight gain, and obesity and the occurrence or recurrence of breast cancer has been reported. High body mass and caloric intake correlate with increased breast cancer risk in Western postmenopausal women,[33-35] especially those with a family breast cancer history.[36] Patients who gain weight during adjuvant treatment of breast cancer may have a poorer prognosis,[37-39] although recent overviews of case-control epidemiological studies do not strongly support the dietary fat–breast cancer hypothesis.[40-42] Vitamin A or carotenoid intake may exert a protective effect.[43-45] Alcohol intake may be correlated with increased breast cancer risk.[46-48] College women who exercise have a lower incidence of breast cancer than those who are sedentary.[49] Because of evidence suggesting possible reductions in rates of breast cancer recurrence and second primary cancers, we recommend that patients follow a low-fat, low-alcohol diet that is high in cruciferous vegetables, that they attempt to lose excess weight and prevent significant weight gain, and that they participate in a regular exercise program. Although these changes may have a relatively small statistical benefit in terms of risk reduction, they clearly improve quality of life and give patients a sense of control over their disease.

SURVEILLANCE FOR TOXICITY AND COMPLICATIONS OF TREATMENT

The benefits of adjuvant therapy for breast cancer are well established. Ongoing research is dedicated to improving the efficacy of treatment and identifying patients most and least likely to benefit from adjuvant therapy. The long-term survivorship of patients with breast cancer justifies research efforts to identify and quantitate treatment-related events and determine how these may affect survival and quality of life.

Surgery and Radiation

Lymphedema

The greatest surgical morbidity after axillary lymphadenectomy is the development of arm lymphedema. Less than 1% of patients who undergo surgical lymphadenectomy alone have severe complications within the first 5 years. Axillary radiation therapy increases the probability of complications when added to lymphadenectomy. The probability of axillary complications can be as high as 34% for combined surgery and radiotherapy at 5 years, although less than 5% of these complications are severe or debilitating.[50] Once lymphedema develops, no interventions are curative. Compressive garments and physical therapy can bring symptomatic relief. Preventive measures include care to avoid wounds and infections in the associated upper limb, since severe infections can promote occlusion of the remaining lymphatic channels after axillary dissection or axillary radiation therapy. Although patients should be counseled to care for upper extremity cuts and infections, there is little evidence that using blood pressure cuffs when drawing blood from or placing intravenous lines in the involved upper extremity actually promotes lymphedema.

Reconstruction

Controversy surrounds immediate breast reconstruction after breast cancer surgery. Although patients with reconstructive complications could suffer a delay in systemic treatment, wound healing associated with immediate reconstruction generally does not significantly delay systemic treatment. An occasional patient who has undergone immediate reconstruction requires unanticipated chest wall irradiation through the flap. Although attempts are made to avoid this situation, it has not been shown to adversely affect overall outcome.

Physicians at the University of Washington Breast Cancer Specialty Center offer immediate reconstruction to patients with noninvasive or early cancers such as ductal carcinoma in situ or T1 (less than 2 cm) invasive cancers. Patients with well-differentiated cancers larger than 2 cm are considered for immediate reconstruction on an individual basis. Immediate reconstruction is avoided in patients who are likely to require chest wall irradiation or aggressive systemic therapy postoperatively.

Radiation

Side effects of radiation include skin changes, increased risk of rib fracture, pneumonitis, and heart toxicity. Cardiac toxicity is directly related to the radiation dose and volume of the heart included in the radiation field. Edge et al. cite studies showing a small risk of ischemic heart disease after left-sided radiation treatment in patients after mastectomy. The risk may be less with modern radiation techniques. Cardiac injury has not been a reported complication of radiation associated with breast-conserving therapy. Although the follow-up period for studies using breast conservation is brief, the heart dose is low with modern breast conservation techniques.[51] Follow-up of the large randomized trials comparing breast-conserving therapy with mastectomy should answer questions about the impact of current techniques on the risk of late cardiac mortality.

Hormone Therapy

Tamoxifen is the most widely prescribed antineoplastic agent for the treatment of breast cancer in the United States.[52] Disease-free and overall survival rates have been increased in patients with estrogen receptor– and progesterone receptor–positive breast tumors irrespective of nodal status when tamoxifen has been used as adjuvant therapy, especially in postmenopausal patients.[53-57] Adjuvant tamoxifen has also been shown to reduce non–breast cancer mortality, primarily as a result of its proestrogenic effects in preserving bone mineral density and reducing cholesterol levels and cardiovascular events.[56,57] In addition, tamoxifen has been reported to reduce the risk of contralateral breast cancers by 35% in women with a history of breast cancer.[58]

Because of tamoxifen's frequent use in patients with breast cancer, a detailed discussion of its potential toxicities, aside from a small increase in endometrial cancer incidence, is warranted. Tamoxifen is well tolerated, with side effects that infrequently necessitate discontinuation of therapy.[54,56,59] The most frequent side effects associated with tamoxifen are hot flashes, mild nausea, vaginal bleeding or discharge, irregular menses, nonspecific central nervous system symptoms, and fluid retention. Although ocular effects have been reported with very high doses of tamoxifen, no data from existing trials have suggested that this is problematic at the current recommended dose of 20 mg/day.[60,61] Routine ophthalmic examination is not warranted during tamoxifen therapy except in patients with preexisting ocular conditions, although tamoxifen should be discontinued if ophthalmic abnormalities are known to exist. Thromboembolic complications of women taking tamoxifen have been reported in 1% to 3% of patients.[53,62,63] Thrombocytopenia and leukopenia may occur transiently during the first few weeks of tamoxifen therapy, but these usually resolve. Although no increase in incidence of liver tumors has been reported in any of the tamoxifen trials, cholestasis, changes of fatty liver, hepatitis, hepatic necrosis, and benign liver cysts have been noted.[64] Periodic liver function tests for women taking tamoxifen are a reasonable addition to follow-up surveillance.

Although all women receiving tamoxifen should undergo an annual gynecological examination, we agree with Edge et al. that no evidence supports routine use of endometrial biopsy or uterine ultrasound. When tamoxifen has been started in patients with widespread bone metastases, significant hypercalcemia has been seen.[65] Therefore we recommend following calcium levels in such patients within the first several weeks after tamoxifen initiation. The optimal duration of adjuvant tamoxifen is not yet defined, but current clinical data favor the use of tamoxifen for 2 to 5 years.[57,66] Use of tamoxifen for greater than 5 years in the adjuvant setting is not justified.[67]

The bulk of published data related to tamoxifen risks and benefits is for postmenopausal women. In premenopausal women treated with tamoxifen, serum estrogen and progesterone levels can be elevated as much as four-fold because of a direct stimulatory effect on the ovaries to produce estrogen.[68,69] We recommend periodically measuring estradiol levels in premenopausal women receiving tamoxifen and would consider discontinuing its use in patients with markedly elevated estradiol levels. Although tamoxifen has been associated with estrogen-like effects on the bone and decreased bone resorption in postmenopausal women,[70] there have also been recent reports of negative effects on the bone in premenopausal women, including increased bone resorption and decreased bone density.[71]

Adjuvant Chemotherapy

Although randomized trials provide reliable estimates of the acute toxicity of adjuvant chemotherapy, less is known about late adverse effects. Chemotherapy-induced premature ovarian failure is a prevalent side effect of adjuvant chemotherapy. Age is a major determinant of premature ovarian failure, which occurs in 30% to 50% of women under the age of 40 and in 90% or more of those over the age of 40.[72-74] Cancer patients with chemotherapy-induced ovarian failure have significant decreases in bone mineral density as compared with matched control subjects in whom ovarian failure does not develop.[75,76] Chemotherapy-induced premature ovarian failure may also increase the risk of cardiovascular disease. Menopausal symptoms may affect quality of life long after successful breast cancer treatment.

Alkylating agents, which are nearly ubiquitous in current adjuvant breast chemotherapy regimens, can cause sublethal mutations or chromosomal loss in hematopoietic stem cell precursors, increasing the risk of leukemia. Acute myeloid leukemia and myelodysplastic syndromes are more common in patients treated with alkylating agents. The risk of acute myeloid leukemia is related to the specific alkylating agent and the total cumulative dose or duration of drug exposure. Adjuvant regimens generally no longer include melphalan, the alkylating agent responsible for the majority of reported cases of treatment-related acute myeloid leukemia in patients with breast cancer.[77-79] The increased relative risk of acute myeloid leukemia after cyclophosphamide in doses commonly given today is only 1.3 to 3.[77,78,80] Combining alkylating-agent chemotherapy and radiation therapy may increase the risk of treatment-related acute myeloid leukemia.[78] Recently reports of topoisomerase inhibitor (etoposide, doxorubicin)–associated secondary leukemias have surfaced.[81-83] These may add to the long-term incidence of myelodysplasia and leukemia in the breast cancer population. Nonetheless, the risk of acute myeloid leukemia after standard-dose adjuvant therapy for breast cancer will probably prove to be very small. Perhaps the more important issue is whether the higher total doses of alkylating agents being administered in current high-dose adjuvant trials will result in a higher risk of acute myeloid leukemia.

Doxorubicin-related congestive heart failure usually occurs within weeks to months after treatment but may be seen up to 3 years later.[84-86] In typical breast cancer adjuvant chemotherapy regimens that include doxorubicin the risk of congestive heart failure is reported to be between 0.1% and 1%.[84,87] This risk is related to the total cumulative dose, particularly when it is greater than 550 mg/m^2.[85,86] Other risk factors for cardiotoxicity relate to the schedule of administration (with higher risks after bolus infusions versus lower risks after low-dose weekly infusions or continuous infusion), older age, and prior history of underlying cardiac disease. Radiation and doxorubicin in combination may increase the risk of cardiotoxicity.[86,88]

High-Dose Chemotherapy and Stem Cell Transplantation

Curing women with advanced breast cancer has been an unmet goal because of limited drug efficacy at conventional doses and the development of drug resistance. The poor results have stimulated interest in alternative approaches, including chemotherapy at doses 5 to 30 times higher than those conventionally used, with or without autologous stem cell support. To date between 15% and 30% of women with metastatic breast cancer have not had progression after treatment with high-dose chemotherapy regimens, with the length of follow-up approaching 3 to 5 years in some studies.[89-91] Preliminary findings suggest that high-dose chemotherapy may also prolong disease-free survival when used as consolidation therapy after standard adjuvant treatment for poor-prognosis patients with stage II and III breast cancer.[92] Ongoing randomized, intergroup trials will help to further define the role of high-dose therapy in the adjuvant setting. High-dose therapy is toxic, with treatment-related mortality rates of 5% to 15% and serious nonfatal complication rates in excess of 30%.[90] The toxicity of these high-dose regimens adds a new dimension to follow-up care of patients with breast cancer. Most side effects and complications of high-dose regimens occur within 1 to 2 months after chemotherapy administration. Delayed complications are seen frequently, however. The organs involved depend on the chemotherapy agents used. These delayed complications include infections (cytomegalovirus, herpes simplex virus, *Pneumocystis carinii* pneumonia, fungus), interstitial pneumonitis (1 to 6 months after treatment), venoocclusive disease of the liver, hemolytic-uremic syndrome, hemorrhagic myocarditis, renal insufficiency, gastrointestinal toxicity, peripheral neurotoxicity, and hemorrhagic cystitis.[92-94] Although peripheral blood stem cell support and colony-stimulating factors have reduced the short-term morbidity and mortality associated with high-dose treatments, intensive long-term surveillance of these patients for evidence of treatment-related complications and disease recurrence is mandatory.

SURVEILLANCE FOR CANCER RECURRENCE

Recurrent breast cancer can manifest itself as local, regional, or distant disease. The major goal of primary therapy for breast cancer is to prevent disease recurrence by careful assessment of recurrence risk and application of appropriate primary and adjuvant therapy. With breast-conserving therapy, physicians accept an increased local cancer recurrence rate that does not affect overall survival if recurrence is properly recognized through careful surveillance and treated using modern methods.[95,96] Regional and chest wall breast cancer recurrences have more significant long-term implications for the patient, although in some cases aggressive treatment at the time of relapse can achieve durable disease control.

Although intensive surveillance and early therapy for distant breast cancer metastases generally have not been shown to prolong overall survival, evidence supports some degree of surveillance intensity for distant recurrence. Data from M.D. Anderson Cancer Center support significant 5- and 10-year disease-free survival in patients with isolated single-site disease at the time of recurrence who are treated with aggressive therapy.[97,98] High-dose chemotherapy regimens with and without stem cell support suggest the promise of achieving durable disease-free survival intervals in a subset of patients with metastatic breast cancer and offer the greatest potential benefit to patients with small tumor burdens and minimal exposure to prior chemotherapy regimens.[89,91] Physicians at the University of Washington Breast Cancer Specialty Center use these data to support a slightly more aggressive approach for surveillance of distant breast cancer recurrence than has been outlined by the Roswell Park Cancer Institute group.

Locoregional Recurrence

Predicting the risk of recurrent disease to maximize primary therapy

Locoregional recurrence after mastectomy occurs less commonly than recurrence after conservative surgery and radiation, although it is associated with a worse prognosis.[99] Less than 5% of patients with breast cancer treated by modified radical mastectomy experience locoregional failure,[100,101] and 80% to 90% of such recurrences occur within 5 years after initial treatment.[102,103] In as many as two thirds of mastectomy patients with subsequent locoregional recurrence, distant disease develops.[102,104]

Locoregional recurrence after breast conservation surgery and radiation therapy occurs in 6% to 15% of patients within 10 years after definitive therapy,[105-108] with 70% to 80% occurring in the first 5 years.[108,109] Most local recurrences after breast-conserving therapy can be treated with salvage mastectomy, although approximately 10% are inoperable.[110] Salvage mastectomy achieves locoregional control in 90% of patients up to 15 years after treatment.[109,111-113] By contrast, surgical procedures less extensive than mastectomy fail to achieve optimal local control in 64% of these patients.[107] Local recurrence after breast-conserving therapy provokes anxiety and distress in patients, and the subsequent mastectomy negates the goal of breast conservation while adding additional surgical and anesthetic risk. For these reasons we strongly encourage minimizing local recurrence rates in breast conservation patients through careful patient selection and appropriate adjuvant treatment.

Factors that increase the risk of locoregional recurrence include tumor size, nuclear and histological grade, hormone receptor status, and axillary nodal status.[100,114] The absolute number of involved axillary lymph nodes has a strong correlation with locoregional recurrence. Because the local recurrence rate approaches 20% in patients with large or node-positive cancers when treated with modified radical mastectomy and adjuvant chemotherapy alone, we recommend adding chest wall and nodal radiation therapy in patients with tumors greater than 5 cm (whether treated by mastectomy or breast conservation) or with four or more positive lymph nodes.[115]

Edge et al. suggest that mammography should be performed after breast-conserving surgery and before radiation therapy to ensure completeness of tumor resection. Postbiopsy mammograms are helpful in cases of ductal carcinoma in situ presenting as microcalcifications if surgical margins are questionable. They are less helpful, however, in cases of mass lesions without microcalcifications because of postsurgical parenchymal changes that often obscure mammographic features. Physicians at the University of Washington Breast Cancer Specialty Center use postoperative mammography selectively when it would clearly have an impact on further surgical therapy. Two-view specimen mammography is preferred at the time of the initial surgery to facilitate the evaluation of adequate excision.

Positive margins, gross multicentricity, and extensive intraductal carcinoma appear to adversely affect local recurrence rates in patients treated with breast conservation.[116] The presence of angiolymphatic invasion within the breast and perineural involvement may be associated with increased recurrence risk. The risk of local recurrences related to these factors can be decreased by increasing the volume of tissue excised.[109] Because of the relationship between surgical margins and outcome,[95,117] physicians at the University of Washington Breast Cancer Specialty Center have adopted a multicolored orienting inking approach. Specimens are inked by the surgeon in the operating room to optimize specimen orientation. Repeat excisions to obtain adequate surgical margins are performed regularly.

Multicentric breast cancer, with distinct foci of in situ or invasive carcinoma in separate quadrants, may have an independent adverse impact on local recurrence.[118,119] When patients have anatomically remote synchronous centers of cancer, mastectomy is generally recommended over breast conservation because of potentially increased local recurrence rates. Extensive intraductal carcinoma may also be associated with an increased local recurrence rate, especially in high-grade, comedo-type ductal carcinoma in situ when primary margins have not been completely excised.[111,120,121] Extensive intraductal carcinoma is not considered an absolute contraindication to breast conservation, but we recommend close attention to surgical margins and careful mammographic or ultrasound assessment of the remainder of the breast to minimize local recurrence risk.

The most common risks for regional nodal failure in breast cancer are the presence and number of histologically positive axillary lymph nodes removed at the initial operation.[50,122,123] The extent of axillary dissection at the initial operation is also an important determinant. Fisher et al.[124] reported an 11% axillary recurrence rate in patients with 5 or fewer lymph nodes removed, compared with less than 1% in patients with 10 or more nodes excised at the initial dissection. Other factors reported to be associated with regional lymph node failure include extracapsular extension of the tumor from the lymph nodes and the size of the metastatic tumor within the lymph nodes removed.

Screening for locoregional recurrence

After mastectomy a chest wall recurrence is most often manifested as small cutaneous or subcutaneous nodules or by subtle erythema of the skin found on routine clinical or self-breast examination. After breast-conserving surgery, breast recurrence is detected in equal numbers by physical examination and routine mammography.[125,126] The most common physical finding suggestive of a breast recurrence is a painless mass at or near the operative site,[127] which may be difficult to distinguish from fat necrosis, radiation changes, or infection. Mammographic changes of recurrence after breast-conserving therapy include new calcifications, a new mass, architectural distortion, or inflammatory skin thickening. Recurrences detected by mammography more often represent in situ disease.[96] Alternative modalities for breast imaging, such as ultrasound and magnetic resonance imaging, are being investigated.

Nodal recurrence can appear as a supraclavicular mass, a symptomatic brachial plexopathy, arm edema, or arm pain. With a regional recurrence in the internal mammary chain the manifestations may include a painless parasternal mass, pleural effusion, bony erosion on x-ray, or superior vena cava syndrome.

When chest wall or regional lymph node recurrence is detected, a metastatic workup, including a computed tomographic scan of the chest and abdomen, is indicated. Without further investigation the extent of disease may be underestimated. With careful staging studies, additional sites of disease are identified in up to 50% of patients with locoregional recurrences.[128,129]

Surveillance in patients with lobular carcinoma in situ

Patients with lobular carcinoma in situ are at increased risk for developing ductal carcinoma in situ or invasive breast cancer in both breasts, but whether lobular carcinoma in situ is itself a cancer is disputed. In contrast to the policy at Roswell Park Cancer Institute, we believe that lobular carcinoma in situ is a very well-differentiated, noninvasive cancer with unique biological properties. Genotyping studies evaluating loss of heterozygosity in lobular carcinoma in situ suggest that it is a malignant precursor to invasive lobular breast cancer in some cases.[130] Epidemiological data suggest that patients diagnosed with lobular carcinoma in situ are specifically predisposed to invasive lobular cancer in the contralateral breast.[131] These results are consistent with the hypothesis that lobular carcinoma in situ can transform into invasive cancer with lobular histology in a small subset of patients.

Despite the association between lobular carcinoma in situ and other types of cancer, at least 65% of women with the former do not later have ductal carcinoma in situ or invasive breast cancer. Physicians at the University of Washington Breast Cancer Specialty Center do not routinely recommend surgical intervention in these patients but do support careful surveillance, including annual mammography and physical examination supplemented with breast ultrasonography and biopsy as indicated. However, patients with lobular carcinoma in situ who have additional risk factors for the development of breast cancer, including a family history of premenopausal breast cancer, may consider bilateral mastectomy in place of intensive screening. Since surgical prophylaxis has not been shown to improve survival over careful surveillance in lobular carcinoma in situ, this approach should be reserved for a small minority of women who have been carefully selected and educated as to the benefits and risks of this highly invasive approach.

Distant Recurrence

Predicting the risk of recurrent disease to maximize primary therapy

Once breast cancer becomes apparent in a distant site, the disease is generally incurable. Systemic therapy at this point does not generally alter overall mortality but can improve length of survival, palliate symptoms, and prevent complications. Decreased metastatic recurrence rates and improved overall survival can be achieved through appropriate adjuvant systemic therapy.

Histological grade, tumor size, and nodal status help stratify risk for distant recurrence. Patients with noninvasive (in situ or intraductal) carcinomas are essentially cured by definitive local therapy. Most node-negative patients are disease free at 10 years, even without adjuvant therapy, although up to 30% have a relapse during that decade. Most node-positive patients with breast cancer have had a relapse within 10 years, even with standard adjuvant therapy.[132] The 1990 National Institutes of Health consensus conference concluded that adjuvant systemic therapy was not indicated for node-negative tumors less than 1 cm in size because of their low recurrence risk.[133]

The presence of estrogen receptors and progesterone receptors in breast cancer cells predicts hormone responsiveness and is of unequivocal value in guiding therapeutic decision making. The value of hormone receptors in the overall prognostic assessment of patients with breast cancer is somewhat more controversial. Many reports that relate outcome to measured concentrations of estrogen receptors and progesterone receptors in breast cancer indicate that the greater the expression of the hormone receptors, the better the outcome.[24,134,135] The lack of receptor expression may be more predictive of early relapse than of absolute long-term relapse.[24] Edge et al. make the statement that estrogen receptor status does not predict the time to relapse or the incidence of distant metastases. In general, reports suggesting a lack of correlation between estrogen receptor expression and survival have been based on the biochemical dextran-coated charcoal-binding assay for determination of the presence of these hormone receptors, a technique prone to inaccuracies. Small tumors, tumor handling at the time of biopsy, a low ratio of malignant to normal breast cells or a high volume of ductal carcinoma in situ compared with invasive tumor, and exogenous or endogenous estrogens can all affect the outcome of this test. Reports evaluating hormone receptor positivity using both dextran-coated charcoal and immunocytochemistry methods have shown that the latter method is more reliable and a better predictor of overall and disease-free survival.[136-138] Immunocytochemistry avoids sampling errors because the pathologist, by visualizing staining under the microscope, can avoid false readings caused by the presence of ductal carcinoma in situ or extraneous tissue and can use normal breast tissue as a positive internal control. At the University of Washington Breast Cancer Specialty Center, physicians perform only immunocytochemistry analysis of estrogen receptors and progesterone receptors and routinely use receptor status in predicting risk of recurrence and determining likelihood of benefit from therapy.

Oncogene and tumor suppressor gene analysis can add clinically relevant prognostic information. Amplification of the protooncogene *HER-2/neu* (c-*erb*B-2) and overexpression of its protein product, seen in up to one third of invasive breast carcinomas, have been implicated as poor prognostic indicators in node-positive and some node-negative breast cancers.[130,139-143] Although *HER-2/neu* overexpression is common in ductal carcinoma in situ (50% to 75% of cases), it has no predictive value for risk of recurrence in the in situ setting.[130,144] *HER-2/neu* appears to correlate with response to therapy. Patients with low levels of *HER-2/neu* may benefit more from methotrexate-based adjuvant therapy than patients with high levels.[141] However, retrospective data from a recent Cancer and Leukemia Group B study suggest that moderate- to high-intensity doxorubicin therapy negated the poor prognosis of *HER-2/neu* overexpression in node-positive women.[145] *HER-2/neu* may also be predictive of resistance to tamoxifen.[146-148] We interpret these studies to suggest that dose-intensive doxorubicin can overcome an inherent tumor resistance to tamoxifen and methotrexate-based adjuvant regimens in *HER-2/neu*-positive tumors and improve long-term prognosis.

Screening for distant recurrence

Although the clinical relevance of early detection of distant breast cancer recurrence is controversial, at the University of Washington Breast Cancer Specialty Center and Fred Hutchinson Cancer Research Center, physicians routinely evaluate and screen for early detection of metastases for several reasons. First, metastases may be more effectively treated if detected earlier. More effective treatment includes improved quality of life, palliation of symptoms, and in some cases prolonged disease-free and overall survival. Although the majority of patients with metastatic breast cancer have evidence of metastasis in multiple sites, in 1% to 10% of patients relapse occurs as an isolated distant lesion that can be eradicated by surgery, irradiation, or both. With integrated aggressive systemic therapy the M.D. Anderson Cancer Center group reports 5- and 10-year disease-free survival rates of 39% and 27%, respectively, in this subset of patients with breast cancer.[97] Thus a subgroup of patients with single-site metastatic disease can have prolonged disease-free intervals when treated promptly. With high-dose chemotherapy regimens offering potential long-term, disease-free survival in a subset of patients with stage IV cancer, future studies may demonstrate a survival benefit with early detection of systemic recurrence. In addition, preventing catastrophic events caused by metastatic disease, such as fractures and spinal cord compression, can help maintain quality of life, even if overall survival remains unchanged. Another benefit of close evaluation and screening is that patients can derive emotional benefit and security from follow-up evaluation. Regular evaluation of patients after primary therapy for breast cancer can provide education and emotional support at a time when patients have suffered psychological stress related to their diagnosis and treatment. Knowing that one remains free of disease can facilitate psychological recovery. Finally, recurrence after primary therapy is an important end point for many investigational therapies, and detection of recurrence on a consistent and timely basis is important for research purposes.

Table 15-11 Follow-up of patients with breast cancer: University of Washington Medical Center/ Fred Hutchinson Cancer Research Center

	YEAR				
	1	2	3	4	5
Office visit*	4	4	3	2	2
Mammography (ipsilateral)	2	2	1	1	1
Mammography (contralateral)	1	1	1	1	1
General health screen†	1	1	1	1	1
Chest x-ray	1	1	1	1	1
CEA‡,§	1	1	1	1	1
CA 27.29 (CA 15-3)‡,§	1	1	1	1	1
Complete blood count§	1	1	1	1	1
Liver function tests§	1	1	1	1	1
Bone scan	¶	¶	¶	¶	¶
Chest computed tomography	¶	¶	¶	¶	¶
Abdominal computed tomography	¶	¶	¶	¶	¶

CEA, Carcinoembryonic antigen.
*Includes history, directed physical examination, and quality-of-life review.
†Includes complete physical examination, pelvic examination, and Pap test.
‡Recommended for intermediate- and high-risk breast cancer patients.
§Frequency based on stage and prior or ongoing treatment.
¶Performed only as clinically indicated.

We recommend regularly scheduled follow-up visits that include a history, physical examination, and quality-of-life review (Table 15-11). The importance of monthly self-examination is also stressed. Two thirds of relapses are detected either by the patient or by the clinician on routine history and physical examination.[149-153] We agree with Edge et al. that routine screening bone scans and computed tomographic scans have not been proved cost effective, especially in low-risk patients. In intermediate- and high-risk patients, annual chest x-rays are recommended. While liver and bone lesions frequently cause symptoms, parenchymal lung metastases are asymptomatic more than 80% of the time.[154] Routine chest x-rays in the higher risk subpopulation of patients with breast cancer can also detect pulmonary complications associated with aggressive, dose-intensive chemotherapy regimens.

The measurement of circulating tumor markers has a relatively well-accepted role in monitoring treatment response in patients with established metastatic disease.[155-157] The serial measurement of markers in disease-free patients at risk for recurrent breast cancer is more controversial. Levels of the mucin-associated antigens CEA, CA 27.29 (also known as the CA 15-3 antigen),[158] and to a lesser extent CA-125 can be elevated in breast cancer, particularly when disease is advanced. Whether prompt treatment of recurrent disease detected with circulating tumor markers can improve overall survival is unknown. Because these tests are inexpensive and noninvasive and because a subset of patients with isolated recurrences may benefit by early detection, physicians obtain tumor markers at periodic intervals in intermediate- and high-risk patients.

CONCLUSIONS AND SURVEILLANCE RECOMMENDATIONS

At the University of Washington Breast Cancer Specialty Center and Fred Hutchinson Cancer Research Center, the follow-up of patients with breast cancer emphasizes reducing the risk of recurrence through carefully evaluated primary and adjuvant treatment, educating and maintaining quality of life for the patient and monitoring for locoregional and metastatic recurrence and toxic effects of therapy through regular follow-up visits that focus on history and physical examination.

Once a locoregional recurrence has been detected, patients are screened for metastatic disease. If none is found, the patient is treated with aggressive local treatment to render the patient disease free and systemic therapy is considered. Although patients with distant disease benefit primarily from palliative measures, select patients with metastatic breast cancer can achieve durable responses to aggressive intervention, such as high-dose chemotherapy, with some hope for long-term disease-free survival. Candidates for aggressive therapy are selected on an individual basis.

The health care professional's role in patient education about follow-up strategies is crucial. Many patients believe (incorrectly) that radiographs, scans, and blood tests are more effective than history and physical examination in detecting disease.[159] Patient education about breast cancer, its treatment, and the appropriate application of follow-up testing can increase patient awareness and may be associated with improved psychological and social functioning.[160,161] We encourage and empower patients to participate in their own follow-up management by emphasizing the value of self-examination, physical examination, and mammography in achieving early detection.

REFERENCES

1. Armstrong BK. Oestrogen therapy after the menopause—boon or bane? Med J Aust 1988;148:213-4.
2. Steinberg KK, Thacker SB, Smith SJ, et al. A meta-analysis of the effect of estrogen replacement therapy on the risk of breast cancer. JAMA 1991;265:1985-90.
3. Colditz GA, Hankinson SE, Hunter DJ, et al. The use of estrogens and progestins and the risk of breast cancer in postmenopausal women. N Engl J Med 1995;332:1589-93.
4. Stanford JL, Weiss NS, Voigt LF, Daling JR, Habel LA, Rossing MA. Combined estrogen and progestin hormone replacement therapy in relation to risk of breast cancer in middle-aged women. JAMA 1995;274:137-42.
5. Stoll BA. Hormone replacement therapy in women treated for breast cancer. Eur J Cancer Clin Oncol 1989;25:1909-13.
6. Wile A, Opfell D, Margileth D, Hoda A. Hormone replacement therapy does not affect breast cancer outcome. Proc Am Soc Clin Oncol 1991;10:58.
7. Cobleigh MA, Berris RF, Bush T, et al. Estrogen replacement therapy in breast cancer survivors: a time for change; Breast Cancer Committees of the Eastern Cooperative Oncology Group. JAMA 1994;272: 540-5.

8. Rosen PP, Groshen S, Kinne DW, Norton L. Factors influencing prognosis in node-negative breast carcinoma: analysis of 767 T1N0M0/T2N0M0 patients with long-term follow-up. J Clin Oncol 1993;11:2090-100.
9. Lebherz TB, French L. Nonhormonal treatment of the menopausal syndrome: a double-blind evaluation of an autonomic system stabilizer. Obstet Gynecol 1969;33:795-9.
10. Nissim R. Natural healing in gynecology. New York: Pandora, 1986.
11. Greenblatt R, Teran A. Advice to postmenopausal women. In: Zichella, Whitehead, van Keep, editors. The climacteric and beyond. United Kingdom: Parthenon, 1987.
12. Leiblum S, Bachmann G, Kemmann E, Colburn D, Swartzman L. Vaginal atrophy in the postmenopausal woman: the importance of sexual activity and hormones. JAMA 1983;249:2195-8.
13. Handa VL, Bachus KE, Johnston WW, Robboy SJ, Hammond CB. Vaginal administration of low-dose conjugated estrogens: systemic absorption and effects on the endometrium. Obstet Gynecol 1994; 84:215-8.
14. Hopkins MP, Androff L, Benninghoff AS. Ginseng face cream and unexplained vaginal bleeding. Am J Obstet Gynecol 1988;159:1121-2.
15. Miksicek RJ. Interaction of naturally occurring nonsteroidal estrogens with expressed recombinant human estrogen receptor. J Steroid Biochem Mol Biol 1994;49:153-60.
16. Manni A, Arafah BM, Pearson OH. Androgen-induced remissions after antiestrogen and hypophysectomy in stage IV breast cancer. Cancer 1981;48:2507-9.
17. Goldenberg IS, Waters N, Ravdin RS, Ansfield FJ, Segaloff A. Androgenic therapy for advanced breast cancer in women: a report of the cooperative breast cancer group. JAMA 1973;223:1267-8.
18. Lober J, Rose C, Salimtschik M, Mouridsen HT. Treatment of advanced breast cancer with progestins. Acta Obstet Gynecol Scand Suppl 1981;101:39-46.
19. Noguchi S, Yamamoto H, Inaji H, Imaoka S, Koyama H. Inability of medroxyprogesterone acetate to down regulate estrogen receptor level in human breast cancer. Cancer 1990;65:1375-9.
20. King RM, Welch RS, Martin JK Jr, Coulam CB. Carcinoma of the breast associated with pregnancy. Surg Gynecol Obstet 1985;160: 228-32.
21. Ribeiro G, Jones DA, Jones M. Carcinoma of the breast associated with pregnancy. Br J Surg 1986;73:607-9.
22. Danforth DN Jr. How subsequent pregnancy affects outcome in women with a prior breast cancer. Oncology 1991;5:23-30.
23. Morris T, Greer HS, White P. Psychological and social adjustment to mastectomy: a two-year follow-up study. Cancer 1977;40:2381-7.
24. McGuire WL. Estrogen receptor versus nuclear grade as prognostic factors in axillary node negative breast cancer. J Clin Oncol 1988;6: 1071-2.
25. Fallowfield LJ, Baum M, Maguire GP. Effects of breast conservation on psychological morbidity associated with diagnosis and treatment of early breast cancer. Br Med J Clin Res Ed 1986;293:1331-4.
26. Fallowfield LJ. Psychosocial adjustment after treatment for early breast cancer. Oncology 1990;4:89-97.
27. Fallowfield L, Hall A, Maguire P, Baum M, A'Hern R. A question of choice: results of a prospective 3-year follow-up study of women with breast cancer. The Breast 1994;3:202-8.
28. Maguire P, Tait A, Brooke M, Thomas C, Sellwood R. Effect of counselling on the psychiatric morbidity associated with mastectomy. Br Med J 1980;281:1454-6.
29. Maunsell E, Brisson J, Deschenes L. Psychological distress after initial treatment of breast cancer: assessment of potential risk factors. Cancer 1992;70:120-5.
30. Ganz PA, Hirji K, Sim MS, Schag CA, Fred C, Polinsky ML. Predicting psychosocial risk in patients with breast cancer. Med Care 1993;31:419-31.
31. Kelsey JL, Berkowitz GS. Breast cancer epidemiology. Cancer Res 1988;48:5615-23.
32. McCredie JA, Inch WR, Alderson M. Consecutive primary carcinomas of the breast. Cancer 1975;35:1472-7.
33. Albanes D. Caloric intake, body weight, and cancer: a review. Nutr Cancer 1987;9:199-217.
34. Lubin F, Ruder AM, Wax Y, Modan B. Overweight and changes in weight throughout adult life in breast cancer etiology: a case-control study. Am J Epidemiol 1985;122:579-88.
35. Ingram D, Nottage E, Ng S, Sparrow L, Roberts A, Willcox D. Obesity and breast disease: the role of the female sex hormones. Cancer 1989;64:1049-53.
36. Sellers TA, Kushi LH, Potter JD, et al. Effect of family history, body-fat distribution, and reproductive factors on the risk of postmenopausal breast cancer. N Engl J Med 1992;326:1323-9.
37. Boyd NF, Campbell JE, Germanson T, Thomson DB, Sutherland DJ, Meakin JW. Body weight and prognosis in breast cancer. J Natl Cancer Inst 1981;67:785-9.
38. Donegan WL, Hartz AJ, Rimm AA. The association of body weight with recurrent cancer of the breast. Cancer 1978;41:1590-4.
39. Tartter PI, Papatestas AE, Ioannovich J, Mulvihill MN, Lesnick G, Aufses AH Jr. Cholesterol and obesity as prognostic factors in breast cancer. Cancer 1981;47:2222-7.
40. Jones DY, Schatzkin A, Green SB, et al. Dietary fat and breast cancer in the National Health and Nutrition Examination Survey I Epidemiologic Follow-up Study. J Natl Cancer Inst 1987;79:465-71.
41. Byers T. Diet and cancer: any progress in the interim? Cancer 1988; 62(Suppl 8):1713-24.
42. Goodwin PJ, Boyd NF. Critical appraisal of the evidence that dietary fat intake is related to breast cancer risk in humans. J Natl Cancer Inst 1987;79:473-85.
43. Paganini-Hill A, Chao A, Ross RK, Henderson BE. Vitamin A, beta-carotene, and the risk of cancer: a prospective study. J Natl Cancer Inst 1987;79:443-8.
44. Graham S, Marshall J, Mettlin C, Rzepka T, Nemoto T, Byers T. Diet in the epidemiology of breast cancer. Am J Epidemiol 1982;116:68-75.
45. Katsouyanni K, Trichopoulos D, Boyle P, et al. Diet and breast cancer: a case-control study in Greece. Int J Cancer 1986;38:815-20.
46. Begg CB, Walker AM, Wessen B, Zelen M. Alcohol consumption and breast cancer. Lancet 1983;1:293-4.
47. La Vecchia C, Decarli A, Franceschi S, Pampallona S, Tognoni G. Alcohol consumption and the risk of breast cancer in women. J Natl Cancer Inst 1985;75:61-5.
48. Schatzkin A, Jones DY, Hoover RN, et al. Alcohol consumption and breast cancer in the epidemiologic follow-up study of the first National Health and Nutrition Examination Survey. N Engl J Med 1987;316:1169-73.
49. Frisch RE, Wyshak G, Albright NL, et al. Lower prevalence of breast cancer and cancers of the reproductive system among former college athletes compared to non-athletes. Br J Cancer 1985;52:885-91.
50. Dewar JA, Sarrazin D, Benhamou E, et al. Management of the axilla in conservatively treated breast cancer: 592 patients treated at Institut Gustave-Roussy. Int J Radiat Oncol Biol Phys 1987;13:475-81.
51. Pierce SM, Recht A, Lingos TI, et al. Long-term radiation complications following conservative surgery (CS) and radiation therapy (RT) in patients with early stage breast cancer. Int J Radiat Oncol Biol Phys 1992;23:915-23.
52. Jaiyesimi IA, Buzdar AU, Decker DA, Hortobagyi GN. Use of tamoxifen for breast cancer: twenty-eight years later. J Clin Oncol 1995;13:513-29.
53. Fisher B, Constantino J, Wickerham L. Adjuvant therapy for node negative breast cancer: an update of NSABP findings. Proc Am Soc Clin Oncol 1993;12:79.
54. Ribeiro G, Swindell R. The Christie hospital adjuvant tamoxifen trial—status at 10 years. Br J Cancer 1988;57:601-3.
55. "Nolvadex" Adjuvant Trial Organisation. Controlled trial of tamoxifen as a single adjuvant agent in the management of early breast cancer. Br J Cancer 1988;57:608-11.
56. Breast Cancer Trials Committee. Adjuvant tamoxifen in the management of operable breast cancer: the Scottish Trial: report from the Breast Cancer Trials Committee, Scottish Cancer Trials Office (MRC), Edinburgh. Lancet 1987;2:171-5.

57. Early Breast Cancer Trialists' Collaborative Group. Systemic treatment of early breast cancer by hormonal, cytotoxic, or immune therapy: 133 randomised trials involving 31,000 recurrences and 24,000 deaths among 75,000 women. Lancet 1992;339:71-85.
58. Nayfield SG, Karp JE, Ford LG, Dorr FA, Kramer BS. Potential role of tamoxifen in prevention of breast cancer. J Natl Cancer Inst 1991; 83:1450-9.
59. Love RR, Cameron L, Connell BL, Leventhal H. Symptoms associated with tamoxifen treatment in postmenopausal women. Arch Intern Med 1991;151:1842-7.
60. Vinding T, Nielsen NV. Retinopathy caused by treatment with tamoxifen in low dosage. Acta Ophthalmol 1983;61:45-50.
61. Griffiths MF. Tamoxifen retinopathy at low dosage. Am J Ophthalmol 1987;104:185-6.
62. Nevasaari K, Heikkinen M, Taskinen PJ. Tamoxifen and thrombosis. Lancet 1978;2:946-7.
63. Lipton A, Harvey HA, Hamilton RW. Venous thrombosis as a side effect of tamoxifen treatment. Cancer Treat Rep 1984;68:887-9.
64. Blackburn AM, Amiel SA, Millis RR, Rubens RD. Tamoxifen and liver damage. Br Med J Clin Res Ed 1984;289:288.
65. Legha SS, Powell K, Buzdar AU, Blumenschein GR. Tamoxifen-induced hypercalcemia in breast cancer. Cancer 1981;47:2803-6.
66. Tormey DC, Rasmussen P, Jordan VC. Long-term adjuvant tamoxifen study: clinical update. Breast Cancer Res Treat 1987;9:157-8.
67. National Cancer Institute. Adjuvant therapy of breast cancer. NCI Clinical Announcement: Tamoxifen Update, 1995.
68. Jordan VC, Fritz NF, Langan-Fahey S, Thompson M, Tormey DC. Alteration of endocrine parameters in premenopausal women with breast cancer during long-term adjuvant therapy with tamoxifen as the single agent. J Natl Cancer Inst 1991;83:1488-91.
69. Yasumura T, Akami T, Mitsuo M, et al. The effect of adjuvant therapy with or without tamoxifen on the endocrine function of patients with breast cancer. Jpn J Surg 1990;20:369-75.
70. Love RR, Mazess RB, Barden HS, et al. Effects of tamoxifen on bone mineral density in postmenopausal women with breast cancer. N Engl J Med 1992;326:852-6.
71. Powles TJ, Hickish T, Kanis JA, Tidy A, Ashley S. Effect of tamoxifen on bone mineral density measured by dual-energy x-ray absorptiometry in healthy premenopausal and postmenopausal women. J Clin Oncol 1996;14:78-84.
72. Bonadonna G, Valagussa P, Rossi A, et al. Ten-year experience with CMF-based adjuvant chemotherapy in resectable breast cancer. Breast Cancer Res Treat 1985;5:95-115.
73. Mehta RR, Beattie CW, Das Gupta TK. Endocrine profile in breast cancer patients receiving chemotherapy. Breast Cancer Res Treat 1992;20:125-32.
74. Richards MA, O'Reilly SM, Howell A, et al. Adjuvant cyclophosphamide, methotrexate, and fluorouracil in patients with axillary node-positive breast cancer: an update of the Guy's/Manchester trial. J Clin Oncol 1990;8:2032-9.
75. Bruning PF, Pit MJ, de Jong-Bakker M, van den Ende A, Hart A, van Enk A. Bone mineral density after adjuvant chemotherapy for premenopausal breast cancer. Br J Cancer 1990;61:308-10.
76. Redman JR, Bajorunas DR, Wong G, et al. Bone mineralization in women following successful treatment of Hodgkin's disease. Am J Med 1988;85:65-72.
77. Curtis RE, Boice JD Jr, Moloney WC, Ries LG, Flannery JT. Leukemia following chemotherapy for breast cancer. Cancer Res 1990;50:2741-6.
78. Curtis RE, Boice JD Jr, Stovall M, et al. Risk of leukemia after chemotherapy and radiation treatment for breast cancer. N Engl J Med 1992;326:1745-51.
79. Greene MH, Harris EL, Gershenson DM, et al. Melphalan may be a more potent leukemogen than cyclophosphamide. Ann Intern Med 1986;105:360-7.
80. Haas JF, Kittelmann B, Mehnert WH, et al. Risk of leukaemia in ovarian tumour and breast cancer patients following treatment by cyclophosphamide. Br J Cancer 1987;55:213-8.
81. Ratain MJ, Rowley JD. Therapy-related acute myeloid leukemia secondary to inhibitors of topoisomerase II: from the bedside to the target genes. Ann Oncol 1992;3:107-11.
82. Nichols CR, Breeden ES, Loehrer PJ, Williams SD, Einhorn LH. Secondary leukemia associated with a conventional dose of etoposide: review of serial germ cell tumor protocols. J Natl Cancer Inst 1993;85:36-40.
83. Sugita K, Furukawa T, Tsuchida M, et al. High frequency of etoposide (VP-16)-related secondary leukemia in children with non-Hodgkin's lymphoma. Am J Pediatr Hematol Oncol 1993;15:99-104.
84. Buzdar AU, Marcus C, Smith TL, Blumenschein GR. Early and delayed clinical cardiotoxicity of doxorubicin. Cancer 1985;55:2761-5.
85. Von Hoff DD, Layard MW, Basa P, et al. Risk factors for doxorubicin-induced congestive heart failure. Ann Intern Med 1979;91:710-7.
86. Allen A. The cardiotoxicity of chemotherapeutic drugs. Semin Oncol 1992;19:529-42.
87. Fisher B, Brown AM, Dimitrov NV, et al. Two months of doxorubicin-cyclophosphamide with and without interval reinduction therapy compared with 6 months of cyclophosphamide, methotrexate, and fluorouracil in positive-node breast cancer patients with tamoxifen-nonresponsive tumors: results from the National Surgical Adjuvant Breast and Bowel Project B-15. J Clin Oncol 1990;8: 1483-96.
88. Recht A, Harris JR, Come SE. Sequencing of irradiation and chemotherapy for early-stage breast cancer. Oncology 1994;8:19-28.
89. Antman K, Ayash L, Elias A, et al. A phase II study of high-dose cyclophosphamide, thiotepa, and carboplatin with autologous marrow support in women with measurable advanced breast cancer responding to standard-dose therapy. J Clin Oncol 1992;10:102-10.
90. Williams SF, Gilewski T, Mick R, Bitran JD. High-dose consolidation therapy with autologous stem-cell rescue in stage IV breast cancer: follow-up report. J Clin Oncol 1992;10:1743-7.
91. Dunphy FR, Spitzer G, Buzdar AU, et al. Treatment of estrogen receptor-negative or hormonally refractory breast cancer with double high-dose chemotherapy intensification and bone marrow support. J Clin Oncol 1990;8:1207-16.
92. Peters WP, Ross M, Vredenburgh JJ, et al. High-dose chemotherapy and autologous bone marrow support as consolidation after standard-dose adjuvant therapy for high-risk primary breast cancer. J Clin Oncol 1993;11:1132-43.
93. Peters WP, Shpall EJ, Jones RB, et al. High-dose combination alkylating agents with bone marrow support as initial treatment for metastatic breast cancer. J Clin Oncol 1988;6:1368-76.
94. Vincent MD, Powles TJ, Coombes RC, McElwain TJ. Late intensification with high-dose melphalan and autologous bone marrow support in breast cancer patients responding to conventional chemotherapy. Cancer Chemother Pharmacol 1988;21:255-60.
95. Fisher B, Anderson S, Fisher ER, et al. Significance of ipsilateral breast tumour recurrence after lumpectomy. Lancet 1991;338:327-31.
96. Dershaw DD, McCormick B, Osborne MP. Detection of local recurrence after conservative therapy for breast carcinoma. Cancer 1992;70:493-6.
97. Holmes FA, Buzdar AU, Kau SW, et al. 10 year results of a combined modality approach for patients (PT) with isolated recurrences of breast cancer (IV-NED). Proc Am Soc Clin Oncol 1990;133:35.
98. Blumenschein G, Buzdar AU, Hortobagyi G, Tashima C. Adjuvant chemoimmunotherapy following regional therapy for initial solitary metastases of breast cancer (stage IV NED). In: Jones, Salmon, editors, Adjuvant therapy for cancer II. New York: Grune & Stratton, 1979.
99. Danoff BF, Coia LR, Cantor RI, Pajak TF, Kramer S. Locally recurrent breast carcinoma: the effect of adjuvant chemotherapy on prognosis. Radiology 1983;147:849-52.
100. Fowble B, Gray R, Gilchrist K, Goodman RL, Taylor S, Tormey DC. Identification of a subgroup of patients with breast cancer and histologically positive axillary nodes receiving adjuvant chemotherapy who may benefit from postoperative radiotherapy. J Clin Oncol 1988;6:1107-17.

101. Sykes HF, Sim DA, Wong CJ, Cassady JR, Salmon SE. Local-regional recurrence in breast cancer after mastectomy and adriamycin-based adjuvant chemotherapy: evaluation of the role of postoperative radiotherapy. Int J Radiat Oncol Biol Phys 1989;16:641-7.
102. Crowe JP Jr, Gordon NH, Antunez AR, Shenk RR, Hubay CA, Shuck JM. Local-regional breast cancer recurrence following mastectomy. Arch Surg 1991;126:429-32.
103. Donegan W. Local and regional recurrence. In: Donegan and Spratt, editors. Cancer of the breast. Philadelphia: WB Saunders Company, 1988.
104. Probstfeld MR, O'Connell TX. Treatment of locally recurrent breast carcinoma. Arch Surg 1989;124:1127-9.
105. Fisher B, Redmond C, Poisson R, et al. Eight-year results of a randomized clinical trial comparing total mastectomy and lumpectomy with or without irradiation in the treatment of breast cancer. N Engl J Med 1989;320:822-8.
106. Clark RM, Wilkinson RH, Miceli PN, MacDonald WD. Breast cancer: experiences with conservation therapy. Am J Clin Oncol 1987;10:461-8.
107. Kurtz JM, Amalric R, Brandone H, et al. Local recurrence after breast-conserving surgery and radiotherapy: frequency, time course, and prognosis. Cancer 1989;63:1912-7.
108. Montague ED, Ames FC, Schell SR, Romsdahl MM. Conservation surgery and irradiation as an alternative to mastectomy in the treatment of clinically favorable breast cancer. Cancer 1984;54(11 Suppl):2668-72.
109. Clarke DH, Le MG, Sarrazin D, et al. Analysis of local-regional relapses in patients with early breast cancers treated by excision and radiotherapy: experience of the Institut Gustave-Roussy. Int J Radiat Oncol Biol Phys 1985;11:137-45.
110. Kurtz JM, Jacquemier J, Brandone H, et al. Inoperable recurrence after breast-conserving surgical treatment and radiotherapy. Surg Gynecol Obstet 1991;172:357-61.
111. Kurtz JM, Spitalier JM, Amalric R, et al. The prognostic significance of late local recurrence after breast-conserving therapy. Int J Radiat Oncol Biol Phys 1990;18:87-93.
112. Fowble B, Solin LJ, Schultz DH, Rubenstein J, Goodman RL. Breast recurrence following conservative surgery and radiation: patterns of failure, prognosis, and pathologic findings from mastectomy specimens with implications for treatment. Int J Radiat Oncol Biol Phys 1990;19:833-42.
113. Osborne MP, Borgen PI, Wong GY, Rosen PP, McCormick B. Salvage mastectomy for local and regional recurrence after breast-conserving operation and radiation therapy. Surg Gynecol Obstet 1992;174:189-94.
114. Bedwinek JM, Fineberg B, Lee J, Ocwieza M. Analysis of failures following local treatment of isolated local-regional recurrence of breast cancer. Int J Radiat Oncol Biol Phys 1981;7:581-5.
115. Pisansky TM, Ingle JN, Schaid DJ, et al. Patterns of tumor relapse following mastectomy and adjuvant systemic therapy in patients with axillary lymph node–positive breast cancer: impact of clinical, histopathologic, and flow cytometric factors. Cancer 1993;72:1247-60.
116. Lagios MD. Pathologic features related to local recurrence following lumpectomy and irradiation. Semin Surg Oncol 1992;8:122-8.
117. Veronesi U, Marubini E, Del Vecchio M, et al. Local recurrences and distant metastases after conservative breast cancer treatments: partly independent events. J Natl Cancer Inst 1995;87:19-27.
118. Recht A, Harris JR. Selection of patients with early-stage breast cancer for conservative surgery and radiation. Oncology 1990;4:23-30.
119. Leopold KA, Recht A, Schnitt SJ, et al. Results of conservative surgery and radiation therapy for multiple synchronous cancers of one breast. Int J Radiat Oncol Biol Phys 1989;16:11-6.
120. Lindley R, Bulman A, Parsons P, Phillips R, Henry K, Ellis H. Histologic features predictive of an increased risk of early local recurrence after treatment of breast cancer by local tumor excision and radical radiotherapy. Surgery 1989;105:13-20.
121. Bartelink H, Borger JH, van Dongen JA, Peterse JL. The impact of tumor size and histology on local control after breast-conserving therapy. Radiother Oncol 1988;11:297-303.
122. Pierquin B, Mazeron JJ, Glaubiger D. Conservative treatment of breast cancer in Europe: report of the Groupe Europeen de Curietherapie. Radiother Oncol 1986;6:187-98.
123. Fowble B, Solin LJ, Schultz DJ, Goodman RL. Frequency, sites of relapse, and outcome of regional node failures following conservative surgery and radiation for early breast cancer. Int J Radiat Oncol Biol Phys 1989;17:703-10.
124. Fisher B, Wolmark N, Bauer M, Redmond C, Gebhardt M. The accuracy of clinical nodal staging and of limited axillary dissection as a determinant of histologic nodal status in carcinoma of the breast. Surg Gynecol Obstet 1981;152:765-72.
125. Stomper PC, Recht A, Berenberg AL, Jochelson MS, Harris JR. Mammographic detection of recurrent cancer in the irradiated breast. AJR Am J Roentgenol 1987;148:39-43.
126. Orel SG, Troupin RH, Patterson EA, Fowble BL. Breast cancer recurrence after lumpectomy and irradiation: role of mammography in detection. Radiology 1992;183:201-6.
127. Jardines L, Callans LS, Torosian MH. Recurrent breast cancer: presentation, diagnosis, and treatment. Semin Oncol 1993;20:538-47.
128. Lindfors KK, Meyer JE, Busse PM, Kopans DB, Munzenrider JE, Sawicka JM. CT evaluation of local and regional breast cancer recurrence. AJR Am J Roentgenol 1985;145:833-7.
129. Rosenman J, Churchill CA, Mauro MA, Parker LA, Newsome J. The role of computed tomography in the evaluation of post-mastectomy locally recurrent breast cancer. Int J Radiat Oncol Biol Phys 1988;14:57-62.
130. Allred DC, Clark GM, Molina R, et al. Overexpression of HER-2/neu and its relationship with other prognostic factors change during the progression of in situ to invasive breast cancer. Hum Pathol 1992;23:974-9.
131. Habel LA, Moe RE, Daling JR, Holte S, Rossing MA, Weiss NS. Risk of contralateral breast cancer among women diagnosed with carcinoma *in situ* of the breast. Ann Surg 1996. In press.
132. Ravdin PM. A practical view of prognostic factors for staging, adjuvant treatment planning, and as baseline studies for possible future therapy. Hematol Oncol Clin North Am 1994;8:197-211.
133. NIH Consensus Development Conference statement on the treatment of early-stage breast cancer. Oncology 1991;5:120-4.
134. Sunderland MC, McGuire WL. Prognostic indicators in invasive breast cancer. Surg Clin North Am 1990;70:989-1004.
135. Glick JH. Adjuvant therapy for node-negative breast cancer: a proactive view. Important Adv Oncol 1990;183-97.
136. Querzoli P, Ferretti S, Marzola A, et al. Clinical usefulness of estrogen receptor immunocytochemistry in human breast cancer. Tumori 1992;78:287-90.
137. Reiner A, Neumeister B, Spona J, Reiner G, Schemper M, Jakesz R. Immunocytochemical localization of estrogen and progesterone receptor and prognosis in human primary breast cancer. Cancer Res 1990;50:7057-61.
138. McCarty KS Jr, Kinsel LB, Georgiade G, Leight G, McCarty KS Sr. Long-term prognostic implications of sex-steroid receptors in human cancer. Prog Clin Biol Res 1990;322:279-93.
139. Kallioniemi OP, Holli K, Visakorpi T, Koivula T, Helin HH, Isola JJ. Association of c-erbB-2 protein over-expression with high rate of cell proliferation, increased risk of visceral metastasis and poor long-term survival in breast cancer. Int J Cancer 1991;49:650-5.
140. Yuan J, Hennessy C, Givan AL, et al. Predicting outcome for patients with node negative breast cancer: a comparative study of the value of flow cytometry and cell image analysis for determination of DNA ploidy. Br J Cancer 1992;65:461-5.
141. Gusterson BA, Gelber RD, Goldhirsch A, et al. Prognostic importance of c-erbB-2 expression in breast cancer. International (Ludwig) Breast Cancer Study Group. J Clin Oncol 1992;10:1049-56.

142. Press MF, Pike MC, Chazin VR, et al. Her-2/neu expression in node-negative breast cancer: direct tissue quantitation by computerized image analysis and association of overexpression with increased risk of recurrent disease. Cancer Res 1993;53:4960-70.
143. Bianchi S, Paglierani M, Zampi G, et al. Prognostic significance of c-erbB-2 expression in node negative breast cancer. Br J Cancer 1993;67:625-9.
144. Lodato RF, Maguire HC Jr, Greene MI, Weiner DB, LiVolsi VA. Immunohistochemical evaluation of c-erbB-2 oncogene expression in ductal carcinoma in situ and atypical ductal hyperplasia of the breast. Mod Pathol 1990;3:449-54.
145. Muss HB, Thor AD, Berry DA, et al. c-erbB-2 expression and response to adjuvant therapy in women with node-positive early breast cancer. N Engl J Med 1994;330:1260-6.
146. Benz CC, Scott GK, Sarup JC, et al. Estrogen-dependent, tamoxifen-resistant tumorigenic growth of MCF-7 cells transfected with HER2/neu. Breast Cancer Res Treat 1993;24:85-95.
147. Wright C, Nicholson S, Angus B, et al. Relationship between c-erbB-2 protein product expression and response to endocrine therapy in advanced breast cancer. Br J Cancer 1992;65:118-21.
148. Klijn JG, Berns EM, Bontenbal M, Foekens J. Cell biological factors associated with the response of breast cancer to systemic treatment. Cancer Treat Rev 1993;19(Suppl B):45-63.
149. Muss HB, McNamara MJ, Connelly RA. Follow-up after stage II breast cancer: a comparative study of relapsed versus nonrelapsed patients. Am J Clin Oncol 1988;11:451-5.
150. Winchester DP, Sener SF, Khandekar JD, et al. Symptomatology as an indicator of recurrent or metastatic breast cancer. Cancer 1979; 43:956-60.
151. Scanlon EF, Oviedo MA, Cunningham MP, et al. Preoperative and follow-up procedures on patients with breast cancer. Cancer 1980; 46(4 Suppl):977-9.

Table 15-12 Follow-up of patients with breast cancer by institution

YEAR/PROGRAM	OFFICE VISIT	LFT	MAMM	PELVIC EXAM	PAP TEST	CHEST X-RAY	BONE SCAN
Year 1							
Memorial Sloan-Kettering	3[a]	3	1[b]	1	1	1	
Roswell Park	4	4[d]	2[e]	1	1	1	[f]
Univ Washington/ Fred Hutchinson	4[h]	1[i]	2 ipsi/ 1 contra	[j]	[j]	1	[f]
Japan: Natl Cancer Ctr I[l]	2	2	1			1	1
Japan: Natl Cancer Ctr II[m]	4	4	1			1[n]	1[n]
UK: Royal Liverpool	2		1[e]				[f]
Year 2							
Memorial Sloan-Kettering	3[a]	3	1[b]	1	1	1	
Roswell Park	2	2[d]	1[e]	1	1	1	[f]
Univ Washington/ Fred Hutchinson	4[h]	1[i]	2 ipsi/ 1 contra	[j]	[j]	1	[f]
Japan: Natl Cancer Ctr I[l]	2	2	1			1	1
Japan: Natl Cancer Ctr II[m]	4	4	1			1[n]	1[n]
UK: Royal Liverpool	2		1[e]				[f]

ABD CT abdominal computed tomography
ABD US abdominal ultrasound
CBC complete blood count
CEA carcinoembryonic antigen
CHEST CT chest computed tomography
ENDO BIOPSY endometrial biopsy
LFT liver function tests
MAMM mammogram

152. Coombes RC, Powles TJ, Gazet JC, et al. Screening for metastases in breast cancer: an assessment of biochemical and physical methods. Cancer 1981;48:310-5.
153. Pandya KJ, McFadden ET, Kalish LA, Tormey DC, Taylor SG 4th, Falkson G. A retrospective study of earliest indicators of recurrence in patients on Eastern Cooperative Oncology Group adjuvant chemotherapy trials for breast cancer: a preliminary report. Cancer 1985;55:202-5.
154. Stierer M, Rosen HR. Influence of early diagnosis on prognosis of recurrent breast cancer. Cancer 1989;64:1128-31.
155. Hayes DF, Zurawski VR Jr, Kufe DW. Comparison of circulating CA15-3 and carcinoembryonic antigen levels in patients with breast cancer. J Clin Oncol 1986;4:1542-50.
156. O'Brien DP, Horgan PG, Gough DB, Skehill R, Grimes H, Given HF. CA15-3: a reliable indicator of metastatic bone disease in breast cancer patients. Ann R Coll Surg Engl 1992;74:9-11.
157. Stahli C, Staehelin T, Miggiano V. Spleen cell analysis and optimal immunization for high-frequency production of specific hybridomas. Methods Enzymol 1983;92:26-36.
158. Muss H, Beveridge R, Chan D, et al. Truquant BR RIA for CA 27.29 antigen is highly predictive of relapse in stage II and II breast cancer. Proc Am Soc Clin Oncol 1996;15:113.
159. Muss HB, Tell GS, Case LD, Robertson P, Atwell BM. Perceptions of follow-up care in women with breast cancer. Am J Clin Oncol 1991;14:55-9.
160. GIVIO (Interdisciplinary Group for Cancer Care Evaluation). What doctors tell patients with breast cancer about diagnosis and treatment: findings from a study in general hospitals. Br J Cancer 1986;54:319-326.
161. Jacobs C, Ross RD, Walker IM, Stockdale FE. Behavior of cancer patients: a randomized study of the effects of education and peer support groups. Am J Clin Oncol 1983;6:347-53.

ABD CT	ABD US	CHEST CT	PELVIC US	ENDO BIOPSY	CEA	CA 15-3	ST439	CBC
					3[c]	3[c]		
f	f	f	f	f	g	g		
f		f			1[k]	1[k] (CA 27.29)		1[i]
	1				2	2	2	
	1[n]				4	4	4	
f	f	f	f	f	g	g		
					3[c]	3[c]		
f	f	f	f	f	g	g		
f		f			1[k]	1[k] (CA 27.29)		1[i]
	1				2	2	2	
	1[n]				4	4	4	
f	f	f	f	f	g	g		

a Clinical follow-up examinations are alternated among the surgeon, radiation oncologist, medical oncologist, and occasionally the primary care physician.
b Yearly mammography is recommended after an initial posttreatment mammogram in the conserved breast.
c Although routine monitoring of CA 15-3 and CEA is not performed on all patients, medical oncologists remain optimistic about the potential impact of therapeutic intervention based solely on rising tumor markers.
d Consists of alkaline phosphatase and lactic dehydrogenase.
e Should begin at 6 months after radiation for breast-conserving therapy.
f Performed if clinically indicated.
g If recurrence is documented, it may be useful for assessing treatment response.
h Includes history, directed physical examination, and quality-of-life review; note that an annual general health screen, which includes a complete physical examination, pelvic examination, and Pap test, is also recommended.
i Frequency based on stage and prior or ongoing treatment.
j In general health examination.
k Recommended for intermediate- and high-risk breast cancer patients; frequency based on stage and prior or ongoing treatment.
l Node negative patients, excluding patients with histological grade 3 tumor or positive p53 expression. Such patients are followed up in the same way as node-positive patients.
m Node-positive and select node-negative patients (those with histological grade 3 tumor or positive p53 expression).
n Performed twice a year for patients whose number of metastatic lymph nodes is at least 10, irrespective of histological grade and c-*erb*B-2 expression, and for patients whose number of metastatic lymph nodes is at least four with c-*erb*B-2 positive expression or histological grade 3 tumor.

Continued.

Table 15-12 Follow-up of patients with breast cancer by institution—cont'd

YEAR/PROGRAM	OFFICE VISIT	LFT	MAMM	PELVIC EXAM	PAP TEST	CHEST X-RAY	BONE SCAN
Year 3							
Memorial Sloan-Kettering	3[a]	3	1[b]	1	1	1	
Roswell Park	2	2[d]	1[e]	1	1	1	[f]
Univ Washington/ Fred Hutchinson	3[h]	1[i]	1 ipsi/ 1 contra	[j]	[j]	1	[f]
Japan: Natl Cancer Ctr I[l]	2	2	1			1	1
Japan: Natl Cancer Ctr II[m]	2	2	1			1	1
UK: Royal Liverpool	2		1[e]				[f]
Year 4							
Memorial Sloan-Kettering	2[a]	2	1[b]	1	1	1	
Roswell Park	2	2[d]	1[e]	1	1	1	[f]
Univ Washington/ Fred Hutchinson	2[h]	1[i]	1 ipsi/ 1 contra	[j]	[j]	1	[f]
Japan: Natl Cancer Ctr I[l]	2	2	1			1	1
Japan: Natl Cancer Ctr II[m]	2	2	1			1	1
UK: Royal Liverpool	1		1[e]				[f]
Year 5							
Memorial Sloan-Kettering	2[a]	2	1[b]	1	1	1	
Roswell Park	2	2[d]	1[e]	1	1	1	[f]
Univ Washington/ Fred Hutchinson	2[h]	1[i]	1 ipsi/ 1 contra	[j]	[j]	1	[f]
Japan: Natl Cancer Ctr I[l]	2	2	1			1	1
Japan: Natl Cancer Ctr II[m]	2	2	1			1	1
UK: Royal Liverpool	1		1[e]				[f]

ABD CT	ABD US	CHEST CT	PELVIC US	ENDO BIOPSY	CEA	CA 15-3	ST439	CBC
					3[c]	3[c]		
[f]	[f]	[f]	[f]	[f]	[g]	[g]		
[f]		[f]			1[k]	1[k] (CA 27.29)		1[i]
	1				2	2	2	
	1				2	2	2	
[f]	[f]	[f]	[f]	[f]	[g]	[g]		
					2[c]	2[c]		
[f]	[f]	[f]	[f]	[f]	[g]	[g]		
[f]		[f]			1[k]	1[k] (CA 27.29)		1[i]
	1				2	2	2	
	1				2	2	2	
[f]	[f]	[f]	[f]	[f]	[g]	[g]		
					2[c]	2[c]		
[f]	[f]	[f]	[f]	[f]	[g]	[g]		
[f]		[f]			1[k]	1[k] (CA 27.29)		1[i]
	1				2	2	2	
	1				2	2	2	
[f]	[f]	[f]	[f]	[f]	[g]	[g]		

CHAPTER 16

Ovarian Carcinoma

Roswell Park Cancer Institute

RAYMOND P. PEREZ

Ovarian cancer remains a significant and deadly disease. It was diagnosed in about 26,600 women and caused the deaths of 14,500 in 1995 in the United States.[1] Although ovarian cancer is only the third most prevalent gynecological malignancy, the annual death toll from this disease in the United States exceeds that of all other gynecological malignancies combined. The majority of patients have advanced, surgically incurable disease at the time of diagnosis. Despite these somber statistics, ovarian cancer typically responds favorably to initial therapies and the majority of treated patients are rendered clinically free of disease.

Unfortunately, most patients with advanced ovarian cancer are also destined to have relapses. This is reflected in the 20% to 30% 5-year survival rate observed among patients with advanced disease and in the potential for relapse to occur 10 or more years after treatment. Whether a significant percentage of these patients are cured of ovarian cancer is unclear. However, most patients experience a clinical disease-free interval measured in months to years. Thus surveillance is an important issue for the majority of patients with ovarian cancer.

Most of this chapter is devoted to the biology, natural history, treatment, and follow-up of common epithelial ovarian carcinoma, by far the most common category of ovarian malignancy. The remainder of the chapter briefly considers the relatively uncommon nonepithelial malignancies.

BIOLOGY AND CLINICAL FEATURES

Approximately 90% of ovarian malignancies arise from the ovarian surface epithelium. These are collectively referred to as common epithelial ovarian carcinoma. Although ovarian carcinogenesis is still incompletely understood, evidence suggests that malignant transformation is related to repetitive trauma to the ovarian surface epithelium.[2] Increasing parity and oral contraceptive use are associated with significantly decreased risk of ovarian carcinoma, whereas nulliparity and the use of fertility-enhancing drugs are associated with increased risk.[3,4] Additional evidence supporting a relationship between trauma to the surface epithelium and malignant transformation comes from an in vitro model in which cultured rat ovarian surface epithelial cells were observed to transform spontaneously with high frequency after repeated passage, conditions under which cells were required to repeatedly grow and divide.[5] These conditions might be considered analogous to the cellular proliferation necessary to repair defects in the ovarian surface epithelium after ovulation. Although additional factors may also influence carcinogenesis, these data support the hypothesis that ovarian surface epithelial proliferation is related to carcinogenesis.

Common epithelial ovarian carcinoma is somewhat unique in that it tends to grow and metastasize primarily within the peritoneum. Tumor cells may be shed from the primary site into the peritoneum, where they circulate in peritoneal fluid and implant diffusely; tumor cells may also disseminate into the retroperitoneal lymphatics that drain the ovary. Visceral metastases tend to occur late if at all. The typ ical pattern of growth and dissemination of the disease is reflected in the staging classification developed by the Federation Internationale de Gynecologie et d'Obstetrique (FIGO) (Table 16-1).

Symptoms are often not noticed until the disease is advanced. Common symptoms include abdominal distention or pain, vaginal bleeding, early satiety, constipation, dysuria, and urinary frequency. One report suggests that many patients with disease found to be localized at laparotomy actually had symptoms for some time before diagnosis.[6] Abdominal swelling, fatigue, and problems with urination were the most common symptoms among early-stage patients. The median delay from the onset of symptoms until seeking medical attention was 4 weeks in this series, with 22.5% of patients delaying more than 3 months. Fear, similarity to a previous benign condition, and the perception that symptoms were "not serious" were the most common reasons given for the delays. The authors suggest that patient education might increase the proportion of patients whose disease is diagnosed at an early stage. This, however, has not been proved. Moreover, most of these symptoms are also found in advanced disease. There are few reliable findings on history or physical examination to discriminate between early- and advanced-stage disease.

Table 16-1 Federation Internationale de Gynecologie et d'Obstetrique staging classification for ovarian cancer

I. Tumor limited to ovaries (one or both)
  A. Tumor limited to one ovary
  B. Tumor limited to both ovaries
  C. Tumor limited to one or both ovaries with any of the following: capsular rupture, tumor on ovarian surface, malignant cells in ascites or peritoneal washings
II. Tumor involves one or both ovaries with pelvic extension
  A. Extension and/or implants on the uterus and/or tubes
  B. Extension to other pelvic tissues
  C. Pelvic extension (IIA or IIB) with malignant cells in ascites or peritoneal washings
III. Tumor involves one or both ovaries with microscopically confirmed peritoneal metastases outside the pelvis and/or regional lymph node metastasis
  A. Microscopic peritoneal metastasis beyond the pelvis
  B. Macroscopic peritoneal metastasis beyond the pelvis 2 cm or less in greatest dimension (prior to debulking)
  C. Peritoneal metastasis beyond the pelvis more than 2 cm in greatest dimension (prior to debulking) and/or regional lymph node metastasis
IV. Distant metastasis (excludes peritoneal metastasis)

From American Joint Committee on Cancer, Beahrs OH, Henson DE, Hutter RVP, Kennedy BJ, editors. Manual for staging of cancer. Philadelphia: JB Lippincott Company, 1992.

MANAGEMENT AND TREATMENT OUTCOMES

Although a detailed discussion of the management of ovarian cancer is beyond the scope of this chapter, management and treatment outcomes provide a framework within which to consider follow-up. Treatment of most patients involves surgery, followed by chemotherapy. Surgical staging and debulking are typically accomplished simultaneously during laparotomy. The goal of debulking is to leave as little post-operative residual disease as possible. Ovarian carcinoma is a relatively chemotherapy-sensitive disease. Alkylating agents, platinum compounds, antimetabolites, taxanes, and other categories of drugs are active agents.

Specific treatment approaches vary somewhat based on the extent of disease found at laparotomy (Table 16-2). Early disease includes completely resected stage I and II categories. These can be further subdivided into low- and high-risk categories based on tumor grade and on the extent of disease within these stages. The role of adjuvant melphalan versus observation in low-risk, early-disease patients was considered in a randomized trial conducted by the Gynecologic Oncology Group (GOG).[7] There was no statistically significant difference in survival between treatment and control groups; approximately 90% survival was observed at 10 years for both treatment groups. No deaths were recorded in either arm of the study after 6 years' follow-up. Thus for low-risk, early-stage patients surgery alone appears to be very effective and the risk of death from relapsed disease appears to be greatest within the first 6 years.

Table 16-2 Gynecologic Oncology Group classification of epithelial ovarian cancer

Early disease—completely resected stage I and II
  Low risk—IA or IB, moderate to well-differentiated grade
  High risk—any of the following: stage IA or IB, poorly differentiated grade; stage IC, all stage II
Advanced disease—incompletely resected stage II, and all stage III-IV
  Optimal stage III—largest residual nodule ≤1 cm following debulking
  Suboptimal stage III—largest residual nodule >1 cm following debulking

Modified from Hoskins WJ. Primary surgical management of advanced epithelial ovarian cancer. In: Rubin SC, Sutton GP, editors. Ovarian cancer. New York: McGraw-Hill, 1993:241-53.

The outcome for patients with high-risk, early disease is not as good as for the low-risk group. The prognosis for these patients is sufficiently poor that adjuvant treatment has routinely been administered. Adjuvant melphalan chemotherapy was compared with intraperitoneal ^{32}P in a GOG randomized trial of high-risk, early-disease patients.[7] No difference in survival was found between treatment groups, although the toxicities of melphalan were greater. Overall, approximately 65% of high-risk, early-disease patients in this trial survived 10 years, with relapses observed at least as late as 8.5 years. An ongoing GOG trial is randomly dividing patients between treatment with intraperitoneal ^{32}P and combination chemotherapy including cyclophosphamide and cisplatin, a regimen shown to benefit patients with advanced disease. Results from this study are pending. Thus, although the optimal adjuvant regimen for high-risk patients with early disease remains to be defined, these patients clearly have a decreased probability of survival and increased likelihood of recurrent disease compared with low-risk patients.

For patients with advanced disease there is little disagreement that the extent of debulking at initial laparotomy is associated with treatment outcome. Overall, patients whose disease can be optimally debulked, defined by most authors as having no residual nodule greater than 2 cm in diameter, have a mean survival of approximately 39 months, compared with 17 months for patients with suboptimally debulked disease.[8] Whether the extent of resection was actually the more important variable in patients with optimally debulked disease or whether these patients had disease with intrinsically favorable biological features, thus permitting debulking, is not clear.

The chemotherapy of advanced disease is currently in evolution, primarily because of the results of recent trials using the drug paclitaxel. Previously, combination chemotherapy regimens for patients with advanced disease generally included an alkylating agent (usually cyclophosphamide) plus either cisplatin or carboplatin, with or without other agents. An overview analysis of all randomized trials of chemotherapy in patients with advanced-stage ovarian cancer, published in 1991, indicated that such platinum-based combination regimens were superior to single-agent chemotherapy and demonstrated a trend toward improved survival compared with non-platinum-based combinations.[9]

Surgical debulking followed by platinum-based chemotherapy has been relatively effective for patients with advanced disease. However, the percentage of patients rendered free of disease by these treatments depends in part on how aggressively one attempts to document residual disease. Approximately 40% to 60% of patients with advanced disease achieve clinically complete response, meaning that no disease is detectable by physical examination, serum markers, or radiographic studies. Only about 30% of patients whose response is evaluated by laparotomy (second-look procedure) are found to have a pathologically complete response to treatment. Thus the majority of patients have detectable residual disease after treatment, although invasive procedures may be required to document it.

In most patients with advanced-stage ovarian carcinoma, clinically apparent recurrent disease eventually develops. The median time to clinical relapse in most contemporary clinical trials is in the range of 1.5 to 2 years. Approximately 20% to 30% of patients with advanced-stage disease survive 5 years from diagnosis, and late relapses occur beyond that time. Long-term follow-up of treated patients with advanced-stage ovarian cancer demonstrates that relapses can occur at least 9 to 10 years after diagnosis and the 10-year survival rate for these patients is only approximately 5%.[10] Given the potential for late relapses, whether any patients with advanced-stage disease are cured is not entirely clear. It is clear, however, that advanced-stage patients without evidence of disease after treatment remain at risk for relapse and are potential candidates for surveillance for at least 10 years after diagnosis.

Given the survival figures just quoted, it is obvious that no curative salvage treatment is available at present. However, second-line chemotherapy can produce objective responses in some patients, offering the potential for significant palliation.[11] Drugs with significant second-line activity include paclitaxel (~30%), ifosfamide (12% to 22%), and hexamethylmelamine (16%). In addition, the probability of response to second-line chemotherapy appears to be related to whether patients previously achieved a complete response and to the disease-free interval. The response rate after treatment with platinum-based combination chemotherapy for patients whose disease recurred within 12 months was 26%, compared with 77% for those with recurrences later than 24 months in one published report.[12] Similar results were reported in an analysis of a series of British phase II trials in patients with relapsed ovarian cancer.[13] In these trials the treatment-free interval and the initial disease stage were the only factors predictive of response to second-line treatment on multivariate analysis. Other authors have also reported a relationship between the disease-free interval and response to subsequent chemotherapy.[14,15] Not surprisingly, the response rates for second-line chemotherapy were extremely low in patients who failed to respond to initial therapy. Such patients are generally considered refractory to chemotherapy.

The activity noted for paclitaxel as second-line chemotherapy suggests that the drug may have utility as part of front-line treatment. The GOG compared the combination of paclitaxel and cisplatin with that of cyclophosphamide and cisplatin, one of the standard treatment regimens, as first-line therapy of patients with poor-prognosis (that is, suboptimally debulked), advanced-stage ovarian cancer in a phase III trial (GOG No. 111).[16,17] Preliminary results of this trial demonstrate significant advantages in the rates of clinical response, pathologically complete response, disease-free survival, and overall survival for patients treated with paclitaxel and cisplatin. The median survival time was over 1 year longer for patients treated with taxol and cisplatin (37.5 months) versus cytoxan and cisplatin (24.5 months). The activity of paclitaxel and cisplatin in good-prognosis patients with advanced-stage ovarian carcinoma is being defined. However, increasing numbers of oncologists now consider paclitaxel plus cisplatin or carboplatin to be the standard front-line chemotherapy regimen for patients with advanced-stage ovarian carcinoma.

Patients with low-risk early disease appear to have excellent outcomes after surgery and rarely have a relapse later than 6 years after diagnosis. In contrast, patients with high-risk early disease and advanced disease have considerably higher probabilities of relapse and remain at risk for relapse more than 10 years after diagnosis. The different outcomes in these groups of patients have implications for surveillance.

CURRENT PRACTICE

Detailed consideration of surveillance in patients with epithelial ovarian cancer is difficult because few formal guidelines exist. Almost no objective data are available regarding the optimal techniques or their timing. Most of the methods available for surveillance are also being evaluated in the screening setting. Data from screening investigations may provide some indication of the sensitivity and specificity of individual tests, although the frequency of positive test results is much higher in a population of patients treated for ovarian cancer because of the much higher prevalence of disease in these patients, compared with a screening population. Risk-benefit and cost-benefit analyses for these tests in either setting are not available.

The objectives of posttreatment surveillance in an ovarian cancer population are not clearly defined. Isolated relapses that can be treated with curative intent are extremely rare, if they occur at all. It is therefore not yet clear that early detection of relapsed disease is beneficial, since surveillance is performed within the context of salvage treatments that produce objective responses but are not curative. The limitations of available second-line treatments suggest the existence of some latitude in the optimal timing for identifying disease recurrence. The optimal time is not necessarily equivalent to the earliest possible time that can be achieved with existing technologies. However, objective responses may provide meaningful palliation. Moreover, since patient performance status is a powerful predictor of response and toxicity after treatment, it is probably desirable to diagnose relapsed disease sufficiently early to allow initiation of second-line treatment before the patient's functional status deteriorates.

Evaluation of the efficacy of any posttreatment surveillance method must necessarily include consideration of the benchmark against which test performance is to be compared. At present there is no agreement as to the most appropriate benchmark in clinically disease-free patients with treated ovarian cancer who are under surveillance. Most of the available data involve comparison of the findings at second-look laparotomy with noninvasive or less invasive techniques. Many of these investigations did not evaluate the serial use of the noninvasive methods, which would be typical in a surveillance setting. In addition, some of the second-look laparotomy studies were confounded by using the results from surveillance tests to trigger laparotomy. Given the absence of curative second-line therapy and the potential for late relapses, a reasonable alternative benchmark might be a prospective evaluation of a test for its ability to detect symptomatic recurrence. Unfortunately, no data of the latter type are currently available.

Second-Look Laparotomy and Laparoscopy

Second-look laparotomy is performed to surgically and pathologically evaluate the disease status of patients who are clinically free of disease after initial therapy. Although the exact timing of the exploration has varied in different investigations, second-look operations are generally performed soon after completion of initial chemotherapy (generally 6 to 12 months after initial diagnosis). Barter and Barnes[18] reviewed the modern (1980-1990) experience with second-look laparotomy, summarizing results on 5,190 patients from 71 reported series. Overall, slightly greater than half of the patients were found to have residual disease at the time of second look, 75% of which was macroscopic. The percentage of patients found to have persistent disease at the time of second look increased with the stage of disease, from 16% for patients with FIGO stage I disease to 67% for FIGO stage IV disease. The risk of subsequent recurrence after second look also increased with disease stage, from 9% (FIGO I and II) to 32% (FIGO III and IV). The majority of recurrences took place within 2 years after negative second look, although later relapses were documented. Median survival times ranged from 11 to 32 months after recurrence in these patients.

The indications for routine use of second-look laparotomy have diminished in recent years. In the past the procedure was commonly performed either to document a complete response to treatment, in which case treatment was discontinued, or to demonstrate that the patient had disease that had failed to respond, in which case treatment was changed. With the widespread availability of a reliable tumor marker, CA-125, the assessment of response to initial therapy is most often made noninvasively. Moreover, the limitations of second-line treatments have become apparent in recent years, so it has become more difficult to justify routine use of second-look procedures to prompt a change in therapy. Second-look laparotomy can be justified in the context of a clinical investigation, where pathological documentation of response may be desirable. Whether the procedure is ever indicated outside of an investigative setting is not clear.

Laparoscopy is a less invasive procedure that has been used to assess disease status and that was initially considered a potential alternative to second-look laparotomy. Laparoscopy offers the potential for direct visualization and biopsy of suspected disease within the peritoneal cavity. Positive findings at laparoscopy may provide valuable confirmation of the presence of persistent or recurrent disease, though this can often be ascertained less invasively by cytological evaluation of aspirated ascites. Unfortunately, the entire peritoneum cannot be visualized by laparoscopy, which probably accounts for the high false-negative rate reported for this procedure; approximately 39% of patients with negative laparoscopies are found to have disease at second-look laparotomy.[18] Overall, because of these limitations, laparoscopy has no defined role in routine surveillance of patients with ovarian cancer.

Noninvasive Surveillance Methods

The applicability of comparisons between positive or negative second-look laparotomies and the results of less invasive modalities is uncertain. As noted previously, such comparisons are limited to a single point in time. The fact that many patients have a relapse after a negative second-look laparotomy has not generally been considered in evaluations of alternative diagnostic methods.

Physical (including pelvic) examination is an inexpensive, noninvasive, and low-risk method for surveillance. As with the initial presentation, relapsed disease often is asymptomatic or produces only subtle symptoms until a considerable tumor burden is present. Although a bulky mass or ascites is usually detectable, smaller volume disease may be missed. It has been estimated that 10,000 annual screening examinations would have to be performed to detect one early-stage ovarian cancer. Recent reports comparing physical examination with imaging modalities have yielded mixed results. In one prospective study of patients with suspected primary or recurrent ovarian cancer the accuracies of computed tomography and magnetic resonance imaging were comparable and both modalities had slightly better accuracy and less interobserver variability than physical examination in a relatively small number of patients.[19] In contrast, Seewalt et al.[20] indicate that physical examination may be comparable or superior to computed tomography for detecting disease recurrence. Computed tomographic scans, physical examinations, and serum markers (CA-125) were obtained in 100 patients referred to the University of Washington for treatment of recurrent or persistent ovarian cancer.

Computed tomography scans were read by radiologists blinded to the results of the other studies. Physical examination detected masses not appreciated by computed tomographic scan in the pelvis and at the vaginal apex, sites visualized poorly by computed tomography. Further comparisons of physical examination and various imaging modalities should clarify the relative utility of these methods. At present the ease of performance and lack of expense of physical examination justify its continued routine use.

Culdocentesis is a technique in which peritoneal fluid is aspirated from the rectouterine cul-de-sac by a vaginal approach. Limited data suggest that negative cytological findings by culdocentesis may correspond to negative findings at second-look laparotomy.[18] Culdocentesis has not been formally evaluated for disease surveillance. Since the technique depends on the presence of free-floating or shed tumor cells in the peritoneal cavity, it seems unlikely that culdocentesis would be sensitive to very small-volume or isolated recurrences. At present the use of culdocentesis for surveillance has not been sufficiently evaluated to justify its routine use outside of an investigative setting.

Ultrasound is a reasonably inexpensive imaging method with the capacity to confirm the presence of bulky relapsed disease or ascites. Unfortunately, it is somewhat operator dependent and also fairly insensitive to small-volume disease. Ultrasound may be more sensitive than physical examination for the detection of small masses in some pelvic locations. However, it has limited sensitivity for peritoneal and pelvic disease, prevertebral lymph nodes less than 3 cm in diameter, omental plaques less than 1.5 cm in diameter, and mesenteric masses less than 5 cm in diameter. Peritoneal masses less than 2 cm in diameter may also not be reliably detected by ultrasound.[18,21,22] In the review by Barter and Barnes[18] the sensitivity of ultrasound ranged from 20% to 89% and its specificity ranged from 75% to 100% in comparison with findings at second-look laparotomy. Many of these studies were initiated some years ago, and ultrasound imaging using more contemporary technology might be slightly more effective at detecting limited amounts of disease.

Ultrasound using high-frequency transvaginal probes produces images with better resolution than conventional transabdominal ultrasound.[22,23] This technology is being evaluated for screening, where its sensitivity and specificity appear to be better than those of conventional ultrasound. In clinical screening studies few small, early-stage lesions have been detected. High-frequency transvaginal ultrasound has not yet been evaluated for utility in the surveillance of patients with ovarian cancer after treatment, so no conclusive recommendations can be made regarding its potential application.

Computed tomography is not generally sufficiently sensitive to detect small-volume disease (resolution 1 to 2 cm). Overall, in comparison with findings at second-look laparotomy, computed tomography has a sensitivity of 44%, specificity of 86%, and overall diagnostic accuracy of 63%.[18] However, computed tomography is widely available, is familiar to clinicians, and produces results that are not subject to substantial interobserver variability. For these reasons computed tomography has been widely used for imaging patients with ovarian cancer. It is probably best suited for serial assessment of disease response in patients with known primary or recurrent disease. It has not been shown to affect the management or clinical outcomes of patients in the surveillance setting. There computed tomography has generally been limited to noninvasive assessment of potential recurrence in patients who are symptomatic or who have rising tumor marker levels.

Magnetic resonance imaging allows ready visualization of masses within the pelvis.[22] Its resolution characteristics are similar to those of computed tomography, with the additional advantage of allowing imaging in several planes. However, few data on the efficacy of this modality in ovarian cancer patients are available. Magnetic resonance imaging is also significantly more expensive than either ultrasound or computed tomography. Thus recommendations regarding the use of magnetic resonance imaging must be deferred pending additional data.

Positron emission tomography is a newer imaging modality that allows visualization of metabolic and biochemical activity. Few studies have been reported regarding its use in patients with ovarian cancer. However, preliminary results suggest that positron emission tomography is an accurate imaging technique that may yield information complementary to other imaging methods such as computed tomography. Positron emission tomography and computed tomography were performed in 51 patients with suspected ovarian cancer before laparotomy.[24] In these patients positron emission tomography had 83% sensitivity, 80% specificity, and 82% accuracy (compared with 82%, 53%, and 72%, respectively, for computed tomography). The positive predictive value for patients in whom both computed tomography and positron emission tomography were positive was 95% and the negative predictive value for patients in whom both studies were negative was 100%. Serial positron emission tomography performed in 14 patients indicated that recurrent or persistent disease could be detected, although no formal comparison between positron emission tomography and other methods was performed. Another group of investigators obtained positron emission tomographic and computed tomographic scans in a small number of patients before second-look laparotomy.[25] Positron emission tomography detected disease not apparent by serum markers, computed tomography, or ultrasound in individual patients, although the small study size did not permit quantitative comparison of these methods. Further investigations should more clearly define whether this modality has utility in the surveillance of patients with ovarian cancer.

Immunoscintigraphy is an imaging technique that uses radionuclide-conjugated monoclonal antibodies to localize sites of disease.[26-28] Recent investigations have focused on the use of ^{111}indium-labeled B72.3 antibodies, which recognize the TAG 72.3 antigen that is frequently expressed on the surface of adenocarcinoma cells. Limited data suggest that immunoscintigraphy may have predictive value comparable to that of computed tomographic scanning.[28] Formal cost-effectiveness analyses have yet to be performed. However, current estimates suggest that immunoscintigraphy may cost slightly less than computed tomography but more than ultrasound.[26] At present data are insufficient to permit firm recommendations about the use of immunoscintigraphy in routine surveillance of patients with ovarian cancer. Ongoing investigations should clarify the utility of this imaging method.

CA-125 is a glycoprotein expressed on the surface of ovarian carcinoma cells that is shed into the peritoneal cavity and circulating blood in the majority of patients.[29] Nearly 90% of patients with advanced ovarian carcinoma have detectable levels of CA-125. Unfortunately, levels are less frequently elevated in patients with small-volume disease; levels are elevated in less than 50% of patients with disease limited to the ovary. The insensitivity of CA-125 in detecting limited-volume disease is apparent from screening studies; early-stage disease is rarely detected. The ability of CA-125 to detect residual disease before second-look laparotomy has been evaluated in numerous studies. Overall, CA-125 has approximately 44% sensitivity, 96% specificity, and 65% accuracy in this setting.[18] These indices are nearly identical to those obtained with computed tomography. The per-test cost of CA-125 determination is considerably less than that of computed tomography. Surveillance using serial assessment of CA-125 levels may permit diagnosis of relapse several months earlier than strategies not using CA-125.[30-34]

The use of CA-125 and other tumor markers was considered in an international consensus conference in 1993.[35] There is currently no consensus regarding the routine use of CA-125 in the follow-up of patients with ovarian cancer. It is recommended that, when used, CA-125 be considered as part of the overall clinical picture. Reinstitution of therapy based solely on changes in the CA-125 level is not recommended. Several other serum tumor markers may be elevated in patients with ovarian carcinoma, including CA 15-3 and TAG 72.3. However, other markers generally lack sufficient predictive value and do not provide information that complements CA-125. Thus the routine use of other markers is not recommended.

Surveillance Recommendations

The lack of sensitivity of available diagnostic methods and the limitations of current second-line treatment regimens make it difficult to justify an aggressive, technology-intensive approach to follow-up. At present a recommendation that patients have periodic physical examinations seems reasonable (Table 16-3). The relative sensitivity and comparatively low cost of CA-125 determination suggest that it is also reasonable to use routinely. Imaging and invasive diagnostic methods should probably be reserved for evaluation of abnormalities identified by changes in symptoms, physical examination, or CA-125 levels. Given the nonspecific nature of ovarian cancer symptoms and signs and the limitations of noninvasive methods for assessment of disease status, histological confirmation of first relapse, when feasible, seems prudent.

Table 16-3 Follow-up of patients with ovarian cancer (epithelial tumors): Roswell Park Cancer Institute

	YEAR				
	1	2	3	4	5
Office visit*	3-4	3-4	3-4	1-2	1-2
CA-125	3-4	3-4	3-4	1-2	1-2
Imaging studies	†	†	†	†	†

*Includes pelvic examination.
†Imaging is indicated to confirm suspected relapse. Specific modalities may vary, depending on suspected site and available technologies. Histological or cytological confirmation of suspected relapse is strongly encouraged, especially for first recurrence.

Patients should probably be followed up most frequently during the first 3 years, since the majority of relapses occur within this time-frame. Reevaluation three or four times a year seems to be a reasonable frequency during the first 2 to 3 years after treatment. Patients who remain clinically free of disease for 3 years can probably be followed up at less frequent intervals subsequently (one to two times per year). Given the rarity of relapse beyond 6 years in patients with low-risk, early-stage disease, surveillance can probably be discontinued in these patients after that time unless ovary-conserving surgery has been performed. In contrast, patients with high-risk, early- and advanced-stage disease remain at risk for relapse for at least 10 years after treatment. Thus surveillance should probably be continued indefinitely in these patients.

Considerable uncertainty persists regarding the optimal methods and timing of surveillance in patients with ovarian cancer. The preceding recommendations will have to be reevaluated as new technologies and treatments emerge. In addition, formal cost-benefit analyses should be considered to determine whether alternative recommendations are justified. Such analyses might reasonably be incorporated into cooperative group therapeutic trials, where defined populations of patients are already being treated and followed up in a uniform manner.

It will be important for such analyses to account for the potential effects of lead-time bias when potential beneficial effects of surveillance are considered. Lead-time bias refers to an apparent improvement in survival among patients in a screening population that is due solely to earlier diagnosis, rather than to a change in the natural history of the disease (that is, patients die of disease at the same time, but they know they have disease for a longer period). This issue is addressed in much greater detail elsewhere.

Several reports indicate that women with ovarian cancer may be at risk for developing second primary malignancies.[36-39] The relative risk of developing acute nonlymphocytic leukemia, carcinomas of the breast, lung, colon, rectum, and urinary system, and malignancies of the nervous system and connective tissues is increased in patients with ovarian cancer compared with the general population. Whether the increased risk for all of these sites is related to treatment or whether increased risk indicates the presence of one or more common risk factors for development of malignancy is not clear. For acute nonlymphocytic leukemia the relationship to treatment is somewhat clearer. Estimates of the relative risk of acute leukemia among patients who have had chemotherapy for ovarian cancer range from 12 to 950 times the risk in the general population.[36,37,39] The risk of leukemia appears to be greatest among patients treated with alkylating agents. Among alkylating agents the highest risks are associated with drugs no longer commonly used, including chlorambucil, melphalan, and thiotepa. The potential for development of second primary malignancies at any of these sites must be considered by the physicians who perform surveillance on patients with ovarian cancer. Surveillance for each of these sites is discussed in detail elsewhere in this volume. At present the risk of second primary malignancies in patients with ovarian cancer is not known to be sufficiently high to justify routine surveillance. However, practitioners should recognize the potential for their occurrence and maintain an appropriate index of suspicion.

Two specific subgroups of patients warrant further comment: patients with familial disease and very young patients. It is estimated that less than 5% of cases of ovarian cancer are familial.[9] As noted previously, three specific familial syndromes are recognized: site-specific, breast-ovarian, and familial adenocarcinoma (Lynch II syndrome). The breast-ovarian syndrome is the most common of these. Currently considerable attention is being devoted to screening investigations in this population. However, no evidence has been found that the natural history of common epithelial ovarian cancer in patients with familial disease differs from that in nonfamilial disease. Thus recommendations for surveillance are as outlined previously.

Recently the breast-ovarian familial syndrome was linked to a gene on chromosome 17q called *BRCA1*.[40,41] It is not yet possible to predict risk or to use *BRCA1* for population screening. However, it is possible that this gene is a molecular marker that might be followed in the surveillance setting. Such specific applications have yet to be tested in the clinic.

Limited data suggest that the clinical features of ovarian cancer in very young women (less than 30 years of age) may be different from those of older patients. In one report, very young patients had lower grade and earlier stage disease than a comparable group of patients aged 30 to 39.[21] In addition, survival was significantly longer in the very young patients. Although these data are retrospective and await confirmation, they suggest that very young patients may have better outcomes, determined primarily by stage and grade. At present no data suggest differences between the biology of ovarian cancer of a given stage and grade in younger versus older patients.

SURVEILLANCE FOR TUMORS OF LOW MALIGNANT POTENTIAL (BORDERLINE TUMORS)

Epithelial tumors of low malignant potential (borderline tumors) contain cells that have many histological features of malignancy but do not invade the ovarian stroma.[42-45] Borderline tumors comprise up to 15% of ovarian tumors. They may be localized to the ovaries or found in locations throughout the peritoneum. Whether these latter lesions represent metastases or multiple primary lesions remains controversial. Borderline tumors are managed primarily by surgical resection. At present there are no data to support the routine use of chemotherapy in patients with these tumors. Overall, they have a much better prognosis than common epithelial ovarian cancer. Survival rates for all stages remain in the range of greater than 95% at 10 years, and an 89% survival rate at 20 years has been reported. The likelihood of relapse and death from disease is influenced by stage. Relapse occurs in approximately 2% to 7% of patients with stage I or II disease, versus 14% to 20% of patients with stage III or IV disease; survival figures are similar. Recurrent disease has generally been managed by repeat resection; prolonged disease-free survival after repeat resection has been observed.

Borderline tumors thus clearly differ from common epithelial ovarian cancer in their indolent natural histories and in their response to surgical therapy alone. Given the potential for surgical salvage of patients with this neoplasm, it would be helpful if specific surveillance modalities were available to detect early recurrence. Unfortunately, data regarding surveillance of these patients are essentially nonexistent. The available clinical data are predominantly retrospective, with most reports including patients diagnosed before the availability of CA-125 and when less sophisticated imaging methods were available. Thus definitive recommendations regarding surveillance cannot be made for this population.

SURVEILLANCE FOR OVARIAN GERM CELL TUMORS

Ovarian germ cell tumors are an uncommon but highly treatable subset of ovarian malignancies.[46] Germ cell tumors in women can be broadly classified as either dysgerminomas or nondysgerminomas. Dysgerminomas, analogous to seminomas in men, tend to be stage I at diagnosis. Surgical resection, alone or followed by adjuvant radiation, is often adequate treatment. Patients with relapse or advanced disease can frequently be cured by platinum-based chemotherapy. Nondysgerminomas tend to be diagnosed at a higher stage, but the outcome for these patients with surgery followed by chemotherapy is also quite good. Ovarian germ cell tumors frequently produce alpha-fetoprotein and beta-human chorionic gonadotropin, which can be monitored in the serum as indicators of tumor burden, response to therapy, and development of recurrent disease. There are few formal guidelines regarding surveillance in these patients and even fewer data regarding optimal methods and timing. At present it is reasonable to propose follow-up similar to that for male patients with germ cell tumors, as outlined elsewhere in this volume.

SURVEILLANCE FOR STROMAL TUMORS

Stromal tumors comprise another uncommon subset of ovarian malignancies, including granulosa cell tumors, theca-fibroma group tumors, Sertoli-Leydig tumors, and steroid cell tumors.[47] Most of these subtypes are sufficiently rare that it is difficult to make any statements regarding follow-up. However, some features of granulosa cell tumors deserve comment.[48-51] Granulosa cell tumors tend to be diagnosed at an early stage and are primarily managed surgically. The serum level of inhibin may be a useful marker of tumor burden or disease recurrence.[52] The use of other potential serum markers, such as progesterone or estradiol levels, is less established.[53,54] Although the majority of patients in some reports had recurrence within 2 years of initial treatment,[49] the disease may have a protracted and indolent natural history. Relapses are documented 20 years or more after diagnosis.[55,56] Recurrences most commonly occur within the peritoneum and may be localized, allowing for surgical salvage. Distant metastases are less frequent. Although no formal guidelines exist, the natural history of the disease suggests that patients with malignant granulosa cell tumors require surveillance for an extended period (perhaps indefinitely). The appearance of new symptoms suggestive of disease (such as pain or abdominal complaints) or a rising inhibin level should prompt reevaluation for disease recurrence.

PSYCHOLOGICAL IMPACT OF SURVEILLANCE IN PATIENTS WITH OVARIAN CANCER

There are essentially no objective data regarding the psychological impact of surveillance in ovarian cancer patients. However, some data reported from screening populations may be relevant. Anecdotal reports about women undergoing screening for hereditary breast cancer or breast-ovarian cancer suggest that persistent fear, anxiety, and apprehension are common and that patients may employ a wide variety of coping strategies.[57] These anecdotal results contrast somewhat with findings from a prospective, controlled psychological assessment of women in an ultrasound screening program for familial ovarian cancer in Britain.[58] This study specifically addressed the impact of false-positive and true-negative ultrasound results on formal assessments of anxiety, depression, and overall well-being. Before scans, high-risk subjects' scores on these assessments did not differ significantly from those of the control group (drawn from the general population, not known to have an increased cancer risk) or from previously established population-based scores. This suggests that patients in the screening population did not experience persistent anxiety, depression, or distress. As expected, true-negative scans resulted in decreased scores on anxiety scales and an improved sense of overall well-being, while false-positive results were associated with increased anxiety and diminished sense of well-being. The changes that occurred in patients with false-positive scans were generally short lived. Whether these results can be applied to other populations is unknown. However, the results imply that while practitioners must remain sensitive to the psychological impact of a prior diagnosis of cancer and the potential for its recurrence, patients under surveillance do not necessarily have severe or debilitating psychological symptoms.

FUTURE PROSPECTS

Surveillance of the patient with ovarian cancer remains a difficult problem. Few established guidelines and essentially no objective data are available regarding comparison of the available methods for surveillance. It is somewhat sobering to recognize that despite advances in imaging technology, serum markers, and understanding of the molecular biology of ovarian cancer, the recommendations proposed in this chapter differ little from those of Griffiths and Parker[59] in 1982 (with the exception of CA-125, which was not then available). Comparison of surveillance methods should be considered within the context of ongoing cooperative group clinical trials, since these will necessarily include defined patient populations that are treated and followed up in a standardized fashion. In particular, cooperative group trials should permit meaningful cost-benefit analyses to be performed. Optimal approaches to surveillance must also be defined in the context of efforts to develop improved treatment strategies for recurrent disease, lest physicians find themselves without effective treatments to offer patients in whom recurrent disease is diagnosed. It is hoped that coordinated efforts to improve surveillance and treatment will have a tangible impact on the survival and quality of life of patients with ovarian cancer.

Fundamental changes in surveillance may flow from a better understanding of mechanisms of disease. Although a detailed discussion of ovarian cancer biology is beyond the scope of this chapter, altered expression of one or more cellular genes is crucial to ovarian carcinogenesis. Increased expression of several protooncogenes *(ras, myc, her-2/neu,)* and deletions or mutations of tumor suppressor genes (p53) have been reported in ovarian carcinoma cell lines and tumor samples.[60-62] Further evidence supporting this contention comes from clinical observations demonstrating that ovarian carcinoma can be transmitted by autosomal-dominant inheritance patterns. Three such familial syndromes have been described: heritable ovarian cancer can occur within site-specific, breast-ovarian, or familial adenocarcinoma (Lynch II) syndromes.[9] Investigation of tissues obtained from some patients in high-risk families has led to the recent identification, cloning, and sequencing of *BRCA1,* a gene associated with familial breast and ovarian cancers.[40,41] Further delineation of the molecular biology of ovarian cancer may identify specific genetic markers that could be used for surveillance of patients after treatment or possibly for early diagnosis and screening.

REFERENCES

1. Wingo PA, Tong T, Bolden S. Cancer statistics, 1995. CA Cancer J Clin 1995;45:8-30.
2. Fathalla M. Factors in the causation and incidence of ovarian cancer. Obstet Gynecol Surv 1973;27:751-68.
3. Negri E, Franceschi S, Tzonou A, et al. Pooled analysis of 3 European case-control studies. I. Reproductive factors and risk of epithelial ovarian cancer. Int J Cancer 1991;49:50-6.
4. Franceschi S, Parazzini F, Negri E, et al. Pooled analysis of 3 European case-control studies of epithelial ovarian cancer. III. Oral contraceptive use. Int J Cancer 1991;49:61-5.
5. Godwin A, Testa J, Handel L, et al. Spontaneous transformation of rat ovarian surface epithelial cells: association with cytogenetic changes and implications of repeated ovulation in the etiology of ovarian cancer. J Natl Cancer Inst 1992;84:592-601.
6. Smith EM, Anderson B. The effects of symptoms and delay in seeking diagnosis on stage of disease at diagnosis among women with cancers of the ovary. Cancer 1985;56:2727-32.
7. Young RC, Walton L, Ellenberg SS, et al. Adjuvant therapy of stage I and stage II epithelial ovarian cancer: results of two prospective randomized trials. N Engl J Med 1990;322:1021-7.
8. Ozols R, Rubin S, Dembo A, Robboy S. Epithelial ovarian cancer. In: Hoskins W, Perez C, Young R, editors. Principles and practice of gynecologic oncology. Philadelphia: JB Lippincott Company, 1992:731-81.
9. Gallion HH, Smith SA. Hereditary ovarian cancer. Semin Surg Oncol 1994;10:249-54.
10. Sutton GP, Stehman FB, Einhorn LH, Roth LM, Blessing JA, Erlich CE. Ten-year follow-up of patients receiving cisplatin, doxorubicin, and cyclophosphamide chemotherapy for advanced epithelial ovarian carcinoma. J Clin Oncol 1989;7:223-9.
11. Thigpen JT, Vance RB, Khansur T. Second-line chemotherapy for recurrent carcinoma of the ovary. Cancer 1993;71(4 Suppl):1559-64.
12. Markman M, Rothman R, Hakes T, et al. Second-line platinum therapy in patients with ovarian cancer previously treated with cisplatin. J Clin Oncol 1991;9:389-93.
13. Khan O, Cosgrove DO, Fried AM, Savage PE. Ovarian carcinoma follow-up: US versus laparotomy. Radiology 1986;159:111-3.
14. Blackledge G, Lawton F, Redman C, Kelly K. Response of patients in phase II studies of chemotherapy in ovarian cancer: implications for patient treatment and the design of phase II trials. Br J Cancer 1989;59:650-3.
15. Hoskins PJ, O'Reilly SE, Swenerton KD. The "failure free interval" defines the likelihood of resistance to carboplatin in patients with advanced epithelial ovarian cancer previously treated with cisplatin; relevance to therapy and new drug testing. Int J Gynecol Cancer 1991;1:205-8.
16. McGuire WP, Hoskins WJ, Brady MF, et al. A phase III trial comparing cisplatin/cytoxan (PC) and cisplatin/taxol (PT) in advanced ovarian cancer (AOC). Proc Am Soc Clin Oncol 1993;12:255 (Abstract).
17. McGuire WP, Hoskins WJ, Brady MF, et al. Taxol and cisplatin (TP) improves outcome in advanced ovarian cancer (AOC) as compared to cytoxan and cisplatin (CP). Proc Am Soc Clin Oncol 1995;14:275(Abstract).
18. Barter JF, Barnes WA. Second-look laparotomy. In: Rubin SC, Sutton GP, editors. Ovarian cancer. New York: McGraw-Hill, 1993: 269-300.
19. Buist MR, Golding RP, Burger CW, et al. Comparative evaluation of diagnostic methods in ovarian carcinoma with emphasis on CT and MRI. Gynecol Oncol 1994;52:191-8.
20. Seewalt VL, Cain JM, Greer BE, Tamimi HK, Figge DC, Livingston RB. Reviving the pelvic examination for evaluating the status of ovarian carcinoma. J Clin Oncol 1995;13:799.
21. Plaxe SC, Braly PS, Freddo JL, McClay E, Kirmani S, Howell SB. Profiles of women age 30-39 and age less than 30 with epithelial ovarian cancer. Obstet Gynecol 1993;81:651-4.
22. Cohen CJ, Jennings TS. Screening for ovarian cancer: the role of noninvasive imaging techniques. Am J Obstet Gynecol 1994;170: 1088-94.
23. Bourne T, Campbell S, Steer C, Whitehead MI, Collins WP. Transvaginal colour flow imaging: a possible new screening technique for ovarian cancer. Br Med J 1989;299:1367-70.
24. Hubner KF, McDonald TW, Niethammer JG, Smith GT, Gould HR, Buonocore E. Assessment of primary and metastatic ovarian cancer by positron emission tomography (PET) using 2-[^{18}F]deoxyglucose (2-[^{18}F]FDG). Gynecol Oncol 1993;51:197-204.
25. Casey MJ, Gupta NC, Muths CK. Experience with positron emission tomography (PET) scans in patients with ovarian cancer. Gynecol Oncol 1994;53:331-8.
26. Delaloye AB, Delaloye B. Immunoscintigraphy in cancer care. Cancer 1994;73:900-4.
27. Krag DN, Ford P, Smith L, et al. Clinical immunoscintigraphy of recurrent ovarian cancer with indium 111-labeled B72.3 monoclonal antibody. Arch Surg 1993;128:819-23.
28. Surwit EA, Childers JM, Krag DN, et al. Clinical assessment of ^{111}In-CYT-103 immunoscintigraphy in ovarian cancer. Gynecol Oncol 1993;48:285-92.
29. Bast RC, Klug TL, St. John E, et al. A radioimmunoassay using a monoclonal antibody to monitor the course of epithelial ovarian cancer. N Engl J Med 1985;309:883-7.
30. Bruzzone MA, Onetto M, Campora E, et al. CA-125 monitoring in the management of ovarian cancer. Anticancer Res 1990;10:1353-60.
31. Hising C, Anjegard IM, Einhorn N. Clinical relevance of the CA 125 assay in monitoring of ovarian cancer patients. Am J Clin Oncol 1991;14:111-4.
32. Kaminska JA, Kowalska MM, Sablinska B, Pietrzak P. Usefulness of determination of CA-125 in monitoring patients with ovarian carcinoma. Eur J Gynaecol Oncol 1993;14(Suppl):128-32.
33. Hogberg T, Kagedal B. Long-term follow-up of ovarian carcinoma with monthly determinations of serum CA 125. Gynecol Oncol 1992; 46:191-8.
34. Crombach G, Zipple HH, Wurz H. Clinical significance of cancer antigen 125 (CA 125) in ovarian cancer. Cancer Detect Prev 1985; 8:135-9.
35. Allen DG, Baak J, Belpomme D, et al. Advanced epithelial ovarian cancer: 1993 consensus statements. Ann Oncol 1993;4(Suppl 4):S83-8.
36. Kaldor JM, Day NE, Petterson F, et al. Leukemia following chemotherapy for ovarian cancer. N Engl J Med 1990;322:1-6.
37. Prior P, Pope DJ. Subsequent primary cancers in relation to treatment of ovarian cancer. Br J Cancer 1989;59:453-9.
38. Schoen RE, Weissfield JL, Kuller LH. Are women with breast, endometrial, or ovarian cancer at increased risk for colorectal cancer? Am J Gastroenterol 1994;89:835-42.
39. Einhorn N, Eklund G, Franzen S, Lambert B, Lindsten J, Soderhall S. Late side effects of chemotherapy in ovarian carcinoma. Cancer 1982;49:2234-41.
40. Black DM, Solomon E. The search for the familial breast/ovarian cancer gene. Trends Genet 1993;9:22-6.
41. Miki Y, Swenson J, Shattuck-Eidens D, et al. A strong candidate for the breast and ovarian cancer susceptibility gene *BRCA1*. Science 1994;266:66-71.
42. Harlow BL, Weiss NS, Lofton S. Epidemiology of borderline ovarian tumors. J Natl Cancer Inst 1987;78:71-4.
43. Nation JG, Krephart GV. Ovarian carcinoma of low malignant potential: staging and treatment. Am J Obstet Gynecol 1986;154:290-3.
44. Leake JF, Currie JL, Rosenshein NB, Woodruff JD. Long-term follow-up of serous ovarian tumors of low malignant potential. Gynecol Oncol 1992;47:150-8.

45. Massad LS, Hunter VJ, Szpak CA, Clarke-Pearson DL, Creasman WT. Epithelial ovarian tumors of low malignant potential. Obstet Gynecol 1991;78:1027-32.
46. Williams SD. Ovarian germ cell tumors. In: Rubin SC, Sutton GP, editors. Ovarian cancer. New York: McGraw-Hill, 1993:391-404.
47. Price FV, Schwartz PE. Management of ovarian stromal tumors. In: Rubin SC, Sutton GP, editors. Ovarian cancer. New York: McGraw-Hill, 1993:405-23.
48. Malmstrom H, Hogberg T, Risberg B, Simonsen E. Granulosa cell tumors of the ovary: prognostic factors and outcome. Gynecol Oncol 1994;52:50-5.
49. Fox H, Agrawal K, Langley FA. A clinicopathologic study of 92 cases of granulosa cell tumor of the ovary with special reference to the factors influencing prognosis. Cancer 1975;35:231-41.
50. Evans AT, Gaffey TA, Malkasian GD, Annegers JF. Clinicopathologic review of 118 granulosa and 82 theca cell tumors. Obstet Gynecol 1980;55:231-8.
51. Pankratz E, Boyes DA, White GW, Galliford BW, Fairey RN, Benedet JL. Granulosa cell tumors: a clinical review of 61 cases. Obstet Gynecol 1978;52:718-23.
52. Lappohn RE, Burger HG, Bouma J, Bangah M, Krans M, de Bruijn HW. Inhibin as a marker for granulosa cell tumors. N Engl J Med 1989;321:790-3.
53. Lomax CW, May HV, Panko WB, Thornton WN. Progesterone production by an ovarian granulosa cell carcinoma. Obstet Gynecol 1977;50(Suppl):S39-40.
54. Kaye SB, Davies E. Cyclophosphamide, adriamycin, and cisplatinum for the treatment of advanced granulosa cell tumor, using serum estradiol as a marker. Gynecol Oncol 1986;24:261-4.
55. Li MK, van der Walt JD. Recurrent granulosa cell tumor of the ovary 22 years after primary excision. J Coll Surg Edinb 1984;29:192-4.
56. Simmons RL, Sciarra JJ. Treatment of late recurrent granulosa cell tumors of the ovary. Surg Gynecol Obstet 1967;124:65-70.
57. Lynch HT, Lynch J, Conway T, Severin M. Psychological aspects of monitoring high risk women for breast cancer. Cancer 1994;74 (3 Suppl):1184-92.
58. Wardle FJ, Collins W, Pernet AL, Whitehead MI, Bourne TH, Campbell S. Psychological impact of screening for familial ovarian cancer. J Natl Cancer Inst 1993;85:653-7.
59. Griffiths CT, Parker LM. Ovarian cancer. In: Eiseman B, Robinson WA, Steele G Jr, editors. Follow-up of the cancer patient. New York: Thieme-Stratton, Inc., 1982:159-68.
60. Perez RP, Godwin AK, Hamilton TC, Ozols RF. Ovarian cancer biology. Semin Oncol 1991;18:186-204.
61. Marks JR, Davidoff AM, Kerns BJ, et al. Overexpression and mutation of p53 in epithelial ovarian cancer. Cancer Res 1991;51:2979-84.
62. Okamoto A, Sameshima Y, Yokayama S, et al. Frequent allelic losses and mutations of the p53 gene in human ovarian cancer. Cancer Res 1991;51:5171-6.
63. Hoskins WJ. Primary surgical management of advanced epithelial ovarian cancer. In: Rubin SC, Sutton GP, editors. Ovarian cancer. New York: McGraw-Hill, 1993:241-53.

➢ COUNTERPOINT

Memorial Sloan-Kettering Cancer Center

NADEEM R. ABU-RUSTUM AND JOHN P. CURTIN

The review of ovarian cancer surveillance after curative intent treatment by Perez is well written and comprehensive. Particularly in regard to the issues of follow-up surveillance using serum tumor markers and medical imaging studies, we agree that in most cases these tests are overused with little value demonstrated in any studies reported to date. However, two areas deserve further comment.

SECOND-LOOK SURGERY

A widely accepted management approach for patients with epithelial ovarian cancer consists of three basic components: initial surgery with complete, thorough staging and debulking of advanced disease, combination platinum-based chemotherapy, and surgical reassessment to determine response to initial therapy.[1,2] Patients who complete an initial course of platinum-based chemotherapy with obvious persistence or progression of disease by clinical examination, imaging studies, or tumor marker (CA-125) have a poor outcome and may be offered investigational or standard salvage chemotherapy, hormone therapy, or no further therapy. Patients who complete their initial chemotherapy with a partial clinical response by physical examination, imaging studies, or tumor marker (CA-125) may also be candidates for investigational or standard salvage therapy with intravenous or intraperitoneal chemotherapy. Their response to salvage treatment can be assessed by serial physical examination, imaging studies, and patterns of change in tumor markers. Deterioration or improvement in symptoms, if initially present, may also be a valuable tool in assessing response to salvage therapy.

The management of patients who complete an initial course of chemotherapy with a complete clinical response remains controversial. This group of patients with epithelial ovarian cancer has better survival times than nonresponders and even a chance for cure. However, most still have subclinical disease that will eventually progress and ultimately result in death. Follow-up varies depending on the institution and the treating physician. Options for follow-up include serial monitoring with physical examinations, tumor markers, and imaging studies (when indicated) or surgical exploration to assess pathological response to therapy (second-look surgery). If the physician and patient decide against second-look surgery, follow-up at 3-month intervals for the first 2 to 3 years and thereafter at 6-month intervals should be considered (Table 16-4). At each visit, a complete physical examination with special attention to the patient's

Table 16-4 Follow-up of patients with ovarian cancer (epithelial tumors after bilateral adnexectomy): Memorial Sloan-Kettering Cancer Center

	YEAR				
	1	2	3	4	5
Office visit	4	4	4	2	2
CA-125*	4	4	4	2	2
Imaging studies†	‡	‡	‡	‡	‡

*Indicated for patients with previously abnormal levels.
†Consists of abdominal computed tomography, pelvic computed tomography, chest x-ray, abdominal ultrasound, pelvic ultrasound, and pelvic magnetic resonance imaging as clinically indicated.
‡Performed as clinically indicated.

symptoms should be performed. Tumor marker (CA-125) determinations should be offered at each visit to patients known to have previously abnormal levels; imaging studies such as computed tomography should be requested only when clinically indicated or to confirm a clinical suspicion of recurrence.

The second-look operation for epithelial ovarian cancer remains the most reliable method for assessing disease status in patients who have completed initial therapy and who have no evidence of persistent disease by physical examination, imaging studies, and tumor markers. Candidates for second-look surgery should be able to tolerate the procedure and also be eligible to receive further chemotherapy, either intravenously or intraperitoneally, as salvage or consolidation, based on the findings at second-look surgery. In selected patients, such as those with early-stage disease, second-look surgery is not indicated.[3] However, given that most patients with epithelial ovarian cancer have stage III or IV disease at diagnosis and because of the relative chemosensitivity of epithelial ovarian cancer, the majority of patients complete the initial course of chemotherapy with no clinical evidence of disease and may be candidates for surgical reassessment.

Second-look operations have been performed in patients with ovarian cancer for the last two decades. The operation itself rarely has therapeutic value; however, it provides the most accurate clinical data regarding response to initial therapy and current status of disease. Patients with platinum-sensitive tumors and small-volume residual disease (less than 0.5 cm) may benefit from further intraperitoneal chemotherapy.[5] Patients with no evidence of disease may be offered investigational consolidation therapy or be observed off therapy. Patients with gross persistent or progressive disease that was missed clinically have a poor prognosis and can be offered investigational or standard salvage chemotherapy or be observed off therapy.

Secondary complete cytoreduction at second-look surgery, which may be accomplished in approximately 32% of patients, may result in improved survival if the residual disease is rendered microscopic by surgical resection.[6] Traditionally the operation is performed through a midline vertical incision to maximize access to intraabdominal and pelvic organs; often these incisions extend near the rib margin to expose the diaphragm. The odds of finding persistent disease are high in patients with advanced disease (stages III and IV), with approximately 45% of these patients having gross residual disease and another 20% having microscopic residual disease.[7,8] The risk of having persistent disease also increases to nearly 77% in patients whose disease was suboptimally debulked before initiation of chemotherapy as compared with 54% of patients who had optimal cytoreduction.[9]

Because of the high incidence of persistent carcinoma, surgeons should consider the least invasive exploratory technique (laparoscopy) to assess for persistent disease and to determine size and distribution. The operation should also provide information on the extent of adhesions in the peritoneal cavity to help identify patients who may be candidates for intraperitoneal therapy. Laparotomy clearly has an advantage over laparoscopy in patients with grossly persistent disease where complete surgical secondary cytoreduction is anticipated in an attempt to improve survival. Reported complications arising from second-look laparotomy include wound infection (12%), urinary tract infections (13%), pulmonary complications (5%), bowel injury (4%), and prolonged ileus (13%).[10]

Laparoscopy has been described as a method for surgical reassessment in patients with ovarian cancer since the early 1970s.[11,12] These early reports were received with limited acceptance of laparoscopy as a replacement for laparotomy. The limitation of laparoscopic practice as described included inadequate visualization in up to 12% of patients,[13] a high false-negative rate of approximately 11% to 55%,[14,15] and a high complication rate (mainly bowel injury) in 2% to 9% of patients.[13,16] In addition, there were limitations in performing extensive laparoscopic sampling of areas of tumor persistence including retroperitoneal lymph nodes.[17] However, several authors have pointed out advantages to the laparoscopic approach, including a reduction in the need for laparotomy in 36% to 50% of cases.[11,14,15,18] The recent improvement in instrumentation and the development of videolaparoscopy have resulted in a renewed interest in minimal access surgery. The safety of this approach has also been documented with minimal intraoperative and postoperative complications.[19] This low complication rate noted in laparoscopic second-look procedures as compared with laparotomy will need to be confirmed in a randomized clinical trial.

With the introduction of videolaparoscopy and the recent developments in laparoscopic surgical equipment, more operative laparoscopic procedures are being performed safely in a variety of patients with gynecological malignancies. The second-look operation is an ideal example, primarily because in the majority of patients the main purpose is to search for residual disease and, less frequently, to perform extensive procedures like secondary debulking, hysterectomy, and reversal of colostomy. With advanced laparoscopic techniques, adhesions can usually be released to improve visualization of peritoneal surfaces, allowing the biopsy of suspect lesions and sampling of areas of tumor persistence, including the pelvic and periaortic lymph nodes. Laparoscopic sampling of these nodal regions is being performed more frequently for restaging and in the second-look setting.[19] Peritoneal washings can be obtained and intraperitoneal catheters can be inserted under direct visualization.

Laparoscopy has limitations, primarily the inability to palpate unvisualized areas and the lack of adequate exposure to the posterior diaphragm behind the liver where disease may be missed in patients with diaphragmatic metastasis. Second-look laparoscopy can be safely performed as an initial procedure using an open technique in most patients. It may also spare approximately 50% of patients the morbidity and charges of laparotomy. The need for conversion to laparotomy because of a lack of gross persistent disease may be reduced if intraoperative cytological consultation is obtained on washings retrieved laparoscopically before conversion to laparotomy, with the understanding that only 22% of patients with microscopically positive second-look operations will have positive cytological findings according to previous publications.[20]

SURVEILLANCE AFTER CONSERVATIVE THERAPY

When a young woman has a suspect adnexal mass and is found to have either a tumor of the ovary with low malignant potential or a well-differentiated tumor confined to one ovary, conservative therapy, which retains both fertility and hormonal function of the ovaries and uterus, is possible. The number of patients with this finding at diagnosis varies from institution to institution. However, approximately 10% of patients with epithelial ovarian cancer have low-malignant potential tumors and approximately 10% of patients with epithelial tumors are less than 35 years of age. When this clinical scenario is encountered, thorough staging is usually indicated. However, complete removal of the uterus, tubes, and ovaries may be avoided in these young women. The question, then, becomes how best to follow these patients after surgical treatment.

Given that these patients have a documented epithelial ovarian cancer, they deserve close clinical follow-up that should at least mimic what is recommended for patients who are at high risk of ovarian cancer because they are members of a family with a hereditary cancer predisposition such as breast/ovarian-specific syndrome, ovarian-specific syndrome, or Lynch II syndrome. These patients should be examined frequently and should undergo transvaginal ultrasound every 6 months as well as measurement of relevant serum tumor markers every 3 months for the first 3 years (Table 16-5). Any rise in CA-125 levels or the appearance of a suspect mass on ultrasound should be an indication for further evaluation.

The question arises as to whether these patients should undergo routine removal of the ovaries after completion of planned childbearing. Few data have been published in the literature to assist the clinician in this clinical decision-making process. If the patient can be assumed to be at risk because she has already demonstrated the presence of one epithelial ovarian tumor arising in an ovary, her risk is at least equal to that of patients who have a positive family history. Once childbearing is completed, the patient should consider elective oophorectomy and hysterectomy. The alternative is to continue long-term close surveillance using transvaginal ultrasound and serum CA-125 testing.

If the patient is found to have a germ cell tumor of the ovary, conservative surgery, followed by adjuvant chemotherapy, is the standard of care. The posttreatment surveillance of these patients should include serum tumor markers as well as physical examination and transvaginal ultrasound in patients with retained ovaries (Table 16-5).

Table 16-5 Follow-up of patients with ovarian cancer (retained adnexae): Memorial Sloan-Kettering Cancer Center

	YEAR				
	1	2	3	4	5
Office visit	4	4	4	2	2
CA-125*	4	4	4	2	2
Beta-human chorionic gonadotropin*,†	4	4	4	2	2
Alpha-fetoprotein*,†	4	4	4	2	2
Transvaginal ultrasound‡	2	2	2	2	2
Abdominal computed tomography	§	§	§	§	§
Pelvic computed tomography	§	§	§	§	§
Pelvic magnetic resonance imaging	§	§	§	§	§

*Indicated for patients with previously abnormal levels.
†Performed for patients with germ cell tumors only.
‡Indicated for patients with a low-malignant-potential tumor or a well-differentiated tumor confined to one ovary.
§Performed as clinically indicated.

Since the known recurrence rate is low in these patients and there does not seem to be a high propensity to bilaterality for most germ cell tumors, elective oophorectomy after childbearing is not usually recommended and these patients should be followed up in a routine fashion.

CONCLUSION

This review has addressed many of the concerns regarding follow-up of patients who have completed therapy. Future studies must focus on appropriate follow-up and should address issues such as the psychological impact of various methods of follow-up, as well as cost-benefit and cost-effectiveness analyses of the various tests and examinations offered to patients. As physicians gain knowledge regarding the genetic aspects of ovarian cancer, there may be more patients who will require close surveillance for the development of ovarian neoplasia. Women who have undergone prophylactic oophorectomy, because they are genetically predisposed to ovarian cancer, constitute another group of interest, since they are at continued, albeit small, risk of peritoneal primary cancers.

REFERENCES

1. Rubin SC. Second-look laparotomy in ovarian cancer. In: Markman M, Hoskins WJ, editors. Cancer of the ovary. New York: Raven Press, 1993:175-85.
2. Morrow CP, Curtin JP, Townsend DE, editors. Synopsis of gynecologic oncology. 4th ed. New York: Churchill Livingstone, 1993:233-74.
3. Rubin SC, Jones WB, Curtin JP, Barakat RR, Hakes TB, Hoskins WJ. Second-look laparotomy in stage I ovarian cancer following comprehensive surgical staging. Obstet Gynecol 1993;82:139-42.
4. Rubin SC, Lewis JL Jr. Second-look surgery in ovarian carcinoma. Crit Rev Oncol Hematol 1988;8:75-91.

5. Markman M, Hakes T, Reichman B, et al. Intraperitoneal therapy in the management of ovarian carcinoma. Yale J Biol Med 1989;62: 393-403.
6. Hoskins WJ, Rubin SC, Dulaney E, et al. Influence of secondary cytoreduction at the time of second-look laparotomy on the survival of patients with epithelial ovarian cancer. Gynecol Oncol 1989;34: 365-71.
7. Copeland LJ, Gershenson DM, Wharton JT, et al. Microscopic disease at second-look laparotomy in advanced ovarian cancer. Cancer 1985;55:472-8.
8. Gershenson DM, Copeland LJ, Wharton JT, et al. Prognosis of surgically determined complete responders in advanced ovarian cancer. Cancer 1985;55:1129-35.
9. Ozols RF, Rubin SC, Dembo AJ, Robboy S. Epithelial ovarian cancer. In: Hoskins WJ, Perez CA, Young RC, editors. Principles and practice of gynecologic oncology. Philadelphia: JB Lippincott Company, 1992:731-81.
10. Janisch H, Schieder K, Koelbl H. Diagnostic versus therapeutic second-look surgery in patients with ovarian cancer. Baillieres Clin Obstet Gynaecol 1989;3:191-200.
11. Rosenoff SH, Young RC, Anderson T, et al. Peritoneoscopy: a valuable staging tool in ovarian carcinoma. Ann Intern Med 1975;83:37-41.
12. Bagley CM Jr, Young RC, Schein PS, Chabner BA, DeVita VT. Ovarian cancer metastatic to the diaphragm—frequently undiagnosed at laparotomy: a preliminary report. Am J Obstet Gynecol 1973;116: 397-400.
13. Quinn MA, Bishop GJ, Campbell JJ, Rodgerson J, Pepperell RJ. Laparoscopic follow-up of patients with ovarian cancer. Br J Obstet Gynaecol 1980;87:1132-9.
14. Xygakis AM, Politis GS, Michalas SP, Kaskarelis DB. Second-look laparoscopy in ovarian cancer. J Reprod Med 1984;29:583-5.
15. Ozols RF, Fisher RI, Anderson T, Makuch R, Young RC. Peritoneoscopy in the management of ovarian cancer. Am J Obstet Gynecol 1981;140:611-9.
16. Berek JS, Griffiths CT, Leventhal JM. Laparoscopy for second-look evaluation in ovarian cancer. Obstet Gynecol 1981;58:192-8.
17. Rutledge FN. The second-look operation for ovarian cancer. Baillieres Clin Obstet Gynaecol 1989;3:175-82.
18. Piver MS, Lele SB, Barlow JJ, Gamarra M. Second-look laparoscopy prior to proposed second-look laparotomy. Obstet Gynecol 1980;55: 571-3.
19. Childers JM, Lang J, Surwit EA, Hatch KD. Laparoscopic surgical staging of ovarian cancer. Gynecol Oncol 1995;59:25-33.
20. Rubin SC, Dulaney ED, Markman M, Hoskins WJ, Saigo PE, Lewis JL Jr. Peritoneal cytology as an indicator of disease in patients with residual ovarian cancer. Obstet Gynecol 1988;71:851-3.

➢ COUNTER POINT

Kyushu University Hospital, Japan

TOSHIHARU KAMURA

Ovarian cancer is uncommon in Japan, but the incidence is increasing. For this reason the Japan Society of Obstetricians and Gynecologists has begun to register patients with ovarian cancer. The rise in incidence of common forms of ovarian cancer in Japan is due to life-style changes among Japanese women. Similar to that of women in Western countries, childbearing occurs at advanced ages and the number of pregnancies is small. In addition, oral contraceptives are still unavailable to women. However, borderline, germ cell, and stromal tumors are still rare. Therefore this counterpoint focuses on invasive common epithelial cancer.

Cisplatin was first used to treat ovarian cancer in Japan in the early 1980s. Previously the prognosis of advanced disease had been poor and 5-year survivors were uncommon. Since the introduction of cisplatin, approximately 30% of patients with advanced ovarian cancer have survived beyond 5 years after initial treatment. Cisplatin, adriamycin, and cyclophosphamide are now commonly used in postoperative chemotherapy.[1] A standard regimen is administered for more than 6 cycles and consists of cisplatin 50 mg/kg, adriamycin 50 mg/kg, and cyclophosphamide 500 mg/kg. Recently carboplatin and 4'-epiadriamycin, analogs of cisplatin and adriamycin, have been used in combination chemotherapy to reduce nephrotoxicity and cardiotoxicity, respectively. A phase II study in Japan showed that paclitaxel or docetaxel achieved approximately a 30% response rate for recurrent or advanced ovarian cancer. The response rate is relatively low when compared with those shown by the Gynecologic Oncology Group and the European Organization for Research and Treatment of Cancer. In Japan, when paclitaxel or docetaxel becomes commercially available, phase III studies will begin, as are already performed in many Western countries.

High-risk ovarian cancer patients include those who have residual disease after initial surgery, high histological tumor grade, or advanced disease.[1,2] In the experience at Kyushu University Hospital, 30% of patients with advanced ovarian cancer had progressive disease, while 27% achieved no evidence of disease (NED) status at 5 years after initial therapy (Figure 16-1). The remaining 43% had recurrence after the NED period. Follow-up after initial therapy in patients who achieve NED status is the focus of this counterpoint.

Second-look laparotomy has been performed on patients with NED to assess the pathological response of chemotherapy quickly, which has contributed to the development of new drug therapies. However, considering its substantially low specificity and the current lack of effective second-line treatments, the benefit of second-look laparotomy in terms of survival is unclear.[3] Treatment should be assessed with the end point of clinical progression-free survival.

Of the patients who had recurrence after achieving NED status, 53% had only peritoneal disease, 33% had peritoneal disease and distant metastases simultaneously, and 14% had only distant metastases when recurrent disease was discovered. Those metastatic sites included the liver, pleura, lung, skin, spleen, brain, and vagina. Because initial recurrence occurs so often in sites other than the peritoneal surface, many physicians have questioned the utility of second-look laparotomy. Physicians at Kyushu University Hospital believe this procedure should be considered experimental and carried out only in controlled trials.

Since initial recurrence tends to appear in distant organs, examination at each follow-up visit should consist of various imaging methods, including chest x-ray, ultrasound, computed tomography, and magnetic resonance imaging, as well

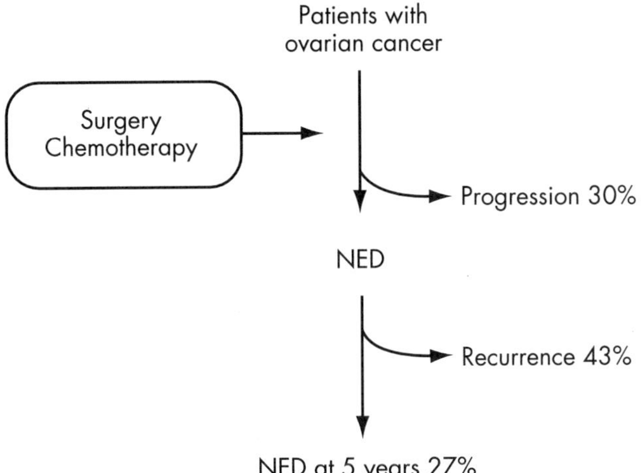

Figure 16-1 Outcome of patients with advanced ovarian cancer at Kyushu University Hospital. *NED,* No evidence of disease.

as physical examination. As described by Perez, both computed tomography and magnetic resonance imaging have limitations in detecting recurrent disease and both are expensive. Tables 16-6 and 16-7 depict the follow-up strategies employed at Kyushu University Hospital. For patients at high risk of recurrence, computed tomography is performed every 3 months (Table 16-7). When the computed tomographic scan shows a small doubtful shadow, physicians repeat scanning at monthly intervals. If the doubtful shadow enlarges, physicians judge that the mass is a recurrent tumor. If there is no change in size, efforts are made to obtain histological or cytological specimens.

Magnetic resonance imaging offers no more information than computed tomography but has the potential to differentiate blood from other serous or mucinous fluids. If a space-occupying lesion is detected with ultrasound or computed tomography, magnetic resonance imaging is occasionally useful. The efficacy of positron emission tomography is uncertain at this time.

Ultrasound is less invasive and expensive than computed tomography or magnetic resonance imaging, but almost all reports of its utility focus on preoperative diagnosis and initial treatment. It is useful to detect recurrence in parenchymal organs such as the liver, kidney, and spleen. However, intraperitoneal masses are difficult to detect with ultrasound and these are common sites of recurrence. An advantage of ultrasound is that if an abnormal mass is detected, an aspiration sample is easy to take under ultrasound guidance.[4] Recently, transvaginal ultrasound has become available. This is easy to use and can reliably detect minimal pelvic ascites accumulations.

The tumor marker CA-125 is the most popular and useful marker to detect recurrent disease.[5] At Kyushu University Hospital the serum CA-125 value is measured biweekly until it decreases to the normal range (below 35 U/ml) after primary surgery. After having decreased to this range, the CA-125 level is monitored monthly during initial chemotherapy. After completion of chemotherapy the level is measured at every follow-up visit.

Table 16-6 Follow-up of patients with ovarian cancer (early-stage, low-risk disease): Kyushu University Hospital, Japan

	YEAR				
	1	**2**	**3**	**4**	**5**
Office visit*	4	4	3	2	2
CA-125	4	4	3	2	2
Transvaginal ultrasound	4	4	3	2	2
Abdominal computed tomography	†	†	†	†	†
Pelvic computed tomography	†	†	†	†	†

*Includes pelvic examination.
†Performed as clinically indicated.

Table 16-7 Follow-up of patients with ovarian cancer (high-risk and advanced disease): Kyushu University Hospital, Japan

	YEAR				
	1	**2**	**3**	**4**	**5**
Office visit*	12	6	3	3	3
CA-125	12	6	3	3	3
Transvaginal ultrasound	12	6	3	3	3
Abdominal computed tomography	4	3	†	†	†
Pelvic computed tomography	4	3	†	†	†

*Includes pelvic examination.
†Performed as clinically indicated.

Among 40 patients with advanced ovarian cancer who were followed according to the protocol dictated in Table 16-7, nine whose CA-125 level normalized within 4 weeks after primary surgery achieved 5-year survival. All patients whose CA-125 level remained higher than 35 U/ml recurred within 2 years, even if the patient had achieved NED status according to all other parameters. In patients whose CA-125 level decreased below 10 U/ml, 36% had recurrence within 2 years. The data suggest that an initial decrease below 35 U/ml within 4 weeks indicates possible long-term survival, while a lesser decrease in the CA-125 level does not. Therefore patients whose CA-125 level does not fall below 35 U/ml should undergo close follow-up. Among patients with recurrence, CA-125 levels were elevated after detection of recurrence in only 21%. Therefore a negative CA-125 value has low sensitivity.

In practice, physicians at Kyushu University Hospital combine some of the methods mentioned previously to detect recurrent cancer as early as possible, particularly in patients at high risk of recurrence. The follow-up protocol for early-stage, low-risk patients consists of CA-125, chest x-ray, transvaginal ultrasound, and pelvic examination (Table 16-6). For high-risk patients, in addition to the preceding examinations, computed tomography is routinely employed for 2 years after treatment to explore the liver, retroperitoneal lymph nodes, and peritoneal surface (Table 16-7).

As stated by Perez, patients who have recurrence rarely achieve long-term survival except for those with low-malignant-potential tumors. Since methods to detect and treat recurrent tumors are so poor, patients always fear recurrence. In this context physicians should make every effort to support patients with ovarian cancer psychologically.

REFERENCES

1. Kamura T, Tsukamoto N, Suenaga T, Kaku T, Matsukuma K, Matsuyama T. [Evaluation of the efficacy of cisplatin-based chemotherapy for epithelial ovarian cancer: comparison with treatments employed before cisplatin era.] (in Japanese) Jpn J Cancer Chemother 1987;14:1260-3.
2. Morikawa Y, Kawai M, Kano T, et al. Clinical remission criteria for epithelial carcinoma of the ovary. Gynecol Oncol 1993;48:342-8.
3. Creasman WT. Second-look laparotomy in ovarian cancer. Gynecol Oncol 1994;55:S122-7.
4. Zanetta G, Brenna A, Pittelli M, Lissoni A, Trio D, Riotta S. Transvaginal ultrasound-guided fine needle sampling of deep cancer recurrence in the pelvis: usefulness and limitations. Gynecol Oncol 1994; 54:59-63.
5. Rosman M, Hayden CL, Thiel RP, et al. Prognostic indicators for poor risk of epithelial ovarian carcinoma. Cancer 1994;74:1323-8.

➢ COUNTERPOINT

University of Washington Medical Center ▪ Fred Hutchinson Cancer Research Center

BARBARA A. GOFF AND BENJAMIN E. GREER

One of the primary goals of postoperative surveillance is to detect recurrence while curative treatment is still an option. Unfortunately, 70% to 80% of patients with ovarian cancer eventually have recurrence and relapses are rarely curable. The medical literature provides very little guidance or consensus as to the appropriate strategies for ovarian cancer surveillance. Even less information is available regarding the cost effectiveness of various surveillance modalities. We agree that there is currently no evidence that intensive monitoring or salvage therapy has a significant impact on overall survival. However, the absence of data does not necessarily mean that a subset of such patients will not benefit from an aggressive surveillance and treatment strategy.[1] Although treatment of relapses rarely yields long-term cures, salvage therapy can produce objective responses, including complete responses. In addition, salvage therapy can reduce symptoms and improve overall quality of life.

Second-look surgery in the management of epithelial ovarian cancer is a controversial topic. Clearly, findings at the time of second-look laparotomy can indicate prognosis and predict the likelihood of ultimate survival, although little evidence has been presented in the literature that survival improves.[2] Unfortunately, studies that find a lack of benefit for this procedure were not designed to specifically evaluate its impact on overall survival.[3] After primary therapy patients with advanced ovarian cancer with tumor marker CA-125 levels less than 35 U/ml will have detectable disease at second-look laparotomy in approximately 50% of cases. Although recurrent disease develops in 30% to 50% of patients with a negative exploration, the value of repeat exploration may be to identify those patients with negative or microscopic residual disease who have drug-responsive tumors and possibly more favorable tumor biology.[4] These patients are ideal candidates for consolidation or dose-intensive therapy and present an opportunity to improve overall survival rates. In a study by Copeland et al.,[4] patients with advanced ovarian cancer who had microscopic residual disease at second-look laparotomy and then went on to receive additional chemotherapy had 2- and 5-year survival rates of 96% and 71%, respectively. At the University of Washington Medical Center and Fred Hutchinson Cancer Research Center the decision for planned reexploration is individualized for each patient. In general, physicians here believe that this procedure should be performed in patients with advanced ovarian cancer who are good candidates for consolidation therapy, especially when opportunities to participate in prospective clinical trials are available.

We agree with Perez that physical examination, especially pelvic examination, is an important component to ovarian cancer surveillance. Surprisingly, pelvic examination is not performed routinely in many centers, despite its proven benefit. Nodularity or small masses at the vaginal apex that can be missed by computed tomography or ultrasound are easily felt by someone with experience in performing pelvic examinations. For patients with a history of epithelial ovarian cancer and an elevated CA-125 level before therapy, this is generally a sensitive marker of recurrent disease. CA-125 can often detect disease before symptoms, physical findings, or radiographic abnormalities.[1] In the group of patients whose CA-125 level and physical examination remain normal, performing additional radiographic studies has no clear benefit. A combination of CA-125 and general physical and pelvic examinations has been shown to detect progressive disease in 90% of patients with recurrent ovarian cancer.[5] In the small group of patients whose CA-125 level or other tumor marker level was not elevated before treatment, routine surveillance by abdominal and pelvic computed tomography may have a role. At this time too few data exist on other imaging modalities to suggest routine use in this population or other groups of patients with ovarian cancer.

Table 16-8 Follow-up of patients with ovarian cancer: University of Washington Medical Center/Fred Hutchinson Cancer Research Center

	YEAR				
	1	2	3	4	5
Office visit*	3-4	3-4	2-3	2-3	2-3
CA-125†	3-4	3-4	2-3	2-3	2-3
Health maintenance‡	1	1	1	1	1
Radiographic studies	§	§	§	§	§

*Includes physical, pelvic, and rectovaginal examinations.
†For patients with elevated pretreatment CA-125 levels.
‡Includes mammogram, stool guaiac testing, and other screening procedures appropriate for the patient.
§Includes chest x-ray, abdominal and pelvic computed tomography, abdominal and pelvic ultrasound, and magnetic resonance imaging. Performed as clinically indicated for symptoms.

Our recommendations for follow-up are similar to those of Perez (Table 16-8). After initial surgery and chemotherapy the decision for second-look laparotomy is individualized in each patient. During the first 2 years patients are followed up every 3 to 4 months and at each visit patients have a complete history and physical, pelvic, and rectovaginal examinations. In addition, for those patients in whom the pretreatment CA-125 level was elevated, CA-125 is checked at each visit. After 2 years follow-up every 4 to 6 months is recommended until 5 years and, subsequently, every 6 to 12 months after the fifth year. In addition, we recommend yearly mammograms, stool guaiac measurement at each visit, and screening for colorectal carcinoma as per the American Cancer Society recommendations.

An area of active research that holds promise for surveillance of ovarian cancer patients is the evaluation of sera for oncoproteins or cytokines that are shed into the blood from the tumor. For example, the *HER-2/neu* oncogene product p185*neu* is a transmembrane protein. The extracellular domain of *neu* can be shed from cancer cells that overexpress *HER-2/neu.* Recent studies have shown that elevated levels of *neu* protein are found in the sera of patients with breast and ovarian cancers.[6] Elevated serum levels correlate with tumor overexpression.[7] Another recent finding is that both tumor necrosis factor and the tumor necrosis factor membrane receptor can be elevated in the sera of patients with ovarian cancer, suggesting that both may be valuable tumor markers.[8,9] In a recent study the tumor necrosis factor soluble receptor was shown to have higher sensitivity, specificity, and positive predictive values for detecting disease than CA-125 in patients with ovarian cancer.[8]

In patients with germ cell malignancies it is important to detect recurrence early, since salvage therapy may achieve a cure. The following tumor markers are usually elevated with germ cell tumors: dysgerminoma, lactate dehydrogenase; endodermal sinus tumor, alpha-fetoprotein; and embryonal tumor, alpha-fetoprotein and beta-human chorionic gonadotropin. These tumor markers are sensitive indicators of recurrence and should be checked every 2 months for the first year. Approximately 75% of recurrences occur within the first year. Tumor markers can be checked every 3 months in the second year. Recurrences after 2 years in this population are rare. Tumor markers are not elevated in all patients with germ cell tumors (immature teratomas and some dysgerminomas). These patients may benefit from radiographic surveillance.

Stromal tumors are rare and in general have a favorable prognosis. We agree that, if possible, serum inhibin levels should be followed in women who have granulosa cell tumors. A rising inhibin level may predict a recurrence before symptoms occur. However, there are no data evaluating whether early detection has an impact on overall survival.

In conclusion, we agree that prospective trials are needed to evaluate the efficacy and costs of various treatment strategies. At present intensive surveillance for epithelial ovarian cancer may not have a role but that is a direct consequence of poor results in treating recurrent disease. As new chemotherapeutic and treatment modalities that are effective against recurrent disease are developed, surveillance strategies for ovarian cancer patients will need to be altered accordingly.

REFERENCES

1. Markman M. Follow-up of the asymptomatic patient with ovarian cancer. Gynecol Oncol 1994;55:S134-7.
2. Creasman WT. Second look laparotomy in ovarian cancer. Gynecol Oncol 1994;55:S122-7.
3. Podratz KC, Cliby WA. Second look surgery in the management of epithelial ovarian cancer. Gynecol Oncol 1994;55:128-33.
4. Copeland LJ, Gershenson DM, Wharton JT. Microscopic disease at second-look laparotomy in advanced ovarian cancer. Cancer 1985; 55:472-8.
5. National Institute of Health Consensus Development Conference Statement. Ovarian cancer: screening, treatment, and follow-up. Gynecol Oncol 1994;55:4-11.
6. McKinzie SJ, DeSombre KA, Bast BS. Serum levels of HER-2/neu (C-*erb*B-2) correlate with overexpression of p185*neu* in human ovarian cancer. Cancer 1993;71:3942-6.
7. Meden H, Marx D, Fattahi A, et al. Elevated serum levels of a C-*erb* B-2 oncogene product in ovarian cancer patients and pregnancy. J Cancer Res Clin Oncol 1994;120:378-81.
8. Grosen EA, Granger GA, Gatanaga M, et al. Measurements of soluble membrane receptors for tumor necrosis factor and lymphotoxin in the sera of patients with gynecologic malignancy. Gynecol Oncol 1993; 50:68-77.
9. Kutteh WH, Kutteh CC. Quantitation of tumor necrosis factor-alpha, interleukin-1beta, and interleukin-6 in the effusions of ovarian epithelial neoplasms. Am J Obstet Gynecol 1992;167:1864-9.

Table 16-9 Follow-up of patients with ovarian cancer by institution

YEAR/PROGRAM	OFFICE VISIT	CA-125	IMAG	B-HCG	AFP
Year 1					
Memorial Sloan-Kettering I[a]	4	4[b]	[c,d]		
Memorial Sloan-Kettering II[e]	4	4[b]		4[b,f]	4[b,f]
Roswell Park[h]	3-4[i]	3-4	[j]		
Univ Washington/ Fred Hutchinson	3-4[k]	3-4[l]			
Japan: Kyushu Univ I[o]	4[i]	4			
Japan: Kyushu Univ II[p]	12[i]	12			
Year 2					
Memorial Sloan-Kettering I[a]	4	4[b]	[c,d]		
Memorial Sloan-Kettering II[e]	4	4[b]		4[b,f]	4[b,f]
Roswell Park[h]	3-4[i]	3-4	[j]		
Univ Washington/ Fred Hutchinson	3-4[k]	3-4[l]			
Japan: Kyushu Univ I[o]	4[i]	4			
Japan: Kyushu Univ II[p]	6[i]	6			
Year 3					
Memorial Sloan-Kettering I[a]	4	4[b]	[c,d]		
Memorial Sloan-Kettering II[e]	4	4[b]		4[b,f]	4[b,f]
Roswell Park[h]	3-4[i]	3-4	[j]		
Univ Washington/ Fred Hutchinson	2-3[k]	2-3[l]			
Japan: Kyushu Univ I[o]	3[i]	3			
Japan: Kyushu Univ II[p]	3[i]	3			
Year 4					
Memorial Sloan-Kettering I[a]	2	2[b]	[c,d]		
Memorial Sloan-Kettering II[e]	2	2[b]		2[b,f]	2[b,f]
Roswell Park[h]	1-2[i]	1-2	[j]		
Univ Washington/ Fred Hutchinson	2-3[k]	2-3[l]			
Japan: Kyushu Univ I[o]	2[i]	2			
Japan: Kyushu Univ II[p]	3[i]	3			

ABD CT abdominal computed tomography
AFP alpha-fetoprotein
B-HCG beta-human chorionic gonadotropin
HEALTH health maintenance
IMAG imaging studies
MRI magnetic resonance imaging
RADIOG radiographic studies
TV US transvaginal ultrasound

TV US	ABD CT	PELVIC CT	PELVIC MRI	HEALTH	RADIOG
2[g]	[d]	[d]	[d]		
				1[m]	[n]
4	[d]	[d]			
12	4	4			
2[g]	[d]	[d]	[d]		
				1[m]	[n]
4	[d]	[d]			
6	3	3			
2[g]	[d]	[d]	[d]		
				1[m]	[n]
3	[d]	[d]			
3	[d]	[d]			
2[g]	[d]	[d]	[d]		
				1[m]	[n]
2	[d]	[d]			
3	[d]	[d]			

a Patients with epithelial tumors after bilateral adnexectomy.
b Indicated for patients with previously abnornal levels.
c Consists of abdominal computed tomography, pelvic computed tomography, chest x-ray, abdominal ultrasound, pelvic ultrasound, and pelvic magnetic resonance imaging as clinically indicated.
d Performed as clinically indicated.
e Patients with retained adnexae.
f Performed for patients with germ cell tumors only.
g Indicated for patients with a low-malignant-potential tumor or a well-differentiated tumor confined to one ovary.
h Patients with epithelial tumors.
i Includes pelvic examination.
j Imaging is indicated to confirm suspected relapse. Specific modalities may vary, depending on suspected site and available technologies. Histological or cytological confirmation of suspected relapse is strongly encouraged, especially for first recurrence.
k Includes physical, pelvic, and rectovaginal examinations.
l For patients with elevated pretreatment CA-125 levels.
m Includes mammogram, stool guaiac testing, and other screening procedures appropriate for the patient.
n Includes chest x-ray, abdominal and pelvic computed tomography, abdominal and pelvic ultrasound, and magnetic resonance imaging. Performed as clinically indicated for symptoms.
o Patients with early-stage, low-risk disease.
p Patients with high-risk and advanced disease.

Continued.

Table 16-9 Follow-up of patients with ovarian cancer by institution—cont'd

YEAR/PROGRAM	OFFICE VISIT	CA-125	IMAG	B-HCG	AFP
Year 5					
Memorial Sloan-Kettering I[a]	2	2[b]	[c,d]		
Memorial Sloan-Kettering II[e]	2	2[b]		2[b,f]	2[b,f]
Roswell Park[h]	1-2[i]	1-2	[j]		
Univ Washington/ Fred Hutchinson	2-3[k]	2-3[l]			
Japan: Kyushu Univ I[o]	2[i]	2			2
Japan: Kyushu Univ II[p]	3[i]	3			3

TV US	ABD CT	PELVIC CT	PELVIC MRI	HEALTH	RADIOG
2[g]	d	d	d		
				1[m]	n
2	d	d			
3	d	d			

CHAPTER 17

Endometrial Carcinoma

University of Washington Medical Center ▪ Fred Hutchinson Cancer Research Center

BENJAMIN E. GREER, BARBARA A. GOFF, AND WUI-JIN KOH

Adenocarcinoma of the endometrium is the most common malignancy of the female genital tract in the United States.[1] It is estimated that 32,800 new cases were diagnosed in 1995, with 5,900 deaths resulting from the disease. In approximately 75% of patients the invasive neoplasm is confined to the uterus at diagnosis.

Because of early symptoms of irregular vaginal bleeding in this predominantly postmenopausal patient population, the often localized nature of the disease, and the generally high survival rate, many physicians have the attitude that adenocarcinoma of the endometrium is a relatively benign disease. However, a critical evaluation of survival data indicates that this concept is erroneous. Although the estimated annual number of new cases of endometrial cancer in the United States has remained constant, the estimated number of deaths more than doubled from 2,900 in 1987 to 5,900 in 1995. This dramatic increase in deaths makes it imperative that physicians identify high-risk patients and tailor appropriate treatment to provide the best opportunity for long-term survival.

The traditionally described patient with endometrial cancer is an obese, hypertensive, postmenopausal woman of low parity. However, approximately 35% of patients are not obese and show no signs of hyperestrogenism.[2] In addition, the proportion of younger patients with endometrial cancer has been increasing.[3] The principal factor that predisposes women to endometrial cancer is chronic, unopposed exposure to estrogen. Endogenous factors that increase estrogen exposure are obesity, chronic anovulation, estrogen-secreting tumors, early menarche, and late menopause. Exogenous factors primarily include the use of unopposed estrogen. In addition, women taking tamoxifen as adjuvant therapy for breast cancer have an increased risk of endometrial cancer similar to those taking unopposed estrogen.[4,5] Other factors that have been associated with an increased risk of endometrial cancer include pelvic radiation therapy, diabetes, and hypertension. Patients with a family history of Lynch II family syndrome are at increased risk of endometrial cancer, as well as colon, breast, and ovarian cancers. Factors that reduce the risk of endometrial cancer include high parity, smoking, and use of combination oral contraceptives.

No satisfactory screening test is available for endometrial cancer. No sampling method or blood test with sufficient sensitivity or specificity has been developed to detect endometrial cancer in asymptomatic individuals. Since the majority of endometrial cancers are stage I at diagnosis and have a relatively favorable outcome, mass screening is unlikely to be cost effective or to increase overall survival rates. Routine cervical cytological examination occasionally leads to the diagnosis of endometrial cancer, but only 30% to 50% of women with endometrial cancer have malignant cells on a Papanicolaou (Pap) smear.[6] Furthermore, patients with suspect or malignant cells on Pap smear are more likely to have deeper myometrial invasion, higher tumor grade, positive peritoneal cytological findings, and more advanced stage of disease.[7] Annual endometrial biopsies cannot be recommended for all women,[8] but endometrial sampling may be justifiable in patients with increased exposure to unopposed estrogens and a strong family history of endometrial, breast, bowel, or ovarian cancers. Ultrasonic measurement of the thickness of the endometrium has been used to evaluate patients with symptoms. When the endometrial stripe is less than 5 mm thick, the incidence of endometrial cancer is very low.[9] If the endometrial stripe exceeds 10 mm, the risk of hyperplasia or endometrial cancer is 10% to 20%. Therefore any patient with a thickened endometrium on ultrasound should undergo endometrial biopsy.

Ninety percent of patients with endometrial carcinoma have abnormal vaginal bleeding. The most common presentation is postmenopausal bleeding. Perimenopausal patients with intermenstrual bleeding or increasingly heavy periods and premenopausal patients with abnormal bleeding, particularly if there is a history of anovulation, are also at risk. Diagnosis can usually be made by an office endometrial biopsy. If an endometrial carcinoma diagnosis is established, endocervical curettage should be performed to evaluate for endocervix involvement. A routine Pap smear cannot be relied on to indicate the presence of endometrial cancer.

The histological information from the endometrial biopsy and endocervical curettage should be sufficient for planning definitive treatment. Office endometrial biopsies have a false-negative rate of about 10%. Thus a negative endometrial biopsy in a symptomatic patient must be followed by a fractional curettage under anesthesia. Hysteroscopy may be helpful in evaluating the endometrium for lesions, such as a polyp, if the patient has persistent or recurrent undiagnosed bleeding.[10] Preoperative evaluation for early-stage endometrial cancer should be limited to complete blood count, electrolytes with blood urea nitrogen and creatinine, liver function tests, electrocardiography, and chest x-ray. Other ancillary tests such as cystoscopy, sigmoidoscopy, ultrasound, computed tomography, and magnetic resonance imaging should be reserved for evaluating clinical symptoms, physical findings, or abnormal laboratory findings as indicated. A recent report of magnetic resonance imaging in 88 patients demonstrated only a 66% sensitivity rate for detection of myometrial invasion, and only 6% of cases were considered adequate for evaluation of paraaortic lymph nodes.[11] Serum CA-125 assay may be helpful in patients with high-grade lesions, papillary serous carcinomas, local extension, or distant metastasis.[12]

STAGING

During the past 25 years two staging systems have been devised by the Federation Internationale de Gynecologie et d'Obstetrique (FIGO). The 1970 criteria for staging endometrial cancer incorporated only information gained from presurgical evaluation including physical examination and diagnostic fractional dilation and curettage (Table 17-1).[13] A significant number of patients at that time were not treated with primary surgery because of obesity or various other medical problems. This staging system should be used if the patient is not a surgical candidate because of advanced disease or severe comorbid medical problems. Over the past 20 years several studies in the literature demonstrated that clinical staging was inaccurate and did not reflect actual disease extent in 15% to 20% of patients.[14-16] This reported understaging and, more important, the ability to identify multiple prognostic factors with full pathological review made possible with surgical staging motivated a change in the staging classification. Therefore in 1988 the Cancer Committee of FIGO introduced a surgical staging system[17] (Table 17-2) that incorporates a complete assessment of pathological data such as histological features, grade, myometrial invasion, and extent and location of extrauterine spread.

Table 17-1 FIGO staging system for endometrial cancer: 1970

Stage I
- Carcinoma is confined to the corpus
  - Stage Ia: Length of uterine cavity is less than or equal to 8 cm
  - Stage Ib: Length of uterine cavity is greater than 8 cm
- Stage I cases should be subgrouped with regard to the histological type of the adenocarcinoma as follows:
  - Grade 1: Highly differentiated adenomatous carcinoma
  - Grade 2: Moderately differentiated adenomatous carcinoma with partly solid areas
  - Grade 3: Predominantly solid or entirely undifferentiated carcinoma

Stage II
- Carcinoma has involved the corpus and cervix but has not extended outside the uterus

Stage III
- Carcinoma has extended outside the uterus but not outside the true pelvis

Stage IV
- Carcinoma has extended outside the true pelvis or has obviously involved the mucosa of the bladder or rectum
- Bullous edema as such does not permit a case to be allotted to stage IV
  - Stage IVa: Spread of the growth to adjacent organs
  - Stage IVb: Spread to distant organs

From Cancer Committee to the General Assembly of F.I.G.O. Int J Gynaecol Obstet 1971;9:172.

TREATMENT

Historically, the treatment of endometrial carcinoma has varied widely. For early-stage disease, treatment has ranged from total abdominal hysterectomy and bilateral salpingo-oophorectomy (TAH-BSO) to preoperative external beam radiation therapy and intracavitary brachytherapy followed in 6 weeks by an adjuvant TAH-BSO. Local and regional bias pertaining to the use of preoperative or postoperative radiation therapy remains. The majority of patients with endometrial carcinoma today undergo primary surgery but not always with complete surgical staging such as nodal dissection or upper abdominal evaluation. The following recommendations for treatment of adenocarcinoma of the endometrium represent a reasonable treatment plan based on recently reported surgicopathological staging data and treatment results.

Clinical Stage I

As noted previously, the majority of patients with endometrial cancer have stage I disease at presentation. The distribution of endometrial carcinoma by clinical stage in a review of 7,663 patients is summarized in Table 17-3.[18] The surgical procedure for the staging of a patient with endometrial cancer clinically confined to the fundal portion of the uterus would be peritoneal lavage for cytology, TAH-BSO, and a biopsy of pelvic and aortic nodes by an abdominal approach. During surgery the abdominal organs including the diaphragm, liver, omentum, and pelvic and bowel peritoneal surfaces should be carefully inspected and palpated. The pathological information obtained provides the optimal basis for the decision and design of adjuvant therapy. Recently, laparoscopic pelvic and paraaortic lymphadenectomy in association with laparoscopically assisted vaginal hysterectomy has been proposed as an alternative surgical approach. Trials evaluating this new method are under way.[19] This potentially less invasive approach should be applied judiciously by experienced practitioners, and long-term follow-up is required to compare its results with that of traditional laparotomy.

Table 17-2 FIGO staging for endometrial cancer: 1988

Stage IA G123	Tumor limited to endometrium
Stage IB G123	Invasion to less than one-half the myometrium
Stage IC G123	Invasion to more than one-half the myometrium
Stage IIA G123	Endocervical glandular involvement only
Stage IIB G123	Cervical stromal invasion
Stage IIIA G123	Tumor invades serosa and/or adnexa, and/or positive peritoneal cytology
Stage IIIB G123	Vaginal metastases
Stage IIIC G123	Metastases to pelvic and/or paraaortic lymph nodes
Stage IVA G12	Tumor invasion of bladder and/or bowel mucosa
Stage IVB	Distant metastases including intraabdominal and/or inguinal lymph nodes

HISTOPATHOLOGY—DEGREE OF DIFFERENTIATION

Cases of carcinoma of the corpus that should be classified (or graded) according to the degree of histological differentiation, as follows:

G1 = 5% or less of a nonsquamous or nonmorular solid growth pattern

G2 = 6% to 50% of a nonsquamous or nonmorular solid growth pattern

G3 = more than 50% of a nonsquamous or nonmorular solid growth pattern

NOTES ON PATHOLOGICAL GRADING

1. Notable nuclear atypia, inappropriate for the architectural grade, raises the grade of a grade 1 or grade 2 tumor by 1.
2. In serous adenocarcinomas, clear-cell adenocarcinomas, and squamous cell carcinomas, nuclear grading takes precedence.
3. Adenocarcinomas with squamous differentiation are graded according to the nuclear grade of the glandular component.

RULES RELATED TO STAGING

1. Because corpus cancer is now staged surgically, procedures previously used for determination of stages are no longer applicable, such as the findings from fractional dilation and curettage to differentiate between stage I and II.
2. It is appreciated that there may be a small number of patients with corpus cancer who will be treated primarily with radiation therapy. If that is the case, the clinical staging adopted by FIGO in 1971 would still apply, but designation of that staging system would be noted.
3. Ideally, width of the myometrium should be measured along with the width of tumor invasion.

From Cancer Committee to the General Assembly of F.I.G.O. Int J Gynaecol Obstet 1989;28:189-90.

Table 17-3 Clinical stage of patients with carcinoma of the endometrium at diagnosis

STAGE	PERCENT
I	74.8
II	11.4
III	10.7
IV	2.9
Undetermined	0.2

From Annual report on the results of treatment in gynaecological cancer. Int J Gynaecol Obstet 1991;36:140.

The most controversial component of surgical staging is the pelvic and aortic lymphadenectomy and whether it should be required for all patients with disease confined to the uterus. Among issues to be considered are surgical skills of the operating surgeon, the required extent of lymphadenectomy, the opinion of some that low-grade and noninvasive endometrial cancers do not justify routine lymphadenectomy, and the reality that some obese patients are not technically suitable for nodal dissection. The incidence of pelvic and aortic node metastasis is related to the grade of tumor and depth of myometrial invasion. Based on retrospective analysis of patients who have undergone full surgicopathological correlation, it has been suggested that patients with grade 1 and 2 tumors and less than one-third myometrial invasion may be spared the risks associated with lymph node dissection, whereas nodal sampling is recommended for all patients with grade 3 tumors, deep myometrial invasion, cervical involvement, or suspect nodes at surgery.

However, other intraoperative and postoperative considerations must be factored into the decision to perform lymphadenectomy. In 15% to 20% of cases the preoperative grade, as assessed by endometrial biopsy or curettage, is upgraded on final fixed pathological evaluation of the hysterectomy specimen.[20] In addition, the intraoperative evaluation of myometrial invasion by gross examination of fresh tissue is increasingly inaccurate as the grade of tumor increases. In one study the depth of invasion was accurately determined by gross examinations in 87.3% of grade 1 lesions, 64.9% of grade 2 lesions, and 30.8% of grade 3 lesions.[21] Further indication for complete surgical staging is suggested in a recent report demonstrating a statistically improved survival in patients with complete node dissection when compared with no node dissection or just node plucking, even when adjusted for other clinicopathological variables.[22] The two confounding surgicopathological variables relating to assessment of grade and myometrial invasion and the potential therapeutic benefit of lymph node dissection make the concept of selective lymph node dissection difficult to apply prospectively with accuracy. Therefore complete surgical

Table 17-4 Extrauterine spread in 621 patients who had endometrial cancer clinically confined to the uterus and underwent complete surgical staging

EXTRAUTERINE SPREAD	PERCENT
Positive peritoneal cytological findings	12
Adnexa involvement	5
Pelvic node metastasis	9
Paraaortic node metastasis	6
Other extrauterine metastasis	6

Data from Creasman WT, Morrow CP, Bundy BN, Homesley HD, Graham JE, Heller PB. Cancer 1987;60(Suppl 8):2035-41.

Table 17-5 Five-year recurrence-free survival rates for surgically staged patients

SURGICAL-PATHOLOGICAL FINDINGS	PERCENT
Tumor entirely confined to uterine corpus and no vascular invasion	92.7
Involvement of isthmus or cervix	69.8
Positive peritoneal cytological findings	56.0
Vascular space invasion	55.0
Pelvic node or adnexal metastasis	57.8
Aortic node metastases or gross laparotomy findings	41.2

From Morrow CP, Bundy BN, Kurman RJ, et al. Gynecol Oncol 1991;40:55-65.

staging to provide full pathological and prognostic data on which to base decisions regarding adjuvant treatment should be advocated for all patients who do not have medical or technical contraindications to lymph node dissection.

Studies by the Gynecologic Oncology Group (GOG) have been instrumental in identifying the prognostically important surgicopathological features of endometrial cancers. The incidence of extrauterine disease in a group of 621 patients with tumors clinically confined to the uterus is shown in Table 17-4.[16] Prognosis is correlated with histological grade and myometrial invasion. Increasing tumor grade and myometrial invasion are associated with an increasing risk of pelvic and paraaortic node metastases, adnexal metastases, positive peritoneal cytological findings, local vault recurrence, and hematogenous spread. Patients with high-grade and deep myometrial invasion often have multiple extrauterine sites of involvement. In grade 1 carcinomas with no myometrial invasion the risk of pelvic or paraaortic lymph node metastases is less than 3%. At the other end of the spectrum, positive pelvic nodes are found in 34% and paraaortic nodes in 23% of patients with grade 3 endometrial cancers that have invaded the myometrium to the outer third.

In a GOG outcome analysis of 895 patients, those patients undergoing complete surgical staging who were found to have endometrial cancer limited to the uterine fundus with pathological risk factors limited to grade and myometrial invasion had a 5-year disease-free interval of 92.7%.[23] A summary of other outcomes based on prognostic factors and risks is provided in Table 17-5. However, these survival data should be viewed in the context of selection bias for adjuvant radiation therapy, which was not prescribed by protocol. Two other conclusions that can be deduced from the data in this report are that locoregional recurrence is reduced by radiation therapy and that malignant cytology is an adverse finding, especially with respect to the risk for abdominopelvic and distant failure.

Other important prognostic factors not included in the GOG data set are age, with younger women (less than 60 years) having a better prognosis; tumor bulk, with tumors larger than 2 cm having a higher incidence of lymph node metastases; and aneuploid tumors, which are associated with a significant increase of recurrence and death.[24-26] In addition, clear cell and papillary serous histological types have a worse prognosis than the more common endometrioid histological type. Patients with uterine papillary serous carcinoma have a high incidence of extrauterine spread.[27]

Clinical Stage II

Clinical stage II endometrial cancer has been traditionally treated with preoperative whole pelvic external beam radiation therapy and brachytherapy followed by a TAH-BSO 6 weeks after completion of radiation.[28] The overall 5-year survival rate of patients with stage II cancer is 59.2%, but it is 69.8% in patients with occult cervical involvement.[23,29] The preceding approach, which combines a full course of radiation therapy followed by adjuvant hysterectomy, precludes complete histological assessment of true cervical involvement, as well as other pathological risk factors, and could compromise patient outcome if extrauterine spread outside the radiation field is detected at surgery. At the University of Washington Medical Center and Fred Hutchinson Cancer Research Center cancer is considered clinical stage II if the cervix is grossly abnormal or if endocervical curettage demonstrates probable cervical stroma invasion. Such a patient will undergo preoperative tandem and ovoids brachytherapy to deliver a point A dose of 2500 to 3000 cGy, followed by TAH-BSO and complete surgical staging surgery within 24 to 48 hours after removal of the implant. Postoperative external beam radiation therapy is then recommended based on full evaluation of pathological risk factors and with the radiation fields tailored to cover the extent of disease.

Using the approach just outlined, a review of 40 patients at University of Washington Medical Center and Fred Hutchinson Cancer Research Center with presumed clinical stage II disease demonstrated only 20% (8 of 40) of the patients to have true pathological stage II disease. Forty-five percent (18 of 40) of the patients did not have evidence of cervical involvement, and most did not require postoperative adjuvant therapy. The remaining 35% had either stage III or IV disease. This is a reasonable approach to clinical stage II endometrial carcinoma. The use of preoperative tandem and ovoids brachytherapy permits adequate dosage to the parametria in patients with true cervical involvement while not limiting postoperative options. It preserves the ability for accurate surgicopathological evaluation of disease extent, permits custom design of postoperative radiation fields, avoids gross undertreatment or overtreatment, and identifies patients requiring more complex treatment strategies. Occasionally in young patients there is a question of primary endometrial versus cervical carcinoma or corpus et colli, in which primary radical hysterectomy and lymph node dissection may be appropriate treatment.

Clinical Stages III and IV

Stage III and IV endometrial carcinomas require individualized treatment planning. They may be diagnosed preoperatively or at the time of exploratory surgery for what was thought to be disease confined to the uterus. Even in advanced cases surgery is often indicated for control of bleeding, relief of obstructive symptoms, and tumor debulking.

The treatment of stage III endometrial carcinoma depends on the distribution of disease and postoperative residual tumor volume. The significance of positive peritoneal cytological findings without other extrauterine risk factors is controversial.[30] Patients with metastatic disease in lymph nodes should receive postoperative radiation therapy designed to cover the nodal areas at risk. This is true even in patients with paraaortic nodal disease that may potentially be cured by extended-field radiation therapy.[23,31,32] Patients with postoperative, residual intraabdominal disease of less than 2 cm confined to the lower abdomen are candidates for whole abdominal radiation therapy.[33-35] Patients with gross parametrial disease or vaginal metastases may require radiation therapy as primary treatment. When residual disease is greater than 2 cm in the abdomen or there is evidence of distant extraabdominal metastases, either hormonal or cytotoxic chemotherapy should be used.

Survival rates for patients with advanced endometrial cancer vary with presentation. In one study the 5-year survival rate for clinical stage III was 16%, as compared with 40% with surgicopathological stage III disease.[36] In another study the 5-year survival rate was 80% when the ovary or fallopian tube was the only extrauterine site of involvement, as compared with 15% when metastasis to other extrauterine structures, such as nodes or intraperitoneal surfaces, was involved.[37] In a recent study the reported survival time in stage IV endometrial carcinoma was poor, with a median of 12 months. Patients who underwent surgical cytoreduction had a median survival time of 18 months, versus 8 months for those without surgery.[38]

Adjuvant Radiation Therapy

The role of postoperative radiation therapy is clear when patients have pathologically documented extrauterine disease and are at risk for recurrence and death. However, adjuvant radiation therapy in patients whose cancers are limited to the uterus is less certain. In a recent large GOG study, 92.7% of patients with negative surgical-pathological findings beyond the uterine corpus had a 5-year disease-free interval, although 42.9% received some form of adjuvant radiation therapy.[23] High-risk patients with poorly differentiated tumors, unusual histological features, lymphovascular space invasion, deep myometrial invasion, and extension to the cervix are candidates for postoperative adjuvant therapy. Brachytherapy delivered to the upper vagina reduces the incidence of vaginal cuff failure but in and of itself may provide inadequate coverage of other pelvic structures. External beam therapy reduces in-field pelvic failures but may not affect overall survival rates.

These observations of improved locoregional tumor control with radiation therapy in high-risk patients, without consistent survival impact, have recently led several clinical investigators to reevaluate external beam pelvic radiation therapy. Insufficient coverage of anatomical volumes at risk has been documented in studies using intraoperative measurements, magnetic resonance imaging, computed tomography, and lymphangiography.[39-43] Therefore the historical outcome data in reference to survival after external beam adjuvant radiation therapy may not be valid because of inadequate field design. Future studies of adjuvant radiation therapy will need to use contemporary field design for adequate coverage of volumes at risk.[44]

Hormonal Therapy and Chemotherapy

Systemic hormonal and cytotoxic agents with identified activity have been used for treating undetected systemic disease in high-risk patients to reduce the risk of distant failure.[45] A survival benefit for these modalities has not been conclusively demonstrated. Hormonal therapy and chemotherapy for advanced or metastatic endometrial cancer are palliative. Objective responses to progestin therapy have been reported in approximately 20% of patients.[46] Single-agent or multiagent cytotoxic chemotherapy, in which cisplatin and doxorubicin have been most widely used, may provide a response in up to 60% of patients. However, complete responses are infrequent and the duration of response and survival in most patients with advanced and metastatic disease is short.[47]

POSTOPERATIVE SURVEILLANCE

The traditional postoperative surveillance protocol for endometrial cancer has been a clinic visit with a physical examination and Pap smear every 3 months for the first year, every 4 months for the second year, and every 6 months for the third, fourth, and fifth years.[48-51] Chest x-rays were usually obtained annually. A recent survey confirms that, with some variations, these follow-up guidelines have been widely practiced.[52] However, the guidelines are arbitrary and have been taught and perpetuated without quantifiable clinical data to support their use.

Two current trends in medicine have motivated the reevaluation of the traditional guidelines and methods of surveillance. The first is the shift to evidence-based medicine.[53] The second is the advent of managed care to improve efficiency and decrease costs. Published studies of randomized trials comparing intensive schedule-based versus patient-initiated follow-up practices in patients with breast cancer demon-

Table 17-6 Clinical stage I and II endometrial cancer: symptomatic and asymptomatic recurrences

AUTHOR	YEAR	NO. OF TREATED PATIENTS	PATIENTS WITH RECURRENCE NO. (%)*	SYMPTOMATIC RECURRENCES NO. (%)†	ASYMPTOMATIC RECURRENCES NO. (%)†
Podczaski et al.[48]	1992	300	47 (16)	23 (49)	24 (51)
Shumsky et al.[49]	1994	317	53 (17)	40 (75)	13 (25)
Berchuck et al.[50]	1995	354	44 (12)	27 (61)	17 (39)
Reddoch et al.[51]	1995	398	44 (11)‡	16 (41)	23 (59)
Total		1,369	188 (14)	106 (58)	78 (42)

*Percent of all patients followed.
†Percent of all documented recurrences.
‡Complete information on 39 patients.

strated that the former may provide earlier detection of recurrence but does not confer an overall survival advantage.[54,55] Similar conclusions have been made in regard to intensive follow-up protocols for colon and rectal carcinomas.[56,57]

Four recent reports in the literature have evaluated the efficacy of routine intensive postoperative surveillance of patients with clinical stage I and II endometrial carcinomas.[48-51] The 1,369 patients in these published series, each with a median at-risk follow-up interval of approximately 5 years, had a recurrence rate of 14% (188 of 1,369). Fifty-eight percent of the patients had symptomatic recurrences, while the remaining 42% had no associated symptoms (Table 17-6). From 70% to 95% of recurrences were diagnosed within 3 years of initial treatment. Of the 188 patients with recurrent disease, 36% (68 of 188) had disease confined to the pelvis and 64% (120 of 188) had some component of distant metastasis.

In the two most recent reports detailed information on the diagnosis of recurrence was available for 83 patients.[50,51] The diagnosis of recurrence was established by physical examination in 63% (52 of 83) of patients. The other recurrences were detected by chest x-ray in 14% (11 of 83), CA-125 in 7% (6 of 83), Pap smear in 5% (4 of 83), computed tomography in 5% (4 of 83), and other tests in 6% (5 of 83). Overall survival in these 83 fully evaluated patients was 13% (11 of 83). The salvage rate for vaginal recurrences was 38% (8 of 21), whereas the salvage rate for distant failure was 5% (3 of 62).

The use of routine radiographic and laboratory tests is questioned, since a careful history and physical examination would lead to identification of most patients with recurrent disease. Two studies have shown no long-term survivors among patients with lung metastases, even in cases of isolated asymptomatic disease diagnosed by chest x-ray only.[49,50] In a prospective, postoperative surveillance study of 266 patients with endometrial cancer, serial CA-125 levels were elevated in 32 patients.[58] The elevation was observed in 19 of 33 patients (58%) with recurrent disease. False elevations were noted in 13 patients, 12 of whom had radiation therapy. In another study the median time from detection of elevated CA-125 level to evidence of frank recurrence was 1.8 months.[12] Therefore the clinical utility of CA-125 remains unverified, since the diagnosis is made at advanced stages of recurrence without long-term salvage potential.

The goal of intensive surveillance after primary therapy is to detect earlier recurrences for which salvage management is presumably more effective. Patients with small-volume recurrent disease limited to the vagina may have salvage rates of 50% or more.[48,50,59] However, those with advanced pelvic disease or extrapelvic metastasis have limited therapeutic options, and long-term survival is rare.[48-51]

Intensive, schedule-based surveillance has not been shown to detect recurrence earlier than patient-initiated follow-up in unselected populations after initial treatment of endometrial cancer.[48-51] There is also no apparent difference in survival after salvage therapy between patients whose recurrences are diagnosed at routine, asymptomatic follow-up and those whose diagnosis is based on development of symptoms.[49]

Patients whose initial surgicopathological evaluation showed higher grade tumor, deep myometrial invasion, and extrauterine involvement are at high risk for recurrence.[23] It has been suggested that to maximize the efficiency of surveillance strategies, intensive follow-up should be limited to this subset of patients. However, two caveats apply. First, although the rate of recurrence is higher in these patients with pathological, high-risk features, the absolute number of recurrences may be the same or higher in patients considered to have low-risk features, since this lower risk group accounts for the great majority of patients with initially diagnosed endometrial cancer.[50] Second, many patients with local high-risk pathological features undergo adjuvant radiation therapy, which significantly alters the pattern, if not the overall incidence, of relapse. Isolated vaginal and pelvic recurrence rates are significantly reduced in patients who receive radiation therapy.[23,48] The use of prior radiation also limits salvage options in patients subsequently found to have local recurrence. Pending the development of more specific and sensitive markers of relapse, as well as better systemic treatment, intensive, schedule-based surveillance may be cost effective only if aimed at identifying early vaginal and pelvic failure in high-risk patients who have not received adjuvant pelvic radiation and who currently represent the only patients for whom curative salvage therapy is reasonably achievable.

Table 17-7 Endometrial cancer surveillance: symptoms to be reported by patients and evaluated

Bleeding (vaginal, bladder, rectum)
Decreased appetite or weight loss
Pain (pelvis, abdomen, hip, back)
Cough or shortness of breath
Swelling (abdomen or leg)
Nausea or vomiting
New mass or skin lesion
Dizziness or "blackouts"

From Reddoch JM, Burke TW, Morris M, Tornos C, Levenback C, Gershenson DM. Gynecol Oncol 1995:59;221-5.

Table 17-8 Follow-up of patients with endometrial cancer*: University of Washington Medical Center/Fred Hutchinson Cancer Research Center

	YEAR				
	1	2	3	4	5
Office visit†	2	2	2	1	1
CA-125‡	2	2	2	1	1
Pap test	1	1	1	1	1
Health maintenance§	1	1	1	1	1

*For patients who have surgically staged endometrial carcinoma treated with curative intent and who remain asymptomatic. Symptomatic patients need evaluation when symptoms appear.
†Includes pelvic examination.
‡If elevated at time of initial treatment or with known extrauterine disease.
§Should include blood pressure, breast examination, mammography as clinically indicated, stool guaiac testing, immunizations, and an opportunity to evaluate other health problems not related to the primary diagnosis of endometrial cancer.

Data from the four published reports provide information for the development of new guidelines for postoperative surveillance in endometrial cancer.[48-51] Based on the findings of these 1,369 patients, certain trends emerge. The majority of patients with recurrence had symptoms. Patient education is imperative. After completion of primary treatment, all patients should receive verbal and written instructions regarding recognition of symptoms of recurrent disease (Table 17-7). Patients with any of these symptoms should seek prompt evaluation and not delay until the next scheduled appointment.

The recommendations for follow-up surveillance of patients with surgically staged endometrial carcinoma treated with curative intent are outlined in Table 17-8. These guidelines are less intensive than the traditional and empirical postoperative surveillance but represent recommendations based on the available data in the literature presented in this chapter and on a consensus of radiation and gynecological oncologists at the University of Washington/Fred Hutchinson Cancer Research Center. Cost-benefit analysis from a recent study revealed that with traditional postoperative surveillance of 354 patients (examinations and Pap smears every 3 to 4 months plus an annual chest x-ray), $700,000 (1995 charge data) was expended to save eight patients.[50] This represents a cost of $87,500 for each life saved. It is unclear whether these patients would have survived without intensive surveillance. Substantial savings can be realized by eliminating the yearly chest x-ray and performing examinations every 6 months rather than every 3 to 4 months. Assuming prompt evaluation and diagnosis of disease in symptomatic patients, this scheme should detect more than 90% of the recurrences. There will be substantial time and cost savings with this less frequent follow-up schedule, as compared with the traditional empirical, intensive surveillance schedule.

In the absence of recurrence, posttreatment surveillance provides psychosocial reassurance and improves the quality of life for patients and their families. Health maintenance has been incorporated into the follow-up schedule and should include blood pressure, breast examination, mammography as clinically indicated, stool guaiac test, immunizations, and an opportunity to evaluate other health problems not related to the primary diagnosis of endometrial cancer.

Further study is required to evaluate if the recommended surveillance schedule in Table 17-8 should be modified for patients at minimal risk of recurrence or for those with high-risk features who have already received maximal adjuvant therapy.

FUTURE PROSPECTS

Recent advances in molecular biology have increased the ability to detect DNA ploidy, oncogenes, and tumor suppressor genes, thereby enhancing the understanding of endometrial cancers. Tumor aneuploidy, p53, *HER-2/neu,* and epidermal growth factor receptor overexpression have been associated with poor prognosis and increased risk of recurrence.[60-63] In the near future, oncogene expression may help to determine which patients should have more aggressive surveillance and which should not. Research is under way in ovarian cancer to evaluate whether oncoproteins in the sera can be used to screen for disease or detect tumor recurrences, and this knowledge may eventually be translated to endometrial cancer.[64,65]

REFERENCES

1. Wingo PA, Tong T, Bolden A. Cancer Statistics 1995. Ca Cancer J Clin 1995;45:8-30.
2. Bokhman JV. Two pathogenetic types of endometrial carcinoma. Gynecol Oncol 1983;15:10-7.
3. Gallup DG, Stock RJ. Adenocarcinoma of the endometrium in women 40 years of age or younger. Obstet Gynecol 1984;64:417-20.
4. Barakat RR, Wong G, Curtin JP, Vlamis V, Hoskins WJ. Tamoxifen use in breast cancer patients who subsequently develop corpus cancer is not associated with a higher incidence of adverse histologic features. Gynecol Oncol 1994;55:164-8.
5. Fisher B, Costantino JP, Redmond CK, Fisher ER, Wickerham DL, Cronin WM. Endometrial cancer in tamoxifen-treated breast cancer patients: findings from the National Surgical Adjuvant Breast and Bowel Project (NSABP) B-14. J Natl Cancer Inst 1994;86:527-37.
6. Gusberg SB, Milano C. Detection of endometrial cancer and its precursors. Cancer 1981;47 Suppl 5:1173-5.

7. DuBeshter B, Warshal DP, Angel C, Dvoretsky PM, Lin JY, Raubertas RF. Endometrial carcinoma: the relevance of cervical cytology. Obstet Gynecol 1991;77:458-62.
8. American College of Obstetricians and Gynecologists. Carcinoma of the endometrium. ACOG Bulletin December 1991;162.
9. Granberg S, Wikland M, Karlsson B, Norstom A, Friberg LG. Endometrial thickness as measured by endovaginal ultrasonography for identifying endometrial abnormality. Am J Obstet Gynecol 1991;164:42-52.
10. Gimpelson RJ, Rappold HO. A comparative study between panoramic hysteroscopy with directed biopsies and dilatation and curettage: a review of 276 cases. Am J Obstet Gynecol 1988;158:489-92.
11. Hricak H, Rubinstein LV, Gherman GM, Karstaedt N. MR imaging evaluation of endometrial carcinoma: results of an NCI cooperative study. Radiology 1991;179:829-32.
12. Duk JM, Aalders JG, Fleuren GJ, de Bruijn HWA. CA 125: a useful marker in endometrial carcinoma. Am J Obstet Gynecol 1986;1097-1102.
13. Cancer Committee to the General Assembly of F.I.G.O. Classification and staging of malignant tumors of the female pelvis. Int J Gynaecol Obstet 1971;9:172.
14. Cowles TA, Magrina JF, Masterson BJ, Capen CV. Comparison of clinical and surgical-staging in patients with endometrial carcinoma. Obstet Gynecol 1985;66:413-6.
15. Boronow RC, Morrow CP, Creasman WT, et al. Surgical staging in endometrial cancer: clinical-pathologic findings of a prospective study. Obstet Gynecol 1984;63:825-32.
16. Creasman WT, Morrow CP, Bundy BN, Homesley HD, Graham JE, Heller PB. Surgical pathologic spread patterns of endometrial cancer: a Gynecologic Oncology Group Study. Cancer 1987;60(Suppl 8): 2035-41.
17. Cancer Committee to the General Assembly of F.I.G.O. Annual report on the results of treatment in gynecologic cancer. Int J Gynaecol Obstet 1989;28:189-90.
18. Annual report on the results of treatment in gynaecological cancer. Int J Gynaecol Obstet 1991;36:140.
19. Childers JM, Brzechffa PR, Hatch KD, Surwit EA. Laparoscopically assisted surgical staging (LASS) of endometrial cancer. Gynecol Oncol 1993;51:33-8.
20. Daniel AG, Peters WA 3d. Accuracy of office and operating room curettage in the grading of endometrial carcinoma. Obstet Gynecol 1988;71:612-4.
21. Goff BA, Rice LW. Assessment of depth of myometrial invasion in endometrial adenocarcinoma. Gynecol Oncol 1990;38:46-8.
22. Kilgore LC, Partridge EE, Alvarez RD, et al. Adenocarcinoma of the endometrium: survival comparisons of patients with and without pelvic node sampling. Gynecol Oncol 1995;56:29-33.
23. Morrow CP, Bundy BN, Kurman RJ, et al. Relationship between surgical-pathological risk factors and outcome in clinical stage I and II carcinoma of the endometrium: a Gynecologic Oncology Group study. Gynecol Oncol 1991;40:55-65.
24. Malkasian GD Jr, Annegers JF, Fountain KS. Carcinoma of the endometrium: stage I. Am J Obstet Gynecol 1980;136:872-88.
25. Schink JC, Lurain JR, Wallemark CB, Chmiel JS. Tumor size in endometrial cancer: a prognostic factor for lymph node metastasis. Obstet Gynecol 1987;70:216-9.
26. Ambros RA, Kurman RJ. Identification of patients with stage I uterine endometrioid adenocarcinoma at high risk of recurrence by DNA ploidy, myometrial invasion, and vascular invasion. Gynecol Oncol 1992;45:235-9.
27. Goff BA, Kato D, Schmidt RA, et al. Uterine papillary serous carcinoma: patterns of metastatic spread. Gynecol Oncol 1994;54:264-8.
28. Reisinger SA, Staros EB, Feld R, Mohiuddin M, Lewis GC. Preoperative radiation therapy in clinical stage II endometrial carcinoma. Gynecol Oncol 1992;45:174-8.
29. Annual Report on the Results of Gynecologic Cancer, Table BIVa. 1992;21:140.
30. Lunian JR. The significance of positive peritoneal cytology in endometrial cancer. Gynecol Oncol 1992;46:143-4.
31. Potish RA, Twiggs LB, Adcock LL, Savage JE, Levitt SH, Prem KA. Paraaortic lymph node radiotherapy in cancer of the uterine corpus. Obstet Gynecol 1985;65:251-6.
32. Hicks ML, Piver MS, Puretz JL, et al. Survival in patients with paraaortic lymph node metastases from endometrial adenocarcinoma clinically limited to the uterus. Int J Radiat Oncol Biol Phys 1993;26: 607-11.
33. Greer BE, Hamberger AD. Treatment of intraperitoneal metastatic adenocarcinoma of the endometrium by the whole-abdomen moving-strip technique and pelvic boost radiation. Gynecol Oncol 1983;16: 365-73.
34. Potish RA. Abdominal radiotherapy for cancer of the uterine cervix and endometrium. Int J Radiat Oncol Biol Phys 1989;16:1453-8.
35. Gibbons S, Martinez A, Schray M, et al. Adjuvant whole abdomino-pelvic irradiation for high risk endometrial carcinoma. Int J Radiat Oncol Biol Phys 1991;21:1019-25.
36. Aalders JG, Abeler V, Kolstad P. Clinical (stage III) as compared to subclinical intrapelvic extrauterine tumor spread in endometrial carcinoma: a clinical and histopathological study of 175 patients. Gynecol Oncol 1984;17:64-74.
37. Bruckman JE, Bloomer WD, Marck A, Ehrmann RL, Knapp RC. Stage III adenocarcinoma of the endometrium: two prognostic groups. Gynecol Oncol 1980;9:12-7.
38. Goff BA, Goodman A, Muntz HG, Fuller AF Jr, Nikrui N, Rice LW. Surgical stage IV endometrial carcinoma: a study of 47 cases. Gynecol Oncol 1994;52:237-40.
39. Greer BE, Koh WJ, Figge DC, Russell AH, Cain JM, Tamimi HK. Gynecologic radiotherapy fields defined by intraoperative measurements. Gynecol Oncol 1990;38:421-4.
40. Russell AH, Walter JP, Anderson MW, Zukowski CL. Sagittal magnetic resonance imaging in the design of lateral radiation treatment portals for patients with locally advanced squamous cancer of the cervix. Int J Radiat Oncol Biol Phys 1992;23:449-55.
41. Kim RY, McGinnis LS, Spencer SA, Meredith RF, Jennelle RL, Salter MM. Conventional four-field pelvic radiotherapy technique without computed tomography–treatment planning in cancer of the cervix: potential geographic miss and its impact on pelvic control. Int J Radiat Oncol Biol Phys 1995;31:109-12.
42. Chun M, Timmerman RD, Mayer R, Ling MN, Sheldon J, Fishman EK. Radiation therapy of external iliac lymph nodes with lateral pelvic portals: identification of patients at risk for inadequate regional coverage. Radiology 1994;194:147-50.
43. Pendlebury SC, Cahill S, Crandon AJ, Bull CA. Role of bipedal lymphangiogram in radiation treatment planning for cervix cancer. Int J Radiat Oncol Biol Phys 1993;27:959-62.
44. Russell AH. Contemporary radiation treatment planning for patients with cancer of the uterine cervix. Semin Oncol 1994;21:30-41.
45. Burke TW, Wolfson AH. Limited endometrial carcinoma: adjuvant therapy. Semin Oncol 1994;21:84-90.
46. Moore TD, Phillips PH, Nerenstone SR, Cheson BD. Systemic treatment of advanced and recurrent endometrial carcinoma: current status and future prospects. J Clin Oncol 1991;9:1071-88.
47. Muss HB. Chemotherapy of metastatic endometrial cancer. Semin Oncol 1994;21:107-13.
48. Podczaski E, Kaminski P, Gurski K, et al. Detection and patterns of treatment failure in 300 consecutive cases of "early" endometrial cancer after primary surgery. Gynecol Oncol 1992;47:323-7.
49. Shumsky AG, Stuart GC, Brasher PM, Nation JG, Robertson DI, Sangkarat S. An evaluation of routine follow-up of patients treated for endometrial carcinoma. Gynecol Oncol 1994;55:229-33.
50. Berchuck A, Anspach C, Evans AC, et al. Postsurgical surveillance of patients with FIGO stage I/II endometrial adenocarcinoma. Gynecol Oncol 1995;59:20-2.
51. Reddoch JM, Burke TW, Morris M, Tornos C, Levenback C, Gershenson DM. Surveillance for recurrent endometrial carcinoma: development of a follow-up scheme. Gynecol Oncol 1995:59;221-5.
52. Barnhill D, O'Connor D, Farley J, Teneriello M, Armstrong D, Park R. Clinical surveillance of gynecologic cancer patients. Gynecol Oncol 1992;46:275-80.

53. Evidence-Based Medicine Working Group. Evidence-based medicine: a new approach to teaching the practice of medicine. JAMA 1992;268:2420-5.
54. Rosselli Del Turco M, Palli D, Cariddi A, Ciatto S, Pacini P, Distante V. Intensive diagnostic follow-up after treatment of primary breast cancer: a randomized trial; National Research Council Project on Breast Cancer follow-up. JAMA 1994;271:1593-7.
55. GIVIO Investigators. Impact of follow-up testing on survival and health-related quality of life in breast cancer patients: a multicenter randomized controlled trial. JAMA 1994;271:1587-92.
56. Patchett SE, Mulcahy HE, O'Donoghue DP. Colonoscopic surveillance after curative resection for colorectal cancer. Br J Surg 1993; 80:1330-2.
57. Steele G Jr. Standard postoperative monitoring of patients after primary resection of colon and rectum cancer. Cancer 1993;71:4225-35.
58. Rose PG, Sommers RM, Reale FR, Hunter RE, Fournier L, Nelson BE. Serial serum CA-125 measurements for evaluation of recurrence in patients with endometrial carcinoma. Obstet Gynecol 1994;84:12-16.
59. Curran WJ Jr, Whittington R, Peters AJ, Fanning J. Vaginal recurrences of endometrial carcinoma: the prognostic value of staging by a primary vaginal carcinoma system. Int J Radiat Oncol Biol Phys 1988;15:803-8.
60. Ito K, Watanabe K, Nasim S, et al. Prognostic significance of p53 overexpression in endometrial cancer. Cancer Res 1994;54:4667-70.
61. Lukes AS, Kohler MF, Pieper CF, et al. Multivariable analysis of DNA ploidy, p53, and HER-2/*neu* as prognostic factors in endometrial cancer. Cancer 1994;73:2380-5.
62. Khalifa MA, Mannel RS, Haraway SD, Walker J, Min KW. Expression of EGFR, HER-2/*neu*, p53, and PCNA in endometrioid, serous papillary, and clear cell endometrial adenocarcinomas. Gynecol Oncol 1994;53;84-92.
63. Saffari B, Jones LA, el-Naggar A, Felix JC, George J, Press MF. Amplification and overexpression of HER-2/*neu* (C-*erb*B2) in endometrial cancers: correlation with overall survival. Cancer Res 1995;55:5693-8.
64. Grosen EA, Granger GA, Gantanaga M, et al. Measurement of the soluble membrane receptors for tumor necrosis factor and lymphotoxin in the sera of patients with gynecologic malignancy. Gynecol Oncol 1993;50:68-77.
65. McKenzie SJ, DeSombre KA, Bast BS, et al. Serum levels of HER-2/*neu* (C-erbB2) correlate with overexpression of p185^{neu} in human ovarian cancer. Cancer 1993;71:3942-6.

➢ COUNTER POINT

Memorial Sloan-Kettering Cancer Center

RICHARD R. BARAKAT

The frequency and extent of follow-up visits and surveillance tests for patients with a history of gynecological cancer have traditionally been based on arbitrary guidelines established and perpetuated at various institutions throughout the United States. Recent changes in medicine occurring throughout the country, however, have led to a reevaluation of standard medical practices. With managed care contracts now being awarded to low-cost providers, there is increased incentive to determine the most cost-effective manner of providing care.

Endometrial cancer is the most common gynecological malignancy in the United States. Approximately 70% to 80% of endometrial cancers are confined to the uterus at initial presentation, and only 10% to 15% of these eventually recur.[1] Since the majority of patients with endometrial cancer do well and no clear evidence has been presented that early detection of disease recurrence improves outcome, reevaluation of the practice of routine intensive surveillance in women with a history of endometrial cancer has become necessary. Although patients with medical complications, unexplained symptoms, or evidence of recurrent tumor require intensive follow-up, guidelines are needed for healthy, asymptomatic women who have been potentially cured and who remain clinically free of disease.

In 1992 Barnhill et al.[2] reported on the clinical surveillance programs used in the follow-up of patients with gynecological cancer as noted from a survey of 94 members of the Society of Gynecologic Oncologists. For asymptomatic patients with no clinical evidence of disease, the majority of respondents reported seeing the patients in the clinic every 3 months for the first year after surgery, every 3 to 4 months the second year, every 6 months for the next 3 years, and annually thereafter. In the majority of cases physical examination included the breasts, abdomen, lymph node regions, and pelvis. In addition to a pelvic examination, 84% reported performing a Pap smear at each visit. In terms of surveillance studies, 72% obtained annual chest x-rays for the first 2 years after surgery, which decreased to approximately 50% for the next 3 years. Computed tomographic scans were obtained annually by approximately one third of respondents for the first 2 years after surgery, a figure that steadily declined thereafter. Although these follow-up practices are used widely, there is no rationale for any particular surveillance protocol based on examination sensitivity, cost effectiveness, or survival benefit.

Several recent publications have attempted to address the issue of postsurgical surveillance in patients with endometrial cancer in an effort to devise a more efficient and cost-effective method of follow-up.[3-6] Specific attention was paid to the value of history and physical examination, Pap smear, chest x-ray, and the CA-125 tumor marker in detecting recurrent disease. A great deal can be learned from these studies and applied to the development of future strategies for follow-up of these patients.

HISTORY AND PHYSICAL EXAMINATION

Combining the data from the four studies, 188 patients (14%) had disease recurrence, with 78 (42%) having no associated symptoms. In 81% of the recurrences the disease was detected because of either symptoms or physical findings. In patients who were asymptomatic at the time of recurrence, approximately 52% had disease detected by physical examination. Therefore only 37 patients (48% of 78) had their recurrent disease detected by other diagnostic tests. In symptomatic patients the most common presenting complaint was pain, either abdominal or pelvic, followed by weight loss, lethargy, and vaginal bleeding. Podczaski et al.[3] reported that only two of 23 symptomatic patients had abnormal bleeding, whereas 19 of 40 patients had vaginal bleeding in the series by Shumsky et al.[4] Clearly patient education regarding the signs and symptoms of recurrent disease should be incorporated into a surveillance program. Physicians should act promptly to evaluate symptomatic patients, targeting diagnostic tests toward the symptoms.

VAGINAL CYTOLOGY

According to Barnhill et al.,[2] 84% of asymptomatic patients being followed for a history of gynecological cancer undergo Pap smears at each visit. Again, reviewing the findings of the four published surveillance series, only 13 of the 188 patients (6.9%) with recurrent disease were found to have vaginal cytological abnormalities. However, this was an isolated finding not associated with an abnormal physical examination or symptoms in only five (2.7%) of these patients. Obtaining Pap smears routinely at each follow-up visit does not appear to be beneficial.

CHEST X-RAYS

Surveillance chest x-rays are obtained by the majority of gynecological oncologists during the first 2 years after surgery for early-stage endometrial cancer. Recurrent disease was detected by chest x-ray in 27 of 188 (14.4%) of the patients reported in the pooled series. Although chest x-rays can document the presence of distant recurrences, their impact is limited by the poor outcome of patients with pulmonary metastases. Virtually all of these patients die of their disease. The intent of routine surveillance is to detect patients who have cancer recurrence after primary treatment for endometrial cancer (10% to 15% of patients treated with curative intent), with the hope that early initiation of therapy will improve the outcome. In view of the lack of effective systemic therapy for endometrial cancer and the poor prognosis of patients with pulmonary metastases, routine surveillance chest x-rays cannot be recommended.

CA-125 TUMOR MARKER

Elevated levels of the tumor-associated antigen CA-125 have been documented in patients with advanced or recurrent endometrial cancer and are correlated with the clinical course of disease.[7] Rose at al.[7] noted that CA-125 levels were elevated in 19 of 33 (58%) patients with recurrent endometrial cancer. Reddoch et al.[6] detected recurrence by an elevated serum CA-125 level in six of 23 (26%) asymptomatic patients. None of the patients achieved long-term survival, which probably reflects the association between an elevated CA-125 level and widespread disease. In view of the short lead time between CA-125 elevation and diagnosis of recurrence, surveillance CA-125 levels have limited value and are best reserved for patients with an elevated level at initial diagnosis.

SUMMARY

Recent changes in health care services throughout the United States have led to a reevaluation of long-standing arbitrary guidelines for follow-up of patients treated for cure of early-stage endometrial cancer. Four recent studies in the literature[3-6] have led to a critical review of these practices and their relative merits. Based on these studies, Greer et al. have proposed a sound, evidence-based strategy for the postoperative surveillance of asymptomatic patients with early-stage endometrial cancer treated with curative intent. Since the majority of recurrences occur within 3 years of surgery, Greer et al. recommend pelvic examinations biannually for 3 years and annually thereafter. Because only 68 of 188 (36%) of the reported recurrences were confined to the pelvis, a complete physical examination should also include the abdomen and lymph node regions, especially the inguinal and supraclavicular areas.

Greer et al. do not include surveillance chest x-rays as part of their recommendations and advocate annual rather than routine Pap smears. In an era in which cost containment is extremely important, this follow-up schema appears to be cost effective and justified by the available literature. There is no evidence in the literature that routine chest x-rays improve survival, and these studies appear to indicate that routine Pap smears do not improve the outcome of patients with isolated vaginal recurrences. Based on the data, obtaining annual Pap smears seems reasonable. Whether this should be continued annually after 3 years is debatable. Alternatively, as more retrospective data emerge, physicians may consider discontinuing annual Pap smears after 3 years in favor of an every-3-year policy.

The recommendation of Greer et al. for serial CA-125 determinations in patients with elevated levels at the time of diagnosis or with known extrauterine disease is also reasonable, but there is no evidence that such monitoring will improve patient outcome. Postoperative follow-up also allows the incorporation of a health maintenance program, including blood pressure evaluation, breast examination, and stool guaiac testing. The postoperative surveillance schedule proposed by Greer et al. appears to be a sound one that is similar to the protocol recently instituted by the Gynecology Service Disease Management Team at Memorial Sloan-Kettering Cancer Center (Table 17-9). One important issue that should be addressed is the psychological support that

Table 17-9 Follow-up of patients with endometrial cancer*: Memorial Sloan-Kettering Cancer Center

	YEAR				
	1	2	3	4	5
Office visit†	2	2	2	1	1
CA-125‡	2	2	2	1	1
Pap test	1	1	1	1	1
Health maintenance§	1	1	1	1	1

*The follow-up strategy I recommend is identical to the strategy recommended by Greer et al. of the University of Washington Medical Center/Fred Hutchinson Cancer Research Center.
†Includes examination of the pelvis, abdomen, and lymph node regions, especially the inguinal and supraclavicular areas.
‡If elevated at time of initial treatment or with known extrauterine disease.
§Should include blood pressure, breast examination, mammography as clinically indicated, stool guaiac testing, immunizations, and an opportunity to evaluate other health problems not related to the primary diagnosis of endometrial cancer.

routine follow-up visits provide for patients with cancer. The value of this support may be impossible to measure objectively. Although the cost savings from less intensive surveillance are substantial, physicians need to continue to provide emotional support and reassurance to their patients. The combination of patient education, phone contact by a nurse at regular intervals, and prompt evaluation of symptoms may be a more cost-effective method of practice that continues to provide the emotional support patients with cancer need and deserve.

REFERENCES

1. Morrow CP, Bundy BN, Kurman RJ, et al. Relationship between surgical-pathological risk factors and outcome in clinical stage I and II carcinoma of the endometrium: a Gynecologic Oncology Group study. Gynecol Oncol 1991;40:55-65.
2. Barnhill D, O'Connor D, Farley J, Teneriello M, Armstrong D, Park R. Clinical surveillance of gynecologic cancer patients. Gynecol Oncol 1992;46:275-80.
3. Podczaski E, Kaminski P, Gurski K, et al. Detection and patterns of treatment failure in 300 consecutive cases of "early" endometrial cancer after primary surgery. Gynecol Oncol 1992;47:323-7.
4. Shumsky AG, Stuart GC, Brasher PM, Nation JG, Robertson DI, Sangkarat S. An evaluation of routine follow-up of patients treated for endometrial carcinoma. Gynecol Oncol 1994;55:229-33.
5. Berchuk A, Anspach C, Evans AC, et al. Postsurgical surveillance of patients with FIGO Stage I/II endometrial adenocarcinoma. Gynecol Oncol 1995;59:20-4.
6. Reddoch JM, Burke TW, Morris M, Tornos C, Levenback C, Gershenson DM. Surveillance for recurrent endometrial carcinoma: development of a follow-up scheme. Gynecol Oncol 1995;59:221-5.
7. Rose PG, Sommers RM, Reale FR, Hunter RE, Fournier L, Nelson BE. Serial serum CA 125 measurements for evaluation of recurrence in patients with endometrial carcinoma. Obstet Gynecol 1994;84:12-6.

➢ COUNTERPOINT

National Cancer Center Hospital, Japan

TAKAHIKO SONODA

When gynecological cancer is found, almost all practicing clinicians in Japan refer patients to a gynecological oncologist at a major cancer center or a university hospital. At present, routine follow-up after primary treatment of gynecological cancer is not standardized. However, knowledge of the natural history and clinical progression of endometrial cancer has quantitatively and qualitatively improved as the incidence of the disease has increased and new medical technology has developed, particularly during the past 10 years. Today the histological classification and staging system for endometrial cancer are established so that the prognosis of patients is easily predicted. Therefore it is proper to recommend a basic follow-up routine for patients with endometrial cancer in Japan, as well as in other countries.

DEMOGRAPHICS

The Japanese female population aged 34 years and younger was 28.60 million and those aged 35 and over was 32.95 million in 1985.[1] Endometrial cancer develops mainly in the latter group. Today the incidence of endometrial cancer is 10.5 per 100,000 of the female population, compared with five per 100,000 about 30 years ago. Westernization of dietary habits, such as a greater intake of fatty foods, and lengthening of the life span of Japanese women have caused a higher incidence of endometrial cancer. The age distribution of patients with endometrial cancer is as follows: younger than 35 years of age, 5.7%; 35 to 39 years of age, 3.5%; 40 to 49 years of age, 18.1%; and ages 50 and over, 79.2%.[2] Although mass screening activity is high, its effect on endometrial cancer prognosis is not yet clear.

SIZE OF THE PROBLEM

The ratio of endometrial cancer to cervical cancer was 1:20 formerly but is now estimated to be three to seven times higher.[3] In 1987 the number of deaths from uterine cancer in Japan was 4,700. Accordingly, the number of patients with endometrial cancer in Japan is estimated at 6,270 with the annual number of deaths at 1,190. Kuramoto et al.[4] reported that endometrial cancer incidence in women between 40 and 49 years of age has been increasing. Between 1987 and 1991, 27% of women with endometrial cancer in their hospital were in this age category. (For the years 1989 to 1991 at the National Cancer Center Hospital, 21% of women with endometrial cancer were between 40 and 49 years of age.) If the frequency of mass screening for the disease is increased, more conclusive data regarding the rate of increase in incidence will become available. The increase in endometrial cancer among women in the prime of life should be stressed.

ECONOMIC IMPLICATIONS

Everyone in Japan has medical insurance in some form. The health insurance law for the aged approved in 1983 includes a no-cost screening visit for endometrial cancer. Japanese insurance plans are divided into three main categories: employee's health insurance (for employees and dependents), national health insurance (mainly for the self-employed), and health insurance for the elderly (which is a supplementary system for those 70 years and over and their dependents). National health insurance generally pays 70% of all medical costs and reimburses the recipient for high-cost medical care such as cancer treatment. Employee-based health insurance covers 90% of medical bills of an employee (insured person only) and 70% of dependents' bills. In 1992, 82.1 million persons in Japan and 42.4 million dependents were covered.[1] A "point" is the unit of payment (10 yen per unit) for the medical care and services provided under "The Table of Points." The Table of Points lists the number of points by type of medical care and services provided. The Table of Points is issued by the Japanese government and revised periodically. The standard medical bill in 1995 U.S. dollars for a patient with endometrial cancer receiving surgical treatment is approximately $12,000, which covers various kinds of examinations, surgical procedures, anesthesia, transfusions, other medical services, and meals during an approximately 6-week hospital stay. The

Table 17-10 Survival rates (%) of patients with endometrial cancer in Japan treated 1966-1976

		YEAR				
STAGE	N	1	2	3	4	5
I	(1,432)	95.4	91.3	89.2	87.6	84.8
G-1	(720)	96.7	93.6	91.9	91.2	89.0
G-2	(240)	94.8	91.7	90.4	86.7	83.0
G-3	(107)	87.2	77.2	68.4	66.9	65.1
G-?	(365)	95.6	90.4	89.0	87.0	83.8
II	(324)	90.5	78.3	71.6	68.8	65.2
III	(164)	73.0	57.8	48.4	44.4	42.6
IV	(63)	38.0	21.6	18.2	13.0	13.0
Overall	(1,983)	87.7	81.4	78.0	75.9	73.3

Data from Japan Society of Obstetrics and Gynecology (The Tumor Committee). Gann Monogr Cancer Res 1995;43:173-5.

Table 17-11 G-3 ratio,* surgical operation rate, and relative 5-year survival rate by stage

	TOTAL				
STAGE	N	(%)	G-3 (%)	SURGICAL OPERATION RATE (%)	5-YEAR SURVIVAL RATE (%)
I	1,432	(72.2)	11.6	94.7	84.8
II	324	(16.3)	16.2	88.0	65.2
III	164	(8.3)	22.5	67.1	42.6
IV	63	(3.2)	37.5	33.3	13.0
Overall	1,983	(100)	14.0	89.4	75.8

Data from Japan Society of Obstetrics and Gynecology (The Tumor Committee). The national survey of uterine corpus cancer in Japan. Vol. 1, 1980.
*Percentage of total with grade 3 neoplasms.

Table 17-12 Percentage of prognostic factors by histological grade

	GRADE		
PROGNOSTIC FACTOR	G-1 (%)	G-2 (%)	G-3 (%)
Lymph node involvement			
0	89.1	86.5	73.9
1	4.7	6.2	6.5
2, 3	4.0	5.1	7.6
4 or more	2.3	2.2	12.0
Depth of muscle invasion			
Superficial	22.1	21.9	12.1
Less than one third	53.2	52.9	43.9
One third or more	12.8	13.9	14.6
Location of the lesion			
Fundus	45.9	45.2	35.9
Side wall	21.2	22.8	16.3
Isthmus	3.9	4.2	6.5
Fundus↔Isthmus	29.2	27.9	41.3
Length of the uterine cavity			
Stage Ia (≥8 cm)	61.5	67.8	68.2
Stage Ib (<8 cm)	32.5	32.3	31.8

Data from Japan Society of Obstetrics and Gynecology (The Tumor Committee). Gann Monogr Cancer Res 1995;43:173-5.

routine follow-up at the National Cancer Center Hospital for 5 years after treatment costs a patient about $2,000, and insurance covers this.

CURRENT PRACTICE

Current follow-up strategies among practicing gynecological oncologists are devised from their clinical experiences and from the few published data relating to follow-up strategy. Data regarding endometrial cancer prognosis indicate that approximately 10% of patients with stage I disease die within 3 years of initial treatment. Approximately 9.5% of patients with stage II disease, 27% of patients with stage III disease, and 62% of patients with stage IV disease die within 1 year after initial treatment. This indicates that a careful follow-up schedule should focus on the first 2 years after treatment (Table 17-10).[5] Prognostic factors are useful in devising cancer follow-up strategy. In endometrial cancer, stage and grade (G-classification) are important factors in devising that strategy. Survival, G-3, and surgical operation by clinical stage are presented in Table 17-11.[2] Surgical operation is carried out even on patients with stage III (67.1%) or IV (33.3%). G-classification correlates with other main prognostic factors except for uterine size (Table 17-12).[2] Stage migration from clinical stage I (cTI) to stage II (pTII) cancer is not uncommon in G-3 cancer, which is often located at the isthmus (Table 17-13).[5]

Recurrence rates based on histological risk factors have been analyzed in patients treated at the National Cancer Center Hospital (Table 17-14). The recurrence rate for patients with G-3 classification is 37.5%; for muscle invasion, 41.0%; for vascular involvement, 29.0%; for lymphatic permeation, 46.0%; and for lymph node involvement, 50.0%. Because of these risk factors, postoperative irradiation is planned for patients with deep muscle invasion, positive lymph nodes, positive vaginal stump, or cervical stromal involvement (if radical hysterectomy was not carried out). Of patients with stage I, class G-3 disease analyzed, 12.8% died of the disease within 1 year. Sites of recurrence and survival time after recurrence of 107 patients are presented in Table 17-15. Their relative survival rates were 82.2% for year 1, 56.6% for year 2, 48.2% for year 3, 35.3% for year 4, and 25.2% for year 5.[2] Local recurrence was effectively controlled by postsurgical radiation therapy (Table 17-16). Distant recurrence by G-classification and postsurgical staging are shown in Tables 17-17 and 17-18. Takeshima et al.[6] studied endometrial cancer recurrence hazard after adequate surgery and stressed that adjuvant therapy for patients with prognostic risk factors should be established. They showed that relapses were rare 5 years after appropriate surgery but did not recommend a specific follow-up strategy. Putative endometrial cancer risk factors, including hypertension (22%), obesity (24%), diabetes (5%), and family history of endometrial cancer,[2] are often observed in Japan and may influence the follow-up strategy to some extent.

The current actual follow-up routine at the National Cancer Center Hospital is almost the same as that employed by Greer et al. (Table 17-19). I consulted several oncologists

Table 17-13 Cervical involvement by clinical staging

	STAGE/GRADE							
	I-G-1	I-G-2	I-G-3	I-G?	II	III	IV	OVERALL
Cervix (−)	628	187	82	284	71	46	8	1,306
Cervix (+)	31	14	8	16	176	47	6	298
(?)	41	19	11	42	40	15	8	176
Cervical involvement ratio	4.8	7.0	8.9	5.3	71.3	51.7	42.9	18.6%

Data from Japan Society of Obstetrics and Gynecology (The Tumor Committee). Gann Monogr Cancer Res 1995;43:173-5.

Table 17-14 Histological risk factors and recurrence rate

RISK FACTORS	RATE (%)	NO. WITH RECURRENCE/ TOTAL EVALUABLE	RISK FACTORS	RATE (%)	NO. WITH RECURRENCE/ TOTAL EVALUABLE
Histological grade			Vascular involvement		
G-1	4.5	4/89	(−)	10.9	13/119
G-2	25.3	21/83	(+)	29.0	29/100
G-3	37.5	6/16	Lymphatic permeation		
Unknown	35.5	11/31	(−)	8.3	13/156
Muscular invasion			(+)	46.0	29/63
One half or more	10.8	17/158	Lymph node involvement		
Less than one half	41.0	25/61	(−)	13.9	26/187
			(+)	50.0	16/32

Data from Chitose K, Sonoda T. Sanfujinka no Sekai 1995;47:117-24.

Table 17-15 Sites of recurrence and survival time after recurrence in 107 patients with stage I (cT1) endometrial cancer

SURVIVAL TIME (MO)	VAGINA	VAGINA/ PERIVAGINA	PELVIS	EXTRAPELVIS	PELVIS/ EXTRAPELVIS	UNKNOWN	TOTAL (%)
0-6	3	7	14	17	10	1	52 (48.6)
7-12	2	1	6	3	6	—	18 (16.8)
13-18	2	1	—	—	1	—	4 (3.7)
19-24	1	2	2	1	1	—	7 (6.5)
25-36	3	2	—	1	—	—	6 (5.6)
37-48	1	1	1	1	1	—	5 (4.7)
49-60	—	—	1	1	—	—	1 (1.9)
61-72	1	—	—	—	—	—	1 (0.9)
73-84	—	—	—	1	—	—	1 (0.9)
85-90	1	—	—	1	—	—	2 (1.9)
Unknown	1	2	1	4	2	—	9 (8.4)
Total	15	16	25	29	21	1	107 (100%)

Data from Japan Society of Obstetrics and Gynecology (The Tumor Committee). The national survey of uterine corpus cancer in Japan. Supplement, 1988.

about endometrial cancer follow-up intervals and examinations, and all concurred. The follow-up intervals are every 1 to 3 months for the first year, every 3 to 4 months for the second year, every 4 to 6 months for the third year, every 6 months for the four and fifth years, and every 6 to 12 months for the sixth year and thereafter. The tests performed during follow-up include pelvic examination, urinalysis, complete blood count, erythrocyte sedimentation rate, liver function tests, and kidney function tests. Fibrin degeneration product and C-reactive protein are periodically evaluated and detect generalized cancer recurrence. Routine chest x-rays are taken every 6 months, and tumor markers such as CA-125, CA 19-9, and CEA are periodically evaluated. An ultrasound-guided scan or computed tomographic scan of the pelvis, aortic region, and upper abdomen may be obtained if necessary.

Table 17-16 Sites of recurrence by postoperative radiation therapy

	POSTOPERATIVE RADIATION THERAPY		
	YES	NO	OVERALL
Number	50	169	219
Local recurrence	0	5	5 (2.3%)
Distant recurrence	19	16	35 (16.0%)
Recurrence rate	38.0%	12.4%	40 (18.3%)

Data from Chitose K, Sonoda T. Sanfujinka no Sekai 1995;47:117-24.

Consensus Among Radiation Oncologists and Gynecologists

Radiation oncologists and gynecologists cooperate from the beginning of treatment of uterine cancer. However, because endometrial adenocarcinoma may possibly be radioresistant, most gynecologists in Japan usually insist on surgery and few patients are referred to radiotherapists. Even patients with stage III endometrial cancer are candidates for surgery (Table 17-11). Although Heyman's Ra packing is not employed in Japan, external and intracavitary radiation therapy is planned for inoperable patients and those whom

Table 17-17 Distant recurrence sites by histological grade

SITE OF RECURRENCE	G-1 (N = 89)	G-2 (N = 83)	G-3 (N = 16)	UNKNOWN (N = 31)	TOTAL (N = 219)
Lung		7	2	2	11
Liver	1	3	1	2	7
Abdominal cavity		2	1	1	4
Urethra or ureterovesical junction		2	2		4
Bone		2	1		3
Supraclavicular nodes	1	2			3
Paraaortic nodes		1			1
Other sites		2			2
Distant recurrence	2	21	7	5	35
Rate	2.2%	25.3%	43.8%	16.1%	16%

Data from Chitose K, Sonoda T. Sanfujinka no Sekai 1995;47:117-24.

Table 17-18 Distant recurrence by postoperative stage (number of survivors)

	STAGE								
SITE	IA	IB	IC	IIA	IIB	IIIA	IIIB	IIIC	SURVIVAL
Lung	1	1 (1)	2 (2)		2	2		4 (1)	4/11
Liver	1	1			1	2		2	0/7
Abdominal tumor		1				1		2	0/4
Urethra or ureterovesical junction			2 (1)					2	1/4
Bone			2					1	0/3
Supraclavicular nodes		1						2 (1)	1/3
Paraaortic nodes								1	0/1
Other sites								2	0/2

Data from Chitose K, Sonoda T. Sanfujinka no Sekai 1995;47:117-24.

Table 17-19 Follow-up of patients with endometrial cancer: National Cancer Center Hospital, Japan

	YEAR				
	1	2	3	4	5
Office visit*	4-12	3-4	2-3	2	2
Pap test	4-12	3-4	2-3	2	2
Complete blood count	4-12	3-4	2-3	2	2
Erythrocyte sedimentation rate	4-12	3-4	2-3	2	2
Liver function tests	4-12	3-4	2-3	2	2
Kidney function tests	4-12	3-4	2-3	2	2
Urinalysis	4-12	3-4	2-3	2	2
CEA	2	2	2	2	2
CA-125	2	2	2	2	2
CA 19-9	2	2	2	2	2
Fibrin degradation products	2	2	2	2	2
C-reactive protein	2	2	2	2	2
Chest x-ray	2	2	2	2	2
Abdominal computed tomography or ultrasound	†	†	†	†	†
Pelvic computed tomography or ultrasound	†	†	†	†	†
Chest computed tomography or ultrasound	†	†	†	†	†
Bone x-ray	†	†	†	†	†
Barium enema	†	†	†	†	†
Drip infusion pyelography	†	†	†	†	†
Bone scan	†	†	†	†	†
Electroencephalography	†	†	†	†	†

CEA, Carcinoembryonic antigen.
*Includes history, physical examination, and pelvic examination.
†Performed as clinically indicated.

the gynecologists consider poor candidates for surgery. Only 82 of 4,497 patients were principally treated by radiation therapy from 1989 to 1991.[3] After evaluation of the surgical specimen, postoperative irradiation is generally performed for high-risk patients (588 of 1,752, 33.6%). Preoperative irradiation is also sometimes used (53 of 1,752, 3.0%).[2]

ROLE OF TUMOR MARKERS

CA-125, CA 15-3, CA 19-9, CEA, tumor polypeptide antigen, and immunosuppressive acid protein are often measured to predict distant endometrial cancer recurrences, although they are not very sensitive even if combined. However, the combination of CA-125 and CA 15-3, for example, caused a reduction in false-positive results of CA-125, with an acceptable sensitivity of 41%. The combination may be used to predict extrauterine spread and to monitor chemotherapy response in endometrial cancer.[7] The elevation of a tumor marker that was positive before treatment and negative after may be an early indicator of recurrent disease, but not all tumor markers are positive before treatment (Table 17-20).

TNM STAGE AND TUMOR GRADE

As mentioned previously, almost all patients with endometrial cancer undergo a hysterectomy at which time pTNM stage and histological grade are determined. Patients who are not surgical candidates are clinically staged (cTNM), and the grading depends on endometrial biopsy. Five-year survival rates by G-classification in the stage I group were as follows: I-G-1, 89.0%; I-G-2, 83.0%; and I-G-3, 65.1% (Table 17-10). The frequency of lymph node involvement by G-classification was as follows: I-G-1, 7.2%; I-G-2, 6.1%; and I-G-3, 14.6%. On the other hand, lymph node involvement of stages II and III was 23.8% and 35.2%, respectively.[2] The data imply that stage I-G-3 should be regarded as advanced cancer, which may possibly develop distant recurrence such as lung and liver metastases, as well as local recurrence in the pelvis. The high-risk patients in stage I-G-3 should have more frequent follow-up and various examinations to discover relapse as early as possible. Sites of recurrence by postoperative radiation therapy, histological grade, and staging (pTN) are shown in Tables 17-16, 17-17, and 17-18, respectively.[8]

ROLE OF IMAGING TESTS AND MARKERS

Before primary treatment, magnetic resonance imaging or computed tomography is indispensable in determining whether radical surgery is indicated. If the muscle invasion depth is more than half the myometrium or cervical stromal invasion is present, radical hysterectomy is performed. Magnetic resonance imaging is not very effective in detecting recurrence. Computed tomography is recommended to detect nodal and upper abdominal metastases. Ultrasound-guided scanning is used more often than computed tomography because of its simplicity.

If tumor markers rise, various tests are performed to evaluate possible sites of relapse. Sato et al.[9] reported that the CA-125 cutoff value to predict recurrence differs according to the risk of the patient: in low-risk patients the cutoff should be less than 17, in the moderate-risk group 18 to 32, and in the high-risk group more than 32. Other markers such as CA 19-9 and CEA are commonly measured in Japan.

Inspection of the vaginal wall sometimes reveals an abnormal mass or atypical colposcopic findings. Vaginal cytological examination is routine but should be followed by biopsy because of the possibility of a false-negative result.

Table 17-20 Percentage of patients with abnormal pretreatment tumor marker levels by stage and G-classification

CUTOFF	CEA >2.7 μg/L	CA-125 >35 U/mL	CA 19-9 >37 U/mL	CA 15-3 >15 U/mL
Stage I	14.0%	8.1%	23.1%	23.5%
II, III, IV	30.0	38.5	30.0	23.1
G classification				
G-1	12.5	0.0	20.0	27.8
G-2, G-3	23.5	32.0	31.3	25.0
Overall	18.2	16.0	15.0	26.7

Data from National Cancer Center Hospital, 1987.

Complete blood count and erythrocyte sedimentation rate are nonspecific but occasionally useful predictors of recurrence. Subtle signs of recurrence such as slight abdominal distention, pain, and ataxia should not be overlooked. Lung metastasis is often so silent that a chest x-ray every 6 months cannot be neglected for at least 3 years after treatment. Liver metastasis does not always cause abnormal liver function, and such complaints as anorexia or easy fatigability should be addressed.

IMPACT OF ADJUVANT THERAPIES

Any therapy may be successful when performed while the recurrent lesion is small and localized. Some recurrent lesions can be surgically removed completely as in the case of colon, solitary nodular lung, or liver metastases. Even a brain tumor metastasis can be effectively treated by surgery. Pelvic exenteration has recently proved successful and safe in well-selected patients. Radiation therapy is rarely employed for disseminated multiple distant metastases. Vaginal recurrence is effectively controlled by intracavitary irradiation. Radiation therapy of bone metastasis is effective for mitigating pain. Hyperthermia as adjuvant therapy is combined with radiation therapy at some institutions. Adjuvant chemotherapy may enhance the outcome after exenteration. A regimen that includes cisplatin is commonly used. Oral etoposide, cyclophosphamide, 5-fluorouracil, and medroxyprogesterone acetate are preferred for outpatients. Some physicians prescribe them as maintenance therapy.

RECURRENCE OF THE INDEX NEOPLASM

Early detection of recurrence is essential, and multimodality treatment is often used. Primary stage IVb cancer has a dismal outlook. However, Goff et al.[10] studied prognostic factors of 47 stage IV patients and concluded that their prognosis may be improved by hysterectomy, if feasible. This shows the efficacy of cytoreduction, which may also be applicable in recurrent endometrial cancer. Chemotherapy often plays a substantial role in the treatment of recurrence after primary surgery and radiation therapy have failed. Although new chemotherapeutic drugs such as paclitaxel and CPT-11 are not encouraging at present, systemic treatment may improve median survival time in selected patients.

FUTURE PROSPECTS

Multiinstitutional, prospective trials are needed, especially when new anticancer drugs or new technologies are put into clinical use. In Japan protocols and results must be examined by the Committee of Anti-Cancer Medicine of the Central Pharmaceutical Affairs Council of the Ministry of Health and Welfare. The Japan Clinical Oncology Group is promoting a prospective randomized trial in accordance with a grant-in-aid for cancer research from the Ministry of Health and Welfare. An ovarian cancer group has recently participated in a study with the Japan Clinical Oncology Group. The Japanese Association of Gynecologic Oncology and Chemotherapy has been promoting prospective, randomized controlled trials of chemotherapy for cervical, endometrial, ovarian, and trophoblastic cancers since 1988. The results are reported annually by the several committees of the association. Meanwhile, the Tumor Committee of the Japanese Society of Obstetrics and Gynecology has planned a second nationwide survey to obtain data about prognostic factors of endometrial cancer, including treatment of relapse. Although the survey is retrospective, it will be followed by a multiinstitutional, controlled trial. The aforementioned trials are feasible, and the results are published by the study group that planned the protocol and analyzed the data. Thus findings of the Japan Clinical Oncology Group trials are published in *Annual Report of Cancer Research* from the Ministry of Health and Welfare, and results of the Japanese Association of Gynecologic Oncology and Chemotherapy trials appear in *Chemotherapy and Oncology* (both printed in Japanese).

Gurpide[11] reviewed studies on oncogenes and steroid receptors of endometrial cancer and suggested that both could play important roles in endometrial cancer control. Exon 7 deletion ER mRNA in endometrial cancer was observed by Kato.[12] These are just a few of the many promising surveillance tests currently in preclinical development. The National Cancer Center Hospital has already begun a clinical test of oncogene-based diagnosis of pancreatic cancer, with a test for endometrial cancer to follow in the future.

REFERENCES

1. Ministry of Health and Welfare. 1994 health and welfare statistics in Japan. Japan: Health and Welfare Statistics Association in Japan, 1994.
2. Japan Society of Obstetrics and Gynecology (The Tumor Committee). The national survey of uterine corpus cancer in Japan. Vol. 1, 1980.
3. Japan Society of Obstetrics and Gynecology (The Tumor Committee). Annual report of uterine cancer. Acta Obstet Gynecol Jpn 1989-1995.
4. Kuramoto et al. [Screening for endometrial cancer—its expected objectives.] (in Japanese) Sanfuijinka no Chiryo 1993;66:174-8.
5. Japan Society of Obstetrics and Gynecology (The Tumor Committee). Registration of gynecologic malignancies: carcinoma of the corpus uteri. Gann Monogr Cancer Res 1995;43:173-5.
6. Takeshima N, Umezawa S, Shimizu Y, et al. Recurrent endometrial cancer after complete surgery. Acta Obstet Gynecol Jpn 1994;46:253-9.
7. Scambia G, Gadducci A, Panici PB, et al. Combined use of CA 125 and CA 15-3 in patients with endometrial carcinoma. Gynecol Oncol 1994;54:292-7.
8. Chitose K, Sonoda T. [Endometrial cancer recurrence after surgery.] (in Japanese) Sanfujinka no Sekai 1995;47:117-24.
9. Sato A, Bo M, Otani T, Mochizuki M. Expression of epidermal growth factor: transforming growth factor-alpha and epidermal growth factor receptor messenger RNA in human endometrium and endometrial carcinoma. Acta Obstet Gynecol Jpn 1995;47:473-8.
10. Goff BA, Goodman A, Muntz HG, Fuller AF Jr, Nikrui N, Rice LW. Surgical stage IV endometrial carcinoma: a study of 47 cases. Gynecol Oncol 1994;52:237-40.
11. Gurpide E. Endometrial cancer: biochemical and clinical correlates. J Natl Cancer Inst 1991;83:405-16.
12. Kato J. Endometrial cancer: epidemiology, early diagnosis, steroid hormone receptor status and aberrant gene expression of the receptors. In: Popkin and Peddle, editors. Women's health today. New York: Parthenon Publishing Group, 1994:119-28.
13. Japan Society of Obstetrics and Gynecology (The Tumor Committee). The national survey of uterine corpus cancer in Japan. Supplement, 1988.

➢ COUNTERPOINT

Roswell Park Cancer Institute

RAYMOND P. PEREZ

Rational consideration of the appropriate follow-up for a given malignancy must take into account the natural history of the disease, the ability to detect recurrence, and the efficacy of existing treatments. Endometrial carcinoma is the most common gynecological malignancy. Despite the absence of effective screening tests, the majority of patients have relatively limited disease at diagnosis. Three fourths of patients have clinical stage I disease (confined to the corpus), and another 11% have disease limited to the corpus and cervix.

STAGING

Greer et al. emphasize the importance of complete surgical staging at the time of initial treatment; disease extent is underestimated in approximately 20% to 25% of patients with clinically early-stage disease. This subgroup of patients is at increased risk of relapse, which has implications for the types and frequency of methods used for surveillance.

Routine surgical staging of patients with clinical stage I disease has been the subject of some debate in recent years. Some retrospective reports have questioned the value of routine surgical staging in this subgroup of patients. In one series[1] pelvic retroperitoneal and paraaortic nodes were removed at the time of hysterectomy only if their involvement was strongly suspected based on operative findings, depth of myometrial invasion, or evidence of extrapelvic extension of disease. Many patients in this series received adjuvant radiation, and some received adjuvant chemotherapy as well. Relapse occurred in 21 patients, and the authors concluded that routine staging lymphadenectomy would not have benefitted these patients based on analysis of the patterns of recurrence and other prognostic factors. In another retrospective analysis, Gal et al.[2] failed to observe a relationship between depth of myometrial invasion and survival in 23 patients with surgical stage I disease. Survival was noted to be significantly better for FIGO stage I disease versus stage III disease. Of note, both retrospective analyses were uncontrolled and conclusions in each were drawn from samples of fewer than 25 patients with relapse.

An argument might be made against routine surgical staging of patients based on a hypothetically increased risk of morbidity or mortality related to operative staging. However, no such increased risk has been observed. Orr et al.[3] documented extrauterine disease by surgical staging in 27.9% of 168 patients with clinically early-stage disease. Overall the rates of serious morbidity were low. One patient died of postoperative aspiration pneumonitis. In another retrospective report, postoperative morbidity was compared in 104 patients treated with hysterectomy alone versus 196 patients who underwent hysterectomy plus staging lymphadenectomy.[4] The addition of staging lymphadenectomy did not significantly increase morbidity.

A number of reports have demonstrated that surgical staging provides potentially valuable prognostic information. Wolfson et al.[5] observed that the surgical stage of disease was the strongest predictor of survival for patients with endometrial carcinoma. Some investigators have observed that individual components of the FIGO staging, such as grade, depth of tumor invasion, and cervical involvement, might be more powerful prognostic factors when entered separately into a predictive model.[6] However, this contention remains to be validated. Accurate knowledge of disease extent based on surgical staging is one of the most important factors in estimating whether a patient will remain disease free and attempting to predict patterns of failure. Greer et al. recommend surgical staging of all patients except when medical contraindications, supported by the available data, are present.

A review of outcomes after surgical staging shows that many patients with endometrial carcinoma have a good prognosis. Greer et al. note that the 5-year disease-free survival rate is approximately 93% for patients with surgical stage I disease and nearly 70% for those with surgical stage II disease. Because of the predominance of early-stage disease at diagnosis, approximately 75% of patients with endometrial carcinoma remain disease free for 5 years or more and are probably cured. Ongoing investigations are attempting to define additional prognostic factors. Some data suggest that specific tumor histological types (such as clear cell and adenosquamous), ploidy, progesterone receptor status, and overexpression of certain oncogenes (such as *HER-2/neu*) may also predict the risk of relapse.[7] Whether such factors provide information independent of that apparent by the current staging system remains to be determined.

ROUTINE SURVEILLANCE

Greer et al. provide some detailed information about timing and patterns of relapse for patients with clinical stage I and II disease (disease confined to the uterus and cervix). The overwhelming majority of relapses (80% to 90%) in this population occur within the first 3 years after treatment.[8,9] Approximately one third of recurrences are in the pelvis, and the remainder are distant metastases.

A number of retrospective analyses have considered the utility of routine surveillance.[10-12] Relapses were often associated with symptoms, with symptomatic relapses occurring in 41% to 75% in various series. None of the published reports demonstrated any difference in rates of detection of potentially curable recurrences between patients under routine surveillance and those seeking treatment of symptoms. No difference in survival was apparent between these two groups.

Results of analyses of the value of surveillance should be considered from a critical perspective. It should be reiterated that the majority of patients with endometrial carcinoma have early-stage disease at diagnosis and that the disease-free and overall survival rates of these patients are relatively high. As a result, improvements in survival resulting from surveillance may be difficult to detect. Moreover, none of the reports provide estimates of the statistical power to detect meaningful effects. None of these reports account for lead time or length bias in their analyses of outcomes. Finally, these comparisons are confounded by the fact that there are not really two groups being compared; all women in these series were under routine surveillance and symptoms developed in a subgroup of patients between surveillance visits. A more valid comparison would have been a prospective, randomized study of surveillance versus patient-initiated contact. Unfortunately, such a comparison might prove difficult to perform because patients and practitioners have preexistent biases regarding the utility of follow-up.

Although the published data on surveillance are limited by the factors noted, no other objective data regarding the value of routine surveillance in endometrial carcinoma are available. The published reports have not demonstrated that routine surveillance is of value. Nonetheless, a practice pattern survey indicated that the majority of gynecological oncologists recommend relatively frequent follow-up visits (including general and pelvic examinations and Pap smear), annual chest radiographs, serial serum tumor marker studies, and mammography.[13] Although some of these procedures might be justified from the standpoint of general screening (such as mammography), many are difficult to justify, especially at the frequencies with which they are performed. Future clinical trials in endometrial carcinoma should include analyses of the cost versus the utility of routine surveillance.

RECURRENCE

One reason that surveillance has not proved beneficial may be the substantial limitations of the available therapies for recurrent disease. This is emphasized by the relatively poor salvage rate of 38% for apparently isolated vaginal recurrences, as noted by Greer et al. The salvage rate for distant metastases is considerably worse (5%). Reasons for the low salvage rate among patients with apparently localized recurrence are not discussed in detail. However, if truly isolated relapse were the rule, the majority of such patients should be salvaged by surgical reexcision. The reported outcomes in these patients suggest that apparently localized relapse is usually the initial indication of extensive disease rather than a potentially curable lesion.

In general terms, relapse occurs in 25% or less of patients with endometrial carcinoma. The best prognosis is observed in patients with isolated recurrence in the pelvis, with vaginal recurrence having the most favorable outlook. Relapse is in the pelvis in only about one third of patients, many of whom do not have isolated vaginal recurrence. Of those with vaginal recurrence, only about one third are saved by current therapies. Simple mathematics would suggest that the number of patients benefitting from routine surveillance is likely to be very small.

The bulk of the discussion by Greer et al. deals with recurrence for disease localized to the uterus and cervix (clinical stage I and II). Detailed data on patterns of failure and results of salvage therapy are not presented for clinical stage III or IV disease. Given the relatively poor prognoses of these patients and the greater difficulty in achieving a disease-free state, few objective data are likely to be available.

One interesting topic that was not directly addressed by Greer et al. is the potential use of molecular markers for disease surveillance. A number of oncogenes have been implicated in endometrial proliferation and in the oncogenesis and progression of endometrial carcinoma, including *HER-2/neu*, c-fms, c-fos, myc, *ras*-family, bFGF, and others.[14] Potential marker proteins have also been described, including CA-125, CA 15-3, and others. Markers specific for endometrial carcinoma have not been identified. However, identification of such markers may lead to powerful

Table 17-21 Follow-up of patients with endometrial cancer*,†: Roswell Park Cancer Institute

	YEAR				
	1	2	3	4	5
Office visit‡	2	2	2	1	1
Serum CA-125§	2	2	2	1	1
Pap test	1	1	1	1	1
Health maintenance¶	1	1	1	1	1

*The follow-up strategy I recommend is identical to the strategy recommended by Greer et al. of the University of Washington Medical Center/Fred Hutchinson Cancer Research Center.
†For surgically staged patients who have asymptomatic endometrial carcinoma treated with curative intent and who remain asymptomatic. Symptomatic patients need evaluation when the symptoms appear.
‡Includes pelvic examination.
§If elevated at time of initial treatment or with known extrauterine disease.
¶Should include blood pressure, breast examination, mammography as clinically indicated, stool guaiac testing, immunizations, and an opportunity to evaluate other health problems not related to the primary diagnosis of endometrial cancer.

methods of detecting recurrent or residual disease, such as the polymerase chain reaction. Detection of minimal disease by polymerase chain reaction is being investigated in several hematological malignancies and solid tumors, such as carcinomas of the prostate, breast, colon, and pancreas, Ewing's sarcoma, and melanoma.[15] Whether molecular approaches can improve on the results obtained by classic surveillance approaches will depend in part on corresponding advances in treatment of recurrent disease and on their clinical validation.

Frequent or technologically intensive surveillance of patients with endometrial carcinoma is difficult to justify. Greer et al. recommend an approach to surveillance that is more restrained than current practice but that seems eminently reasonable given the available data (Table 17-21). It is imperative that surveillance be critically evaluated in the context of careful prospective clinical investigations, since such data are currently not available. Only then can the utility of routine surveillance in the management of patients with endometrial carcinoma be unequivocally defined.

Table 17-22 Follow-up of patients with endometrial cancer by institution

YEAR/PROGRAM	OFFICE VISIT	SERUM CA-125	PAP TEST	HEALTH	CBC	ESR	LFT	KFT	URIN	CEA
Year 1										
Memorial Sloan-Kettering[a]	2[b]	2[c]	1	1[d]						
Roswell Park[e]	2[f]	2[c]	1	1[d]						
Univ Washington/ Fred Hutchinson[g]	2[f]	2[c]	1	1[d]						
Japan: Natl Cancer Ctr	4-12[h]	2	4-12		4-12	4-12	4-12	4-12	4-12	2
Year 2										
Memorial Sloan-Kettering[a]	2[b]	2[c]	1	1[d]						
Roswell Park[e]	2[f]	2[c]	1	1[d]						
Univ Washington/ Fred Hutchinson[g]	2[f]	2[c]	1	1[d]						
Japan: Natl Cancer Ctr	3-4[h]	2	3-4		3-4	3-4	3-4	3-4	3-4	2
Year 3										
Memorial Sloan-Kettering[a]	2[b]	2[c]	1	1[d]						
Roswell Park[e]	2[f]	2[c]	1	1[d]						
Univ Washington/ Fred Hutchinson[g]	2[f]	2[c]	1	1[d]						
Japan: Natl Cancer Ctr	2-3[h]	2	2-3		2-3	2-3	2-3	2-3	2-3	2

ABD CT abdominal computed tomography
ABD US abdominal ultrasound
BONE bone scan
CBC complete blood count
CEA carcinoembryonic antigen
C-REAC PROTEIN C-reactive protein
CXR chest x-ray
DRIP PYE drip infusion pyelography
EEG electroencephalography
ESR erythrocyte sedimentation rate
FIBRIN fibrin
HEALTH health maintenance
KFT kidney function test
LFT liver function test
URIN urinalysis

REFERENCES

1. Belinson JL, Lee KR, Badger GJ, Pretorius RG, Jarrell MA. Clinical stage I adenocarcinoma of the endometrium—analysis of recurrences and the potential benefit of staging lymphadenectomy. Gynecol Oncol 1992;44:17-23.
2. Gal D, Recio FO, Zamurovic D. The new International Federation of Gynecology and Obstetrics surgical staging and survival rates in early endometrial carcinoma. Cancer 1992;69:200-2.
3. Orr JW, Holloway RW, Orr PF, Holimon JL. Surgical staging of uterine cancer: an analysis of perioperative morbidity. Gynecol Oncol 1991;42:209-12.
4. Homesley HD, Kadar N, Barrett RJ, Lentz SS. Selective pelvic and periaortic lymphadenectomy does not increase morbidity in surgical staging of endometrial carcinoma. Am J Obstet Gynecol 1992;167: 1225-8.
5. Wolfson AH, Sightler SE, Markoe AM, et al. The prognostic significance of surgical staging for carcinoma of the endometrium. Gynecol Oncol 1992;45:142-6.
6. Kadar N, Malfetano JH, Homesley HD. Determinants of survival of surgically staged patients with endometrial carcinoma histologically confined to the uterus: implications for therapy. Obstet Gynecol 1992;80:655-9.
7. Gusberg SB. Virulence factors in endometrial cancer. Cancer 1993; 71:1464-6.
8. Greven KM, Lanciano RM, Corn B, Case D, Randall ME. Pathologic stage III endometrial carcinoma: prognostic factors and patterns of recurrence. Cancer 1993;71:3697-702.
9. Berchuck A, Anspach C, Evans AC, et al. Postsurgical surveillance of patients with FIGO stage I/II endometrial adenocarcinoma. Gynecol Oncol 1995;59:20-4.
10. Podczaski E, Kaminski P, Gurski K, et al. Detection and patterns of treatment failure in 300 consecutive cases of "early" endometrial cancer after primary surgery. Gynecol Oncol 1992;47:323-7.
11. Shumsky AG, Stuart GC, Brasher PM, Nation JG, Robertson DI, Sangkarat S. An evaluation of routine follow-up of patients treated for endometrial carcinoma. Gynecol Oncol 1994;55:229-33.
12. Reddoch JM, Burke TW, Morris M, Tornos C, Levenback C, Gershenson DM. Surveillance for recurrent endometrial carcinoma: development of a follow-up scheme. Gynecol Oncol 1995;59:221-5.
14. Barnhill D, O'Connor D, Farley J, Teneriello M, Armstrong D, Park R. Clinical surveillance of gynecologic cancer patients. Gynecol Oncol 1992;46:275-80.
15. Gurpide E. Endometrial cancer: biochemical and clinical correlates. J Natl Cancer Inst 1991;83:405-16.
16. Johnson PW, Burchill SA, Selby PJ. The molecular detection of circulating tumour cells. Br J Cancer 1995;72:268-76.

CA 19-9	FIBRIN	C-REAC PROTEIN	CXR	ABD CT/US	PELVIC CT/US	CHEST CT/US	BONE X-RAY	BARIUM ENEMA	DRIP PYE	BONE	EEG
2	2	2	2	i	i	i	i	i	i	i	i
2	2	2	2	i	i	i	i	i	i	i	i
2	2	2	2	i	i	i	i	i	i	i	i

a The follow-up strategy this author recommends is identical to the strategy recommended by Greer et al. of the University of Washington Medical Center/Fred Hutchinson Cancer Research Center.
b Includes examination of the pelvis, abdomen, and lymph node regions, especially the inguinal and supraclavicular areas.
c If elevated at time of initial treatment or with known extrauterine disease.
d Should include blood pressure, breast examination, mammography as clinically indicated, stool guaiac testing, immunizations, and an opportunity to evaluate other health problems not related to the primary diagnosis of endometrial cancer.
e For surgically staged asymptomatic patients who have endometrial carcinoma treated with curative intent and who remain asymptomatic. Symptomatic patients need evaluation when the symptoms appear.
f Includes pelvic examination.
g For patients who have surgically staged endometrial carcinoma treated with curative intent and who remain asymptomatic. Symptomatic patients need evaluation when symptoms appear.
h Includes history, physical examination, and pelvic examination.
i Performed as clinically indicated.

Continued.

Table 17-22 Follow-up of patients with endometrial cancer by institution—cont'd

YEAR/PROGRAM	OFFICE VISIT	SERUM CA-125	PAP TEST	HEALTH	CBC	ESR	LFT	KFT	URIN	CEA
Year 4										
Memorial Sloan-Kettering[a]	1[b]	1[c]	1	1[d]						
Roswell Park[e]	1[f]	1[c]	1	1[d]						
Univ Washington/ Fred Hutchinson[g]	1[f]	1[c]	1	1[d]						
Japan: Natl Cancer Ctr	2[h]	2	2		2	2	2	2	2	2
Year 5										
Memorial Sloan-Kettering[a]	1[b]	1[c]	1	1[d]						
Roswell Park[e]	1[f]	1[c]	1	1[d]						
Univ Washington/ Fred Hutchinson[g]	1[f]	1[c]	1	1[d]						
Japan: Natl Cancer Ctr	2[h]	2	2		2	2	2	2	2	2

CA 19-9	FIBRIN	C-REAC PROTEIN	CXR	ABD CT/US	PELVIC CT/US	CHEST CT/US	BONE X-RAY	BARIUM ENEMA	DRIP PYE	BONE	EEG
2	2	2	2	i	i	i	i	i	i	i	i
2	2	2	2	i	i	i	i	i	i	i	i

CHAPTER 18

Prostate Carcinoma

Roswell Park Cancer Institute

ROBERT P. HUBEN

The impact of prostate cancer on the health and well-being of men in the United States is enormous. Approximately 200,000 new cases of prostate cancer will be detected in 1997, and about 35,000 to 40,000 will die of this disease.[1] The number of new cases of prostate cancer detected has also increased dramatically, largely because of better public awareness of prostate cancer and screening undertaken to diagnose the disease at an early and potentially curable stage, since it is asymptomatic at onset. As a consequence, the number of men undergoing radical prostatectomy in the United States has shown a corresponding increase. Definitive radiation therapy remains an alternative therapy for localized prostate cancer for many men. How should these patients be followed up after completion of therapy? Many patients appear to be followed in an arbitrary fashion as far as follow-up laboratory tests or imaging studies are concerned. Although the frequency and intensity of follow-up depend on the clinical situation, it is reasonable to address the issue of follow-up studies on the basis of their potential cost-benefit considerations. In the case of prostate cancer, one specific marker, serum prostate specific antigen (PSA), is probably the most valuable and reliable of all tumor markers used routinely for any cancer at present in the United States. Use of this test has simplified the follow-up of patients after completion of definitive treatment for localized prostate cancer, although questions remain regarding the interpretation of PSA level changes that occur after treatment.

In this review treatment options for prostate cancer and pretreatment studies routinely performed in staging patients before definitive therapy are discussed. The role of PSA is examined closely, since it is the crux of both follow-up and evaluation of treatment outcomes. Management of patients with PSA elevations after both radical prostatectomy and definitive radiation therapy is discussed, with emphasis on the role of adjuvant therapies when available. Finally, some thoughts about future directions in both follow-up and adjuvant therapy are offered.

STAGING AND TREATMENT OF LOCALIZED PROSTATE CANCER

Tumor Markers for Prostate Cancer

Prostate specific antigen

The development and subsequent widespread application of PSA level determinations have had a profound impact on the diagnosis and management of prostate cancer. As Stamey[2] has suggested, PSA may be the most meaningful and useful tumor marker in all of cancer biology. PSA was initially isolated in 1979 at Roswell Park Cancer Institute by Wang et al.,[3] who demonstrated its prostatic tissue specificity. The purified antigen was determined to be distinct from prostatic acid phosphatase. With the development of an enzyme-linked immunoabsorbant assay procedure, it was possible to detect a PSA level as low as 0.1 ng/ml.[4] PSA levels can be measured reliably by either a monoclonal immunoradiometric assay or a polyclonal radioimmunoassay, both of which are commercially available. The former is used by 95% of commercial and research laboratories in the United States, and the reference range for PSA using this assay is zero to 4 ng/ml.[5]

PSA is a kallikrein-like serine protease that is produced exclusively by the epithelial cells of all types of prostatic tissue, benign and malignant.[5] Its biological function appears to be the liquefaction of the seminal coagulum. Concentrations of PSA have been reported to be the same per gram of tissue in normal, hyperplastic, and cancerous prostatic tissue.[6] Although false-positive PSA elevations may occur, they are organ specific. Spurious elevations of PSA have been documented after digital rectal examination, cystoscopic examination, and prostate biopsy.[7] Other organ-specific causes of false elevations of PSA include bacterial prostatitis and acute urinary retention.[2] From a practical point of view, bacterial prostatitis is the condition that most frequently presents a dilemma in management, and a fall in PSA level after initiation of antibiotic therapy for suspected prostatitis is usually diagnostic. A background of low-grade chronic bacterial prostatitis may be responsible for some of the fluctuations in PSA level commonly seen in patients observed for a known prostate cancer or as part of a routine check. About 25% of patients with prostatic hyperplasia only have an elevated PSA level.[5]

Although the role of PSA in routine screening for prostate cancer is highly controversial, its value in the routine follow-up of patients after definitive therapy for prostate cancer is irrefutable. It has obviated the need for most if not all other tests or procedures. However, what to do about a climbing PSA level after definitive therapy remains an entirely different controversy.

Prostatic acid phosphatase

Since the introduction of PSA determinations, the clinical value of routine determinations of prostatic acid phosphatase levels has declined dramatically. When compared under defined clinical conditions, PSA has proved consistently more sensitive, specific, and reliable and has accurately predicted the course of subsequent clinical events in patients with prostate cancer. In a report by Ercole et al.,[8] PSA level was elevated in 98% of 86 men with active stage D2 disease, whereas prostatic acid phosphatase level was elevated in only 76% of the patients. Therefore PSA was the only elevated marker in 22% of patients, whereas prostatic acid phosphatase was the only elevated marker in 1%. Only one patient had negative PSA and prostatic acid phosphatase levels. Comparison of presurgery PSA levels and subsequent pathological findings showed a good correlation of elevated PSA levels with extracapsular disease in this series. Moreover, PSA measurements after surgery either reflected or predicted clinical status in more than 90% of the patients on subsequent follow-up. The superiority of PSA when compared with prostatic acid phosphatase in accurately reflecting clinical outcome in patients after definitive therapy has been confirmed in numerous studies.[5,9,10] In fact, routine prostatic acid phosphatase determinations add so little to the management of patients with prostate cancer that physicians at Roswell Park Cancer Institute stopped doing these studies about 5 years ago. Since then, there has not been a single instance in which prostatic acid phosphatase measurements were considered necessary in making a major clinical decision. In contrast, PSA levels are used to make treatment recommendations on a daily basis.

Other Pretreatment Staging Procedures

After the diagnosis of prostate cancer is made, a number of tests are commonly performed in addition to PSA and digital rectal examination. These two studies, however, are undoubtedly the most useful in determining the extent of disease and ultimate outcome.

Bone scanning is generally performed after diagnosis of prostate cancer, regardless of the PSA level. Bone scans are rarely positive with a PSA level less than 20 ng/ml, but bone scanning is still performed routinely to rule out occult metastatic disease when radical prostatectomy is being contemplated.[5] If bone scans were obtained only when the PSA level was greater than 20 ng/ml, this would significantly reduce the cost of pretreatment staging, but my impression is that relatively few urologists are willing to proceed with surgery without having a negative bone scan as a reassurance. Accurate pretreatment staging is presumed to affect the design of any posttreatment surveillance strategy, as well as surveillance costs and utility.

Computed tomography and to a lesser extent magnetic resonance imaging are commonly performed in the staging of newly diagnosed prostate cancer, although the rationale for their use is somewhat unclear. Computed tomography provides little if any useful information about the local extent of disease, and its usefulness in detecting large nodes appears questionable at best. Since I see many patients for second opinions at Roswell Park Cancer Institute, I have noted that about 80% of patients who come in for a second opinion have had computed tomography of the pelvis and often the abdomen as part of their pretreatment staging.

Based on the preceding observation I reviewed the results of computed tomography in the staging of patients before radical prostatectomy.[11] At Roswell Park Cancer Institute, physicians stopped performing computed tomography of the pelvis in patients before radical prostatectomy approximately 5 years ago. A retrospective study of the last 158 radical prostatectomies performed at Roswell Park Cancer Institute was conducted, including 65 patients who had computed tomography performed and 93 patients who did not have it as part of their preoperative staging. In the 65 patients whose computed tomographic scans were reported negative for metastatic disease, four (6.1%) had positive nodes at surgery, while four of the 93 patients (4.3%) who did not have computed tomography were found to have positive nodes as well. Disease was microscopic in both groups, suggesting that routine computed tomography contributes little to the decision-making process for patients who are potential candidates for radical prostatectomy. I believe that computed tomography will continue to be performed as part of routine staging for patients before radical prostatectomy, although this practice is highly questionable on the basis of cost-benefit considerations.

Lymphangiography and intravenous pyelography are no longer recommended for patients before definitive therapy for localized prostate cancer. Since the yield of these studies is extremely low, they are rarely performed today. The staging system for prostate cancer of the American Joint Committee on Cancer is shown in Table 18-1.[12]

Treatment Options for Localized Prostate Cancer

Surveillance as a treatment option

The dramatic increase in the number of radical prostatectomies being performed in the United States over the past decade has raised reasonable concerns about possible overtreatment of patients with prostate cancer. A number of series have revealed a high incidence of so-called occult or incidental adenocarcinoma of the prostate, and about 10% of men who undergo a transurethral resection of the prostate gland for presumed benign prostatic hyperplasia are found to have prostate cancer.[13,14] In addition, the extreme variability of the natural history of prostate cancer is well recognized, although stage and grade provide solid information about prognosis.

One stage of disease for which observation is a recognized option is so-called stage A1 prostate cancer (TNM stage T1a). Although variably defined, it refers to focal low-grade adenocarcinoma of the prostate, which is usually detected at the time of transurethral resection of the prostate gland. In such patients PSA level has been a useful predictor of the extent and clinical significance of residual disease after transurethral resection of the prostate. A PSA level of less than 1 ng/ml after transurethral resection of the prostate

Table 18-1 Staging of prostate cancer

PRIMARY TUMOR (T)	
TX	Primary tumor cannot be assessed
T0	No evidence of primary tumor
T1	Clinically inapparent tumor not palpable or visible by imaging
T1a	Tumor incidental histological finding in 5% or less of tissue resected
T1b	Tumor incidental histological finding in more than 5% of tissue resected
T1c	Tumor identified by needle biopsy (e.g., because of elevated prostate specific antigen)
T2	Palpable tumor confined within prostate*
T2a	Tumor involves half of a lobe or less
T2b	Tumor involves more than half of a lobe but not both lobes
T2c	Tumor involves both lobes
T3	Tumor extends through the prostatic capsule†
T3a	Unilateral extracapsular extension
T3b	Bilateral extracapsular extension
T3c	Tumor invades seminal vesicle(s)
T4	Tumor is fixed or invades adjacent structures other than seminal vesicles
T4a	Tumor invades external sphincter, bladder neck, or rectum
T4b	Tumor invades levator muscles or is fixed to pelvic wall
LYMPH NODES (N)	
NX	Regional lymph nodes cannot be assessed
N0	No regional lymph node metastasis
N1	Metastasis in a single lymph node, 2 cm or less in greatest dimension
N2	Metastasis in a single lymph node, more than 2 cm but not more than 5 cm in greatest dimension, or multiple lymph nodes, none more than 5 cm in greatest dimension
N3	Metastasis in a lymph node more than 5 cm in greatest dimension
DISTANT METASTASIS (M)‡	
MX	Presence of distant metastasis cannot be assessed
M0	No distant metastasis
M1	Distant metastasis
M1a	Nonregional lymph nodes
M1b	Bone
M1c	Other sites

From American Joint Committee on Cancer, Beahrs OH, Henson DE, Hutter RVP, Kennedy BJ, editors. Manual for staging of cancer. Philadelphia: JB Lippincott Company, 1992.

*Tumor found in one or both lobes by needle biopsy, but not palpable or visible by imaging, is classified as T1c.

†Invasion into the prostatic apex or into (but not beyond) the prostatic capsule is not classified as T3, but as T2.

‡When more than one site of metastasis is present, the most advanced category (pM1c) is used.

in which prostate cancer is an incidental finding reliably predicts a residual tumor volume of less than 0.5 cm^3 on the subsequent surgical specimen.[13,14] Approximately 30% to 40% of patients with A1 prostate cancer have PSA levels of less than 1 ng/ml after transurethral resection of the prostate.[14] Patients with a PSA level more than 10 ng/ml generally have residual tumor volumes greater than 0.5 cm^3. Patients with stage A1 tumors and PSA levels between 1 and 10 ng/ml may continue to present a management problem, although factors such as age and general health are also important considerations. In this situation changes in the PSA levels and the rapidity with which PSA increases may be more critical factors in determining subsequent therapy.

A conservative approach to management of clinically localized prostate cancer was supported by the clinical study of Chodak et al.,[15] who performed a metaanalysis of 828 case records from six nonrandomized studies of men who were treated conservatively for clinically localized prostate cancer. In this series disease-specific survival 10 years after diagnosis of prostate cancer was 87% for men with grade 1 or 2 tumors and 34% for those with grade 3 tumors. Metastasis-free survival among men who had not died of other causes was 81% for grade 1, 58% for grade 2, and 26% for grade 3 disease. Although this was a nonrandomized study, the authors concluded that conservative management is a reasonable approach for patients with grade 1 or 2 prostate cancers that are clinically localized, particularly for men who have an average life expectancy of 10 years or less. Use of PSA level as a monitoring mechanism for stage A1 prostate cancer or in patients who have palpable disease that is low grade and not associated with an elevated PSA level allows some measure of comfort for patients and physicians alike, as long as the PSA level remains stable.

Radical prostatectomy

The most striking trend in the management of localized prostate cancer has been the dramatic increase in the number of radical prostatectomies performed annually in the United States. The past decade has seen a more than fivefold increase in the number of radical prostatectomies, since the number of newly diagnosed prostate cancers, particularly in young men, has increased dramatically.[16-18] The number of new cases of prostate cancer, in turn, reflects widespread availability and acceptance of routine PSA determinations to screen for otherwise asymptomatic disease.[19,20] As previously noted, this translates into approximately 200,000 new cases of prostate cancer diagnosed annually in the United States.[1]

Another factor that has undoubtedly increased the acceptance of radical prostatectomy as a treatment option for localized prostate cancer is the description by Walsh et al.[21,22] of the nerve-sparing radical prostatectomy, which demonstrates that the majority of men sexually active before surgery can maintain potency. The impotence that universally occurred before the description of this technique had been a major obstacle to acceptance of radical prostatectomy as a treatment option, particularly for younger men. Other potential complications of radical prostatectomy include urinary incontinence, which occurs in 2% to 10% of patients, and the risk of perioperative complications such as deep venous thrombosis and myocardial infarction.

Long-term results in large series of patients undergoing radical prostatectomy show excellent control of disease in most cases. Zincke et al.[23] from the Mayo Clinic recently reported on a series of 1,143 consecutive patients who underwent radical prostatectomy for clinically localized prostate cancer at that institution. Only 113 (10%) died of prostate cancer and 177 (15%) had metastases. The 10- and 15-year crude survival rates were 75% and 60%, respectively. Cause-specific survival rates were 90% and 83%, respectively. For the last 1,000 patients in this series there were no hospital mortalities and severe incontinence occurred in 1.4%.

In a series of 925 consecutive patients undergoing radical prostatectomy for TNM stage T1 and T2 prostate cancer reported by Catalona and Smith,[24] the overall probability of nonprogression at 5 years was 78%. Overall, 115 patients (12%) had evidence of cancer recurrence after radical prostatectomy in this series. PSA relapse was the only indication of recurrence in 78 patients (68%), while 30 (26%) had local recurrence or distant metastases in addition to PSA evidence of relapse. The interval to detection of recurrent disease after surgery ranged from 1 to 100 months and averaged 24 months. As might be expected, outcome correlated closely with pathological tumor stage. There was no evidence of recurrence in 91% of patients with organ-confined disease, in 74% with positive margins or microscopic capsular penetration, and in 32% with seminal vesicle invasion.

Definitive radiation therapy

Although the percentage of patients with newly diagnosed prostate cancer undergoing definitive radiation therapy for localized prostate cancer is smaller because of the surging popularity of radical prostatectomy, radiation remains an important and effective option for patients with localized prostate cancer. In the past the early response to definitive radiation therapy was often difficult to assess, since some practitioners have considered even positive biopsies after completion of radiation therapy to be of questionable biological significance. However, the advent of PSA determination has provided much clearer answers about both early and long-term response to radiation therapy. It has been suggested that radiation therapy and radical prostatectomy are equally effective for early-stage prostate cancer.[25] For tumors confined to the prostate gland the survival figures generally quoted for 5, 10, and 15 years after radiation therapy are 80%, 60%, and 40%, respectively.[26,27] These results are similar to those reported for surgery, although other studies have suggested a better 15-year survival for men who undergo surgery.[28,29] The advent of PSA determinations has made prediction of treatment failure possible much earlier than before. For patients with extracapsular extension of prostate cancer, survival rates after completion of definitive radiation at 5, 10, and 15 years are usually in the range of 60%, 40%, and 20%, respectively.[30,31]

Complications from radiation therapy vary with such factors as the age and general health of the patient and the total dose of radiation delivered, but they are generally quite low. Chronic complications such as radiation proctitis or cystitis are reported to occur in less than 10% of patients, while impotence occurs in about 30% in most series.[26,27] Mild diarrhea and a sense of tiredness or fatigue may occur during the course of radiation, but these usually subside after completion of therapy. The incidence of life-threatening complications from radiation therapy is extremely low. For this reason radiation therapy can be offered as a relatively safe alternative when radical prostatectomy is not feasible because of the patient's age or general health problems. This difference in patient selection is just one reason that the results of radiation therapy and radical prostatectomy for localized disease are difficult if not impossible to compare.

Surgery versus radiation

Comparison of the reported results of radical prostatectomy and radiation therapy in the management of localized prostate cancer is fraught with difficulties.[16] As noted, patients for whom radiation therapy is recommended are generally older and sicker. I do not recommend radical prostatectomy at Roswell Park Cancer Institute for men older than 70 years of age, for example. While this may represent yet another bias in certain circumstances, considerations of life expectancy and increased surgical risk are not unreasonable deterrents to surgery. A history of significant cardiac or pulmonary disease generally excludes patients from surgery, which is another obvious selection bias. Most important, patients considered to be poor candidates for radical prostatectomy, based on the local extent of disease as assessed by digital rectal examination or the degree of PSA elevation, are often referred for radiation therapy as a result. Since these factors, particularly pretreatment PSA levels, have been shown time and again to be the most reliable predictors of treatment outcome, it is not surprising that such differences in outcomes between surgery and radiation are observed.

In balancing any real or apparent benefits from a surgical approach, one must also weigh the risks associated with the procedure. Several recent reports have suggested that complications of radical prostatectomy, in particular incontinence and impotence, occur more frequently after radical prostatectomy than has been generally reported.[32-34] These studies suggest that patients are reporting higher rates of complications and lower rates of satisfaction than their surgeons are. Whether these should be evaluated differently during follow-up after these alternate forms of primary therapy is not known.

An obvious and crucial difference between radical prostatectomy and radiation therapy series is the inherent noncomparability of clinical and pathological stage. Critical staging factors, such as seminal vesicle or capsular invasion and lymph node status, are available in surgical series but not in radiation series. Clinicopathological correlations show understaging in 50% to 80% of clinically staged patients.[24,29] These differences in patient selection and stage of disease make attempts at meaningful comparison of the results of radiation and surgery risky at best.

Cryosurgery of the prostate

An emerging treatment option for localized prostate cancer is radical cryosurgical ablation of the prostate gland, which involves in situ freezing of the entire gland, periprostatic tissue, neurovascular pedicles, and proximal seminal vesicles.[35] Cryoablation was attempted in the past and has been given new life because of improvements in imaging and access to the prostate.

In brief the technique involves the insertion of up to five cryoprobes into the prostate gland using guidewires and dilators under transrectal ultrasound (TRUS) guidance. Once proper position of the cryoprobes is confirmed by ultrasound, liquid nitrogen is circulated within the probes, creating an "ice ball" in the prostate that can be monitored by ultrasound. The goal of the freezing process is to observe the rim of the freeze zone passing through the prostatic capsule without reaching the rectal wall. A percutaneously inserted suprapubic tube, which is placed immediately before cryosurgery, is removed when the postvoid residual is less than 100 ml.

In a preliminary report by Onik et al.,[35] 23 patients were divided into two groups based on the number of cryoprobes used. The first and earlier group of patients was treated by freezing the prostate gland with two cryoprobes placed multiple times, while the second group of patients was treated with five cryoprobes placed simultaneously. Treatment response was determined by the PSA level and by both selected and random biopsies 3 months after cryosurgery. Residual disease was detected in three of the eight patients in the first group (37.5%) and in one of the 15 patients in the second group (6.7%), for a combined response rate of 82.6%. Complications have been reported for the entire group of 55 patients treated to date. These included freezing of the rectum in four patients (5.9%), which resulted in urethrorectal fistula in two. Sloughing of prostatic urethral tissue occurred in three patients (4.4%). Limited follow-up of patients who were potent before cryosurgery indicated that five of 14 patients (35%) retained potency after the procedure. Obviously it will take more patients and more time before the role of cryosurgical ablation of the prostate becomes apparent, and the optimal follow-up strategy is unknown. An area in which this technique may have more application and acceptance is the treatment of patients who still have localized disease after definitive radiation therapy, since other treatment options have serious limitations, as will be discussed.

FOLLOW-UP PROCEDURES

Follow-Up After Radical Prostatectomy

After radical prostatectomy, serial determination of PSA is the most critical indicator of tumor recurrence and thus patient outcome. Stated simply, the PSA should fall to an undetectable level after total removal of the prostate gland. Remnants of cloacogenic glandular epithelium in normal urethral and anal glands contain PSA-secreting cells, but this is unlikely to be a significant cause of PSA elevation in this clinical setting.[36] A small amount of benign prostatic tissue could have been left behind at surgery, particularly in patients whose surgery predated the more anatomical approach to radical prostatectomy that is now accepted, but the number of patients in this category is extremely small. With either of the two commercially available assays generally used, a PSA level greater than 0.4 ng/ml strongly suggests the presence of residual disease.[37,38] Although PSA measurements have simplified the follow-up of patients after radical prostatectomy and obviated the need for most or all other studies, a number of issues are unresolved. These include whether early detection of recurrent disease, as heralded by a postoperative PSA elevation, will result in an ultimate survival advantage if adjuvant therapy is recommended and promptly initiated. How can one determine whether a postoperative PSA elevation indicates local recurrence or occult distant spread? What other tests if any are helpful in answering this question? Does a PSA elevation after radical prostatectomy necessarily indicate that clinical evidence of recurrence will develop, or do other factors predict reliably which patients will have rapid progression? Who or what is being treated—the patient or the PSA level? PSA determinations have answered a lot of questions, but they have also raised many that are even more difficult to answer at present.

One of the earliest reports examining both preoperative and postoperative PSA levels in patients undergoing radical prostatectomy was that of Oesterling et al.[39] from the Johns Hopkins Hospital. The preoperative PSA level was significantly and positively related to final pathological stage when all 178 patients were examined as a group by logistic regression analysis. However, the preoperative PSA level was unable to predict final pathological stage on an individual basis because of the high number of false-positive and false-negative results, an observation that has been made repeatedly over the years. Postoperative PSA determinations were performed in a group of 127 patients, with a mean follow-up duration of 2 years. Of the 101 patients who had organ-confined cancer or capsular penetration only, 92 (91%) had a follow-up antigen concentration of less than 0.2 ng/ml, while only five of 26 men (19%) with either seminal vesicle involvement or lymph node involvement had an antigen level less than 0.2 ng/ml. Eight of the 127 patients (6%) had a documented clinical recurrence, and all had elevated follow-up PSA levels. Only four of the eight patients (50%) with documented tumor recurrence had an elevated prostatic acid phosphatase level. Most authors have concluded that PSA level is the most effective tool in follow-up after radical prostatectomy.

A recent update of the Johns Hopkins experience has examined timing of PSA elevations and development of clinical disease, as well as the results of expectant management of patients who have an elevated PSA level after radical prostatectomy.[38] There were 875 men who had PSA determinations within the first year after surgery. Of these, 112 (13%) had detectable PSA levels as their first manifestation of disease recurrence. This occurred within a year of surgery in eight men (4.3%) and in an additional 30 and 21 men within the second and third postoperative years, respectively. This disease progression occurred in 60% of men who had a detectable PSA level within the first year after surgery, compared with 28% and 25% of those whose PSA level became detectable in years 2 and 3, respectively. Disease recurrence within the first year was local in two cases and distant in 21.

Most of the patients with elevated PSA level as the first sign of disease recurrence in this series were managed expectantly. There were 101 men who were followed without radiation or hormonal therapy for an average of about 2½ years after detection of PSA. Twenty-one men subsequently received either hormonal or radiation therapy before any sign of progression, and one man was lost to follow-up. Of the 79 remaining men who have been followed up with no treatment until progression, 12 have had local recurrence, 30 have had distant metastases, and 57 still have isolated elevation of PSA as their only sign of recurrence. Therefore a postoperative PSA elevation was not a harbinger of clinically significant disease in the majority of patients in this series during the follow-up period.

The often striking discrepancy between PSA elevation after radical prostatectomy and the development of clinical evidence of recurrent disease was also illustrated in the report by Frazier et al.[40] In a group of 226 patients who underwent radical perineal prostatectomy for organ-confined prostate cancer, clinical failure (defined by elevation of serum acid phosphatase level, biopsy-proven local recurrence, or evidence of malignant disease on bone scan) occurred in 3.9% of patients with organ-confined tumors, 7% with specimen-confined tumors, and 13.2% with positive margins. When a PSA elevation of greater than 0.5 ng/ml was used as the indicator of failure, however, the failure rates rose to 9.8% for the organ-confined group, 39.4% for the specimen-confined group, and 66% for the margin-positive group. The interval from initial elevation of postoperative PSA to clinical detection of failure ranged from 2 to 28 months, with a median of 16 months. Of the 73 patients in whom a postoperative PSA level greater than 0.5 ng/ml was found, 11 have been followed up for more than 36 months without clinical evidence of failure in this series.

A number of other factors have been examined in an effort to distinguish between local recurrence and distant metastases when a PSA elevation occurs postoperatively. It has been suggested that a combination of Gleason score, pathological stage, and rate of change of PSA level or PSA level 1 year after surgery can be helpful in this distinction.[37] If a patient has an isolated elevation of PSA within a year after surgery and had either positive seminal vesicles or lymph nodes at the time of surgery or a Gleason score of 8 for tumors, we believe the PSA elevation most likely indicates distant metastases, for which hormonal therapy is generally recommended.[37] However, a PSA elevation that occurs more than 1 year after surgery in a patient with normal seminal vesicles and lymph nodes at surgery and a tumor with a Gleason score of 7 or less most likely indicates a local recurrence, for which radiation therapy to the prostatic bed may be a more appropriate therapy.

In patients with an elevated PSA level after radical prostatectomy, the PSA doubling time may also indicate whether they are likely to benefit from adjuvant therapy when it can be reliably determined that a PSA elevation is not due to the development of distant metastases. In the report by Trapasso et al.,[34] postprostatectomy PSA doubling times were significantly different in patients who ultimately had progression to distant metastases when compared with those in whom either clinical local recurrence or PSA elevation was the sole indicator of recurrence. The median PSA doubling time in those patients who ultimately had bone metastases was 4.3 months, compared with 11.7 months in patients without evidence of progression to metastatic disease. All patients with metastases in this report had PSA doubling times of less than 12 months.

It would be reasonable to anticipate that patients with positive surgical margins would be at high risk for local recurrence after radical prostatectomy. There is a rather striking discrepancy, however, between the presence of positive surgical margins and the development of subsequent evidence of disease progression. In several series only 30% to 40% of patients with focally positive margins had progression by 5 years postoperatively.[41] Several possible explanations for this phenomenon have been suggested. Possibly these patients will ultimately demonstrate evidence of progressive disease, although the long length of follow-up and exquisite sensitivity of the PSA assay argue against this possibility. It is also possible that focally positive margins consisting of relatively few neoplastic glands are destroyed by the local inflammatory response at a surgical site. A final and perhaps most likely explanation for the discrepancy between positive margins and progression is a technical one. False-positive margins may be due to artifactual problems, rather than identifying patients at risk for local recurrence.[41] The finding that a surprisingly large number of patients with focally positive margins at the time of surgery fail to develop clinical evidence of local progression argues strongly against local adjuvant therapy without confirmation by a subsequent PSA elevation.

As might be expected, PSA determinations are not foolproof in detecting recurrent disease after radical prostatectomy. There have been sporadic anecdotal reports of patients in whom recurrent disease developed despite very low or undetectable PSA levels. In my experience such patients usually have very high-grade or anaplastic tumors. Goldrath and Messing[42] reported on two patients with documented progression of disease in whom PSA level was undetectable. One patient had an abnormal rectal examination, an elevated prostatic acid phosphatase level, and a subsequent positive needle biopsy despite an undetectable PSA level, while the second patient had progressive bone metastases on bone scan despite an undetectable PSA level. In a patient described by Takayama et al.,[43] a painful induration developed at the urethrovesical anastomosis after radical prostatectomy, which revealed adenocarcinoma on an ultrasound-guided needle biopsy despite an undetectable PSA level. This situation occurs so infrequently, however, that other diagnostic tests beyond PSA determination and rectal examination appear unwarranted on a cost-effectiveness basis.

Is TRUS beneficial in detecting local recurrence after radical prostatectomy? In a report of 20 patients with suspected local recurrence after either radical prostatectomy or cystoprostatectomy, TRUS verified the presence of recurrence in 19 patients (95%), as confirmed by biopsy of the visualized lesions.[44] Of these 19 recurrences, 14 had a hypoechoic appearance, while in the remaining five patients the echo pattern was isoechoic. However, these patients were a highly selected group, since they were suspected of having local recurrence on the basis of an abnormal rectal examination.

More recently the use of TRUS for detecting local recurrence in patients with detectable PSA levels after radical prostatectomy and no identifiable distant metastases has been suggested.[45] Of 20 patients who underwent TRUS combined with biopsies, nine (45%) were found to have histological evidence of local recurrence at the initial assessment. TRUS displayed abnormalities in 12 of the 20 patients, seven of whom had positive biopsies. Random biopsies of the vesicourethral junction were positive in two of eight patients with negative ultrasound findings and an unremarkable digital rectal examination. The authors concluded that TRUS-guided biopsy is a useful diagnostic approach in patients suspected to have local failure when the digital rectal examination is unremarkable.

"Ultrasensitive" assays have been developed that will allow for earlier indication of treatment failure after radical prostatectomy.[36,46] These newer techniques still cannot distinguish between local recurrence and distant metastases. Such refinements in laboratory technique will be of real clinical benefit only if early indication of recurrent or persistent disease and prompt initiation of adjuvant therapy are associated with longer survival than in patients whose disease recurrence is detected at a later date. How should a PSA elevation after radical prostatectomy be treated, if at all? To answer this question, it is necessary to look at the role of adjuvant therapy, particularly irradiation of the prostate bed, in patients with an elevated PSA level after radical prostatectomy.

Role of Adjuvant Radiation Therapy After Radical Prostatectomy in the Management of Prostate Specific Antigen Elevation

Careful surveillance of patients who have undergone radical prostatectomy for localized prostate cancer would be particularly critical if there was evidence that early additional or adjuvant therapy would cause the PSA level to fall to an undetectable range and effect a cure of the disease that was not a result of surgery. Several large series have looked at the effect of adjuvant radiation therapy on patients with a PSA elevation after radical prostatectomy. As discussed previously, a number of clinical clues may provide information regarding the site of recurrent disease, that is, whether an elevated PSA level after radical prostatectomy is due to local recurrence or occult distant spread. The experience at Roswell Park Cancer Institute is probably fairly typical of the reported outcomes. I conducted a retrospective review of 22 patients who received adjuvant radiation therapy after radical retropubic prostatectomy because of a postoperative elevation in PSA.[47] PSA declined to an undetectable level in 11 of these patients (50%) but subsequently rose in six over an average follow-up period of 28 months. Five of the patients (23%) have had a persistently undetectable PSA level during this follow-up period. As in other reports, adjuvant radiation therapy appears to be remarkably well tolerated, despite the potential for radiation injury to either the bladder or rectum in a postsurgical field. None of the patients had any significant complications from adjuvant radiation therapy, although most experienced the transient bowel and bladder irritability that are not uncommon in patients receiving definitive radiation therapy.

In the report by Lange et al.[48] the stored sera from 15 patients who had an elevated PSA level after radical prostatectomy but before radiation therapy were analyzed and PSA levels were found to decrease by more than 50% in 12 of the 15 patients (80%) and to undetectable levels in 53% of patients. An additional 29 men were studied prospectively when they showed increasing levels of PSA from 9 to 95 months after radical prostatectomy. Of the 29, 19 had positive random needle biopsies of the urethrovesical anastomosis. In 82% of patients the PSA level decreased by more than 50% after radiation and fell to an undetectable range in 43%. Side effects of radiation therapy were reported to be minimal. One of the interesting aspects of this report is that the response to radiation therapy did not correlate with the results of the preradiation biopsy of the urethrovesical anastomosis. Even when the biopsy was negative, adjuvant radiation therapy decreased PSA levels in 70% of the patients and to undetectable levels in 30%, while the comparable figures were 89% and 50% in patients with positive biopsies of the anastomotic site.

Hudson and Catalona[49] reported decline of a persistently detectable PSA level to an undetectable range in six of 21 patients (29%) who received postoperative radiation therapy after radical prostatectomy, and all patients remained free of evidence of tumor recurrence, with a mean follow-up of 12.6 months. Seven of 13 patients whose PSA levels remained detectable after adjuvant radiation therapy had clinical evidence of tumor recurrence.

In a subsequent report by the same authors the results of early versus delayed adjuvant radiation therapy after radical prostatectomy were analyzed in terms of PSA response.[50] The indications for adjuvant radiation therapy in 64 patients were pathological stage C disease in 27, a detectable PSA level in 11, or both in 26. Of the 27 patients treated prophylactically for pathological stage C disease, 18 (67%) had no evidence of recurrence after radiation therapy within the first 6 months postoperatively, with a median follow-up of 40 months. Of the 22 men who were treated for PSA elevation after surgery, 15 (68%) had no evidence of recurrence, with a median follow-up of 27.5 months. Of 15 men treated within the first 6 months after radical prostatectomy for persistently detectable PSA levels, eight (53%) had an initial decrease in PSA level to an undetectable range and only five (33%) had a persistently undetectable PSA level, with a median follow-up of 36 months. The authors concluded that there was no apparent difference in treatment outcome between patients receiving early postoperative adjuvant radiation therapy and those for whom radiation therapy was delayed until an elevation of PSA was detected. Therefore it seems reasonable to defer adjuvant radiation therapy until a rise in PSA level occurs in patients at risk for local recurrence after radical prostatectomy. As previously noted the presence of positive surgical margins often fails to predict the development of local recurrence. This finding also calls into question the necessity or advantage of progressively more sensitive assays for PSA after radical prostatectomy, since it appears that those patients who will ultimately benefit from adjuvant radiation therapy in this setting will do so even when such therapy is delayed.

Follow-Up After Definitive Radiation Therapy

As in the case of patients undergoing radical prostatectomy for localized prostate cancer, postradiation PSA level is the single most important measure for evaluating response to therapy. Similarly, there is convincing evidence that pretreatment PSA level is the single most important prognostic factor in predicting response to radiation therapy, as well as in predicting response to patients undergoing radical prostatectomy.[51] Stated simply, a rising PSA level after definitive radiation therapy indicates disease recurrence and a rising PSA level often predates clinical recurrence by months or years.[52] Again, as in the case of patients who undergo radical prostatectomy, PSA testing permits detection of persistence or recurrence of disease at an earlier time than with any other method. However, the impact of subsequent therapy and the clinical significance of the elevated PSA level itself after radiation therapy are both uncertain.

Since normal prostatic epithelium remains after definitive radiation, PSA levels remain detectable in most cases after definitive radiation therapy. The initial rate of response to radiation therapy, as heralded by PSA level decline, appears to be extremely high, and more than 90% of patients receiving definitive radiation therapy will demonstrate an initial decline in PSA level in most series.[52,53] The lowest level to which the PSA drops and the time interval that it takes to achieve that nadir level may have important prognostic significance.

An early series of patients who received definitive radiation therapy and in whom posttreatment serial PSA levels were measured was reported by Stamey et al.[54] at Stanford. There were 183 men in this series, of whom 163 had received external beam radiation therapy totaling 7,000 cGy and 20 had undergone I-125 seed implantation. With a mean follow-up interval of 5 years, only 11% of the 183 patients had undetectable PSA levels. Multiple PSA determinations were performed in 124 of the 183 patients. PSA levels were declining in 82% of patients during the first year after completion of radiation therapy, but only 8% continued to decline beyond the first year. Of 80 patients observed more than 1 year after completion of radiation therapy, 51% had increasing PSA levels, while the PSA level was stable in 41%. The authors were also able to demonstrate that increasing PSA levels after radiation therapy correlated with progression to metastatic disease and residual cancer on prostate biopsy, which has always been a controversial issue. Lastly, total serum acid phosphatase levels were demonstrated to be only poorly correlated with both PSA and subsequent clinical progression and provided no useful additional information.

The Stanford group also examined the role of TRUS-guided biopsy and PSA level in patients who had undergone definitive radiation therapy. They examined the results in 27 men who underwent TRUS-guided needle biopsies more than 18 months after completion of radiation therapy for localized prostate cancer.[55] The mean interval after completion of therapy was more than 5 years. This was not a randomly selected group, however. Fifteen of the 27 patients were selected at random, but 12 of the 27 were encouraged to undergo biopsy based on either elevated or increasing PSA levels. The biopsies performed were extremely thorough in each case and included those directed at any hypoechoic areas, as well as systemic biopsies performed from apex to base bilaterally and biopsy of the seminal vesicles, even when they appeared grossly normal by ultrasound. Overall, 25 of the 27 patients (93%) had postradiation biopsies that were positive for cancer, including all five patients with prostatic induration and 20 of 22 patients (91%) with normal postirradiation digital rectal examination. Ultrasound findings correlated poorly with pathological findings, as did the results of digital rectal examination. Ten of 12 patients (83%) with PSA levels less than 10 ng/ml had positive biopsies, as did all 15 patients whose PSA levels were greater than 10 ng/ml.

Recently several large series of patients who have undergone definitive radiation therapy have been reported in which both pretreatment and posttreatment PSA levels were shown to provide important prognostic information. Zagars[53] has reported on the experience at M.D. Anderson Cancer Center, which involved a group of 423 patients who received definitive radiation therapy for localized prostate cancer. Stage distribution was stage A2 in 122 patients, stage B in 143, and stage C in 148 patients. Of the total group, 42 patients (10%) sustained a disease relapse, which was local in 32 cases, distant in 12, and nodal in three. In 96 patients (23%) a rising PSA level was detected, and 104 (25%) have either had relapse or developed a rising PSA profile. Of note is a fall in PSA level in relation to its pretreatment value in 96% of the patients in this series. The doubling times of PSA levels after radiation appeared to be substantially shorter than those reported for untreated patients under observation, suggesting that a more aggressive cell population remained after completion of radiation therapy, which was associated with more rapidly rising PSA levels. Patients were investigated for evidence of spread of disease once the PSA level exceeded 10 ng/ml, largely because of patient anxiety about documentation of metastatic disease. I recommend androgen ablation for patients who have a rising PSA level after definitive radiation therapy.

In the study just described, the author was able to show a strong correlation between PSA levels at 6 months and treatment outcome. In a similar report patients were stratified according to the highest PSA level recorded for each patient at 6 to 60 months after completion of treatment.[56] A sharp cutoff in overall response rate was seen in patients whose PSA level exceeded 4 ng/ml at 6 months after completion of therapy. Patients with a highest late PSA level of less than 4 ng/ml had a 20% incidence of relapse or rising PSA level at 4 years, while patients with a highest late PSA level of greater than 4 ng/ml had a 90% incidence of relapse or rising PSA level at 3 years. Therefore it appears that patients whose PSA level exceeds 4 ng/ml at 6 months after completion of radiation therapy are destined to have a poor outcome from their radiation therapy.

Zagars[51] has also examined PSA level as an outcome variable for patients with T1 and T2 prostate cancers treated by definitive radiation therapy. There were 269 patients followed for 9 to 73 months after completion of external beam radiation therapy for clinical stage T1 or T2 tumors. The actual incidence of increasing PSA levels was 30% at 5 years and the incidence of relapse or increasing PSA levels was 36% at the same time. A direct correlation was again shown with pretreatment PSA levels. Relapse occurred in 14% of patients with a PSA level less than 4 ng/ml, in 33% of patients whose PSA level was between 4 and 10 ng/ml, in 55% of patients with a PSA level between 10 and 30 ng/ml, and in more than 80% of patients whose initial PSA level was more than 30 ng/ml. However, the nadir PSA value was the most significant aspect of the assay and was typically achieved 6 to 12 months after completion of radiation therapy. Patients in whom the nadir PSA level fell to less than 1 ng/ml had only a 12% relapse rate at 5 years, while approximately two thirds of patients with a nadir exceeding 4 ng/ml failed by 2 years. The author concluded that complete irradiation of all localized prostate cancer is considerably more difficult to achieve than has traditionally been believed, based on posttreatment PSA data.

The study by Goad et al.[52] at Baylor also demonstrated the strong predictive value of postirradiation PSA levels and subsequent clinical course. In this series 76 patients received definitive irradiation and 68 patients were treated with interstitial radioactive gold seed implantation combined with external beam therapy. The remaining eight patients received standard external beam irradiation to a minimum dose of 7000 cGy. The nadir, or lowest level of PSA after radiation therapy, was classified as undetectable (less than or equal to 0.4 ng/ml in this report), detectable and within normal range (0.5 to 4 ng/ml), or greater than normal (greater than 4 ng/ml). Twenty-eight patients achieved a nadir PSA level in an undetectable range, but this did not preclude subsequent progression, since three patients had clinical evidence of progressive disease and another had a PSA elevation only, for an overall progression rate of 14%. All six patients in whom the PSA nadir exceeded 4 ng/ml had clinical evidence of disease progression. If the PSA level failed to return to normal, all patients manifested failure of therapy within 2 years.

The length of time necessary to achieve nadir PSA levels may also have predictive value, although the time necessary to achieve the nadir levels seems to vary considerably. In a large study by Landmann and Hunig[28] it was determined that PSA values that failed to normalize 6 months after completion of treatment were associated with high risk of recurrence. However, in the series by Goad et al.,[52] 11 of 28 patients (39%) who achieved an undetectable PSA level did so more than 12 months after radiation. It seems likely therefore that the extent of decline, rather than the rate of decline, is the more important indicator.

As previously noted the biological significance of a climbing PSA level after definitive radiation therapy continues to be debated. However, it appears that a rising PSA value indicates treatment failure and subsequent clinical relapse. It is the subsequent rate of progression of disease that is difficult to predict because of the extremely variable natural history of prostate cancer. In a study by Kabalin et al.[55] from Stanford, increasing PSA levels were detected in 44 of 117 patients who received definitive radiation therapy for localized prostate cancer. Clinical relapse occurred in 30 of these 44 patients (68%), with a mean interval of 156 days.

Salvage Prostatectomy for Radiation Failure

A potential option for selected patients who show clinical or biochemical evidence of treatment failure is salvage radical prostatectomy, but the selection issue is an important one. In a report by Pontes et al.,[57] salvage surgery was performed in 43 patients who failed definitive radiation therapy, entailing prostatectomy in 35 patients and cystoprostatectomy in eight. As might be anticipated from the dangers inherent in operating in a previously irradiated field, complications of surgery were considered significant in this report. There were four rectal injuries, one ureteral injury, and one perioperative death. Ten of the 35 patients (30%) who underwent salvage prostatectomy were incontinent. Discouragingly, only 30% of the whole group had negative surgical margins. Ten of the patients have had no evidence of recurrence of disease in follow-up ranging from 1 to 10 years. Whether earlier consideration of salvage prostatectomy based on early PSA level results after radiation therapy would be associated with better outcome or a lower rate of complications is a provocative but unanswered question.

Follow-Up of Patients Undergoing Hormonal Therapy for Prostate Cancer

PSA level is also the most sensitive and reliable indicator of response to hormonal therapy in any form, although recent evidence suggests that PSA expression may be under hormonal regulation and may therefore not reflect the clinical course of disease.[58] Despite this concern, PSA level can generally predict the course of disease after initiation of hormone therapy and is the earliest indicator of the development of hormonal resistance.

Stamey et al.[59] reported on the response of PSA level to the initiation of hormonal therapy in 45 patients who received such therapy in various forms. With a mean interval of 2 years after initiation of therapy, this study showed that 9% had undetectable PSA levels, and 22% were within normal range. Fall in PSA level was most pronounced in the 6 months after initiation of treatment and 21 of 29 patients (72%) had increasing PSA levels after 6 months. The level to which PSA falls after initiation of hormonal therapy may also have important prognostic significance. In a report by Miller et al.,[60] patients whose posttreatment nadir PSA level decreased to less than 4 ng/ml had a significantly longer remission than those whose nadir PSA level remained elevated.

The issue of whether PSA level adequately and accurately reflects clinical status in patients receiving hormonal therapy was raised by Leo et al.,[58] who found that PSA levels were significantly lower in hormonally treated men with metastatic prostate cancer, despite symptoms and bone scan findings similar to those for patients with metastatic disease who had not received hormonal therapy. In a group of 43 patients who had received no prior therapy the median PSA level was 96.0 ng/ml, while in 38 men who had started hormonal therapy an average of 14 months before evaluation the median PSA level was 16.5 ng/ml. Thirteen men (34%) in the latter group had a PSA level less than 4.0 ng/ml. However, it is usually the trend in PSA levels, rather than the absolute number, that is a reliable predictor of stabilization or progression in patients receiving hormonal therapy.

In patients who are not responding to hormonal therapy consisting of a luteinizing hormone–releasing hormone analog and the antiandrogen flutamide, cessation of flutamide is associated with a fall in PSA level in a significant number of patients.[61]

Surveillance Strategies

A schema for the follow-up evaluation of patients after either radical prostatectomy or definitive radiation therapy for the treatment of localized prostate cancer is shown in Table 18-2. Initial PSA evaluation is done at 1 month after completion of therapy, although the significance of this value depends on the treatment received. The PSA level should have returned to an undetectable range in men treated by radical prostatectomy, and failure to do so indicates a dire prognosis. The PSA level should be decreased from baseline in men treated by radiation therapy, although

Table 18-2 Follow-up of patients with prostate cancer: Roswell Park Cancer Institute

	YEAR				
	1	2	3	4	5
Office visit*	5	3	2	2	2
Prostate specific antigen	5	3	2	2	2
Complete blood count	1	0	0	0	0
Multichannel blood tests†	1	0	0	0	0
Bone scan	‡	‡	‡	‡	‡
Pelvic computed tomography	‡	‡	‡	‡	‡

*Includes digital rectal examination.
†Consists of sodium, potassium, chloride, carbon dioxide, blood urea nitrogen, creatinine, and glucose.
‡Performed if clinically indicated.

more time will be necessary to determine the nadir value and to predict outcome. A significant increase in PSA level in men treated by radiation therapy indicates progressive metastatic disease.

Thereafter PSA and digital rectal examination are performed every 3 months for the first year after completion of therapy and every 4 months for the second year. In the majority of patients treated by either radical prostatectomy or radiation therapy the outcome of therapy can be predicted with some confidence, since most patients in whom either therapy is unsuccessful have elevated or rising PSA values at this time. PSA and digital rectal examination are performed every 6 months thereafter until 5 years after therapy, at which point I recommend yearly testing.

The role of other studies in routine follow-up is extremely limited. Complete blood count and serum chemistry values are obtained 1 month after completion of therapy to rule out the possibility of any hematological problem or other problems related to therapy. The proposed schedules of PSA and physical examinations also seem appropriate in terms of patient history and in determining whether any significant side effects of therapy have resulted. That is, questions regarding continence or potency can be discussed with the patient at these same intervals, while the issues of bladder or bowel irritative symptoms and potency can be discussed with patients after radiation therapy. After 2 years following completion of therapy, 6-month intervals between evaluations are recommended.

Other diagnostic or imaging studies, such as bone scans and computed tomographic scans, are not recommended for routine follow-up. The only indication for these studies is if clinical symptoms suggestive of recurrent or progressive disease develop, although the likelihood of this occurring in the absence of a significant change in PSA level is remote. This is why these studies are of no value on a routine basis. If a patient has an increase in PSA level and adjuvant therapy is being considered, the policy at Roswell Park

Cancer Institute has been to obtain a bone scan to rule out occult metastatic spread. Computed tomography has no practical value in detecting the site of recurrence in patients with an elevated PSA level after definitive therapy, so its role in this setting must be questioned. While patients should be evaluated on an individual basis, the above schema is adequate and appropriate for the majority of patients.

FUTURE PROSPECTS

If further improvements are to be made in the treatment and outcome of patients with localized prostate cancer, efforts might be better directed to the areas of initial therapy and patient selection than to improvements in surveillance modalities. PSA is close to an ideal tumor marker after completion of definitive therapy for prostate cancer, since many of the problems in diagnosis or staging encountered with this test are obviated when the diagnosis of prostate cancer has been established. Further refinements in the sensitivity of the PSA assay would appear to be of limited benefit unless a resultant treatment strategy is defined. Similarly, there appears to be no role at present for multiinstitutional follow-up trials for prostate cancer unless the role of PSA level in this setting is seriously challenged. Although tremendous advances are being made in the field of molecular genetics, these advances are unlikely to have a significant impact on the follow-up of patients with prostate cancer in the near future.

Since it is often "microscopic" factors that determine outcome in the treatment of patients with localized prostate cancer, refinements in existing imaging modalities will probably not greatly improve the ability to stage patients before therapy or assist in detecting recurrence as a routine surveillance measure. Perhaps techniques such as radioactive labeling of tumor-specific antigens may be helpful in the future, but progress in this area has been slow.

PSA determinations are the basis of follow-up for patients after treatment for localized prostate cancer. This assay has allowed the early detection of persistent or recurrent prostate cancer, but the issue of subsequent therapy, as discussed, is unresolved.

REFERENCES

1. Parker SL, Tong T, Bolden S, Wingo PA. Cancer statistics, 1997. CA Cancer J Clin 1997;47:5-27.
2. Stamey TA. Prostate specific antigen in the diagnosis and treatment of adenocarcinoma of the prostate. Monogr Urol 1989;10:49.
3. Wang MC, Valenzuela LA, Murphy GP, Chu TM. Purification of a human prostate specific antigen. Invest Urol 1979;17:159-63.
4. Myrtle JF. Normal levels of prostate-specific antigen (PSA). In: Clinical aspects of prostate cancer. New York: Elsevier Science Publishing Co., 1989: 83.
5. Oesterling JE. Prostate specific antigen: a critical assessment of the most useful tumor marker for adenocarcinoma of the prostate. J Urol 1991;145:907-23.
6. Bruce AW, Choe BK. Tumor markers in prostatic disease. In: Adenocarcinoma of the prostate. New York: Springer-Verlag, 1987:196.
7. Armitage TG, Cooper EH, Newling WW, Robinson MR, Appleyard I. The value of the measurement of serum prostate specific antigen in patients with benign prostatic hyperplasia and untreated prostate cancer. Br J Urol 1988;62:584-9.
8. Ercole CJ, Lange PH, Mathisen M, Chiou RK, Reddy PK, Vessella RL. Prostatic specific antigen and prostatic acid phosphatase in the monitoring and staging of patients with prostatic cancer. J Urol 1987; 138:1181-4.
9. Lange PH, Ercole CJ, Lightner DJ, Fraley EE, Vessella R. The value of serum prostate specific antigen determinations before and after radical prostatectomy. J Urol 1989;141:873-9.
10. Seamonds B, Yang N, Anderson K, Whitaker B, Shaw LM, Bollinger JR. Evaluation of prostate-specific antigen and prostatic acid phosphatase as prostate cancer markers. Urology 1986;28:472-9.
11. Auriemma PR, Huben RP. Evaluating the role of CT scans in the staging of newly diagnosed prostate cancer. Submitted for publication.
12. American Joint Committee on Cancer, Beahrs OH, Henson DE, Robert VP, Kennedy BJ, editors. Manual for staging of cancer. 4th ed. Philadelphia: JB Lippincott Company, 1992.
13. Austenfeld MA. Treatment of stage A1 prostate cancer: the case for observation. Semin Urol 1993;11:58-63.
14. Bahnson RR. Treatment of stage A1 prostate cancer: the case for treatment. Semin Urol 1993;11:54-7.
15. Chodak GW, Thisted RA, Gerber GS, et al. Results of conservative management of clinically localized prostate cancer. N Engl J Med 1994;330:242-8.
16. Kantoff PW, Talcott JA. The radical prostatectomy series: apples are not oranges. J Clin Oncol 1994;12:2243-5.
17. Lu-Yao GL, McLerran S, Wasson J, Wennberg JE. An assessment of radical prostatectomy: time trends, geographic variation, and outcomes. JAMA 1993;269:2633-6.
18. Reynolds T. Prostate cancer rates climbed sharply in 1990. J Natl Cancer Inst 1993;85:947-8.
19. Lee F, Littrup PJ, Torp-Pederson ST, et al. Prostate cancer: comparison of transrectal US and digital rectal examination for screening. Radiology 1988;168:389-94.
20. Mettlin C, Jones GW, Murphy GP. Trends in prostate cancer care in the United States, 1974-1990: observations from the patient care evaluation studies of the American College of Surgeons Commission on Cancer. CA Cancer J Clin 1993;43:83-91.
21. Walsh PC, Donker PJ. Impotence following radical prostatectomy: insight into etiology and prevention. J Urol 1982,128:492-7.
22. Walsh PC, Lepor H, Eggleston JC. Radical prostatectomy with preservation of sexual function: anatomical and pathological considerations. Prostate 1983;4:473-85.
23. Zincke H, Bergstralh EJ, Blute ML, et al. Radical prostatectomy for clinically localized prostate cancer: long-term results of 1,143 patients from a single institution. J Clin Oncol 1994;12:2254-63.
24. Catalona WJ, Smith DS. 5-year tumor recurrence rates after anatomical radical retropubic prostatectomy for prostate cancer. J Urol 1994;152:1837-42.
25. National Institutes of Health Consensus Development Conferences Statement, June 15-17, 1987. The management of clinically localized prostate cancer. J Urol 1987;138:1369-75.
26. Bagshaw MA. Potential for radiotherapy alone in prostate cancer. Cancer 1985;55:2079-85.
27. Kaplan ID, Cox RS, Bagshaw MA. Prostate specific antigen after external beam radiotherapy for prostatic cancer: follow-up. J Urol 1993;149:519-22.
28. Landmann C, Hunig R. Prostatic specific antigen as an indicator of response to radiotherapy in prostate cancer. Int J Radiat Oncol Biol Phys 1989;17:1073-6.
29. Stamey TA, Ferrari MK, Schmid HP. The value of serial prostate specific antigen determinations 5 years after radiotherapy: steeply increasing values characterize 80% of patients. J Urol 1993;150: 1856-9.
30. Hanks GE, Asbell A, Krall JM, et al. Outcome for lymph node dissection negative T-1b, T-2 (A-2, B) prostate cancer treated with external beam radiation therapy in RTOG 77-06. Int J Radiat Oncol Biol Phys 1991;21:1099-103.
31. Hanks GE, Martz KL, Diamond JJ. The effect of dose on local control of prostate cancer. Int J Radiat Oncol Biol Phys 1988;5:1299-305.

32. Fowler F Jr, Barry MJ, Lu-Yao G, Roman A, Wasson J, Wennberg JE. Patient-reported complications and follow-up treatment after radical prostatectomy: the national Medicare experience; 1988-1990. Urology 1993;42:622-9.
33. Talcott JA, Rieker P, Propert K, et al. Complications of treatment for early prostate cancer: a prospective, multi-institutional outcomes study. Proc Annu Meet Am Soc Clin Oncol 1994;13:A711.
34. Trapasso JG, DeKernion JB, Smith RB, Dorey F. The incidence and significance of detectable levels of serum prostate specific antigen after radical prostatectomy. J Urol 1994;152:1821-5.
35. Onik GM, Cohen JK, Reyes GD, Rubinsky B, Chang Z, Baust J. Transrectal ultrasound-guided percutaneous radical cryosurgical ablation of the prostate. Cancer 1993;72:1291-9.
36. Stamey TA, Graves HC, Wehner N, Ferrari M, Freiha FS. Early detection of residual prostate cancer after radical prostatectomy by an ultrasensitive assay for prostate specific antigen. J Urol 1993;149: 787-92.
37. Partin AW, Pearson JD, Landis PK, et al. Evaluation of serum prostate-specific antigen velocity after radical prostatectomy to distinguish local recurrence from distant metastases. Urology 1994;43:649-59.
38. Partin AW, Pound CR, Clemens JQ, Epstein JI, Walsh PC. Serum PSA after anatomic radical prostatectomy: the Johns Hopkins experience after 10 years. Urol Clin North Am 1993;20:713-25.
39. Oesterling JE, Chan DW, Epstein JI, et al. Prostate specific antigen in the preoperative and postoperative evaluation of localized prostatic cancer treated with radical prostatectomy. J Urol 1988;139:766-72.
40. Frazier HA, Robertson JE, Humphrey PA, Paulson DF. Is prostate specific antigen of clinical importance in evaluating outcome after radical prostatectomy? J Urol 1993;149:516-8.
41. Epstein JI. Surgical margins in patients with carcinoma of the prostate. AUA Update Series 1994;13:53.
42. Goldrath DE, Messing EM. Prostate specific antigen: not detectable despite tumor progression after radical prostatectomy. J Urol 1989;142:1082-4.
43. Takayama TK, Krieger JN, True LD, Lange PH. Recurrent cancer despite undetectable prostate specific antigen. J Urol 1992;148:1541-2.
44. Parra RO, Wolf RM, Huben RP. The use of transrectal ultrasound in the detection and evaluation of local pelvic recurrences after a radical urological pelvic operation. J Urol 1990;144:707-9.
45. Abi-Aad AS, MacFarlane MT, Stein A, DeKernion JB. Detection of local recurrence after radical prostatectomy by prostate specific antigen and transrectal ultrasound. J Urol 1992;147:952-5.
46. Takayama TK, Vessella RL, Brawer MK, Noteboom J, Lange PH. The enhanced detection of persistent disease after prostatectomy with a new prostate specific antigen immunoassay. J Urol 1993;150:374-8.
47. Raminski DA, Huben RP. Adjuvant radiation therapy in the treatment of adenocarcinoma of the prostate following radical prostatectomy. Submitted for publication.
48. Lange PH, Lightner DJ, Medini E, Reddy PK, Vessella RL. The effect of radiation therapy after radical prostatectomy in patients with elevated prostate specific antigen levels. J Urol 1990;144:927-32.
49. Hudson MA, Catalona WJ. Effect of adjuvant radiation therapy on prostate specific antigen following radical prostatectomy. J Urol 1990;143:1174-7.
50. McCarthy JF, Catalona WJ, Hudson MA. Effect of radiation therapy on detectable serum prostate specific antigen levels following radical prostatectomy: early versus delayed treatment. J Urol 1994;151:1575-8.
51. Zagars GK. Prostate specific antigen as an outcome variable for T1 and T2 prostate cancer treated by radiation therapy. J Urol 1994;152:1786-91.
52. Goad JR, Chang SJ, Ohori M, Scardino PT. PSA after definitive radiotherapy for clinically localized prostate cancer. Urol Clin North Am 1993;20:727-36.
53. Zagars GK. Serum PSA as a tumor marker for patients undergoing definitive radiation therapy. Urol Clin North Am 1993;20:737-47.
54. Stamey TA, Kabalin JN, Ferrari M. Prostate specific antigen in the diagnosis and treatment of adenocarcinoma of the prostate. III. Radiation treated patients. J Urol 1989;141:1084-7.
55. Kabalin JN, Hodge KK, McNeal JE, Freiha FS, Stamey TA. Identification of residual cancer in the prostate following radiation therapy: role of transrectal ultrasound guided biopsy and prostate specific antigen. J Urol 1989;142:326-31.
56. Zagars GK. The prognostic significance of a single serum prostate-specific antigen value beyond six months after radiation therapy for adenocarcinoma of the prostate. Int J Radiat Oncol Biol Phys 1993;27:39-45.
57. Pontes JE, Montie J, Klein E, Huben R. Salvage surgery for radiation failure in prostate cancer. Cancer 1993;71(3 Suppl):976-80.
58. Leo ME, Bilhartz DL, Bergstralh EJ, Oesterling JE. Prostate specific antigen in hormonally treated stage D2 prostate cancer: is it always an accurate indicator of disease status? J Urol 1991;145:802-6.
59. Stamey TA, Kabalin JN, Ferrari M, Yang N. Prostate specific antigen in the diagnosis and treatment of adenocarcinoma of the prostate. IV. Anti-androgen treated patients. J Urol 1989;141:1088-90.
60. Miller JI, Ahmann FR, Drach GW, Emerson SS, Bottaccini MR. The clinical usefulness of serum prostate specific antigen after hormonal therapy of metastatic prostate cancer. J Urol 1992;147:956-61.
61. Scher HI, Kelly WK. Flutamide withdrawal syndrome: its impact on clinical trials in hormone-refractory prostate cancer. J Clin Oncol 1993;11:1566-72.

➢ COUNTER POINT

Memorial Sloan-Kettering Cancer Center

GUIDO DALBAGNI AND WILLIAM R. FAIR

Prostate carcinoma is one of the most common cancers. It has been estimated that in 1995 there were 244,000 cases with 40,400 deaths in the United States.[1] Many uncertainties surround prostate cancer. The natural history of the disease is not known. Some tumors behave in an indolent fashion, while others metastasize early. There are uncertainties surrounding the optimal management of prostate cancer as well. Modification of the current modalities of treatment are under way to improve results. Neoadjuvant hormonal treatment has been introduced to improve the rate of organ-confined disease after radical prostatectomy in an attempt to influence final outcome. Three-dimensional conformal radiation therapy has been introduced to enhance results by increasing the dose delivery without increasing morbidity.

PROSTATE SPECIFIC ANTIGEN AND RADICAL PROSTATECTOMY

Radical prostatectomy offers the best chance of cure for clinically localized prostate cancer, especially in men not older than 70 years of age and in otherwise good general health, with a life expectancy of at least 10 years. Overall, survival rates in studies involving highly selected series of patients have been comparable to those in age-matched control patients without prostate cancer.[2]

In a proportion of patients with prostate carcinoma, local recurrence or distant metastasis develops. Epstein et al.[3] followed up 507 men who underwent radical prostatectomy for clinical stages A and B for a mean of 3.9 years (range 1 to 10 years). Of the 507 men, 4.8% had distant metastasis alone,

Table 18-3 Incidence of detectable prostate specific antigen after radical prostatectomy

AUTHORS	ORGAN CONFINED	CAPSULAR PENETRATION	SEMINAL VESICLES INVOLVED	LYMPH NODES INVOLVED	FOLLOW-UP[a] DURATION RANGE	FOLLOW-UP[a] DURATION MEAN	UPPER LIMIT OF NORMAL PSA LEVEL (ng/ml)
Oesterling et al.[4]	4/81 (5%)	5/20 (20%)	21/26[b] (81%)		2-1032	24	0.2
Stamey et al.[5]	3/48 (6%)	2/31 (6.5%)	2/10 (20%)	8/13[c] (61.5%)	4-27	13	0.3[d]
Stein et al.[6]	16/98 (16%)	20/55 (36%)	12/19 (63%)	11/18 (61%)	3-162	45	0.4
Frazier et al.[7]	10/102 (9.8%)	28/71[e] (39.4%)	35/53[f] (66%)		N/A	N/A	0.5
Partin et al.[8]	17/356 (4.8%)	22/194 (11.2%)[g]	34/66 (66%)	54/71 (76%)	12-120[h]	66	0.2

[a]Follow-up in months.
[b]Includes positive seminal vesicles and positive lymph nodes.
[c]The five patients with normal prostate specific antigen levels had either orchiectomy or radiation.
[d]Pros-check.
[e]Includes specimen-confined tumors.
[f] Includes margin-positive tumors.
[g] Established capsular penetration low-grade: 32 of 189 patients (17%). Established capsular penetration high-grade: 26 of 79 (33%).
[h] Follow-up duration for patients without evidence of recurrence is 49 months (range 12 to 120 months).

2% had distant metastasis with local recurrence, and 2.4% experienced only local recurrence. Because of the generally indolent course of prostate cancer, these figures might be an underestimate of the potential failure rate after radical prostatectomy. Indeed, the incidence of recurrences as detected by a rise in the PSA level after surgery is higher.[4-8] Since PSA is produced mainly by the prostatic epithelial cells, a radical prostatectomy eliminates the source of PSA. This results in a decline of the serum level of PSA to an undetectable level if all prostatic tissue including prostatic cancer has been removed. Thus a rise in PSA level indicates residual disease that will eventually manifest itself clinically.

The incidence of biochemical failure as determined by a rise in PSA level occurs in a significant proportion of patients treated by radical prostatectomy, ranging from 19% to 38%. Considering an elevated PSA level as an indication of recurrence, Epstein et al.[3] noted that 23.8% of patients had progressive disease after surgery, with an elevated PSA level as the only evidence of progression in 64% of these men.

In the study by Oesterling et al.,[4] 127 patients underwent radical retropubic prostatectomy and were followed postoperatively with PSA measurements. The interval between surgery and determination of serum PSA levels ranged from 2 months to 8.6 years. A value of less than 0.2 ng/ml was used as reference, since this value represented the upper limit of the female range. Seventy-seven of 81 men with organ-confined prostate cancer had undetectable PSA levels. Fifteen of 20 patients with capsular penetration had undetectable PSA levels. Twenty-one of 26 men with seminal vesicle or lymph node involvement had a PSA value of less than 0.2 ng/ml.

Hudson et al.[9] evaluated the clinical use of postoperative PSA measurements to monitor response to therapy after radical prostatectomy. PSA decreased to an undetectable level (less than 0.6 ng/ml) in 89% of the patients with organ-confined disease, in 87% of those with microscopically positive margins only, and in only 34% of patients with seminal vesicle involvement or positive lymph nodes. The PSA level was obtained within 6 months in 93 patients and more than 6 months after radical prostatectomy in 81 patients, suggesting the possibility that the proportion of patients with an undetectable PSA level after radical prostatectomy might be lower and that those values were inflated by a subset of patients in whom a rising PSA level developed after an initial decrease to an undetectable level. Clinical recurrent disease developed in 80% of patients with a postoperative PSA level greater than 10 ng/ml, while only one patient with an undetectable PSA level has had recurrent disease.

Stamey et al.[5] reported the postoperative PSA values of 97 patients who underwent radical prostatectomy. Eighty-two patients (85%) reached an undetectable level within 3 weeks after radical prostatectomy. PSA was measured by the Yang Pros-Check polyclonal radioimmunoassays, and the undetectable reference range was set at 0.3 ng/ml. With a mean follow-up of 12 months the proportion of patients with biochemical failure increased (Table 18-3).

Frazier et al.[7] noted the presence of biochemical failure in 9.8% of patients with organ-confined disease, 39.4% of patients in the specimen-confined group, and 66% in the margin-positive group. Clinical failure occurred in 3.9% of the first group, 7% of the second group, and 13.2% of the third group. Of the patients who had relapse, the interval from the initial elevation of PSA level to clinical recurrence ranged from 2 to 28 months (median 16 months). Among the patients with a high postoperative PSA level who did not have recurrence the follow-up ranged from 4 to 46 months. Thus the percentage of patients with an elevated postoperative PSA level among those with specimen-confined and margin-positive cancers is similar to the 10-year failure rate in long-term follow-up.

In another study, Stein et al.[10] studied 230 patients who had radical prostatectomy between 1972 and 1989 and whose median follow-up time was only 4 years. Fifty-five patients having surgery were excluded from the study because of node-positive disease. An analysis of patients with node-negative disease was presented. Patients who had pathologically organ-confined disease did extremely well, with an overall actuarial survival rate of 80% at 10 years. However, patients whose tumor involved the capsule or seminal vesicles had a significantly reduced survival rate. Most important in this study, however, was the observation that the clinical disease-free survival rate was significantly altered depending on whether the results of PSA testing were considered in the definition of disease-free survival. If a measurable PSA level is considered an indicator of residual disease, the overall disease-free survival rate is approximately half of that determined by physical examination or imaging studies only. In this group the 5- and 10-year disease-free survival rates were 61% and 41%, respectively. Thus almost 60% of the patients undergoing radical prostatectomy who are found to have pT1 through T3N0M0 disease will have recurrence within 10 years.

Similar results were obtained in a recently published French study by Fendler et al.[11] In this study a detectable PSA level after radical prostatectomy was taken as an indicator of progression. In patients with pathologically staged pT2 disease only 17% had evidence of progression 5 years after surgery. However, in those with disease beyond the prostatic capsule (pT3), 70% had evidence of progression. Thus it is evident that disease beyond the confines of the prostatic capsule indicates an increased risk of progression, which at 5 years after surgery may be in the range of 50% to 70%.

An excellent study addressing this question was published by Morton et al.[12] from the Johns Hopkins Hospital. The investigators reported the rate of clinical failure as determined by standard physical examination and imaging studies and the rate of biological failure, which included PSA values, in a large number of patients after radical prostatectomy. In patients with pathological organ-confined disease at the time of radical prostatectomy, follow-up ranged from 1 to 8.5 years, with a median of 4 years. In 337 patients whose disease was organ confined pathologically, only 3% had evidence of clinical failure with a median 4-year follow-up. However, the failure rate doubled to 6% when a detectable PSA value was included as evidence of biological failure. In 122 patients whose disease was beyond the organ but confined to the specimen the clinical failure rate was 10%. However, the biological failure rate, which included both clinical and PSA end points, was 26%. Most disturbing was that of 254 patients whose disease involved the margin of the specimen, 38% had evidence of failure by standard clinical measurements during the follow-up period. However, when a detectable PSA level was considered as evidence of recurrent disease, 79% of patients with margin-positive disease had evidence of a biological failure.

Partin et al.[8] reported the Johns Hopkins experience, in which 955 men underwent radical prostatectomy with bilateral pelvic lymph node dissection, with an average follow-up time of 4.1 years (range 1 to 10 years) for those without recurrence and 5.6 years (range 1 to 10 years) for those with disease progression. The failure rate was 4.8% for patients with organ-confined disease, 11.2% for patients with focal capsular penetration, 17% for those with established capsular penetration (low-grade), 23% for those with capsular penetration (high-grade), 52% for those with seminal vesicle invasion, and 76% for those with lymph node involvement. Seventy-nine men were followed expectantly until progression for an average of 2.6 years (range 1 to 8 years). Twelve of these patients have local recurrence, 30 have distant metastases, and 57 still have elevations of PSA as the only sign of recurrence. All patients with a clinical recurrence had a detectable PSA level. The reference range for PSA was greater than 0.2 ng/ml.[8]

A close correlation exists between biochemical failure and clinical failure. The lag time between biochemical and clinical failure ranges from a few months to almost 10 years. Several reports in the literature suggest the presence of a direct correlation between the timing of PSA detectability relative to the radical prostatectomy and the detection of local recurrence or distant metastasis. In the study by Hudson et al.,[13] 14 of 93 evaluable patients had a detectable PSA level. Seven patients had a PSA level greater than 0.6 ng/ml at 6 months after surgery, including three (43%) who had clinical recurrence at less than 1 year. Conversely, only one of seven patients (14%) with a detectable PSA level during year 1 of follow-up had a documented clinical recurrence.

In the series by Lange et al.,[14] distant metastasis occurred in six of 59 patients and the PSA level steadily increased 12 to 43 months before metastases were clinically detectable. There was a direct correlation between the PSA level at 3 to 6 months and the disease-free interval. In the two patients with an initial PSA level of less than 0.2 ng/ml, metastasis was found at 54 and 71 months, respectively, while objective recurrence occurred at 11, 13, and 33 months in the patients with an initial PSA level greater than 0.5 ng/ml. Similarly, in the series by Stein et al.,[6] by analyzing the Kaplan-Meier curve in which time to progression in patients with a 6-month detectable PSA value is compared with progression in patients with an undetectable PSA value at 6 months, it was estimated that 70% of patients with early positive PSA values would have progression of disease within the first 3 years.[6]

Similar results were obtained from an excellent study by Frazier et al.[7] at Duke University. The authors also contrasted the clinical failure and PSA (biological failure) at various time points. At a mean follow-up time of slightly greater than 3 years, patients with organ-confined disease at the time of radical prostatectomy had only a 3.9% failure rate; however, the PSA failure rate was more than double the

Table 18-4 Follow-up of patients with prostate cancer: Memorial Sloan-Kettering Cancer Center

	YEAR				
	1	2	3	4	5
Office visit*	4	2	2	2	2
Prostate specific antigen	4	2	2	2	2
Bone scan	†	†	†	†	†
Abdominal computed tomography	†	†	†	†	†
Pelvic computed tomography	†	†	†	†	†

*Includes digital rectal examination.
†Performed if a detectable prostate specific antigen level after radical prostatectomy indicates recurrence.

clinical failure rate (9.8%). As in the Johns Hopkins series, in patients whose disease was specimen confined but beyond the prostatic capsule, 39% had evidence of detectable clinical or PSA failure after radical prostatectomy. In the group with margin-positive disease, although only 13% had clinical evidence of failure after surgery, 68% had a detectable PSA level, indicating a biological failure within the follow-up period. What is most interesting in the studies from Duke University is that the investigators were able to show that the biological or PSA failure rate at 2 years was essentially the same as the clinical failure rate as measured by physical examination or imaging study at 10 years.[15] These data are compelling evidence that early signs of biological failure will translate into clinical evidence of disease progression if follow-up is long enough.

Stein et al.[6] measured PSA levels in 190 patients after radical prostatectomy. None of the patients with an undetectable PSA level have had clinical recurrence within a follow-up period of 41 months, whereas 20 of 59 patients with a detectable PSA level after surgery had clinical progression, with a mean time to progression of 37 months. Once the PSA level becomes detectable, pathological stage and Gleason score no longer provide any prognostic information.

CURRENT PRACTICE

PSA clearly plays a major role in follow-up of patients after a radical prostatectomy at Memorial Sloan-Kettering Cancer Center (Table 18-4). All patients undergo digital rectal examination and serum PSA measurement at 3-month intervals during the first year and at 6-month intervals thereafter. A detectable PSA level after radical prostatectomy is an indication of recurrence, and those patients are evaluated with bone scan or computed tomography of the abdomen and pelvis. If either shows evidence of metastatic disease, the patient receives hormonal therapy. If the metastatic workup is negative, a biopsy of the anastomotic site is performed. If the biopsy is positive, the patient is considered for radiation therapy. However, if the biopsy is negative, hormonal therapy or observation is offered.

Despite the increased enthusiasm for radical prostatectomy, significant clinical understaging exists. Of 139 patients whose disease was detected solely as a result of an elevated PSA evaluation on routine examination or an abnormality in transrectal ultrasound with no concomitant abnormality in digital rectal examination (stage T1c), less than half (49%) were found to have disease confined to the prostate.[16] In a compilation of five series involving almost 1,500 patients with clinical T1 or T2 carcinoma of the prostate (clinically organ-confined disease) who had radical prostatectomy, only 680 (47%) were found to have a tumor confined to the prostate on pathological examination.[4-8] Rosen et al.[17] found that only 37% of 98 patients with clinical stage T2 disease had pathological pT2 disease. In three series with clinical stage B2 disease involving 310 patients the results were even more alarming in that only 87 of 310 patients (28%) had organ-confined disease at the time of radical prostatectomy.[18,19] In summary, then, 53% of tumors thought to be clinically localized (T1 or T2) are beyond the prostate at the time of radical prostatectomy and only 28% of those thought to be clinically B2 are confined to the prostate.

NEOADJUVANT HORMONAL THERAPY BEFORE RADICAL PROSTATECTOMY

PSA elevation after radical prostatectomy often translates into clinical failure, and a significant proportion of patients undergoing radical prostatectomy have extracapsular disease. Moreover, there is a low incidence of biochemical failure after surgery for pathologically organ-confined tumors. By decreasing the understaging errors, physicians could improve the long-term results of radical prostatectomy.

The challenge to the surgeon is to improve the rate of organ-confined disease at the time of radical prostatectomy. Clearly, detection at an earlier stage of the disease when the tumor is confined within the prostate would help in this regard. With the currently available modalities, physicians are unlikely to detect the majority of prostate cancer at a time when the disease is totally confined to the prostate. The alternative strategy would be to downstage the tumor.

The role of preoperative hormonal treatment has been recently addressed. In a nonrandomized trial, Monfette et al.[20] reported on 34 patients who received a luteinizing hormone–releasing hormone (LH-RH) analog in combination with an antiandrogen 3 months before radical prostatectomy. They noted a 30% to 50% reduction in blood loss, as well as a reduction in the size of the prostate. No malignant cells could be detected in 10 specimens. However, this study did not address pathological downstaging. Although some nonrandomized studies have not shown significant downstaging,[21,22] most data show that neoadjuvant hormonal therapy results in pathological downstaging.

Fair et al.[23] reported their results in 69 patients. All patients were treated with goserelin (Zoladex) and flutamide for 3 months before radical prostatectomy. The majority of patients had organ-confined disease (10% had T1 lesions; 71%, T2 tumors; 4%, T3 tumors; and 13%, T2/T3 tumors).

Of those patients, 3 (4%) had no tumors in the specimens and 48 (70%) had organ-confined disease. These results compared favorably with a concurrent control group, with 48% organ-confined disease. The margin positive rate was 10% in patients on the neoadjuvant regimen compared with 33% in the untreated group.

Labrie et al.[24] reported a significant downstaging in patients receiving neoadjuvant therapy with flutamide and leuprolide (Lupron). The controlled randomized trial included 142 patients. Positive surgical margins were reduced from 68.5% in the control arm to 13% in the treatment arm.

Haggman et al.[25] reported the effect of 3 months of LH-RH analog treatment (cyproterone acetate) on pathological stage after radical prostatectomy. This study included 40 patients, 26 with clinical organ-confined disease and 14 with T3 tumors. Eighteen patients (46%) had organ-confined disease and 69% had negative surgical margins. These results compared favorably with those in a group of patients who did not receive the neoadjuvant regimen, 19% of whom had organ-confined disease. Solomon et al.[26] reported a decrease in the positive-margin rate from 35.3% in patients undergoing prostatectomy alone to 11.5% in patients who were treated with 3 months of LH-RH analog with an antiandrogen before surgery. Civantos et al.[27] noted the presence of positive surgical margins in 19% of the specimens exposed to total androgen blockade versus 43% in the untreated group. Furthermore, prostate intraepithelial neoplasia was seen in 35% of patients compared with 82% in the untreated prostate glands.

Whether the neoadjuvant regimen before radical prostatectomy will result in an improvement in the organ-confined and specimen-confined rates will require more clinical investigation. In addition, whether such improvements will translate into an improvement in survival will require a longer follow-up.

THREE-DIMENSIONAL CONFORMAL RADIATION THERAPY

There is significant hazard of local progression after radiation therapy for clinically localized prostate cancer. Perez et al.[28] reported their results on 577 patients who received definitive radiation therapy. All patients were followed for a minimum of 3 years, with a median of 6.5 years. The local failure rate was 12% in stage A2 (five of 41), 17% in stage B (31 of 185), 28% in stage C (93 of 328), and 48% in stage D1 (11 of 23). Shipley et al.[29] reported on 370 patients who were followed for a minimum of 5 years. They showed a 28% incidence of local recurrence by 8 years in patients with stages T3 and T4, while the local recurrence was 8% for stage T2. Local control has also been shown to correlate with survival. Perez et al.[30] have shown that the 10-year survival in patients with stage C disease was 40% in 110 patients with no evidence of recurrence versus 20% in 94 patients with local recurrence alone or combined with distant metastasis.

A significant proportion of patients after radiation therapy will have positive biopsies. Kabalin et al.[31] performed systematic biopsies in 27 men 18 months or more after completion of radiation therapy for localized prostate cancer and correlated their findings with the PSA level. Overall, 93% of the patients had positive biopsies. Eighty-three percent (10 of 12) of the patients with a PSA level less than 10 ng/ml had positive biopsies along with 100% (15 of 15) of the patients with a PSA level exceeding 10 ng/ml.

Dugan et al.[32] performed postirradiation biopsies in 37 men who initially had T3 adenocarcinoma of the prostate. All biopsies were performed in men with no evidence of clinical local failure 24 months or more after completion of external beam radiation. Thirty-eight percent of the patients had positive biopsies. Twenty-one percent of the patients with a PSA level less than 2.5 ng/ml had positive biopsies compared with 71% of patients with a PSA level exceeding 2.5 ng/ml. The predictive value of a positive biopsy on clinical local recurrence or distant metastasis was not available because of the short follow-up period.

The significance of a positive biopsy after radiation therapy is controversial. It is associated with a worse clinical outcome than a negative biopsy, particularly if combined with a rising PSA level. Goad et al.[33] reported on 76 patients treated with interstitial gold seed implantation with external beam therapy (68 patients) or external beam radiation alone (eight patients). Fifty-six percent of the patients had a positive postradiation biopsy, and 18% had progression after a median follow-up time of 27 months (range 6 to 60 months). Clinical progression was detected in 46% of patients (12 of 26) with a positive biopsy and a rising PSA level. Furthermore, Stamey et al.[34] reported on 113 patients in whom PSA was tested after radiation therapy. At a mean follow-up of 5 years, 78% had a rising PSA level. They concluded that only a small proportion of patients with localized cancer can be cured by radiation therapy.

The technique of irradiation does play an important role in clinical local control. Perez et al.[30] have shown that patients with stage C disease receiving doses higher than 6,500 cGy had a probability of failure of 25% compared with 44% in patients receiving 6,000 to 6,500 cGy. Thus a higher dose results in better local control.

Three-dimensional conformal therapy has been introduced to increase the accuracy of dose delivery to the prostate and at the same time avoid normal tissues through the use of multiple beam angles. This approach allows an increase in the dose delivered, enhancing local tumor control without significantly increasing the complication rate. Leibel et al.[35] presented preliminary results of a phase I dose-escalation study using three-dimensional conformal radiation therapy in localized prostate cancer. One hundred twenty-three patients were treated, with 28 receiving 75.6 Gy. The median follow-up was 15.2 months. The radiation was well tolerated; only 32% of patients had grade 2 and 3 morbidity. The PSA level normalized in 67% of patients within 14 months. More recently Leibel et al.[36] reported an update of their initial results, showing that the 3-year actuarial probability of survival with a normal PSA level was 97% for T1c and T2a tumors, 86% with T2b, 60% with T2c, and 43% for T3 disease. Whether three-dimensional conformal therapy will result in improvement in local control after radiation therapy will require further clinical investigations and a longer follow-up.

After three-dimensional conformal radiation therapy, patient follow-up is similar to that recommended after radical prostatectomy. Bone scanning and computed tomography are performed if the PSA level rises. If the bone or computed tomographic scan shows evidence of metastatic disease, the patient is started on hormonal therapy. If the metastatic workup is negative, TRUS with biopsy is performed. If the biopsy is negative, the patient is offered hormonal therapy or observation. If the biopsy is positive, hormonal therapy, observation, or cryosurgical ablation of the prostate is considered.

REFERENCES

1. Wingo PA, Tong T, Bolden S. Cancer statistics 1995. CA Cancer J Clin 1995;45:8-30.
2. Gibbons RP, Correa RJ Jr, Brannen GE, Mason JT. Total prostatectomy for localized prostatic cancer. J Urol 1984;131:73-6.
3. Epstein JI, Pizov G, Walsh PC. Correlation of pathologic findings with progression after radical retropubic prostatectomy. Cancer 1993;71:3582-93.
4. Oesterling JE, Chan DW, Epstein JI, et al. Prostate specific antigen in the preoperative and postoperative evaluation of localized prostatic cancer treated with radical prostatectomy. J Urol 1988;139:766-72.
5. Stamey TA, Kabalin JN, McNeal JE, et al. Prostate specific antigen in the diagnosis and treatment of adenocarcinoma of the prostate. II. Radical prostatectomy treated patients. J Urol 1989;141:1076-83.
6. Stein A, deKernion JB, Dorey F. Prostatic specific antigen related to clinical status 1 to 14 years after radical prostatectomy. Br J Urol 1991;67:626-31.
7. Frazier HA, Robertson JE, Humphrey PA, Paulson DF. Is prostate specific antigen of clinical importance in evaluating outcome after radical prostatectomy. J Urol 1993;149:516-8.
8. Partin AW, Pound CR, Clemens JQ, Epstein JI, Walsh PC. Serum PSA after anatomic radical prostatectomy: the Johns Hopkins experience after 10 years. Urol Clin North Am 1993;20:713-25.
9. Hudson MA, Bahnson RR, Catalona WJ. Clinical use of prostate specific antigen in patients with prostate cancer. J Urol 1989;142:1011-7.
10. Stein A, deKernion JB, Smith RB, Dorey F, Patel H. Prostate specific antigen levels after radical prostatectomy in patients with organ confined and locally extensive prostate cancer. J Urol 1992;147:942-6.
11. Fendler JP, Dujardin T, Bringeon G, Adeleine P, Devonec M, Perrin P. [Progression after radical prostatectomy of cancer of the prostate: prognostic criteria and the role of PSA in monitoring.] (in French) Prog Urol 1992;2:58-65.
12. Morton RA, Steiner MS, Walsh PC. Cancer control following anatomical radical prostatectomy: an interim report. J Urol 1991;145:1197-200.
13. Lange PH, Ercole CJ, Lightner DJ, Fraley EE, Vessella RL. The value of serum prostate specific antigen determinations before and after radical prostatectomy. J Urol 1989;141:873-9.
14. Paulson DF, Moul JW, Walther PJ. Radical prostatectomy for clinical stage T1-2N0M0 prostatic adenocarcinoma: long-term results. J Urol 1990;145:1180-4.
15. Epstein JI, Walsh PC, Carmichael M, Brendler CB. Pathologic and clinical findings to predict tumor extent of nonpalpable (Stage T1c) prostate cancer. JAMA 1994:271:368-74.
16. Rosen MA, Goldstone L, Lapin S, Wheeler T, Scardino PT. Frequency and location of extracapsular extension and positive surgical margins in radical prostatectomy specimens. J Urol 1992;148:331-7.
17. Catalona WJ, Bigg SW. Nerve-sparing radical prostatectomy: evaluation of results after 250 patients. J Urol 1990;143:538-44.
18. Walsh PC, Lepor H. The role of radical prostatectomy in the management of prostatic cancer. Cancer 1987;60(3 Suppl):526-37.
19. Monfette G, Dupont A, Labrie F. Temporary combination therapy with flutamide and tryptex as adjuvant to radical prostatectomy for the treatment of early stage prostate cancer. In: Labrie F, editor. Early stage prostate cancer: diagnosis and choice of therapy. New York: Elsevier Science Publishers B.V., 1989:41.
20. Schulman CC, Sassine AM. Neoadjuvant hormonal deprivation before radical prostatectomy. Eur Urol 1993;24:450-5.
21. MacFarlane MT, Abi-Aad A, Stein A, Danella J, Belldegrun A, deKernion JB. Neoadjuvant hormonal deprivation in patients with locally advanced prostate cancer. J Urol 1993;150:132-4.
22. Fair WR, Aprikian AG, Cohen D, Sogani P, Reuter V. Use of neoadjuvant androgen deprivation therapy in clinically localized prostate cancer. Clin Invest Med 1993;16:516-22.
23. Labrie F, Dupont A, Cusan L, et al. Downstaging of localized prostate cancer by neoadjuvant therapy with flutamide and lupron: the first controlled and randomized trial. Clin Invest Med 1993;16:499-509.
24. Haggman M, Hellstrom M, Aus G, et al. Neoadjuvant GnRH-agonist treatment (triptorelin and cyproterone acetate for flare protection) and total prostatectomy. Eur Urol 1993;24:456-60.
25. Solomon MH, McHugh TA, Dorr RP, Lee F, Siders DB. Hormone ablation therapy as neoadjuvant treatment to radical prostatectomy. Clin Invest Med. 1993;16:532-8.
26. Civantos F, Marcial MA, Banks ER, et al. Pathology of androgen deprivation therapy in prostate carcinoma: a comparative study of 173 patients. Cancer 1995;75:1634-41.
27. Perez CA, Pilepich MV, Garcia D, Simpson JR, Zivnuska F, Hederman MA. Definitive radiation therapy in carcinoma of the prostate localized to the pelvis: experience at the Mallinckrodt Institute of Radiology. NCI Monogr 1988;7:85-94.
28. Shipley WU, Prout Jr GR, Coachman NM, et al. Radiation therapy for localized prostate carcinoma: experience at the Massachusetts General Hospital (1973-1981). NCI Monogr 1988;7:67-73.
29. Perez CA, Pilepich MV, Zivnuska F. Tumor control in definitive irradiation of localized carcinoma of the prostate. Int J Radiat Oncol Biol Phys 1986;12:523-31.
30. Kabalin JN, Hodge KK, McNeal JE, Freiha FS, Stamey TA. Identification of residual cancer in the prostate following radiation therapy: role of transrectal ultrasound guided biopsy and prostate specific antigen. J Urol 1989;142:326-31.
31. Dugan TC, Shipley WU, Young RH, et al. Biopsy after external beam radiation therapy for adenocarcinoma of the prostate: correlation with original histological grade and current prostate specific antigen levels. J Urol 1991;146:1313-6.
32. Goad JR, Chang SJ, Ohori M, Scardino PT. PSA after definitive radiotherapy for clinically localized prostate cancer. Urol Clin North Am 1993;20:727-36.
33. Stamey TA, Ferrari MK, Schmid HP. The value of serial prostate specific antigen determinations 5 years after radiotherapy: steeply increasing values characterize 80% of patients. J Urol 1993;150: 1856-9.
34. Leibel SA, Heimann R, Kutcher GJ, et al. Three-dimensional conformal radiation therapy in locally advanced carcinoma of the prostate: preliminary results of a phase I dose-escalation study. Int J Radiat Oncol Biol Phys 1993;28:55-65.
35. Leibel SA, Zelefsky MJ, Kuthcher GJ, Burman CM, Kelson S, Fuks Z. Three-dimensional conformal radiation therapy in localized carcinoma of the prostate: interim report of a phase 1 dose-escalation study. J Urol 1994;152:1792-8.

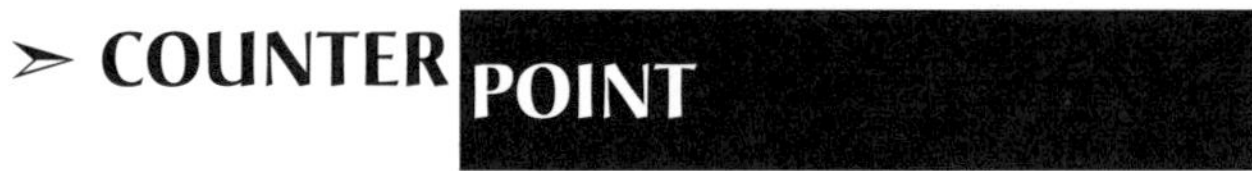

➢ COUNTERPOINT

National Cancer Center Hospital, Japan

TADAO KAKIZOE

Prostate cancer is common in Western countries but has been relatively uncommon in Asia[1] (Figures 18-1 and 18-2). Now, however, a sharp increase in prostate cancer is developing in Japan[1] (Table 18-5, Figure 18-3). This has been attributed to the rapidly increasing number of elderly and to a change from a traditional Japanese diet to a Western diet. In addition, increasing public awareness of prostate cancer and traditional screening efforts targeted at early detection of gastric, cervical, pulmonary, mammary, and colon cancers in Japan may be having an effect on the number of reported cases. Consequently the prevention, diagnosis, treatment, and follow-up of prostate cancer have come to constitute one of the most important health issues in Japan.

Until recently the diagnosis of prostate cancer in Japan relied on digital rectal examination, the assay of serum prostatic acid phosphatase, and the blind, finger-guided core needle biopsy procedure. Recent improvements in the methods of diagnosis include assay for serum PSA,[2] digital rectal examination, TRUS, and TRUS-guided core needle biopsy using a biopsy gun. Random biopsy of a digital rectal examination–indicated nodule-free prostate is now commonly conducted for patients over 55 who have elevated PSA levels. As a consequence the diagnostic procedure for determining the presence of prostate cancer has become much more precise and systematic. However, accurate determination of the stage of development of prostate cancer is still imperfect. The follow-up of prostate cancer has also changed remarkably. Patient age, stage of cancer at the time of treatment, and grade of primary tumor are important in the design of follow-up strategies.

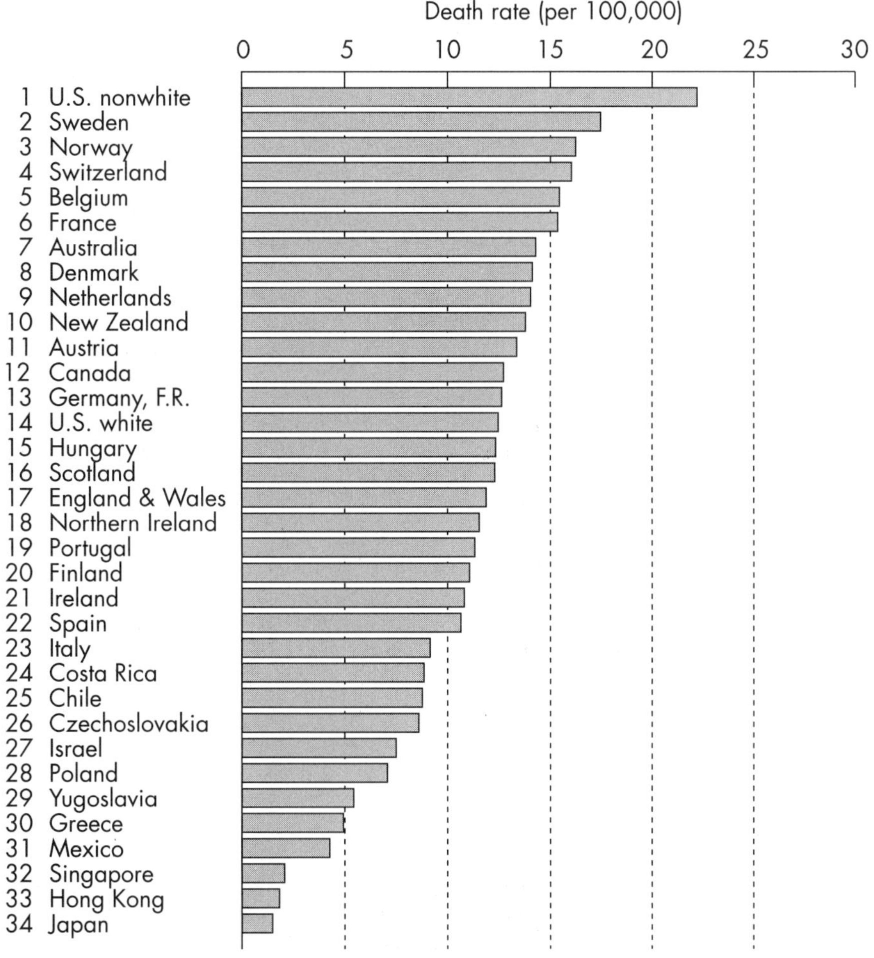

Figure 18-1 Age-adjusted death rates of prostate cancer in 1963-1967. (From Tominaga S, Aoki K, Hanai A, Kurihara N, editors. White paper on cancer statistics. Tokyo: Shinohara Press, 1993.)

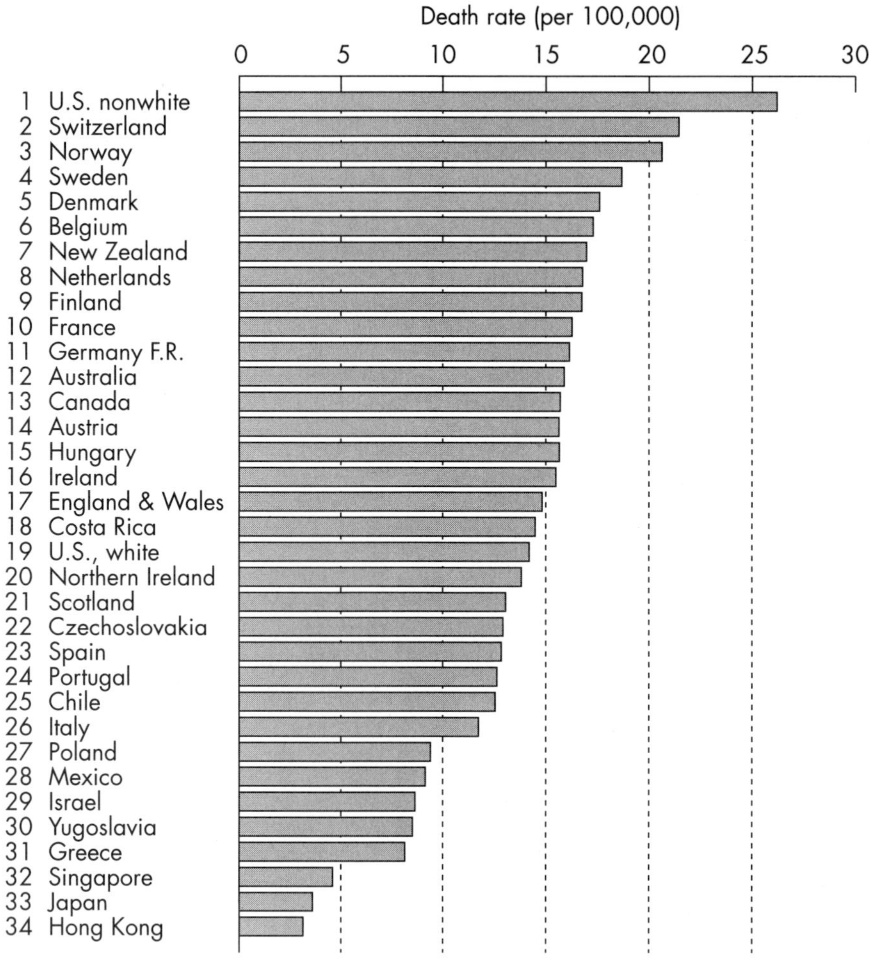

Figure 18-2 Age-adjusted death rates of prostate cancer in 1983-1987. (From Tominaga S, Aoki K, Hanai A, Kurihara N, editors. White paper on cancer statistics. Tokyo: Shinohara Press, 1993.)

Table 18-5 Prostate cancer mortality statistics in Japan (1950-1990)

YEAR	NO. OF DEATHS	CRUDE DEATH RATE PER 100,000	AGE-ADJUSTED DEATH RATE PER 100,000*	AVERAGE AGE AT DEATH IN YEARS	YEAR	NO. OF DEATHS	CRUDE DEATH RATE PER 100,000	AGE-ADJUSTED DEATH RATE PER 100,000*	AVERAGE AGE AT DEATH IN YEARS
1950	83	0.2	0.5	66.5	1971	886	1.7	3.0	72.6
1951	128	0.3	0.6	64.5	1972	975	1.9	3.3	72.8
1952	147	0.4	0.8	67.5	1973	1,107	2.1	3.6	73.5
1953	196	0.5	1.0	67.6	1974	1,179	2.2	3.7	73.3
1954	235	0.5	1.2	65.8	1975	1,267	2.3	3.8	73.7
1955	273	0.6	1.3	68.1	1976	1,296	2.3	3.8	73.7
1956	305	0.7	1.5	69.3	1977	1,448	2.6	4.1	74.5
1957	358	0.8	1.8	69.6	1978	1,499	2.7	4.0	74.5
1958	431	1.0	2.1	70.6	1979	1,666	2.9	4.4	74.9
1959	453	1.0	2.2	70.9	1980	1,736	3.0	4.4	75.0
1960	480	1.1	2.2	71.0	1981	1,866	3.2	4.6	75.4
1961	487	1.1	2.3	71.8	1982	2,053	3.5	4.8	75.7
1962	578	1.2	2.5	70.5	1983	2,168	3.7	4.9	76.1
1963	599	1.3	2.6	71.1	1984	2,315	3.9	5.1	76.3
1964	703	1.5	3.0	72.4	1985	2,640	4.5	5.6	76.8
1965	683	1.4	2.8	71.1	1986	2,756	4.6	5.6	76.4
1966	717	1.5	2.9	72.2	1987	2,969	5.0	5.8	76.9
1967	730	1.5	2.9	72.0	1988	3,035	5.1	5.7	77.0
1968	825	1.7	3.1	72.2	1989	3,420	5.7	6.1	76.6
1969	937	1.9	3.4	72.3	1990	3,460	5.8	6.0	77.2
1970	883	1.8	3.2	72.6					

From Tominaga S, Aoki K, Hanai A, Kurihara N, editors. White paper on cancer statistics. Tokyo: Shinohara Press, 1993.
*Standardized on the age distribution of the model population for the year 1985 in Japan.

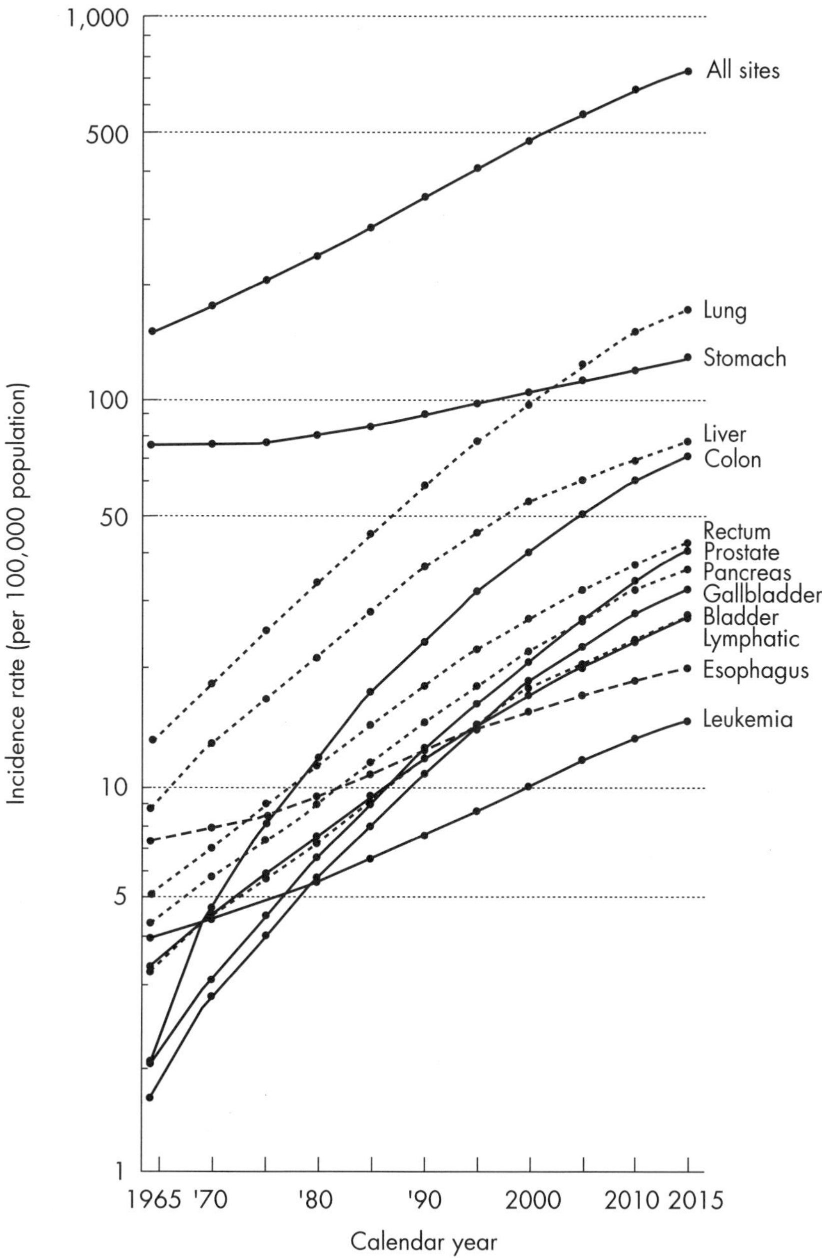

Figure 18-3 Prediction of crude incidence rates according to primary site for men in Japan. (From Tominaga S, Aoki K, Hanai A, Kurihara N, editors. White paper on cancer statistics. Tokyo: Shinohara Press, 1993.)

DIAGNOSIS

The staging system commonly used in Japan is the Japanese Urological Association (JUA) system,[3] adapted from the TNM and Whitmore-Jewett systems. Hereafter the TNM system is used for description. The JUA grading system, which uses the three classification criteria of well-, moderately, and poorly differentiated, is used in the text. Various PSA assay procedures are used in Japan, and a comparison[4] of these is provided in Table 18-6. Patients usually visit a urology clinic because of difficulty in voiding or are referred by a general practitioner who has detected an elevated PSA level.

When an abnormal nodule, increased consistency of the prostate, or an irregular prostatic capsule is detected by digital rectal examination or if the PSA level or TRUS findings are abnormal, TRUS-guided core biopsies are performed. Sextant biopsies are used at many institutions. Patients with elevated PSA levels but no abnormal digital rectal examination findings are also examined by means of TRUS-guided core biopsies, usually sextant biopsies. Once a diagnosis of prostate cancer is established by histological examination, the spread of the disease is ascertained by chest x-ray, bone scintigraphy, abdominal and pelvic computed tomography, complete blood count, and biochemistry, including total pro-

Table 18-6 Comparison of assay systems for detecting serum prostate specific antigen values

ASSAY SYSTEM	1 MARKIT-F PA	2 MARKIT-M PA	3 EIKEN PA	4 WAKO PA
Production	Dai-nihon Pharmaceutical	Dai-nihon Pharmaceutical	EIKEN Chemical	Wako Fine Chemical
Distributor	Dai-nihon Pharmaceutical	Dai-nihon Pharmaceutical	EIKEN Chemical	Wako Fine Chemical
Principle	EIA competition	EIA one-step sandwich	RIA double antibody	EIA one-step sandwich
	PoAb	MoAb	PoAb	MoAb
	Anti rabbit-IgG	MoAb	Anti rabbit-IgG	PoAb
	β-Gal	HRP	^{125}I	HRP
Detection range (ng/ml)	1.5-300	0.5-100	1.0-100	10-320
Normal level (ng/ml)	3.6	3.6	3.0	19.0

From Kuriyama M, Akimoto S, Akaza H, et al. Jpn J Clin Oncol 1992;22:393-9.
EIA, Enzyme immunoassay; *RIA*, radioimmunoassay; *TRFIA*, time-resolved fluoroimmunoassay; *PoAb*, polyclonal antibody; *MoAb*, monoclonal antibody; *IgG*, immunoglobulin G; *HRP*, horseradish peroxide; *ALP*, alkaline phosphatase; *Eu*, europium.

tein, albumin, blood urea nitrogen, creatinine, alkaline phosphatase, and liver function tests. For T4 disease, drip infusion pyelography is also included for evaluation of the upper urinary tract. Pyelography is usually omitted for other stages.

Although lymph node status is generally evaluated by pelvic computed tomography, this examination has limited diagnostic value except when lymph nodes are grossly enlarged. Consequently lymph node status is also frequently examined by laparoscopic surgery, minilaparotomy, or ordinary lymph node dissection by open surgery. Lymphangiography is not commonly performed because of the technical difficulty involved and low sensitivity.

TREATMENT

Prostate cancer is characterized by the extreme variability of its natural history and the heterogeneity of its histological pattern. Currently stage and grade provide the most reliable prognostic information.

T1a prostate cancer (focal low-grade adenocarcinoma of the prostate) is usually detected at the time of transurethral resection of the enlarged prostate gland because of difficulty in voiding. The treatment of patients with T1a prostate cancer and postoperative PSA levels between 1 and 10 is open to question.[5] In such circumstances rapidity of change in the PSA level is a critical factor in determining subsequent treatment. The age and general health of a patient are also important factors. Patients who have a life expectancy of 10 years or less usually are followed up by surveillance alone.

Patients who have high-grade T1b, T1c, or T2 prostate cancer are usually treated by radical prostatectomy. Ten years ago radical prostatectomy was a rather rare operation in Japan. With the dramatic increase in patient load and modernization of diagnostic procedures, however, radical prostatectomy is becoming common.

Definitive radiation therapy has not gained popularity in Japan. One reason is that surgical treatment traditionally has been the most powerful modality[6]; another reason is the unsatisfactory centralization of radiation equipment. As a consequence, radiation therapy is most frequently used for palliation of painful bone metastases. Radiation therapy is carried out with curative intent for T1 and T2 prostate cancer patients at a limited number of institutions. Radiation therapy, with or without endocrine therapy, is common for patients with T3 prostate cancer or N-positive prostate cancer.

Researchers at the National Cancer Center Hospital organized a randomized clinical trial involving 100 patients undergoing neoadjuvant endocrine therapy and either radical prostatectomy or definitive radiotherapy, followed by a resumption of endocrine therapy for T2C and T3 lesions.[7] Neoadjuvant endocrine therapy for 2 months resulted in shrinkage of the prostate and lowering of PSA levels. With the exception of two patients, one of whom died from progression of the disease and the other dying because of a separate and subsequent cancer, all the patients are alive, with an average follow-up period of 25 (range 3 to 53) months. Another 5 years is required for the study to mature.

Endocrine treatment is usually used for patients with T4, N-positive, or M1 prostate cancer. In past decades the treatment of choice was orchiectomy with or without diethylstilbestrol diphosphate. Estrogen therapy was not toxic and did not appear to have as many adverse effects in Japanese patients as in Western patients. However, the number of patients with such complications is now increasing in Japan. Again, change in diet from traditional Japanese to Western may be responsible. Consequently the popularity of estrogen therapy is now on the decrease. Physicians at the National Cancer Center Hospital now have a wide selection of such endocrine therapies as antiandrogens, LH-RH agonists, and total androgen blockade using a combination of

5 BALL ELSA PSA	6 E-TEST TOSOH II PA	7 PROS-CHECK PSA	8 DELFIA PSA	9 TANDEM-R PSA
CIS Bio (France)	Tosoh	Yang Laboratory (USA)	Pharmacia (Sweden)	Hybritec (USA)
CIS Japan	Tosoh	Fuji Chemical	Pharmacia Japan	Baxter
IRMA one-step sandwich	EIA one-step sandwich	RIA double antibody	TRFIA sandwich	IRMA sandwich
MoAb	MoAb	PoAb	MoAb	MoAb
MoAb	MoAb	Anti rabbit-IgG	MoAb	MoAb
^{125}I	Magnet-ALP	^{125}I	Eu	^{125}I
0.2-130	0.5-33.1	0.5-50	0.1-500	0.2-100
2.0	2.0	2.5	11.7	4.0

Table 18-7 Medical costs (charges) of prostate cancer management procedures

PROCEDURE	COST (U.S. $)*
Radical prostatectomy	2,130
Transurethral resection	1,090
High-energy radiation therapy	95/session
Orchiectomy	220
Luteinizing hormone–releasing hormone agonist	752/injection
Diethylstilbestrol	1/tablet
Antiandrogen	2/tablet
Computed tomographic scan	110
Bone scintigram	250
Prostate specific antigen	28
Transrectal ultrasound	50
Frozen histopathology	250

*Calculated at Y100 = U.S. $1.00.

Table 18-8 Follow-up of patients with prostate cancer: National Cancer Center Hospital, Japan

	YEAR				
	1	2	3	4	5
Office visit*	5	4	4	3	3
Prostate specific antigen	5	4	4	3	3
Complete blood count	2	1	1	1	2
Multichannel blood tests†	2	1	1	1	1
Urinalysis	2	1	1	1	1
Alpha-fetoprotein	1	1	1	1	1
CEA	1	1	1	1	1
CA 19-9	1	1	1	1	1
Chest x-ray	1	1	1	1	1
Bone scan	‡	‡	‡	‡	‡
Abdominal computed tomography	‡	‡	‡	‡	‡
Pelvic computed tomography	‡	‡	‡	‡	‡
X-ray of kidneys, ureter, and bladder with drip infusion pyelography	‡	‡	‡	‡	‡

CEA, Carcinoembryonic antigen.
*Includes digital rectal examination.
†Consists of total protein, albumin, total bilirubin, blood urea nitrogen, creatinine, sodium, potassium, chloride, calcium, glutamic-oxaloacetic transaminase, glutamic-pyruvic transaminase, alkaline phosphatase, and lactic dehydrogenase.
‡Performed only if clinically indicated or if prostate specific antigen levels increase.

such therapies. In such circumstances PSA level is useful in monitoring therapy effectiveness. The frequent use of LH-RH agonists, which are expensive, may have a strong influence on medical expenditures and Japan's national medical health insurance system.

FOLLOW-UP

The frequency and intensity of follow-up studies are rather arbitrarily determined by urologists in Japan without serious consideration of the cost effectiveness of each examination. This is because all patients are primarily covered by some type of health insurance. Patients with prostate cancer are followed up for various reasons. For patients who have received radical prostatectomy, early detection of local recurrences[8,9] will possibly provide an opportunity for subsequent radiation therapy[10] to the prostatic bed. For patients who have received definitive radiation therapy for localized disease, local recurrence could be the target for salvage prostatectomy.[11] For patients undergoing continued endocrine therapy for advanced disease, evidence of exacerbation would provide an opportunity to either modify endocrine therapy or add radiation therapy. For patients with T1a prostate cancer simply under surveillance the addition of endocrine therapy, surgery, or radiation therapy could be considered; for patients initially treated by various modalities the detection of metastases at any stage indicates the possibility for endocrine therapy or radiation therapy.

PSA measurements have significantly simplified the follow-up of patients after various treatments and obviated the necessity for almost all other examinations. After radical prostatectomy and definitive radiation therapy for localized prostate cancers, serial determination of PSA levels and repeated digital rectal examination are the most critical indicators of tumor recurrence and distant metastases. PSA measurement and digital rectal examination are carried out every 3 months in the initial year, every 4 months in the second and third years, and every 6 months thereafter through the fifth to perhaps the tenth years. Complete blood count and liver function tests are performed throughout the same period. Bone scintigraphy and computed tomography are conducted when PSA levels begin to rise or when specific signs or symptoms indicate their necessity. After endocrine therapy commences, PSA measurement is the most sensitive and reliable procedure for follow-up examination.

Medical expenses for typical procedures conducted in the management of prostate cancer in Japan are listed in Table 18-7. Patients pay 10% to 30% of these charges, depending on the type of insurance they have, and the rest is covered by insurance. Reimbursement for such charges is extremely low, leading to pressure from the JUA and Japanese Hospital Association on the Ministry of Health and Welfare of Japan for upward revisions. Thus cost considerations affect follow-up decision making at several levels.

The number of times each modality should be requested each year for prostate cancer patients for follow-up after definitive therapy is indicated in Table 18-8. The strategy is similar to that at Roswell Park Cancer Institute. An exception is the effort to detect second malignancies, which was previously described. Routine practice at the National Cancer Center Hospital in Tokyo includes complete blood count, chemistries, and urinalysis as part of the general health checkup. Studies with tumor markers such as alpha-fetoprotein, carcinoembryonic antigen, and CA 19-9, as well as chest x-rays, are performed annually for the detection of second malignancies. Liver, colon, pancreas, and lung cancers have sharply increased in Japanese men recently, and approximately 10% of patients treated for primary cancer at the National Cancer Center Hospital have second malignancies. Bone scanning; computed tomography; x-ray of the kidney, ureter, and bladder with drip infusion pyelography; and other examinations are used only when clinically indicated or when PSA levels increase for the detection of recurrences or metastases of prostate cancer.

REFERENCES

1. Tominaga S, Aoki K, Hanai A, Kurihara N, editors. [White paper on cancer statistics.] (in Japanese) Tokyo: Shinohara Press, 1993.
2. Wang MC, Valenzuela LA, Murphy GP, Chu TM. Purification of a human prostate specific antigen. Invest Urol 1979;17:159-63.
3. Japanese Urological Association, The Japanese Pathological Society: general rules for clinical and pathological studies on prostate cancer. Tokyo: Kanehara Press, 1985.
4. Kuriyama M, Akimoto S, Akaza H, et al. Comparison of various assay systems for prostate-specific antigen standardization. Jpn J Clin Oncol 1992;22:393-9.
5. Partin AW, Pound CR, Clemens JQ, Epstein JI, Walsh PC. Serum PSA after anatomic radical prostatectomy: the Johns Hopkins experience after 10 years. Urol Clin North Am 1993;20:713-25.
6. Figures on cancer in Japan. Kakizoe T, editor. Tokyo Foundation for Promotion of Cancer Research. 1993:18.
7. Isaka S, Shimazaki J, Akimoto S, et al. A prospective randomized trial for treating stages B2 and C prostate cancer: radical surgery or irradiation with neoadjuvant endocrine therapy. Jpn J Clin Oncol 1994;24:218-23.
8. Catalona WJ, Smith DS. 5-Year tumor recurrence rates after anatomical radical retropubic prostatectomy for prostate cancer. J Urol 1994;152:1837-42.
9. Stamey TA, Graves HC, Wehner N, Ferrari M, Freiha FS. Early detection of residual prostate cancer after radical prostatectomy by an ultrasensitive assay for prostate specific antigen. J Urol 1993;149:787-92.
10. Lange PH, Lightner DJ, Medini E, Reddy PK, Vessella RL. The effect of radiation therapy after radical prostatectomy in patients with elevated prostate specific antigen levels. J Urol 1990;144:927-32.
11. Pontes JE, Montie J, Klein E, Huben R. Salvage surgery for radiation failure in prostate cancer. Cancer 1993;71:976-80.

➢ COUNTER POINT

University of Washington Medical Center

THOMAS K. TAKAYAMA AND PAUL H. LANGE

The primary chapter is divided into three main sections: staging, treatment, and follow-up of prostate carcinoma. In the first section Huben presents basic information regarding the uses of PSA, digital rectal examination, prostatic acid phosphatase, bone scan, computed tomography, and lymphangiography in the diagnosis and staging of prostate carcinoma. Subsequently therapeutic options are presented, including radical prostatectomy, radiation therapy, and cryosurgery. In the second section, follow-up procedures including the use of PSA level, TRUS-guided needle biopsy of the urethrovesical anastomosis, and bone scan are discussed.

DIAGNOSIS AND STAGING

It is now evident that the use of PSA has significantly improved physicians' ability to diagnose prostate cancer. However, a slightly elevated PSA level (PSA less than 10 ng/ml) is still unable to distinguish accurately between prostate cancer and benign enlargement of the prostate. Alternatives including PSA density, PSA velocity, age-specific PSA, and various molecular forms of PSA have addressed this problem.[1-5] Unfortunately, these methods are not foolproof and are generally used only as rough guidelines in the evaluation of a particular patient. In the future, better diagnostic tests and tumor markers, including those based on molecular biology,[6] may improve the ability not only to detect cancer, but also to understand its potential for developing metastatic disease.

Once the diagnosis of prostate cancer has been made, staging of disease can be viewed in two separate ways: classic staging or evaluation of possible spread of disease outside of the prostate versus determination of whether the cancer is significant with high risk of progression or insignificant with no effect on survival or quality of life. With regard to classic staging, Huben describes the significant information available on the use of PSA levels. Other tests besides PSA can be performed in the staging of prostate cancer. We agree with Huben that computed tomography or magnetic resonance imaging should not be included in the routine evaluation of men with prostate cancer. We would also add bone scanning to this list because the chance of detecting metastatic disease by these methodologies is infinitely small if the PSA level is below 10 ng/ml, the tumor is low to moderate grade, and digital rectal examination demonstrates less than stage C disease.[7-10] Therefore only when PSA levels are greater than or equal to 10 ng/ml or the patient has high-grade disease or evidence of stage T3 (or greater) disease would a bone scan for staging be recommended.

The question of whether a cancer is clinically significant is an entirely different aspect of staging. Small, low-grade cancers are generally believed to be insignificant, based primarily on autopsy data. However, the true natural history of these low-grade cancers is not known and may change with time. Many of the currently detected cancers are small and of low or moderate tumor grade. Unfortunately, current technology cannot clearly separate these tumors into those that will subsequently metastasize and those that will never spread. Recently investigators from the Mayo Clinic devised a nomogram that could help predict clinically insignificant prostate cancer.[11] To use this nomogram, the patient's age, initial cancer volume, pathological Gleason grade, and tumor doubling time are required. With an arbitrary doubling time of 3 years, the authors found that only 3.9% of 337 patients who underwent radical prostatectomy in their series would have been considered to have clinically insignificant tumors. These investigators made several arguable assumptions. For example, a tumor volume of 20 cm^3 was chosen as the end point for significant tumor size at the end of one's life expectancy. Clearly, further research is necessary to determine the efficacy of such nomograms. Nevertheless, such studies are essential for predicting which patients with prostate cancer would benefit from therapeutic intervention. The various issues regarding screening of the normal population for prostate cancer are complex and beyond the scope of this commentary.[12]

TREATMENT OPTIONS

The therapeutic options for prostate cancer are evolving, and the correct choice or appropriate therapy may be controversial. For example, for localized low- to moderate-grade cancers, many investigators are asking whether watchful waiting or therapeutic intervention is better. The discussions on both sides of this argument are beyond the scope of this commentary, but because of lack of prospective randomized trials neither side has definitive proof. For this reason the Prostate Cancer Intervention Versus Observation Trial that is currently under way should be supported.[12]

The data supporting either radical prostatectomy or radiation therapy for the management of localized cancer are also complex. In general, radiation therapy is recommended for patients who are poor candidates for radical prostatectomy. Consequently, comparing the efficacy of these modalities in retrospective studies in the past is often unreliable. Furthermore, since patients treated by primary radiation therapy do not have complete pathological data, the precise staging of the patients is difficult. Recent studies have used preoperative PSA levels to help predict patients who are more likely to be cured with either modality.[13,14] As expected, patients with PSA levels greater than 10 to 13 ng/ml tend to have a greater risk of recurrence than those with lower PSA levels, regardless of the therapy. Although the most recent data on survival without evidence of disease after radical prostatectomy versus radiation therapy suggest a significant advantage of the former treatment, more data are needed to confirm this result. Careful analysis of patients stratified by pretreatment PSA levels would allow improved comparison of surgery versus radiation therapy in the future. We agree with Huben that radiation therapy could be recommended as a safe alternative to radical prostatectomy in certain cases, especially for patients who may have medical contraindications to surgery or who have a less than 10-year life expectancy.

In addition to radical prostatectomy or radiation therapy alone, other options are worth consideration. In some patients cryosurgery is said to be an attractive alternative because it may lack some of the major complications encountered in the above procedures. The long-term results are still unavailable, although preliminary results are promising.[15,16] Combination therapy may be recommended in patients who are at higher risk of therapeutic failure. For example, neoadjuvant androgen withdrawal therapy before definitive radiation therapy is being evaluated by the Radiation Therapy Oncology Group in a prospective randomized study for patients with bulky tumors or advanced-stage disease.[17] Results suggest improvement in relapse-free survival (including relapse detected by PSA level alone), but more time is necessary to confirm these data. Another alternative is neoadjuvant androgen withdrawal therapy before radical prostatectomy.[18-22] For bulky or advanced-stage disease, most studies thus far do not show any significant stage reduction by this treatment, despite a noticeable decrease in tumor and prostate size. For patients with localized tumors (stages T1 and T2), results are more encouraging.

FOLLOW-UP PROCEDURES

In general a reasonable method of following patients after primary therapy for prostate cancer would include mea-

Table 18-9 Follow-up of patients with prostate cancer: University of Washington Medical Center

	YEAR				
	1	2	3	4	5
Office visit*	4	3	2	1	1
Prostate specific antigen	4	3	2	1	1
Complete blood count	1	0	0	0	0
Electrolytes	1	0	0	0	0
Liver function tests	1	0	0	0	0
Kidney function tests	1	0	0	0	0
Needle biopsy†	‡	‡	‡	‡	‡
Bone scan	‡	‡	‡	‡	‡
Pelvic computed tomography	‡	‡	‡	‡	‡
Pelvic magnetic resonance imaging	‡	‡	‡	‡	‡

*Includes digital rectal examination.
†Prostate or urethrovesical anastomosis.
‡Performed if clinically indicated.

suring serum PSA levels (Table 18-9) and performing a digital rectal examination to rule out obvious local recurrence, although digital rectal examination may not be necessary in the future because it rarely gives unique information. If the PSA level begins to rise, a bone scan is indicated. If the bone scan is negative, TRUS-guided prostate needle biopsy or needle biopsy of the urethrovesical anastomosis is warranted. If these are negative, the physician may simply follow PSA levels.

A major question after treatment of prostate cancer is why follow-up is needed if subsequent treatment is not effective. Recent data suggest that early diagnosis and treatment of recurrent disease have advantages, that adjuvant radiation therapy and salvage surgery in select cases may be helpful, and that patients have the right to know whether they have evidence (such as an elevated PSA level) of recurrent disease. Huben correctly points out that no definitive proof exists that early detection and treatment of persistent disease after initial therapy improve survival. However, he does recommend treatment in two specific situations. First, if the patient (with T3c or higher stage or a Gleason score of 8 or more) has an isolated elevation of PSA levels within 1 year of surgery, Huben would institute hormonal therapy. On the other hand, radiation therapy would be recommended for patients with lower risk of recurrence and a PSA elevation more than 1 year after surgery.

While we agree with instituting adjuvant radiation therapy for localized disease and hormonal therapy for metastatic disease, distinguishing these two situations is much more complex. Physicians need to consider all of the risk factors for disease persistence, not just tumor grade and pathological stage. For example, the age of the patient and life expectancy, tumor volume, DNA ploidy, and presurgery and postsurgery PSA patterns should be taken into account.[23] Furthermore, physicians need to understand the utility of TRUS and needle biopsy of the anastomosis in determining local versus distant disease.[24-26] It is widely accepted now that needle biopsy is far superior to digital rectal examination in detecting local recurrence. However, a negative result by this modality may still be due to sampling error. Another consideration is how the pattern of increase in PSA levels after surgery predicts local versus metastatic disease.[23] For example, persistently elevated PSA levels after surgery usually suggest disseminated disease, whereas a gradual increase in postoperative decreased PSA levels suggests local recurrence.

Regardless of the rate of increase in PSA levels or other risk factors, a positive needle biopsy of the anastomosis in the face of a negative bone scan suggests the possibility that the disease is still localized. Physicians must consider all these factors when deciding to institute additional therapy such as adjuvant radiation therapy after radical prostatectomy.

Proper follow-up of patients after therapy for prostate cancer requires a basic understanding of the value of the PSA assay before and after therapy (needle biopsy after surgery or TRUS-guided biopsy of the prostate after radiation therapy), the risk factors for treatment failure, and the therapeutic options once recurrence (persistence may be a more accurate term) has been detected. Huben has addressed these issues separately for the three main treatments: radical prostatectomy, radiation therapy, and hormonal therapy.

Follow-Up After Radical Prostatectomy

Although we agree with Huben that the PSA assay is the most reliable method of follow-up of patients after radical prostatectomy, elevated PSA level is often not immediately reflective of overt clinical disease. The demonstration of the utility of PSA after radical prostatectomy dates back to earlier studies comparing PSA with prostatic acid phosphatase levels after surgery.[27-29] A retrospective analysis of stored sera from patients who had radical prostatectomy at the University of Washington Medical Center demonstrated unequivocal progressive elevation of PSA levels after reaching greater than 0.4 ng/ml by the then-available Tandem-R assay (Hybritech, San Diego). All of these patients eventually manifested clinical evidence of disease and almost all patients who had clinical disease recurrence initially had a progressive rise in PSA levels.[29] Therefore the patients who seemingly do not have clinical recurrence are often not followed up long enough to demonstrate clinical disease.

How high should the PSA level reach after surgery before physicians consider this abnormal? It is currently believed that 0.1 ng/ml indicates disease recurrence. In the future, with better PSA assays, this level may be less than 0.01 ng/ml.

Adjuvant Radiation Therapy

Definitive evidence that adjuvant radiation therapy improves survival is not currently available, but this modality does have certain benefits. For example, local recurrence rates after surgery have clearly been decreased by radiation.[14,23,30-32]

This is significant because local recurrence is a major source of morbidity for patients after surgery. Despite a lack of prospective randomized studies, which are certainly needed, evidence suggests a potential survival advantage with the use of adjuvant radiation therapy. For example, many patients with elevated PSA levels after surgery who are treated with adjuvant radiation therapy tend to respond with subsequent drops in their PSA levels.[33] This effect can be seen even in patients with negative needle biopsy of the urethrovesical anastomosis, suggesting that the recurrence was still local.[33] Furthermore, patients with lower PSA levels generally respond better than those with higher levels. It is here that the ultrasensitive PSA assay may offer some advantage. This result resembles that of primary radiation therapy, which is more effective for low-volume disease as well.

Whether a combination of hormonal therapy with adjuvant radiation therapy confers additional benefit is unknown but remains an attractive possibility. The prospective randomized study of adjuvant hormonal therapy with primary radiation therapy mentioned previously would support this idea. Theoretically, hormonal therapy could better sensitize tumor cells to respond to radiation therapy or sterilize tumor clones that are resistant to radiation but sensitive to hormonal therapy. Nevertheless, treating patients in a controlled study is better than having a nihilistic attitude about the possible lack of survival advantage of adjuvant radiation therapy in these patients.

Based on the preceding considerations the University of Washington Medical Center has developed tentative recommendations[23] for the use of adjuvant radiation therapy when participation in randomized studies is not possible. High-risk patients (for example, patients with a high Gleason score, high pathological stage, or unequivocal residual disease at surgery), especially if they are young with initially undetectable PSA levels, should receive adjuvant radiation therapy before any rise in postoperative PSA levels because low-volume disease may best respond to this therapy. For patients with rapidly rising or initially detectable postoperative PSA levels and negative needle biopsy results, the disease most likely already exists at distant sites, and we would therefore initiate therapy aimed at systemic disease. For patients with rapidly rising postoperative PSA levels and positive needle biopsy findings, local irradiation is recommended. If the postoperative PSA levels rise gradually, we would initiate adjuvant radiation therapy regardless of the needle biopsy result because of the possibility of biopsy sampling error and the fact that the gradual increase in PSA level suggests that the disease is still local. Obviously these recommendations must be individualized by the peculiarities of the patient and disease and by the availability of newer radiation therapy.[34]

Follow-Up After Primary Radiation Therapy

Follow-up after primary radiation therapy for prostate cancer requires an understanding of the risk factors for recurrence, monitoring procedures, and subsequent treatment options. As in patients undergoing radical prostatectomy, the risk factors for this group include tumor grade and stage, preradiation and postradiation PSA patterns, and the patient's life expectancy.[13,35,36] PSA levels after radiation therapy generally follow a biphasic response: a rapid fall during the initial 3 months followed by a more gradual fall in the next 9 months.[37] The nadir PSA level (0.5 to 1.0 ng/ml) is usually reached within 12 months after therapy.[35] The best prognostic factor is the pretreatment PSA level.[13] Posttreatment PSA levels, especially the nadir level and length of time to reach the nadir, may be additional factors.[13,35,36]

The significance of a positive prostate biopsy after treatment must also be considered. Although some argue that a positive biopsy may simply reflect tumor cells in dormancy, others have shown that prostatic epithelial cells of irradiated patients can grow in tissue culture.[38] Some investigators have found a strong correlation between poor outcome and positive biopsy results.[39] At present most agree that if the PSA level is elevated and the biopsy is positive, the patient has significant persistent or recurrent disease. On the other hand, if the PSA measurement is negative despite a positive biopsy, the clinical importance of the persistent or recurrent disease is controversial.

A major consideration is whether the patient can tolerate salvage surgery after radiation therapy. Recent studies have shown acceptable levels of morbidity resulting from surgery. Patients with incontinence may require cystoprostatectomy with continent diversion.[40] This more extensive procedure may also offer the best chance for cure because of the extra tissue margins that are removed. The specific indications, risks, and benefits of salvage surgery are discussed elsewhere.[41,42]

Follow-Up After Hormonal Therapy

Follow-up procedures after hormonal therapy for prostate cancer appear less complex, partly because of the lack of subsequent therapeutic options. Most alternative treatments such as chemotherapy have not demonstrated any significant survival benefit for advanced disease, and the responses are of short duration.[43-46] Intermittent androgen therapy in the future may offer patients prolonged survival, but data are still lacking.[47,48] With this newer therapy, monitoring (especially with PSA levels) is more frequent. Patients with rising PSA levels probably should have periodic bone scans, which might predict, for example, subsequent cord compression.[49] Any bone involvement can also be serially followed for progression or response to hormonal therapy along with the rising PSA slope.

SURVEILLANCE PROTOCOL

In general we agree with the surveillance protocol suggested by Huben, with minor differences (Table 18-9). Because the majority of patients (92%) who have undetectable PSA levels over 3 years after surgery are essentially cured,[50,51] we recommend annual measurement of PSA levels rather than every 6 months beyond the initial 3-year period if the PSA level remains negative. If the PSA level is progressively positive at any time, a bone scan is recommended. If the PSA level is negative or equivocal, a needle biopsy should be performed to document local disease.

FUTURE PROSPECTS

For future prospects we agree with Huben that improvements in initial therapy would be helpful. However, better detection of the difference between biologically significant and insignificant tumors is just as important. Testing the advantages of various therapies and comparing the results with expectant therapy in randomized trials require physician support as well. Many agree that the PSA assay has revolutionized the management of prostate cancer both in the initial diagnosis and in the early detection of persistent disease after therapy. The less obvious advantage of PSA is the improvement in physicians' ability to evaluate the variety of treatment modalities. Pretreatment PSA levels can better stratify patients into specific risk categories, and posttreatment PSA levels can identify treatment failures more quickly than other methods that identify only overt clinical disease. Clinicians have the responsibility to be constantly aware of advances in the use of the PSA assay, as well as other modalities that will help in managing patients.

SUMMARY

Follow-up of patients after primary therapy for prostate carcinoma requires an understanding of the risk factors for failure of primary treatment, advances in surveillance modalities, and the subsequent treatment options once disease recurrence is identified. Although the PSA assay is the best current method for early detection of disease recurrence, lack of prospective randomized studies has hampered the demonstration of any survival benefit from subsequent therapeutic interventions. Nevertheless, certain treatments such as adjuvant radiation therapy after radical prostatectomy may decrease the morbidity of recurrent disease. Regardless of whether these treatments are initiated, the patient has the right to know whether the disease has recurred. Future improvements in the management of patients with prostate cancer require physician participation in well-controlled studies to determine both diagnostic and therapeutic efficacies.

REFERENCES

1. Oesterling JE, Cooner WH, Jacobsen SJ, Guess HA, Lieber MM. Influence of patient age on the serum PSA concentration: an important clinical observation. Urol Clin North Am 1993;20:671-80.
2. Tchetgen MB, Oesterling JE. The role of prostate-specific antigen in the evaluation of benign prostatic hyperplasia. Urol Clin North Am 1995;22:333-44.
3. Benson MC, Whang IS, Pantuck A, et al. Prostate specific antigen density: a means of distinguishing benign prostatic hypertrophy and prostate cancer. J Urol 1992;147:815-6.
4. Lilja H, Christensson A, Dahlen U, et al. Prostate-specific antigen in serum occurs predominantly in complex with alpha 1-antichymotrypsin. Clin Chem 1991;37:1618-25.
5. Stenman UH, Leinonen J, Alfthan H, Rannikko S, Tuhkanen K, Alfthan O. A complex between prostate-specific antigen and alpha 1-antichymotrypsin is the major form of prostate-specific antigen in serum of patients with prostatic cancer: assay of the complex improves clinical sensitivity for cancer. Cancer Res 1991;51:222-6.
6. Williams BJ, Jones E, Zhu XL, et al. Evidence for a tumor suppressor gene distal to BRCA1 in prostate cancer. J Urol 1996;155:720-5.
7. Huncharek M, Muscat J. Serum prostate-specific antigen as a predictor of radiographic staging studies in newly diagnosed prostate cancer. Cancer Invest 1995;13:31-5.
8. Levran Z, Gonzalez JA, Diokno AC, Jafri SZ, Steinert BW. Are pelvic computed tomography, bone scan and pelvic lymphadenectomy necessary in the staging of prostatic cancer? Br J Urol 1995;75:778-81.
9. Oesterling JE. Using PSA to eliminate the staging radionuclide bone scan: significant economic implications. Urol Clin North Am 1993; 20:705-11.
10. Oesterling JE. Using prostate-specific antigen to eliminate unnecessary diagnostic tests: significant worldwide economic implications. Urology 1995;46(3 Suppl A):26-33.
11. Dugan JA, Bostwick DG, Myers RP, Qian J, Bergstralh EJ, Oesterling JE. The definition and preoperative prediction of clinically insignificant prostate cancer. JAMA 1996;275:288-94.
12. Lange PH. Future studies in localized prostate cancer: what should we think? what can we do? J Urol 1994;152:1932-8.
13. Zagars GK, Pollack A, von Eschenbach AC. Prostate cancer and radiation therapy—the message conveyed by serum prostate-specific antigen. Int J Radiat Oncol Biol Phys 1995;33:23-35.
14. Partin AW, Pound CR, Clemens JQ, Epstein JI, Walsh PC. Serum PSA after anatomic radical prostatectomy: the Johns Hopkins experience after 10 years. Urol Clin North Am 1993;20:713-25.
15. Bahn DK, Lee F, Solomon MH, Gontina H, Klionsky DL, Lee FT Jr. Prostate cancer: US-guided percutaneous cryoablation; work in progress. Radiology 1995;194:551-6.
16. Zippe CD. Cryosurgical ablation for prostate cancer: a current review. Semin Urol 1995;13:148-56.
17. Pilepich MV, Krall J, Al-Sarraf M, et al. A phase III trial of androgen suppression before and during radiation therapy for locally advanced prostatic carcinoma: preliminary report of RTOG protocol 8610 (abstract). Proc Am Soc Clin Oncol 1993;12:229.
18. Armas OA, Aprikian AG, Melamed J, et al. Clinical and pathobiological effects of neoadjuvant total androgen ablation therapy on clinically localized prostatic adenocarcinoma. Am J Surg Pathol 1994; 18:979-91.
19. Cher ML, Shinohara K, Breslin S, Vapnek J, Carroll PR. High failure rate associated with long-term follow-up of neoadjuvant androgen deprivation followed by radical prostatectomy for stage C prostatic cancer. Br J Urol 1995;75:771-7.
20. Fair WR, Aprikian AG, Cohen D, Sogani P, Reuter V. Use of neoadjuvant androgen deprivation therapy in clinically localized prostate cancer. Clin Invest Med 1993;16:516-22.
21. Schulman CC. Neoadjuvant androgen blockade prior to prostatectomy: a retrospective study and critical review. Prostate Suppl 1994;5:9-14.
22. Debruyne FM, Witjes WP, Schulman CC, van Cangh PJ, Oosterhof GO. A multicentre trial of combined neoadjuvant androgen blockade with Zoladex and flutamide prior to radical prostatectomy in prostate cancer: the European Study Group on Neoadjuvant Treatment. Eur Urol 1994;26(Suppl 1):4.
23. Takayama TK, Lange PH. Radiation therapy for local recurrence of prostate cancer after radical prostatectomy. Urol Clin North Am 1994;21:687-700.
24. Kapoor DA, Wasserman NF, Zhang G, Reddy PK. Value of transrectal ultrasound in identifying local disease after radical prostatectomy. Urology 1993;41:594-7.
25. Lightner DJ, Lange PH, Reddy PK, Moore L. Prostate specific antigen and local recurrence after radical prostatectomy. J Urol 1990;144:921-6.

26. Abi-Aad AS, Macfarlane MT, Stein A, deKernion JB. Detection of local recurrence after radical prostatectomy by prostate specific antigen and transrectal ultrasound. J Urol 1992;147:952-5.
27. Stamey TA, Yang N, Hay AR, McNeal JE, Freiha FS, Redwine E. Prostate-specific antigen as a serum marker for adenocarcinoma of the prostate. N Engl J Med 1987;317:909-16.
28. Hudson MA, Bahnson RR, Catalona WJ. Clinical use of prostate specific antigen in patients with prostate cancer. J Urol 1989;142:1011-7.
29. Lange PH, Ercole CJ, Lightner DJ, Fraley EE, Vessella R. The value of serum prostate specific antigen determinations before and after radical prostatectomy. J Urol 1989;141:873-9.
30. Eisbruch A, Perez CA, Roessler EH, Lockett MA. Adjuvant irradiation after prostatectomy for carcinoma of the prostate with positive surgical margins. Cancer 1994;73:384-7.
31. Zietman AL, Coen JJ, Shipley WU, Althausen AF. Adjuvant irradiation after radical prostatectomy for adenocarcinoma of prostate: analysis of freedom from PSA failure. Urology 1993;42:292-8.
32. Cheng WS, Frydenberg M, Bergstralh EJ, Larson-Keller JJ, Zincke H. Radical prostatectomy for pathologic stage C prostate cancer: influence of pathologic variables and adjuvant treatment on disease outcome. Urology 1993;42:283-91.
33. Lange PH, Lightner DJ, Medini E, Reddy PK, Vessella RL. The effect of radiation therapy after radical prostatectomy in patients with elevated prostate specific antigen levels. J Urol 1990;144:927-32.
34. Sandler HM, McLaughlin PW, Ten Haken RK, Addison H, Forman J, Lichter A. Three dimensional conformal radiotherapy for the treatment of prostate cancer: low risk of chronic rectal morbidity observed in a large series of patients. Int J Radiat Oncol Biol Phys 1995;33: 797-801.
35. Pisansky TM, Cha SS, Earle JD, et al. Prostate-specific antigen as a pretherapy prognostic factor in patients treated with radiation therapy for clinically localized prostate cancer. J Clin Oncol 1993;11:2158-66.
36. Stamey TA, Ferrari MK, Schmid HP. The value of serial prostate specific antigen determinations 5 years after radiotherapy: steeply increasing values characterize 80% of patients. J Urol 1993;150: 1856-9.
37. Zagars GK, Sherman NE, Babaian RJ. Prostate-specific antigen and external beam radiation therapy in prostate cancer. Cancer 1991; 67:412-20.
38. Musselman PW, Tubbs R, Connelly RW, et al. Biological significance of prostatic carcinoma after definitive radiation therapy. J Urol 1987;137:114A.
39. Scardino PT, Frankel JM, Wheeler TM, et al. The prognostic significance of post-irradiation biopsy results in patients with prostatic cancer. J Urol 1986;135:510-6.
40. Pontes JE. Role of surgery in managing local recurrence following external-beam radiation therapy. Urol Clin North Am 1994;21:701-6.
41. Younes E, Haas GP, Montie JE, Smith JB, Powell IJ, Pontes JE. Value of preoperative PSA in predicting pathologic stage of patients undergoing salvage prostatectomy. Urology 1994;43:22-5.
42. Brenner PC, Russo P, Wood DP, Morse MJ, Donat SM, Fair WR. Salvage radical prostatectomy in the management of locally recurrent prostate cancer after ^{125}I implantation. Br J Urol 1995;75:44-7.
43. Maulard C, Richaud P, Droz JP, Jessueld D, Dufour EF, Housset M. Phase I-II study of the somatostatin analogue lanreotide in hormone-refractory prostate cancer. Cancer Chemother Pharmacol 1995;36:259-62.
44. Brandes LJ, Bracken SP, Ramsey EW. N,N-diethyl-2-[4-(phenylmethyl)phenoxy] ethanamine in combination with cyclophosphamide: an active, low-toxicity regimen for metastatic hormonally unresponsive prostate cancer. J Clin Oncol 1995;13:1398-403.
45. Kelly WK, Curley T, Leibretz C, Dnistrian A, Schwartz M, Scher HI. Prospective evaluation of hydrocortisone and suramin in patients with androgen-independent prostate cancer. J Clin Oncol 1995;13:2208-13.
46. Akimoto S, Ohki T, Akakura K, Masai M, Shimazaki J. Chemotherapy for endocrine-therapy-refractory prostate cancer. Cancer Chemother Pharmacol 1994;35(Suppl):S18-S22.
47. Goldenberg SL, Bruchovsky N, Gleave ME, Sullivan LD, Akakura K. Intermittent androgen suppression in the treatment of prostate cancer: a preliminary report. Urology 1995;45:839-44.
48. Bruchovsky N, Goldenberg SL, Rennie PS, Gleave M. [Theoretical considerations and initial clinical results of intermittent hormone treatment of patients with advanced prostatic carcinoma]. Urologe A 1995;34:389-92.
49. Osborn JL, Getzenberg RH, Trump DL. Spinal cord compression in prostate cancer. J Neurooncol 1995;23:135-47.
50. deKernion JB, Franklin JR, Belldegrun A, Smith RB. Surgery from a US perspective. Cancer Surv 1995;23:315-20.
51. deKernion JB. What is the value of radical prostatectomy for localized prostate cancer? AUA Today 1995;8:23-4.

Table 18-10 Follow-up of patients with prostate cancer by institution

YEAR/PROGRAM	OFFICE VISIT[a]	PSA	CBC	MCBT	BONE	PELVIC CT	ABD CT	URIN
Year 1								
Memorial Sloan-Kettering	4	4			[b]	[b]	[b]	
Roswell Park	5	5	1	1[c]	[d]	[d]		
Univ Washington	4	4	1		[d]	[d]		
Japan: Natl Cancer Ctr	5	5	2	2[f]	[g]	[g]	[g]	2
Year 2								
Memorial Sloan-Kettering	2	2			[b]	[b]	[b]	
Roswell Park	3	3			[d]	[d]		
Univ Washington	3	3			[d]	[d]		
Japan: Natl Cancer Ctr	4	4	1	1[f]	[g]	[g]	[g]	1
Year 3								
Memorial Sloan-Kettering	2	2			[b]	[b]	[b]	
Roswell Park	2	2			[d]	[d]		
Univ Washington	2	2			[d]	[d]		
Japan: Natl Cancer Ctr	4	4	1	1[f]	[g]	[g]	[g]	1
Year 4								
Memorial Sloan-Kettering	2	2			[b]	[b]	[b]	
Roswell Park	2	2			[d]	[d]		
Univ Washington	1	1			[d]	[d]		
Japan: Natl Cancer Ctr	3	3	1	1[f]	[g]	[g]	[g]	1
Year 5								
Memorial Sloan-Kettering	2	2			[b]	[b]	[b]	
Roswell Park	2	2			[d]	[d]		
Univ Washington	1	1			[d]	[d]		
Japan: Natl Cancer Ctr	3	3	2	1[f]	[g]	[g]	[g]	1

ABD CT abdominal computed tomography
AFP alpha-fetoprotein
BIOPSY needle biopsy
BONE bone scintigraphy
CBC complete blood count
CEA carcinoembryonic antigen
CXR chest x-ray
ELE electrolytes
KFT kidney function test
KUB x-ray of kidneys, ureter, bladder with drip pyelography
LFT liver function tests
MCBT multichannel blood tests
MRI magnetic resonance imaging
PSA prostate specific antigen
URIN urinalysis

AFP	CEA	CA 19-9	CXR	KUB	ELE	LFT	KFT	BIOPSY	PELVIC MRI
					1	1	1	d,e	d
1	1	1	1	g					
								d,e	d
1	1	1	1	g					
								d,e	d
1	1	1	1	g					
								d,e	d
1	1	1	1	g					
								d,e	d
1	1	1	1	g					

a Includes digital rectal examination.
b Performed if a detectable prostate specific antigen level after radical prostatectomy indicates recurrence.
c Consists of sodium, potassium, chloride, carbon dioxide, blood urea nitrogen, creatinine, and glucose.
d Performed if clinically indicated.
e Prostate or urethrovesical anastomosis.
f Consists of total protein, albumin, total bilirubin, blood urea nitrogen, creatinine, sodium, potassium, chloride, calcium, glutamic-oxaloacetic transaminase, glutamic-pyruvic transaminase, alkaline phosphatase, and lactic dehydrogenase.
g Performed only if clinically indicated or if prostate specific antigen levels increase.

CHAPTER 19

Testicular Carcinoma

Roswell Park Cancer Institute

Derek Raghavan

In the past 20 years dramatic progress has been made in the management of testicular cancer, so that the physician's entire approach has changed. The major developments that have effected these changes have been an improvement in understanding of the biology of the disease (including a clearer definition of patterns of spread and prognostic determinants) and the introduction of combination chemotherapy as curative treatment for patients with metastatic disease. Because cure is now the expectation after treatment of testicular cancer of all stages, defined protocols for long-term follow-up of these patients are needed, especially since the potential exists for unexpected late side effects of treatment. A plan of follow-up must take into consideration the characteristics of the typical patient with testicular cancer, the patterns of spread of the disease, the potential for early or late relapse, and possible adverse consequences of treatment. Since this is a curable cancer of young men, each with the potential for another 50 to 60 years of life, the importance of appropriate follow-up is self-evident.

BIOLOGY OF TESTICULAR CANCER

The majority of testicular cancers are germ cell tumors originating from primordial germ cells that arise in the genital ridges. These tumors have the capacity to differentiate along two major lines: seminoma and nonseminoma.[1] The most common type of seminoma is the classic variant, which is composed of uniform round or polygonal cells with abundant cytoplasm and a centrally placed nucleolus. Less commonly, spermatocystic and anaplastic variants have been described, although it should be noted that the anaplastic variant sometimes represents a misdiagnosed nonseminoma germ cell tumor.[2] Several histological variants are in the group of nonseminoma germ cell tumors, including embryonal carcinoma, mature and immature teratoma, endodermal sinus tumor, and choriocarcinoma.[3] Frequently nonseminoma germ cell tumor is composed of several of these elements and may consist of elements of undifferentiated cancer, trophoblastic tissue, and varying components of somatic differentiation.[1,3] Less than 5% of testicular cancers consist of lymphomas and other non–germ cell tumors.[4] These are not covered in this chapter.

In Western society the incidence of testicular cancer is three to six new cases per 100,000 males per year, representing one of the most common malignancies in young men. Furthermore, evidence indicates that the incidence of testicular cancer is rising, especially in Scandinavia, although the reasons remain unknown. Other population groups, such as Asians, Africans, and African-Americans, have a relatively low incidence of this disease.

Substantial similarities exist in the characteristics of seminomas and nonseminoma germ cell tumors.[1,3] Both occur predominantly in younger men, usually in the age range of 18 to 35 years. They usually follow an orderly pattern of spread, from the testis to the surrounding supportive tissues or up the spermatic cord to regional and distant lymphatics, and sometimes to visceral sites via blood-borne metastasis. Both are characterized by the elaboration of tumor markers: alpha-fetoprotein and human chorionic gonadotropin in the case of nonseminoma germ cell tumor and human chorionic gonadotropin in the case of seminoma. In addition, they are characterized by common etiological associations, including a characteristic marker on the short arm of chromosome 12,[5] testicular maldescent, carcinoma in situ of the testis,[6] and a less clearly explained association with the syndrome of multiple atypical nevi.[7] Both tumors are also sensitive to chemotherapy.[8,9]

Some important differences between seminoma and nonseminoma germ cell tumor do exist, including a somewhat older age range for patients with seminoma, a higher prevalence of second primary tumors in men with seminoma, different patterns of metastasis, and substantial radiosensitivity in seminoma, in contrast to marked radioresistance in nonseminoma germ cell tumor. As a consequence, the patterns of diagnosis and management differ somewhat, although the expectation is to achieve cure in each instance.

CURRENT APPROACHES TO TREATMENT

Early-Stage Disease

Primary surgery

Inguinal orchiectomy is the treatment of choice for primary testicular cancer, allowing both diagnosis and definitive treatment to be effected in one step. The details of the surgical procedure are beyond the scope of this chapter; however, certain principles bear emphasis.

The diagnosis should be clear on clinical grounds before surgery. Alternative diagnoses, such as testicular torsion and orchitis, should be excluded if possible. To aid in this process, a careful history and examination, testicular ultrasonography, and (where possible) rapid assay of the tumor markers alpha-fetoprotein and human chorionic gonadotropin may be helpful. Important features in the history that may suggest the presence of a testicular germ cell tumor include the onset, nature, and duration of the symptoms, family history, prior maldescent of the testicle(s), recent development of gynecomastia, history of infertility, and prior history of testicular cancer. On physical examination, enlargement of the testis, often with induration and a craggy quality, raises suspicion of tumor. Other classic features that increase the level of suspicion include physical features of metastatic disease, such as an abdominal mass, supraclavicular adenopathy, or the dyspnea associated with lung metastases. It has been suggested that germ cell tumors may be associated with congenital musculoskeletal anomalies[1] and with multiple atypical nevi,[7] which should also increase suspicion of an underlying testicular germ cell tumor, depending on the clinical context.

When orchiectomy is anticipated, the correct surgical approach requires inguinal exploration with soft clamp control of the spermatic cord before manipulation to avoid the potential for tumor cell dissemination. If not previously done, blood should be drawn for measurement of routine hematological and biochemical indices and for estimation of serum tumor markers. Because the differences among the various histological patterns may be subtle, having a specialist in tumor pathology is important in making the correct diagnosis.[10] Accordingly, the specimen should be sent for extramural review if such a specialist is not available on site, with an emphasis on accurate histological definition and T staging of the tumor (including the definition of vascular and lymphatic involvement). Immunohistochemical staining for alpha-fetoprotein or human chorionic gonadotropin gives further information about the nature of the tumor.

On occasion, when the diagnosis is truly in doubt, inguinal exploration with spermatic cord control and careful examination with or without a frozen section may define the diagnosis. Rarely, bivalving the testis may be helpful, although there is no guarantee that the testis will function normally if bivalved and then sutured and returned to the scrotum without orchiectomy. In my view it is a fundamental error to return the testis to the scrotum without performing some type of biopsy, even if the surgeon is confident that no clinical evidence of cancer is visible on direct viewing.

In the vast majority of cases transscrotal incision is contraindicated because of the risk of local or distant tumor dissemination, and it is generally recommended that transscrotal needle aspiration be avoided unless there is an unequivocal diagnosis of hydrocele without underlying cancer.

Staging

Either before definitive surgery, when the diagnosis of cancer is anticipated, or after the procedure a formal staging process is mandatory to define the extent of disease and thus determine the treatment required. In addition to the usual clinical staging process, which includes a careful history and physical examination, other investigations are required.

Routine blood work is necessary, including a complete blood count to determine whether associated infection or marrow infiltration is present; this is uncommon unless the tumor is a testicular lymphoma. Also required is a biochemical screen to look for renal dysfunction (such as obstruction of ureters from a lymph node mass) or hepatic involvement, which is also uncommon. Since there is a high frequency of hypercholesterolemia in treated patients with germ cell tumors,[11] pretreatment serum lipids should be measured.

The serum tumor markers alpha-fetoprotein and human chorionic gonadotropin should also be measured. Ideally the first specimens should be obtained before primary surgery. Alpha-fetoprotein normally has a half-life in the circulation of 5 to 7 days, and human chorionic gonadotropin has a half-life of 24 to 36 hours.[12] Prolongation of tumor marker elevations after orchiectomy usually indicates occult metastatic disease and implies the need for further investigation and treatment.[12]

Chest x-rays, both posteroanterior and lateral, are necessary to exclude large pulmonary metastases or evidence of mediastinal lymph node involvement. Occasionally, pectus excavatum is associated with germ cell tumors of the testis. An abdominal plain radiograph (if computed tomography is not available) may indicate loss of the psoas shadow. This may be due to massive abdominal lymphadenopathy.

Computed tomographic scans of the abdomen and pelvis are often used to define the extent of lymph node enlargement. If systemic therapy is not anticipated, computed tomography of the chest may indicate the presence of occult pulmonary deposits not visualized on the plain chest x-ray.

More recently magnetic resonance imaging has become available for the assessment of metastatic involvement. However, whether this technology offers any benefit over computed tomography in the routine workup of a patient with testicular cancer is not yet clear.

Computed tomography or magnetic resonance imaging of the brain is not routinely necessary unless symptoms of intracranial metastasis are present or unless the predominant histological type of the primary tumor is choriocarcinoma, which has a tendency to metastasize to the brain. In patients with multiple pulmonary metastases, a computed tomographic scan or magnetic resonance imaging of the brain is prudent.

On completion of the staging protocol a stage classification can be assigned to the tumor. Three systems of classification are commonly used in clinical practice, each having been developed to allow accurate prognostication and the allocation of appropriate treatment to the individual patient with a specific stage of disease (Table 19-1).

Table 19-1 Stage classification of testicular cancer

DESCRIPTION	ROYAL MARSDEN HOSPITAL*	CONVENTIONAL U.S. SYSTEM	AJCC CLASSIFICATION†
Cancer limited to testis	I	A	I
Cancer in abdominal nodes	II	B	II
Involved mediastinal supradiaphragmatic lymph nodes	III	C	III
Visceral metastases	IV	C	III

*Subclassifications A-B-C, depending on volume of disease (Peckham et al.[9]).
†Fourth edition, AJCC.[44]

Treatment After Orchiectomy

Stage I(A) tumors: seminoma

The type of tumor and extent of disease determine the requirements for optimal treatment. In the case of stage I seminoma the conventional approach has been to irradiate the draining ipsilateral pelvic lymph nodes and paraaortic nodes with a dose of 25 to 30 Gy. With this therapy the cure rate is approximately 90%, with only occasional tumors relapsing outside the field of irradiation.[13] This pattern of relapse can usually be predicted by risk factors such as the T stage or presence of lymphatic or vascular invasion within the primary tumor. If an elevated, circulating level of alpha-fetoprotein is identified in a patient with seminoma, management should be predicated as if the patient had nonseminoma germ cell tumor,[2] as outlined later.

More recently the policy of active surveillance, in which patients undergo a meticulous program of scrutiny without additional adjuvant therapy after inguinal orchiectomy, has been applied to patients with stage I seminoma.[14] This program requires repeated office visits, with regular monitoring of tumor markers and radiological screening for the development of metastases (reviewed in greater detail in the ensuing section on nonseminoma germ cell tumor). Although initial reports suggested that this approach might not be safe because of an insidious pattern of spread of seminoma, with advanced-stage disease being documented at the time of first relapse, more recent experience has shown that the outcomes are comparable to those achieved with adjuvant radiation therapy.[14] Although the relapse rate is higher without elective radiation therapy, the total survival rates are similar because of the efficacy of either radiation therapy or chemotherapy for the treatment of relapsed seminoma.

Stage I(A) tumors: nonseminoma germ cell tumors

In the case of stage I nonseminoma germ cell tumor, the choice of treatment rests between retroperitoneal lymph node dissection and a policy of active surveillance. Since the demonstration that adjuvant radiation therapy has little role in the management of stage I nonseminoma germ cell tumor,[9] retroperitoneal lymph node dissection has been regarded as the standard of treatment. This approach gives diagnostic and prognostic information and provides definitive treatment for patients with micrometastatic nodal involvement. Initial techniques of surgical dissection, which required virtually complete resection of all retroperitoneal lymph node tissue, were associated with incompetent ejaculation and associated infertility, a high price for a young man to pay. There was also the potential for other complications of major abdominal surgery, including the formation of adhesions, the occurrence of pulmonary emboli or wound infections, and the occasional development of a lymphocele or lymphatic leakage. More recently, modified nerve-sparing techniques, with a less thorough dissection of the retroperitoneum, have allowed maintenance of ejaculatory function in most patients. In some centers laparoscopic lymph node dissection is being investigated, with the intention of further reducing the morbidity of surgery. Whether this will produce the same cure rates will require time to decide, since the ultimate local relapse rate has not yet been defined.

The policy of active surveillance was first implemented for patients with stage I nonseminoma germ cell tumor. The initial programs called for careful staging and meticulous follow up.[15,16] The initial protocols required monthly follow-up visits for the first 6 to 12 months after orchiectomy, with careful physical examination, measurement of tumor markers, and alternating chest x-rays and computed tomographic scans of the chest, abdomen, and pelvis. The frequency of visits decreased over the ensuing 3 to 5 years.

Relapse rates in the range of 17% to 40% have been identified, with a cumulative relapse rate of approximately 25% in the experience with more than 1,000 patients with stage I nonseminoma germ cell tumor. Series with relapse rates at the higher end of the spectrum may well represent inappropriate selection of cases or an absence of review of the histological or staging investigations from outside centers. More than 50% of first relapses occur in the retroperitoneal lymph nodes, and the majority have been associated with elevations of serum tumor marker levels. Marker-only relapses (elevated tumor marker levels without an obvious site of recurrence) or pulmonary metastases are less frequent.[15,16] Since patterns of spread and relapse have been defined in an accumulated experience of more than 1,000 cases undergoing active surveillance, the frequency of follow-up visits and computed tomographic scans has been reduced. However, this should not be done in an unsupervised or unstructured fashion because investigators at several referral centers have begun to see patients with advanced-stage (bad-prognosis) disease at the time of first relapse after active surveillance.

Early studies of the treatment of stage I testicular cancer revealed a series of adverse prognostic factors, including advanced T stage[17,18] and vascular-lymphatic infiltration.[19] From the studies of active surveillance much additional information has been gleaned regarding the natural history of testicular cancer and patterns of relapse. In addition, it has become clear that late relapses (beyond 5 years) may occur, particularly with immature teratoma (teratocarcinoma), vascular-lymphatic invasion,[15,20-24] and advanced T stage.[15,16] It has also been suggested that embryonal cancer histology is an adverse prognostic determinant[15,20] and that the presence of endodermal sinus tumor is a favorable prognostic factor,[20] although this has not been maintained in multivariate analyses.

Investigational protocols using adjuvant chemotherapy have been developed to prevent recurrence in high-risk groups.[25,26] Although the early results suggest a marked reduction in relapse rates, longer follow-up will be required before such treatment can be defined as standard, particularly in view of the potential late complications of systemic chemotherapy.

Small-volume lymph node metastases

On completion of a staging workup, evidence of small-volume lymph node involvement is occasionally found. In the case of seminoma, such patients are usually treated by radiation therapy to the ipsilateral lymph nodes in the pelvis, with extension to the paraaortic chain (including the involved nodes).[13] Although there has been a tendency toward dose reduction, most clinicians use a relatively standard dose of 30 to 35 Gy to ensure local tumor control.

In the case of nonseminoma germ cell tumor, the optimal management of early stage II (stage B, N1, or N2) disease is controversial. Clinicians generally agree that radiation therapy has no role. However, there are proponents of retroperitoneal lymph node dissection who advocate a standard surgical approach that offers both diagnosis and definitive treatment. These proponents cite surgical cure rates of up to 50%, particularly in patients with only microscopic evidence of lymph node involvement. With this approach chemotherapy can be used to save most patients with relapse.

The alternative approach is to offer first-line cytotoxic chemotherapy to patients with early stage II disease, based on cure rates approaching 100% for patients with small-volume metastases limited to the retroperitoneal nodes. The attraction of this approach is that it limits the morbidity of surgery. However, this may be offset by the acute toxicity of chemotherapy and the potential for late complications. To date, no randomized trial has attempted to resolve this issue and the decision is usually predicated on the biases of the clinician and preferences of the patient. The issue was addressed in one important randomized trial, in which 195 patients with stage II nonseminoma germ cell tumor were randomly allocated to receive two cycles of adjuvant chemotherapy or to undergo a program of observation with salvage chemotherapy at the time of relapse.[27] It should be remembered that the group of patients included cases of N2 or N3 disease. Of the 98 patients who were observed, nearly 48 (49%) had relapse, but the majority were saved with chemotherapy and 93 were alive and disease free at the time of reporting. Conversely, of 97 patients allocated to adjuvant chemotherapy, six had relapse, although only one of these had actually received the chemotherapy before the recurrence and 94 of the 97 survived. It was concluded that there was no statistically significant difference in outcome.[27]

Another controversial issue is the management of the patient with marker-only disease (that is, without evidence of specific lymph node or other metastases but with persistent elevation of serum marker levels after orchiectomy). Retroperitoneal lymph node dissection identifies a proportion of cases with occult lymphatic involvement and achieves cure in some of them. However, up to 50% of the patients undergoing surgery eventually require chemotherapy. Here the cure rates with cytotoxic chemotherapy are close to 100%, although there is significant risk of additional late toxicity as compared with surgery alone. In the situation of marker-only disease my practice has been to use initial combination chemotherapy, reserving surgery for the occasional patient in whom persistent lymph node enlargement is subsequently identified on scan.

Advanced Lymph Node Involvement and Distant Metastases

For patients with lymph node metastases greater than 5 cm in diameter (stage II C, B2, B3, N2, or N3 disease) and for those with visceral metastases (lung, liver, bone, and so on), the treatment of choice is systemic chemotherapy. Apparent cure was achieved in up to 70% of cases with the use of the early combinations of cisplatin, vinblastine, and bleomycin.[8,9] With increased experience it became possible to allocate prognostic categories requiring more intensive chemotherapeutic regimens based on inferior outcomes with standard cisplatin-based chemotherapy.[28-30] Adverse prognostic factors include greatly elevated serum tumor marker levels,[22,28,30,31] bulky disease,[28,29] the number of pulmonary metastases,[22,31] and sites of involvement.[22,28,31] Metastatic disease in brain, liver, and possibly bone also connotes a worse prognosis with standard therapy.[22] At Memorial Sloan-Kettering Cancer Center a numerical algorithm for attribution of prognosis has been developed, predicated on tumor marker levels and extent of disease,[30] and has been used to identify patients requiring specific dose-intensive treatment strategies.[32] Most systems classify these tumors into similar prognostic groups, and attempts are being made to develop a single classification system that will ensure uniform reporting of the results of treatment.

Randomized clinical trials have resulted in the replacement of vinblastine by etoposide in combination chemotherapy with consequent reduction of acute toxicity and retention of high cure rates. However, recent studies

Table 19-2 Late toxicity of treatment for testicular cancer

ORGAN SYSTEM OR PROBLEM	POTENTIAL ISSUE	FOLLOW-UP
Cardiovascular	Hypertension	Blood pressure check
	Coronary artery disease	H&P; EKG; stress test?
	Peripheral vascular disease	H&P
	Cerebrovascular disease	H&P; Doppler study
	Raynaud's phenomenon	H&P
	Hyperlipidemia	Biochemical screen for lipids
Gastrointestinal	Peptic ulceration	H&P; endoscopy?; barium study
	Abdominal pain/diarrhea	H&P; relevant radiology
Neurological	Peripheral neuropathy	H&P; nerve conduction testing
	Autonomic neuropathy	H&P; blood pressure
	Hearing loss	H&P; audiogram
Psychosocial	Marital problems	History/interview
	Infertility	History/interview
	Employment problems	History/interview
	Legal/sociopathic problems	History/interview
Pulmonary	Pneumonitis/fibrosis	H&P; chest x-ray; DLCO?; PFTs?
Renal	Renal failure/nephritis	H&P; biochemical screen; creatinine clearance
	Hypomagnesemia	H&P; biochemical screen
	Hyperuricemia	H&P; biochemical screen
Second malignancies	Leukemia	H&P; CBC
	Melanoma/dysplastic nevi	H&P; dermatology consult?
	Other solid tumors	H&P; screening tests?

H&P, History and physical examination; *EKG,* electrocardiogram; *DLCO,* carbon monoxide diffusing capacity; *PFTs,* pulmonary function tests; *CBC,* complete blood count.

have shown occasional cases of acute leukemia in patients who have received etoposide-containing regimens and this policy requires further review. An attempt was made to reduce toxicity by deleting bleomycin, but this resulted in lower cure rates[33] and has been abandoned. Maintaining caution and vigilance is important in the development of new trials having the reduction of side effects of therapy as a primary end point, since there is risk of reducing cure rates in the attempt to ameliorate the toxicity of treatment.

CHRONIC TOXICITY OF TREATMENT: IMPLICATIONS FOR FOLLOW-UP

A detailed review of the toxicity of treatment is beyond the scope of this chapter and has been covered elsewhere.[34] In particular a discussion of acute side effects of treatment is not relevant to the current topic. However, the chronic or delayed side effects of treatment now constitute one of the major targets of a program of long-term follow-up; accordingly, these are summarized in brief. More detail is available in several reviews.[13,34]

Surgery

Most of the side effects of retroperitoneal surgery are acute and self-limited.[35,36] Nevertheless, in patients who have undergone extensive retroperitoneal dissection, especially if radiation therapy or chemotherapy has also been used, the potential for extensive adhesions and chronic lymphatic obstruction exists. In addition, the potential for long-term infertility resulting from incompetent ejaculatory function has been well characterized.

Radiation Therapy

With current schedules and dosimetry of irradiation, few major toxic side effects are seen, apart from the risk of induced second malignancies.[13] However, it should not be forgotten that many patients are alive and require follow-up after receiving some of the now outmoded schedules of treatment in which higher dosages were used. Patients who have undergone higher dose radiation to the retroperitoneal nodes may have peptic ulcers, intraabdominal adhesions, irregularity of bowel function, chronic myelosuppression, and renal dysfunction caused by nephritis.[37,38]

Until the mid-1970s patients commonly received radiation therapy to pulmonary or mediastinal deposits or consolidative irradiation after chemotherapy to large residual masses. Intraabdominal adhesions or significant pulmonary scarring may develop, especially if bleomycin and radiation were both used. Late cardiac disease may also occur.[39]

Chemotherapy

Curative chemotherapy for metastatic testicular cancer has been available only for the past 20 years, so knowledge regarding late toxicity is still evolving. Nevertheless, chart surveys and prospective clinical studies have provided detailed preliminary information about the patterns of late toxicity in patients treated with cisplatin-based combination chemotherapy.[34] This information is helpful in defining some of the end points of a protocol for follow-up (Table 19-2).

The cardiovascular system may be affected by a range of late side effects, including hypertension, ischemic heart disease and other forms of vascular occlusion, peripheral vascular disorders, Raynaud's phenomenon, cerebrovascular disease, and hypercholesterolemia.[34] Renal failure, hypomagnesemia, and hyperuricemia can probably be attributed to the renal toxicity of cisplatin, since these complications appear less frequently among patients treated with carboplatin-based regimens.

After intensive treatment with bleomycin, pulmonary damage may develop in some patients. This is often diagnosed because of impairment in carbon monoxide diffusing capacity. Severe oxygen toxicity may develop during anesthesia if high inspired oxygen concentrations are used. However, these pulmonary toxicities are usually not a problem if the clinical state of the patient and the lung's diffusing capacity for carbon monoxide are monitored during treatment and bleomycin is discontinued quickly if abnormalities occur. However, as noted previously, an attempt to eliminate pulmonary toxicity by deleting bleomycin completely from standard chemotherapy results in a reduced cure rate.[33] Clinically significant pulmonary dysfunction appears to occur only in patients who continue to smoke cigarettes.[40]

Neurological side effects are surprisingly common if specific provocative tests, such as nerve conduction studies and audiometry, are used.[40] However, except for occasional patients with persistent paresthesias or autonomic neuropathy (found especially if cisplatin or a vinca alkaloid has been given), neurological side effects are uncommon.

The development of second malignancies is a serious risk. In about 4% of patients with testicular cancer a second primary tumor of the testis develops, especially in males with seminoma as the primary tumor. However, more recent follow-up studies have also shown an increased incidence of other solid tumors among long-term survivors with testicular cancer.[41] Of particular concern has been a series of reports that alkylating agents and etoposide may cause acute leukemia in this patient population.[42] In most instances etoposide-related leukemia appears to be a function of high dosage, although Segelov et al.[43] reported a case in which acute leukemia developed after only four courses of cisplatin, etoposide, and bleomycin.

The increased risk of malignant melanoma among patients with testicular cancer[41] may be due to the apparent association between multiple atypical cutaneous nevi and germ cell tumors of the testis.[7] As a consequence the skin of such patients should be monitored to identify atypical nevi and affected patients should then be offered regular dermatological surveillance.

As yet it is not clear whether patients are at increased risk for solid tumors that may be due to specific carcinogens. For example, it is not known whether patients treated

Table 19-3 Long-term follow-up program for testicular cancer

Knowledge of pattern of relapse
Knowledge of common late effects and potential therapy
Mechanism to identify patients
Mechanism to recall patients for follow-up
Scheduling system
Mechanism to identify and pursue defaulting patients
Documentation of action for defaulting patients
Plan for appropriate referral if necessary
Documentation for initial treatment center

for advanced germ cell tumors who continue to smoke are at increased risk for lung carcinoma, as compared with smokers who have not had previous chemotherapy. Follow-up programs should monitor such patients and provide data on their fate, in addition to treating late relapses of cancer or complications of therapy.

REQUIREMENTS FOR A LATE FOLLOW-UP PROTOCOL

Certain characteristics are associated almost exclusively with patients who have testicular cancer. In addition to the youth of the patients and hence the need for protracted follow-up, a proportion of patients with germ cell tumors of the testis have an unusual personality, verging on the sociopathic. These patients have a characteristic unreliability with respect to health care issues and follow-up and a substantial distaste for the authority figures who represent the health care delivery system. They may default from the planned treatment program and often require additional, meticulous efforts to ensure adequate follow-up. This commonly means a specific mechanism to detect missed office visits, with subsequent telephone calls and similar measures to reschedule the requisite clinical visits (Table 19-2). Because of the potential for iatrogenic disorders associated with the treatment of testicular cancer,[34] these patients must be surveyed for the range of potential problems outlined previously, including the complications of surgery, radiation therapy, or chemotherapy and the late sequelae of the disease itself.

Since some of the disease- and treatment-associated disorders have been identified in surveys of patients only 5 to 10 years after treatment, it is possible that the reported prevalence figures are low and will increase with longer follow-up or that other unsuspected problems will emerge even later. As a consequence, the continuation of careful and focused follow-up is essential for these patients (Table 19-3).

Despite the problems, a sense of perspective must be maintained. Testicular cancer was formerly a relentless killer of young men, and immense progress has been made in only 20 years. Physicians should not make the mistake of modifying or delaying effective treatment to avoid the small risk of late complications. Instead, the logical approach is to offer curative therapy for patients with a curable cancer and

Table 19-4 Follow-up of patients with testicular cancer (stage A): Roswell Park Cancer Institute

	YEAR				
	1	2	3	4	5
Office visit	6	4	2	2	2
Alpha-fetoprotein	6	4	2	2	2
Human chorionic gonadotropin	6	4	2	2	2
Lactic dehydrogenase	6	4	2	2	2
Complete blood count	5	2	2	2	2
Multichannel blood tests*	5	2	2	2	2
Chest x-ray	4	4	2	2	2
Abdominal computed tomography	3	2	2	1	1†
Chest computed tomography	2	‡	‡	‡	‡

*Consists of creatinine and alkaline phosphatase.
†After 5 years performed as clinically indicated, especially for patients with immature teratoma.
‡Performed as clinically indicated.

Table 19-5 Follow-up of patients with testicular cancer (stages B and C): Roswell Park Cancer Institute

	YEAR				
	1	2	3	4	5
Office visit	5	3	2	2	2
Alpha-fetoprotein	5	3	2	2	2
Human chorionic gonadotropin	5	3	2	2	2
Lactic dehydrogenase	5	3	2	2	2
Complete blood count	4	2	2	2	2
Multichannel blood tests*	4	2	2	2	2
Chest x-ray	3	3	2	2	2
Abdominal computed tomography	3	2	1	1	0†
Chest computed tomography	2	1	‡	‡	‡

*Consists of creatinine and alkaline phosphatase.
†After 5 years performed as clinically indicated, especially for patients with immature teratoma.
‡Performed as clinically indicated.

then follow up in a structured fashion, allowing appropriate diagnosis and early management of any complications that ensue. The follow-up strategies for patients with testicular cancer used at Roswell Park Cancer Institute are described in Tables 19-4 and 19-5.

REFERENCES

1. Raghavan D, Neville AM. The biology of testicular tumours. In: Innes-Williams D, Chisholm G, editors. Scientific foundations of urology. 2nd ed. London: William Heinemann Medical Books, 1992:785-96.
2. Raghavan D, Sullivan AL, Peckham MJ, Neville AM. Elevated serum alphafetoprotein and seminoma: clinical evidence for a histologic continuum? Cancer 1982;50:982-9.
3. Mostofi FK, Price EB Jr. Tumors of the male genital system: atlas of tumor pathology. 2nd series. Washington: Armed Forces Institute of Pathology, 1979:1-175.
4. Hamilton CR, Horwic A. Rare tumours of the testis and paratesticular tissues. In: Williams CJ, Krikorian J, Green MR, Raghavan D, editors. Textbook of uncommon cancer. New York: Wiley Liss, Chichester, 1988:225-48.
5. Rodriguez E, Mathew S, Reuter V, Ilson DH, Bosl GJ, Chaganti RS. Cytogenetic analysis of 124 prospectively ascertained male germ cell tumors. Cancer Res 1992;52:2285-91.
6. Skakkebaek NE. Carcinoma in situ of the testis: frequency and relationship to invasive germ cell tumours in infertile men. Histopathology 1978;2:157-70.
7. Raghavan D, Zalcberg J, Grygiel JJ, et al. Multiple atypical nevi: a cutaneous marker of germ cell tumors. J Clin Oncol 1994;12:2284-7.
8. Einhorn LH. Testicular cancer as a model for a curable neoplasm: the Richard and Hinda Rosenthal Foundation Award Lecture. Cancer Res 1981;41:3275-80.
9. Peckham MJ, Barrett A, McElwain TJ, Hendry WF, Raghavan D. Non-seminoma germ cell tumours (malignant teratoma) of the testis: results of treatment and an analysis of prognostic factors. Br J Urol 1981;53:162-72.
10. Segelov E, Cox KM, Raghavan D, McNeil E, Lancaster L, Rogers J. The impact of histological review on clinical management of testicular cancer. Br J Urol 1993;71:736-8.
11. Raghavan D, Cox K, Childs A, Grygiel J, Sullivan D. Hypercholesterolemia after chemotherapy for testis cancer. J Clin Oncol 1992; 10:1386-9.
12. Lange PH, Raghavan D. Clinical applications of tumor markers in testicular cancer. In: Donohue JP, editor. The management of testicular cancer. Baltimore: Williams & Wilkins, 1983:111-30.
13. Gospodarowicz M, Warde PR. Early stage seminoma. In: Raghavan D, Scher HI, Leibel S, Lange PH, editors. Principles and practice of genitourinary oncology. Philadelphia: JB Lippincott Company. In press.
14. Gospodarowicz M, Warde PR, Catton CN, et al. The Princess Margaret Hospital experience with surveillance following orchiectomy for stage I testicular seminoma. Proc Am Soc Clin Oncol 1995. In press.
15. Hoskin P, Dilly S, Easton D, et al. Prognostic factors in stage I non-seminomatous germ cell tumors managed by orchiectomy and surveillance: implications for adjuvant chemotherapy. J Clin Oncol 1986;4:1031-6.
16. Raghavan D, Colls B, Levi J, et al. Surveillance for stage I non-seminomatous germ cell tumours of the testis: the optimal protocol has not yet been defined. Br J Urol 1988;61:522-6.
17. Raghavan D, Peckham MJ, Heyderman E, et al. Prognostic factors in clinical stage I non-seminomatous germ-cell tumours of the testis. Br J Cancer 1982;45:167-73.
18. Raghavan D, Vogelzang NJ, Bosl GJ, et al. Tumor classification and size in germ-cell testicular cancer: influence on the occurrence of metastases. Cancer 1982;50:1591-5.
19. Sandeman TF, Matthews JP. The staging of testicular tumors. Cancer 1979;43:2514-24.
20. Freedman LS, Parkinson MC, Jones WG, et al. Histopathology in the prediction of relapse of patients with stage I testicular teratoma treated by orchiectomy alone. Lancet 1987;2:294-8.
21. Klepp O, Olsson AM, Henrikson H, et al. Prognostic factors in clinical stage I nonseminomatous germ cell tumors of the testis: multivariate analysis of a prospective multicenter study. J Clin Oncol 1990;8:509-18.
22. Mead GM, Stenning SP, Parkinson MC, et al. The Second Medical Research Council study of prognostic factors in nonseminomatous germ cell tumors: Medical Research Council Testicular Tumour Working Party. J Clin Oncol 1992;10:85-94.

23. Moriyama N, Daly JJ, Keating MA, Lin CW, Prout GR Jr. Vascular invasion as a prognosticator of metastatic disease in nonseminomatous germ cell tumors of the testis. Cancer 1985;56:2492-8.
24. Vaeth M, Schultz HP, von der Maase H, et al. Prognostic factors in testicular germ cell tumours. Acta Radiol Oncol Biol Phys 1984;23: Fasc.4:271-85.
25. Pont J, Holtl W, Kosak D, et al. Risk-adapted treatment choice in stage I nonseminomatous testicular germ cell cancer by regarding vascular invasion in the primary tumor: a prospective trial. J Clin Oncol 1990;8:16-20.
26. Sandeman TF, Yang C. Results of adjuvant chemotherapy for low-stage nonseminomatous germ cell tumors of the testis with vascular invasion. Cancer 1988;62:1471-5.
27. Williams SD, Stablein DM, Einhorn LH, et al. Immediate adjuvant chemotherapy versus observation with treatment at relapse in pathological stage II testicular cancer. N Engl J Med 1987; 317:1433-8.
28. Bajorin D, Katz A, Chan E, Geller N, Vogelzang N, Bosl GJ. Comparison of criteria for assigning germ cell tumor patients to "good risk" and "poor risk" studies. J Clin Oncol 1988;6:786-92.
29. Birch R, Williams S, Cone A, et al. Prognostic factors for favorable outcome in disseminated germ cell tumors. J Clin Oncol 1986;4:400-7.
30. Bosl GJ, Geller NL, Cirrincione C, et al. Multivariate analysis of prognostic variables in patients with metastatic testicular cancer. Cancer Res 1983;43:3404-7.
31. Levi JA, Thomson D, Sandeman T, et al. A prospective study of cisplatin-based combination chemotherapy in advanced germ cell malignancy: role of maintenance and long-term follow-up. J Clin Oncol 1988;6:1154-60.
32. Bosl GJ, Geller NL, Vogelzang NJ, et al. Alternating cycles of etoposide plus cisplatin and VAB-6 in the treatment of poor-risk patients with germ cell tumors. J Clin Oncol 1987;5:436-40.
33. Levi JA, Raghavan D, Harvey V, et al. The importance of bleomycin in combination chemotherapy for good-prognosis germ cell carcinoma: Australasian Germ Cell Trial Group. J Clin Oncol 1993;11: 1300-5.
34. Boyer M, Raghavan D. Toxicity of treatment of germ cell tumors. Semin Oncol 1992;19:128-42.
35. Donohue JP, Rowland RG. Complications of retroperitoneal lymph node dissection. J Urol 1981;125:338-40.
36. Whitmore WF Jr. Surgical treatment of clinical stage I nonseminomatous germ cell tumors of the testis. Cancer Treat Rep 1982;66:5-10.
37. Aass N, Fossa SD, Aass M, Lindegaard MW. Renal function related to different treatment modalities for malignant germ cell tumours. Br J Cancer 1990:62:842-6.
38. Hamilton CR, Horwich A, Bliss JM, Peckham MJ. Gastrointestinal morbidity of adjuvant radiotherapy in stage I malignant teratoma of the testis. Radiother Oncol 1987;10:85-90.
39. Lederman GS, Sheldon TA, Chaffey JT, Herman TS, Gelman RS, Coleman CN. Cardiac disease after mediastinal irradiation for seminoma. Cancer 1987;60:772-6.
40. Boyer M, Raghavan D, Harris PJ, et al. Lack of late toxicity in patients treated with cisplatin-containing combination chemotherapy for metastatic testicular cancer. J Clin Oncol 1990;8:21-6.
41. Kaldor JM, Day NE, Band P, et al. Second malignancies following testicular cancer, ovarian cancer, and Hodgkin's disease: an international collaborative study among cancer registries. Int J Cancer 1987;39:571-85.
42. Pedersen-Bjergaard J, Daugaard G, Hansen SW, Philip P, Larsen SO, Rorth M. Increased risk of myelodysplasia and leukemia after etoposide, cisplatin and bleomycin for germ-cell tumours. Lancet 1991;338:359-63.
43. Segelov E, Raghavan D, Coates A, Kronenberg H. Acute leukemia following chemotherapy including etoposide for testicular carcinoma. Aust N Z J Med 1993;23:718-9.
44. American Joint Committee on Cancer, Beahrs OH, Henson DE, Robert VP, Kennedy BJ, editors. Manual for staging of cancer. 4th ed. Philadelphia: JB Lippincott Company, 1992:187-9.

➢ COUNTER POINT

Memorial Sloan-Kettering Cancer Center

JOEL SHEINFELD

Approximately 6,600 new cases of testicular cancer and 350 deaths from the disease are estimated to have occurred in the United States in 1993.[1] The 5-year survival for testicular cancer has increased dramatically over the past three decades, from 63% in the 1960s to 93% at present.[1] This has been commonly attributed to effective cisplatin-based chemotherapy and surgery, the advent of computed tomography and reliable tumor markers, refined clinical staging, and follow-up modalities.[2]

Given the high probability of cure that is now possible, the current focus is on individualizing therapy for specific patients so that survival is not compromised, morbidity is minimized, and quality of life is maintained. The cornerstone of this approach is the reliable prediction of each patient's prognosis.[3,4]

NATURAL HISTORY

A number of features regarding the natural history of germ cell tumor have influenced the successful management of this disease. These features include germ cell origin, which is associated with sensitivity to irradiation and a variety of chemotherapeutic agents and with the potential for spontaneous or induced differentiation to histologically benign teratoma; rapid growth rate; the production of specific tumor markers; occurrence in young men without significant comorbid conditions who are capable of tolerating intensive therapy if necessary; and a predictable and systematic pattern of metastatic spread from the primary site to the retroperitoneal lymph nodes and subsequently to the lung or posterior mediastinum.[5,6]

Lymphatic tumor spread is common to all forms of germ cell tumor, and understanding the testicular lymphatic drainage has sharpened the focus of clinical staging and follow-up by identifying the most likely sites of metastatic disease. A detailed anatomical description is beyond the scope of this discussion, but several important concepts should be established. First, the primary landing zone draining the right testis is within the interaortocaval region, while that of the left testicle is the paraaortic and preaortic lymph nodes. In addition, contralateral spread is more common with right-sided tumors, rare with left-sided tumors, and usually associated with advanced disease.[2,5,7]

CURRENT APPROACHES TO TREATMENT

There is no controversy regarding the role of an inguinal orchiectomy in the treatment of germ cell tumor of the testis. Orchiectomy enables histopathological diagnosis, gives information needed for tumor, nodes, metastases (TNM) categorization, and is associated with minimal morbidity, no mortality, and small functional sacrifice. It provides local control of the tumor with virtual 100% effectiveness. Furthermore, a select subset of patients may be cured by orchiectomy alone.[2,6] Subsequent therapy and follow-up depend on the histological features of the primary tumor, the natural history of the disease, the accuracy of clinical staging, the existence of therapeutic alternatives, and awareness of patterns of relapse.[2,6]

CLINICAL STAGING

Meticulous pathological evaluation of the orchiectomy specimen is critical given the prognostic implications of various histological variables such as local extent of tumor, presence of vascular or lymphatic invasion, and proportion of histological subtypes of tumors.[8-19] After a radical orchiectomy, clinical staging includes physical examination, radiographic evaluation of the abdomen, retroperitoneum, and chest, and measurement of the serum tumor markers alpha-fetoprotein and beta-human chorionic gonadotropin, as well as lactic dehydrogenase.

The most effective imaging modality to evaluate retroperitoneal lymph nodes is computed tomography, with an overall sensitivity approaching 80%.[2,5,20,21] An abdominal computed tomographic scan is normal in 70% of patients with newly diagnosed seminomas and approximately 35% of those with newly diagnosed nonseminoma germ cell tumors. Lymph nodes in the primary landing zones measuring 1 to 2 cm contain metastatic deposits approximately 70% of the time.[21,22] Adequate opacification of the duodenum and jejunum is important. In the postchemotherapy setting a computed tomographic scan is not able to distinguish among residual viable disease, teratoma, and necrosis. Furthermore, a normal computed tomographic scan does not preclude the presence of disease. Magnetic resonance imaging adds little to the management of most patients with germ cell tumor. However, occasionally it provides valuable preoperative information regarding patency and involvement of the great vessels in patients with bulky disease.

Routine chest x-rays detect lung metastasis in approximately 10% to 15% of patients with nonseminoma germ cell tumor and 5% of those with pure seminoma. Computed tomography of the chest is more sensitive than chest x-ray but less specific, since nodules as small as 2 mm can be identified, most of which are benign and unrelated to the tumor, particularly in seminoma.

Serum tumor markers are critically important for diagnosis, staging, predicting the prognosis, monitoring response to therapy, and monitoring for relapse.[23] Serum levels of beta-human chorionic gonadotropin are elevated in 40% to 60% of patients with testicular cancer, including 10% to 25% of patients with pure seminoma.[24] Serum levels of alpha-fetoprotein are elevated in 50% to 70% of patients with nonseminoma germ cell tumor. An elevated alpha-fetoprotein level is incompatible with the diagnosis of seminoma, regardless of histological findings.[23] Approximately 60% of patients with clinical stage I disease, 70% with stage II, and 90% with stage III have an elevation of either alpha-fetoprotein or beta-human chorionic gonadotropin levels at presentation.[23] The magnitude of marker elevation has significant prognostic implications, since it reflects tumor burden.[15,25-28] Measuring the rate of decline of serum markers (the serum half-life) by serial determinations has been shown to be predictive of response to therapy.[11,29-32]

NONSEMINOMA GERM CELL TUMORS

Clinical Stage I

In the United States and most parts of Europe the standard approach to clinical stage I nonseminoma germ cell tumor is retroperitoneal lymph node dissection (RPLND), and it remains the standard against which most alternatives are judged.[2,3,32] RPLND provides the most accurate staging of the retroperitoneal nodes, which are the first site of metastatic spread in 85% to 90% of patients with germ cell tumor. Despite improved computed tomography methodology, 15% to 40% of patients are clinically understaged.[2] RPLND is curative in the majority of patients with pathological stage I (N0) disease. Relapse rates average about 10%, and disease-free survival approximates 100%.[33-40]

Treatment failures in the retroperitoneum are rare after a properly completed RPLND, regardless of pathological findings. Relapses are usually serological or in the pulmonary parenchyma or mediastinum, where early detection by periodic serum marker determinations and chest x-ray is likely and cure by appropriate chemotherapy is probable.[37] These should be performed monthly during the first year, bimonthly the second year, quarterly the third year, every 4 months the fourth year, biannually the fifth year, and yearly thereafter (Table 19-6). Baseline computed tomographic scans of the abdomen and pelvis are usually obtained 3 to 4 months postoperatively and on a yearly basis thereafter. Routine computed tomography of the chest is not necessary unless suspicion is raised by the chest x-ray. Elevation of serum tumor markers should prompt a thorough and complete staging workup.

Although RPLND is a major operative procedure, it is associated with acceptable morbidity and a mortality rate of less than 1% in tertiary centers. Major and minor complication rates have averaged about 15% and are reviewed elsewhere.[2,41-47] The most important long-term sequela of a bilateral RPLND has been the loss of ejaculation and consequently potential fertility.[2,47-49] The incidence of this complication is related to the extent of the dissection. Recent modifications based on surgical mapping studies of the pattern of retroperitoneal metastases[2,50-52] and a better understanding of the neuroanatomy of seminal emission and ejaculation have improved the preservation of ejaculatory capacity without compromising the efficacy of the procedure.[2] A detailed description of nerve-sparing RPLND and modified templates is beyond the scope of this discussion but is reviewed elsewhere.

The justification for surveillance rests with improved accuracy of clinical staging and follow-up technique and the availability of effective therapy for early failures. Moreover,

Table 19-6 Follow-up of patients with testicular cancer (stage I nonseminoma germ cell tumor): Memorial Sloan-Kettering Cancer Center

	YEAR				
	1	2	3	4	5
Office visit	12	6	4	3	2
Chest x-ray	12	6	4	3	2
Alpha-fetoprotein	12	6	4	3	2
Beta-human chorionic gonadotropin	12	6	4	3	2
Lactic dehydrogenase	12	6	4	3	2
Abdominal computed tomography*	5†	3	2	2	2
Pelvic computed tomography*	5†	3	2	2	2
Chest computed tomography	‡	‡	‡	‡	‡

*Performed biannually in year 1 and annually thereafter for patients with stage N0 nonseminoma germ cell tumor or patients with stage I N1 or N2a nonseminoma germ cell tumor who have not undergone adjuvant chemotherapy.
†Includes one test performed at baseline.
‡Indicated if abnormality is detected on chest x-ray.

Table 19-7 Follow-up of patients with testicular cancer (stage II N1, N2a, N2b, or N3 nonseminoma germ cell tumor after retroperitoneal lymph node dissection*): Memorial Sloan-Kettering Cancer Center

	YEAR				
	1	2	3	4	5
Office visit	6	3	2	2	2
Chest x-ray	6	3	2	2	2
Alpha-fetoprotein	6	3	2	2	2
Beta-human chorionic gonadotropin	6	3	2	2	2
Lactic dehydrogenase	6	3	2	2	2
Abdominal computed tomography	1	0	0	0	0
Pelvic computed tomography	1	0	0	0	0
Chest computed tomography	†	†	†	†	†

*Assuming postoperative chemotherapy is performed.
†Indicated if abnormality is detected on chest x-ray.

the probability of avoiding therapy beyond orchiectomy, given that approximately 70% of patients with clinical stage I disease are cured by orchiectomy, makes subsequent treatment of any kind (surgery, chemotherapy, or radiation) unnecessary.[53]

Patient compliance cannot be overemphasized. Relapse occurs in approximately 25% to 30% of patients who are observed.[8-19,54-57] The retroperitoneum alone is the site of relapse in approximately 50% of patients, the lungs in about 20%, and both sites in another 10%. Elevation of serum tumor markers is noted in 15% to 20% of cases as the only evidence of tumor relapse. The median time to relapse exceeds 4 years, and Freedman et al.[9] noted a 4% annual relapse rate for the third and fourth years. Given the rapid growth rates of most tumors and the short recurrence interval, close observation is mandatory during the first 2 years and with a decreasing probability of relapse the evaluation intervals are then prolonged.[53] A physical examination, chest x-ray, and determination of alpha-fetoprotein, beta-human chorionic gonadotropin, and lactic dehydrogenase levels are required at monthly intervals during the first year, every other month the second year, quarterly in the third year, every 4 months the fourth year, and biannually thereafter. A computed tomographic scan of the abdomen is necessary at baseline, as well as every 3 months the first year, every 4 months the second year, and every 6 months thereafter (Table 19-6).

Marker-only disease

The current recommendation for patients with marker-only disease after orchiectomy despite a thorough clinical and radiographic evaluation is primary chemotherapy. Many of these patients have systemic disease and have persistently elevated markers after RPLND, regardless of pathological findings. Although survival is excellent whether patients undergo primary RPLND or primary chemotherapy, the latter approach minimizes the therapeutic burden.[58,59]

Clinical Stage II

Clinical stage II nonseminoma germ cell tumor refers to metastatic disease confined to the retroperitoneum and is divided into IIa (nodes less than 2 cm in diameter), IIb (nodes 2 to 5 cm in diameter), and IIc (nodes greater than 5 cm in diameter). Induction chemotherapy is the treatment of choice for patients with high-volume disease (stage IIc).[2]

The traditional approach to patients with stage IIa and IIb tumors has been RPLND with subsequent pathological classification (Table 19-7). Adjuvant therapy is unnecessary for patients with stage N0 disease, given the excellent prognosis with surgery alone.[33-36] The overall risk of relapse in patients with positive nodes is about 50%.

Prognostic factors predictive of relapse after complete resection of clinical stage IIa or IIb have been evaluated. With the exception of the Testicular Cancer Intergroup Study, most investigators have noted that the risk of relapse is related to the size and number of positive nodes found at RPLND. Patients with pathological stage N1 or N2a (fewer than six nodes involved and none greater than 2 cm in diameter) have a low risk of relapse. Therefore careful surveillance is the treatment of choice, assuming patient compliance can be ensured and no undue psychological factors are present. Three or four cycles of cisplatin-based therapy are required at relapse. Most relapses occur within the first 2 years and are evidenced by an elevation in serum tumor marker levels or by pulmonary or mediastinal masses, thus dictating the appropriate follow-up regimen (Table 19-7).

Table 19-8 Follow-up of patients with testicular cancer (stage III nonseminoma germ cell tumor after retroperitoneal lymph node dissection and chemotherapy*): Memorial Sloan-Kettering Cancer Center

	YEAR				
	1	2	3	4	5
Office visit	4	3	2	2	2
Chest x-ray	4	3	2	2	2
Alpha-fetoprotein	4	3	2	2	2
Beta-human chorionic gonadotropin	4	3	2	2	2
Lactic dehydrogenase	4	3	2	2	2
Abdominal computed tomography†	1	0	0	0	0
Pelvic computed tomography†	1	0	0	0	0
Chest computed tomography	‡	‡	‡	‡	‡

*Assuming no viable cancer is detected.
†Performed annually if teratoma is detected in the retroperitoneum.
‡Indicated if abnormality is detected on chest x-ray.

Table 19-9 Follow-up of patients with testicular cancer (stage I, IIA, or IIB seminoma): Memorial Sloan-Kettering Cancer Center

	YEAR				
	1	2	3	4	5
Office visit	4	3	2	2	2
Chest x-ray	4	3	2	2	2
Alpha-fetoprotein	4	3	2	2	2
Beta-human chorionic gonadotropin	4	3	2	2	2
Lactic dehydrogenase	4	3	2	2	2
Abdominal computed tomography	2	1	1	1	1
Pelvic computed tomography	2	1	1	1	1
Chest computed tomography	*	*	*	*	*

*Indicated if abnormality is detected on chest x-ray.

Patients with completely resected N2b or N3 disease have a relapse probability of at least 50% and thus should receive two cycles of adjuvant cisplatin-based therapy. Relapses after adjuvant therapy in this setting are extremely rare (less than 1%), and survival is virtually universal. Patients with incompletely resected disease (N4) should receive standard induction chemotherapy with consideration of postchemotherapy surgery, depending on the clinical response and radiographic findings.

Clinical Stage III

There is universal agreement that the initial treatment for patients with advanced germ cell tumor is cisplatin-based chemotherapy, and multiple regimens have been developed over the past 20 years.[60-64] As it became clear that a large proportion of patients with advanced disease can achieve durable complete remission while others are refractory to conventional therapy, clinical investigation began to focus on identifying prognostic variables that could reliably segregate individual patients according to risk (probability of achieving complete remission) and thus could refine therapy accordingly.[3,4] For good-risk patients the goal has become minimizing treatment-related morbidity without compromising cure, while for poor-risk patients the goal is to improve complete remission rates with investigational regimens that increase the hazards of therapy.[2,5]

In general, the extent of disease has been shown to correlate with response to therapy and survival. A number of prognostic variables thought to reflect tumor burden have been evaluated, including serum levels of beta-human chorionic gonadotropin,[25-27] alpha-fetoprotein,[26-28] and lactic dehydrogenase,[26,27] visceral metastasis,[27] and number and size of pulmonary nodules.[29] Tumor histology[28] and rate of marker decline have also been extensively studied.[29-31,65]

Several predictive models have been developed for risk stratification[27-29] and are beyond the scope of this discussion. The role of bleomycin remains controversial. Three randomized clinical trials have evaluated the elimination of bleomycin from etoposide- and cisplatin-containing regimens. No differences in response or survival rates were noted in two trials,[63,66] while the third trial reported an increased number of adverse events in the 2-day arm.[67]

Surgery remains an integral part in the management of patients with advanced germ cell tumor. Earlier reports indicated that the pathological findings at surgery were necrosis, teratoma, or persistent malignancy, each in approximately one third of cases.[68] More recent series have noted a decrease in the proportion of patients with viable cancer[69-72] and have attributed this to improved staging techniques and more effective chemotherapy regimens. Current reviews report that necrosis and fibrosis comprise 40% of resected specimens, teratoma 40%, and viable germ cell tumor the remaining 20%.[68-72] Patient prognosis is directly related to the histopathological features of the resected specimen, with the finding of residual viable cancer associated with a significantly lower relapse-free survival rate than if teratoma or necrosis is found. Patients with residual malignancy that has been completely resected should undergo two additional cycles of chemotherapy (Table 19-8).

Despite the histologically benign nature of teratoma, complete resection has significant advantages. First, teratoma may grow, obstruct, or invade local structures and become unresectable.[73-74] Second, there is the risk of malignant transformation or nongerminal carcinomatous malignant elements, which occur in 8% to 11% of cases, with a recurrence rate of 58% to 86%.[75-76] Teratoma may also remain dormant and result in late recurrence, often after 2 years but sometimes as long as 16 years after resection.[77-78] Furthermore, several studies confirm the need to resect all sites of residual disease (lung, mediastinum, supraclavicular area, or retroperitoneum), since pretreatment findings are not predictive of subsequent histological changes and an approximately 35% discordance in pathological features has been noted between resected specimens from different sites.[79]

SEMINOMA

The management of clinical stages I, IIa, and IIb is radiation therapy, with protocols and fractionation adjusted appropriately to individual patients. Prophylactic radiation to the mediastinum is contraindicated, since it results in chemotherapy intolerance and, consequently, higher morbidity and mortality rates. Relapse rates for clinical stage I disease range from 2% to 9%, while those for clinical stages IIa and IIb range from 5% to 15%. Relapses occur rarely in the irradiated field, and most develop as a supraclavicular or mediastinal mass.[80-82] Consequently, follow-up must pay particular attention to these areas with serial physical examinations and chest x-rays (Table 19-9).

The treatment for bulky (clinical stage IIc) or metastatic seminoma (stage III) is cisplatin-based systemic chemotherapy. The management of postchemotherapy residual masses in this setting is somewhat controversial given the higher morbidity of surgery resulting from the technical demands of dealing with the severe desmoplastic reaction, the rare finding of teratoma, and the overall incidence of viable seminoma. The policy at Memorial Sloan-Kettering Cancer Center is to resect postchemotherapy masses less than 3 cm, since most residual viable seminomas fall in this group.

Given the dramatic improvement in survival of patients with testicular cancer, there has been an increasing awareness and appropriate emphasis on the surveillance and management of the chronic and delayed sequelae of therapy. These are elegantly outlined by Raghavan with pertinent reviews cited.

REFERENCES

1. Boring CC, Squires TS, Tong T. Cancer statistics, 1993. CA Cancer J Clin 1993;43:7-26.
2. Sheinfeld J. Nonseminomatous germ cell tumors of the testis: current concepts and controversies. Urology 1994;44:2-14.
3. Hesketh PJ, Krane RJ. Prognostic assessment in nonseminomatous testicular cancer: implications for therapy. J Urol 1990;144:1-9.
4. Bosl GJ, Geller NL, Bajorin D, et al. A randomized trial of etoposide + cisplatin versus vinblastine + bleomycin + cisplatin + cyclophosphamide + actinomycin in patients with good prognosis germ cell tumors. J Clin Oncol 1988;6:1231-8.
5. Richie JP. Neoplasms of the testis. In: Walsh PC, Retik AB, Stamey TA, et al., editors. Campbell's urology, 6th ed. Philadelphia: WB Saunders Company, 1992:1222-63.
6. Whitmore WF Jr. Surgical treatment of clinical stage I nonseminomatous germ cell tumors of the testis. Cancer Treat Rep 1982;66:5-10.
7. Sogani PC. Evolution of the management of stage I nonseminomatous germ-cell tumors of the testis. Urol Clin North Am 1991;18:561-73.
8. Sogani PC, Fair WR. Surveillance alone in the treatment of clinical stage I nonseminomatous germ cell tumor of the testis (NSGCT). Semin Urol 1988;6:53-6.
9. Freedman LS, Parkinson MC, Jones WG, et al. Histopathology in the prediction of relapse of patients with stage I testicular teratoma treated by orchiectomy alone. Lancet 1987;2:294-8.
10. Hoskin P, Dilly S, Easton D, Horwich A, Hendry W, Peckham MJ. Prognostic factors in stage I non-seminomatous germ-cell testicular tumors managed by orchiectomy and surveillance: implications for adjuvant chemotherapy. J Clin Oncol 1986;4:1031-6.
11. Dunphy CH, Ayala AG, Swanson DA, Ro JY, Logothetis C. Clinical stage I nonseminomatous and mixed germ cell tumors of the testis: a clinicopathologic study of 93 patients on a surveillance protocol after orchiectomy alone. Cancer 1988;62:1202-6.
12. Rorth M, von der Maase H, Nielsen ES, Pedersen M, Schultz H. Orchidectomy alone versus orchidectomy plus radiotherapy in stage I nonseminomatous testicular cancer: a randomized study by the Danish Testicular Carcinoma Study Group. Int J Androl 1987;10: 255-62.
13. Pizzocaro G, Zanoni F, Milani A, et al. Orchiectomy alone in clinical stage I nonseminomatous testis cancer: a critical appraisal. J Clin Oncol 1986;4:35-40.
14. Fung CY, Kalish LA, Brodsky GL, Richie JP, Garnick MB. Stage I nonseminomatous germ cell testicular tumor: prediction of metastatic potential by primary histopathology. J Clin Oncol 1988;6:1467-73.
15. Javadpour N, Young JD Jr. Prognostic factors in nonseminomatous testicular cancer. J Urol 1986;135:497-9.
16. Raghavan D, Peckham MJ, Heyderman E, Tobias JS, Austin DE. Prognostic factors in clinical stage I non-seminomatous germ-cell tumours of the testis. Br J Cancer 1982;45:167-72.
17. Gelderman WA, Schraffordt Koops H, Sleijfer DT, et al. Orchiectomy alone in stage I nonseminomatous testicular germ cell tumors. Cancer 1987;59:578-80.
18. Moriyama N, Daly JJ, Keating MA, Lin CW, Prout GR Jr. Vascular invasion as a prognosticator of metastatic disease in nonseminomatous germ cell tumors of the testis: importance in "surveillance only" protocols. Cancer 1985;56:2492-8.
19. Moul JW, McCarthy WF, Fernandez EB, Sesterhenn IA. Percentage of embryonal carcinoma and of vascular invasion predicts pathological stage in clinical stage I nonseminomatous testicular cancer. Cancer Res 1994;54:362-4.
20. Husband, JE, Peckham MJ, MacDonald JS, Hendry WF. The role of computed tomography in the management of testicular teratoma. Clin Radiol 1979;30:243-52.
21. Lien HH, Stenwig AE, Ous S, Fossa SD. Influence of different criteria for abnormal lymph node size on reliability of computed tomography in patients with nonseminomatous testicular cancer. Acta Radiol (Diagn) 1986;27:199-203.
22. Fernandez EB, Moul JW, Foley JP, Colon E, McLeod DG. Retroperitoneal imaging with third and fourth generation computed axial tomography in clinical stage I nonseminomatous germ cell tumors. Urology 1994;44:548-52.
23. Klein EA. Tumor markers in testis cancer. Urol Clin North Am 1993;20:67-73.
24. Lange PH, Nochomovitz LE, Rosai J. Serum alpha-fetoprotein and human chorionic gonadotropin in patients with seminoma. J Urol 1980;124:472-8.
25. Levi JA, Thomson D, Sandeman T, et al. A prospective study of cisplatin-based combination chemotherapy in advanced germ cell malignancy: role of maintenance and long-term follow-up. J Clin Oncol 1988;6:1154-60.
26. Birch R, Williams S, Cone A, et al. Prognostic factors for favorable outcome in disseminated germ cell tumors. J Clin Oncol 1986;4:400-7.
27. Bosl GJ, Geller NL, Cirrincione C, et al. Multivariate analysis of prognostic variables in patients with metastatic testicular cancer. Cancer Res 1983;43:3403-7.
28. Stoter G, Sylvester R, Sleijfer DT, et al. Multivariate analysis of prognostic factors in patients with disseminated nonseminomatous testicular cancer: results from a European Organization for Research on Treatment of Cancer Multiinstitutional Phase III Study. Cancer Res 1987;47:2714-8.

29. Vogelzang NJ, Lange PH, Goldman A, Vessel RH, Fraley EE, Kennedy BJ. Acute changes of alpha-fetoprotein and human chorionic gonadotropin during induction chemotherapy of germ cell tumors. Cancer Res 1982;42:4855-61.
30. Picozzi VJ Jr, Freiha FS, Hannigan JF Jr, Torti FM. Prognostic significance of a decline in serum human chorionic gonadotropin levels after initial chemotherapy for advanced germ-cell carcinoma. Ann Intern Med 1984;100:183-6.
31. Toner GC, Geller NL, Tan C, Nisselbaum J, Bosl GJ. Serum tumor markers half-life during chemotherapy allows early prediction of complete response and survival in nonseminomatous germ cell tumors. Cancer Res 1990;50:5904-10.
32. Sternberg CN. Role of primary chemotherapy in stage I and low-volume stage II nonseminomatous germ-cell testis tumors. Urol Clin North Am 1993;20:93-109.
33. Johnson DE, Bracken RB, Blight EM. Prognosis for pathologic stage I nonseminomatous germ cell tumors of the testis managed by retroperitoneal lymphadenectomy. J Urol 1976;116:63-5.
34. Bredael JJ, Vugrin D, Whitmore WF Jr. Recurrences in surgical stage I nonseminomatous germ cell tumors of the testis. J Urol 1983;130:476-8.
35. Walsh PC, Kaufman JJ, Coulson WF, Goodwin WE. Retroperitoneal lymphadenectomy for testicular tumors. JAMA 1971;217:309-12.
36. Staubitz WJ, Early KS, Magoss IV, Murphy GP. Proceedings: surgical treatment of non-seminomatous germinal testis tumors. Cancer 1973;32:1206-11.
37. Donohue JP, Thornhill JA, Foster RS, Rowland RG, Bihrle R. Retroperitoneal lymphadenectomy for clinical stage A testis cancer (1965 to 1989): modifications of technique and impact on ejaculation. J Urol 1993;149:237-43.
38. Richie JP, Kantoff PW. Is adjuvant chemotherapy necessary for patients with stage B1 testicular cancer? J Clin Oncol 1991;9:1393-6.
39. Hartlapp JH, Weissbach L, Bussar-Maatz R. Adjuvant chemotherapy in nonseminomatous testicular tumour stage II. Int J Androl 1987; 10:277-84.
40. Socinski MA, Garnick MB, Stomper PC, Fung CY, Richie JP. Stage II nonseminomatous germ cell tumors of the testis: an analysis of treatment options in patients with low-volume retroperitoneal disease. J Urol 1988;140:1437-41.
41. Skinner DG, Melumed A, Lieskovsky G. Complications of thoracoabdominal retroperitoneal lymph node dissection. J Urol 1982;127: 1107-10.
42. Waters WB, Garnick MB, Richie JP. Complications of retroperitoneal lymphadenectomy in the management of nonseminomatous tumors of the testis. Surg Gynecol Obstet 1982;154:501-4.
43. Donohue JP, Rowland RG. Complications of retroperitoneal lymph node dissection. J Urol 1981;125:338-40.
44. Bihrle R, Donohue JP, Foster RS. Complications of retroperitoneal lymph node dissection. Urol Clin North Am 1988;15:237-42.
45. Sago AL, Ball TP, Novicki DE. Complications of retroperitoneal lymphadenectomy. Urology 1979;13:241-3.
46. Babaian RJ, Bracken RB, Johnson DE. Complications of transabdominal retroperitoneal lymphadenectomy. Urology 1981;17:126-8.
47. Lange PH, Chang WY, Fraley EE. Fertility issues in the therapy of nonseminomatous testicular tumors. Urol Clin North Am 1987;14: 731-47.
48. Moul JW, Robertson JE, George SL, Paulson DF, Walther PJ. Complications of therapy for testicular cancer. J Urol 1989;142:1491-6.
49. Lange PH, Narayan P, Fraley EE. Fertility issues following therapy for testicular cancer. Semin Urol 1984;2:264-74.
50. Lange PH, Narayan P, Vogelzang NJ, Shafer RB, Kennedy BJ, Fraley EE. Return of fertility after treatment for nonseminomatous testicular cancer: changing concepts. J Urol 1983;129:1131-5.
51. Donohue JP, Zachary JM, Maynard BR. Distribution of nodal metastases in nonseminomatous testis cancer. J Urol 1982;128:315-20.
52. Ray B, Hajdu SI, Whitmore WF Jr. Proceedings: distribution of retroperitoneal lymph node metastases in testicular germinal tumors. Cancer 1974;33:340-8.
53. Lowe BA. Surveillance versus nerve-sparing retroperitoneal lymphadenectomy in stage I nonseminomatous germ-cell tumors. Urol Clin North Am 1993;20:75-83.
54. Gels ME, Hoekstra HJ, Sleijfer DT, et al. Detection of recurrence in patients with clinical stage I nonseminomatous testicular germ cell tumors and consequences for further follow-up: a single-center 10-year experience. J Clin Oncol 1995;13:1188-94.
55. Read G, Stenning SP, Cullen MH, et al. Medical Research Council prospective study of surveillance for stage I testicular teratoma: Medical Research Council Testicular Tumors Working Party. J Clin Oncol 1992;10:1762-8.
56. Nicolai N, Pizzocaro G. A surveillance study of clinical stage I nonseminomatous germ cell tumors of the testis: 10-year followup. J Urol 1995;154:1045-9.
57. Pont J, Holtl W, Kosak D, et al. Risk-adapted treatment choice in stage I nonseminomatous testicular germ cell cancer by regarding vascular invasion in the primary tumor: a prospective trial. J Urol 1990;8:16-20.
58. Nichols CR, Foster RS, Messemer JE, Donohue JP, Einhorn LH. The management of patients with clinical stage I testicular nonseminomatous germ cell tumors (NSGCT) and persistently elevated serologic markers [abstract]. Proc Am Soc Clin Oncol 1995;14:230.
59. Davis BE, Herr HW, Fair WR, Bosl GJ. The management of patients with nonseminomatous germ cell tumors of the testis with serologic disease only after orchiectomy. J Urol 1994;152:111-4.
60. Einhorn LH, Donohue J. Cis-diaminedichloroplatin, vinblastine, and bleomycin combination chemotherapy in disseminated testicular cancer. Ann Intern Med 1977;871:293-8.
61. Vugrin D, Herr HW, Whitmore WF Jr, Sogani PC, Golbey RB. VAB-6 combination chemotherapy in disseminated cancer of the testis. Ann Intern Med 1981;95:59-61.
62. Einhorn LH, Williams SD. Chemotherapy of disseminated testicular cancer. Cancer 1980;46:1339-44.
63. Bajorin DF, Geller NL, Weisen SF, Bosl GJ. Two-drug therapy in patients with metastatic germ cell tumors. Cancer 1991;67:28-32.
64. Peckham MJ, Barrett A, Liew KH, et al. The treatment of metastatic germ-cell testicular tumours with bleomycin, etoposide and cis-platin (BEP). Br J Cancer 1983;47:613-9.
65. Logothetis CJ, Samuels ML, Trindade A, Grant C, Gomez L, Ayala A. The prognostic significance of endodermal sinus tumor histology among patients treated for stage III non-seminomatous germ cell tumors of the testes. Cancer 1984;53:122-8.
66. Stoter G, Kaye SB. Prognostic factors and treatment options in disseminated nonseminomatous testicular cancer. International Testicular & Prostate Cancer Conference, Toronto, Canada 1990;40.
67. Loehrer PJ Sr, Johnson D, Elson P, Einhorn LH, Trump D. Importance of bleomycin in favorable-prognosis disseminated germ cell tumors: an Eastern Cooperative Oncology Group Trial. J Clin Oncol 1995;13:470-6.
68. Donohue JP, Rowland RG, Kopecky K, et al. Correlation of computerized tomographic changes and histological findings in 80 patients having radical retroperitoneal lymph node dissection after chemotherapy for testis cancer. J Urol 1987;137:1176-9.
69. Gelderman WA, Koops HS, Sleijfer DT, Oosterhuis JW, Oldhoff J. Treatment of retroperitoneal residual tumor after PVB chemotherapy of nonseminomatous testicular tumors. Cancer 1986;58:1418-21.
70. Harding MJ, Brown IL, MacPherson SG, Turner MA, Kaye SB. Excision of residual masses after platinum based chemotherapy for non-seminomatous germ cell tumours. Eur J Cancer Clin Oncol 1989;25:1689-94.
71. Toner GC, Panicek DM, Heelan RT, et al. Adjunctive surgery after chemotherapy for nonseminomatous germ cell tumors: recommendations for patient selection. J Clin Oncol 1990;8:1683-94.
72. Mulder PF, Oosterhof GO, Boetes C, de Mulder PH, Theeuwes AG, Debruyne FM. The importance of prognostic factors in the individual treatment of patients with disseminated germ cell tumours. Br J Urol 1990;66:425-9.
73. Logothetis CJ, Samuels ML, Trindade A, Johnson DE. The growing teratoma syndrome. Cancer 1982;50:1629-35.

74. Logothetis CJ, Samuels ML. Surgery in the management of stage III germinal cell tumors: observations on the M.D. Anderson Hospital experience, 1971-1979. Cancer Treat Rev 1984;11:27-37.
75. Ahmed T, Bosl GJ, Hajdu SI. Teratoma with malignant transformation in germ cell tumors in men. Cancer 1985;56:860-3.
76. Ahlgren AD, Simrell CR, Triche TJ, Ozols R, Barsky SH. Sarcoma arising in a residual testicular teratoma after cytoreductive chemotherapy. Cancer 1984;54:2015-8.
77. Gelderman WA, Scraffordt Koops H, Sleijfer DT, Oosterhuis JW, Oldhoff J. Late recurrence of mature teratoma in nonseminomatous testicular tumors after PVB chemotherapy and surgery. Urology 1989;33:10-4.
78. Loehrer PJ Sr, Hui S, Clark S, et al. Teratoma following cisplatin-based combination chemotherapy for nonseminomatous germ cell tumors: a clinicopathological correlation. J Urol 1986;135:1183-6.
79. Tiffany P, Morse MJ, Bosl G, et al. Sequential excision of residual thoracic and retroperitoneal masses after chemotherapy for stage III germ cell tumors. Cancer 1986;57:978-83.
80. Thomas GM, Rider WD, Dembo AJ, et al. Seminoma of the testis: results of treatment and patterns of failure after radiation therapy. Int J Radiat Oncol Biol Phys 1982;8:165-74.
81. Willan BD, McGowan DG. Seminoma of the testis: a 22-year experience with radiation therapy. Int J Radiat Oncol Biol Phys 1985;11:1769-75.
82. Hanks GE, Herring DF, Kramer S. Patterns of care outcome studies: results of the national practice in seminoma of the testis. Int J Radiat Oncol Biol Phys 1981;7:1413-7.

➢ COUNTERPOINT

National Cancer Center Hospital, Japan

TADAO KAKIZOE

Dramatic progress has been achieved during the past 20 years in the management of testicular cancer in such areas as understanding the biology of this disease; precisely evaluating the spread of the disease by computed tomography, magnetic resonance imaging, ultrasound, and other appropriate modalities; monitoring the therapeutic effect with such tumor markers as alpha-fetoprotein and beta-human chorionic gonadotropin; and introducing effective chemotherapeutic drugs such as cisplatin and etoposide. Consequently, physicians are able to adopt a logical approach and can plan a strict strategy for the management and follow-up of patients with testicular cancer.

Testicular cancer is unique in that patients are usually young, occasionally pay little attention to issues of their own health care, and sometimes are emotionally labile. Most patients expect a cure even when the disease is found at an advanced stage. Long-term follow-up is necessary with regard to possible recurrences, late sequelae of treatment, and the development of contralateral testicular cancer and secondary malignancy. If the patient is single at the time of treatment, consultation is required with respect to future marriage and the possibility of fathering a child.

Since Raghavan has extensively described the management and follow-up of testicular cancer, this counterpoint includes only what is characteristic in Japan and specific procedures initiated at the National Cancer Center Hospital in Tokyo.

CHARACTERISTICS OF TESTICULAR CANCER IN JAPAN

The incidence of testicular cancer in Japan is relatively low. The Japanese Urological Association initiated a nationwide bladder cancer registry system in 1982, but the registration of testicular cancer has yet to begin. The incidence of testicular cancer in Japan has been steady since 1975. On the basis of the Osaka Cancer Registry,[1] the estimated number of new cases in 1984 was 836. The incidence of testicular cancer in the 25- to 30-year age group is 3.9 per 100,000 population, making it the most common malignancy in this age group.

Yoshida et al.[2] surveyed patients with testicular cancer at the major Japanese institutions and collected 505 cases.

Table 19-10 Stage classification by the Japanese Urological Association

STAGE	DESCRIPTION
I	No evidence of metastasis
II	Lymph node metastasis beneath diaphragm only
II A	Retroperitoneal lymph node metastasis less than 5 cm in longest diameter
II B	Palpable abdominal tumor or retroperitoneal lymph node metastasis larger than 5 cm in longest diameter
III	Distant metastasis
III 0	Tumor marker is positive, but metastatic site is unidentified
III A	Mediastinal or supraclavicular lymph node metastasis
III B	Pulmonary metastasis
B1	Number of metastases at least equal to 4 and longest diameter of each metastasis less than 2 cm
B2	Number of metastases equal to or more than 5 and longest diameter more than 2 cm
III C	Metastasis other than lung

From Japanese Urologic Association, Japanese Pathologic Society. [General rule for clinical and pathological studies on testicular tumors.] (In Japanese) Tokyo: Kanehara Press, 1984.

Table 19-11 Histological classification of germ cell tumors

A. Tumors of one histological type
  1. Seminoma
    a. Typical seminoma
    b. Anaplastic seminoma
    c. Spermatocytic seminoma
  2. Embryonal carcinoma
  3. Yolk sac tumor
  4. Choriocarcinoma
  5. Teratoma
    a. Mature
    b. Immature
    c. With malignant transformation
  6. Polyembryoma

B. Tumors of more than one histological type
  1. Embryonal carcinoma and teratoma (teratocarcinoma)
  2. Choriocarcinoma and any other types
  3. Other combinations

From Japanese Urologic Association, Japanese Pathologic Society. [General rule for clinical and pathological studies on testicular tumors.] (In Japanese) Tokyo: Kanehara Press, 1984.

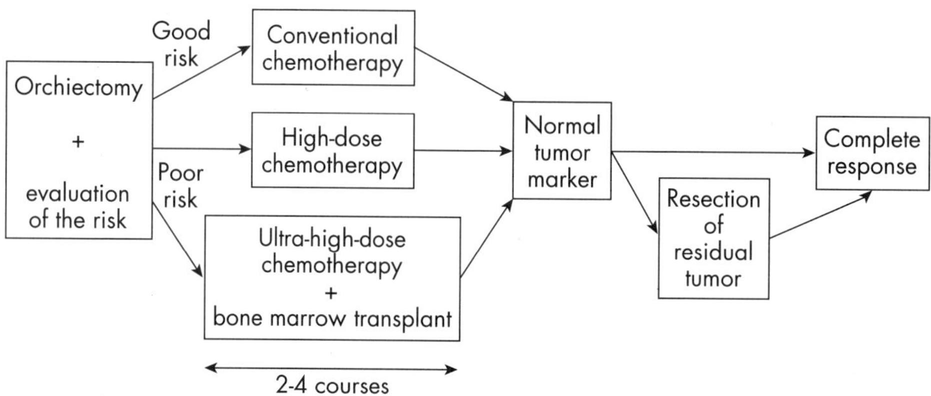

Figure 19-1 A schematic outline of the treatment for advanced nonseminoma germ cell tumor.

		Day				
DRUG	DOSAGE	1	2	3	4	5
Cisplatin	120 mg/m^2	↓				
Etoposide	100 mg/m^2	↓	↓	↓	↓	↓

Figure 19-2 Protocol of chemotherapy used as a first-line treatment at the National Cancer Center Hospital, Tokyo.

According to their report, 71% of the patients were between the ages of 15 and 44 and 32% were between 25 and 34. Seminoma accounted for 43% of the cases, and nonseminoma germ cell tumors accounted for 57%. The distribution of seminoma stages I, II, and III (Walter Reed classification) was, respectively, 78.3%, 14.8%, and 6.9%. However, the distribution of NSGCT stages I, II, and III was, respectively, 56.6%, 15.4%, and 27.9%, indicating higher percentages of advanced-stage nonseminoma germ cell tumor.

STAGING SYSTEM USED IN JAPAN

In 1984 the Japanese Urological Association published the booklet *General Rules for Clinical and Pathological Studies on Testicular Tumors,*[3] which has been used throughout Japan as a guide for the management of patients with testicular cancer. The staging system used is shown in Table 19-10, and the pathological classifications appear in Table 19-11. This publication includes descriptions of the history, occupation, and education of new patients; results of initial workup; typical demonstrations of computed tomography, magnetic resonance imaging, ultrasound, and lymphangiography at each specific stage; and examples of the pathological and histological features of each histological classification. It is useful for both the urologist and the pathologist and has greatly contributed to accurate descriptions, both clinical and pathological, of patients with testicular cancer.

INITIAL WORKUP AND MANAGEMENT STRATEGY

When a new patient with testicular cancer is seen at the National Cancer Center Hospital in Tokyo, an inguinal orchiectomy under spinal anesthesia is performed that same day or the following day at the latest. While the official pathology report based on step-section examination of the specimen is awaited, the initial workup of the spread of disease is conducted by preoperative measurement of alpha-

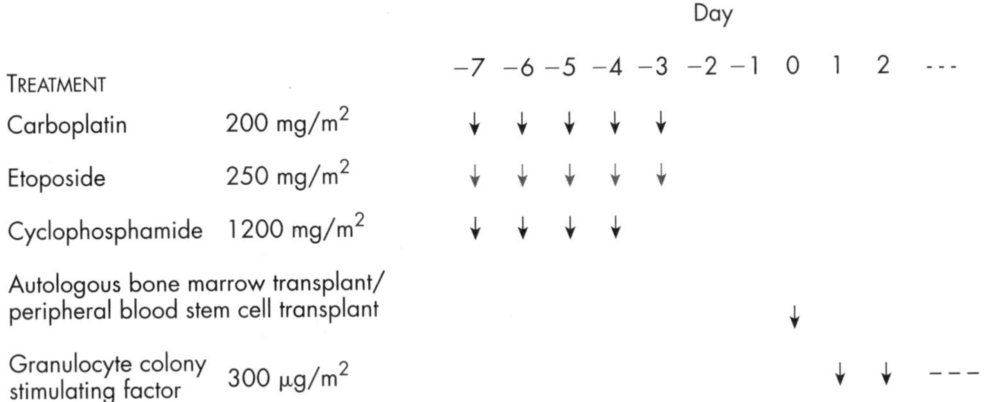

Figure 19-3 Investigational protocol for advanced nonseminoma germ cell tumor by a combination of high-dosage chemotherapy and autologous bone marrow transplantation, including carboplatin and cyclophosphamide.

Table 19-12 Follow-up of patients with testicular cancer (stage I seminoma treated by prophylactic retroperitoneal irradiation): National Cancer Center Hospital, Japan

	YEAR				
	1	2	3	4	5
Office visit*	2	2	2	1	1
Chest x-ray	2	2	2	1	1
Complete blood count	2	2	2	1	1
Multichannel blood tests†	2	2	2	1	1
Abdominal ultrasound‡	2	2	1	1	1
Abdominal computed tomography‡	2	2	1	0	0
Alpha-fetoprotein	2	2	0	0	0
Beta-human chorionic gonadotropin	2	2	0	0	0

*Includes physical examination of the contralateral testis and supraclavicular lymph nodes.
†Include total protein, albumin, total bilirubin, blood urea nitrogen, creatinine, sodium, potassium, chloride, glutamic-oxaloacetic transaminase, glutamic-pyruvic transaminase, alkaline phosphatase, lactic dehydrogenase, and beta$_2$-microglobulin.
‡Computed tomography and ultrasound of the abdomen are considered equivalent. Either (not both) can be used.

Table 19-13 Follow-up of patients with testicular cancer (stage I nonseminoma germ cell tumor without retroperitoneal lymph node dissection and stage II seminoma and nonseminoma germ cell tumor): National Cancer Center Hospital, Japan

	YEAR				
	1	2	3	4	5
Office visit*	12†	6†	4†	2	2
Alpha-fetoprotein	12	6	4	2	2
Beta-human chorionic gonadotropin	12	6	4	2	2
Complete blood count	4	4	4	2	2
Multichannel blood tests‡	4	4	4	2	2
Chest x-ray	4	4	3	2	2
Abdominal computed tomography§	2	2	2	1	1
Abdominal ultrasound§	2	2	2	1	1
Helical computed tomography	¶	¶	¶	¶	¶

*Includes physical examination of the contralateral testis and supraclavicular lymph nodes.
†Performed four times per year for stage II seminoma and nonseminoma germ cell tumor.
‡Include total protein, albumin, total bilirubin, blood urea nitrogen, creatinine, sodium, potassium, chloride, glutamic-oxaloacetic transaminase, glutamic-pyruvic transaminase, alkaline phosphatase, lactic dehydrogenase, and beta$_2$-microglobulin.
§Computed tomography and ultrasound of the abdomen are considered equivalent. Either (not both) can be used.
¶Performed if indicated by other test results.

fetoprotein and beta-human chorionic gonadotropin, complete blood count, blood chemistry including renal and liver function tests, chest x-ray, helical computed tomography of the lungs and mediastinum, and computed tomography of the retroperitoneal lymph nodes and liver. Helical computed tomography of the lungs is useful for detecting occult pulmonary deposits not visualized by plain chest x-ray and is used when markers alone are positive or findings in the latter case are indefinite. Physical examination includes status of the contralateral testicle and supraclavicular lymph nodes, palpation of the abdomen, and neurological examination for possible brain metastasis.

On receipt of the official pathology report, a treatment strategy is planned, based on whether the tumor is a pure seminoma or nonseminoma germ cell tumor and the clinical stage. The plan is then explained to the patient in detail. Should the disease be advanced, this explanatory process is particularly important for successful accomplishment of the entire course of treatment. A schematic outline of the treat-

Table 19-14 Follow-up of patients with testicular cancer (stage III seminoma and nonseminoma germ cell tumor): National Cancer Center Hospital, Japan

	YEAR				
	1	2	3	4	5
Office visit*	12	4	4	2	2
Alpha-fetoprotein	12	4	4	2	2
Beta-human chorionic gonadotropin	12	4	4	2	2
Complete blood count	4	4	4	2	2
Multichannel blood tests†	4	4	4	2	2
Chest x-ray	4	4	3	2	2
Abdominal computed tomography‡	2	2	2	1	1
Abdominal ultrasound‡	2	2	2	1	1
Helical computed tomography	§	§	§	§	§
Brain computed tomography or magnetic resonance imaging	§	§	§	§	§

*Includes physical examination of the contralateral testis and supraclavicular lymph nodes.
†Include total protein, albumin, total bilirubin, blood urea nitrogen, creatinine, sodium, potassium, chloride, glutamic-oxaloacetic transaminase, glutamic-pyruvic transaminase, alkaline phosphatase, lactic dehydrogenase, and beta$_2$-microglobulin.
‡Computed tomography and ultrasound of the abdomen are considered equivalent. Either (not both) can be used.
§Performed if indicated by other test results.

ment for nonseminoma germ cell tumor is illustrated in Figure 19-1.

When chemotherapy is indicated, physicians at the National Cancer Center Hospital use a combination of cisplatin and etoposide as first-line chemotherapy (Figure 19-2). When a large tumor mass places the patient at high risk, the present investigational protocol is high-dosage chemotherapy followed by autologous bone marrow transplantation (Figure 19-3).

FOLLOW-UP AFTER COMPLETE RESPONSE

Once complete response has been achieved, follow-up of the patient commences at the outpatient clinic. The intervals and thoroughness of examination depend on the initial clinical stage and histological type. The points of follow-up are early detection of metastasis or relapse; evaluation of treatment-related complications of bone marrow, pulmonary, renal, and residual testicular functions; evaluation of the status of the contralateral testicle; and early detection of secondary malignancy. Various follow-up tests depending on clinical stage and histological type are performed (Tables 19-12 through 19-14). Because of the possibility of brain metastasis in stage III testicular carcinoma, whenever patients complain of a headache or any type of focal symptoms of the brain, computed tomography or magnetic resonance imaging of the brain is recommended.

REFERENCES

1. Tominaga S, Aoki K, Fujimoto I, Kurihara M, editors. Cancer mortality and morbidity statistics. Gann Monogr on Cancer Res 41. Tokyo: Japan Scientific Society Press, 1994:126-7.
2. Yoshida O, Kiriyama T, Miyakawa M, et al. [Clinical statistics on testicular tumors in the Japanese during the 1970s.] (In Japanese with English abstract) Acta Urol Jpn 1985;31:337-56.
3. Japanese Urologic Association, Japanese Pathologic Society. [General rule for clinical and pathological studies on testicular tumors.] (In Japanese) Tokyo: Kanehara Press, 1984.

➢ COUNTER POINT

University of Washington Medical Center

CELESTIA S. HIGANO AND PAUL H. LANGE

The importance of appropriate follow-up of testicular cancer has been succinctly described by Raghavan. Affected patients are frequently in the midst of their productive years, and unlike many other cancers, recurrent testicular cancer can be successfully treated and cured in the majority of cases.

In follow-up of patients with testicular cancer, it is worthwhile to make the distinction between patients with low-stage disease who opt for no further therapy and those who receive additional therapy. Patients with what appears to be clinical stage I seminoma or nonseminomatous germ cell tumor may choose surveillance and forego further therapy after orchiectomy. Since there is a reasonable chance that orchiectomy alone will be curative and recurrences usually occur within 2 years of diagnosis, more intense scrutiny during that time is required.

Physicians at the University of Washington Medical Center differ slightly from Raghavan's stage A follow-up regimen and recommend a more classic schedule (Table 19-15). During the first year follow-up includes a history, physical examination, chest x-ray, and serum markers including alpha-fetoprotein, beta-human chorionic gonadotropin, and lactic dehydrogenase every month, as well as computed tomography of the abdomen and pelvis every other month. During the second year visits take place every 2 months, with computed tomography performed every 4 months. From years 3 to 5, visits and computed tomography take place every 6 months, and thereafter visits are annual. Raghavan has suggested that the frequency of surveillance testing can be decreased from previous practices because the patterns of spread and relapse have now been established. Although different surveillance schedules may be studied prospectively in academic centers, we believe the established surveillance

Table 19-15 Follow-up of patients with testicular cancer (stage I after orchiectomy alone): University of Washington Medical Center

	YEAR				
	1	2	3	4	5
Office visit	12	6	2	2	2
Chest x-ray	12	6	2	2	2
Alpha-fetoprotein	12	6	2	2	2
Beta-human chorionic gonadotropin	12	6	2	2	2
Lactic dehydrogenase	12	6	2	2	2
Abdominal computed tomography	6	3	2	2	2
Pelvic computed tomography	6	3	2	2	2

Table 19-16 Follow-up of patients with testicular cancer (stages I and II after retroperitoneal lymph node dissection): University of Washington Medical Center

	YEAR				
	1	2	3	4	5
Office visit	12	6	3	3	3
Chest x-ray	12	6	3	3	3
Alpha-fetoprotein	12	6	3	3	3
Beta-human chorionic gonadotropin	12	6	3	3	3
Lactic dehydrogenase	12	6	3	3	3
Abdominal computed tomography	1*	0	0	0	0
Pelvic computed tomography	1*	0	0	0	0

*Baseline computed tomography indicated postoperatively.

schedule should be followed until reports of outcomes with less frequent testing have been published.

The history should include asking the patient about a personal assessment of the remaining testicle (that is, whether the patient is performing self-examinations) and the presence of breast tenderness or any symptoms suggestive of lung or abdominal disease such as cough or abdominal discomfort. The physical examination should include lymph nodes (supraclavicular nodes are important), lungs, breasts, abdomen, and the remaining testicle. Chest x-ray is performed, and serum markers should be drawn.

As opposed to surveillance for high-risk disease, follow-up testing after a patient has chosen to proceed with additional primary treatment for low-risk disease is not as frequent because the likelihood of relapse after the additional therapy is low. Tables 19-16 through 19-19 outline various recommended schedules for follow-up. Routine computed

Table 19-17 Follow-up of patients with testicular cancer (stage II after adjuvant chemotherapy): University of Washington Medical Center

	YEAR				
	1	2	3	4	5
Office visit	4	2	1	1	1
Chest x-ray	4	2	1	1	1
Alpha-fetoprotein	4	2	1	1	1
Beta-human chorionic gonadotropin	4	2	1	1	1
Lactic dehydrogenase	4	2	1	1	1
Complete blood count	4	2	1	1	1
Liver function tests	4	2	1	1	1
Abdominal computed tomography	2-3	2-3	0	0	0
Pelvic computed tomography	2-3	2-3	0	0	0

Table 19-18 Follow-up of patients with testicular cancer (stage III after chemotherapy, complete response): University of Washington Medical Center

	YEAR				
	1	2	3	4	5
Office visit	6	3	1	1	1
Chest x-ray	6	3	1	1	1
Alpha-fetoprotein	6	3	1	1	1
Beta-human chorionic gonadotropin	6	3	1	1	1
Lactic dehydrogenase	6	3	1	1	1
Complete blood count	6	3	1	1	1
Liver function tests	6	3	1	1	1
Abdominal computed tomography	2-3	2-3	0	0	0
Pelvic computed tomography	2-3	2-3	0	0	0

Table 19-19 Follow-up of patients with testicular cancer (seminoma after orchiectomy and radiation therapy): University of Washington Medical Center

	YEAR				
	1	2	3	4	5
Office visit	6	3	2	1	1
Chest x-ray	6	3	2	1	1
Alpha-fetoprotein	6	3	2	1	1
Beta-human chorionic gonadotropin	6	3	2	1	1
Lactic dehydrogenase	6	3	2	1	1
Abdominal computed tomography	2-3	2-3	0	0	0
Pelvic computed tomography	2-3	2-3	0	0	0

tomography is generally not performed if the patient has undergone a retroperitoneal lymph node dissection because recurrence in the retroperitoneum is rare in that setting. However, a baseline postoperative computed tomographic scan can be helpful in the event that computed tomography is needed in the future. In the follow-up of patients who have received chemotherapy, periodic complete blood counts and liver function tests are also recommended. The practice at the University of Washington Medical Center is to obtain computed tomographic scans every 4 to 6 months

Table 19-20 Follow-up of patients with testicular cancer by institution

YEAR/PROGRAM	OFFICE VISIT	AFP	HCG/B-HCG	LDH	CBC	MCBT
Year 1						
Memorial Sloan-Kettering I[a]	12	12	12	12		
Memorial Sloan-Kettering II[e]	6	6	6	6		
Memorial Sloan-Kettering III[f]	4	4	4	4		
Memorial Sloan-Kettering IV[h]	4	4	4	4		
Roswell Park I[i]	6	6	6	6	5	5[j]
Roswell Park II[k]	5	5	5	5	4	4[j]
Univ Washington I[l]	12	12	12	12		
Univ Washington II[m]	12	12	12	12		
Univ Washington III[o]	4	4	4	4	4	
Univ Washington IV[p]	6	6	6	6	6	
Univ Washington V[q]	6	6	6	6		
Japan: Natl Cancer Ctr I[r]	2[s]	2	2		2	2[t]
Japan: Natl Cancer Ctr II[v]	12[w,x]	12	12		4	4[t]
Japan: Natl Cancer Ctr III[z]	12[w]	12	12		4	4[t]

ABD CT abdominal computed tomography
ABD US abdominal ultrasound
AFP alpha-fetoprotein
CBC complete blood count
CHEST CT chest computed tomography
CT computed tomography
CXR chest x-ray
HCG/B-HCG human chorionic gonadotropin/beta-human chorionic gonadotropin
HEL CT helical computed tomography
LDH lactate dehydrogenase
LFT liver function tests
MCBT multichannel blood tests
MRI magnetic resonance imaging

for the first 2 years after chemotherapy or radiation therapy, but no data exist to support this approach.

Occasionally patients report symptoms that require additional testing such as a bone scan, computed tomography, or magnetic resonance imaging of the brain. These tests are not part of routine follow-up. The importance of late sequelae, including relapse and complications of chemotherapy, radiation, or surgery, has been underscored by Raghavan. Although the likelihood of cure is high after 5 years, annual follow-up examinations for life are recommended.

CXR	ABD CT	CHEST CT	PELVIC CT	HEL CT	BRAIN CT/MRI	ABD US	LFT
12	5[b,c]	[d]	5[b,c]				
6	1	[d]	1				
4	1[g]	[d]	1[g]				
4	2	[d]	2				
4	3	2					
3	3	2					
12	6		6				
12	1[n]		1[n]				
4	2-3		2-3				4
6	2-3		2-3				6
6	2-3		2-3				
2	2[u]					2[u]	
4	2[u]			y		2[u]	
4	2[u]			y	y	2[u]	

a Patients with stage I nonseminoma germ cell tumor.
b Performed biannually in year 1 and annually thereafter for patients with stage N0 nonseminoma germ cell tumor or patients with stage I N1 or N2a nonseminoma germ cell tumor who have not undergone adjuvant chemotherapy.
c Includes one test performed at baseline.
d Indicated if abnormality is detected on chest x-ray.
e Patients with stage II N1, N2a, N2b, or N3 nonseminoma germ cell tumor (assuming postoperative chemotherapy is performed) after retroperitoneal lymph node dissection.
f Patients with stage III nonseminoma germ cell tumor after retroperitoneal lymph node dissection and chemotherapy (assuming no viable cancer is detected).
g Performed annually if teratoma is detected in the retroperitoneum.
h Patients with stage I, IIA, or IIB seminoma.
i Patients with stage A testicular cancer.
j Consists of creatinine and alkaline phosphatase.
k Patients with stages B and C testicular cancer.
l Stage I after orchiectomy alone.
m Stages I and II after retroperitoneal lymph node dissection.
n Baseline computed tomography indicated postoperatively.
o Stage II after adjuvant chemotherapy.
p Stage III after chemotherapy, complete response.
q Patients with seminoma after orchiectomy and radiation therapy.
r Stage I seminoma treated by prophylactic retroperitoneal irradiation.
s Includes physical examination of the contralateral testis and supraclavicular lymph nodes.
t Include total protein, albumin, total bilirubin, creatinine, sodium, potassium, chloride, glutamic-oxaloacetic transaminase, glutamic-pyruvic transaminase, alkaline phosphatase, lactic dehydrogenase, and beta$_2$-microglobuin.
u Computed tomography and ultrasound of the abdomen are considered equivalent. Either (not both) can be used.
v Stage I nonseminoma germ cell tumor without retroperitoneal lymph node dissection and stage II seminoma and nonseminoma germ cell tumor.
w Includes physical examination of the contralateral testis and supraclavicular lymph nodes.
x Performed four times per year for stage II seminoma and nonseminoma germ cell tumor.
y Performed if indicated by other test results.
z Stage III seminoma and nonseminoma germ cell tumor.
aa Performed as clinically indicated.
bb After 5 years performed as clinically indicated, especially for patients with immature teratoma.

Continued.

Table 19-20 Follow-up of patients with testicular cancer by institution—cont'd

YEAR/PROGRAM	OFFICE VISIT	AFP	HCG/B-HCG	LDH	CBC	MCBT
Year 2						
Memorial Sloan-Kettering I[a]	6	6	6	6		
Memorial Sloan-Kettering II[e]	3	3	3	3		
Memorial Sloan-Kettering III[f]	3	3	3	3		
Memorial Sloan-Kettering IV[h]	3	3	3	3		
Roswell Park I[i]	4	4	4	4	2	2[j]
Roswell Park II[k]	3	3	3	3	2	2[j]
Univ Washington I[l]	6	6	6	6		
Univ Washington II[m]	6	6	6	6		
Univ Washington III[o]	2	2	2	2	2	
Univ Washington IV[p]	3	3	3	3	3	
Univ Washington V[q]	3	3	3	3		
Japan: Natl Cancer Ctr I[r]	2[s]	2	2		2	2[t]
Japan: Natl Cancer Ctr II[v]	6[w,x]	6	6		4	4[t]
Japan: Natl Cancer Ctr III[z]	4	4	4		4	4[t]
Year 3						
Memorial Sloan-Kettering I[a]	4	4	4	4		
Memorial Sloan-Kettering II[e]	2	2	2	2		
Memorial Sloan-Kettering III[f]	2	2	2	2		
Memorial Sloan-Kettering IV[h]	2	2	2	2		
Roswell Park I[i]	2	2	2	2	2	2[j]
Roswell Park II[k]	2	2	2	2	2	2[j]
Univ Washington I[l]	2	2	2	2		
Univ Washington II[m]	3	3	3	3		
Univ Washington III[o]	1	1	1	1	1	
Univ Washington IV[p]	1	1	1	1	1	
Univ Washington V[q]	2	2	2	2		
Japan: Natl Cancer Ctr I[r]	2[s]				2	2[t]
Japan: Natl Cancer Ctr II[v]	4[w,x]	4	4		4	4[t]
Japan: Natl Cancer Ctr III[z]	4[w]	4	4		4	4[t]

CXR	ABD CT	CHEST CT	PELVIC CT	HEL CT	BRAIN CT/MRI	ABD US	LFT
6	3[b]	d	3[b]				
3		d					
3	g	d	g				
3	1	d	1				
4	2	aa					
3	2	1					
6	3		3				
6							
2	2-3		2-3				2
3	2-3		2-3				3
3	2-3		2-3				
2	2[u]					2[u]	
4	2[u]			y		2[u]	
4	2[u]			y	y	2[u]	
4	2[b]	d	2[b]				
2		d					
2	g	d	g				
2	1	d	1				
2	2	aa					
2	1	aa					
2	2		2				
3							
1							1
1							1
2							
2	1[u]					1[u]	
3	2[u]			y		2[u]	
3	2[u]			y	y	2[u]	

Continued.

Table 19-20 Follow-up of patients with testicular cancer by institution–cont'd

YEAR/PROGRAM	OFFICE VISIT	AFP	HCG/B-HCG	LDH	CBC	MCBT
Year 4						
Memorial Sloan-Kettering I[a]	3	3	3	3		
Memorial Sloan-Kettering II[e]	2	2	2	2		
Memorial Sloan-Kettering III[f]	2	2	2	2		
Memorial Sloan-Kettering IV[h]	2	2	2	2		
Roswell Park I[i]	2	2	2	2	2	2[j]
Roswell Park II[k]	2	2	2	2	2	2[j]
Univ Washington I[l]	2	2	2	2		
Univ Washington II[m]	3	3	3	3		
Univ Washington III[o]	1	1	1	1	1	
Univ Washington IV[p]	1	1	1	1	1	
Univ Washington V[q]	1	1	1	1		
Japan: Natl Cancer Ctr I[r]	1[s]				1	1[t]
Japan: Natl Cancer Ctr II[v]	2[w]	2	2		2	2[t]
Japan: Natl Cancer Ctr III[z]	2[w]	2	2		2	2[t]
Year 5						
Memorial Sloan-Kettering I[a]	2	2	2	2		
Memorial Sloan-Kettering II[e]	2	2	2	2		
Memorial Sloan-Kettering III[f]	2	2	2	2		
Memorial Sloan-Kettering IV[h]	2	2	2	2		
Roswell Park I[i]	2	2	2	2	2	2[j]
Roswell Park II[k]	2	2	2	2	2	2[j]
Univ Washington I[l]	2	2	2	2		
Univ Washington II[m]	3	3	3	3		
Univ Washington III[o]	1	1	1	1	1	
Univ Washington IV[p]	1	1	1	1	1	
Univ Washington V[q]	1	1	1	1		
Japan: Natl Cancer Ctr I[r]	1[s]				1	1[t]
Japan: Natl Cancer Ctr II[v]	2[w]	2	2		2	2[t]
Japan: Natl Cancer Ctr III[z]	2[w]	2	2		2	2[t]

CXR	ABD CT	CHEST CT	PELVIC CT	HEL CT	BRAIN CT/MRI	ABD US	LFT
3	2[b]	d	2[b]				
2		d					
2	g	d	g				
2	1	d	1				
2	1	aa					
2	1	aa					
2	2		2				
3							
1							1
1							1
1							
1						1[u]	
2	1[u]			y		1[u]	
2	1[u]			y	y	1[u]	
2	2[b]	d	2[b]				
2		d					
2	g	d	g				
2	1	d	1				
2	1[bb]	aa					
2	bb	aa					
2	2		2				
3							
1							1
1							1
1							
1						1[u]	
2	1[u]			y		1[u]	
2	1[u]			y	y	1[u]	

CHAPTER 20

Urinary Bladder Carcinoma

Memorial Sloan-Kettering Cancer Center

HARRY W. HERR

Urinary bladder cancer is the fourth most common cancer among men and the eighth most common cancer among women in the United States, with more than 52,000 new cases and 11,000 deaths in 1994. The incidence of bladder cancer has increased 36% over the past decade; however, mortality rates have declined by 20%. This is attributed to better detection of carcinoma in situ and improved treatments of localized and regional disease.

Approximately 80% of bladder cancers are confined to the epithelium or submucosa (superficial tumors), and 20% invade the bladder muscle, perivesical fat, or pelvic lymph nodes (locally advanced tumors). Local tumor extent is assessed by an evaluation under anesthesia and transurethral endoscopic resection of the tumor. A transurethral endoscopic resection is both therapeutic and diagnostic for superficial tumors and is predominantly diagnostic for invasive tumors. Depth of tumor infiltration defines T stage, prognosis, and subsequent therapy. Clinical follow-up of bladder tumors is determined by the patterns of failure and the short- and long-term consequences of therapy.[1]

The current practice of treating urinary bladder cancer evolved with the cystoscope and the recognition that depth of invasion of the primary tumor is important to the success or failure of treatment. Since most bladder tumors are superficial, endoscopic management with transurethral endoscopic resection is usually successful. Intravesical (topical) therapy is often used after a transurethral endoscopic resection to reduce the rate of tumor recurrence. Transurethral endoscopic resection is generally not accepted therapy for tumors that invade the muscle wall owing to the inadequacy of complete tumor resection. Total cystectomy is required for most deeply invasive neoplasms. Radiation therapy alone does not cure invasive tumors or prevent local bladder recurrences. Half of patients with muscle-invasive bladder cancer die within 5 years of distant metastases unrecognized at the time of cystectomy. Patients at highest risk of systemic disease have primary tumors that have spread beyond the bladder to involve perivesical soft tissue or pelvic lymph nodes. This has led to combination chemotherapy regimens with surgery to reduce distant metastases and improve survival. The optimal multimodality strategy for invasive bladder cancer is still evolving.

General consensus exists among urologists, radiation oncologists, and medical oncologists regarding treatment and follow-up strategies for both superficial and muscle-invasive bladder tumors. Current interest in bladder preservation portends future changes in treatment priorities.

SUPERFICIAL BLADDER TUMORS

Transurethral endoscopic resection is the standard initial treatment for superficial bladder tumors. Despite complete resection, new bladder tumors (tumor recurrence) develop in most patients who undergo this procedure. In the majority of cases the recurrence is superficial, but in 10% to 30% of patients a tumor occurs with invasion into the muscle layer of the bladder (tumor progression). Once the tumor has penetrated the muscle, there is a substantial risk of metastases and death. This grim prognosis for muscle-invasive disease has led to a strategy of vigilant follow-up and repeat transurethral endoscopic resections of recurrent superficial tumors.

Papillary neoplasms may involve only the mucosa (papilloma, Ta) or submucosa (T1) and are either low (G1) or high (G3) grade. Carcinoma in situ (Tis) is a flat, high-grade, often diffuse, and poorly defined tumor. Most superficial tumors are multifocal and recur within 1 to 2 years of initial diagnosis. More important, up to one third of such tumors progress within 5 years to muscle infiltration. T1G3 tumors and diffuse Tis are evaluated frequently, since they are most likely to invade. Papillomas and TaG1 tumors tend to recur in clusters every 1 to 3 years, have long disease-free intervals, pose little risk of progression, and require less frequent evaluation.[2]

Generally, patients undergo outpatient flexible cystoendoscopy under local (topical) anesthesia every 3 months for the first 2 years, every 4 months for years 3 and 4, every 6 months for the fifth year, and annually thereafter for life.[3] Voided urine is obtained at each office visit for cytological examination and flow cytometry if available. Cystoscopy every 3 to 4 months is continued as long as the patient has tumor recurrences.

The incidence of tumors involving the upper collecting system (ureter and renal pelvis) among patients with recurrent superficial bladder tumors is 15% at 3 years, 20%

Table 20-1 Follow-up of patients with urinary bladder cancer (superficial bladder tumors): Memorial Sloan-Kettering Cancer Center

	YEAR				
	1	2	3	4	5
Office visit*	4	4	3	3	2
Cystoscopy†	4	4	3	3	2
Urine cytology	4	4	3	3	2
Intravenous pyelography	1	1	1	1	1

*Symptoms assessed at each visit are hematuria, dysuria, and frequency.
†For patients with papilloma TaG1, cystoscopy is performed every 6 months for the first 3 years and annually thereafter. For patients with TaG2 focal tissue Tis, it is performed every 3 months for the first 2 years, every 6 months for years 3 and 4, and annually thereafter. For patients with T1G2,3 diffuse Tis, cystoscopy is performed every 3 months for the first 2 years, every 4 months for years 3 and 4, every 6 months for year 5, and annually thereafter. Follow-up intervals may shift according to changes in patterns of recurrence. With every recurrence patients return to cystoscopy every 3 months for at least the following year.

within 5 years, and up to 30% between 5 and 10 years. Intravenous pyelography is recommended every year for at least 10 years and probably for life.[4] Table 20-1 shows my approach to follow-up of superficial bladder tumors, as well as modifications for specific tumor types based on risk of tumor progression.

INVASIVE BLADDER CANCER: FOLLOW-UP AFTER CYSTECTOMY

Radical cystectomy, with or without chemotherapy, is the treatment of choice for invasive bladder cancer. The urinary tract is diverted to the skin as an ileal conduit or continent stoma or to the urethra via an orthotopic neobladder.

In most patients with solid tumors follow-up studies after surgery are aimed at the detection of local recurrence or metastasis. The results of salvage therapy are generally poor. Enthusiasm for close follow-up is tempered by the lack of effective treatment. Recurrent bladder cancer, however, responds well to salvage treatment. Urethral or ureteral carcinoma, which is highly curable if detected at an early stage, may develop. In addition, technical or physiological consequences of the urinary diversion can lead to late effects that must be monitored.

The follow-up program after cystectomy has three facets: detection of "new" urothelial tumors, detection of a local recurrence or metastasis, and monitoring of the effects of urinary diversion. Table 20-2 outlines a follow-up strategy for patients after cystectomy. Modifications are often necessary.

Table 20-2 Follow-up of patients with urinary bladder cancer (after cystectomy): Memorial Sloan-Kettering Cancer Center

	YEAR				
	1	2	3	4	5
Office visit*	5	3	2	2	2
Complete blood count	5	3	2	2	2
Electrolytes	5	3	2	2	2
Multichannel blood tests†	5	3	2	2	2
Liver function tests	5	3	2	2	2
Voided urine or ileal conduit cytology‡	5	3	2	2	2
Urethral washings§	4-5	3-4	3-4	2	2
Abdominal computed tomography¶	3	2	1	1	1
Pelvic computed tomography¶	3	2	1	1	1
Chest x-ray	2	2	1	1	1
Intravenous pyelography or renal ultrasound	2	1	1	1	1

*Symptoms assessed at each visit are urinary, stoma, and hematuria, sexual, abdominal pain, weight loss, and back pain. Office visit should include physical examination of the abdomen, groin, lymph nodes, stoma, urethra, penis, and perirectal lymph nodes and digital rectal examination.
†Consists of blood urea nitrogen and creatinine.
‡For patients receiving an orthotopic internal reservoir to the urethra.
§The first urethral wash should be obtained 4 to 8 weeks after cystectomy.
¶The first computed tomographic scan should be obtained at 3 months.

UROTHELIAL RECURRENCE

Urethra

The entire penile urethra in males is usually not excised during a radical cystectomy and thus remains a site for recurrence or new lesions. Patients at risk have multifocal carcinoma of the bladder involving the bladder neck and transitional cell carcinoma extending into the prostatic urethra and ducts. Urethral relapse occurs in 5% to 10% of patients, primarily within the first 2 to 3 years after cystectomy. Follow-up observation of the urethra should therefore be most diligent during this period. Results of delayed therapeutic urethrectomy for urethral cancer are excellent if the recurrence is discovered by urethral washing and if only carcinoma in situ is present. If urethrectomy is prompted by symptoms such as urethral bleeding or pain, invasion is commonly present and survival is poor. Fortunately, urethral washing is easy and effective.[5]

A small catheter is passed to the end of the urethra, and 20 to 30 ml of sterile saline is flushed in pulses through the catheter. The fluid draining around the catheter at the meatus is collected and sent for cytological examination. The presence of atypical or malignant cells on a urethral wash or evidence of bleeding from the meatus is an indication for urethroscopy, often followed by urethrectomy. A urethral wash is obtained 4 to 8 weeks after cystectomy, every 3 to 4 months thereafter for the first 3 years, and every 6 months for the next 2 years. In the absence of symptoms no further examination beyond 5 years is warranted. Patients receiving an orthotopic internal reservoir to the urethra (either males or females) are monitored by voided urine cytology. Direct urethroscopy may also be useful.

Ureters and Renal Pelvis

The incidence of upper tract cancer in all patients after cystectomy is approximately 2% to 4% within 5 years, but patients remain at risk for life. Patients at risk include those with extensive Tis disease in the bladder and distal ureter. If Tis is also present in the prostatic urethra, the lifetime risk for upper tract carcinoma increases to 20%.

Follow-up of the upper tracts is based on imaging and cytological evaluation of the urine. Intravenous pyelography allows visualization of the collecting system for either obstruction or filling defects. A retrograde pyelogram of an ileal conduit is useful to define an area of obstruction more precisely, but it is a more invasive procedure and is performed only in the event of an abnormality on the intravenous pyelogram. Urine cytology remains valuable even after urinary diversion, although more atypical results are likely owing to confusion of ileal or colonic mucosal cells with malignant transitional cells. False-positive results, however, do not generally occur, and positive cytological findings reliably indicate the presence of upper tract cancer.

Local Pelvic Recurrence or Metastases

The overall relapse rate after cystectomy for muscle-invasive cancer varies between 30% and 80%. Of these, 70% occur within the first 2 years, 20% in the third year, and 10% between the fourth and fifth years. Pelvic recurrence occurs in 10% to 20% of patients with bladder-confined cancer, in 30% to 40% of patients with extravesical disease, and in up to 50% of patients with pelvic node metastasis. Ten percent of patients die of locoregional disease alone, although metastases are present in 90% of such patients. In decreasing order of frequency, distant disease appears in the lung, nodes, bone, and liver. After 5 years patients are considered cured of their bladder neoplasm. Early detection of pelvic recurrences or distant metastases after cystectomy is important, since this may translate into cure. Patients with limited-organ metastases, pelvic recurrence, or isolated positive retroperitoneal nodes respond well to cisplatin-based (methotrexate, vinblastine, doxorubicin, and cisplatin) chemotherapy, and 18% remain alive and disease free beyond 5 years.[6]

After cystectomy, baseline abdominal and pelvic computed tomographic scans with contrast are obtained at 3 months. Computed tomography of the pelvis provides optimal imaging of the sites of local recurrence not accessible by physical examination. Computed tomography and chest x-rays are repeated every 6 months for the first 2 years and then once every year for 5 years.

CONSEQUENCES OF URINARY DIVERSION

The urinary reconstruction necessary after cystectomy adds another feature to follow-up. Complications from the diversion and anticipated metabolic complications must be monitored. The use of alternative forms of diversion other than the standard ileal conduit has been a recent trend, and the late sequelae of cutaneous or orthotopic urinary reservoirs may not be manifest until longer follow-up is available.

Technical Complications

Follow-up after urinary diversion requires periodic assessment of the status of the upper tracts. The serum creatinine level monitors total renal function, but an imaging study is valuable to identify hydronephrosis and calculi before severe renal damage and to evaluate conduit or reservoir function. Intravenous pyelography fulfills this role adequately.

The major problem related to an ileal conduit is obstruction of the ureteral-intestinal anastomosis. This produces hydronephrosis in 5% to 10% of patients (4.8% on the right, 8.3% on the left, and 2.4% bilateral), pyelonephritis or urinary tract infection in 10%, renal deterioration after 5 years in 10%, and loss of a kidney in 5%. Other problems include renal calculi in 5% to 10% and stoma problems (hernia, stenosis, and prolapse) in 5%.[7]

Patients with an ileal conduit should be followed up routinely by an enterostomal therapist. Stoma complications can be prevented by proper creation of an everted "rosebud" stoma and meticulous stomal care. Early recognition and care of peristomal skin conditions and proper application of the stoma appliance avoid potentially serious and long-term problems.

Metabolic Consequences

Metabolic consequences after a standard ileal conduit are negligible unless a technical complication occurs. However, continent diversion uses larger segments of the bowel and raises the potential for functional disturbances.[8]

Use of an ileocolic segment for either a continent cutaneous or an orthotopic reservoir removes a portion of the terminal ileum and cecum, exposing the patient to potential malabsorption of vitamin B_{12}. Low vitamin B_{12} levels occur in 25% of patients and may result in neurological symptoms. Measurement of vitamin B_{12} levels during routine follow-up after ileocolic diversion appears appropriate. Diarrhea or steatorrhea may also be troublesome.

Ileal reservoirs using 50 to 70 cm of ileum have not been consistently associated with metabolic abnormalities based on modest follow-up. Diarrhea and malabsorption of fat and bile salts may be seen on occasion, more commonly in patients with previous radiation therapy or other bowel disease. A chronic metabolic (hyperchloremic) acidosis may occur and adversely affect calcium balance and skeletal mineralization. Particularly in women, changes in calcium metabolism may have important long-term sequelae not evident for many years.

The primary long-term problem associated with continent external or orthotopic pouches is chronic distention and larger capacities that potentiate malabsorption. This occurs because of incomplete emptying, as a result of problems with catheterization, mucous obstruction, or inadequate emptying during voiding, leading to a buildup of residual urine. Careful intake and output records need to be maintained by the patient. Patients are also taught intermittent self-catheterization, which should be done at least 2 to 3 times a week to avoid overdistention and subsequent decompensation of the reservoir. The average neobladder capacity is 400 ml, but it is not uncommon after 5 years or more to see reservoir capacity in excess of 1 L, which is dangerously high. Hydronephrosis owing to reflux from overdistention may contribute to deterioration of renal function.

Follow-up of an ileal neobladder at Memorial Sloan-Kettering Cancer Center is as follows: every 2 months for year 1, every 4 months for years 2 and 3, every 6 months for years 4 and 5, and annually thereafter. Urine culture, sensitivity, and cytological studies are obtained every 6 months; voided urine for cytological examination is obtained during every office visit. An intravenous pyelogram is obtained at 6 months for the first 2 years and annually thereafter. Abdominal and pelvic computed tomographic scans with contrast are obtained at 3 months for year 1, every 6 months for years 2 and 3, and annually thereafter. At each visit serum electrolytes, blood urea nitrogen, and creatinine are checked. At designated intervals the residual urine is checked. At each visit the patient is evaluated for continence and bladder emptying.

Malignancy in Bowel Segments

The experience gained with ureterosigmoidostomy demonstrates that the risk of colon cancer is increased 400-fold.[9] Standard practice is for a patient to undergo colonoscopy annually beginning 5 to 10 years after ureterosigmoidoscopy. The potential risk for carcinoma imposed by incorporation of colonic segments into the urinary tract without admixture of the fecal and urinary streams is poorly defined. Anecdotal cases of adenocarcinoma in a reservoir have been noted, but the magnitude of the risk imposed is unclear. Currently, periodic pouchoscopy to monitor for bowel carcinomas is not advised.

FUTURE PROSPECTS

Tumor Markers

Molecular biology has contributed to the identification of numerous tumor markers currently under investigation in the treatment and follow-up of bladder tumors. These include DNA analysis, blood group antigens (LeX), epidermal growth factor, monoclonal antibodies to tumor-associated antigens, and tumor suppressor gene products (p53 and Rb). However, none has been validated in a prospective clinical study. Each marker or combination of markers holds promise as a prognostic variable for identifying risk of tumor progression and directing alternative treatments, but none is currently used or advocated in the routine follow-up of patients with bladder tumor.

Clinical Studies

Multiinstitutional, prospective clinical trials are needed and have proved successful in bladder cancer research. Issues being addressed in such trials are reduction in tumor recurrence and progression of superficial bladder tumors with novel intravesical agents, neoadjuvant and adjuvant chemotherapy regimens to improve survival (especially among patients with locally advanced and node-positive bladder cancer), and multimodal treatment strategies aimed at bladder preservation and improved quality of life of patients with bladder cancer.

REFERENCES

1. Yoshida O, Bono A, Braeckman J, et al. Clinical follow-up. Prog Clin Biol Res 1986;287:287-93.
2. Herr HW, Laudone VP, Whitmore WF Jr. An overview of intravesical therapy for superficial bladder tumors. J Urol 1987;138:1363-8.
3. Herr HW. Outpatient flexible cystoscopy and fulguration of recurrent superficial bladder tumors. J Urol 1990;144:1365-6.
4. Schwalb DM, Herr HW, Sogani PC, et al. Positive urinary cytology following a complete response to intravesical bacillus Calmette-Guerin therapy: pattern of recurrence. J Urol 1994;152:382-7.
5. Hardeman SW, Soloway MS. Urethral recurrence following radical cystectomy. J Urol 1990;144:666-9.
6. Sternberg CM, Yagoda A, Scher HI, et al. Methotrexate, vinblastine, doxorubicin and cisplatin for advanced transitional cell carcinoma of the urothelium: efficacy and patterns of response and relapse. Cancer 1989;64:2448-58.
7. Sullivan JW, Grabstald H, Whitmore WF Jr. Complications of ureteroileal conduit with radical cystectomy: review of 336 cases. J Urol 1980;124:797-801.
8. McDougal WS. Metabolic complications of urinary intestinal diversion. J Urol 1992;147:1199-208.
9. Filmer RB, Spencer JR. Malignancies in bladder augmentations and intestinal conduits. J Urol 1990;143:671-8.

➢ COUNTERPOINT

National Cancer Center Hospital, Japan

TADAO KAKIZOE

Herr presents a strategy for follow-up of patients with bladder cancer that takes into account the risk of multiple tumor development in the upper urinary tract and urethra. Herr also appropriately covers the evaluation of patients with urinary diversion after cystectomy. I agree almost entirely with the recommended strategies. The surveillance schedules followed by physicians at the National Cancer Center Hospital are presented in Tables 20-3 and 20-4, with minor modifications added.

Table 20-3 Follow-up of patients with urinary bladder cancer (superficial bladder tumors): National Cancer Center Hospital, Japan

	YEAR				
	1	2	3	4	5
Office visit*	4	3	3	2	2
Cystoscopy†	4	3	3	2	2
Urine cytology†	4	3	3	2	2
Intravenous pyelography	1	1	1	1	1

*Symptoms assessed at each visit are hematuria, dysuria, and frequency.
†Follow-up intervals may shift according to the cystoscopic and cytological findings, particularly for patients with T1G3 disease.

Table 20-4 Follow-up of patients with urinary bladder cancer (after cystectomy): National Cancer Center Hospital, Japan

	YEAR				
	1	2	3	4	5
Office visit*	6	5	3	2	2
Complete blood count	6	5	3	2	2
Multichannel blood tests†	6	5	3	2	2
Voided urine or ileal conduit cytology‡	6	5	3	2	2
Urethral washings	2	2	2	2	2
Chest x-ray	2	2	2	2	1
Abdominal computed tomography	2	2	1	1	1
Pelvic computed tomography	2	2	1	1	1
Intravenous pyelography	1	1	1	1	1
Urodynamic study‡	1	0	0	0	0
Radiological and nuclear medicine studies	§	§	§	§	§

*Symptoms assessed at each visit are urinary, stomal, and sexual function and the presence of hematuria, fever, abdominal pain, weight loss, thirst, and back pain. The office visit should include physical examination of the abdomen, stoma, urethra, rectum, and inguinal supraclavicular nodes.
†Consists of blood urea nitrogen and creatinine.
‡For patients receiving an orthotopic neobladder.
§Bone x-ray, bone scintigram, and liver and brain computed tomographic scans are obtained when indicated by symptoms or signs.

URETHRAL RECURRENCE

When deciding to use an ileal conduit or continent reservoir for reconstruction of the urinary tract after cystectomy, physicians at the National Cancer Center Hospital carefully evaluate the characteristics of the resected bladder cancer for factors that increase the risk of urethral recurrence. If widespread carcinoma in situ in the bladder or cancer in the bladder neck, prostatic urethra, or prostatic tissue is identified by cystoscopy or biopsy, urethrectomy is performed simultaneously with cystectomy.[1] If the urethra is left intact after cystectomy because preoperative evaluation indicates a low risk for urethral recurrence, physicians question the patient about urethral discharge, particularly bloody discharge, at each office visit after cystectomy. If a patient has such symptoms, urethral washings and retrograde urethrography are indicated. Even when patients do not have such symptoms, urethral washings are obtained twice a year.

In female patients the most important risk factor for urethral involvement appears to be bladder neck involvement by bladder cancer.[2] Creation of an orthotopic neobladder anastomosed to the urethra has been performed in six female patients with low risk of urethral recurrence and good functional results. Based on current selection criteria for creation of an orthotopic neobladder, urethral recurrence is rare.

VOIDING FUNCTION OF ORTHOTOPIC NEOBLADDER

Orthotopic ileal neobladder is offered to both male and female patients when clinically indicated.[2,3] Voiding difficulty (sometimes requiring intermittent self-catheterization) is the major problem, rather than incontinence. Consequently a urodynamic study of the neobladder is performed 2 to 3 months after its construction.

REFERENCES

1. Tobisu K, Tanaka Y, Mizutani T, Kakizoe T. Transitional cell carcinoma of the urethra in men following cystectomy for bladder cancer: multivariate analysis for risk factors. J Urol 1991;146:1551-4.
2. Coloby PJ, Kakizoe T, Tobisu K, Sakamoto M. Urethral involvement in female bladder cancer patients: mapping of 47 consecutive cysto-urethrectomy specimens. J Urol 1994;152:1438-42.
3. Tobisu K, Coloby PJ, Fujimoto H, Mizutani T, Kakizoe T. An ileal neobladder for a female patient after a radical cystectomy to ensure voiding from the urethra: a case report. Jpn J Clin Oncol 1992;22:359-64.

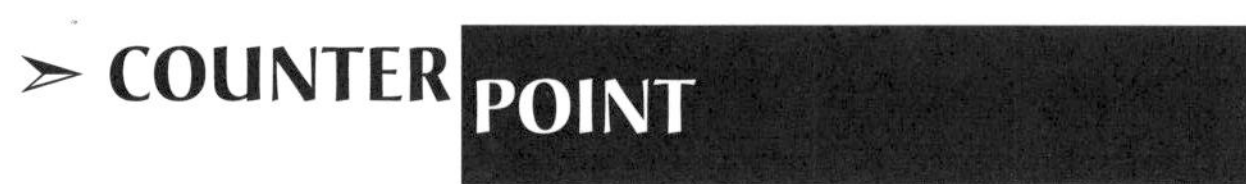

Roswell Park Cancer Institute

ROBERT P. HUBEN

An optimal follow-up strategy for patients with superficial or invasive bladder cancer is extremely difficult to define because of the many permutations in clinical presentation, natural history, and treatment history that would influence the extent and frequency of follow-up studies. The studies recommended by Herr for the follow-up of patients with both superficial and invasive bladder cancer seem to strike a reasonable balance and allow some modification based on tumor grade or stage in the case of superficial tumors. For this latter group of patients, physicians at Roswell Park Cancer Institute have a somewhat different schedule of cystoscopy, as shown in Table 20-5. The presence of atypical cytological features triggers the return to 3-month intervals between evaluations, and positive cytological findings lead to a full workup, including cystoscopy with bladder biopsies, selective upper tract cytological studies, and biopsy of the prostatic urethra.

The recommendation at Roswell Park Cancer Institute is annual intravenous pyelography in patients with superficial tumors and after cystectomy for invasive tumors to monitor the upper tracts. Physicians at Roswell Park Cancer Institute perform retrograde pyelography (loopogram) commonly in patients who have undergone cystectomy and ileal conduit urinary diversion, since about one in five patients reports a previous allergic reaction to the contrast media used in intravenous pyelography. Patients routinely take an oral fluoroquinolone antibiotic the night before and the morning of the procedure. Retrograde pyelography is still an invasive procedure, as noted, and the risk of septic complications is real despite such precautions.

Table 20-5 Follow-up of patients with urinary bladder cancer (superficial bladder tumors): Roswell Park Cancer Institute

	YEAR				
	1	2	3	4	5
Office visit	4	3	2	2	2
Cystoscopy	4	3	2	2	2
Urine cytology	4	3	2	2	2
Intravenous pyelography	1	1	1	1	1

Table 20-6 Follow-up of patients with urinary bladder cancer (after cystectomy): Roswell Park Cancer Institute

	YEAR				
	1	2	3	4	5
Office visit*	4	3	2	2	2
Complete blood count	4	3	2	2	2
Electrolytes	4	3	2	2	2
Multichannel blood tests†	4	3	2	2	2
Liver function tests	4	3	2	2	2
Voided urine or ileal conduit cytology‡	4	3	2	2	2
Urethral washings§	4	3	2	2	2
Chest x-ray	2	2	1	1	1
Intravenous pyelography or retrograde pyelogram¶	2	1	1	1	1

*Symptoms assessed at each visit are urinary, stomal, and hematuria, sexual, abdominal pain, weight loss, and back pain. The office visit should include physical examination of the abdomen, groin lymph nodes, stoma, urethra, and penis and digital rectal examination.
†Consists of blood urea nitrogen and creatinine.
‡For patients receiving an orthotopic internal reservoir to the urethra.
§The first urethral wash should be obtained 4 to 8 weeks after cystectomy.
¶Retrograde pyelography performed only for patients with a previous allergic reaction to the contrast media used in intravenous pyelography.

As stated by Herr, urethral washings are an important but often overlooked part of the routine follow-up in men after radical cystectomy and urinary diversion. I strongly recommend prophylactic urethrectomy in patients when the final pathology report shows involvement of the prostatic urethra.

I disagree with the recommendation regarding the performance of routine computed tomography in patients with a history of invasive bladder cancer. The ultimate issue is whether obtaining routine computed tomographic scans in the follow-up of asymptomatic patients improves patient outcome. This seems unlikely, but a more scientific way to resolve the issue would be a prospective study in which patients are randomly assigned to different follow-up strategies. Determination of both tumor recurrence detection rates and subsequent outcome should show which studies are warranted. At Roswell Park Cancer Institute computed tomography is performed only if indicated by history or physical findings. Such indications include liver function abnormalities, abdominal or pelvic pain, unilateral leg swelling, or findings on rectal examination that prompt suspicion. Otherwise the follow-up schema is similar to the one proposed by Herr (Table 20-6). An exception to this approach is in patients who receive adjuvant chemotherapy for positive lymph nodes or extravesical extension of disease. In this situation a pretreatment baseline computed tomographic scan is obtained and patients are followed up with routine computed tomography every 6 months for 2 years after completion of chemotherapy.

➢ COUNTER POINT

University of Washington Medical Center

WILLIAM J. ELLIS AND PAUL H. LANGE

Herr provides an excellent overview of the follow-up of carcinoma of the urinary bladder. The principles embodied in the chapter reflect the current standard of care. However, several modifications can probably be made in the proposed scheme that would decrease costs without increasing risk to the patient (Tables 20-7 and 20-8).

The intensity of cystoscopic follow-up in patients with superficial bladder tumors may be decreased, as outlined in Table 20-7. The length of follow-up may also be decreased. Herr recommends endoscopic follow-up for life. As the cycle restarts after recurrence, this is often the case. However, some patients, particularly those with TaG1 tumors, never have recurrences. Abel[1] has suggested that patients with these low-risk tumors need be checked only once per year. A more reasonable approach is to continue endoscopic evaluation for 10 years.[2] After 10 years without recurrence patients can be followed up with annual urinalysis and voided urine cytology. The bladder tumor antigen test, discussed later, may also be of benefit in these patients. If hematuria, malignant cytology, or an abnormal bladder tumor antigen test is discovered, reevaluation with cystoscopy and intravenous pyelography is indicated. Longer term endoscopic follow-up may be indicated in patients who continue to smoke, those with high-grade lesions, and those treated with bacillus Calmette-Guerin.

Although voided urine cytological examination is recommended, bladder barbitage cytology is superior for the detection of cytologically atypical cells.[3] Because patients are evaluated with cystoscopy anyway, there is no added cost to the patient. One drawback to bladder barbitage is that the upper tracts may not be evaluated. This problem may be circumvented by performing the barbitage initially on entering the bladder, before draining the residual urine. Alternatively, a urine sample may be obtained before bladder barbitage.

The bladder tumor antigen test is a new examination that detects basement membrane complexes in the urine through

Table 20-7 Follow-up of patients with urinary bladder cancer (superficial bladder tumors): University of Washington Medical Center

	YEAR				
	1	2	3	4	5
Office visit*	4	2	1	1	1
Bladder tumor antigen	4	2	1	1	1
Cystoscopy†	4	2	1	1	1
Bladder barbitage cytology‡	4	2	1	1	1
Intravenous pyelography	1	0	1	0	1

*Symptoms assessed at each visit are hematuria, dysuria, and frequency.
†For patients with papilloma TaG1, cystoscopy is performed at 3 months, 6 months, 1 year, and annually thereafter. Follow-up of all other tumors adheres to the intervals listed in the table. Follow-up intervals may shift according to changes in patterns of recurrence. For every recurrence patients restart the cycle and return to the follow-up provided in year 1. Follow-up beyond 10 years consists of urinalysis, bladder tumor antigen test, and voided urine cytology.
‡Performed in conjunction with cystoscopy.

a latex agglutination assay. The test is designed to be performed in an office setting. A recent study found this test to be more sensitive than voided urine cytology in diagnosing malignancy, particularly grade 1 and 2 noninvasive tumors for which the sensitivity of urine cytology is low.[4] The test does not replace cystoscopy or urine cytology. However, it will probably serve as a useful adjunct to these studies. A particular advantage of this test is that the results can be available before cystoscopy.

The stated incidence of tumors of the upper collecting system in patients with superficial bladder cancer recurrence is high. An upper tract recurrence rate of less than 5% is more realistic. Oldenbring et al.[5] noted upper tract tumors in 1.7% of patients in a cohort followed for an average of 7 years. Walzer and Soloway[6] noted a similar incidence of upper tract tumors in patients with superficial bladder tumors. Patients at highest risk for upper urothelial malignancies are those with multiple bladder tumors or tumors involving the ureteral orifices.[5] The figures quoted by Herr are more representative of patients with bladder carcinoma in situ that does not respond to intravesical bacillus Calmette-Guerin therapy.[7] In patients without recurrent bladder tumors the benefit of annual intravenous pyelography in the absence of hematuria and with negative cytological findings is small. After initial screening, intravenous pyelography every 2 to 3 years is reasonable. The development of hematuria unexplained by bladder findings or recurrent tumors warrants repeat upper tract evaluation.

Although computed tomography is recommended to evaluate for local recurrence after radical cystectomy, the value of this approach has not been proved. As noted by Herr, the vast majority of patients with locoregional recurrences of transitional cell carcinoma have other metastases that will be detected by chest x-ray or liver function tests. Alkaline phosphatase can assist in screening for both liver

Table 20-8 Follow-up of patients with urinary bladder cancer (after cystectomy): University of Washington Medical Center

	YEAR				
	1	2	3	4	5
Office visit*	5	3	2	2	2
Multichannel blood tests†	5	3	2	2	2
Liver function tests	5	3	2	2	2
Bladder tumor antigen	5	3	2	2	2
Urine cytology‡	5	3	2	2	2
Urethral washings	5	3	2	2	2
Abdominal computed tomography§	3	2	2	1	1
Pelvic computed tomography§	3	2	2	1	1
Chest x-ray	2	2	2	1	1
Intravenous pyelography or renal ultrasound¶	2	1	1	1	1
Vitamin B_{12}	0	2	2	2	2

*Symptoms assessed at each visit are urinary, stoma and hematuria, sexual, abdominal pain, weight loss, and back pain. The office visit should include physical examination of the lymph nodes, abdomen, groins, stoma, urethra, penis, and rectum.
†Consists of serum sodium, potassium, chloride, bicarbonate, blood urea nitrogen, and creatinine.
‡Voided specimen for patients with orthotopic reservoirs. Fresh catch for patients with ileal conduits. Catheterized specimens for patients with continent urinary reservoirs.
§The first computed tomographic scan should be obtained at 3 months.
¶The first upper tract study should be approximately 6 weeks after cystectomy to rule out obstruction. A renogram may be substituted for this first test.

and bony metastases. However, the primary reason for our weak endorsement of computed tomography in postcystectomy follow-up is the lack of proven long-term benefit with early treatment of locoregional recurrences.

Low vitamin B_{12} levels are a potential problem in patients whose terminal ileum is diverted from the gastrointestinal tract. Patients with ileal conduits rarely develop vitamin B_{12} deficiencies. When larger segments of the terminal ileum are removed, particularly with diversions using the ileal-cecal segment, the risk of vitamin B_{12} deficiency is more substantial.[8] Measurement of vitamin B_{12} levels in only years 2 through 5 after cystectomy should be adequate to detect most patients in whom vitamin B_{12} deficiency will develop. Most patients have adequate vitamin B_{12} stores to last at least 2 years. If the deficiency does not develop within 5 years, the patient probably has sufficient functioning ileum to adequately absorb vitamin B_{12}.

The follow-up of urothelial malignancies will continue to evolve. Current research efforts directed toward understanding the genetics of tumorigenesis and progression should improve the stratification of urothelial tumors into high- and low-risk categories. This stratification should decrease the cost of bladder cancer follow-up by decreasing the intensity of follow-up in low-risk patients. In addition, these studies may provide cancer detection tests that will render many current practices obsolete.

REFERENCES

1. Abel PD. Follow-up of patients with "superficial" transitional cell carcinoma of the bladder: the case for a change in policy. Br J Urol 1993;72:135-42.
2. Holmang S, Hedelin H, Anderstrom C, Johansson SL. The relationship among multiple recurrences, progression and prognosis of patients with stages TA and T1 transitional cell cancer of the bladder followed for at least 20 years. J Urol 1995;153:1823-7.
3. Murphy WM, Crabtree WN, Jukkola AF, Soloway MS. The diagnostic value of urine versus bladder washing in patients with bladder cancer. J Urol 1981;126:320-2.
4. Sarosdy MF, deVere White RW, Soloway MS, et al. Results of a multicenter trial using the BTA test to monitor for and diagnose recurrent bladder cancer. J Urol 1995;154:379-84.
5. Oldenbring J, Glifberg I, Mikulowski P, Hellsten S. Carcinoma of the renal pelvis and ureter following bladder carcinoma: frequency, risk factors, and clinicopathological findings. J Urol 1989;141:1311-3.
6. Walzer Y, Soloway MS. Should the follow-up of patients with bladder cancer include routine excretory urography? J Urol 1983;130:672-3.
7. Schwalb MD, Herr HW, Sogani PC, Russo P, Sheinfeld J, Fair WR. Positive urinary cytology following a complete response to intravesical bacillus Calmette-Guerin therapy: pattern of recurrence. J Urol 1994; 152:382-7.
8. Steiner MS, Morton RA, Marshall FF. Vitamin B_{12} deficiency in patients with ileocolic neobladders. J Urol 1993;149:255-7.

Table 20-9 Follow-up of patients with urinary bladder cancer by institution

YEAR/PROGRAM	OFFICE VISIT	CYSTOS	URINE CYT	IVP	CBC	ELE	MCBT	LFT	VU/ICC
Year 1									
Memorial Sloan-Kettering I[b]	4[c]	4[d]	4	1					
Memorial Sloan-Kettering II[e]	5[f]				5	5	5[g]	5	5[h]
Roswell Park I[b]	4	4	4	1					
Roswell Park II[e]	4[f]				4	4	4[g]	4	4[h]
Univ Washington I[b]	4[c]	4[k]		1					
Univ Washington II[e]	5[m]		5[n]				5[o]	5	
Japan: Natl Cancer Ctr I[b]	4[c]	4[q]	4[q]	1					
Japan: Natl Cancer Ctr II[e]	6[r]			1	6		6[g]		6[s]
Year 2									
Memorial Sloan-Kettering I[b]	4[c]	4[d]	4	1					
Memorial Sloan-Kettering II[e]	3[f]				3	3	3[g]	3	3[h]
Roswell Park I[b]	3	3	3	1					
Roswell Park II[e]	3[f]				3	3	3[g]	3	3[h]
Univ Washington I[b]	2[c]	2[k]							
Univ Washington II[e]	3[m]		3[n]				3[o]	3	
Japan: Natl Cancer Ctr I[b]	3[c]	3[q]	3[q]	1					
Japan: Natl Cancer Ctr II[e]	5[r]			1	5		5[g]		5[s]
Year 3									
Memorial Sloan-Kettering I[b]	3[c]	3[d]	3	1					
Memorial Sloan-Kettering II[e]	2[f]				2	2	2[g]	2	2[h]
Roswell Park I[b]	2	2	2	1					
Roswell Park II[e]	2[f]				2	2	2[g]	2	2[h]
Univ Washington I[b]	1[c]	1[k]		1					
Univ Washington II[e]	2[m]		2[n]				2[o]	2	
Japan: Natl Cancer Ctr I[b]	3[c]	3[q]	3[q]	1					
Japan: Natl Cancer Ctr II[e]	3[r]			1	3		3[g]		3[s]

ABD CT abdominal computed tomography
B12 vitamin B_{12}
BBC bladder barbitage cytology
BTA bladder tumor antigen
CBC complete blood count
CXR chest x-ray
CYSTOS cystoscopy
ELE electrolytes
IVP intravenous pyelography
IVP/RENAL US intravenous pyelography/renal ultrasound
IVP/RETRO intravenous pyelography or retrograde pyelography
LFT liver function test
MCBT multichannel blood tests
RAD NUC radiological and nuclear medicine studies
URETH WASH urethral washings
URINE CYT urine cytology
URODYN urodynamic study
VU/ICC voided urine/ileal conduit cytology

URETH WASH	CXR	IVP/ RETRO[a]	ABD CT	PELVIC CT	IVP/ RENAL US	URODYN	RAD NUC	BTA	BBC	B12
4-5[i]	2		3[j]	3[j]	2					
4[i]	2	2								
								4	4[l]	
5	2		3[j]	3[j]	2[p]			5		
2	2		2	2		1[s]	[t]			
3-4[i]	2		2[j]	2[j]	1					
3[i]	2	1								
								2	2[l]	
3	2		2[j]	2[j]	1[p]			3		2
2	2		2	2			[t]			
3-4[i]	1		1[j]	1[j]	1					
2[i]	1	1								
								1	1[l]	
2	2		2[j]	2[j]	1[p]			2		2
2	2		1	1			[t]			

a Retrograde pyelography performed only for patients with a previous allergic reaction to intravenous pyelography contrast media.
b Patients with superficial bladder tumors.
c Symptoms assessed at each visit are hematuria, dysuria, and frequency.
d For patients with papilloma TaG1, cytoscopy is performed every 6 months for the first 3 years and annually thereafter. For patients with TaG2 focal tissue Tis, it is performed every 3 months for the first 2 years, every 6 months for years 3 and 4, and annually thereafter. For patients with T1G2,3 diffuse Tis cystoscopy is performed every 3 months for the first 2 years, every 4 months for years 3 and 4, every 6 months for year 5, and annually thereafter. Follow-up intervals may shift according to changes in patterns of recurrence. With every recurrence, patients return to cystoscopy every 3 months for at least the following year.
e After cystectomy.
f Symptoms assessed at each visit are urinary stoma and hematuria, sexual, abdominal pain, weight loss, and back pain. The office visit should include physical examination of the abdomen, groin lymph nodes, stoma, urethra, penis, and perirectal lymph nodes by digital rectal examination.
g Consists of blood urea nitrogen and creatinine.
h For patients receiving an orthotopic internal reservoir to the urethra.
i The first urethral wash should be obtained 4 to 8 weeks after cystectomy.
j The first computed tomographic scan should be obtained at 3 months.
k For patients with papilloma TaG1, cystoscopy is performed at 3 months, 6 months, 1 year, and annually thereafter. Follow-up of all other tumors adheres to the intervals listed in the table. Follow-up intervals may shift according to changes in patterns of recurrence. For every recurrence, patients restart the cycle and return to the follow-up provided in year 1. Follow-up beyond 10 years consists of urinalysis, bladder tumor antigen test, and voided urine cytology.
l Performed in conjunction with cystoscopy.
m Symptoms assessed at each visit ar urinary, stoma and hematuria, sexual, abdominal pain, weight loss, and back pain. The office visit should include physical examination of the lymph nodes, abdomen, groins, stoma, urethra, penis, and rectum.
n Voided specimen for patients with orthotopic reservoirs. Fresh catch for patients with ileal conduits. Catheterized specimens for patients with continent urinary reservoirs.
o Consists of serum sodium, potassium, chloride, bicarbonate, blood urea nitrogen, and creatinine.
p The first upper tract study should be approximately 6 weeks after cystectomy to rule out obstruction. A renogram may be substituted for this first test.
q Follow-up intervals may shift according to the cystoscopic and cytological findings, particularly for patients with T1G3 disease.
r Symptoms assessed at each visit are urinary function, stoma function, sexual function, and the presence of hematuria, fever, abdominal pain, weight loss, thirst, and back pain. The office visit should include physical examination of the abdomen, stoma, urethra, rectum, and inguinal supraclavicular nodes.
s For patients receiving an orthotopic neobladder.
t Bone x-ray, bone scintigram, and liver and brain computed tomographic scans are performed when indicated by symptoms or signs.

Continued.

Table 20-9 Follow-up of patients with urinary bladder cancer by institution—cont'd

YEAR/PROGRAM	OFFICE VISIT	CYSTOS	URINE CYT	IVP	CBC	ELE	MCBT	LFT	VU/ICC
Year 4									
Memorial Sloan-Kettering I[b]	3[c]	3[d]	3	1					
Memorial Sloan-Kettering II[e]	2[f]				2	2	2[g]	2	2[h]
Roswell Park I[b]	2	2	2	1					
Roswell Park II[e]	2[f]				2	2	2[g]	2	2[h]
Univ Washington I[b]	1[c]	1[k]							
Univ Washington II[e]	2[m]		2[n]				2[o]	2	
Japan: Natl Cancer Ctr I[b]	2[c]	2[q]	2[q]	1					
Japan: Natl Cancer Ctr II[e]	2[r]			1	2		2[g]		2[s]
Year 5									
Memorial Sloan-Kettering I[b]	2[c]	2[d]	2	1					
Memorial Sloan-Kettering II[e]	2[f]				2	2	2[g]	2	2[h]
Roswell Park I[b]	2	2	2	1					
Roswell Park II[e]	2[f]				2	2	2[g]	2	2[h]
Univ Washington I[b]	1[c]	1[k]	1						
Univ Washington II[e]	2[m]		2[n]				2[o]	2	
Japan: Natl Cancer Ctr I[b]	2[c]	2[q]	2[q]	1					
Japan: Natl Cancer Ctr II[e]	2[r]			1	2		2[g]		2[s]

URETH WASH	CXR	IVP/ RETRO[a]	ABD CT	PELVIC CT	IVP/ RENAL US	URODYN	RAD NUC	BTA	BBC	B12
2[i]	1		1[j]	1[j]	1					
2[i]	1	1								
								1	1[l]	
2	1		1[j]	1[j]	1[p]			2		2
2	2		1	1			[t]			
2[i]	1		1[j]	1[j]	1					
2[i]	1	1								
								1	1[l]	
2	1		1[j]	1[j]	1[p]			2		2
2	1		1	1			[t]			

CHAPTER 21

Renal Cell Carcinoma

Memorial Sloan-Kettering Cancer Center

PAUL RUSSO

In 1995 an estimated 28,800 new cases of renal cell carcinoma (61% in males and 39% in females) were diagnosed in the United States and 11,700 deaths from the disease occurred. Renal cell carcinoma accounts for 2% to 3% of malignancies in adults and causes 2.3% of cancer deaths in the United States annually.[1] Approximately 2% of cases of renal cell carcinoma are bilateral. Data from more than 10,000 cases of renal cancer entered in the Connecticut Tumor Registry suggest an increase in the incidence of renal cancer between 1935 and 1989. The incidence increased from 0.7 to 4.2 per 100,000 in females and from 1.6 to 9.6 per 100,000 in males.[2] Factors implicated in the development of renal cell carcinoma include cigarette smoking, exposure to petroleum products, obesity, diuretic use, cadmium exposure, and ionizing radiation.[3-6] No data are available in the recent literature regarding the economic impact of renal cell carcinoma in the United States.

CLINICAL PRESENTATION, DIAGNOSIS, AND EXTENT OF DISEASE EVALUATION

The differential diagnosis of a renal mass includes benign cysts (simple or complex), pseudotumors (column of Bertin), angiomyolipomas, oncocytoma, urothelial carcinoma, renal cell carcinoma, lymphoma, and metastatic tumor. Approximately 85% of solid renal masses prove to be renal cell carcinoma on pathological examination.[7] Imaging of the kidney with computed tomography, ultrasound, and magnetic resonance imaging has led to the classification of complex renal masses and excluded some (fat-containing angiomyolipomas) from surgical resection.[8] These improved methods of kidney imaging have also markedly increased the incidental diagnosis of renal cell carcinoma from between 10% and 15% to between 25% and 50% over the last 20 years. Today less than 10% of patients have the classic triad of hematuria, pain, and flank mass. Those with metastatic or locally advanced disease at diagnosis make up approximately 30% of the population.[9]

Incidentally discovered renal tumors are confined within the renal capsule (pT2 or less) in 75% of cases and are associated with a 5-year survival rate of 75%.[10-13] Incidentally discovered renal cell carcinoma, when compared with symptomatic renal cell carcinoma, is significantly smaller (mean 5 cm), has a lower T stage, and is associated with a higher likelihood of survival. Analysis of histological grade and DNA ploidy pattern reveals no difference between incidental and symptomatic renal cell carcinoma.[14] This stage migration has resulted in a decrease in the incidence of metastatic disease at presentation to less than 20% and has improved 5-year survival.[15] The incidental discovery of smaller renal carcinomas has also encouraged the more liberal application of partial nephrectomy (nephron-sparing surgery).[16]

Renal cell carcinoma is associated with a wide array of systemic symptoms, including anemia, polycythemia, hypercalcemia, weight loss, acute varicocele, and fever.[17] Physical examination is performed with special attention to supraclavicular and cervical nodes for signs of adenopathy and the presence of a palpable abdominal mass, a bruit, lower extremity edema, varicocele, subcutaneous nodules, or penile or vaginal metastases. Laboratory evaluation should include a complete blood count, serum calcium, liver function tests, and serum creatinine.

The extent of disease evaluation should include chest x-ray and abdominal computed tomography to focus on the lung and regional nodes, the most common sites of metastatic disease.[18] The T stage can be correctly predicted by abdominal computed tomography in 80% of cases.[19] If a nodule is observed on chest x-ray, a computed tomographic scan of the chest is indicated to rule out multiple pulmonary metastases. Computed tomography of the chest has a greater yield of finding metastatic nodules in patients with large primary tumors.[20] Bone scanning is not routinely performed unless the patient has an elevated alkaline phosphatase level or complains of bone pain.[18] If computed tomography raises the possibility of extension to the renal vein or inferior vena cava, Doppler ultrasound or magnetic resonance imaging is performed to define the uppermost level of the thrombus.[21] Computed tomography of the brain is not routinely performed unless the patient complains of a headache or manifests a neurological deficit. Angiography is used in selected cases if partial nephrectomy is planned and the tumor is centrally located.

STAGING AND PROGNOSTIC FACTORS

Surgical resection remains the only effective therapy for clinically localized renal cell carcinoma. Before operation a tumor stage is assigned. Two staging systems, the Robson system and the International Union Against Cancer tumor, nodes, metastases (TNM) classification, are used in renal cell carcinoma.[22,23] Descriptive limitations in the Robson system include regional node involvement and renal vein or inferior vena cava involvement. The TNM staging system more explicitly describes the extent of local and regional disease and thus is preferred at Memorial Sloan-Kettering Cancer Center. One of the most important prognostic determinants of 5-year survival is the local extent of the tumor (organ-confined disease with TNM stage T1 or T2 or Robson stage I [70% to 80%] or a tumor extending into perinephric fat with TNM stage T3a or Robson stage II [60% to 70%]). The presence of regional nodal metastases, whether single, multiple, contralateral, fixed, or juxtaregional, with Robson stage IIIb or TNM stage N1, N2, N3, or N4 (5% to 20%) is another prognostic determinant. The presence of metastatic disease at presentation with Robson stage IVb or TNM stage M1 (5% or less) is a third important predictor of 5-year survival. Other adverse prognostic indicators, usually associated with locally advanced or metastatic tumors, include high pathological grade, sarcomatoid histological findings, large tumor size (greater than 10 cm), weight loss, hypercalcemia, and an elevated sedimentation rate.[24] Controversy exists concerning whether renal vein invasion is predictive of poor outcome independent of tumor size and regional nodal status. Two recent studies using multivariate analysis failed to show renal vein invasion as an independent risk factor.[25,26]

Bilateral renal cell carcinoma, synchronous or asynchronous, occurs in 2% to 4% of patients with renal cell carcinoma. With the advent of improved imaging modalities and associated stage migration this percentage may increase. Patients with synchronous tumors have a better overall 5-year survival (78%) than those with asynchronous tumors (38%). In general, prognostic factors described above relative to grade and stage of the individual tumor resected predict overall survival in the cases of bilateral renal cell carcinoma. Decisions concerning the surgical treatment of bilateral renal cell carcinoma (that is, partial nephrectomy and radical nephrectomy alone or in combination) are made after a complete assessment of overall renal function and the size and location of the tumors involved.[27,28]

Inferior vena cava extension, in the absence of regional nodal or distant metastatic disease and after complete surgical resection, is associated with adjusted 5- and 10-year survival rates in the range of 50%.[29] Hatcher et al.[30] described the important difference for prognosis between inferior vena cava invasion and free-floating extension into the inferior vena cava. In a series of 44 patients those with free-floating extension of the tumor into the inferior vena cava had a 69% 5-year survival (median 9.9 years), whereas those with direct inferior vena cava invasion had a 25% 5-year survival (median 1.2 years), which could be improved to 57% if the involved segment of the inferior vena cava wall could be resected completely. Prognosis did not seem to depend on the level of inferior vena cava involvement up to and including the right atrium. In patients with inferior vena cava involvement and other adverse prognostic indicators (extrafascial spread or lymph node or distant metastases), 5-year survival was 18% (median less than 0.9 year).[30] The importance of the presence or absence of metastatic disease at the time of diagnosis of renal cell carcinoma invading the venous system is provided by Libertino et al.[29] in an update of a 24-year experience with 100 patients with renal cell carcinoma extending into the renal vein, vena cava, or right atrium. Of the 72% of patients with no metastatic disease at the time of diagnosis and complete resection, median survival time was 21.1 years, with a 5-year survival rate of 64% and 10-year survival rate of 57%. Patients whose tumors were resected but who were found to have metastatic disease had a median survival time of 2.5 years and a 5-year survival rate of 20%, with no survivors beyond 8 years.[31]

SURGICAL TREATMENT OF RENAL CELL CARCINOMA

Surgical treatment, including the resection of vena caval thrombi, is the only effective treatment for clinically localized renal cell carcinoma. In highly selected cases surgical treatment of locally recurrent renal cell carcinoma and limited metastatic disease has been employed.

In 1969 Robson et al.[22] reported the results of radical nephrectomy, which they defined as perifascial resection of the kidney, perirenal fat, regional lymph nodes, and ipsilateral adrenal gland. Over the last 25 years modifications to this approach have gained acceptance. These modifications include performing adrenalectomy only on patients with large tumors involving the entire kidney or upper pole,[32] the need for and extent of regional lymphadenectomy (particularly in the era of incidental detection of renal cell carcinoma),[33,34] and the evolution of partial nephrectomy for small, clinically localized tumors.[16,22,35-39]

Inconsistencies exist in the literature concerning the components of radical nephrectomy (that is, limits of regional lymph node dissection), which often make comparisons of results among institutions difficult to interpret. Although randomized studies have not been performed to confirm the value of the various components of radical nephrectomy or that radical nephrectomy is more effective than simple nephrectomy alone, this operation remains the gold standard approach to clinically localized renal cell carcinoma.[22,40,41]

The indications for nephron-sparing surgery for renal cell carcinoma include situations in which standard radical nephrectomy would render the patient functionally anephric, thus necessitating dialysis. These situations include renal cell carcinoma in a solitary kidney, renal cell carcinoma in one kidney with inadequate contralateral renal function (for example, because of hypertension, renal calculus disease, or reflux), and bilateral synchronous renal cell carcinoma. A functioning renal remnant of at least 20% is needed to maintain adequate renal function. Partial nephrectomy, particularly in patients with large (greater than 4 cm), centrally located tumors for which resection enters the renal collecting system, is associated with a temporary urinary fistula rate of 17%. Ischemia time of greater than 60 minutes is associated with an increased risk of temporary acute renal failure (11% of patients) and chronic renal insufficiency necessitating long-term dialysis (3.4% of patients).[42] Surgical complications lead to an adverse clinical outcome in 3.1% of patients undergoing partial nephrectomy. Enucleation of kidney tumors, as opposed to partial nephrectomy, is discouraged because tumor cells in the pseudocapsule lead to a high likelihood of local recurrence.[43,44]

A study from the Cleveland Clinic of 216 patients with sporadic renal cell carcinoma undergoing partial nephrectomy supports the effectiveness of this approach. In its report, 47 patients had bilateral synchronous tumors, 95 patients had renal cell carcinoma in a solitary kidney, 57 patients had associated azotemia or medical or urological disease necessitating renal preservation, and 17 patients had tumors with a normal opposite kidney. Eighty-three percent of patients had T1,2 or T3a tumors. The 5-year cancer-specific survival rate in this series was 87% (T1,2 94% and T3a 79%). Survival was 95% in patients with unilateral renal cell carcinoma, 85% in those with synchronous renal cell carcinoma, and 73% in those with asynchronous bilateral renal cell carcinoma. Local recurrence developed in nine of 216 patients (4%). The local recurrence rate was higher in large, symptomatic tumors (6.7%) than in small, incidentally discovered tumors (1.1%).[45] Partial nephrectomy, with low perioperative morbidity and low recurrence rates, represents a significant improvement in the surgical management of renal cell carcinoma.

For renal cell carcinoma invading the inferior vena cava and right atrium, resection can be associated with long-term survival despite a perioperative mortality approaching 10%, depending on the local extent of the primary tumor and the level of vena caval extension.[22,27,28,46-49] Vena cavotomy or vena caval resection often requires the assistance of cardiovascular surgeons and may require the techniques of venovenous bypass[46] or cardiopulmonary bypass with or without circulatory arrest.[47] The prognosis in tumors involving the vena cava depends on the T stage of the tumor and whether the thrombus is floating free within the caval lumen (69% 5-year survival) or directly invading the caval wall (26% 5-year survival).

Reports from several centers have described a preliminary experience with laparoscopic radical and partial nephrectomy for the resection of small renal tumors. The techniques, as described, offer the patient a shorter postoperative recovery and hospital stay but lead to long operations, even when performed by the few expert laparoscopic surgeons inclined to develop this approach. Concerns have been voiced regarding the appropriateness of therapeutic laparoscopy in cancer surgery, particularly in regard to morcellation of the specimen required for its removal and the potential for intraoperative tumor spillage with peritoneal and operating portal wound seeding. Based on these concerns it is unlikely that laparoscopic nephrectomy, as currently practiced, will supplant standard open surgical nephrectomy.[50-52]

Local recurrence is rarely an isolated clinical event and is usually associated with the development of metastatic disease. Local recurrences are more common in patients with large, locally advanced tumors with regional nodal metastases. Historically, local recurrences in the renal bed without metastatic disease were reported in approximately 5% of patients undergoing radical nephrectomy.[53] With the advent of computed tomography, early detection of a local recurrence can be observed in up to 30% of patients undergoing radical nephrectomy and 5% of patients selected for partial nephrectomy.[54,55] After a complete evaluation of extent of disease and in the absence of effective, systemic treatment, resection of the local recurrence remains the treatment of choice. Operation for local recurrence is a formidable procedure that may necessitate en bloc resection of the adjacent muscle, bowel, spleen, pancreas, or liver. Because of insufficient patient numbers, data are not available to determine if such resections improve survival.[56] Radiation therapy for palliation of symptoms from a local recurrence or observation alone also remains a reasonable option for treatment in selected patients.

In the absence of effective systemic therapy for metastatic renal cell carcinoma,[57] aggressive resection of pulmonary metastases has been undertaken. In highly selected patients with solitary metastases and long disease-free intervals before resection (greater than 3 years), 5-year survival in the range of 36% has been reported.[58] Surgical resection of residual tumors of the lung, kidney, and retroperitoneum after partial response to biological response modifiers has also been undertaken with encouraging short-term results. Patients with metastatic disease not responding to initial systemic therapy should not undergo delayed nephrectomy.[59] It must be remembered that renal cell carcinoma has a long and often unpredictable natural history and that reports of survival after surgical resection of metastatic renal cell carcinoma may still fit within the time-frame of this natural history.[60,61] Randomized trials of resection of metastatic disease versus observation alone would be needed to clarify this issue.

SYSTEMIC THERAPY FOR METASTATIC RENAL CELL CARCINOMA

Metastatic renal cell carcinoma is not a chemotherapy-responsive tumor. Yagoda et al.[62] reviewed more than 3,500 patients treated with one of 72 chemotherapeutic agents and found objective responses in only 5% of patients. Trials of drugs in combination have also demonstrated the ineffectiveness of standard chemotherapy.[63] The nearly uniform expression of P-glycoprotein in renal cell carcinoma[64] has raised the possibility that reversal of the multidrug-resistant gene activity by agents such as dexverapamil may increase the chemosensitivity of renal cell carcinoma.[65] To date, however, no effective systemic chemotherapy regimen for metastatic renal cell carcinoma has been identified.

Extensive work with immunotherapeutic agents, including interleukin 2 (IL-2), interferon-alpha, and adoptive immunotherapy with IL-2/lymphokine-activated killer cells and IL-2/tumor-infiltrating lymphocyte cells, has demonstrated objective partial and complete response rates in the 10% to 30% range.[66-70] Although dramatic and durable remissions have been observed in some patients, overall results are not significantly better than single agent IL-2 or interferon-alpha therapy. A search for novel agents, alone or in combination, is ongoing, making entry into clinical trials an option for patients with metastatic renal cell carcinoma. A recent report by Motzer et al.[71] describes one such new approach, combining interferon-alpha and 13-cis-retinoic acid, which yielded an overall response rate of 30%. Randomized trials are under way to further evaluate this and other regimens.

STRATEGIES FOR FOLLOW-UP

No guidelines have been established for the follow-up of patients who have undergone surgical treatment of renal cell carcinoma. Urological surgeons have different philosophies regarding the management of isolated metastases or local recurrences after radical or partial nephrectomy and the referral to medical or radiation oncologists for the treatment of metastatic disease. The intensity of follow-up and tests ordered during follow-up also vary from center to center.[72] In the absence of effective systemic therapies for metastatic disease, overly compulsive follow-up may diagnose asymptomatic, metastatic disease earlier but may not necessarily provide a therapeutic advantage. Excessive costs and patient anxiety may also occur unnecessarily during follow-up.

Follow-up strategies were proposed from a contemporary radical nephrectomy series by Sandock et al.[73] after a detailed analysis of the pattern of disease progression, sites of metastatic failure, and the efficiency of tests required to diagnose relapse. These investigators reviewed 137 patients with node-negative, nonmetastatic renal cell carcinoma who underwent radical nephrectomy between 1979 and 1993 at Case Western affiliated hospitals. Recurrence correlated closely with the clinical stage of the tumor at the time of diagnosis. Relapse occurred in no stage T1 patients, 15% of stage T2 patients, and 53% of stage T3 patients. Of the 19 patients in whom pulmonary metastases developed, 14 (74%) had cough, dyspnea, pleuritic chest pain, or hemoptysis. In all patients with pulmonary metastases the metastatic disease was diagnosed by plain chest x-ray. Of the 13 in whom intraabdominal metastatic disease developed, 12 (92%) complained of abdominal symptoms or had abnormal liver function tests that led to the diagnosis. One patient was found on routine computed tomographic scan to have an isolated liver metastasis, which did not, however, cause abnormal liver function tests. All 10 patients in whom bone metastases developed complained of new bone pain, leading to plain bone films or bone scans confirming the diagnosis. Only one patient had an isolated brain metastasis, which was associated with central nervous system symptoms and was confirmed by computed tomography. Two patients had unusual cutaneous soft tissue recurrences noted on physical examination. Despite the often unpredictable natural history of renal cell carcinoma, 85% of patients who had a relapse did so during the first 3 years after radical nephrectomy, with the remaining relapses occurring between 3.4 and 11.4 years.

Table 21-1 Follow-up of patients with renal cancer: Memorial Sloan-Kettering Cancer Center

	YEAR				
	1	2	3	4	5
Office visit	2	2	2	2	2
Creatinine clearance, urine*	2	2	2	2	2
Protein, urine (24-hour)*	2	2	2	2	2
Renal ultrasound†	2	2	2	2	2
Abdominal computed tomography†	2	2	2	2	2
Pelvic computed tomography†	2	2	2	2	2
Liver function tests‡	2	2	2	1	1
Chest x-ray‡	2	2	2	1	1

*For patients who have undergone partial nephrectomy.
†For asymptomatic patients with von Hippel-Lindau disease.
‡For patients with T2 and T3 disease.

Based on these findings, a recommendation for follow-up of clinically localized renal cell carcinoma after radical nephrectomy is proposed as follows (Table 21-1). For T1 tumors a history and physical examination every 6 months are recommended. For T2 and T3 tumors a history and physical examination every 6 months are recommended, as well as liver function tests, and posteroanterior and lateral chest x-rays every 6 months for 3 years, then annually. Specialized scans such as bone scans, plain bone x-rays, and computed tomographic scans of the abdomen, pelvis, and brain are not routinely recommended unless directed by specific patient symptoms or signs.

Renal cell carcinoma is notorious for unusual, late, symptomatic metastatic recurrences in organs such as the pancreas, thyroid, skin, duodenum, and adrenal glands. These recurrences are often evaluated and treated as primary tumors, and aggressive surgical resection is undertaken.[74-76]

The increased use of partial nephrectomy requires special follow-up of the previously operated kidney and if necessary the normal contralateral kidney. Satellite, or secondary, smaller renal cell carcinomas may be clinically undetected at the time of partial nephrectomy. The incidence of satellite tumors seems to increase with the size of the index tumor. In a clinical pathological study addressing this issue in nephrectomy specimens, the rate of satellite tumors was approximately 10% in the 257 kidney tumors less than 5 cm in size.[77] Whether each satellite tumor, many of which are microscopic in nature, has the capacity to develop into a clinically evident local recurrence was not addressed in this study. The search for satellite tumors depends to a large extent on the compulsiveness of the pathological prosection.[78] Intraoperative ultrasound, performed at the time of partial nephrectomy, may assist the surgeon in locating satellite tumor nodules and deep, nonpalpable parenchymal lesions and can safely guide an initial nephrotomy.[79,80]

Patients left with less than one functional kidney must be carefully followed up to prevent deterioration of renal function. Novick et al.[81] reported on the development of segmental nephrosclerosis leading to proteinuria, renal insufficiency, and end-stage renal disease in certain patients without a history of preoperative renal disease but with greater than a 50% reduction in functioning renal mass. A 24-hour urine test for creatinine clearance and protein should be done at least biannually in the follow-up of patients after partial nephrectomy. Patients who have proteinuria (greater than 150 mg/day) can benefit from a low-protein diet and angiotensin-converting enzyme inhibitor therapy to prevent glomerulopathy in this setting.[82,83]

Careful follow-up is appropriate in patients predisposed to renal cell carcinoma, such as patients with end-stage renal disease, a condition that affects more than 200,000 Americans. Acquired renal cystic disease, a condition defined as multiple cysts involving greater than 25% of the kidney, is most likely the precursor lesion to renal cell carcinoma in patients with end-stage renal disease. Acquired renal cystic disease occurs in 80% to 95% of patients undergoing hemodialysis and 30% to 45% of patients undergoing peritoneal dialysis and has also been reported in kidney transplant recipients. Acquired renal cystic disease affects 45% of patients within the first 3 years of dialysis.[84-86] The percentage of patients undergoing dialysis with acquired renal cystic disease in whom renal cell carcinoma develops ranges from 5% to 30%, making these patients 30 times more likely to have renal cell carcinoma than a member of the general population.[87] Fifteen percent of these patients have metastatic disease at presentation.[88] Patients in whom acquired renal cystic disease develops in kidney transplant allografts may be at increased risk for the development of a more aggressive form of renal cell carcinoma in the setting of immunosuppression.[89,90] In patients undergoing dialysis and transplant recipients, all episodes of gross or microscopic hematuria should be aggressively evaluated. Annual upper tract imaging, usually with initial renal ultrasound, is recommended. With improved medical management of patients with end-stage renal disease and improved survival, renal cell carcinoma is expected to be an increasingly important problem in this patient population.

Von Hippel-Lindau disease is an autosomal dominant disease with nearly complete penetrance by the age of 60.[91] Renal cell carcinoma that is often bilateral and multicentric develops in approximately 50% of patients with von Hippel-Lindau disease. Upper tract imaging studies (ultrasound or computed tomography) are performed at biannual intervals on asymptomatic patients with the clinical stigmata of von Hippel-Lindau disease. Molecular genetic screening of completely asymptomatic family members is now being done with careful upper tract imaging in anticipation of the development of renal cell carcinoma.[92,93]

When bilateral renal cell carcinoma is encountered in patients with von Hippel-Lindau disease, the treatment options include bilateral nephrectomy and dialysis or bilateral partial nephrectomy with careful surveillance for local recurrence. Novick and Streem[94] reviewed nine patients with von Hippel-Lindau disease treated with partial nephrectomy. One patient died of metastatic disease at 43 months, and one patient was alive without evidence of disease at 74 months. The remaining seven patients had local recurrences in the operated kidney requiring reoperation, and only three are not receiving hemodialysis. This experience suggests that partial nephrectomy in the setting of von Hippel-Lindau disease is not as effective an alternative as it is in sporadic renal cell carcinoma, and despite careful follow-up in the setting of bilateral disease, nephrectomies and hemodialysis may be required.

FUTURE PROSPECTS

Insight into the genetic basis of renal cell carcinoma, including sporadic, familial, and hereditary forms, has been facilitated in the last 15 years by the development of modern molecular biology techniques. Work on von Hippel-Lindau disease provided the first insight into the hereditary aspects of renal cell carcinoma.[91] In patients with von Hippel-Lindau disease a variety of tumors of neuroectodermal origin develop, including retinal hemangiomas, cerebellar, medullary, and spinal hemangioblastomas, pheochromocytoma, and bilateral renal cell carcinoma. It is estimated that only one of 12 cases of von Hippel-Lindau disease is due to a spontaneous mutation, while the remainder are familial. The diagnosis of von Hippel-Lindau disease is made if a patient exhibits two or more of these conditions or one condition in the context of a positive family history. Renal cell carcinoma, which tends to be multicentric and bilateral, develops in approximately 50% of patients with von Hippel-Lindau disease. Although this was originally described as a less malignant variant of renal cell carcinoma, that is no longer believed to be the case, since 50% of patients with von Hippel-Lindau disease and renal cell carcinoma eventually have metastatic disease. With better treatment of the central nervous system aspects of von Hippel-Lindau disease, renal cell carcinoma has become the most common cause of death in these patients.[91]

Recently the von Hippel-Lindau tumor suppressor gene, located on chromosome 3 (3p25-p26), was identified.[95-97] Germline mutations were identified in 39% of families with von Hippel-Lindau disease, 33% of those with sporadic renal cell carcinoma, and 100% of renal cell carcinoma cell lines. Mutations consisted of deletions, insertions, splice-site mutations, and missense and non-sense mutations. Analysis of 180 sporadic nonrenal tumor types showed no detectable mutations.[98] The von Hippel-Lindau gene is evolutionarily conserved and encodes two widely expressed transcripts of 6 and 6.5 kb. Restriction fragment length polymorphism analysis in patients with von Hippel-Lindau disease demonstrated rearrangements in 28 of 221 von Hippel-Lindau kindreds, with 18 rearrangements caused by deletions in the candidate gene.

Investigation of families with clusters of multifocal and bilateral renal cell carcinoma, without the stigmata of von Hippel-Lindau disease, suggests that "familial renal cell carcinoma" is also associated with the loss of tumor suppressor genes. Additional chromosomal abnormalities involving chromosome 3 (balanced translocation between the short arm of chromosome 3 and the long arm of chromosome 8 and a translocation from chromosome 3 to 11) have been reported.[99-101] Interestingly, investigators found no evidence of loss of heterozygosity in 3p in more than three generations of a family affected with papillary-type renal cell carcinoma, suggesting that other tumor suppressor genes not located on 3p can predispose patients to the papillary variant of renal cell carcinoma.[102] Allelic loss of 3p was also not associated with sporadic cases of papillary renal cell carcinoma.[103] Other molecular genetic studies performed on papillary renal cell carcinoma have demonstrated a loss of the Y chromosome and trisomy 3q,7,8,12,16,17,20. Chromophobe renal cell carcinoma is characterized by a highly specific combination of loss of chromosomes 1, 2, 6, 10, 13, 17, and 21 and gross rearrangement of mitochondrial DNA.[104] Other variant forms of sporadic renal cell carcinoma, such as oncocytic, non–clear cell, papillary tumors, also were found not to have allelic loss of 3p.[105]

Further investigations on sporadic forms of renal cell carcinoma have demonstrated that the region of 3p affected by familial translocation is not identical to the region of 3p most frequently deleted in sporadic cases of renal cell carcinoma.[106] Anglard et al.[107] identified loss of heterozygosity at one or more of 10 loci tested on the short arm of chromosome 3. This group also confirmed a loss of heterozygosity on 3p in 25 of 28 (89%) cell lines derived from nonpapillary forms of renal cell carcinoma with localization of the putative tumor suppressor gene to d3S18.[108] Other abnormalities involving loss of heterozygosity on chromosomes 3, 5, 9, 11, 13, 17, and 22 have been observed in sporadic renal cell carcinoma.[109-111] Investigation of the p53 region of chromosome 17 revealed 14 of 29 (48%) cell lines with a loss of heterozygosity. This loss did not correlate with 3p loss or histological subtype, suggesting that this may be a secondary event associated with the progression of renal cell carcinoma.[112] Other studies using immunohistochemistry have also implicated the mutated form of p53 as a poor prognostic indicator in renal cell carcinoma.[113] In addition, mutations involving neighboring regions in one or more tumor suppressor genes (3p13-p24) may be involved in sporadic renal cell carcinoma.

Improved understanding of the genetic defects of renal cell carcinoma may eventually lead to the early identification of asymptomatic family members of index cases in familial renal cell carcinoma. The liberal use of renal ultrasound as a screening tool has already been effective in diagnosing subclinical renal tumors in von Hippel-Lindau disease families.[92,93] The role molecular genetics will play in staging, prognosis, and screening in sporadic cases of renal cell carcinoma remains to be defined.

CONCLUSION

There has been increased understanding of the genetic defects associated with renal cell carcinoma. Molecular biological probes are already being used to detect subclinical cases of renal cell carcinoma in family members of patients with von Hippel-Lindau disease or familial renal cell carcinoma. Careful surveillance of patients with acquired renal cystic disease is indicated. The widespread availability of abdominal ultrasound, magnetic resonance imaging, and computed tomography has increased the number of incidentally discovered cases of renal cell carcinoma to approximately 30%, resulting in stage migration to smaller tumors with better overall prognosis. Use of partial nephrectomy as a treatment option has also increased, resulting in low rates of local recurrence, even in the presence of a normal contralateral kidney. Despite extensive research into systemic therapy for renal cell carcinoma, surgical resection is the only effective treatment. Partial nephrectomy, radical nephrectomy, vena caval resection, resection of isolated local recurrence, and resection of isolated metastatic disease all remain viable options for the treatment of renal cell carcinoma.

Prognosis depends on the size of the primary tumor and regional nodal status. Follow-up strategies for patients with small, incidentally discovered tumors can be simplified to biannual chest x-rays, liver function tests, and physical examination. Routine use of bone scans, abdominal computed tomography, or brain scans is not necessary, since symptoms usually declare the presence of metastatic disease to these sites. Patients undergoing partial nephrectomy have approximately a 5% chance of a local recurrence in the operated kidney, necessitating annual imaging studies (ultrasound or computed tomography) in addition to the above. High-risk patients such as members of von Hippel-Lindau disease families or patients with end-stage renal disease also require annual upper tract imaging.

REFERENCES

1. Wingo PA, Tong T, Bolden S. Cancer statistics, 1995. Ca Cancer J Clin 1995;45:8-30.
2. Katz DL, Zheng T, Holford TR, Flannery J. Time trends in the incidence of renal carcinoma: analysis of Connecticut Tumor Registry data, 1935-1989. Int J Cancer 1994;58:57-63.
3. Kreiger N, Marrett LD, Dodds L, Hilditch S, Darlington GA. Risk factors for renal cell carcinoma: results of a population-based case-control study. Cancer Causes Control 1993;4:101-10.
4. Finkle WD, Mclaughlin JK, Rasgon SA, Yeoh HH, Low JE. Increased risk of renal cell cancer among women using diuretics in the United States. Cancer Causes Control 1993;4:555-8.
5. McCredie M, Stewart JH. Risk factors for kidney cancer in New South Wales. I. Cigarette smoking. Eur J Cancer 1992;28A:2050-4.
6. Mellemgaard A, Engholm G, McLaughlin JK, Olsen JH. Risk factors for renal cell carcinoma in Denmark: role of weight, physical activity, and reproductive factors. Int J Cancer 1994;56:66-71.
7. Morash C, Russo P. Pathologic findings after nephrectomy for presumed renal cell carcinoma. J Urol 1995;153:438A.
8. Bosniak MA. Problems in the radiologic diagnosis of renal parenchymal tumors. Urol Clin North Am 1993;20:217-30.

9. Mevorach RA, Segal AJ, Tersegno ME, Frank IN. Renal carcinoma: incidental diagnosis and natural history: review of 235 cases. Urology 1992;39:519-22.
10. Tsukamoto T, Kumamoto Y, Yamazaki K, et al. Clinical analysis of incidentally found renal carcinomas. Eur Urol 1991;19:109-13.
11. Aslaksen A, Gothlin JH. Imaging of solid renal masses. Curr Opin Radiol 1991;3:654-62.
12. Aso Y, Homma Y. A survey on incidental renal cell carcinoma in Japan. J Urol 1992;147:340-3.
13. Porena M, Vespasiani G, Rosi P, et al. Incidentally detected renal cell carcinoma: role of ultrasonography. J Clin Ultrasound 1992;20:395-400.
14. Sasaki Y, Homma Y, Hosaka Y, Tajima A, Aso Y. Clinical and flow cytometric analyses of renal cell carcinomas with reference to incidental or non-incidental detection. Jpn J Clin Oncol 1994;24:32-6.
15. Kessler O, Mukamel E, Hadar H, Gillon G, Konechezky M, Servadio C. The impact of the improved diagnosis of renal cell carcinoma on the course of the disease. J Surg Oncol 1994;57:201-4.
16. Novick AC. Renal-sparing surgery for renal cell carcinoma. Urol Clin North Am 1993;20:277-82.
17. Skinner DG, Colvin RB, Vermillion CD, Pfister RC, Leadbetter WF. Diagnosis and management of renal cell carcinoma: a clinical and pathological study of 309 cases. Cancer 1971;28:1165-77.
18. Newhouse JH. The radiologic evaluation of the patient with renal cancer. Urol Clin North Am 1993;20:231-46.
19. Tammela TL, Leinonen AS, Kontturi MJ. Comparison of excretory urography, angiography, ultrasound and computed tomography for T category staging of renal cell carcinoma. Scand J Urol Nephrol 1991;25:283-6.
20. Lim DJ, Carter MF. Computerized tomography in the preoperative staging for pulmonary metastases in patients with renal cell carcinoma. J Urol 1993;150:1112-4.
21. Myneni L, Hricak H, Carroll PR. Magnetic resonance imaging of renal carcinoma with extension into the vena cava: staging accuracy and recent advances. Br J Urol 1991;68:571-8.
22. Robson CJ, Churchill BM, Andersen W. The results of radical nephrectomy for renal cell carcinoma. J Urol 1969;101:297-301.
23. The UICC TNM classification. In: Harmen MH, editor. TNM classification of malignant tumours. Geneva: Union Internationale Contre le Cancer, 1978.
24. Thrasher JB, Paulson DF. Prognostic factors in renal cancer. Urol Clin North Am 1993;20:247-62.
25. Boxer RJ, Waisman J, Lieber MM, Mampaso FM, Skinner DG. Renal carcinoma: computer analysis of 96 patients treated by nephrectomy. J Urol 1979;122:598-601.
26. Selli C, Hinshaw WM, Woodard BH, Paulson DF. Stratification of risk factors in renal cell carcinoma. Cancer 1983;52:899-903.
27. McDonald MW. Current therapy for renal cell carcinoma. J Urol 1982;127:211-7.
28. Zincke H, Swanson SK. Bilateral renal cell carcinoma: influence of synchronous and asynchronous occurrence on patient survival. J Urol 1982;128:913-5.
29. Libertino JA, Zinman L, Watkins E Jr. Long-term results of resection of renal cell carcinoma with extension into the inferior vena cava. J Urol 1987;137:21-4.
30. Hatcher PA, Anderson EE, Paulson DF, Carson CC, Robertson JE. Surgical management and prognosis of renal cell carcinoma invading the vena cava. J Urol 1991;145:20-4.
31. Swierewski DJ, Swierewski MJ, Libertino JA. Radical nephrectomy in patients with renal cell carcinoma with venous, venal caval, and atrial extension. Am J Surg 1994;168:205-9.
32. Sagalowsky AI, Kadesky KT, Ewalt DM, Kennedy TJ. Factors influencing adrenal metastasis in renal cell carcinoma. J Urol 1994;151: 1118-4.
33. Herrlinger JA, Schrott KM, Schott G, Sigel A. What are the benefits of extended dissection of the regional lymph nodes in the therapy of renal cell carcinoma? J Urol 1991;146:1224-7.
34. Ditonno P, Traficante A, Battaglia M, Grossi FS, Selvagi FP. Role of lymphadenectomy in renal cell carcinoma. Prog Clin Biol Res 1992; 378:169-74.
35. Licht MR, Novick AC. Nephron sparing surgery for renal cell carcinoma. J Urol 1993;145:1-7.
36. Steinbach F, Stockle M, Muller SC, et al. Conservative surgery of renal cell tumors in 140 patients: 21 years of experience. J Urol 1992;148:24-30.
37. Thrasher JB, Robertson JE, Paulson DF. Expanding indications for conservative renal surgery in renal cell carcinoma. Urology 1994; 43:160-8.
38. Butler BP, Novick AC, Miller DP, Campbell SA, Light MR. Management of small unilateral renal cell carcinomas: radical versus nephron-sparing surgery. Urology 1995;45:34-41.
39. Herr HW. Partial nephrectomy for renal cell carcinoma with a normal opposite kidney. Cancer 1994;73:160-2.
40. Patel NP, Lavengood RW. Renal cell carcinoma: natural history and results of treatment. J Urol 1978;119:722-6.
41. Sene AP, Hunt L, McMahon RF, Carroll RN. Renal carcinoma in patients undergoing nephrectomy: analysis of survival and prognostic factors. Br J Urol 1992;70:125-34.
42. Campbell SC, Novick AC, Streem SB, Klein E, Licht M. Complications of nephron-sparing surgery for renal tumors. J Urol 1994; 151:1177-80.
43. Marshall FF, Taxy JB, Fishman EK, Chang R. The feasibility of surgical enucleation for renal cell carcinoma. J Urol 1986;135:231-4.
44. Blackley SK, Ladaga L, Woolfitt RA, Schellhammer PF. Ex situ study of the effectiveness of enucleation in patients with renal cell carcinoma. J Urol 1988;140:6-10.
45. Licht MR, Novick AC, Goormastic M. Nephron-sparing surgery in incidental versus suspected renal cell carcinoma. J Urol 1994;152:39-42.
46. Burt M. Inferior vena caval involvement by renal cell carcinoma: use of venovenous bypass as adjunct during resection. Urol Clin North Am 1991;18:437-44.
47. Klein EA, Kaye MC, Novick AC. Management of renal cell carcinoma with vena caval thrombi via cardiopulmonary bypass and deep hypothermic circulatory arrest. Urol Clin North Am 1991;18:445-7.
48. Langenburg SE, Blackbourne LH, Sperling JW, et al. Management of renal tumors involving the inferior vena cava. J Vasc Surg 1994;20: 385-8.
49. Montie JE, el Ammar R, Pontes JE, et al. Renal cell carcinoma with inferior vena cava tumor thrombi. Surg Gynecol Obstet 1991;173: 107-15.
50. Biquet P, Balde S, Andrianne R. Experience prelimininaire de la nephrectomie laparoscopique. Acta Urol Belg 1994;62:11-5.
51. Kerbl K. Clayman RV, McDougall EM, Kavoussi LR. Laparoscopic nephrectomy: the Washington University experience. Br J Urol 1994;73:231-6.
52. McDougall EM, Clayman RV, Anderson K. Laparoscopic wedge resection of a renal tumor: initial experience. J Laparoendosc Surg 1993;3:577-81.
53. Rafla S. Renal cell carcinoma: natural history and results of treatment. Cancer 1970;25:26-40.
54. Parienty RA, Richard F, Pradel J, Vallancien G. Local recurrence after nephrectomy for primary renal cancer: computerized tomography recognition. J Urol 1984;13:246-9.
55. Campbell SC, Novick AC. Management of local recurrence following radical nephrectomy or partial nephrectomy. Urol Clin North Am 1994;21:593-9.
56. Esrig D, Ahlering TE, Lieskovsky G, Skinner DG. Experience with fossa recurrence of renal cell carcinoma. J Urol 1992;147:1491-4.
57. Frank W, Stuhldreher D, Saffrin R, Shott S, Guinan P. Stage IV renal cell carcinoma. J Urol 1994;152:1998-9.
58. Cerfolio RJ, Allen MS, Deschamps C, et al. Pulmonary resection of metastatic renal cell carcinoma. Ann Thorac Surg 1994;57:339-44.
59. Kim B, Louie AC. Surgical resection following interleukin 2 therapy for metastatic renal cell carcinoma prolongs remission. Arch Surg 1992;127:1343-9.
60. Ruiz JL, Vera C, Server G, Osca JM, Boronat F, Jimenez Cruz JF. Renal cell carcinoma: late recurrences in 2 cases. Eur Urol 1991; 20:167-9.
61. Rackley R, Novick A, Klein E, Bukowski R, McLain D, Goldfarb D. The impact of adjuvant nephrectomy on multimodality treatment of metastatic renal cell carcinoma. J Urol 1994;152:1399-403.

62. Yagoda A, Petrylak D, Thompson S. Cytotoxic chemotherapy for advanced renal cell carcinoma. Urol Clin North Am 1993;20:303-21.
63. Harris DT. Hormonal therapy and chemotherapy of renal-cell carcinoma. Semin Oncol 1983;10:422-30.
64. Thiebaut F, Tsuruo T, Hamada H, Gottesman MM, Pastan I, Willingham MC. Immunohistochemical localization in normal tissues of different epitopes in the multidrug transport protein P170: evidence for localization in brain capillaries and cross reactivity of one antibody with a muscle protein. J Histochem Cytochem 1989;37:159-64.
65. Motzer RJ, Lyn P, Fischer P, et al. Phase I/II trial of dexverapamil plus vinblastine for patients with advanced renal cell carcinoma. J Clin Oncol 1995;13:1958-65.
66. Rosenberg SA. The development of new immunotherapies for the treatment of cancer using interleukin-2: a review. Ann Surg 1988; 208:121-35.
67. Rosenberg SA, Lotze MT, Muul LM, et al. A progress report on the treatment of 157 patients with advanced cancer using lymphokine-activated killer cells and interleukin-2 or high-dose interleukin-2 alone. N Engl J Med 1987;316:889-97.
68. Wirth MP. Immunotherapy for metastatic renal cell carcinoma. Urol Clin North Am 1993;20:283-95.
69. Minasian LM, Motzer RJ, Gluck L, Mazumdar M, Vlamis V, Krown SE. Interferon alfa-2a in advanced renal cell carcinoma: treatment results and survival in 159 patients with long-term follow-up. J Clin Oncol 1993;11:1368-75.
70. Ilson DH, Motzer RJ, Kradin RL, et al. A phase II trial of interleukin-2 and interferon alfa-2a in patients with advanced renal cell carcinoma. J Clin Oncol 1992;10:1124-30.
71. Motzer RJ, Schwartz L, Law TM, et al. Interferon alfa-2a and 13-cis-retinoic acid in renal cell carcinoma: antitumor activity in a phase II trial and interactions in vitro. J Clin Oncol 1995;13:1950-7.
72. Montie JE. Follow-up after partial or total nephrectomy for renal cell carcinoma. Urol Clin North Am 1994;21:589-92.
73. Sandock DS, Seftel AD, Resnick MI. A new protocol for the follow up of renal cell carcinoma based on pathological stage. J Urol 1995;154:28-31.
74. McNichols DW, Segura JW, DeWeerd JH. Renal cell carcinoma: long-term survival and late recurrence. J Urol 1981;126:17-23.
75. Takatera H, Maeda O, Oka T, et al. Solitary late recurrence of renal cell carcinoma. J Urol 1986;136:799-800.
76. Freedman AI, Tomaszewski JE, Van Arsdalen KN. Solitary late recurrence of renal cell carcinoma presenting as a duodenal ulcer. Urology 1992;39:461-3.
77. Jacqmin D, Saussine C, Roca D, Roy C, Bollack C. Multiple tumors in the same kidney: incidence and therapeutic implications. Eur Urol 1992;21:32-4.
78. Lee SE, Kim HH. Validity of kidney-preserving surgery for localized renal cell carcinoma. Eur Urol 1994;25:204-8.
79. Gilbert BR, Russo P, Zirinsky K, Kazam E, Fair WR, Vaughn ED Jr. Intraoperative sonography: application in renal cell carcinoma. J Urol 1988;139:582-4.
80. Assimos DG, Boyce H, Woodruff RD, Harrison LH, McCullough DL, Kroovand RL. Intraoperative renal ultrasonography: a useful adjunct to partial nephrectomy. J Urol 1991;146:1218-20.
81. Novick AC, Gephardt G, Guz B, Steinmuller D, Tubbs RR. Long-term follow-up after partial removal of a solitary kidney. N Engl J Med 1991;325:1058-62.
82. Brenner BM. Hemodynamically mediated glomerular injury and progressive nature of kidney disease. Kidney Int 1983;23:647-55.
83. Meyer TW, Anderson S, Rennke HG, Brenner BM. Converting enzyme inhibitor therapy limits progressive glomerular injury in rats with renal insufficiency. Am J Med 1985;79(Suppl 3):31-6.
84. Dunnill MS, Millard PR, Oliver D. Acquired cystic disease of the kidneys: a hazard of long-term intermittent maintenance hemodialysis. J Clin Pathol 1977;30:868-77.
85. Katz A, Sombolos K, Oreopoulos DG. Acquired cystic disease of the kidney in association with chronic ambulatory peritoneal dialysis. Am J Kidney Dis 1987;9:426-9.
86. Gehrig JJ Jr, Gottheiner JI, Swenson RS. Acquired cystic disease of the end-stage kidney. Am J Med 1985;79:609-20.
87. Matson MA, Cohen EP. Acquired cystic kidney disease: occurrence, prevalence, and renal cancers. Medicine 1990;69:217-26.
88. Sasagawa I, Nakada T, Kubota Y, Suzuki Y, Ishigooka M, Terasawa Y. Renal cell carcinoma in dialysis patients. Urol Int 1994;53:79-81.
89. Pope JC, Koch MO, Bluth RF. Renal cell carcinoma in patients with end-stage renal disease: a comparison of clinical significance in patients receiving hemodialysis and those with renal transplants. Urology 1994;44:497-501.
90. Williams JC, Merguerian PA, Schned AR, Morrison PM. Acquired renal cystic disease and renal cell carcinoma in an allograft kidney. J Urol 1995;153:395-6.
91. Maher ER, Yates JW, Harries R, et al. Clinical features and natural history of von Hippel-Lindau disease. Q J Med 1990;77:1151-63.
92. Glenn GM, Linehan WM, Hosoe S, et al. Screening for von Hippel-Lindau disease by DNA polymorphism analysis. JAMA 1992;267: 1226-31.
93. Maher ER, Bentley E, Payne SJ, et al. Presymptomatic diagnosis of von Hippel-Lindau disease with flanking DNA markers. J Med Genet 1992;29:902-5.
94. Novick AC, Streem SB. Long-term follow up after nephron-sparing surgery for renal cell carcinoma in von Hippel-Lindau disease. J Urol 1992;147:1488-90.
95. Seizinger BR, Rouleau GA, Ozelius LJ, et al. Von Hippel-Lindau disease maps to the region of chromosome 3 associated with renal cell carcinoma. Nature 1988;332:268-9.
96. Tory K, Brauch H, Linehan M, et al. Specific genetic change in tumors associated with von Hippel-Lindau disease. J Natl Cancer Inst 1989;81:1097-101.
97. Latif F, Tory K, Gnarra J, et al. Identification of the von Hippel-Lindau disease tumor suppressor gene. Science 1993;260:1317-20.
98. Whaley JM, Naglich J, Gelbert L, et al. Germ-line mutations in the von Hippel-Lindau tumor-suppressor gene are similar to somatic von Hippel-Lindau aberrations in sporadic renal cell carcinoma. Am J Hum Genet 1994;55:1092-102.
99. Cohen AJ, Li FP, Berg S, et al. Hereditary renal-cell carcinoma associated with a chromosomal translocation. N Engl J Med 1979; 301:592-5.
100. Pathak S, Strong LC, Ferrell RE, Trindade A. Familial renal cell carcinoma with a 3:11 chromosomal translocation limited to tumor cells. Science 1982;217:939-41.
101. Zbar B, Brauch H, Talmadge C, Linehan M. Loss of alleles of loci on the short arm of chromosome 3 in renal cell carcinoma. Nature 1987;327:721-4.
102. Zbar B, Tory K, Merino M, et al. Hereditary papillary renal cell carcinoma. J Urol 1994;151:561-6.
103. Foster K, Crossey PA, Cairns P, et al. Molecular genetic investigation of sporadic renal cell carcinoma: analysis of allele loss on chromosomes 3p,5q,11p,17, and 22. Br J Cancer 1994;69:230-4.
104. Kovacs G. The value of molecular genetic analysis in the diagnosis and prognosis of renal cell tumors. World J Urol 1994;12:64-8.
105. Presti JC, Rao PH, Chen Q, et al. Histopathological, cytogenetic, and molecular characterization of renal cortical tumors. Cancer Res 1991;51:1544-52.
106. Boldog F, Arheden K, Imreh S, et al. Involvement of 3p deletions in sporadic and hereditary forms of renal cell carcinoma. Genes Chromosom Cancer 1991;3:403-6.
107. Anglard P, Tory K, Brauch H, et al. Molecular analysis of genetic changes in the origin and development of renal cell carcinoma. Cancer Res 1991;51:1071-7.
108. Anglard P, Trahan E, Liu S, et al. Molecular and cellular characterization of human renal cell carcinoma cell lines. Cancer Res 1992; 52:348-56.
109. Ogawa O, Habuchi T, Kakehi Y, Koshiba M, Sugiyama T, Yoshida O. Allelic losses at chromosome 17p in human renal cell carcinoma are inversely related to allelic losses at chromosome 3p. Cancer Res 1992;52:1881-5.
110. Cairns P, Tokino K, Eby Y, Sidransky D. Localization of tumor suppressor loci on chromosome 9 in primary human renal cell carcinomas. Cancer Res 1995;55:224-7.

111. Kovacs G, Kiechle-Schwarz M, Scherer G, Kung HF. Molecular analysis of the 11p region in renal cell carcinomas. Cell Mol Biol 1992;38:59-62.
112. Reiter RE, Anglard P, Liu S, Gnarra JR, Linehan WM. Chromosome 17p deletions and p53 mutations in renal cell carcinoma. Cancer Res 1993;53:3092-7.
113. Uhlman DL, Nguyen PL, Manivel JC, et al. Association of immunohistochemical staining for p53 with metastatic progression and poor survival in patients with renal cell carcinoma. J Natl Cancer Inst 1994;86:1470-5.

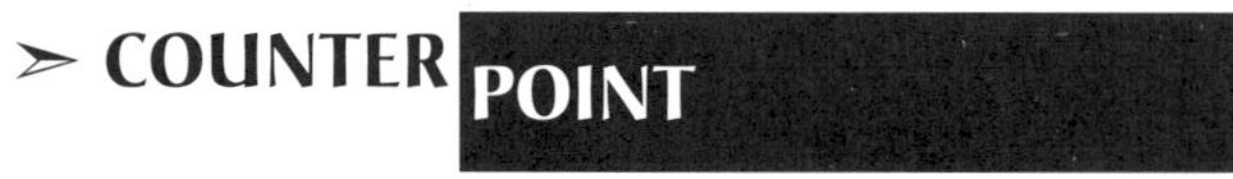

➢ COUNTER POINT

National Cancer Center Hospital, Japan

TADAO KAKIZOE

Russo provides a comprehensive description of contemporary renal cell carcinoma management, including incidence, molecular background, clinical evaluation, staging, surgical treatment, systemic therapy, and strategies for follow-up. I present an opinion, based on experience at the National Cancer Center Hospital in Tokyo, that differs slightly from Russo's.

STATISTICS

There is no nationwide registration for renal cell carcinoma in Japan. According to the official mortality statistics for this disease in Osaka, the calculated death rate for renal cell carcinoma per 100,000 population in Japan was 1.2 in 1970 and 2.5 in 1990 and is expected to increase to 3.0 by 2010[1] (Figure 21-1). Renal cell carcinoma is one of the cancers, similar to lung, liver, colorectal, breast, and prostate cancers, that are expected to increase in incidence in Japan. A nationwide survey by Aso and Homma[2] documented a dramatic increase in the incidence of renal cell carcinoma from 20 cases in 1980 to 338 cases in 1988 in an analysis of 1,428 cases from 116 collaborating institutions. Detection occurred at routine health checkup in 32.8% of the cases and during examinations for unrelated disease in the remainder.

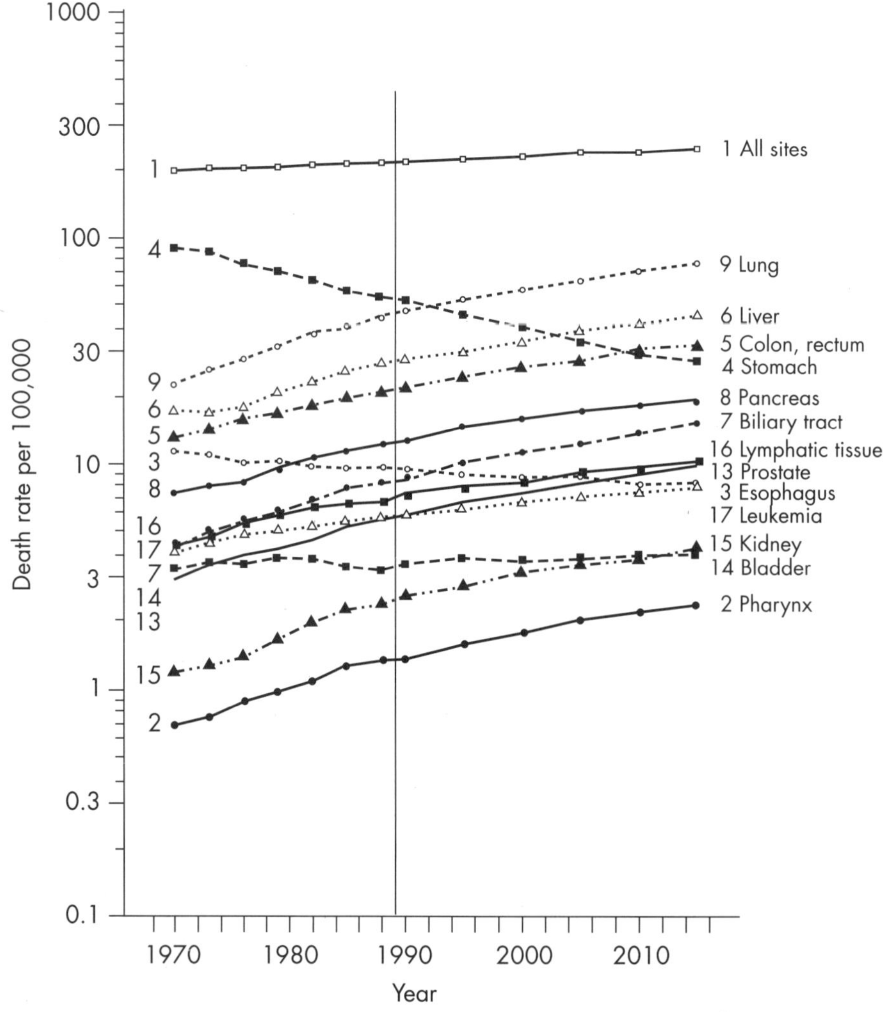

Figure 21-1 Calculated death rate for renal cell carcinoma per 100,000 population in Japan. (From Tominaga S, Aoki K, Hanai A, Kurihara N, editors. White paper on cancer statistics. Tokyo: Shinohara Press, 1993.)

The methods of detection were ultrasound (68%), computed tomography (22%), and excretory urography (6%). The 5-year survival rate was 96.5%, indicating that incidental renal cell carcinoma detection may improve the prognosis of this disease. According to a survey by Okajima (unpublished manuscript), an analysis of 1,100 cases collected from five institutions including the National Cancer Center Hospital during 1984 and 1993 also indicated a marked increase in the incidence of renal cell carcinoma (Figure 21-2). The increased rate of detection of renal cell carcinoma as an incidental finding is closely related to the follow-up strategies for this disease.

STAGING

Staging of renal cell carcinoma is conducted in Japan based on the guidebook *General Rules for Clinical and Pathological Studies on Renal Cell Carcinoma,*[3] published by the Japanese Urological Association, Japanese Pathological Society, and Japan Radiological Society. Since this staging system is almost the same as the TNM system, no new information can be added here.

SURGICAL TREATMENT

Modification of the surgical treatment of small renal cell carcinoma detected incidentally, as described by Russo, has also emerged in Japan. The increasing trend toward partial nephrectomy for small renal cell carcinoma, bilateral cancer, and cancer in the solitary kidney has an impact on the strategies for follow-up of this disease.

TREATMENT OF METASTATIC DISEASE

Metastatic disease from renal cell carcinoma is most commonly treated with interferon-alpha in Japan, and the objective response rate is 10% to 30%, as reported by Russo. Physicians at the National Cancer Center Hospital previously analyzed the survival rate of 174 patients who underwent nephrectomy for renal cell carcinoma to evaluate the effectiveness of surgical treatment of metastases.[4] In 34 of

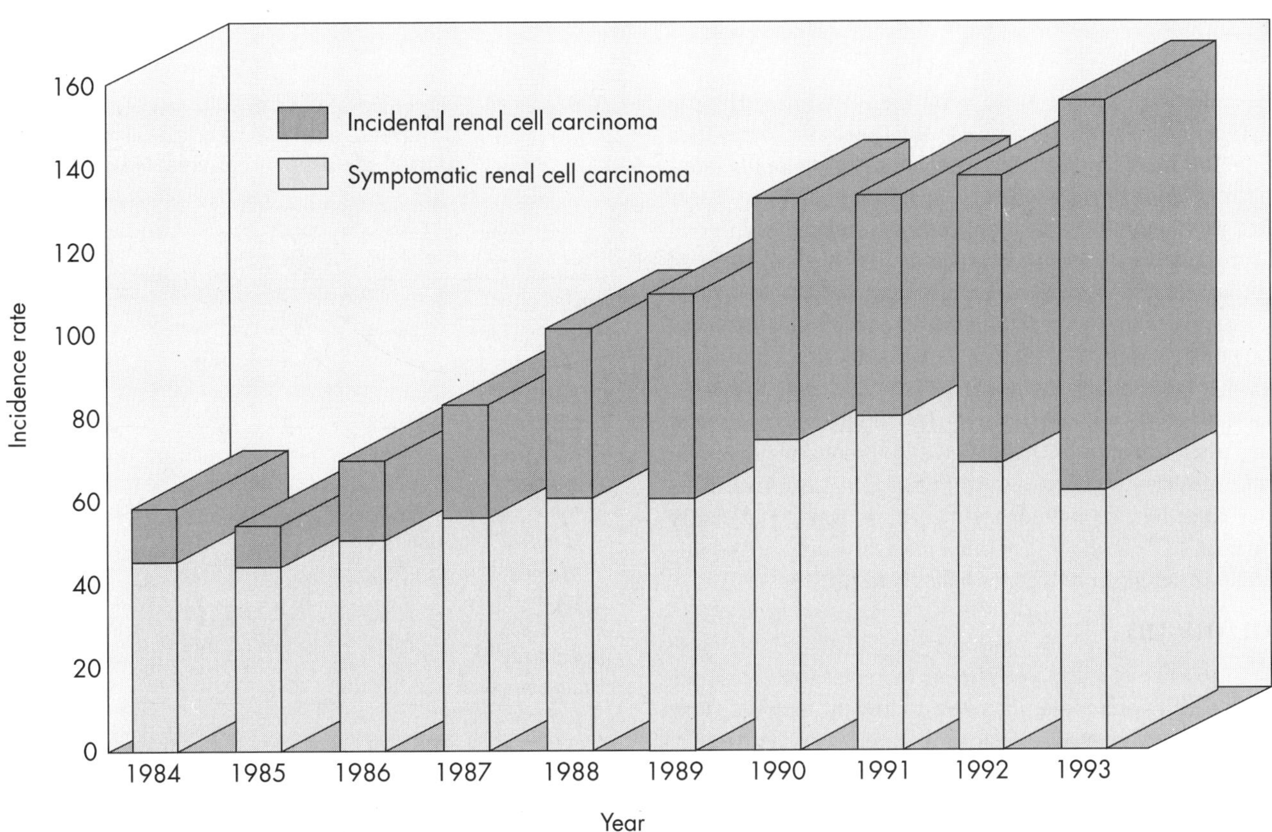

Figure 21-2 Chronological increase of incidental renal cell carcinoma. Data collected from five institutions in Japan during 1984 and 1993. (Data from Okajima, unpublished manuscript. Management of incidentally detected small renal cell carcinoma. Multi-institutional study supported by a grant from the Ministry of Health and Welfare of Japan.)

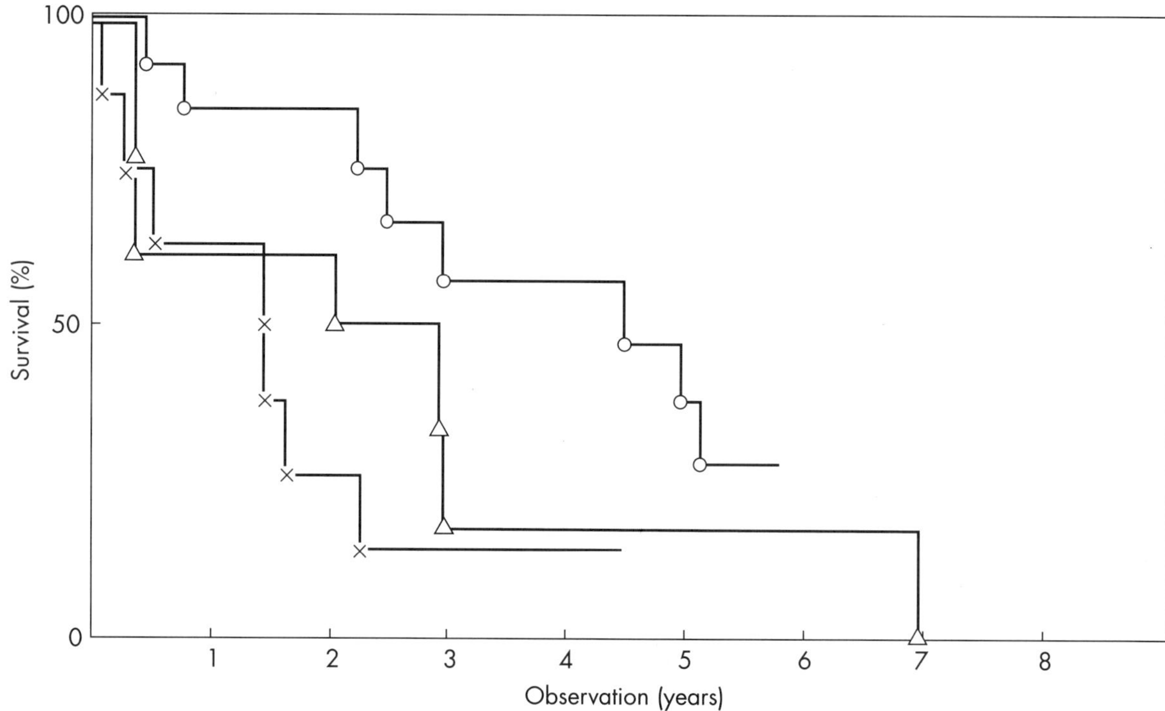

Figure 21-3 Survival rates after surgery for metastases in patients with pulmonary resections *(open circles)*, bone resections *(open triangles)*, and brain resections *(Xs)*. (From Tobisu K, Kakizoe T, Takai K, Tanaka Y, Mizutani T. J Clin Oncol 1990;20:263-7.)

the patients resections were performed concurrently with nephrectomy. For 38 patients 44 resections were performed in the follow-up period after nephrectomy. Apparently curative resections of metastases at the time of nephrectomy or after nephrectomy were significantly correlated with good survival after surgery, irrespective of the number of metastatic foci. Aggressive surgical treatment was beneficial in patients with a longer tumor-free period after nephrectomy or with stable disease for about 6 months after surgical treatment, although this might simply be a reflection of a natural disease course in this group of patients. Survival rates after resection in patients with pulmonary, bone, and brain metastases are shown in Figure 21-3. Survival time after resection for pulmonary metastasis was significantly better ($p < .05$) than that for brain metastasis, but not significantly different from that for bone metastasis.

FOLLOW-UP

In the absence of effective systemic therapies for metastases of renal cell carcinoma, intensive follow-up may diagnose asymptomatic metastases earlier but may not necessarily provide a therapeutic advantage. Follow-up of clinically localized renal cell carcinoma after radical nephrectomy is conducted based on pathological stage at the National Cancer Center Hospital (Table 21-2). Patients who have had partial nephrectomy require a special follow-up program focusing on the previously operated kidney for the development of new tumors or recurrence and function of the

Table 21-2 Follow-up of patients with renal cancer (T1 disease after radical or partial nephrectomy): National Cancer Center Hospital, Japan

	YEAR				
	1	2	3	4	5
Office visit*	3	2	2	2	2
Complete blood count	3	2	2	2	2
Multichannel blood tests†	3	2	2	2	2
Chest x-ray	3	2	2	2	2
Enhanced renal computed tomography‡	1	1	1	1	1
Abdominal ultrasound or computed tomography§	1	1	1	0	0
Bone scan	¶	¶	¶	¶	¶
Bone x-ray	¶	¶	¶	¶	¶
Brain computed tomography	¶	¶	¶	¶	¶

*Includes history and physical examination of the supraclavicular lymph nodes and abdomen.
†Consists of blood urea nitrogen and creatinine.
‡For patients who have undergone partial nephrectomy.
§Test selection based on cost and availability.
¶Performed when indicated by history or physical examination.

Table 21-3 Follow-up of patients with renal cancer (T2 and T3 disease after radical nephrectomy or T4 disease after resection of metastases simultaneous with or subsequent to radical nephrectomy): National Cancer Center Hospital, Japan

	YEAR				
	1	2	3	4	5
Office visit*	4	3	3	2	2
Complete blood count	4	3	3	2	2
Multichannel blood tests†	4	3	3	2	2
Chest x-ray	4	3	3	2	2
Abdominal ultrasound or computed tomography‡	1	1	1	1	1
Bone scan	§	§	§	§	§
Bone x-ray	§	§	§	§	§
Helical chest computed tomography	§	§	§	§	§
Brain computed tomography	§	§	§	§	§
Brain magnetic resonance imaging	§	§	§	§	§

*Includes history and physical examination. After year 5, office visits are annual until year 10.
†Consists of blood urea nitrogen, creatinine, and calcium.
‡Test selection based on cost and availability.
§Performed when indicated by history or physical examination.

residual kidney tissue. Follow-up for patients with T2 and T3 disease who have undergone radical nephrectomy or those with T4 disease who have undergone resections of metastases simultaneously with or subsequent to radical nephrectomy is summarized in Table 21-3.

REFERENCES

1. Tominaga S, Aoki K, Hanai A, Kurihara N, editors. [White paper on cancer statistics.] (in Japanese) Tokyo: Shinohara Press, 1993.
2. Aso Y, Homma Y. A survey of incidental renal cell carcinoma in Japan. J Urol 1992;147:340-3.
3. Japanese Urological Association, Japanese Pathological Society, and Japan Radiological Society. General rules for clinical and pathological studies on renal cell carcinoma. Tokyo: Kanehara Press, 1983.
4. Tobisu K, Kakizoe T, Takai K, Tanaka Y, Mizutani T. Surgical treatment of metastatic renal cell carcinoma. Jpn J Clin Oncol 1990;20:263-7.

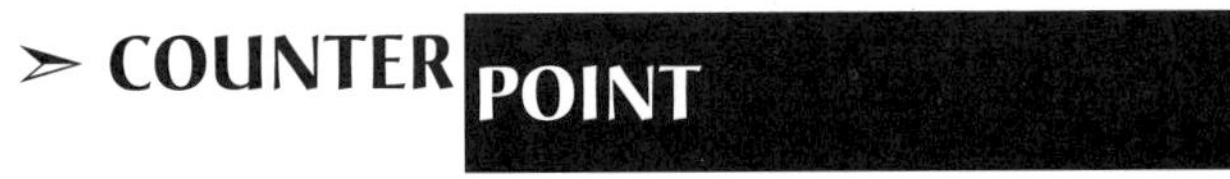

Roswell Park Cancer Institute

ROBERT P. HUBEN

Russo provides a thorough, practical review of the natural history and follow-up of patients who have undergone nephrectomy for renal cell carcinoma. The recommendations regarding specific means of monitoring postoperative status are those recently proposed by Sandock et al.[1] Such retrospective analyses of the apparent clinical benefit versus the costs of laboratory and other diagnostic studies are sorely needed to determine optimum follow-up strategies. Russo recommends a careful history and physical examination, liver function tests, and chest x-ray every 6 months for 3 years and yearly thereafter in patients with a history of T2 and T3 lesions. Patients with a history of T1 tumors are followed up with history and physical examination only at the same intervals. Computed tomographic scans are not recommended as routine. At Roswell Park Cancer Institute physicians follow a similar schema with minor modifications (Table 21-4), although several issues in the follow-up of patients with renal cell carcinoma warrant additional comment or emphasis.

Table 21-4 Follow-up of patients with renal cancer: Roswell Park Cancer Institute

	YEAR				
	1	2	3	4	5
Office visit	2	2	2	1	1
Chest x-ray*	2	2	2	1	1
Multichannel blood tests†	2	2	2	1	1

*Posteroanterior and lateral. Not performed for patients with T1 lesions.
†Consists of blood urea nitrogen and creatinine.

The importance of a careful history and physical examination in the follow-up of patients with renal cell carcinoma has been emphasized. Loss of appetite, unexplained weight loss, and symptoms suggestive of intermittent small bowel obstruction are common harbingers of recurrence. Patients with a history of fever of unknown origin or hypercalcemia before radical nephrectomy often have a return of these markers at recurrence. As in the study by Sandock et al.,[1] it is the clinical impression at Roswell Park Cancer Institute that patients with recurrent metastatic renal cell carcinoma are likely to have symptoms related to recurrence fairly early in their course and that the yield of routine diagnostic studies in asymptomatic patients is low.

In regard to laboratory studies, it has been routine at this institution to check renal function rather than liver function at the time of yearly examinations for patients with all stages of renal cell carcinoma. The rationale for monitoring the function of the contralateral kidney is to rule out other renal diseases such as nephrosclerosis, particularly in older patients. Concern about the status of the contralateral kidney is often expressed by the patient and physicians at this institution, who have believed that a yearly check of renal function is useful in allaying this anxiety. However, the cost-benefit ratio of this practice has not been analyzed.

I share Russo's skepticism regarding the long-term benefit of resecting locally recurrent renal cell carcinoma, since such lesions are rarely well defined at operation and, as stated, resection of other organs, particularly small bowel segments that had become involved with the tumor mass, is often necessary. Skepticism extends to the likelihood of long-term benefit from resection of metastatic renal cell carcinoma in general. Although resection of metastatic renal cell carcinoma, particularly solitary lesions, has been reported to be associated with 5-year survival rates of up to 50%, this figure seems overly optimistic in my experience. In a review conducted at Roswell Park Cancer Institute the estimated overall survival rate in 29 patients who underwent excision of a solitary metastasis was only 41% at 2 years and 13% at 5 years.[2] With experience, one's enthusiasm for resecting locally recurrent renal cell carcinoma often wanes.

As discussed by Russo, renal cell carcinoma often follows an unpredictable course and has a highly variable natural history. This variability is manifested by occasional recurrences despite favorable prognostic factors and prolonged survival despite unfavorable prognostic indicators. As noted further, renal cell carcinoma is notorious for its tendency to recur late after radical nephrectomy, although this remains relatively uncommon and should not significantly affect the nature or frequency of follow-up.

Lastly, I agree with Russo that the absence of relatively effective treatments for recurrent renal cell carcinoma weighs against extensive follow-up studies in patients who have undergone radical nephrectomy for localized renal cell carcinoma. As noted in this review, earlier diagnosis of recurrence in an asymptomatic patient does not necessarily translate into a higher probability of response to subsequent therapy.

REFERENCES

1. Sandock DS, Seftel AD, Resnick MI. A new protocol for the follow-up of renal cell carcinoma based on pathological stage. J Urol 1995; 154:28-31.
2. Dineen MK, Pastore RD, Emrich LJ, Huben RP. Results of surgical treatment of renal cell carcinoma with solitary metastasis. J Urol 1988;140:277-9.

➢ COUNTER POINT

University of Washington Medical Center

John A. Thompson and Paul H. Lange

Renal cell carcinoma has long fascinated physicians because of its variable natural history, association with several paraneoplastic syndromes, and response, albeit variable, to immunotherapy. Russo provides an excellent summary of the epidemiology, diagnosis, and treatment of renal cell carcinoma and introduces and interprets the diverse and often conflicting opinions regarding the evaluation and follow-up of patients with renal cell carcinoma. His reviews of the management strategies for patients with von Hippel-Lindau disease and for patients who undergo nephron-sparing surgery are particularly valuable.

Guidelines for follow-up of patients after initial surgery for renal cell carcinoma should emphasize early detection of treatable recurrent disease and should be cost effective. Russo's recommended follow-up is based on the assumption that surgical resection is the only effective treatment. However, systemic immunotherapy regimens including IL-2 or interferon-alpha are capable of inducing durable complete remissions in patients with recurrent or metastatic renal cell carcinoma. At the University of Washington Medical Center between 1988 and 1995, 120 patients with metastatic renal cell carcinoma were treated with a variety of regimens of high-dose continuous intravenous IL-2 with lymphokine-activated killer cells.[1,2] Sixteen of these patients have achieved complete remission (duration between 1 and 8+ years), and only one complete responder has had a relapse. Rosenberg et al.,[3] as well as other groups,[4] have also reported durable complete remissions in patients with metastatic renal cell carcinoma. Hence a combined modality approach is often indicated for the treatment of recurrent, metastatic disease.

The approach taken at the University of Washington Medical Center for patients with recurrent, metastatic renal cell carcinoma after nephrectomy is dictated by the patient's age and performance status and the location of the metastases. The rates of response to therapy with high-dose continuous infusion IL-2 for different sites of metastases are as follows: lung with soft tissue only (40%), liver (20%), bone (20%), and renal fossa (less than 5%). Thus for patients with metastatic disease to lung, bone, or liver, initial systemic IL-2-based therapy should be considered. Patients who achieve partial response may later be rendered free of disease by consolidative surgery. The advantage of this approach is that it permits therapy of occult micrometastatic, as well as macroscopic, disease. By contrast, the use of surgery as initial therapy in patients with metastatic renal cell carcinoma requires a delay in the initiation of systemic treatment. In a series of 54 patients with metastatic renal cell carcinoma who underwent cytoreductive nephrectomy before immunotherapy, 20 were unable to receive immunotherapy as a direct result of the surgery or the delay caused by the nephrectomy.[5] The role of debulking cytoreductive surgery before immunotherapy is therefore being challenged. Response rates to IL-2-based immunotherapy for renal fossa recurrences are discouraging. For isolated recurrences in the renal fossa, surgical resection may be the preferred approach to initial therapy. The multimodality treatment plan in these situations often includes preoperative arterial embolization and intraoperative radiation therapy.

The conventional radiological methods used for postoperative follow-up (chest x-ray, computed tomography, and magnetic resonance imaging) provide good spatial resolution of recurrent lesions but do not give information about tumor cell viability or metabolic activity. The use of positron emission tomography may provide important information in the postoperative evaluation of selected patients with documented or suspected recurrent renal cell carcinoma.[6] Positron emission tomography produces tomographic images based on photon emissions from radiolabeled molecules such as ^{18}F-fluorodeoxyglucose. ^{18}F-fluorodeoxyglucose is relatively concentrated in renal cell carcinoma tumor deposits because of the higher metabolic activity of tumor cells, which results in increased glucose utilization, the greater affinity for ^{18}F-fluorodeoxyglucose relative to glucose because of differences in glucose transport mechanisms between renal cell carcinoma and normal tissues, and the increased delivery of tracer because of increased blood flow to hypervascular renal cell carcinoma deposits. Positron emission tomography can provide a total body scan to search for occult foci of abnormal metabolic activity. It can also be used to quantitate the metabolic activity at discrete foci, which may allow the assessment of response to therapy. Positron emission tomography is of particular benefit in evaluating patients who have demonstrated stable disease or partial response after systemic therapy. Residual lesions identified by computed tomography or magnetic resonance imaging may be characterized as metabolically inert (residual fibrosis) or metabolically active. Positron emission tomography may also be used to characterize lesions in anatomical sites where a biopsy is difficult.

Table 21-5 summarizes postoperative surveillance guidelines for nonhereditary renal cell carcinoma. Detailed preoperative assessment is also important. This assessment should comprise complete history and physical examination and laboratory tests including urinalysis, complete blood count, creatinine, electrolytes, serum glutamic-oxaloacetic transaminase, lactic dehydrogenase, alkaline phosphatase, and calcium. Because renal cell carcinoma occurs frequently in older patients with an extensive smoking history, preoperative pulmonary function testing and cardiology evaluation may be indicated if chronic obstructive pulmonary disease or atherosclerotic vascular disease is suspected. Chest and abdominal computed tomography or magnetic resonance imaging is recommended, as well as a bone scan if the patient reports bone pain or if the alkaline phosphatase level is elevated. Computed tomography of the brain is indicated if there are unexplained neurological signs or symptoms.

Systemic immunotherapy should be considered as initial therapy if patients are found to have metastatic disease at presentation. Radical nephrectomy may be reserved for consolidation therapy in patients who demonstrate response to systemic therapy at metastatic sites. Exceptions to this approach include patients who have gross hematuria with associated obstructive symptoms or pain related to the primary tumor, as well as protocol settings that require primary tumor tissue, such as tumor-infiltrating lymphocyte protocols.

Radical nephrectomy remains the standard surgical approach for patients without evidence of metastatic disease at preoperative evaluation. Russo describes clinical settings in which a nephron-sparing approach may be preferable, such as renal cell carcinoma in a single kidney, renal cell carcinoma in one kidney with inadequate contralateral renal function, and bilateral synchronous renal cell carcinoma.

Table 21-5 Follow-up of patients with renal cancer*: University of Washington Medical Center

	YEAR				
	1	2	3	4	5
Office visit†	2	2	2	1	1
Liver function tests‡	2	2	2	1	1
Chest x-ray	2	2	2	1	1
Urinalysis	2	2	2	1	1
Abdominal computed tomography§	2	2	0	0	0
Bone scan	1¶	¶	¶	¶	¶
Chest computed tomography**	1	0	0	0	0
Creatinine††	1	0	0	0	0

*This follow-up schema assumes that the preoperative evaluation includes history and physical examination, liver function tests, chest x-ray, bone scan, chest and abdominal computed tomography, urinalysis, and creatinine.
†Directed history includes assessment of pain, weight loss, fever, night sweats, polyuria, and hematuria. Directed physical examination includes soft tissue, lymph node, and abdominal examinations.
‡Includes serum glutamic-oxaloacetic transaminase, alkaline phosphatase, and lactic dehydrogenase.
§Performed on all patients preoperatively. For patients with T2N0 disease, performed once at 6 months. For patients with T3, T4, and N+ disease, performed every 6 months for 2 years.
¶Performed at baseline. If no evidence of metastasis exists at baseline, repeat bone scan only if bone pain or an elevated alkaline phosphatase level is detected.
**Performed on patients with T3N+ and T4N+ disease.
††Performed on patients with less than 50% residual renal mass postoperatively.

The risk of recurrence of localized renal cell carcinoma is highest in the first 3 years after surgery. In a retrospective series of 137 patients with localized renal cell carcinoma, 85% of recurrences occurred within 3 years of surgery.[7] Furthermore, the majority of recurrences were heralded by the development of symptoms such as cough, pain, fever, or weight loss before documentation by laboratory or radiological means. Thus the recommendations shown in Table 21-5 represent the minimal suggested follow-up. The development of new signs or symptoms of recurrence should be promptly investigated. The postoperative follow-up outlined in Table 21-5 allows flexibility depending on the risk of recurrence. Patients with pT1,2N0M0 primary cancers have a low risk of recurrence after radical nephrectomy.

The largest study of patterns of failure after surgical resection of unilateral, nonmetastatic renal cell carcinoma included 172 consecutive patients treated at Memorial Sloan-Kettering Cancer Center between 1978 and 1988. Only 10 of the 172 patients had pT1 lesions, and none had relapse. Of the 172, 99 had pT2N0 lesions and nine had relapse (three in the renal fossa and six at distant sites). For patients with pT2N0 disease there was a 27% actuarial risk of recurrence within 7 years.[8] Thus for the patients with pT1N0 lesions, which have a relatively good prognosis, the recommended follow-up is simple and consists of history and physical examination, chest x-ray, liver function tests, and urinalysis every 6 months for 3 years and annually thereafter. Follow-up for pT2N0 lesions is the same, except that computed tomography of the abdomen is recommended at the 6-month follow-up visit. Patients with positive nodes or pT3 or pT4 primary tumors have a higher risk of recurrence, often in the liver or renal fossa. For this reason computed tomography of the abdomen is indicated every 6 months for the first 2 postoperative years.

Nephrotoxic contrast agents should be used with caution. The administration of both iodinated and noniodinated contrast reagents within 2 to 4 weeks of IL-2 therapy may cause a delayed IL-2 recall syndrome of severe hypotension, capillary leak, and transient renal failure.[9] Patients who have less than 50% of normal renal mass postoperatively are at increased risk for the development of progressive renal disease related to hyperfiltration. Renal function should be carefully evaluated in these patients before the use of contrast agents. For patients with significantly diminished renal mass or intrinsic renal disease, alternative imaging modalities such as magnetic resonance imaging or positron emission tomography may be preferable. If the decision is made to use contrast agents in patients with diminished renal function, the administration of 1 to 2 L of 0.45% saline during or immediately after the contrast infusion may ameliorate renal toxicity.[10]

The follow-up guidelines set forth here emphasize the use of currently available conventional imaging techniques. Rapidly increasing understanding of the molecular changes associated with renal cell carcinoma may open the door to more sensitive and specific means of diagnosis and early detection. Mutations in the von Hippel-Lindau gene have been detected in DNA from formalin-fixed tumor tissue from 57% of patients with nonhereditary renal cell carcinoma.[11] Identification of the somatic mutation in the von Hippel-Lindau gene in a patient's primary tumor may permit polymerase chain reaction–based testing to detect tumor cells in the circulating blood or urine. This approach has the potential to provide earlier detection of recurrence or persistent disease than do currently available tests.[12]

Table 21-6 Follow-up of patients with renal cancer by institution

YEAR/PROGRAM	OFFICE VISIT	CXR	MCBT	CREAT	PROT U	LFT	CBC	RENAL US	ABD CT
Year 1									
Memorial Sloan-Kettering	2	2[a]		2[b,c]	2[c]	2[a]		2[d]	2[d]
Roswell Park	2	2[e]	2[f]						
Univ Washington[g]	2[h]	2		1[i]		2[j]			2[k]
Japan: Natl Cancer Ctr I[n]	3[o]	3	3[f]				3		
Japan: Natl Cancer Ctr II[r]	4[s]	4	4[t]				4		
Year 2									
Memorial Sloan-Kettering	2	2[a]		2[b,c]	2[c]	2[a]		2[d]	2[d]
Roswell Park	2	2[e]	2[f]						
Univ Washington[g]	2[h]	2		[i]		2[j]			2[k]
Japan: Natl Cancer Ctr I[n]	2[o]	2	2[f]				2		
Japan: Natl Cancer Ctr II[r]	3[s]	3	3[t]				3		

ABD CT abdominal computed tomography
ABD US abdominal ultrasound
BRAIN CT brain computed tomography
BRAIN MRI brain magnetic resonance imaging
CBC complete blood count
CHEST CT chest computed tomography
CREAT creatinine
CXR chest x-ray
ENH REN CT enhanced renal computed tomography
HEL CHE CT helical chest computed tomography
LFT liver function test
MCBT multichannel blood tests
PROT U urinary protein (24-hour)
RENAL US renal ultrasound
URIN urinalysis

REFERENCES

1. Thompson JA, Shulman KL, Benyunes MC, et al. Prolonged continuous intravenous infusion interleukin-2 and lymphokine-activated killer cell therapy for metastatic renal cell carcinoma. J Clin Oncol 1992;10:960-8.
2. Thompson J, Nemunaitis J, Vogelzang N, et al. Phase I trial of CT1501R in cancer patients receiving high-dose interleukin-2. Proc Am Soc Clin Oncol 1994;13:977.
3. Rosenberg SA, Yang JC, Topalian SL, et al. Treatment of 283 consecutive patients with metastatic melanoma or renal cell cancer using high-dose bolus interleukin-2. JAMA 1994;271:907-13.
4. Fyfe G, Fisher RI, Rosenberg SA, Sznol M, Parkinson DR, Louie AC. Results of treatment of 255 patients with metastatic renal cell carcinoma who received high-dose recombinant interleukin-2 therapy. J Clin Oncol 1995;13:688-96.
5. Robertson CN, Linehan WM, Pass HI. Preparative cytoreductive surgery in patients with metastatic renal cell carcinoma treated with adoptive immunotherapy with interleukin-2 or interleukin-2 plus lymphokine activated killer cells. J Urol 1990;144:614-8.
6. Wahl RL, Hutchins GD, Buchsbaum DJ, Liebert M, Grossman HB, Fisher S. ^{18}F-2-deoxy-fluoro-D-glucose uptake into human tumor xenografts: feasibility studies for cancer imaging with positron-emission tomography. Cancer 1991;67:1544-50.
7. Sandock DS, Seftel AD, Resnick MI. A new protocol for the follow-up of renal cell carcinoma based on pathologic stage. J Urol 1995;154:28-31.
8. Rabinovitch RA, Zelefsky MJ, Gaynor JJ, Fuks Z. Patterns of failure following surgical resection of renal cell carcinoma: implications for adjuvant local therapy and systemic therapy. J Clin Oncol 1994;12:206-12.
9. Shulman KL, Thompson JA, Benyunes MC, Winter TC, Fefer A. Adverse reactions to intravenous contrast media in patients treated with interleukin-2. J Immunother 1993;13:208-12.
10. Solomon R, Werner C, Mann D, D'Elia J, Silva P. Effects of saline, mannitol, and furosemide to prevent acute decreases in renal function induced by radiocontrast agents. N Engl J Med 1994;331:1416-20.
11. Gnarra JR, Tory K, Weng Y, et al. Mutation of the VHL tumour suppressor gene in renal carcinoma. Nat Genet 1995;7:85-90.
12. Linehan WM, Lerman MI, Zbar B. Identification of the von Hippel-Lindau (VHL) gene: its role in kidney cancer. JAMA 1995;273:564-70.

PELVIC CT	ENH REN CT	ABD US OR CT	BONE SCAN	BONE X-RAY	BRAIN CT	HEL CHE CT	BRAIN MRI	URIN	CHEST CT
2[d]									
			1[l]					2	1[m]
	1[b]	1[p]	q	q	q				
		1[p]	q	q	q	q	q		
2[d]									
			l					2	m
	1[b]	1[p]	q	q	q				
		1[p]	q	q	q	q	q		

a For patients with T2 and T3 disease.
b Urine.
c For patients who have undergone partial nephrectomy.
d For asymptomatic patients with von Hippel-Lindau disease.
e Posteroanterior and lateral. Not performed for patients with T1 lesions.
f Consists of blood urea nitrogen and creatinine.
g This follow-up schema assumes that the preoperative evaluation includes history and physical examination, liver function tests, chest x-ray, bone scan, chest and abdominal computed tomography, urinalysis, and creatinine.
h Directed history includes assessment of pain, weight loss, fever, night sweats, polyuria, and hematuria. Directed physical examination includes soft tissue, lymph node, and abdominal examinations.
i Performed on patients with less than 50% residual renal mass postoperatively.
j Includes serum glutamie-oxaloacetic transaminase, alkaline phosphatase, and lactic dehydrogenase.
k Performed on all patients preoperatively. For patients with T2N0 disease, performed once at 6 months. For patients with T3, T4, and N+ disease, performed every 6 months for 2 years.
l Performed at baseline. If no evidence of metastasis exists at baseline, repeat bone scan only if bone pain or an elevated alkaline phosphatase level is detected.
m Performed on patients with T3N+ and T4N+ disease.
n Patients with T1 disease after radical or partial nephrectomy.
o Includes history and physical examination of the supraclavicular lymph nodes and abdomen.
p Test selection based on cost and availability.
q Performed when indicated by history or physical examination.
r T2 and T3 disease after radical nephrectomy or T4 disease after resection of metastases simultaneous with or subsequent to radical nephrectomy.
s Includes history and physical examination. After year 5, office visits are annual until year 10.
t Consists of blood urea nitrogen, creatinine, and calcium.

Continued.

Table 21-6 Follow-up of patients with renal cancer by institution—cont'd

YEAR/PROGRAM	OFFICE VISIT	CXR	MCBT	CREAT	PROT U	LFT	CBC	RENAL US	ABD CT
Year 3									
Memorial Sloan-Kettering	2	2[a]		2[b,c]	2[c]	2[a]		2[d]	2[d]
Roswell Park	2	2[e]	2[f]	2[a]					
Univ Washington[g]	2[h]	2		[i]		2[j]			[k]
Japan: Natl Cancer Ctr I[n]	2[o]	2	2[f]				2		
Japan: Natl Cancer Ctr II[r]	3[s]	3	3[t]				3		
Year 4									
Memorial Sloan-Kettering	2	1[a]		2[b,c]	2[c]	1[a]		2[d]	2[d]
Roswell Park	1	1[e]	1[f]						
Univ Washington[g]	1[h]	1		[i]		1[j]			[k]
Japan: Natl Cancer Ctr I[n]	2[o]	2	2[f]				2		
Japan: Natl Cancer Ctr II[r]	2[s]	2	2[t]				2		
Year 5									
Memorial Sloan-Kettering	2	1[a]		2[b,c]	2[c]	1[a]		2[d]	2[d]
Roswell Park	1	1[e]	1[f]						
Univ Washington[g]	1[h]	1		[i]		1[j]			[k]
Japan: Natl Cancer Ctr I[n]	2[o]	2	2[f]				2		
Japan: Natl Cancer Ctr II[r]	2[s]	2	2[t]				2		

PELVIC CT	ENH REN CT	ABD US OR CT	BONE SCAN	BONE X-RAY	BRAIN CT	HEL CHE CT	BRAIN MRI	URIN	CHEST CT
2[d]									
			l					2	m
	1[b]	1[p]	q	q	q				
		1[p]	q	q	q	q	q		
2[d]									
			l					1	m
	1[b]		q	q	q				
		1[p]	q	q	q	q	q		
2[d]									
			l					1	m
	1[b]		q	q	q				
		1[p]	q	q	q	q	q		

CHAPTER 22

Lymphoma

University of Washington Medical Center ▪ Fred Hutchinson Cancer Research Center

DAVID G. MALONEY AND FREDERICK R. APPELBAUM

Increasing numbers of patients with Hodgkin's disease and non-Hodgkin's lymphoma become long-term survivors after treatment. Advances have been most encouraging in the management of Hodgkin's disease and the aggressive non-Hodgkin's histological types, in which the majority of patients, especially those with early-stage disease, appear to be cured. After successful induction of remission, patients generally are followed up by physical examination, laboratory tests, and selected imaging studies. The frequency and specific tests critical to the management of asymptomatic patients after treatment for lymphoma have been neither firmly established nor rigorously tested in clinical trials. Most physicians are guided by their own experience and the outcomes of clinical trials reporting the comparison of treatment regimens. Despite the limited data available, evaluation of patients after treatment for lymphoma must be performed with clear objectives in mind. Goals of follow-up evaluation include identification of disease recurrence, acute toxic effects of treatment, and late complications. The relative importance of each of these goals differs depending on the clinical situation. Prognostic features both at disease presentation and during treatment, as well as long-term risks from the specific treatment, must be considered when planning follow-up evaluations.

Surveillance studies to detect recurrent disease may be more important when an effective salvage treatment applicable to the clinical situation is available. Patients with Hodgkin's disease or aggressive non-Hodgkin's lymphoma generally are initially treated with curative intent. Patients with relapse may still have an opportunity for long-term survival after subsequent treatment. In this population detection of recurrent disease may prompt immediate consideration of aggressive therapy. In contrast, although patients with "low-grade" lymphomas usually respond to many forms of therapy, most patients ultimately have a recurrence and are not considered curable with current conventional therapy. When recurrent disease is detected in this population, therapy is often used to control the symptoms of disease with palliative rather than curative intent. The intensity of surveillance for disease recurrence may therefore be different in these populations.

Lymphoma treatment, whether successful or not, is associated with side effects and toxicity that may be life threatening. At completion of the planned therapy, patients are still at risk for late side effects from the treatment regimen. These may be manifest as direct damage to organ systems by chemotherapy or radiation therapy or as a predisposition to other chronic diseases or secondary malignancies. Examples include infertility, thyroid insufficiency, and pulmonary or cardiac toxicity. Breast carcinoma may occur in a patient years after mediastinal radiation therapy and be detected at an early curable stage by surveillance. The clinical situation of the patient and the type of lymphoma therapy given greatly influence the types and frequencies of complications for which the patient is at risk and the studies that may be included for follow-up. In some situations, when the risk of relapse is low, the long-term toxicity of the treatment regimen or secondary malignancy exceeds the risk of recurrent disease as the cause of death. Depending on the clinical situation the posttreatment evaluation must be aimed at detecting and managing these additional problems.

In this chapter general and specific approaches for the follow-up of patients treated for Hodgkin's disease, aggressive non-Hodgkin's lymphoma (intermediate and high grade), and low-grade non-Hodgkin's lymphoma are discussed. Considered first are the general outcomes of current therapy that can be expected based on known prognostic factors, the patterns of disease recurrence, the prognosis and applicability of salvage treatment, and the current practice of follow-up. Second, specific tests to detect disease recurrence are analyzed. Third, complications of treatment and recommended methods of follow-up are discussed. Because few studies have formally demonstrated the utility (or lack thereof) of most follow-up modalities, two types of guidelines can be offered, those that reflect the general recommendations made by experts and those that are actually data driven. As clinical investigators begin to look at the costs and benefits of many of these studies (and appropriately so), recommendations may well change.

HODGKIN'S DISEASE

The treatment of Hodgkin's disease represents one of the true successes in oncology. Although a relatively rare disease, with an estimated 7,800 new cases diagnosed in the United States in 1995,[1] this lymphoma was universally fatal before radiation therapy[2] and the pioneering development of the MOPP (mechlorethamine, oncovin, procarbazine, and prednisone) combination chemotherapy regimen in the 1960s.[3] At present nearly 75% of patients can be cured with irradiation, chemotherapy, or combined-modality therapy. An even higher success rate has been observed in the treatment of patients whose disease is diagnosed and treated in earlier stages. The incidence of Hodgkin's disease has a bimodal peak, occurring more frequently in young adults and in the elderly. As more young patients become long-term survivors and are followed up for extended periods, complications and late toxic effects of treatment are becoming increasingly evident. In groups with a favorable prognosis the risk of dying from a late toxic effect of therapy exceeds the risk of relapse. New approaches in the treatment of favorable-stage patients have focused on reducing the acute and long-term toxicity of the treatment while maintaining a high level of disease-free survival.[4] Improved treatment is still needed for patients with advanced-stage, unfavorable-prognosis Hodgkin's disease. Current approaches include aggressive high-dose therapy with hematological stem cell transplantation in attempts to further improve long-term survival.[5]

Pretreatment Risk Features

The pretreatment prognosis of patients with Hodgkin's disease can be influenced by a number of factors, although as treatment has improved, they have a lesser effect on overall survival. Four major histological subtypes of Hodgkin's disease have been identified. In a series of 1,770 patients followed up at Stanford the most common histological type was nodular sclerosing (75%), followed by mixed cellularity (15%), lymphocyte predominant (5%), and lymphocyte depleted subtypes (1%), with 4% unclassified. With current therapy the overall survival of patients with all histological subtypes is similar, although the risk of relapse may be different. In the Stanford series there was an 88% freedom from relapse for lymphocyte predominant, 76% for mixed cellularity, and 72% for nodular sclerosing Hodgkin's disease. Overall survival at 20 years was 59% to 68%. Careful staging of disease remains important in planning the treatment. Other prognostic factors include the presence or absence of bulky disease and B symptoms and patient age at presentation. The most important factor appears to be age, with a 97% freedom from relapse for patients less than 10 years of age, 72% to 74% for patients ages 10 to 60, and only 47% for patients more than 60 years of age.[6]

Current Treatment

The general approaches to the treatment of Hodgkin's disease are only summarized here, since a thorough discussion of the treatment of each clinical presentation of Hodgkin's disease is beyond the scope of this chapter. Patients with early-stage Hodgkin's disease can be cured by treatment with irradiation alone.[7] At least 36 Gy is usually delivered to involved regions and to extended prophylactic fields in nodal regions at risk for occult disease. In children a combined-modality regimen using chemotherapy with low-dose involved-field irradiation is now used because of severe effects on bone and muscle development and growth observed with high-dose irradiation.[4,8] Careful staging is critical. Patients with advanced-stage Hodgkin's disease are treated with multiagent chemotherapy with or without low-dose irradiation. The use of MOPP alone has been replaced by ABVD (adriamycin, bleomycin, vinblastine, and dacarbazine) or a MOPP/ABVD or MOPP/ABV hybrid, each of which has been shown to be superior to MOPP in randomized trials.[9] These newer regimens are associated with a lower rate of infertility and decreased risk of secondary leukemia. Patients with extensive unfavorable disease may be candidates for early treatment or consolidation with high-dose therapy and hematological stem cell support.[5]

Patterns of Relapse After Initial Treatment for Hodgkin's Disease

Hodgkin's disease can recur after initial irradiation in irradiated or nonirradiated sites. Although late relapses are seen, most relapses occur during the first 6 years of follow-up. When patients are staged with laparotomy, relapses are rarer and usually regional, while patients treated after clinical staging often have relapse in distant, nonirradiated sites, reflecting understaging of the initial disease using clinical evaluation.[10] Relapses in patients with laparotomy-staged I and IIA disease treated with irradiation fields limited to the mantle regions (omitting paraaortic fields) generally occur in nonirradiated nodal regions below the diaphragm.[11] Patients treated with combination chemotherapy for advanced-stage disease generally have relapse in previous sites of disease, most often nodal regions.[12] The use of adjuvant irradiation to all nodal sites of disease in chemotherapy-treated patients decreases the risk of relapse.[13]

Management of Recurrent Disease After Primary Therapy

Patients with relapse after initial irradiation are usually treated with multiagent combination chemotherapy, with 55% to 60% becoming long-term disease-free survivors.[14,15] Relapses after primary therapy with MOPP or combined modality therapy can be treated with additional chemotherapy regimens, such as ABVD,[16] etoposide, vinblastine, and doxorubicin,[17] or high-dose therapy with autologous or allogeneic stem cell transplantation.[18] The duration of remission produced by the primary therapy predicts the response to second-line chemotherapy. In one series patients with a first remission of less than 1 year had a 17% likelihood of disease-free survival 4 years later after salvage chemotherapy and thus are considered candidates for innovative, high-dose treatment approaches.[17] Disease sensitivity to cytoreductive therapy before high-dose regimens and tumor bulk are important factors determining outcome and are frequently used as selection criteria for aggressive treatment.[19,20] In general, studies suggest that transplantation is more effective if performed earlier

Table 22-1 Working Formulation classification of non-Hodgkin's lymphoma

PROGNOSTIC GROUP	PERCENT OF PATIENTS†	MEDIAN SURVIVAL TIME* (YR)	5-YEAR SURVIVAL RATE (%)
LOW GRADE			
Small lymphocytic	3.6	5.8	59
Follicular small cleaved cell	22.5	7.2	70
Follicular mixed small and large cell	7.7	5.1	50
INTERMEDIATE GRADE			
Follicular large cell	3.8	3.0	45
Diffuse small cleaved cell	6.9	3.4	33
Diffuse mixed small and large cell	6.7	2.7	38
Diffuse large cell	19.7	1.5	35
HIGH GRADE			
Large cell immunoblastic	7.9	1.3	32
Lymphoblastic	4.2	2.0	26
Small noncleaved cell	5.0	0.7	23

From Non-Hodgkin's Lymphoma Pathologic Classification Project. Cancer 1982;49:2112-35.
*Survival based on patients with disease diagnosed between July 1971 and December 1975.
†Percentage of the 1,014 patients included in the original cohort.

after relapse and in patients with chemotherapy-sensitive, minimal disease.[18]

Current Follow-Up Practice for Patients with Hodgkin's Disease

At most centers an aggressive follow-up schedule is used after treatment for Hodgkin's disease. At Stanford, after irradiation, patients have clinic visits every 2 months for year 1, every 3 months during year 2, every 4 months during year 3, every 6 months during years 4 and 5, and annually thereafter.[7] Evaluations include physical examination, complete blood count, erythrocyte sedimentation rate, lactic dehydrogenase and alkaline phosphatase levels, and chest x-ray. Yearly thyroid function studies with measurement of thyroxine and thyroid-stimulating hormone are obtained. Early posttreatment computed tomographic scans of the chest are obtained to assess response and to provide a baseline for future evaluation. In a series from Boston, when mantle field irradiation alone was used, long-term surveillance of abdominal and pelvic nodes with abdominal and pelvic computed tomographic or gallium scans every 6 to 12 months for the first 5 years was done.[11]

After chemotherapy or combined modality treatment for bulky or advanced-stage Hodgkin's disease the Stanford group uses the same schedule of follow-up with complete blood count, chemistry panel with lactic dehydrogenase and alkaline phosphatase, erythrocyte sedimentation rate, and chest x-ray. Abdominal films for evaluation of lymphangiograms at each visit or computed tomographic scans of the abdomen and pelvis are repeated at the end of years 1 or 2 if no residual lymphangiographic contrast material is present.[21]

Unfortunately, few studies have examined the utility of aggressive follow-up in detecting recurrent Hodgkin's disease after treatment. A recent abstract detailed 2,512 outpatient visits over 5 years for the follow-up of 210 patients in complete remission after treatment with combination chemotherapy with or without low-dose irradiation.[22] Thirty-seven relapses were detected, and 30 of 37 patients had symptoms of disease, with 15 patients requesting unscheduled evaluation. Only four asymptomatic relapses were detected through physical examination (enlarged nodes in two patients) or chest x-ray (two patients). Detailed evaluation of the efficacy of follow-up to detect asymptomatic disease recurrence has not been reported from other centers. Most physicians who follow a large number of patients can recall cases in which recurrent disease was found on imaging studies or as a result of screening tests, although this appears to occur in a minority of cases.

NON-HODGKIN'S LYMPHOMA

Histological Classification

An estimated 51,000 cases of non-Hodgkin's lymphoma were diagnosed in the United States in 1995.[1] Several systems developed in Europe and the United States have been used to categorize subtypes of non-Hodgkin's lymphoma based on histological appearance. A working formulation was proposed as a framework to provide communication among users of these classification systems and to group histological types as low, intermediate, or high grade based on natural history.[23] Recent advances using genetic analysis, molecular markers, and immunophenotyping have led to the proposal of a new classification system that includes several entities not included in the working formulation.[24] Analysis and long-term follow-up of clinical outcomes will be required to determine whether this categorization will add useful information for planning therapy. However, a basic understanding of the working formulation is necessary to

Table 22-2 International index and age-adjusted index of prognostic factors for patients with aggressive non-Hodgkin's lymphoma

RISK GROUP	NO. OF FACTORS	CR RATE (%)	5-YEAR RFS RATE OF PATIENTS ACHIEVING CR (%)	5-YEAR SURVIVAL RATE (%)
OVERALL GROUP				
Low	0 or 1	87	70	73
Low-intermediate	2	67	50	51
High-intermediate	3	55	49	43
High	4 or 5	44	40	26
AGE-ADJUSTED INDEX FOR PATIENTS LESS THAN 60 YEARS OF AGE				
Low	0	92	86	83
Low-intermediate	1	78	66	69
High-intermediate	2	57	53	46
High	3	46	58	32
AGE-ADJUSTED INDEX FOR PATIENTS 60 YEARS OF AGE OR OLDER				
Low	0	91	46	56
Low-intermediate	1	71	45	44
High-intermediate	2	56	41	37
High	3	36	37	21

From International Non-Hodgkin's Lymphoma Prognostic Factors Project. N Engl J Med 1993;329:987-94.
CR, Complete remission; *RFS,* relapse-free survival.
For overall group, factors are based on age 60 or older, stage III or IV, extranodal sites greater than 1, elevated serum lactic dehydrogenase level, and nonambulatory performance status.

direct a rational surveillance strategy. An outline of the working formulation is given in Table 22-1.

The low-grade histological types include the small lymphocytic, the follicular small cell cleaved, and follicular mixed small cell and large cell types. They are characterized by occurrence in a middle-aged to elderly population, with advanced, widespread disease at diagnosis that is generally slow growing and with median survival times ranging from 8 to 10 years.[25] Although the disease is usually responsive to a wide variety of treatments, patients have continued episodes of relapse and are not considered curable with standard treatment regimens. Histological transformation to an intermediate- or high-grade non-Hodgkin's lymphoma may occur at any time, with an estimated rate of 40% to 70% at 8 to 10 years.[25]

The aggressive intermediate- and high-grade categories include large cell, small noncleaved cell, and immunoblastic histological types. These diseases are more often localized but have an aggressive clinical course. In contrast to the indolent histological types, these cancers can be cured by multiagent chemotherapy alone or combined with radiation therapy in the majority of patients with early-stage disease and in 30% to 40% of patients with advanced-stage disease.[9,26] Salvage high-dose therapy may be curative in patients with relapse after initial therapy.[19,20]

Aggressive Non-Hodgkin's Lymphoma

Prognostic features and current treatment

Between 36% and 90% of patients with stage I through IV large cell lymphoma achieve complete remission after aggressive multiagent chemotherapy alone or in combination with radiation therapy. An international index based on the outcomes of therapy in more than 2,031 patients has been formulated and used to estimate the prognosis of patients with aggressive non-Hodgkin's lymphoma. An age-adjusted index was also derived for patients older or younger than 60 years of age. This index places patients into four risk groups based on four features: stage III or IV disease, elevated serum lactic dehydrogenase level, nonambulatory performance status, and more than one extranodal site of involvement.[27] An outline of this index is presented in Table 22-2 along with the likelihood of complete remission, the percentage of patients with a durable complete remission at 5 years, and overall survival at 5 years. Patients under the age of 60 with none of the risk factors have a 92% chance of complete remission and an 83% 5-year survival rate. In contrast, patients under the age of 60 in the highest risk group with four risk factors have only a 46% chance of complete remission and a 32% 5-year survival rate. When the index is applied to patients over the age of 60, similar response rates are observed, but with lower 5-year survival rates of 56% for good risk factors and 21% for patients with the highest risk factors. Interestingly, the decreases in relapse-free survival observed in the older patients were most striking in the low and low-intermediate risk groups. Additional factors shown to provide prognostic information that are not included in this index include measures of proliferation, cytogenetic abnormalities, beta$_2$-microglobulin levels, major histocompatibility complex molecule expression, and CD44 expression.[28] Knowledge of the patient's pretreatment risk features is important in predicting the likelihood of disease relapse and can be used in planning patient follow-up.

Further information can be obtained from treatment-related prognostic factors. The disease's intrinsic susceptibility to chemotherapy influences response to treatment. In one study patients requiring more than five cycles of chemotherapy to achieve complete remission had a 40% disease-free survival, while patients achieving complete remission in three or fewer cycles had an 80% disease-free survival at 2 years.[29] Similar results have been obtained using gallium scans after four to six cycles of therapy. Patients who had persistent uptake midway through chemotherapy achieved less durable complete remission.[30] Although the issue of dose intensity is still debated, the inability to treat patients with full doses on schedule is clearly associated with a poor prognosis.[31,32]

All stages of aggressive large cell lymphoma are treated with multiagent chemotherapy. Low-dose irradiation is usually added to initial sites of disease for early-stage disease and to areas of prior bulky disease.[9] Significant survival advances were made with the addition of the anthracycline doxorubicin in the 1970s. Since then a number of second- and third-generation combination chemotherapy regimens have been developed and used. Despite dramatic differences between regimens in pilot and phase I and II clinical trials, randomized clinical trials have shown the regimens to be nearly equivalent in efficacy. A national high-priority study has compared the outcomes of the newer generation regimens—bleomycin, doxorubicin, cyclophosphamide, vincristine, dexamethasone, methotrexate, and calcium leucovorin rescue; methotrexate, calcium leucovorin rescue, doxorubicin, cyclophosphamide, vincristine, bleomycin, and prednisone; and cyclophosphamide, doxorubicin, etoposide, prednisone, cytarabine, bleomycin, vincristine, methotrexate, and calcium leucovorin rescue—and the first-generation regimen of cyclophosphamide, doxorubicin, vincristine, and prednisone as initial therapy for patients with advanced-stage aggressive lymphoma. Further follow-up of the study continues to demonstrate no significant difference in survival among the four regimens, with lower cost and less toxicity observed in the cyclophosphamide, doxorubicin, vincristine, and prednisone arm.[26] With a median follow-up of 4 years the overall disease-free survival is 43%.[33] Additional prospective, randomized trials have yielded similar results.[34,35]

Patterns of relapse

Typical patterns of disease relapse can also be used to identify follow-up studies likely to detect recurrent disease. Disease relapse is most frequent within the first 3 years, with rare relapses occurring after 5 years.[27] Several series analyzing sites of relapse have been reported. In one study 139 of 215 patients (65%) with stage II through IV large cell lymphoma treated with the regimen of bleomycin, doxorubicin, cyclophosphamide, vincristine, dexamethasone, methotrexate, and calcium leucovorin rescue achieved complete remission and were monitored for relapse.[36] Recurrent disease developed in 36 patients. Of these, 67% had recurrence detected in new sites, 25% of which were in new sites only and 42% of which were in both new sites and sites of previous disease. The pattern of disease presentation was also mirrored in the relapse pattern. Most patients with only nodal disease at presentation had relapse in nodal areas, and patients with extranodal disease at presentation had relapses involving extranodal sites. In this study tests not targeting specific disease sites such as physical examination, serum lactic dehydrogenase level, and gallium scan were the most sensitive for the detection of recurrent disease. Another group found that 80% of patients with relapse had disease in new sites (56% new only) and that the initial pattern of disease presentation was not associated with sites of relapse.[37]

Disease bulk has been associated with a decreased chance of complete remission and increased chance of relapse,[28] and patients often receive adjuvant radiation therapy to sites of bulky disease after treatment. However, patients with bulky stage II through IV disease have relapse in both new and old sites.[38] Thus, even when bulky disease is present, evaluation of the patient in complete remission should be directed accordingly, using studies not directed only at sites of prior disease.

Current clinical practice of follow-up evaluation

The greatest risk for disease relapse occurs in the first 2 to 3 years after the induction of complete remission, with rare relapses occurring after 5 years. After most clinical trials patients are evaluated every 2 to 3 months for the first year, every 3 to 6 months for the next 4 years, and annually thereafter. Typical evaluations comprise physical examination and laboratory tests, including complete blood count, serum lactic dehydrogenase level, and at least one directed radiographic study every 3 months for the first year and every 6 months for the next 1 to 2 years.[36] Examples of radiographic studies include chest x-ray, computed tomography, and magnetic resonance imaging. At some centers scintigraphy with gallium-67 (Ga-67) has proved useful in detecting recurrent disease and plays a prominent role in follow-up. This is discussed in detail later in the chapter.

Treatment of relapse

Selected patients with aggressive non-Hodgkin's lymphoma who have relapse after primary treatment may still achieve long-term disease-free survival following salvage therapy. Currently most approaches involve high-dose chemotherapy with or without total body radiation followed by either autologous or allogeneic bone marrow or peripheral blood stem cell support. In the treatment of selected patients as many as 50% may be long-term survivors.[19,20] In a randomized trial, high-dose therapy for patients with recurrent aggressive non-Hodgkin's lymphoma resulted in a survival advantage compared with conventional chemotherapy.[39] The use of this therapy in first remission for high-risk patients is less clear. In one series high-dose therapy appeared useful for patients at highest risk for relapse but did not benefit the overall population.[40] Despite these promising results, applicability of this form of therapy is limited by patient age and performance status and is usually restricted to patients with chemotherapy-responsive disease. In most series patients with minimal disease have a better outcome, which suggests but does not prove that earlier detection of recurrent disease in a patient population eligible for aggressive therapy may be beneficial. An additional factor to consider at the time of recurrent disease detection is the potential for obtaining a tumor-free stem cell source for use with subsequent high-dose therapy. Early detection of relapse may allow harvesting of bone marrow or stem cells before significant tumor involvement.

Low-Grade Non-Hodgkin's Lymphoma

Prognostic features and current therapy

In contrast to Hodgkin's disease and aggressive non-Hodgkin's lymphoma, little change in long-term survival has been observed in the treatment of patients with low-grade non-Hodgkin's lymphoma in the past 20 years.[25] The histological subtypes according to the working formulation are given in Table 22-1. The follicular histological types are the most common and have a characteristic t(14:18) chromosomal translocation, which results in the overexpression of the bcl-2 protein. Expression of this protein protects cells from programmed cell death. Prognostic factors for poor outcome include older age, advanced stage, poor performance status, presence of B symptoms, bulky disease, bone marrow involvement, and high serum lactic dehydrogenase or beta$_2$-microglobulin levels.[25] The international index for aggressive non-Hodgkin's lymphoma (Table 22-2) has been applied to a group of patients with low-grade non-Hodgkin's lymphoma, with stratification into three prognostic groups.[41] The low-risk group had a 10-year survival rate of 75% with a time to treatment failure of more than 7 years, while the high-risk group had no 10-year survivors (median survival time less than 3 years) and a time to treatment failure of less than 2 years. The high-risk group contained 11% of the population evaluated. The intermediate-risk group was defined by combining the high-to-intermediate- and the low-to-intermediate-risk groups for a 10-year survival rate of 50% and a time to treatment failure of less than 3 years. The chance of complete remission after therapy was 60% in the intermediate-risk and 21% in the high-risk groups.

Low-grade non-Hodgkin's lymphoma is rarely localized at disease presentation, and stages III and IV with bone marrow involvement are common. When disease is localized, treatment with extensive field irradiation with or without chemotherapy may provide 10-year disease-free survival in 30% to 50% of patients, although late relapses may be observed.[42] Treatment of advanced-stage disease may range from observation alone for asymptomatic patients to aggressive combined modality therapy. Randomized studies have generally not shown a survival advantage for any single treatment approach.[25,43] In nearly all studies a continuous pattern of relapse is suggested, without an apparent long-term plateau in disease-free survival. The addition of interferon to the treatment regimen and after therapy may improve disease-free survival and possibly overall survival.[44] However, the side effects of interferon may outweigh the minimal beneficial effects observed in some but not all studies. It is too early to know the impact of high-dose therapy with autologous hematopoietic stem cell transplantation in low-grade histological types, although a number of studies have been reported.[45] In those with the longest follow-up, late relapses are being observed and overall survival has not yet been improved, although disease-free survival may be better than with a matched historical cohort.[46] Further follow-up should determine the applicability of this approach in selected patients. The use of allogeneic marrow transplantation in patients with low-grade non-Hodgkin's lymphoma has been limited, although it appears to promote long-term disease-free survival, presumably because of the addition of a graft-versus-lymphoma effect.[47]

Patients with relapse after a response to initial therapy are likely to respond to either retreatment or additional agents with a shorter duration of subsequent remissions.[48] Median survival time after first relapse ranges from 2 to 6 years in most studies. Treatment-related poor prognostic factors include a duration of remission after first treatment of less than 12 months.[49] In 30% to 60% of patients with low-grade non-Hodgkin's lymphoma the disease is transformed to an aggressive histological pattern at some time during its course.[25] Histological transformation requires aggressive therapy and usually results in a short survival time.[50]

Current practice of follow-up

Most patients with low-grade non-Hodgkin's lymphoma experience relapse, and further treatment is often delayed until clear disease progression or the development of symptoms. Early detection of disease recurrence has not been shown to make a difference in overall survival. Follow-up of most patients in remission includes physical examinations and blood tests every 3 to 6 months. Frequently used blood tests include white blood cell count and platelets to evaluate marrow function and serum tests to measure renal and hepatic function. Patients with symptoms or palpable adenopathy should undergo periodic imaging studies to identify disease areas that may soon cause complications. Examples include bulky nodal disease causing hydronephrosis, pain, or other neurological symptoms. Intensive screening of patients in remission is probably not warranted except in study circumstances or when early intervention with additional treatments is planned. Treatment options for patients with relapsed low-grade non-Hodgkin's lymphoma include standard chemotherapy or high-dose therapy with hematological stem cell support, new drugs or immunotherapy with vaccines, and monoclonal antibodies alone or labeled with radioisotopes or toxins. Support of clinical trials evaluating these approaches is important, since they will eventually improve the overall survival and quality of life of patients with low-grade non-Hodgkin's lymphoma.

USE OF SPECIFIC TESTS TO DETECT DISEASE RECURRENCE

Imaging Modalities

Most physicians use some form of site-directed radiographic study in the follow-up of patients in remission. The most frequently used studies are chest x-rays and computed tomographic scans of previously involved sites of disease. The value of routine screening for disease relapse in asymptomatic patients has not been rigorously tested.[51] In the study reported by Weeks et al.[36] the value of follow-up tests for patients with aggressive non-Hodgkin's lymphoma was examined in 36 patients with relapse. Despite close follow-up, only two of 36 relapses were detected before the development of symptoms, and routine radiological evaluation detected only one recurrence. At the time of recurrent disease patients had been evaluated by examination, complete blood count, lactic dehydrogenase level, and chest x-ray within the previous 2 to 3 months. Those with relapse detected by computed tomography had been screened with a computed tomographic scan a median of 5.6 months earlier. Thus even with conscientious follow-up the majority of patients with relapse of large cell lymphoma returned for unscheduled or scheduled visits with new symptoms of disease, most frequently a palpable tumor mass. In this study screening radiological imaging had a poor sensitivity (14% during screening and 55% during restaging) but a high specificity (94%) in detecting recurrent disease, especially when the patient had signs or symptoms indicating relapse. New sites of disease involvement are frequently seen at relapse after treatment for aggressive non-Hodgkin's lymphoma, and thus site-directed evaluation of prior disease regions has a low sensitivity. Patients with bulky aggressive non-Hodgkin's lymphoma who are in remission also have recurrence in new and old areas of disease.[38]

Patients treated for Hodgkin's disease usually are followed up with chest x-rays and periodic computed tomography. Interpretation of posttreatment images is often difficult because of residual masses and post–radiation therapy scarring of the lungs and mediastinum.[52] Baseline studies are frequently obtained 4 to 6 months after treatment to be used in future evaluation.[7] As described later, gallium scintigraphy or magnetic resonance imaging may provide information on persistent viable tumor tissue. The lymphangiogram is a sensitive method to detect Hodgkin's disease or non-Hodgkin's lymphoma in the lower paraaortic and pelvic lymph nodes.[6] When it is used, patients often have residual contrast medium for 1 to 2 years and a plain film of the abdomen provides excellent surveillance of these areas. This may be particularly important in patients with Hodgkin's disease treated with limited field irradiation protocols.[11] Unfortunately, lymphangiography requires considerable experience in administration and interpretation, so it has largely been replaced by computed tomography or magnetic resonance imaging. Despite these excellent imaging modalities, most patients with Hodgkin's disease have symptomatic recurrence and return for unscheduled visits.[22]

Magnetic resonance imaging may provide additional information by distinguishing active disease from posttreatment residual scarring[53] and in detecting disease processes involving bone marrow[54] when compared with computed tomography. Most studies have focused on initial staging and on evaluating a posttreatment residual mass. Whether the routine use of magnetic resonance imaging after treatment will increase ability to detect disease relapse remains to be seen.

High-dose Ga-67 and single photon emission computed tomography scintigraphy have been widely used in patients with aggressive non-Hodgkin's lymphoma and Hodgkin's disease. Uptake of Ga-67 depends on viable tissue, since necrotic or fibrotic areas are not imaged. Quantitative analysis of the Ga-67 signal has been used to differentiate normal lymph nodes from those involved by lymphoma. In a recent study the test was able to separate lymphoma and normal nodes with a sensitivity of 90%, a specificity of 93%, a positive predictive value of 84%, and a negative predictive value of 96%.[55] At diagnosis most patients with Hodgkin's disease or aggressive non-Hodgkin's lymphoma have gallium-avid tumors. When positive at diagnosis, follow-up scans can be useful in determining the response to therapy and in detecting recurrent disease.[30] Gallium avidity of a residual mass at the completion of therapy correlates with the probability of finding viable tumor on biopsy and subsequent relapse.[56]

The routine use of gallium scanning as a posttreatment screening method to detect recurrent disease is more limited. Weeks et al.[36] found the test to be sensitive (90%) for the detection of aggressive non-Hodgkin's lymphoma during restaging studies after clinical relapse and to have a 90% specificity in control patients in continuous complete remission, but not enough patients had the test in the 3 months before relapse to allow determination of its ability to detect recurrent disease. In a second study 32 patients in whom recurrent disease eventually developed were studied at an average interval of 8.7 months after completion of treatment.[57] At relapse the sensitivity was 95% with a specificity of 89%. In 10 patients the scan was positive an average of 6.8 months before clinical relapse in areas where recurrent disease eventually developed. This group used Ga-67 scintigraphy at 6 and 12 months after complete remission and once a year thereafter.[56]

In some centers Ga-67 scintigraphy has clearly been shown to be useful in directing treatment decisions. However, the test depends on technical expertise in both its method of administration and its interpretation. The routine use of gallium scintigraphy to detect recurrent disease in asymptomatic patients treated for Hodgkin's disease with a low risk for relapse is likely to have low utility.

Somatostatin receptor scintigraphy using ^{111}In-labeled octreotide (a somatostatin analog) can detect somatostatin receptors in activated lymphocytes and in Hodgkin's disease and non-Hodgkin's lymphoma. In one series 98% of patients with Hodgkin's disease and 85% of patients with non-Hodgkin's lymphoma had positive scans.[58] The results of the test were in agreement with conventional imaging in 57% of patients, superior in 35%, and inferior in 8%. Another series showed a 94% true-positive rate and a 6% false-negative rate. These scans detected more lesions than did computed tomographic scans in 52% of cases and fewer lesions in 10%.[59] Other studies of this approach have not been as successful,[60] and the applicability of the approach to the surveillance of asymptomatic patients remains to be determined.

Total body positron emission tomography with fluorine-18 fluoro-2-deoxy-D-glucose has been used to detect the metabolic activity of lymphomatous tissue. The test had a sensitivity of 98% during staging of 58 patients with Hodgkin's disease or non-Hodgkin's lymphoma and a specificity of 95%. It reliably predicted complete remission in patients with persisting abnormal computed tomographic scans.[61] Of note, false-positive inflammatory reactions during therapy and immediately after treatment were observed and had resolved on confirmatory scans.

As previously discussed, an elevated lactic dehydrogenase level at presentation is a poor prognostic feature. In a follow-up of patients with aggressive non-Hodgkin's lymphoma in complete remission, monitoring of lactic dehydrogenase was the only test sensitive to preclinical disease relapse.[36] The lactic dehydrogenase level was elevated in five of 12 patients tested in the 3 months before clinical relapse. In this small sample of patients the sensitivity for preclinical disease was 42%. Interestingly, the elevated test value did not lead to further diagnostic studies until the development of symptoms.

When evaluated in a similar group of 46 patients in durable complete remission, the specificity of an elevation at a point 4 months or more after treatment was 85%. However, half of the patients had an elevated lactic dehydrogenase level in the first month after chemotherapy. This decreased to a median of 15% of patients with an elevation in one 3-month interval over the next 2 years. Once clinical relapse had occurred, lactic dehydrogenase was elevated in 20 of 31 patients for a sensitivity of 65%. Based on lactic dehydrogenase testing the probability of relapse can be adjusted by applying Bayes' theorem. In stage II patients in this study there was a low constant risk of relapse of 2.1% per year. In contrast, patients with stage III or IV disease had a 13.3% per year relapse rate for the first 2 years, a 7.7% risk per year for years 3 through 5, and a 1.6% risk per year thereafter. An elevated lactic dehydrogenase level increased the probability of relapse in any setting, and a normal level decreased the probability of eminent relapse within the next 3 months. For example, in the highest risk groups of stage III and IV patients, within 2 years of treatment the risk of relapse in a 3-month period was 3.3%; the risk was 1.8% with a normal lactic dehydrogenase level and 6.7% with an abnormal level. Although this risk would probably not be high enough to prompt treatment, it could be used to identify patients who should undergo further diagnostic evaluation. In another series elevated lactic dehydrogenase levels were seen in only six of 53 patients before clinical relapse, with false-positive elevations observed in two of 85 patients in remission.[37]

An elevated serum level of beta$_2$-microglobulin is an indicator of poor prognosis in patients with low-grade[62] and aggressive non-Hodgkin's lymphoma[63,64] and may be useful in detecting preclinical relapse. In one series 160 patients in complete remission from aggressive non-Hodgkin's lymphoma were followed up with serial beta$_2$-microglobulin and lactic dehydrogenase levels.[37] Relapse eventually occurred in 53 patients, and abnormal levels of beta$_2$-microglobulin were observed 3 to 23 months before relapse in 49% of the patients. Evaluation at the time of test elevation did not detect recurrent disease. Six patients had elevated levels of both lactic dehydrogenase and beta$_2$-microglobulin, and all had relapse. If this study can be confirmed by others, it may provide a test with sufficient lead time to allow a trial of early chemotherapy in a population destined for disease progression.

The erythrocyte sedimentation rate is frequently monitored in the routine follow-up of patients with Hodgkin's disease. In one retrospective study a persistently elevated value after treatment was associated with a high risk of early or late relapse with aggressive disease.[65] However, the sensitivity and specificity of a positive test in this setting have not been defined, and prospective studies are needed. Other tests, including soluble interleukin-2 (IL-2) receptor, IL-2, IL-6, IL-8, and many others, are being analyzed for their ability to predict relapse or survival in Hodgkin's disease and non-Hodgkin's lymphoma. At this time none has been sufficiently validated.

COMPLICATIONS OF TREATMENT

As more patients with non-Hodgkin's lymphoma and Hodgkin's disease become long-term survivors, an increasing number of patients manifest acute and chronic toxic effects. Survival may be compromised by a number of late complications. These include damage to the cardiopulmonary system from irradiation and exposure to chemotherapy resulting in chronic pulmonary or premature heart disease. Late secondary malignancies such as leukemia and solid tumors are observed in long-term survivors and are related to the timing and type of therapy given for Hodgkin's disease or non-Hodgkin's lymphoma. Early detection of these conditions may allow successful treatment. Many do not become evident until 5 to 20 years after curative lymphoma treatment, making follow-up difficult. However, knowledge of the types and pattern of post-treatment complications is essential in evaluating patients and their symptoms in follow-up.

Infertility

Infertility is a common complication of chemotherapy and has been associated with the use of alkylating agents, cisplatin, procarbazine, or vincristine.[66] In males the risk is dose dependent and the condition can occur with minimal exposure even at a young age. In females the risks of chemotherapy are more unpredictable. The rate of amenorrhea appears to increase rapidly over the age of 25 to 30 years. In the treatment of Hodgkin's disease the use of limited cycles of MOPP chemotherapy or alternative use of other regimens such as ABVD has significantly decreased the risk of treatment-induced infertility.[6] Brief, intensive treatment regimens such as Stanford V are being tested in young patients with advanced disease. Using these combinations of drugs and low-dose irradiation to decrease cardiopulmonary complications and infertility has shown early success.[21] Male patients treated with multiagent chemotherapy who wish to father children after therapy should undergo pretreatment sperm banking.[67] The use of cryopreserved sperm does not appear to increase the risks of congenital abnormalities or spontaneous abortions. Female patients in remission from Hodgkin's disease who regain fertility do not appear to be at increased risk from a subsequent pregnancy, nor are there apparent risks to the health of the child.[68] However, longer follow-up is necessary to rule out the possibility of long-term late effects, and patients and physicians should not assume that infertility is assured after lymphoma therapy.

Cardiac Complications

Most cardiac complications of lymphoma treatment are related to the use of anthracyclines or to acute and chronic effects of radiation therapy. Radiation therapy may cause acute or delayed pericarditis, pericardial effusions or fibrosis, valvular heart disease, conduction abnormalities, and early coronary heart disease.[69] In the follow-up of patients with Hodgkin's disease treated at Stanford a threefold increase in the relative risk of cardiac death occurred, which was exceeded only by death from Hodgkin's disease and other cancers.[70] Mediastinal irradiation was implicated as increasing the risk of cardiac causes of death. The risk was increased by higher radiation doses, less cardiac blocking, treatment at a young age, and longer duration of follow-up. The majority of deaths from heart disease were caused by acute myocardial infarction (63%), and the remainder were due to congestive heart failure, pericarditis, cardiomyopathy, or valvular heart disease. Coronary artery disease has been observed in young patients after mantle field irradiation.[71] The Stanford authors are considering routine electrocardiography and exercise echocardiography at 5-year intervals after therapy to screen patients for significant coronary artery disease. Chest pain in a young patient who otherwise looks well but has a history of mediastinal irradiation must be evaluated thoroughly.

Limiting the cumulative dose of anthracyclines in chemotherapy regimens to 550 mg/m^2 has greatly reduced the risks of acute cardiomyopathy. However, recent observations that late-occurring cardiac failure may develop in young patients after curative treatment for Wilms' tumor and that 25% of patients had echocardiographic abnormalities despite limited cumulative dose exposure are worrisome. Longer follow-up may reveal further chronic toxicity.[72] Although specific recommendations of follow-up have not been made, attention to cardiovascular symptoms in these patients should be a part of their regular care, as should close attention to standard cardiovascular risk factors such as control of smoking, hypertension, and serum lipids.

Pulmonary Complications

Pulmonary complications after treatment of lymphoma are caused primarily by use of the drugs bleomycin or bischloroethylnitrosourea or by radiation therapy. Radiation damage to the lung is related to the dose and field size of treatment. The most common complication is radiation pneumonitis occurring 1 to 3 months after treatment. This may cause dyspnea, cough, or chest pain in 5% of patients and in severe cases requires treatment with corticosteroids followed by gradual withdrawal.[7] Radiographic changes are usually characteristic, although infection or drug toxicity must also be considered in the differential diagnosis. Radiation-induced pulmonary fibrosis typically occurs 6 months after irradiation and stabilizes at 12 to 18 months. Chest x-ray after mantle field irradiation is usually abnormal and complicates the evaluation for treatment response and detection of relapse.[52] Although lung volumes are decreased because of scarring from irradiation, these changes are usually clinically insignificant.

The use of bleomycin in the popular ABVD regimen for advanced Hodgkin's disease has increased the frequency of pulmonary complications. Bleomycin causes acute and chronic pulmonary damage that may be idiosyncratic or related to cumulative dose in excess of 200 units per square meter. Additional bleomycin is contraindicated in patients with pulmonary toxicity. Greater pulmonary toxicity is observed with older patients, concomitant irradiation, or the use of oxygen therapy.

Abnormal pulmonary function has been reported after treatment for Hodgkin's disease or non-Hodgkin's lymphoma. A recent report comparing treatments containing bleomycin with or without mediastinal irradiation found significant changes after treatment that largely resolved by 3 years, with greater effects and less recovery in patients receiving mediastinal radiation.[73] Longer follow-up will be required to determine the eventual consequences of pulmonary damage.

Thyroid Effects

Thyroid dysfunction from treatment for Hodgkin's disease or non-Hodgkin's lymphoma appears to be primarily a complication of radiation therapy. In 20% to 50% of patients with Hodgkin's disease or non-Hodgkin's lymphoma treated with mantle field irradiation, hypothyroidism develops because of primary thyroid failure from the irradiation, occurring as late as 26 years after treatment.[74] The effect on the thyroid is related to the dose of radiation and field size and may be increased by prior lymphangiogram. With close follow-up most hypothyroidism can be detected at an early compensated stage manifest only by elevated levels of thyroid-stimulating hormone. If the disease is undetected, patients may develop myxedema or even die of cardiac failure. Most clinicians recommend yearly monitoring of serum thyroxine and thyroid-stimulating hormone levels, with replacement therapy given when an elevated thyroid-stimulating hormone level is detected.[7] Other thyroid diseases observed after irradiation include Graves' disease (1% to 3% actuarial risk at 10 years) and thyroid nodules including papillary or follicular cancers.[74] Detection and management of thyroid dysfunction are important in prolonged routine follow-up of patients exposed to mediastinal or neck irradiation.

Secondary Malignancies

As more patients become long-term survivors of treated Hodgkin's disease or aggressive non-Hodgkin's lymphoma, late posttreatment second malignancies have become the most serious complication of therapy. In a series of 2,037 patients treated for Hodgkin's disease at Stanford, the actuarial risk of all cancers was 25.5% at 20 years.[6] This included a 3.6% actuarial risk of leukemia at 10 years, a 4.5% risk of secondary non-Hodgkin's lymphoma at 18 years, and a 18.6% risk of other cancers at 20 years. The risk of myelodysplasia and acute myelogenous leukemia appears to be related to prior exposure to chemotherapy, while secondary solid cancers are related to prior treatment with radiation. It is often difficult to determine whether the secondary malignancy is a result of the prior treatment, is a property of the underlying malignancy, or is caused by an inherent genetic defect in the patient. Many of the risks for secondary solid malignancies are not apparent for the first 15 years of observation and are only now being appreciated. A component of the follow-up evaluation of patients treated for Hodgkin's disease or aggressive non-Hodgkin's lymphoma should be directed toward the detection of secondary malignancies at an early, treatable stage.

Myelodysplastic syndrome and acute myeloid leukemia

An increased risk of therapy-related myelodysplasia and acute myelogenous leukemia has been observed in patients with Hodgkin's disease or non-Hodgkin's lymphoma treated with multiple cycles of alkylating agents. The actuarial risk is 10% over a period of 2 to 10 years. The risk appears to be directly related to the cumulative dose and increases exponentially with age.[75] The majority of patients (70%) go through a preleukemic or myelodysplastic phase before the development of acute leukemia, and most exhibit cytogenetic abnormalities often associated with the loss of portions of chromosomes 5, 7, or 17.[76,77] In patients with Hodgkin's disease the greatest risk appears to be due to the use of mechlorethamine in the MOPP chemotherapy regimen, whereas patients treated with irradiation alone have minimal risk. Additional factors include multiple courses of chemotherapy, advanced-stage disease, age over 40 years at Hodgkin's disease diagnosis, and prior splenectomy.[78] The introduction in the 1980s of alternative chemotherapy using ABVD, the MOPP/ABVD hybrid, or similar regimens that limited the exposure to mechlorethamine appears to have decreased the risk of secondary myelodysplasia and acute myelogenous leukemia from 6.4% to 2.1% cumulative risk at 10 years.[79] Most cases of myelodysplasia or acute myelogenous leukemia occur 1 to 9 years after treatment, with the greatest risk in years 4 and 5. A different form of secondary acute myelogenous leukemia has become evident in patients treated with high doses of doxorubicin or with the epipodophyllotoxins VP-16 or VM-26. This form of secondary acute myelogenous leukemia is not associated with a preleukemia phase, is usually of M4 or M5 morphology, and is associated with chromosomal translocations involving bands 11q23 or 21q22.[76] Myelodysplasia and acute myelogenous leukemia have also been the subject of several recent reports after high-dose chemotherapy and autologous marrow or stem cell transplantation, with a reported actuarial incidence of 6% to 18% at 5 years.[80-82] Interestingly, they are rare after allogeneic transplant and may be related to damage occurring to the bone marrow from prior chemotherapy.

Treatment options for the majority of patients with myelodysplasia or acute myelogenous leukemia are limited, and median survival is 4 to 6 months after the development of leukemia.[78] Those who are young and otherwise healthy and for whom a human lymphocyte antigen–matched family member or unrelated donor can be found are candidates for allogeneic bone marrow transplantation. Although experience is limited, transplantation early in the course of secondary myelodysplasia or acute myelogenous leukemia appears to be associated with a greater chance of survival.[83,84] Patients in remission from their underlying malignancy in whom cytopenias develop should have a bone marrow biopsy with cytogenetic analysis to rule out this complication. In older patients transfusion support or use of growth factors may provide transient improvement.

Other secondary tumors

A variety of secondary malignancies have been observed in long-term survivors of Hodgkin's disease and non-Hodgkin's lymphoma. These have been most strongly associated with prior irradiation for Hodgkin's disease and include secondary non-Hodgkin's lymphoma, sarcoma, head and neck cancer, melanoma, and carcinomas of the lung, breast, colon, cervix, and ovary.[6] In contrast to the acute leukemias the incidence of secondary solid cancers continues to increase more than 15 years after treatment.

Patients treated for Hodgkin's disease have an increased risk for the development of secondary non-Hodgkin's lymphoma, most frequently of the diffuse large cell histological type.[79] In one study the risk was 4.1% at 20 years with the greatest increase in risk occurring 10 to 14 years after treatment.[6] The cause is unknown and may be related to immunosuppression from the treatment or to the underlying immunosuppression associated with Hodgkin's disease. Successful treatment options must be individualized based on considerations of the clinical situation and prior Hodgkin's disease therapy.

An increase in breast cancer has been observed in women with Hodgkin's disease treated at a young age with mantle field irradiation. Twenty-six breast cancers were found in 885 women treated for Hodgkin's disease at Stanford.[85] The risk was strongly associated with treatment age and occurred in women treated under the age of 30, with an even greater risk for patients treated under the age of 15. The incidence increased continually after 15 years of follow-up. Most cancers occurred within or at the edge of the radiation field in the medial quadrants of the breast and were of the infiltrating ductal carcinoma histological type. Of these, 14 were identified by physicians during routine follow-up, four by self-examination, and three by symptoms. Four were identified by mammography alone. The authors also note that five of 18 mammograms performed to evaluate clinically suspicious nodules were negative when subsequent biopsy documented malignancy. Cases were mainly stage I or II and were successfully treated in 16 of 26 patients. Most studies recommend routine follow-up examination including breast palpation for women treated under the age of 30, and some have advised routine mammography over the age of 35.[79] Biopsy of clinically suspect lesions should be performed.

The risk of other solid tumors is increased by irradiation treatment for Hodgkin's disease. Most occur within radiation fields and have a latency consistent with experimental models of radiation-induced malignancies. In an earlier series from Stanford the majority of solid tumors were lung cancers that developed in smokers treated with irradiation.[86] Other solid malignancies with an increased incidence include soft tissue sarcoma, head and neck cancer, melanoma, and cancers of the colon, cervix, and ovary, as well as basal cell carcinoma of the skin.[79] No studies have reported effective screening strategies for these late-occurring second malignancies, most of which are detected with the onset of symptoms.

MOLECULAR MARKERS OF DISEASE

More than 80% of follicular non-Hodgkin's lymphoma and 30% of large cell non-Hodgkin's lymphoma express the t(14:18) translocation resulting in the juxtaposition of the joining region of the immunoglobulin heavy chain gene to the bcl-2 protooncogene sequence. This sequence is a specific marker for the malignant clone and can be detected at a level of one cell in 1 million by using the polymerase chain reaction. This is several logs more sensitive than other methods using histology or flow cytometry. Polymerase chain reaction has been used extensively to monitor patients with low-grade follicular non-Hodgkin's lymphoma for residual disease after aggressive therapy and to assess measures to purge tumor from autologous hematopoietic grafts.[87] Several studies have suggested that patients with low-grade follicular non-Hodgkin's lymphoma treated with standard chemotherapy remain positive for t(14:18) on polymerase chain reaction, even when in complete clinical remission lasting more than 10 years.[88] It is not clear if the detected tumor cells have clonogenic potential or may possibly be under some form of host control. Other studies have demonstrated that patients reverting to polymerase chain reaction positivity after treatment with high-dose chemotherapy and hematopoietic stem cell rescue are at increased risk of relapse.[89] Also confounding the interpretation of these studies is the finding of the t(14:18) abnormality in normal individuals, which increases in incidence with age.[90] The consequences of detecting t(14:18) after treatment for non-Hodgkin's lymphoma have not yet been well defined, nor have the treatments been established. The majority of patients with t(14:18) have low-grade non-Hodgkin's lymphoma and will have relapse after standard therapy. Earlier detection of relapse is currently not useful in disease management but may become so with the development of additional low-risk treatments such as immunotherapy with antibodies or vaccines. Further studies and treatments are required before t(14:18) will become a useful surrogate marker for disease relapse.

Most aggressive non-Hodgkin's lymphomas do not have the t(14:18) abnormality but can be detected by developing patient-specific polymerase chain reaction assays based on the clonally restricted B cell immunoglobulin or T cell antigen receptor variable regions. Detection of persistent or recurrent disease in this population may prompt consideration of further curative therapy. This strategy may improve the outcomes of patients with non-Hodgkin's lymphoma if treatments given at a time of molecular relapse are more successful than when given at clinical relapse. Such a strategy will have to be tested in prospective, randomized clinical trials. Much work remains before molecular detection of minimal residual disease will be used routinely to determine complete remission or disease relapse.

RECOMMENDATIONS FOR FOLLOW-UP EVALUATION

Because of the great differences observed in the risk of relapse and in the risk of posttreatment complications in patients with Hodgkin's disease or non-Hodgkin's lymphoma, it is difficult to outline global recommendations for follow-up. Few studies have compared the utility of specific tests, and none have done so in a randomized prospective fashion. A compelling argument for the early detection of recurrent disease could be made if treatments were available that were substantially better if used early instead of delayed until symptomatic relapse. Clinical trials suggest that salvage treatment for Hodgkin's disease or aggressive non-Hodgkin's lymphoma is more effective when patients have

Table 22-3 Follow-up of patients with lymphoma (Hodgkin's lymphoma or aggressive non-Hodgkin's lymphoma in complete remission): University of Washington Medical Center/Fred Hutchinson Cancer Research Center

	YEAR				
	1	2	3	4	5
Office visit	4	4	3	2	2
Lactic dehydrogenase	4	4	3	2	2
Complete blood count	4	4	3	2	2
$Beta_2$-microglobulin*	4	4	3	2	2
Erythrocyte sedimentation rate†	4	4	3	1	1
Alkaline phosphatase†	4	4	3	1	1
Chest x-ray	2	2	2	2	2
Thyroid profile‡	1	1	1	1	1
Site computed tomography or magnetic resonance imaging§	1-2	0-2	0-2	0-1	0-1
Gallium scan§	1-2	0-2	0-2	0-1	0-1

*For patients with aggressive non-Hodgkin's lymphoma.
†For patients with Hodgkin's lymphoma.
‡For patients treated with mediastinal or neck irradiation.
§Indicated if lactic dehydrogenase and $beta_2$-microglobulin levels become abnormal in the absence of detectable disease.

minimal disease than when they have bulky disease. However, no trial has demonstrated an advantage for treatment when disease is detected by screening in these patients.

Patients with Hodgkin's disease or aggressive non-Hodgkin's lymphoma are generally treated with curative intent. Those with relapse may be cured by salvage treatment. Recommended scheduled follow-up and specific tests for asymptomatic patients in complete remission are outlined in Table 22-3. These recommendations are based on the current clinical practice in most centers treating large numbers of patients and must be modified based on patient characteristics and the type of treatment given. In general, patients should have a directed physical examination, serum tests (lactic dehydrogenase or $beta_2$-microglobulin for non-Hodgkin's lymphoma and lactic dehydrogenase, alkaline phosphatase, and erythrocyte sedimentation rate for Hodgkin's disease), and routine complete blood count at each evaluation. If the lactic dehydrogenase and $beta_2$-microglobulin levels become abnormal in the absence of detectable disease, further investigation with computed tomography, magnetic resonance imaging, or gallium scintigraphy should occur. However, even with this level of scrutiny the few studies available indicate that most patients will have symptomatic relapses that are identified at scheduled or unscheduled visits.

Site-directed imaging modalities should be used depending on the clinical situation. Patients with a prior mediastinal mass or treatment with mediastinal irradiation should have periodic chest x-rays. Evaluation by computed tomography or magnetic resonance imaging may be useful in monitoring residual masses. Gallium scintigraphy can detect preclinical relapse and is especially useful in the chest. However, the test requires considerable expertise to administer and interpret and may not be widely available. Because these tests are expensive, most physicians use them only periodically or to investigate symptoms or laboratory test results suggestive of disease recurrence. Further clinical trials are needed to evaluate the utility and predictive value of these studies for screening asymptomatic patients.

The number of tests used to screen for recurrent disease should also be modified by the availability and applicability of subsequent salvage treatment for that patient. Patients with high-risk non-Hodgkin's lymphoma who are young enough for high-dose therapy with hematopoietic stem cell support should be more closely monitored than patients in whom subsequent therapy will be only palliative. Evaluation of patients after clinical protocols may require more aggressive scheduled follow-up. Knowledge of the timing and pattern of disease relapse can be critical in evaluating new drug combinations for efficacy and toxicity.

Patients in remission with low-grade non-Hodgkin's lymphoma should receive a similar schedule of follow-up with close attention to signs and symptoms of disease. The use of frequent imaging tests to detect disease recurrence in asymptomatic patients is not useful outside the setting of clinical trials and probably should be reserved to investigate symptoms or laboratory abnormalities. Enrollment of patients in clinical trials is essential.

Identification and management of acute and long-term complications of treatment are also goals of the follow-up visit. Again, the specific type of treatment given will influence the types of complications observed. Patients treated with mediastinal irradiation should have yearly thyroid function tests and attention to the detection of late solid secondary malignancies. Women irradiated when less than 30 years of age have a significantly increased risk of breast cancer. They should have regular physical examinations and may benefit from periodic mammograms after the age of 35. Complaints of chest pain should be taken seriously and cardiovascular disease ruled out, even in otherwise healthy young patients. Similarly, pulmonary and cardiovascular risk factors should be reduced by control of smoking, hypertension, and serum lipids. A complete blood count may be used to detect disease relapse or posttreatment marrow failure. The cost effectiveness of these approaches has not yet been studied, and the utility of follow-up to detect both disease and complications awaits further systematic analysis.

FUTURE PROSPECTS

Ultimately, disease relapse of non-Hodgkin's lymphoma and possibly Hodgkin's disease may be detected at an early stage before development of clinical symptoms by use of sensitive molecular techniques. As data regarding the consequences of molecular monitoring for early relapse accumulate, clinical trials can be instituted to test the impact of conventional and novel treatments given during a time of minimal residual disease. These tests may someday replace current nonspecific tests such as lactic dehydrogenase, beta$_2$-microglobulin, erythrocyte sedimentation rate, and possibly routine imaging using computed tomography, magnetic resonance imaging, or gallium scintigraphy to detect clinical relapse. Clinical trials further defining the role of molecular markers in patients with Hodgkin's disease or non-Hodgkin's lymphoma seem preferable to expensive studies documenting the clinical utility (or lack thereof) of disease detection using current nonspecific tests.

As survival from non-Hodgkin's lymphoma continues to improve, the long-term consequences of therapy will become more apparent and the need to modify treatment regimens to decrease toxicity while maintaining clinical efficacy will be increasingly recognized. Detection of the widely disparate late complications of therapy is necessary for the development and conduct of such clinical trials and requires committed, long-term follow-up by health care providers.

The follow-up of asymptomatic patients with Hodgkin's disease or aggressive non-Hodgkin's lymphoma in complete remission after therapy must take into account the likelihood of cure from the given treatment and the types of posttreatment complications to which the long-term survivor will be exposed. Knowledge of pretreatment risks and treatment-related prognostic factors is essential in designing follow-up evaluations to detect recurrent disease. Relapse in this population should trigger the institution of salvage therapy in attempts to provide long-term disease-free survival. Patients with low-grade non-Hodgkin's lymphoma should be monitored for the development of signs or symptoms of disease progression. Treatment based on carefully designed clinical trials should be encouraged. It is hoped that the future for these patients will one day be as bright as that for patients with early-stage Hodgkin's disease or aggressive non-Hodgkin's lymphoma.

REFERENCES

1. Wingo PA, Tong T, Bolden S. Cancer statistics, 1995. CA Cancer J Clin 1995;45:8-30.
2. Kaplan HS. The radical radiotherapy of regionally localized Hodgkin's disease. Radiology 1962;78:553-61.
3. DeVita VJ, Serpick AA, Carbone PP. Combination chemotherapy in the treatment of advanced Hodgkin's disease. Ann Intern Med 1970;73:881-95.
4. Rosenberg SA. Modern combined modality management of Hodgkin's disease. Curr Opin Oncol 1994;6:470-2.
5. Armitage JO. Early bone marrow transplantation in Hodgkin's disease. Ann Oncol 1994;5(Suppl 2):S161-3.
6. Rosenberg SA. The treatment of Hodgkin's disease. Ann Oncol 1994;5(Suppl 2):17-21.
7. Hoppe RT. The contemporary management of Hodgkin's disease. Radiology 1988;169:297-304.
8. Donaldson SS. Hodgkin's disease in children. Semin Oncol 1990; 17:736-48.
9. Bonadonna G. Modern treatment of malignant lymphomas: a multidisciplinary approach? Ann Oncol 1994;5(Suppl 2):S5-16.
10. Russell KJ, Donaldson SS, Cox RS, Kaplan HS. Childhood Hodgkin's disease: patterns of relapse. J Clin Oncol 1984;2:80-7.
11. Mauch PM, Canellos GP, Shulman LN, et al. Mantle irradiation alone for selected patients with laparotomy-staged IA to IIA Hodgkin's disease: preliminary results of a prospective trial. J Clin Oncol 1995; 13:947-52.
12. Young RC, Cannellos GP, Chabner BA, et al. Patterns of relapse in advanced Hodgkin's disease treated with combination chemotherapy. Cancer 1978;42:1001-7.
13. Yahalom J, Ryu J, Straus DJ, et al. Impact of adjuvant radiation on the patterns and rate of relapse in advanced-stage Hodgkin's disease with alternating chemotherapy combinations. J Clin Oncol 1991;9:93-201.
14. Roach M 3d, Brophy N, Cox R, Varghese A, Hoppe RT. Prognostic factors for patients relapsing after radiotherapy for early-stage Hodgkin's disease. J Clin Oncol 1990;8:623-9.
15. Healey EA, Tarbell NJ, Kalish LA, et al. Prognostic factors for patients with Hodgkin's disease in first relapse. Cancer 1993;71: 2613-20.
16. Santoro A, Bonfante V, Bonadonna G. Salvage chemotherapy with ABVD in MOPP-resistant Hodgkin's disease. Ann Intern Med 1982;96:139-43.
17. Canellos GP, Petroni GR, Barcos M, Duggan DB, Peterson BA. Etoposide, vinblastine, and doxorubicin: an active regimen for the treatment of Hodgkin's disease in relapse following MOPP. J Clin Oncol 1995;13:2005-11.
18. Anderson JE, Litzow MR, Appelbaum FR, et al. Allogenic, syngeneic, autologous marrow transplantation for Hodgkin's disease: the 21-year Seattle experience. J Clin Oncol 1993;11:2342-50.
19. Weaver CH, Petersen FB, Appelbaum FR, et al. High-dose fractionated total-body irradition, etoposide, and cyclophosphamide followed by autologous stem-cell support in patients with malignant lymphoma. J Clin Oncol 1994;12:2559-66.
20. Horning SJ, Negrin RS, Chao JC, Dong GD, Hoppe RT, Blume KG. Fractionated total-body irradiation, etoposide, and cyclophosphamide plus autografting in Hodgkin's disease and non-Hodgkin's lymphoma. J Clin Oncol 1994;12:2552-8.
21. Bartlett NL, Rosenberg SA, Hoppe RT, Hancock SL, Horning SJ. Brief chemotherapy, Stanford V, and adjuvant radiotherapy for bulky or advanced-stage Hodgkin's disease: a preliminary report. J Clin Oncol 1995;13:1080-8.
22. Radford JA, Eardley A, Woodman C, Crowther D. Routine outpatient (OP) review following treatment for Hodgkin's disease (HD): is it an efficient way of detecting relapse? Proc Am Soc Clin Oncol 1995;14:386.
23. The Non-Hodgkin's Lymphoma Pathologic Classification Project. National Cancer Institute sponsored study of classifications of non-Hodgkin's lymphomas: summary and description of a working formulation for clinical usage. Cancer 1982;49:2112-35.
24. Harris NL, Jaffe ES, Stein H, et al. A revised European-American classification of lymphoid neoplasms: a proposal from the International Lymphoma Study Group. Blood 1994;84:1361-92.
25. Horning SJ. Natural history of and therapy for the indolent non-Hodgkin's lymphomas. Semin Oncol 1993;20(Suppl 5):75-88.
26. Fisher RI, Gaynor ER, Dahlberg S, et al. Comparison of a standard regimen (CHOP) with three intensive chemotherapy regimens for advanced non-Hodgkin's lymphoma. N Engl J Med 1993;328:1002-6.
27. The International Non-Hodgkin's Lymphoma Prognostic Factors Project. A predictive model for aggressive non-Hodgkin's lymphoma. N Engl J Med 1993;329:987-94.
28. Shipp MA. Prognostic factors in aggressive non-Hodgkin's lymphoma: who has "high-risk" disease? Blood 1994;83:1165-73.
29. Armitage JO, Weisenburger DD, Hutchins M, et al. Chemotherapy for diffuse large-cell lymphoma—rapidly responding patients have more durable remissions. J Clin Oncol 1986;4:160-4.
30. Kaplan WD, Jochelson MS, Herman TS, et al. Gallium-67 imaging: a predictor of residual tumor viability and clinical outcome in patients with diffuse large-cell lymphoma. J Clin Oncol 1990;8:1966-70.

31. Kwak LW, Halpern J, Olshen RA, Horning SJ. Prognostic significance of actual dose intensity in diffuse large-cell lymphoma: results of a tree-structured survival analysis. J Clin Oncol 1990;8:963-77.
32. Coiffier B, Gisselbrecht C, Herbrecht R, Tilly H, Bosly A, Brousse N. LNH-84 regimen: a multicenter study of intensive chemotherapy in 737 patients with aggressive malignant lymphoma. J Clin Oncol 1989;7:1018-26.
33. Fisher RI, Gaynor ER, Dahlberg S, et al. A phase III comparison of CHOP vs. m-BACOD vs. ProMACE-CytaBOM vs. MACOP-B in patients with intermediate- or high-grade non-Hodgkin's lymphoma: results of SWOG-8516 (Intergroup 0067), the National High-Priority Lymphoma Study. Ann Oncol 1994;2:91-5.
34. Sertoli MR, Santini G, Chisesi T, et al. MACOP-B versus ProMACE-MOPP in the treatment of advanced diffuse non-Hodgkin's lymphoma: results of a prospective randomized trial by the Non-Hodgkin's Lymphoma Cooperative Study Group. J Clin Oncol 1994;12:1366-74.
35. Cooper IA, Wolf MM, Robertson TI, et al. Randomized comparison of MACOP-B with CHOP in patients with intermediate-grade non-Hodgkin's lymphoma: the Australian and New Zealand Lymphoma Group. J Clin Oncol 1994;12:769-78.
36. Weeks JC, Yeap BY, Canellos GP, Shipp MA. Value of follow-up procedures in patients with large-cell lymphoma who achieve a complete remission. J Clin Oncol 1991;9:1196-203.
37. Aviles A, Narvaez BR, Diaz MJ, et al. Value of serum beta 2 microglobulin as an indicator of early relapse in diffuse large cell lymphoma. Leuk Lymphoma 1993;9:377-80.
38. Shipp MA, Klatt MM, Yeap B, et al. Patterns of relapse in large-cell lymphoma patients with bulk disease: implications for the use of adjuvant radiation therapy. J Clin Oncol 1989;7:613-8.
39. Philip T, Guglielmi C, Chauvin F, et al. Autologous bone marrow transplantation (ABMT) versus conventional chemotherapy (DHAP) in relapsed non-Hodgkin's lymphoma (NHL): final analysis of the PARMA randomized study (216 patients). Proc Am Soc Clin Oncol 1995;14:390a.
40. Haioun C, Lepage E, Gisselbrecht C, et al. Comparison of autologous bone marrow transplantation with sequential chemotherapy for intermediate-grade and high-grade non-Hodgkin's lymphoma in first complete remission: a study of 464 patients: Groupe d'Etude des Lymphomes de l'Adulte. J Clin Oncol 1994;12:2543-51.
41. Lopez-Guillermo A, Montserrat E, Bosch F, Terol MJ, Campo E, Rozman C. Applicability of the International Index for aggressive lymphomas to patients with low-grade lymphoma. J Clin Oncol 1994;12:1343-8.
42. Vaughan Hudson B, Vaughan Hudson G, MacLennan KA, Anderson L, Linch DC. Clinical stage 1 non-Hodgkin's lymphoma: long-term follow-up of patients treated by the British National Lymphoma Investigation with radiotherapy alone as initial therapy. Br J Cancer 1994;69:1088-93.
43. Young RC, Longo DL, Glatstein E, Ihde DC, Jaffe ES, DeVita VT Jr. The treatment of indolent lymphomas: watchful waiting vs. aggressive combined modality treatment. Semin Hematol 1988;25(Suppl 2):11-6.
44. Solal-Celigny P, Lepage E, Brousse N, et al. Recombinant interferon alfa-2b combined with a regimen containing doxorubicin in patients with advanced follicular lymphoma: Groupe d'Etude des Lymphomes de l'Adulte. N Engl J Med 1993;329:1608-14.
45. Armitage JO. Bone marrow transplantation for indolent lymphomas. Semin Oncol 1993;20(suppl 5):136-42.
46. Rohatiner AZ, Johnson PW, Price CG, et al. Myeloablative therapy with autologous bone marrow transplantation as consolidation therapy for recurrent follicular lymphoma. J Clin Oncol 1994;12: 1177-84.
47. van Besien KW, Khouri IF, Giralt SA, et al. Allogeneic bone marrow transplantation for refractory and recurrent low-grade lymphoma: the case for aggressive management. J Clin Oncol 1995;13:1096-102.
48. Johnson PW, Rohatiner AZ, Whelan JS, et al. Patterns of survival in patients with recurrent follicular lymphoma: a 20-year study from a single center. J Clin Oncol 1995;13:140-7.
49. Weisdorf DJ, Andersen JW, Glick JH, Oken MM. Survival after relapse of low-grade non-Hodgkin's lymphoma: implications for marrow transplantation. J Clin Oncol 1992;10:942-7.
50. Yuen AR, Kamel OW, Halpern J, Horning SJ. Long-term survival after histologic transformation of low-grade follicular lymphoma. J Clin Oncol 1995;13:1726-33.
51. Kagan AR, Steckel RJ. Post-treatment surveillance studies for lymphoma patients. Invest Radiol 1992;27:543-7.
52. Radford JA, Cowan RA, Flanagan M, et al. The significance of residual mediastinal abnormality on the chest radiograph following treatment for Hodgkin's disease. J Clin Oncol 1988;6:940-6.
53. Hill M, Cunningham D, MacVicar D, et al. Role of magnetic resonance imaging in predicting relapse in residual masses after treatment of lymphoma. J Clin Oncol 1993;11:2273-8.
54. Hoane BR, Shields AF, Porter BA, Shulman HM. Detection of lymphomatous bone marrow involvement with magnetic resonance imaging. Blood 1991;78:728-38.
55. Even-Sapir E, Bar-Shalom R, Israel O, et al. Single-photon emission computed tomography quantitation of gallium citrate uptake for the differentiation of lymphoma from benign hilar uptake. J Clin Oncol 1995;13:942-6.
56. Front D, Israel O. The role of Ga-67 scintigraphy in evaluating the results of therapy of lymphoma patients. Semin Nucl Med 1995;25:60-71.
57. Front D, Bar-Shalom R, Epelbaum R, et al. Early detection of lymphoma recurrence with gallium-67 scintigraphy. J Nucl Med 1993;34:2101-4.
58. van den Anker-Lugtenburg PJ, Krenning EP, Oei HY, et al. The role of somatostatin receptor scintigraphy in the initial staging of Hodgkin and non-Hodgkin lymphomas. Blood 1994;84(Suppl 1):233a.
59. Vassilakos P, Zikos P, Pagonis S, et al. The contribution of scintigraphic imaging with ^{111}In octreotide in the staging of lymphomas: a comparison to other imaging modalities. Blood 1994;84(Suppl 1):233a.
60. Lipp RW, Silly H, Ranner G, et al. Radiolabeled octreotide for the demonstration of somatostatin receptors in malignant lymphoma and lymphadenopathy. J Nucl Med 1995;36:13-8.
61. Bangerter M, Kocher F, Binder T, et al. Total body positron emission tomography (PET) for staging and follow-up of lymphoma. Proc Am Soc Clin Oncol 1995;14:386a.
62. Litam P, Swan F, Cabanillas F, et al. Prognostic value of serum beta-2 microglobulin in low-grade lymphoma. Ann Intern Med 1991;114:855-60.
63. Aviles A, Zepeda G, Diaz MJ, et al. Beta-2 microglobulin level as an indicator of prognosis in diffuse large cell lymphoma. Leuk Lymphoma 1992;7:135-8.
64. Johnson PW, Whelan J, Longhurst S, et al. Beta-2 microglobulin: a prognostic factor in diffuse aggressive non-Hodgkin's lymphomas. Br J Cancer 1993;67:792-7.
65. Henry-Amar M, Friedman S, Hayat M, et al. Erythrocyte sedimentation rate predicts early relapse and survival in early-stage Hodgkin disease: the EORTC Lymphoma Cooperative Group. Ann Intern Med 1991;114:361-5.
66. Bokemeyer C, Schmoll HJ, van Rhee J, Kuczyk M, Schuppert F, Poliwada H. Long-term gonadal toxicity after therapy for Hodgkin's and non-Hodgkin's lymphoma. Ann Hematol 1994;68:105-10.
67. Sanger WG, Olson JH, Sherman JK. Semen cryobanking for men with cancer—criteria change. Fertil Steril 1992;58:1024-7.
68. Mulvihill JJ, McKeen EA, Rosner F, Zarrabi MH. Pregnancy outcome in cancer patients: experience in a large cooperative group. Cancer 1987;60:1143-50.
69. Stewart JR, Fajardo LF. Radiation-induced heart disease: an update. Prog Cardiovasc Dis 1984;27:173-94.

70. Hancock SL, Tucker MA, Hoppe RT. Factors affecting late mortality from heart disease after treatment of Hodgkin's disease. JAMA 1993;270:1949-55.
71. Hancock SL, Donaldson SS, Hoppe RT. Cardiac disease following treatment of Hodgkin's disease in children and adolescents. J Clin Oncol 1993;11:1208-15.
72. Sorensen K, Levitt G, Sebag-Montefiore D, Bull C, Sullivan I. Cardiac function in Wilms' tumor survivors. J Clin Oncol 1995;13:1546-56.
73. Horning SJ, Adhikari A, Rizk N, Hoppe RT, Olshen RA. Effect of treatment for Hodgkin's disease on pulmonary function: results of a prospective study. J Clin Oncol 1994;12:297-305.
74. Hancock SL, Cox RS, McDougall IR. Thyroid diseases after treatment of Hodgkin's disease. N Engl J Med 1991;325:599-605.
75. van Leeuwen FE, Chorus AM, van den Belt-Dusebout AW, et al. Leukemia risk following Hodgkin's disease: relation to cumulative dose of alkylating agents, treatment with teniposide combinations, number of episodes of chemotherapy, and bone marrow damage. J Clin Oncol 1994;12:1063-73.
76. Pedersen-Bjergaard J, Philip P, Larsen SO, Jensen G, Byrsting K. Chromosome aberrations and prognostic factors in therapy-related myelodysplasia and acute nonlymphocytic leukemia. Blood 1990;76:1083-91.
77. Rosenbloom B, Schreck R, Koeffler HP. Therapy-related myelodysplastic syndromes. Hematol Oncol Clin North Am 1992;6:707-22.
78. Levine EG, Bloomfield CD. Leukemias and myelodysplastic syndromes secondary to drug, radiation, and environmental exposure. Semin Oncol 1992;19:47-84.
79. van Leeuwen FE, Klokman WJ, Hagenbeek A, et al. Second cancer risk following Hodgkin's disease: a 20-year follow-up study. J Clin Oncol 1994;12:312-25.
80. Darrington DL, Vose JM, Anderson JR, et al. Incidence and characterization of secondary myelodysplastic syndrome and acute myelogenous leukemia following high-dose chemoradiotherapy and autologous stem-cell transplantation for lymphoid malignancies. J Clin Oncol 1994;12:2527-34.
81. Miller JS, Arthur DC, Litz CE, Neglia JP, Miller WJ, Weisdorf DJ. Myelodysplastic syndrome after autologous bone marrow transplantation: an additional late complication of curative cancer therapy. Blood 1994;83:3780-6.
82. Stone RM, Neuberg D, Soiffer R, et al. Myelodysplastic syndrome as a late complication following autologous bone marrow transplantation for non-Hodgkin's lymphoma. J Clin Oncol 1994;12:2535-42.
83. Anderson JE, Appelbaum FR, Fisher LD, et al. Allogeneic bone marrow transplantation for 93 patients with myelodysplastic syndrome. Blood 1993;82:677-81.
84. De Witte T, Gratwohl A. Bone marrow transplantation for myelodysplastic syndrome and secondary leukaemias. Br J Haematol 1993; 84:361-4.
85. Hancock SL, Tucker MA, Hoppe RT. Breast cancer after treatment of Hodgkin's disease. J Natl Cancer Inst 1993;85:25-31.
86. Tucker MA, Coleman CN, Cox RS, Varghese A, Rosenberg SA. Risk of second cancers after treatment for Hodgkin's disease. N Engl J Med 1988;318:76-81.
87. Gribben JG, Neuberg D, Barber M, et al. Detection of residual lymphoma cells by polymerase chain reaction in peripheral blood is significantly less predictive for relapse than detection in bone marrow. Blood 1994;83:3800-7.
88. Price CG, Meerabux J, Murtagh S, et al. The significance of circulating cells carrying t(14;18) in long remission from follicular lymphoma. J Clin Oncol 1991;9:1527-32.
89. Gribben JG, Neuberg D, Freedman AS, et al. Detection by polymerase chain reaction of residual cells with the bcl-2 translocation is associated with increased risk of relapse after autologous bone marrow transplantation for B-cell lymphoma. Blood 1993;81:3449-57.
90. Liu Y, Hernandez AM, Shibata D, Cortopassi GA. BCL2 translocation frequency rises with age in humans. Proc Natl Acad Sci U S A 1994;91:8910-4.

➢ COUNTER POINT

Memorial Sloan-Kettering Cancer Center

DAVID J. STRAUS

Maloney and Appelbaum provide an excellent review of follow-up policies developed for patients with malignant lymphomas at Fred Hutchinson Cancer Research Center. Only a few points are added in this discussion. Follow-up policies differ slightly at different centers and are admittedly arbitrary. The policies for follow-up in lymphoma practice at Memorial Sloan-Kettering Cancer Center are also described.

HODGKIN'S DISEASE

A number of prognostic factors in Hodgkin's disease in addition to age, stage, and presence or absence of bulky disease and B symptoms have been reported in the literature. For patients with early-stage Hodgkin's disease, particularly if treated primarily only with radiation therapy, erythrocyte sedimentation rate has been reported to be a powerful adverse prognostic factor, based on experience with a large number of patients treated in protocols of the European Organization for the Research and Treatment of Cancer.[1] Elevation of erythrocyte sedimentation rate during or after treatment was also found to be predictive of recurrence.[2]

In a multivariate analysis using the proportional hazards model, a group of physicians at Memorial Sloan-Kettering Cancer Center found five pretreatment baseline patient characteristics to have an adverse effect on the survival of patients treated for advanced Hodgkin's disease with alternating chemotherapy regimens and adjunctive radiation therapy. The five characteristics are an age of 45 years or older, serum lactic dehydrogenase level greater than 400 U/L (two times normal), low hematocrit, inguinal nodal involvement (a reflection of extensive retroperitoneal involvement in this patient population), and mediastinal mass measuring greater than 45% of thoracic diameter.[3] A number of prognostic factors have been proposed, many of which are probably different expressions of the same biological phenomena. They are classified into four categories[4]:

1. Factors relating to the biology of the disease: advanced age, mixed cellularity, and lymphocyte-depleted histological features
2. Factors relating to indirect or inflammatory effects of the disease, possibly resulting from cytokine production: anemia, low serum albumin, elevated serum alkaline phosphatase, and erythrocyte sedimentation rate
3. Factors relating to tumor burden: massive mediastinal disease, inguinal node involvement, number of nodal or extranodal sites, and serum lactic dehydrogenase

Table 22-4 Follow-up of patients with lymphoma (Hodgkin's lymphoma in complete remission): Memorial Sloan-Kettering Cancer Center

	YEAR				
	1	2	3	4	5
Office visit	4	3	3	2	1
Complete blood count	4	3	3	2	1
Chest x-ray	4	3	3	2	1
Liver function tests	4	3	3	2	1
Erythrocyte sedimentation rate	4	3	3	2	1
Thyroid profile	2	2	2	2	1
Abdominal computed tomography	2	2	2	2	1
Pelvic computed tomography	2	2	2	2	1
Mammography*	0	1	1	1	1

*Performed for female patients over the age of 30 who have received mantle irradiation.

4. Factors relating to treatment: alternating or hybrid versus single chemotherapy regimens, addition of adjuvant radiation therapy, and rapidity of response to chemotherapy

Patients with multiple adverse factors are at particular risk for relapse and thus should be followed up especially carefully. Follow-up policies for patients after primary treatment of Hodgkin's disease at Memorial Sloan-Kettering Cancer Center have been based on relapse experience. The period of greatest risk for relapse appears to be the first 36 to 72 months after completion of treatment.[5,6] Patients are routinely seen every 3 months during the first year, every 4 months during the second and third years, every 6 months during the fourth year, and annually thereafter (Table 22-4). Patients with multiple risk factors are sometimes followed up more frequently. Physical examination, complete blood count, erythrocyte sedimentation rate, liver function tests, and chest x-ray are performed at each follow-up visit. Measurement of serum thyroid-stimulating hormone and thyroxine levels and computed tomography of the abdomen and pelvis with oral and intravenous contrast media are performed every 6 to 8 months during the first 4 years and annually thereafter. Because of the increased risk of breast carcinoma at an early age, female patients over the age of 30 who have received mantle irradiation undergo annual mammography.[7] All patients with compensated thyroid insufficiency who have an elevated thyroid-stimulating hormone level and normal thyroxine level receive levothyroxine for thyroid suppression to prevent hypothyroidism and to reduce the risk of thyroid carcinoma in an overstimulated thyroid gland.[8] Gallium scanning, computed tomography of the chest, and repeat lymphangiography are not routinely performed as follow-up procedures.

Table 22-5 Follow-up of patients with lymphoma (intermediate- or high-grade non-Hodgkin's lymphoma in complete remission): Memorial Sloan-Kettering Cancer Center

	YEAR				
	1	2	3	4	5
Office visit	4*	3	3	2	1
Complete blood count	4*	3	3	2	1
Chest x-ray	4*	3	3	2	1
Liver function tests	4*	3	3	2	1
Abdominal computed tomography	2-3	2	2	2	1
Pelvic computed tomography	2-3	2	2	2	1

*Performed every 2 months for patients with high-grade non-Hodgkin's lymphoma.

NON-HODGKIN'S LYMPHOMA

The review of non-Hodgkin's lymphoma provided by Maloney and Appelbaum is highly detailed and well referenced. A major point that should be emphasized is that the risks of relapse for intermediate- or high-grade and low-grade non-Hodgkin's lymphoma differ. Patients with intermediate- or high-grade non-Hodgkin's lymphoma are at greatest risk for recurrence during the first year (small, noncleaved cell lymphomas) to the fifth year (diffuse, large cell lymphomas).[9,10] With standard combination chemotherapy, relapses are seen with lesser frequency in patients with intermediate-grade histological types between 5 and 8 years after treatment.[11,12] Patients with low-grade lymphomas seem to be at continuous risk for recurrence, even after 10 years.[13]

This difference has determined the follow-up policies developed at Memorial Sloan-Kettering Cancer Center. Patients with high-grade non-Hodgkin's lymphoma are usually examined every 2 months and those with intermediate-grade non-Hodgkin's lymphoma every 2 to 3 months during the first year after the completion of treatment (Table 22-5). As with Hodgkin's disease, follow-up visits are usually scheduled every 4 months during the second and third years, every 6 months in the fourth year, and annually thereafter. Patients with low-grade non-Hodgkin's lymphoma are followed up with a frequency similar to those with intermediate- or high-grade histological types during the first 5 years but are then followed up every 6 months for life because of their continuous risk for recurrence. Physical examination, complete blood count, chest x-ray, and liver function tests are performed at each visit. Computed tomography of the abdomen and pelvis with oral and intravenous contrast media is performed every 4 to 6 months during the first year in patients with intermediate- and high-grade non-Hodgkin's lymphoma, every 6 to 8 months for the second through fourth years, and annually thereafter through 7 to 8 years for those with intermediate-grade non-Hodgkin's lymphoma.

Patients with low-grade non-Hodgkin's lymphoma have computed tomography of the abdomen and pelvis performed

Table 22-6 Follow-up of patients with lymphoma (low-grade non-Hodgkin's lymphoma in complete remission): Memorial Sloan-Kettering Cancer Center

	YEAR				
	1	2	3	4	5
Office visit	4	3	3	2	2
Complete blood count	4	3	3	2	2
Chest x-ray	4	3	3	2	2
Liver function tests	4	3	3	2	2
Abdominal computed tomography	2	2	2	2	2
Pelvic computed tomography	2	2	2	2	2

every 6 months for at least 10 years (Table 22-6). Extranodal sites of initial involvement are also monitored. Initial gastrointestinal tract disease warrants endoscopy or barium studies, and initial bone involvement may require plain x-rays or magnetic resonance imaging. The gastrointestinal tract is also scanned in patients with initial presentations in Waldeyer's ring, since this site is at risk for relapse.[14]

REFERENCES

1. Tubiana M, Henry-Amar M, Burgers MV, van der Werf-Messing B, Hayat M. Prognostic significance of erythrocyte sedimentation rate in clinical stages I-II of Hodgkin's disease. J Clin Oncol 1984;2:194-200.
2. Henry-Amar M, Friedman S, Hayat M, et al. Erythrocyte sedimentation rate predicts early relapse and survival in early-stage Hodgkin's disease: the EORTC Lymphoma Cooperative Group. Ann Intern Med 1991;114:361-5.
3. Straus DJ, Gaynor JJ, Myers J, et al. Prognostic factors among 185 adults with newly diagnosed advanced Hodgkin's disease treated with alternating potentially noncross-resistant chemotherapy and intermediate-dose radiation therapy. J Clin Oncol 1990;8:1173-86.
4. Straus DJ. High-risk Hodgkin's disease prognostic factors. Leuk Lymphoma 1995;15(Suppl 1):41-2.
5. Koziner B, Myers J, Cirrincione C, et al. Treatment of stages I and II Hodgkin's disease with three different therapeutic modalities. Am J Med 1986:80:1067-78.
6. Yahalom J, Ryu J, Straus DJ, et al. Impact of adjuvant radiation on the patterns and rate of relapse in advanced-stage Hodgkin's disease treated with alternating chemotherapy combinations. J Clin Oncol 1991;9:2193-201.
7. Dershaw DD, Yahalom J, Petrek JA. Breast carcinoma in women previously treated for Hodgkin disease: mammographic evaluation. Radiology 1992;184:421-3.
8. Hancock SL, Cox RS, McDougall IR. Thyroid diseases after treatment of Hodgkin's disease. N Engl J Med 1991;325:599-605.
9. Straus DJ, Wong GY, Liu J, et al. Small non-cleaved-cell lymphoma (undifferentiated lymphoma, Burkitt's type) in American adults: results with treatment designed for acute lymphoblastic leukemia. Am J Med 1991;90:328-37.
10. Fisher RI, Gaynor ER, Dahlberg S, et al. Comparison of a standard regimen (CHOP) with three intensive chemotherapy regimens for advanced non-Hodgkin's lymphoma. N Engl J Med 1993;328:1002-6.
11. Jones SE, Grozea PN, Miller TP, et al. Chemotherapy with cyclophosphamide, doxorubicin, vincristine, and prednisone alone or with levamisole or with levamisole plus BCG for malignant lymphoma: a Southwest Oncology Group study. J Clin Oncol 1985;3:1318-24.
12. Gaynor ER, Ultmann JE, Golomb HM, Sweet DL. Treatment of diffuse histiocytic lymphoma (DHL) with COMLA (cyclophosphamide, oncovin, methotrexate, leucovorin, cytosine arabinoside): a 10-year experience in a single institution. J Clin Oncol 1985;3:1596-604.
13. Horning SJ. Natural history of and therapy for the indolent non-Hodgkin's lymphomas. Semin Oncol 1993;20(5 Suppl 5):75-88.
14. Rudders RA, Ross ME, DeLellis RA. Primary extranodal lymphoma: response to treatment and factors influencing prognosis. Cancer 1978;42:406-16.

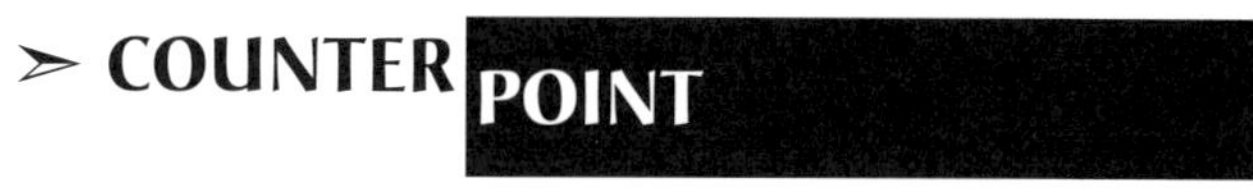

➢ COUNTERPOINT

National Kyushu Cancer Center, Japan

NAOKUNI UIKE

I generally agree with the follow-up methodology described by Maloney and Appelbaum. Additional data are provided concerning the follow-up schedule and future prospects at National Kyushu Cancer Center in Japan.

The incidence of malignant lymphoma is lower in Japan than in Europe or the United States, mainly because of the relatively lower incidence of B cell non-Hodgkin's lymphoma and Hodgkin's disease.[1] The relative frequency of T cell lymphoma in non-Hodgkin's lymphoma is 30% to 70% in Japan,[2] which is approximately three times as high as that in Europe and the United States (10% to 20%).[3,4] National Kyushu Cancer Center is in the Kyushu district, a southern part of Japan that is an endemic area of adult T cell leukemia/lymphoma. At National Kyushu Cancer Center there were 509 patients with non-Hodgkin's lymphoma from 1977 to 1995. Of these 509 patients, 206 (40.5%) had T cell lymphomas, of which 114 (55.3%) were adult T cell leukemia/lymphoma. Adult T cell leukemia/lymphoma is associated with human T cell leukemia virus type I infection and has a poor prognosis. The few patients with adult T cell leukemia/lymphoma who achieve complete remission have to be carefully followed up thereafter for the development of recurrent disease.

FOLLOW-UP CARE

An increased concentration of soluble interleukin-2 receptor (sIL-2R) has been found in patients with diverse diseases, including malignant lymphoma. This relates to a poor prognosis in some patients with lymphoma.[5,6] The increase of sIL-2R seems to be the consequence of a release either directly by tumor cells or indirectly by activated nonmalignant T cells.[7,8] Serial measurements of sIL-2R as a tumor marker are of clinical importance especially in patients with aggressive non-Hodgkin's lymphoma[9] and adult T cell leukemia/lymphoma.[10,11] Serum sIL-2R level seems to be important in detecting disease relapse and may be more useful than beta$_2$-microglobulin or lactic dehydrogenase because the difference in serum sIL-2R levels between normal control subjects and patients with lymphoma is greater than that of beta$_2$-microglobulin or lactic dehydrogenase. Moreover, serum

Table 22-7 Follow-up of patients with lymphoma (Hodgkin's lymphoma or aggressive non-Hodgkin's lymphoma in complete remission): National Kyushu Cancer Center, Japan

	YEAR				
	1	2	3	4	5
Office visit	4	4	3	2	2
Lactic dehydrogenase	4	4	3	2	2
Complete blood count	4	4	3	2	2
Beta$_2$-microglobulin*	4	4	3	2	2
Soluble interleukin-2 receptor	4	4	3	2	2
Erythrocyte sedimentation rate†	4	4	3	1	1
Alkaline phosphatase†	4	4	3	1	1
Chest x-ray	2	2	2	2	2
Thyroid profile‡	1	1	1	1	1
Site computed tomography or magnetic resonance imaging§,¶	1-2	0-2	0-2	0-1	0-1
Gallium scan§	1-2	0-2	0-2	0-1	0-1

*For patients with aggressive non-Hodgkin's lymphoma.
†For patients with Hodgkin's lymphoma.
‡For patients treated with mediastinal or neck irradiation.
§Indicated if lactic dehydrogenase and beta$_2$-microglobulin levels become abnormal in the absence of detectable disease.
¶Test selection based on availability of magnetic resonance imaging.

sIL-2R levels are less affected by renal or hepatic function than are beta$_2$-microglobulin or lactic dehydrogenase, respectively. Therefore monitoring of serum sIL-2R levels should be added to the follow-up methodology (Table 22-7). Further studies are necessary to confirm its sensitivity and specificity for predicting relapse.

FUTURE PROSPECTS

Secondary myelodysplasia/acute myelogenous leukemia is one of the most serious complications because its outcome is so poor and it is rapidly fatal. The only way to cure patients with this complication is to perform allogeneic bone marrow transplantation if possible.

Maloney and Appelbaum emphasize that to detect clinical relapse, a sensitive molecular marker might someday replace current nonspecific tests. The WT1 gene is a tumor suppressor gene that plays a key role in the carcinogenesis of Wilms' tumor.[12,13] Recently expression of the WT1 gene was examined in human hematological malignancies. Significant levels of the gene were expressed in all types of leukemias but not in non-Hodgkin's lymphoma. By using polymerase chain reaction, WT1 could become a new prognostic factor and a new marker for the detection of minimal residual disease in leukemias.[14] WT1 is not useful in detecting disease activity of malignant lymphomas but is a sensitive molecular marker for early recognition of secondary myelodysplasia/acute myelogenous leukemia.

A distinct form of secondary acute myelogenous leukemia that follows chemotherapy with DNA-topoisomerase II inhibitors, especially epipodophyllotoxins (VP-16 and VM-26), is increasingly reported.[15,16] The majority of this form of secondary acute myelogenous leukemia is associated with balanced translocations involving band 11q23. A polymerase chain reaction method has also become available to find the specific fusion sequence of the leukemic clone.[17] Patients with malignant lymphoma treated with chemotherapeutic drugs targeting DNA-topoisomerase II, who are at high-risk for 11q23 leukemia, should be followed to detect the 11q23 fusion gene as early as possible. When the disease develops, some patients can be cured by allogeneic bone marrow transplantation. The application of molecular markers to the early recognition not only of recurrent disease but also of secondary myelodysplasia/acute myelogenous leukemia may give patients a greater chance of survival.

REFERENCES

1. International Agency for Research on Cancer. In: Parkin DM, Muir CS, Whelan SL, Gao YT, Ferlay J, Powell J, editors. Cancer incidence in five continents, Vol. 6. Lyon: World Health Organization, 1992:988-91.
2. The T- and B-Cell Malignancy Study Group. Statistical analysis of immunologic, clinical and histopathologic data on lymphoid malignancies in Japan. Jpn J Clin Oncol 1981;11:15-38.
3. Lennert K, Feller AC. Histopathology of non-Hodgkin's lymphomas (based on the updated Kiel Classification) with a section on clinical therapy by Engelhard M. Brittnger. 2nd ed. New York: Springer, 1992:165-261.
4. Lukes RJ, Parker JW, Taylor CR, Tindle BH, Cramer AD, Lincoln TL. Immunologic approach to non-Hodgkin lymphomas and related leukemias: analysis of the results of multiparameter studies of 425 cases. Semin Hematol 1978;15:322-51.
5. Wagner DK, Kiwanuka J, Edwards BK, et al. Soluble interleukin-2 receptor levels in patients with undifferentiated and lymphoblastic lymphomas: correlation of survival. J Clin Oncol 1987;5:1262-74.
6. Pui CH, Ip SH, Kung P, et al. High serum interleukin-2 receptor levels are related to advanced disease and a poor outcome in childhood non-Hodgkin's lymphoma. Blood 1987;70:624-8.
7. Weiss LM, Michie SA, Mederois LJ, et al. Expression of Tac antigen by non-Hodgkin's lymphomas. Am J Clin Pathol 1987;88:483-5.
8. Chilosi M, Semenzato G, Vinante F, et al. Increased levels of soluble interleukin-2 receptor in non-Hodgkin's lymphomas. Am J Clin Pathol 1989;92:186-91.
9. Stasi R, Zinzani PL, Galieni P, et al. Detection of soluble interleukin-2 receptor and interleukin-10 in the serum of patients with aggressive non-Hodgkin's lymphoma: identification of a subset at high risk of treatment failure. Cancer 1994;74:1792-800.
10. Marcon L, Rubin LA, Kurman CC, et al. Elevated serum levels of soluble Tac peptide in adult T cell leukemia: correlation with clinical status during chemotherapy. Ann Intern Med 1988;109:274-9.
11. Kamihira S, Atogami S, Sohda H, Momita S, Yamoda Y, Tomonaga M. Significance of soluble interleukin-2 receptor levels for evaluation of the progression of adult T-cell leukemia. Cancer 1994;73:2753-58.
12. Call KM, Glaser T, Ito CY, et al. Isolation and characterization of a zinc finger polypeptide gene at the human chromosome 11 Wilms' tumor locus. Cell 1990;60:509-20.
13. Gessler M, Poustka A, Cavenee W, Neve RL, Orkin SH, Bruns GA. Homozygous deletion in Wilms tumours of a zinc-finger gene identified by chromosome jumping. Nature 1990;343:774-8.

14. Inoue K, Sugiyama H, Ogawa H, et al. WT1 as a new prognostic factor and a new marker for the detection of minimal residual disease in acute leukemia. Blood 1994;84:3071-9.
15. Hunger SP, Tkachuk DC, Amylon MD, et al. HRX involvement in de novo and secondary leukemias with diverse chromosome 11q23 abnormalities. Blood 1993;81:3197-203.
16. Felix CA, Winick NJ, Negrini M, Bowman WP, Croce CM, Lange BJ. Common region of ALL-1 gene disrupted in epipodophyllotoxin-related secondary acute myeloid leukemia. Cancer Res 1993;53:2954-6.
17. Yamamoto K, Seto M, Iida S, et al. Analysis of chimeric mRNAs in leukemia with 11q23 translocation. Int J Hematol 1994;59:131.

➢ COUNTERPOINT

Royal Liverpool University Hospital, UK

RICHARD E. CLARK

The evolution of the treatment of lymphomas during this century represents one of the triumphs of modern medicine. The first use of x-rays in treatment was almost 100 years ago,[1] although responses to early radiation treatment were often only temporary. As radiation therapy technology improved, so did clinical outcomes, so that by 1950 survival rates of up to 88% were reported for localized Hodgkin's disease.[2] With the introduction of combination chemotherapy in the 1960s, clinical results improved in advanced lymphomas. Advanced Hodgkin's disease, a condition previously regarded as fatal, could be cured by a regimen of nitrogen mustard, vincristine, procarbazine, and prednisone.[3] Similarly, the related regimen of cyclophosphamide, doxorubicin, vincristine, and prednisone was shown to produce durable remissions and cures in advanced, diffuse, large cell non-Hodgkin's lymphoma.[4] Newer and less toxic, although equally effective, cytotoxic agents have subsequently been introduced, and effective first-line chemotherapy schedules can now safely be given in the outpatient clinic, even for patients with advanced disease.

The development of techniques for the harvesting and manipulation of hematopoietic stem cells has allowed the escalation of chemotherapy schedules to myeloablative doses. After completion of high-dose chemotherapy the patient is rescued from the otherwise inevitable severe and prolonged blood cytopenias by reinfusion of previously harvested bone marrow. Peripheral blood stem cells, obtained by leukapheresis after mobilization of marrow stem cells into the circulation as a result of chemotherapy or hematopoietic growth factors, may lead to more rapid hematopoietic reconstitution than conventional bone marrow, although no evidence has been presented that patients with peripheral blood stem cell transplants have a better disease outcome than recipients of bone marrow. High-dose chemotherapy with autologous peripheral blood stem cell or bone marrow transplant has become widely used in the treatment of relapsed lymphoma.

The purpose of this counterpoint is not to review all aspects of lymphoma follow-up, but rather to provide additional relevant information and to highlight areas in which British practice may differ from that in the United States.

OPTIMAL INITIAL TREATMENT

What role do treatment modalities have in the modern treatment of lymphoma? The majority of patients with early Hodgkin's disease or aggressive non-Hodgkin's lymphoma can be cured by local radiation therapy. A substantial proportion of those with more advanced disease may also be cured by chemotherapy of an intensity safely given on an outpatient basis. Patients who have intermediate- or high-grade non-Hodgkin's lymphoma with poor prognostic features, such as high serum lactic dehydrogenase levels, poor performance status, and extensive disease,[5] and who respond well to initial conventional chemotherapy schedules might benefit from early autologous bone marrow transplanation, and this approach is under investigation. The role of early bone marrow transplant in advanced Hodgkin's disease is not clear, in part because of disagreement about prognostic factors in Hodgkin's disease.

Although a huge body of information on lymphoma treatment is now available, a decision about initial management of newly diagnosed Hodgkin's disease or non-Hodgkin's lymphoma can be difficult. The optimal treatment may vary according to host features such as age and disease features such as histological type, immunological and molecular characteristics, and extent (clinical staging and localization). For patients with relapse the choice of optimal treatment may also depend on the degree and duration of response to previous treatment. For newly diagnosed Hodgkin's disease and aggressive non-Hodgkin's lymphoma requiring chemotherapy, debate continues on the optimal schedule, although in the case of aggressive non-Hodgkin's lymphoma the regimen containing cyclophosphamide, doxorubicin, vincristine, and prednisone is the gold standard against which to compare new regimens.[4] While the recent important proposal for a revised European-American lymphoma histological classification[6,7] may be helpful for lymphoma pathologists, whether its subgroups define distinct clinical entities remains to be seen. Decisions on the management of non-Hodgkin's lymphoma therefore still depend on the Working Formulation classification.[8]

The generally accepted initial management of patients with newly diagnosed lymphoma in the United Kingdom does not differ significantly from the U.S. practice, as expressed by Maloney and Appelbaum. In the United Kingdom current clinical research on the initial treatment of lymphoma focuses particularly on situations in which the optimal treatment is unclear. Examples include the role of early autologous bone marrow transplantation in poor-risk, large cell or lymphoblastic non-Hodgkin's lymphoma responding to initial conventional chemotherapy, the use of limited chemotherapy as well as radiation therapy in localized Hodgkin's disease and early aggressive non-Hodgkin's lymphoma, and the role of surgery and therapy directed against the microorganism *Helicobacter pylori* in the initial management of non-Hodgkin's lymphoma affecting the gastrointestinal tract.

MANAGEMENT OF PATIENTS WITH RELAPSE

For patients with localized relapse, local radiation therapy may still be curative. Patients with more generalized relapse may be cured by conventional chemotherapy schedules. For many patients with relapse, autologous bone marrow transplantation may be the optimal curative option. In relapsed intermediate- or high-grade non-Hodgkin's lymphoma the results of autografting depend on whether the disease remains chemosensitive at the time of transplantation.[9] In Hodgkin's disease, by contrast, bone marrow transplantation in combination with BEAM (carmustine, etoposide, cytosine arabinoside, and melphalan) conditioning may produce lengthy relapse-free survival in patients refractory to the intensive schedule of mini-BEAM, which includes the same drugs as BEAM but in a lower dosage.[10]

In patients with relapse of extensive Hodgkin's disease or aggressive non-Hodgkin's lymphoma, standard practice is to give preliminary conventional chemotherapy to test disease sensitivity. Some institutions, including Royal Liverpool University Hospital, are reluctant to offer autologous bone marrow transplantation to patients with chemoresistant non-Hodgkin's lymphoma (although not Hodgkin's disease).[11] The optimal number of courses of conventional chemotherapy before bone marrow transplantation is unknown, and the possible benefit of reducing disease bulk before autografting must be balanced against the risk of compromising later attempts at stem cell or marrow harvesting. For patients with relapse after high-dose chemotherapy, further treatment occasionally produces durable responses[12] and may ameliorate symptoms and improve quality of life.

SECONDARY MALIGNANCY AFTER LYMPHOMA TREATMENT

A tragic realization of recent years is that a proportion of patients cured of lymphoma may later have a second malignancy. Myeloid malignancy is the most frequent second tumor, and this may manifest as myelodysplasia or acute myelogenous leukemia. There is also an increased incidence of secondary non-Hodgkin's lymphoma and breast, lung, and bladder cancers.[13] The reported incidence of secondary myelodysplasia/acute myelogenous leukemia in patients with lymphoma has varied[13-15] but may approach a relative risk of 16 for all leukemias, with a maximal incidence at 3 to 7 years after completion of treatment. The risk may be greater in Hodgkin's disease than in non-Hodgkin's lymphoma. Patients treated initially by radiation therapy and later with salvage chemotherapy may be at greatest risk. Myelodysplasia/acute myelogenous leukemia may also develop after autografting for lymphoma. A recent report from the European Bone Marrow Transplant Registry suggests that this may occur in approximately 4% of bone marrow transplant recipients.[16]

Secondary myelodysplasia/acute myelogenous leukemia in lymphoma survivors is likely to be due to genetic damage in a primitive hematopoietic stem cell. Epidemiological data support the view that this damage is caused by therapy, rather than being part of the natural history of the underlying lymphoma. An alternative possibility is that quiescent myeloid stem cells bearing infrequent mutations may be recruited into the cell cycle during the marrow recovery phase after myelosuppressive treatment for lymphoma, when they might possess a growth advantage over normal stem cells. As this expanding abnormal population acquires further mutations, a frankly leukemic clone may eventually achieve clonal dominance. The emergence of clinically apparent myeloid malignancy is likely to be the cumulative result of several oncogene mutations, although little is known of the nature or sequence of such lesions.

In a study of 70 hematologically normal patients previously treated successfully for lymphoma, *ras* and *fms* oncogene mutations were identified in some patients[17,18] and hematopoiesis in some patients was clonal.[19] In some patients high levels of chromosomal damage persist several years after successful lymphoma treatment.[20] Myelodysplasia/acute myelogenous leukemia arising after therapy for cancer has a higher incidence of karyotypic abnormalities (especially of chromosomes 5q and 7) and a less favorable prognosis than does de novo disease.[15]

FOLLOW-UP

In contrast to the considerable information available on the treatment of active lymphoma, virtually no data are available on the optimal follow-up arrangements for patients with lymphoma. Patients should remain under the care of a team with special expertise in the management of hematological malignancy. In some centers this may occur in dedicated lymphoma clinics, staffed by both radiotherapists and medical oncologists or hematologists. The United Kingdom differs from many other countries in that the majority of patients with lymphoma are treated and followed up by hematologists rather than by general medical oncologists.

No formal studies have examined the optimal duration of follow-up after completion of treatment. Similarly, no information is available on what procedures or investigations are worthwhile at each follow-up visit. A history inquiring about B symptoms and other symptoms of disease activity is simple and obvious. A complete blood count (incorporating hemoglobin concentration, mean red cell corpuscular volume, platelet count, white blood cell count, and differential) to detect secondary myeloid malignancy is also essential and should be performed for several years after the completion of treatment. However, it is not known whether additional blood tests such as the serum lactic dehydrogenase level or routine surveillance of disease by computed tomography lead to earlier diagnosis of relapse or have any effect on ultimate patient outcome. Overt changes in these parameters may occur after the development of symptoms.[21]

Routine clinical examination is complicated by the fact that many patients in remission have significant fibrotic masses at the sites of previous active disease, which may

Table 22-8 Follow-up of patients with lymphoma (in complete remission): Royal Liverpool University Hospital, UK

	YEAR				
	1	2	3	4	5
Office visit	6-8	4	4	2-3	2-3
Complete blood count	6-8	4	4	2-3	2-3
Chest computed tomography*	2†	‡	‡	‡	‡
Abdominal computed tomography*	2†	‡	‡	‡	‡
Pelvic computed tomography*	2†	‡	‡	‡	‡

*For patients with residual chest, abdominal, or pelvic masses.
†Performed biannually to quarterly for patients with Hodgkin's disease or intermediate- or high-grade non-Hodgkin's lymphoma with a residual bulky mediastinal, pulmonary, or abdominal mass who are otherwise in remission.
‡Performed as clinically indicated by first-year findings.

wax and wane in size without necessarily indicating relapse. Routine clinical examination for lymphadenopathy may be less useful for diagnosing relapse than an inquiry about the presence of symptoms of disease activity or the patient's own observations. Carefully performed studies of the usefulness of each of these ingredients of lymphoma follow-up might yield helpful information, particularly regarding the optimal use of expensive resources such as computed tomography.

Despite the lack of published information a consensus of routine practice for the follow-up of lymphoma in the United Kingdom has emerged. At each visit a simple history is taken, focusing on symptoms suggestive of relapse. A clinical examination of the typical areas of lymphoma involvement is performed, and the complete blood count result is reviewed. Patients who have achieved complete, unambiguous clinical and radiological remission are seen at intervals of 6 to 8 weeks for the first year after completing treatment, 3-month intervals for years 2 and 3, 4- to 6-month intervals for years 4 and 5, and annually thereafter (Table 22-8). Physicians at Royal Liverpool University Hospital do not perform routine radiological surveillance in this group in the absence of symptoms.

Patients with low-grade non-Hodgkin's lymphoma, for whom the aim is to detect progression of disease rather than relapse, are followed up similarly. Patients with Hodgkin's disease or intermediate- or high-grade non-Hodgkin's lymphoma with a residual bulky mediastinal, pulmonary, or abdominal mass who otherwise are in remission are followed up at the same intervals but with the addition of regular computed tomography of the relevant mass initially at 3- to 6-month intervals (Table 22-8). A significant, definite increase in the size of the mass, especially if coupled with recurrence of B symptoms, is taken as evidence of relapse without the need for formal biopsy.

The use of molecular markers for monitoring cancers in remission has attracted considerable interest. For example, several reports have suggested that the monitoring of BCR/abl transcript levels by the reverse-transcriptase polymerase chain reaction after allografting in chronic myeloid leukemia may be used to diagnose relapse earlier than conventional methods.[22] This might be clinically useful, since further treatment with infusions of donor leukocytes may be more effective if given early.[23] In lymphoma, to be of clinical use in detecting early relapse, measurements of lesions such as t(14;18) or immunoglobulin gene rearrangement should become positive significantly before conventional tests. With the exception of monitoring the effectiveness of bone marrow/peripheral blood stem cell purging strategies, molecular monitoring has not yet been shown to be of clinical use and is not routinely used in follow-up. A further problem in interpretation is that bone marrow involvement by lymphoma is variable and often patchy. A negative molecular investigation on blood or marrow would therefore not rule out active disease.

PREEMPTIVE HEMATOPOIETIC CELL HARVESTING

Either bone marrow or peripheral blood stem cells may be collected from patients in remission 2 to 3 weeks after completion of chemotherapy in case future autologous transplantation is needed. A myeloid growth factor (granulocyte colony–stimulating factor or granulocyte-macrophage colony–stimulating factor) usually is used to maximize the yield of peripheral blood stem cells. The rationale for collecting hematopoietic material is that a proportion of patients will experience relapse and the disease might then involve the marrow, making late harvests more likely to be contaminated with lymphoma. Furthermore, adequate hematopoietic cells (especially peripheral blood stem cells) may be more difficult to obtain in heavily pretreated patients.[24] However, only about one third of patients with lymphoma in remission ultimately become candidates for autologous bone marrow transplantation. Routine harvesting from all patients in remission would mean a large number of unnecessary procedures, with significant cost implications (such as staff, access to a cell separator, and additional cryopreservation facilities). The policy at Royal Liverpool University Hospital is to restrict preemptive harvesting to patients at higher risk of relapse, such as those with poor prognostic features at diagnosis or those for whom remission has been difficult to achieve.

CONCLUSION

Unlike patients with most other tumors, many patients with relapse of lymphoma may be offered useful further treatment, often with curative intent. It could be argued that careful follow-up of patients with lymphoma is more important than for many other tumor types, since potentially effective further therapy should not be delayed. It is therefore a surprise that little information has been published on optimal follow-up strategies for patients with lymphoma. Follow-up procedures in lymphoma clinics tend to be based on historical practice, clinical acumen, and common sense, rather than on strategies proved to be clinically effective. These historically based habits may be set to change as physicians' ability to monitor minimal residual disease at the molecular level improves, although the impact of measuring minimal residual disease on outcome is not yet known in lymphoma.

REFERENCES

1. Pusey WA. Cases of sarcoma and of Hodgkin's disease treated by exposures to x-rays: a preliminary report. JAMA 1902;38:166-9.
2. Peters MV. A study in survivals in Hodgkin's disease treated radiologically. AJR Am J Roentgenol 1950;63:299-311.
3. DeVita VT Jr, Serpick AA, Carbone PP. Combination chemotherapy in the treatment of advanced Hodgkin's disease. Ann Intern Med 1970;73:881-95.
4. Gaynor ER, Fisher RI. What is the best treatment for diffuse large cell lymphoma? In: Armitage J, Newland A, Keating A, Burnett A, editors. Haematological oncology. Vol. 4. Cambridge, United Kingdom: Cambridge University Press, 1995:119-34.
5. Coiffier B, Gisselbrecht C, Vose JM, et al. Prognostic factors in aggressive malignant lymphomas: description and validation of a prognostic index that could identify patients requiring a more intensive therapy: the Groupe d'Etudes des Lymphomas Agressifs. J Clin Oncol 1991;9:211-9.
6. Harris NL, Jaffe ES, Stein H, et al. A revised European-American classification of lymphoid neoplasms: a proposal from the International Lymphoma Study group. Blood 1994;84:1361-92.
7. Harris NL, Jaffe ES, Stein H, et al. Lymphoma classification proposal: clarification. Blood 1995;85:857-60.
8. Mason DY, Gatter KC. Not another lymphoma classification! Br J Haematol 1995;90:493-7.
9. Philip T, Armitage JO, Spitzer G, et al. High-dose therapy and autologous bone marrow transplantation after failure of conventional chemotherapy in adults with intermediate-grade or high-grade non-Hodgkin lymphoma. N Engl J Med 1987;316:1493-8.
10. Chopra R, Linch DC, McMillan AK, et al. Mini-BEAM followed by BEAM and ABMT for very poor risk Hodgkin's disease. Br J Haematol 1992;81:197-202.
11. Freedman AS, Nadler LM. Which patients with relapsed non-Hodgkin's lymphoma benefit from high-dose therapy and hematopoietic stem-cell transplantation? J Clin Oncol 1993;11:1841-3.
12. Vose JM, Bierman PJ, Anderson JR, et al. Progressive disease after high-dose therapy and autologous transplantation for lymphoid malignancy: clinical course and patient follow-up. Blood 1992; 80:2142-8.
13. Kaldor JM, Day NE, Band P, et al. Second malignancies following testicular cancer, ovarian cancer, and Hodgkin's disease: an international collaborative study among cancer registries. Int J Cancer 1987;39:571-85.
14. Swerdlow AJ, Douglas AJ, Hudson GV, Hudson BV, Bennett MH, MacLennan KA. Risk of second primary cancers after Hodgkin's disease by type of treatment: analysis of 2846 patients in the British National Lymphoma Investigation. Br Med J 1992;304:1137-43.
15. Kantarjian HM, Keating MJ, Walters RS, et al. Therapy-related leukaemia and myelodysplastic syndrome: clinical, cytogenetic, and prognostic features. J Clin Oncol 1986;4:1748-57.
16. Milligan DW, Kolb HJ, Pearce R, Taghipour G, Goldstone AH. MDS after autografting for lymphoma: a retrospective analysis of the EBMT registry. Bone Marrow Transplant 1996;17(Suppl 1):S148.
17. Carter G, Hughes DC, Clark RE, et al. RAS mutations in patients following cytotoxic therapy for lymphoma. Oncogene 1990;5:411-6.
18. Baker A, Cachia P, Ridge S, et al. FMS mutations in patients following cytotoxic therapy for lymphoma. Leuk Res 1995;19:309-18.
19. Cachia PG, Calligan DJ, Clark RE, Whittaker JA, Jacobs A, Padua RA. Clonal haemopoiesis following cytotoxic therapy for lymphoma. Leukemia 1993;7:795-800.
20. White AD, Jones BM, Clark RE, Jacobs A. Chromosome aberrations following cytotoxic therapy in patients in complete remission from lymphoma. Carcinogenesis 1992;13:1095-9.
21. Weeks JC, Yeap BY, Canellos GP, Shipp MA. Value of follow-up procedures in patients with large-cell lymphoma who achieve a complete remission. J Clin Oncol 1991;9:1196-203.
22. Cross NC, Feng L, Chase A, Bungey J, Hughes TP, Goldman JM. Competitive polymerase chain reaction to estimate the number of BCR-ABL transcripts in chronic myeloid leukaemia patients after bone marrow transplantation. Blood 1993;82:1929-36.
23. Mackinnon S, Papadopoulos EB, Carabasi MH, et al. Donor leucocyte infusions for molecular or cytogenetic relapse of CML following allogeneic BMT: graft-versus leukemia responses with minimal toxicity. Blood 1995;86(Suppl 1):566a.
24. Derigs HG, Peschel C, Huber C, Kolbe K. Mobilisation of peripheral blood stem cells (PBSC) with chemotherapy followed by IL-3 and G-CSF in heavily pretreated patients. Bone Marrow Transplant 1996; 17(Suppl 1):S51.

➢ COUNTERPOINT

Roswell Park Cancer Institute

MYRON S. CZUCZMAN

Maloney and Appelbaum provide a concise and thorough review of the natural history, treatment options, potential complications, and recommended follow-up of patients with Hodgkin's disease or non-Hodgkin's lymphoma. In recent years a limited number of articles have specifically addressed the issue of posttreatment follow-up of patients with these diseases.[1-4] Since I agree with the majority of issues addressed in the primary chapter, this counterpoint serves largely to reemphasize certain important points and expand on others.

The first point is that patients with intermediate- or high-grade non-Hodgkin's lymphoma who respond rapidly to therapy are believed to have a better prognosis than slow responders.[5-7] A recent article by Verdonck et al.[8] evaluated whether patients with aggressive non-Hodgkin's lymphoma and slowly responding disease (to the combination of cyclophosphamide, doxorubicin, vincristine, and prednisone [CHOP]) had a better outcome with autologous bone marrow transplantation or five additional cycles of CHOP. The authors concluded that bone marrow transplant did not confer any significant clinical benefit as compared with additional CHOP chemotherapy. Several questions regarding study design, conditioning regimen for ABMT, definition of partial response, inhomogeneous population, and staging techniques used in this study have been raised. For example, the valuable technique of gallium-67 scintigraphy was not included. It is possible that a significant number of patients with residual masses on computed tomographic scan after three cycles of CHOP and classified as partial responders

Table 22-9 Follow-up of patients with lymphoma (Hodgkin's lymphoma or non-Hodgkin's lymphoma in complete remission): Roswell Park Cancer Institute

	YEAR				
	1	2	3	4	5
Office visit	4	4	2	2	1
Lactic dehydrogenase	4	4	2	2	1
Complete blood count	4	4	2	2	1
Beta$_2$-microglobulin*	4	4	2	2	1
Erythrocyte sedimentation rate†	4	4	2	2	1
Alkaline phosphatase†	4	4	2	2	1
Chest x-ray	2	2	2	2	1
Thyroid profile‡	1	1	1	1	1
Site computed tomography or magnetic resonance imaging§,¶	1-2	0-2	0-2	0-1	0-1
Gallium scan§	0-1	0-1	0-1	0-1	0-1

*For patients with non-Hodgkin's lymphoma and elevated level before treatment.
†For patients with Hodgkin's lymphoma.
‡For patients treated with mediastinal or neck irradiation.
§Indicated if lactic dehydrogenase and beta$_2$-microglobulin levels become abnormal in the absence of detectable disease.
¶Test selection based on the modality that gave optimal tumor visualization at time of presentation.

might actually have been shown to have had complete responses if serial gallium scanning had been performed and had demonstrated conversion from positive to negative. These patients with complete responses would not have gone on to random assignment between ABMT and further CHOP chemotherapy, which would not only have changed the database, but quite possibly the final conclusions of this trial. Gallium-67 scintigraphy is a powerful tool for detecting residual or recurrent non-Hodgkin's lymphoma or Hodgkin's disease in patients with gallium-avid disease and plays a prominent role in the follow-up of patients at Roswell Park Cancer Institute and other centers (Table 22-9).

Several papers have demonstrated the clinical utility of using gallium-67 scanning in the initial evaluation and follow-up of patients with non-Hodgkin's lymphoma and Hodgkin's disease.[9-16] In recent years the sensitivity of gallium-67 scintigraphy has been improved by the injection of larger doses of radionuclide (8 to 10 mCi) and the use of triple-energy-peak gamma camera acquisition and single photon emission computed tomography imaging. Pretreatment gallium scans are positive in the majority of patients with intermediate- or high-grade non-Hodgkin's lymphoma and Hodgkin's disease but are positive in only a minority of patients with low-grade non-Hodgkin's lymphoma. For many patients routine staging evaluation of lymphoma includes pretreatment gallium imaging, history and physical examination, computed tomographic scans of the chest, abdomen, and pelvis, complete blood count with differential, full chemistry profile, erythrocyte sedimentation rate, chest x-ray, histological analysis of bilateral bone marrow aspirate and biopsy specimens, and (when appropriate) flow cytometry and molecular studies including B or T cell gene rearrangement and bcl-2 analysis by polymerase chain reaction. Additional studies, including magnetic resonance imaging, bone scan, computed tomography of the brain and neck, and lumbar puncture, may be performed on individual patients depending on clinical presentation.

Patients with non-Hodgkin's lymphoma or Hodgkin's disease who are gallium positive before treatment and are left with residual tissue after treatment should be assessed by repeat gallium scintigraphy. After completion of therapy, persistence of gallium positivity has been shown to correspond to residual viable tumor[17] and a worse prognosis[15,16] compared with patients who become gallium negative.

In general, interim restaging analysis of patients with lymphoma midway through a planned course of therapy should include gallium imaging (if positive at pretreatment) and repeat computed tomographic scanning of involved areas. Patients with persistent gallium avidity of residual tissue are considered at increased risk for refractory or recurrent disease and are more likely to require additional chemotherapy or more aggressive intervention (ABMT) than patients who revert to gallium negativity midway through treatment.

Magnetic resonance imaging is routinely used to evaluate and follow the response of patients with lymphoma involving the spine, brain, and occasionally bone. Recent research suggests that magnetic resonance imaging may be useful in predicting relapse in residual masses after therapy,[18] but because of poor sensitivity (45%) and subjective interpretation of inhomogeneous signals it is not likely to gain broad acceptance for this indication. On the other hand, bone marrow magnetic resonance imaging may someday prove useful as an adjunct to bone marrow aspirate and biopsy in detecting lymphomatous marrow involvement.[19,20] Maloney and Appelbaum briefly mention two new techniques, somatostatin receptor scintigraphy and positron emission tomography, which are being studied for their utility in the initial evaluation and follow-up of lymphomatous lesions. Another technique under investigation is radioimmunoscintigraphy of non-Hodgkin's lymphoma with ^{99m}technetium-labeled LL2 (anti-CD22) monoclonal antibody Fab' fragment.[21,22] Since antibody scans are not dependent on tumor cell metabolism or uptake of reagents into cells but instead on surface antigen expression, they may someday prove to be an important noninvasive adjunct in the restaging of non-Hodgkin's lymphoma (including low-grade histological types). The clinical utility of these new techniques has not been determined and will depend largely on the results of future studies.

The prognostic value of elevated lactic dehydrogenase, beta$_2$-microglobulin, and erythrocyte sedimentation rate levels is thoroughly discussed in the primary chapter. These tests are typically used for posttreatment surveillance of patients with non-Hodgkin's lymphoma and Hodgkin's disease if levels were elevated before treatment. Because of an increased risk of secondary malignancies after primary cancer therapy, routine follow-up after 5 years normally includes a yearly complete blood count with differential (owing to the risk of myelodysplasia and acute myelogenous leukemia), chest x-ray (to detect lung cancer), gynecological examination, Papanicolaou smear, and mammography in young women starting 10 years after completion of mantle radiation therapy or age 35, whichever is first (to detect breast cancer), thyroid function tests (to detect thyroid dysfunction after head and neck radiation therapy), as well as a thorough physical examination and attention to any complaints disclosed from a full interim history and review of systems.

Sensitive molecular techniques such as polymerase chain reaction are opening the door to an exciting area of cancer research, the study of minimal residual disease and its relationship to clinical relapse. The molecular marker most widely studied by polymerase chain reaction is bcl-2 t(14;18), which is seen in greater than 80% of patients with follicular and 30% of patients with large cell non-Hodgkin's lymphoma. Lymphoma research at Roswell Park Cancer Institute includes studying the effectiveness of various therapies (chemotherapy and immunotherapy) on clearing bcl-2 positivity from the patient's blood and marrow and its relationship to disease recurrence.[23-25] The significance of this result on disease-free and overall survival in patients with low-grade non-Hodgkin's lymphoma is as yet undetermined.

Furthermore, to reemphasize a point made by Maloney and Appelbaum, since most patients with non-Hodgkin's lymphoma do not have the bcl-2 translocation, development of patient-specific clonal B cell gene rearrangement or T cell antigen receptor markers may improve evaluation of the clinical significance of minimal residual disease in patients with aggressive non-Hodgkin's lymphoma.

Table 22-9 outlines the follow-up studies recommended for patients with non-Hodgkin's lymphoma and Hodgkin's disease after treatment. This list should serve only as a general template for the timing of restaging studies. The actual restaging tests performed and intervals used by clinicians should be modified by the patient's complaints, abnormalities found on routine physical examination and by laboratory studies, the availability of various restaging modalities at a given medical center, and the patient's overall clinical status. Follow-up strategies are also affected by personal preference between pursuing potentially curative treatment or simply palliative salvage therapy if relapsed disease is discovered. Future clinical trials should evaluate and compare the utility of the aforementioned modalities, as well as new ones used in screening asymptomatic patients after therapy, so that a more definitive set of specific guidelines may be developed for the routine follow-up of patients with non-Hodgkin's lymphoma and Hodgkin's disease.

REFERENCES

1. Kagan AR, Steckel RJ. Post-treatment surveillance studies for lymphoma patients. Invest Radiol 1992;27:543-7.
2. Radford JA, Eardley A, Woodman C, Crowther D. Routine outpatient review following treatment for Hodgkin's disease: is it an efficient way of detecting relapse? Proc Am Soc Clin Oncol 1995;14:386.
3. Weeks JC, Yeap BY, Canellos GP, Shipp MA. Value of follow-up procedures in patients with large-cell lymphoma who achieve a complete remission. J Clin Oncol 1991;9:1196-203.
4. Stomper PC. Cancer imaging manual. Philadelphia: JB Lippincott Company, 1993:127-56.
5. Armitage JO, Weisenburger DD, Hutchins M, et al. Chemotherapy for diffuse large-cell lymphoma—rapidly responding patients have more durable remissions. J Clin Oncol 1986;4:160-4.
6. Coiffier B, Bryon PA, Berger F, et al. Intensive and sequential combination chemotherapy for aggressive malignant lymphomas (protocol LNH-80). J Clin Oncol 1986;4:147-53.
7. Haw R, Sawka CA, Franssen E, Berinstein NL. Significance of a partial or slow response to front-line chemotherapy in the management of intermediate-grade or high-grade non-Hodgkin's lymphoma: a literature review. J Clin Oncol 1994;12:1074-84.
8. Verdonck LF, van Putten WL, Hagenbeek A, et al. Comparison of CHOP chemotherapy with autologous bone marrow transplantation for slowly responding patients with aggressive non-Hodgkin's lymphoma. N Engl J Med 1995;332:1045-51.
9. Front D, Bar-Shalom R, Epelbaum R, et al. Early detection of lymphoma recurrence with gallium-67 scintigraphy. J Nucl Med 1993; 34:2101-4.
10. Anderson KC, Leonard RC, Canellos GP, Skarin AT, Kaplan WD. High-dose gallium imaging in lymphoma. Am J Med 1983;75:327-31.
11. Front D, Israel O, Epelbaum R, et al. Ga-67 SPECT before and after treatment of lymphoma. Radiology 1990;175:515-9.
12. Front D, Ben-Haim S, Israel O, et al. Lymphoma: predictive value of Ga-67 scintigraphy after treatment. Radiology 1992;182:359-63.
13. Even-Sapir E, Bar-Shalom R, Israel O, et al. Single-photon emission computed tomography quantification of gallium citrate uptake for differentiation of lymphoma from benign hilar uptake. J Clin Oncol 1995;13:942-6.
14. Gasparini MD, Balzarini L, Castellani MR, et al. Current role of gallium scan and magnetic resonance imaging in the management of mediastinal Hodgkin's lymphoma. Cancer 1993;72:577-82.
15. King SC, Reiman RJ, Prosnitz LR. Prognostic importance of restaging gallium scans following induction chemotherapy for advanced Hodgkin's disease. J Clin Oncol 1994;12:306-11.
16. Kaplan WD, Jochelson MS, Herman TS, et al. Gallium-67 imaging: a predictor of residual tumor viability and clinical outcome in patients with diffuse large-cell lymphoma. J Clin Oncol 1990;8:1966-70.
17. Front D, Israel O. The role of Ga-67 scintigraphy in evaluating the results of therapy of lymphoma patients. Semin Nucl Med 1995;25: 60-71.
18. Hill M, Cuningham D, MacVicar D, et al. Role of magnetic resonance imaging in predicting relapse in residual masses after treatment of lymphoma. J Clin Oncol 1993;11:2273-8.
19. Hoane BR, Shields AF, Porter BA, Shulman HM. Detection of lymphomatous bone marrow involvement with magnetic resonance imaging. Blood 1991;78:728-38.
20. Schilder R, Padavic-Shaller K, Schaer A, et al. Lymphoma staging with bone marrow MRI. Proc Am Soc Clin Oncol 1995;14:390.
21. Murthy S, Sharkey RM, Goldenberg DM, et al. Lymphoma imaging with a new technetium-99m labelled antibody, LL2. Eur J Nucl Med 1992;19:394-401.
22. Gasparini M, Bombardieri E, Tondini C, et al. Clinical utility of radioimmunoscintigraphy of non-Hodgkin's lymphoma with radiolabelled LL2 monoclonal antibody, lymphoscan: preliminary results. Tumori 1995;81:173-8.
23. Gribben JG, Freedman AS, Woo SD, et al. All advanced stage non-Hodgkin's lymphomas with a polymerase chain reaction amplifiable breakpoint of bcl-2 have residual cells containing the bcl-2 rearrangement at evaluation and after treatment. Blood 1991;78:3275-80.
24. Czuczman MS, Grillo-Lopez AJ, Jonas C, et al. IDEC-C2B8 and CHOP chemotherapy of low-grade lymphoma. Blood 1995;86(Suppl 1):55a.
25. Rogers J, Ward P, Jackson J, et al. Analysis of bcl-2 t(14;18) translocation in relapsed B-cell lymphoma patients treated with the chimeric anti-CD20 antibody IDEC-C2B8. Cancer Res 1996. Submitted abstract

Table 22-10 Follow-up of patients with lymphoma by institution

YEAR/PROGRAM	OFFICE VISIT	LDH	CBC	BETA 2	ESR	ALP	CXR
Year 1							
Memorial Sloan-Kettering I[a]	4		4		4		4
Memorial Sloan-Kettering II[c]	4[d]		4[d]				4[d]
Memorial Sloan-Kettering III[e]	4		4				4
Roswell Park[f]	4	4	4	4[g]	4[h]	4[h]	2
Univ Washington/Fred Hutchinson[l]	4	4	4	4[m]	4[h]	4[h]	2
Japan: National Kyushu[l]	4	4	4	4[m]	4[h]	4[h]	2
UK: Royal Liverpool[o]	6-8		6-8				
Year 2							
Memorial Sloan-Kettering I[a]	3		3		3		3
Memorial Sloan-Kettering II[c]	3		3				3
Memorial Sloan-Kettering III[e]	3		3				3
Roswell Park[f]	4	4	4	4[g]	4[h]	4[h]	2
Univ Washington/Fred Hutchinson[l]	4	4	4	4[m]	4[h]	4[h]	2
Japan: National Kyushu[l]	4	4	4	4[m]	4[h]	4[h]	2
UK: Royal Liverpool[o]	4		4				
Year 3							
Memorial Sloan-Kettering I[a]	3		3		3		3
Memorial Sloan-Kettering II[c]	3		3				3
Memorial Sloan-Kettering III[e]	3		3				3
Roswell Park[f]	2	2	2	2[g]	2[h]	2[h]	2
Univ Washington/Fred Hutchinson[l]	3	3	3	3[m]	3[h]	3[h]	2
Japan: National Kyushu[l]	3	3	3	3[m]	3[h]	3[h]	2
UK: Royal Liverpool[o]	4		4				
Year 4							
Memorial Sloan-Kettering I[a]	2		2		2		2
Memorial Sloan-Kettering II[c]	2		2				2
Memorial Sloan-Kettering III[e]	2		2				2
Roswell Park[f]	2	2	2	2[g]	2[h]	2[h]	2
Univ Washington/Fred Hutchinson[l]	2	2	2	2[m]	1[h]	1[h]	2
Japan: National Kyushu[l]	2	2	2	2[m]	1[h]	1[h]	2
UK: Royal Liverpool[o]	2-3		2-3				

ABD CT abdominal computed tomography
ALP alkaline phosphatase
BETA 2 $beta_2$-microglobulin
CBC complete blood count
CHEST CT chest computed tomography
CXR chest x-ray
ESR erythrocyte sedimentation rate
LDH lactic dehydrogenase
LFT liver function tests
MAMM mammogram
SIL-2R soluble interleukin-2 receptor

THYROID	SITE CT/MRI	GALLIUM	LFT	ABD CT	PELVIC CT	MAMM	SIL-2R	CHEST CT
2			4	2	2	[b]		
			4[d]	2-3	2-3			
			4	2	2			
1[i]	1-2[j,k]	0-1[j]						
1[i]	1-2[j]	1-2[j]						
1[i]	1-2[j,n]	1-2[j]					4	
				2[p,q]	2[p,q]			2[p,q]
2			3	2	2	1[b]		
			3	2	2			
			3	2	2			
1[i]	1-2[j,k]	0-1[j]						
1[i]	0-2[j]	0-2[j]						
1[i]	0-2[j,n]	0-2[j]					4	
				[p,r]	[p,r]			[p,r]
2			3	2	2	1[b]		
			3	2	2			
			3	2	2			
1[i]	1-2[j,k]	0-1[j]						
1[i]	0-2[j]	0-2[j]						
1[i]	0-2[j,n]	0-2[j]					3	
				[p,r]	[p,r]			[p,r]
2			2	2	2	1[b]		
			2	2	2			
			2	2	2			
1[i]	0-1[j,k]	0-1[j]						
1[i]	0-1[j]	0-1[j]						
1[i]	0-1[j,n]	0-1[j]					2	
				[p,r]	[p,r]			[p,r]

a Patients with Hodgkin's lymphoma in complete remission.
b Performed for female patients over the age of 30 who have received mantle irradiation.
c Patients with intermediate- or high-grade non-Hodgkin's lymphoma in complete remission.
d Performed every 2 months for patients with high-grade non-Hodgkin's lymphoma.
e Patients with low-grade non-Hodgkin's lymphoma in complete remission.
f Patients with Hodgkin's lymphoma or non-Hodgkin's lymphoma in complete remission.
g For patients with non-Hodgkin's lymphoma and elevated level before treatment.
h For patients with Hodgkin's lymphoma.
i For patients treated with mediastinal or neck irradiation.
j Indicated if lactic dehydrogenase and beta$_2$-microglobulin levels become abnormal in the absence of detectable disease.
k Test selection based on the modality that gave optimal tumor visualization at time of presentation.
l Patients with Hodgkin's lymphoma or aggressive non-Hodgkin's lymphoma in complete remission.
m For patients with aggressive non-Hodgkin's lymphoma.
n Test selection based on availability of magnetic resonance imaging.
o Patients in complete remission.
p For patients with residual chest, abdominal, or pelvic masses.
q Performed biannually to quarterly for patients with Hodgkin's disease or intermediate- or high-grade non-Hodgkin's lymphoma with a residual bulky mediastinal, pulmonary, or abdominal mass who are otherwise in remission.
r Performed as clinically indicated by first-year findings.

Continued.

Table 22-10 Follow-up of patients with lymphoma by institution—cont'd

YEAR/PROGRAM	OFFICE VISIT	LDH	CBC	BETA 2	ESR	ALP	CXR
Year 5							
Memorial Sloan-Kettering I[a]	1		1		1		1
Memorial Sloan-Kettering II[c]	1		1				1
Memorial Sloan-Kettering III[e]	2		2				2
Roswell Park[f]	1	1	1	1[g]	1[h]	1[h]	1
Univ Washington/Fred Hutchinson[l]	2	2	2	2[m]	1[h]	1[h]	2
Japan: National Kyushu[l]	2	2	2	2[m]	1[h]	1[h]	2
UK: Royal Liverpool[o]	2-3		2-3				

THYROID	SITE CT/MRI	GALLIUM	LFT	ABD CT	PELVIC CT	MAMM	SIL-2R	CHEST CT
1			1	1	1	1[b]		
			1	1	1			
			2	2	2			
1[i]	0-1[j,k]	0-1[j]						
1[i]	0-1[j]	0-1[j]						
1[i]	0-1[j,n]	0-1[j]					2	
				[p,r]	[p,r]			[p,r]

CHAPTER 23

Stem Cell Transplantation

University of Washington Medical Center ▪ Fred Hutchinson Cancer Research Center

Keith M. Sullivan and Muriel F. Siadak

The past decade has witnessed a rapid increase in the use of hematopoietic stem cell transplantation.[1] With increasing numbers of marrow and blood stem cell transplantations for breast cancer and solid tumors, long-term care of these patients is no longer the sole domain of the hematologist. Data from the Autologous Blood and Marrow Transplant Registry, which is composed of 128 centers in North America, show that use of high-dose chemotherapy and autologous transplantation is growing rapidly and is now more common than allogeneic marrow transplantation (Figure 23-1). Similar growth has been observed in Western Europe, where in several countries stem cell transplantation appears to be more widely available than in the United States.[2]

With the first recipients now 25 years from marrow transplantation,[3] the health care of an increasing number of transplant recipients is given by a broad spectrum of providers. The successful outcome of this procedure, however, may depend on late complications arising months to years after transplantation.[4] Late events may arise from chemoradiation therapy–associated organ toxicity, immunodeficiency, infection, chronic graft-versus-host disease, or recurrent or secondary neoplasms. Table 23-1 lists potential complications, and Figures 23-2 and 23-3 illustrate the interrelationships and time of onset of these late events.[4,5] To provide optimal care for an increasing number of patients, physicians require familiarity with the long-term follow-up care of hematopoietic cell recipients. The following details key areas for follow-up of these patients.

AMBULATORY CARE AND LONG-TERM MONITORING

The role of ambulatory care of the stem cell transplant recipient is expanding. Many services traditionally given on inpatient wards can now be provided in less expensive outpatient settings.[6-9] Although debate surrounds the rapid dissemination of high-dose chemotherapy and stem cell transplantation into community practice outside established transplant centers, follow-up monitoring and reporting of the results of all transplantations are essential for accurate assessment of outcome.[10-12]

Over the past two decades long-term monitoring at Fred Hutchinson Cancer Research Center has undergone testing and refinement.[7] More than 2,500 patients are actively monitored, with tracking performed in several ways. On-site examination of returning patients is conducted at the first and selected subsequent anniversaries of transplantation and includes detailed medical, hematological, and immunological evaluations. Questionnaires are sent to referring physicians initially at 6 months and then at each anniversary of transplantation. The questionnaire is a detailed medical survey succinct enough to ensure a high rate of return on the first mailing (see Appendix A at the end of the chapter). Survival data are reported to the date of last contact, including a standardized rating of the current functional performance (Table 23-2). Yearly questionnaires are also sent to each patient eliciting information about functional performance, symptoms, and medical complications (see Appendix B at the end of the chapter). Prospective coding and key entry of all incoming information in the long-term follow-up office (questionnaires, office and telephone records, and return visits) are performed within 48 hours of receipt, using modified codes of the Systemized Nomenclature of Medicine (College of American Pathologists). This broad-based approach, performed by patients and physicians who are highly interested in remaining in contact with the transplant center, provides reliable lifelong medical updates. With this system all but 4% to 8% of surviving patients were contacted for updates within the last 2-year period.

REGIMEN-RELATED TOXICITIES

Standardized criteria for grading acute effects after high-dose chemoradiation therapy have been reported and are useful in reporting regimen-related toxicities.[13] Potential late effects of high-dose pretransplantation conditioning include the following.

Cataract Formation

Corticosteroids and total body irradiation (TBI) are known cataractogenic agents. Physicians at Fred Hutchinson Cancer Research Center recently reported an analysis of risk factors for cataracts in 492 adults after a median of 6 (range 1 to 18) years after marrow transplantation.[14] During this period of observation cataracts developed in 159 patients

(32%). The probability of cataract formation at 11 years after transplantation was 85%, 50%, 34%, and 19% for patients receiving 10 Gy single-dose TBI, greater than 12 Gy fractionated TBI, 12 Gy fractionated TBI, and no TBI, respectively (p <.0001). Among those developing cataracts the severity was greater in patients given single-dose TBI (59% probability of surgical extraction) than those given greater than 12 Gy fractionated TBI, 12 Gy fractionated TBI, or no TBI (33%, 22%, and 23% probability, respectively). As shown in Figure 23-4, patients given corticosteroids after transplantation had a higher probability of cataracts (45%) than those without steroids (38%) (p <.0001). The median time for cataract development was 2 to 5 years, and all groups reached a plateau at 7 years after transplantation. Thereafter the development of cataracts was unlikely.

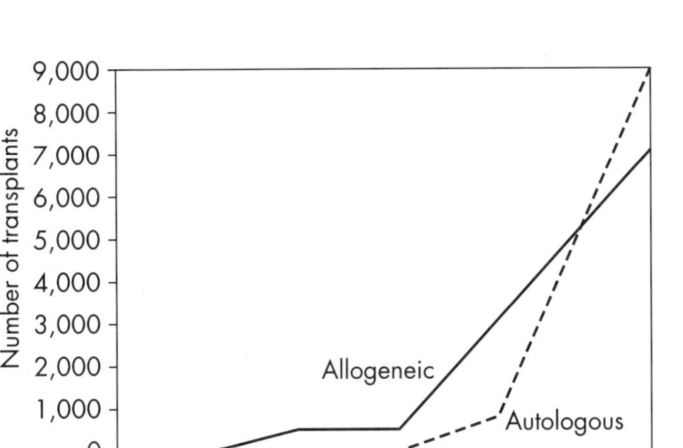

Figure 23-1 Growth of hemopoietic stem cell transplantation (annual number from 1970 to 1993). (From Armitage JO. Autologous Blood and Marrow Registry Newsletter, November 1994, p 2.)

Table 23-1 Late complications of stem cell transplantation

Regimen-related toxicity
Cataracts
Neurological conditions
Gonadal conditions
Endocrine conditions
Growth and development
Immunodeficiency
Infection
Chronic graft-versus-host disease
Bone disease
Relapse of malignancy
Secondary malignancy

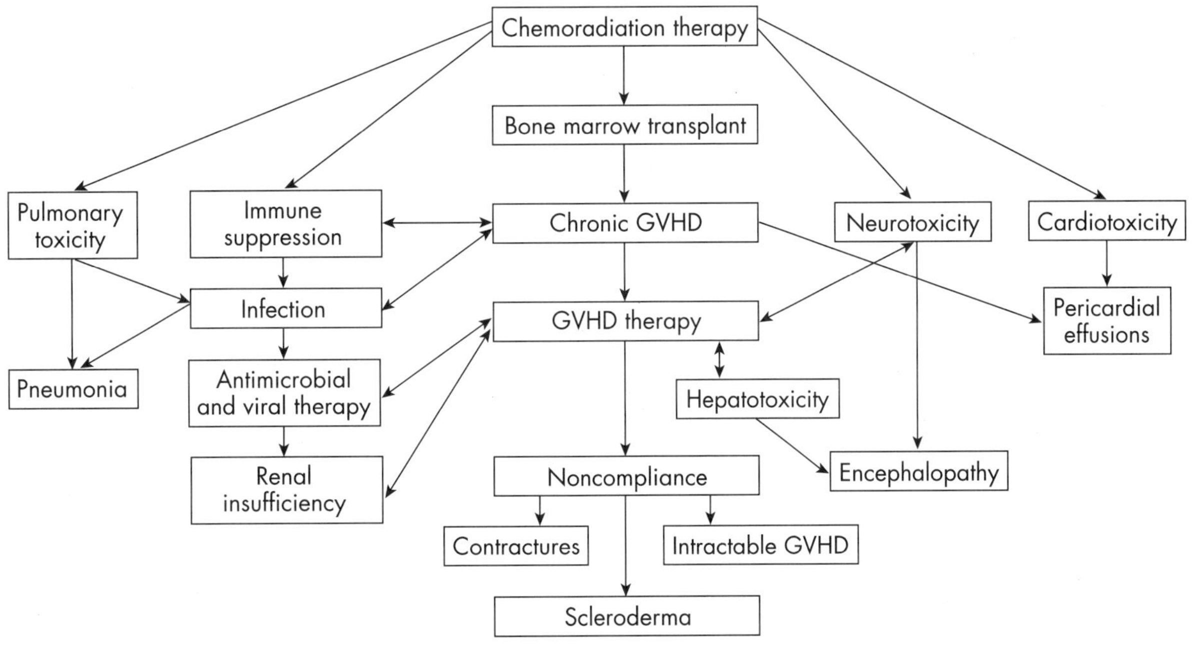

Figure 23-2 Interrelationships of late complications after stem cell transplantation. *GVHD*, Graft-versus-host disease. (From Nims JW. Late effects of bone marrow transplantation: a nursing perspective. In: Kasprisin CA, Snyder EL, editors. Bone marrow transplantation: a nursing perspective. Bethesda, Md: American Association of Blood Banks, 1990:45-57.)

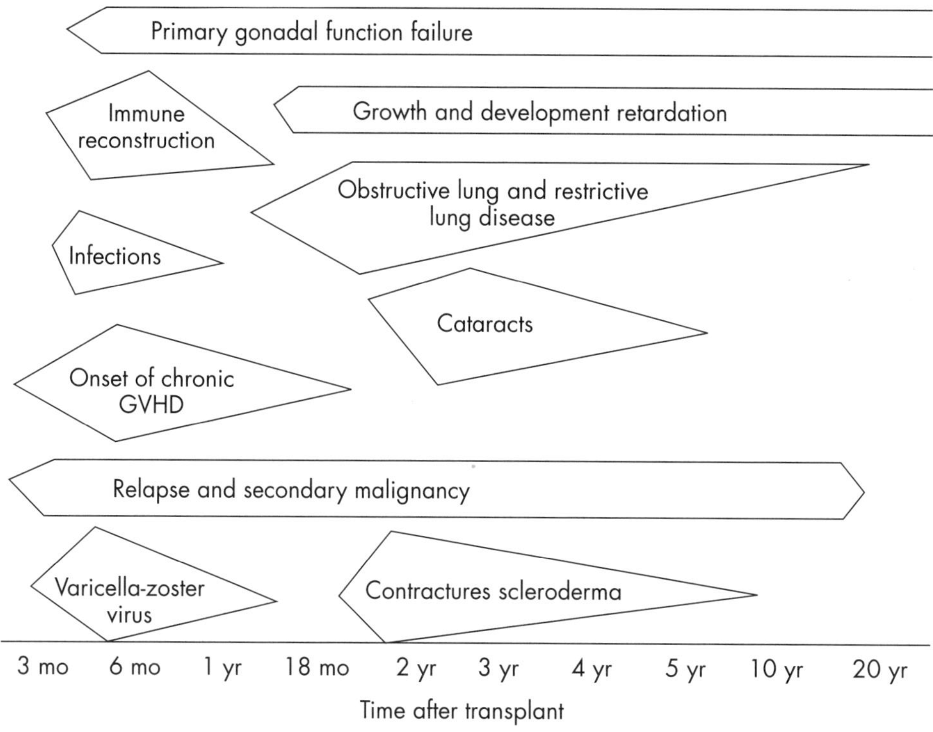

Figure 23-3 Time of onset of late complications. (From Nims JW. Late effects of bone marrow transplantation: a nursing perspective. In: Kasprisin CA, Snyder EL, editors. Bone marrow transplantation: a nursing perspective. Bethesda, Md: American Association of Blood Banks, 1990:45-57.)

Table 23-2 Karnofsky Performance Scale and Lansky Play-Performance Scale

KARNOFSKY PERFORMANCE SCALE* *(For use with persons ages ≥17 years)*			MODIFIED LANSKY PLAY-PERFORMANCE SCALE† *(For use with persons ages 1 through 16 years)*		
100%	=	Normal; no complaints; no evidence of disease	100%	=	Fully active, normal
90%	=	Able to carry on normal activity; minor signs or symptoms of disease	90%	=	Minor restrictions in physically strenuous activity
80%	=	Normal activity with effort; some signs or symptoms of disease	80%	=	Active, but tires more quickly
70%	=	Cares for self; unable to carry on normal activity or to do active work	70%	=	Both greater restriction of, and less time spent in, play activities
60%	=	Requires occasional assistance, but is able to care for most of own needs	60%	=	Up and around, but minimal active play; keeps busy with quieter activities
50%	=	Requires considerable assistance and frequent medical care	50%	=	Gets dressed but lies around much of the day; no active play; able to participate in all quiet play and activities
40%	=	Disabled; requires special care and assistance	40%	=	Mostly in bed; participates in quiet activities
30%	=	Severely disabled; hospitalization is indicated although death is not imminent	30%	=	Often sleeping; play entirely limited to very passive activities
20%	=	Hospitalization necessary; very sick; active supportive treatment necessary	20%	=	No play; does not get out of bed
10%	=	Moribund; fatal processes progressing rapidly	10%	=	Unresponsive
0%	=	Dead	0%	=	Dead

*From Karnofsky DA, Burchenal JH. The clinical evaluation of chemotherapeutic agents in cancer. In: MacLeod CM, editor. Evaluation of chemotherapeutic agents. New York: Columbia University Press, 1949:199-205.

†From Lansky SB, List MA, Lansky LL, Ritter-Sterr C, Miller DR. Cancer 1987;60:1651-6.

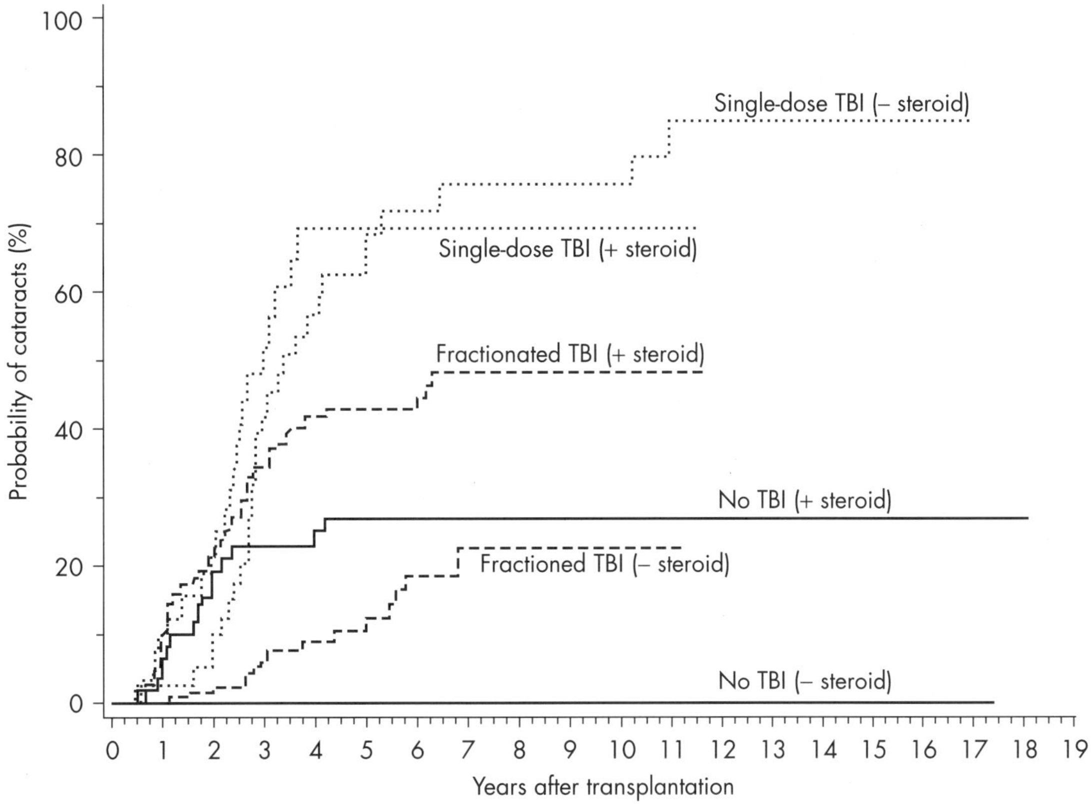

Figure 23-4 Probability of cataracts in patients who received 10 Gy total body irradiation *(TBI)* as a single dose *(bulleted line)* (+) with steroids ($n = 33$) or (–) without steroids ($n = 41$); greater than or equal to 12 Gy of fractionated TBI *(broken line)* (+) with steroids ($n = 250$) or (–) without steroids ($n = 128$); no TBI *(solid line)* (+) with steroids ($n = 60$) or (–) without steroids ($n = 25$). (From Benyunes MC, Sullivan KM, Deeg HJ, et al. Int J Radiat Oncol Biol Phys 1995;32:661-70.)

Neurological Complications

Late neurological complications may result from prior cranial irradiation, recurrent malignancy, intrathecal chemotherapy, or other drug toxicities. Leukoencephalopathy has been noted in 7% of patients who received either cranial irradiation or intrathecal chemotherapy before TBI and transplantation.[15] Mechlorethamine used as a preparative regimen and cyclosporine used as prophylaxis against or treatment of graft-versus-host disease have been associated with neurotoxicity.[16-18]

Endocrine and Growth Abnormalities

Overt hypothyroidism, compensated hypothyroidism, thyroiditis, and thyroid neoplasms may develop after irradiation of the thyroid gland.[19] Patients should be evaluated yearly with physical examinations and thyroid function tests. Thyroid deficiency was noted in 31% to 43% of patients after single-fraction TBI.[19,20] Fractionated TBI has decreased the incidence of compensated hypothyroidism from between 30% and 60% to between 15% and 25%.[19,21]

Growth hormone deficiency has not been observed after high-dose cyclophosphamide chemotherapy.[22] Some children with chronic graft-versus-host disease treated with corticosteroids may have growth arrest followed by normal growth after resolution of chronic graft-versus-host disease and discontinuation of steroid therapy. Busulfan is a preparative conditioning agent known to cross the blood-brain barrier. Growth hormone and growth rate deficiencies have been noted in children prepared with busulfan and cyclophosphamide; accordingly, these children may require growth hormone therapy.[23,24] Growth hormone deficiency has also been reported after TBI, and the incidence may exceed 90% in children prepared with TBI who received prior additional cranial irradiation for central nervous system leukemia.[24,25] Follow-up monitoring is vital so that these deficiencies can be detected early, since final height achieved with growth hormone replacement is inversely related to patient age at the onset of treatment.

Gonadal Dysfunction and Fertility

Gonadal dysfunction is a frequent result of high-dose chemoradiation therapy. In patients who receive only cyclophosphamide-containing regimens, most postpubertal males and females less than 26 years of age will regain gonadal function.[26] In contrast, patients prepared with TBI-containing regimens rarely have return of fertility.[27] Children age 8 years and older should be examined annually and assessed by Tanner Development Scores for grading of secondary sexual development.[28] Those with gonadal failure and delayed development of secondary sexual characteristics appear to benefit from sex hormone replacement therapy (combined with growth hormone supplements if indicated). Among men receiving busulfan-containing regimens, return of gonadal function has been noted in rare individuals as early as 2 years after transplantation. No return of gonadal function has been noted to date in women receiving busulfan-containing regimens.[24]

Gynecological and Obstetrical Care

Gynecological follow-up of postpubertal women studied 1 to 13 years after allogeneic transplantation showed atrophic abnormalities in 33 of 36 recipients of TBI regimens.[29] Recognition of these climacteric abnormalities can lead to early hormone replacement with long-term estrogen and progesterone supplements, thereby alleviating unnecessary discomfort, reducing the risk of osteoporosis, and improving the well-being of the transplant recipient. Obstetrical follow-up of stem cell transplant recipients requires careful attention to potential complications.[30] A review of pregnancies developing after stem cell transplantation in Seattle showed a 28% incidence of preterm delivery, a figure significantly higher than the expected incidence of 8% to 10%.[31] Low birth weight (1.5 to 2.5 kg) or very low birth weight (less than 1.5 kg) infants were observed in 29% of the deliveries, also higher than the expected incidence of 6.5%. The incidence of congenital abnormalities did not appear to differ from the 13% incidence of single congenital anomalies reported for the general population. However, longer follow-up is required to monitor for possible adverse effects of parental exposure to high-dose chemotherapy.

IMMUNODEFICIENCY AND IMMUNIZATION

All stem cell recipients experience immunological impairment for 6 to 12 months after transplantation.[32,33] The tempo of immunological recovery is prolonged by increasing human lymphocyte antigen disparity with the allogeneic donor and development of chronic graft-versus-host disease leading to both cellular and humoral immune defects.[34,35] Hypogammaglobulinemia may develop, and monitoring of serum immunoglobulin G levels and repletion with intravenous immunoglobulin are important to decrease the risk of infection.[36-38]

Reestablishment of immune function permits adoptive transfer of donor-derived, allergen-specific food or drug allergies.[39] Augmentation of disease-specific protective immunity should be given as booster immunizations for patients with low or absent antibody titers at 1 year after transplantation. At the first year, patients free of chronic graft-versus-host disease are likely to respond to booster immunizations with pneumococcal, inactivated polio, influenza, diphtheria, pertussis, tetanus toxoid, hepatitis B, and *Haemophilus influenzae* type B vaccines (Table 23-3). Antibody titers can be tested 2 and 4 weeks after vaccination to evaluate efficacy, and patients should be given the current influenza vaccine each November. Live virus biological vaccines (Sabin oral polio, measles-mumps-rubella, bacille Calmette-Guerin, and oral typhoid vaccines) carry risk in the immunocompromised host, but measles-mumps-rubella can be safely given more than 2 years after transplantation in patients free of chronic graft-versus-host disease and immunosuppressive drug treatment.[40] Contacts and family members should not receive oral polio vaccine during the first year after transplantation, since the patient may be at risk from live virus shedding. This may occur for up to 12 weeks after immunization of family members.

Table 23-3 Recommended immunizations after hematopoietic transplantation

Year 1*	Diphtheria-pertussis-tetanus *Haemophilus influenzae* conjugate Hepatitis B Influenza (repeat every November) Salk poliovirus (inactivated vaccine)
Year 2†	Measles-mumps-rubella
Family member	No Sabin poliovirus during year 1 (Measles-mumps-rubella does not pass to others)

*Patients with chronic graft-versus-host disease may not benefit.
†Only in patients free of chronic graft-versus-host disease and immunosuppressive treatment.

INFECTION

Prior studies have shown that chronic graft-versus-host disease is the major determinant of late infection after allogeneic transplantation and that encapsulated gram-positive organisms are common pathogens.[35,41-44] Physicians at Fred Hutchinson Cancer Research Center recently reported the incidence of late infection in 364 patients given human lymphocyte antigen–identical marrow and 79 patients given autologous marrow from 1985 to 1989.[4] Figure 23-5 depicts the time to first pulmonary infection after discharge. At 5 years after transplantation there was a highly significant difference in pulmonary infection: 52% in patients with chronic graft-versus-host disease, 24% in allograft recipients without chronic graft-versus-host disease, and 3% in autograft recipients. Similarly, the probability of developing sinusitis or otitis media was significantly increased in allogeneic compared with autologous recipients (Figure 23-6).

Varicella-zoster virus infection is seen in 30% to 45% of patients within the first year after stem cell transplantation.[45,46] Risk factors for varicella-zoster virus include allogeneic transplantation, graft-versus-host disease, and chronic immunosuppressive therapy. Cytomegalovirus disease is unusual past 100 days after transplantation. Although patients may excrete cytomegalovirus, clinically apparent late disease is uncommon. Improved supportive care with prophylactic antibiotics, antiviral agents, and, if indicated,

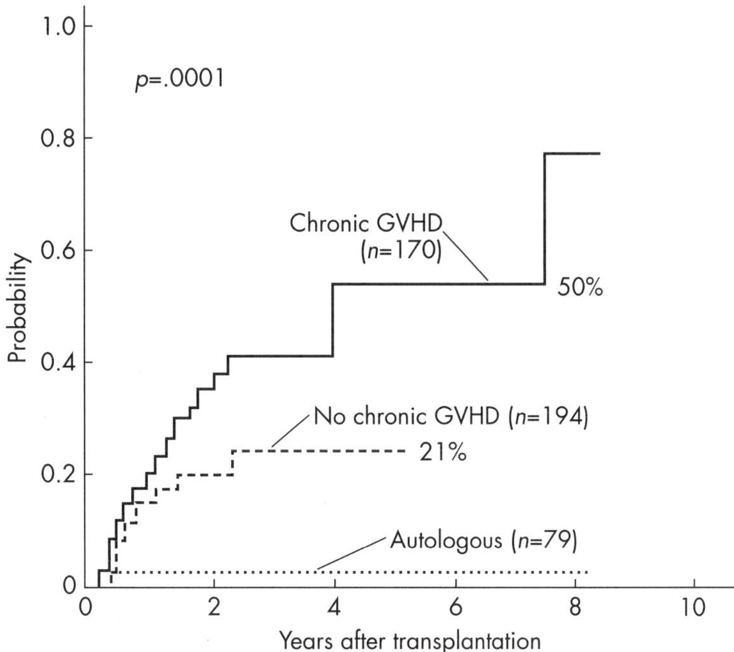

Figure 23-5 Probability of pulmonary infection after discharge home. Between 1985 and 1989, 364 human lymphocyte antigen–identical and 79 autologous marrow recipients returned home a median of 99 days after transplantation. *GVHD,* Graft-versus-host disease. (From Sullivan KM, Mori M, Sanders J, et al. Bone Marrow Transplant 1992;10:127-34.)

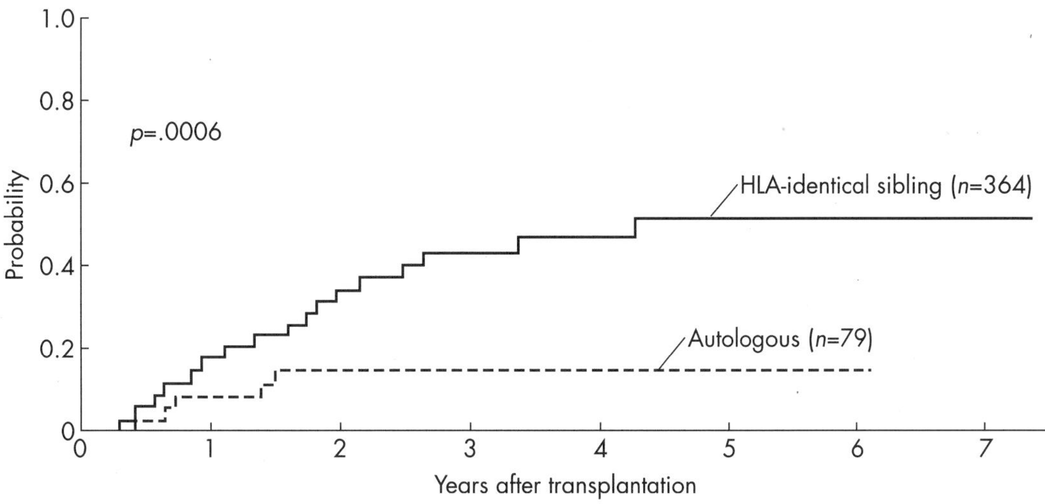

Figure 23-6 Probability of sinusitis or otitis media infection after discharge home. Between 1985 and 1989, 364 human lymphocyte antigen–identical and 79 autologous marrow recipients returned home a median of 99 days after transplantation. (From Sullivan KM, Mori M, Sanders J, et al. Bone Marrow Transplant 1992;10:127-34.)

intravenous immunoglobulin repletion has improved management of these patients.

CHRONIC GRAFT-VERSUS-HOST DISEASE

Chronic graft-versus-host disease is a pleiotropic disorder with clinical and pathological findings resembling several naturally occurring autoimmune diseases. Chronic graft-versus-host disease develops in approximately 33% of related human lymphocyte antigen–matched transplant recipients and 50% to 70% of unrelated or related mismatched recipients within 3 to 18 months after allogeneic transplantation.[47] In decreasing order of frequency, organ involvement includes the skin, mouth, eyes, sinuses, gastrointestinal tract, lungs, muscles, tendons, serous surfaces, and vagina.[48] Two clinical types of chronic graft-versus-host disease have been recognized. Patients with limited disease affecting only the skin and liver have a favorable untreated course; in contrast, those with extensive multiorgan disease have an unfavorable natural course.[49]

Chronic graft-versus-host disease is the major cause of transplantation-related morbidity and mortality after allogeneic stem cell transplantation. Morbidity is highest in patients with the progressive onset of chronic graft-versus-host disease directly following the acute form, intermediate in those with a quiescent onset after resolution of acute graft-versus-host disease, and lowest in patients with a de novo onset.[50,51] A prior study showed that without treatment only 18% of patients with extensive chronic graft-versus-host disease survived free of major disability.[49] Given late in the course of disease, prednisone or antithymocyte globulin appeared little better than no treatment, whereas early prednisone therapy appeared encouraging. In standard-risk patients (platelet counts greater than 100,000/µl), early treatment with prednisone alone improved outcome (21% mortality) to a greater degree than prednisone and azathioprine (40% mortality) because of an increased rate of infection in the azathioprine group.[52] In patients with high-risk disease (platelet counts less than 100,000/µl) survival after treatment with prednisone alone was only 26%. The addition of cyclosporine to an alternating-day regimen of prednisone has improved survival to 52% in high-risk patients.[53] However, mortality continues to be higher than in standard-risk patients because of increased rates of infection. New approaches to treatment include the use of FK506, thalidomide,[54] and phototherapy.[55] Bile acid displacement with ursodeoxycholic acid has been used as secondary treatment of refractory hepatic chronic graft-versus-host disease.[56] Other supportive care measures include long-term administration of trimethoprim-sulfamethoxazole to reduce the risk of bacterial and *Pneumocystis* infection and intravenous immunoglobulin repletion in patients with hypogammaglobulinemia.[57-59] Long-term administration of intravenous immunoglobulin in the absence of serum immunoglobulin G levels less than 500 mg/dl has not been beneficial.[60]

BONE DISEASE

Bone disease is a known complication of solid organ transplantation. The development of avascular necrosis, osteoporosis, and fractures after marrow transplantation is not uncommon, although the incidence and cause of bone disease are not well characterized.[61] Physicians at Fred Hutchinson Cancer Research Center recently reported on nine adult patients who were treated with prednisone and cyclosporine for chronic graft-versus-host disease and were evaluated for biochemical factors associated with skeletal turnover at initiation of immunosuppressive therapy and 9 months later.[62] Single and dual photon absorptiometry of the wrist and spine and dual energy x-ray absorptiometry of the spine were used to evaluate bone mineral density over time. Results showed a significant (greater than 2.5 times the test precision) decrease over 9 months in bone mineral density in three of five evaluable males and all three females. The findings indicated increased collagen and bone turnover, increased urinary magnesium and calcium excretion, and a significant risk of osteoporosis in patients receiving corticosteroid treatment for chronic graft-versus-host disease.

SECONDARY MALIGNANCY

TBI, immunodeficiency, infection, immunosuppression, chronic graft-versus-host disease, and antigenic stimulation and genetic factors have all been postulated to be involved in the development of secondary (new) malignancies in transplant recipients.[63-66] Physicians at Fred Hutchinson Cancer Research Center reported the cumulative incidence of secondary cancers in 330 patients with aplastic anemia who received cyclophosphamide alone as pretransplantation conditioning.[67] As shown in Figure 23-7, the cumulative incidence at 5 years was 0.4% (95% confidence interval 0 to 1.1), at 10 years was 1.4% (0 to 3.4), and at 15 years was 4.2% (0.9 to 8.6).

Data from European groups indicated a higher rate of neoplasms, suggesting that pretransplantation irradiation was a major determinant of late malignancies in patients with aplastic anemia.[68] To further define these interactions, 700 patients with severe aplastic anemia treated with allogeneic marrow transplantation in Seattle or in Paris were reviewed.[69] A malignancy developed in 23 patients 1.4 to 221 (median 91) months after transplantation, for a Kaplan-Meier estimate of 14% (confidence interval 4 to 24) at 20 years. Proportional hazards models indicated that azathioprine therapy ($p < .0001$) and the diagnosis of Fanconi's anemia ($p < .0001$) were significant factors for development of secondary malignancies for all patients. Irradiation was a significant factor ($p = .004$) only if the time-dependent variable azathioprine was not included in the analysis. If only non–Fanconi's anemia patients were considered, azathioprine ($p = .0043$), age ($p = .025$), and irradiation ($p = .042$) were independent risk factors for late secondary neoplasms.

RECURRENT MALIGNANCY

Prior experience has indicated poor survival in patients with recurrence of original malignancy after marrow transplantation.[70] In some patients relapsed leukemia has been successfully treated with second transplantations, but resistant disease and regimen-related toxicities generally lead to high mortality.[71] With the introduction of molecular probes to detect minimal residual malignant disease, new approaches for follow-up are being applied. For patients with chronic myelogenous leukemia, routine monitoring includes marrow and peripheral blood molecular determinations every 6 months after transplantation through year 3, then annual evaluations through year 5. Polymerase chain reaction detection of the BCR/abl fusion transcript 6 or more months after transplantation appears to predict risk of sub-

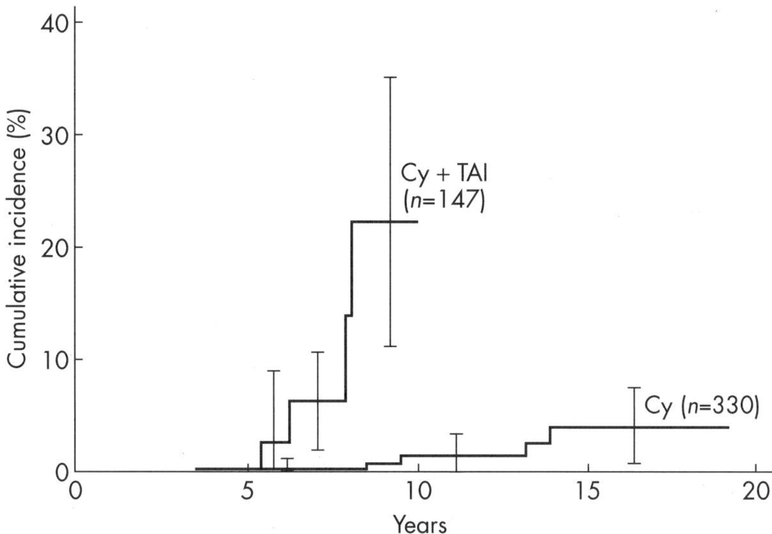

Figure 23-7 Cumulative incidence of secondary malignancy in 330 patients with aplastic anemia given marrow transplantations from family members. Brackets indicate the 5th through 95th percentile confidence intervals. *Cy,* Cyclophosphamide; *TAI,* thoracoabdominal irradiation. (From Witherspoon RP, Storb R, Pepe M, Longton G, Sullivan KM. Blood 1992;79:289.)

sequent relapse.[72] These patients with residual disease could be considered for treatment with alpha-interferon during early molecular or cytogenetic relapse.[73]

Recurrent leukemia after allogeneic transplantation may also be successfully treated with donor leukocyte infusions. This benefit derives from an apparent graft-versus-leukemia effect associated with allogeneic stem cells that recognize and destroy host histocompatibility antigens or tumor-associated antigens.[74,75] Donor leukocyte infusions have been used successfully to treat patients with recurrent leukemia and Epstein-Barr virus–associated lymphoproliferative disorders.[76,77] Thus follow-up monitoring for malignancy as outlined in this and other chapters is an integral part of the care of these patients with cancer.

QUALITY OF LIFE

Recovery from a transplantation is a dynamic process in which physical and psychosocial aspects are joined. Quality of life is a multidimensional construct composed minimally of four domains: physical function, psychological function, social role function, and disease and treatment symptoms. Recent studies examining the medical and psychosocial sequelae of marrow transplantation have reported that most survivors do relatively well, while a smaller group continues to experience less than optimal quality of life.[78-82] Many of these cross-sectional studies have been limited by lack of pretransplantation baseline assessments, small sample sizes, limited scope, and follow-up of less than 5 years. Physicians at Fred Hutchinson Cancer Research Center conducted a prospective analysis of 67 adults before and after allogeneic transplantation.[83] Physical function was most impaired at 90 days after transplantation, with a return to pretransplantation levels of functioning in most areas by 1 year. By 2 years after transplantation 68% of patients had returned to full-time work, and only 9% of 4-year survivors failed to return to full-time occupations. Before transplantation 27% of patients reported depression and 41% reported elevated anxiety. Mean levels of anxiety and depression did not change during the first year. In a multivariate analysis greater emotional distress at 1 year was predicted by pretransplantation family conflict and nonmarried status. Impaired physical recovery at 1 year was predicted by more severe chronic graft-versus-host disease, pretransplantation physical impairment, and family conflict. Family relationships appeared to be important determinants of recovery. The large majority of long-term survivors returned to full-time employment with normal physical and psychosocial functioning, although recovery took longer than 1 year for approximately 40% of patients.

In another study physicians at Fred Hutchinson Cancer Research Center reported a cross-sectional analysis of 125 adults surviving a mean of 10 (range 6 to 18) years after allogeneic (87%) or autologous/syngeneic (13%) transplantation.[84] Seven wide-ranging tests measured physical, psychological, social functioning, and disease and treatment symptoms. Eight percent rated their quality of life as good to excellent, and 5% rated it as poor. The most frequently cited problem during recovery was a perceived lack of social support from family and friends. Although lingering complaints such as fatigue, sexual dysfunction, and sleep disturbances were noted, most survivors judged these to be of low severity and 88% of the 125 patients said the benefits of transplantation outweighed the side effects.

Table 23-4 Quality-of-life ratings

YEARS AFTER BMT	SURVEYS (N)	PATIENTS (N)	PATIENT SELF-RATING (1-10) (s.d.) PSYCHOLOGICAL HEALTH	MEMORY TBI	MEMORY (AGE > 20) NO TBI	OVERALL HEALTH	PHYSICIAN RATING LPPS OR KPS (s.d.)
1-2	1,228	802	8.1 (1.9)	7.7 (2.0)	7.6 (2.1)	7.9 (1.9)	92.1 (12.8)
3-5	907	576	8.5 (2.2)	7.9 (2.0)	7.6 (2.2)	8.4 (1.7)	96.0 (8.8)
6-9	619	375	8.6 (1.8)	7.9 (2.1)	7.9 (1.9)	8.5 (1.7)	96.7 (8.5)
10+	607	312	8.3 (1.9)	7.6 (2.3)	7.9 (2.3)	8.2 (2.1)	95.7 (9.9)

From Campbell J, Sullivan KM, Leisenring W, et al. Blood 1995;86:620a.
BMT, Bone marrow transplantation; *TBI,* total body irradiation; *LPPS,* Lansky Play-Performance Score; *KPS,* Karnofsky Performance Score.

Table 23-5 Follow-up of patients after stem cell transplantation (adults in complete remission): University of Washington Medical Center/Fred Hutchinson Cancer Research Center

	YEAR 1	2	3	4	5
Office visit	9-18*	3-6	2-4	1-2	1-2
Karnofsky Performance Scale evaluation	1	1	1	1	1
Ophthalmological evaluation†	1	1	1	1	1
Oral medicine evaluation	1	1	1	1	1
Engraftment status‡	1	1	1	1	1
Gynecological evaluation§	1	1	1	1	1
Mammogram¶	1	1	1	1	1
Endocrine evaluation**	1	1	1	1	1
Monitoring for malignancy††	1	1	1	1	1
Pulmonary function tests	1	0	0	0	1
Immunizations‡‡	1	0	0	0	0

*Performed between 3 and 12 months after transplantation and discharge home.
†Ophthalmological evaluation consists of a comprehensive examination including slit lamp biomicroscopy and Schirmer's test.
‡Engraftment status assessment comprises complete blood count and markers for donor origin hematopoiesis, including DNA polymorphism studies for sex-matched donor/recipient pairs or cytogenetic or in situ hybridization studies for Y body determination in sex-mismatched pairs.
§Gynecological evaluation includes pelvic examination, Papanicolaou smear, breast examination, and endocrine evaluation, which involves the tests listed below.
¶For total body irradiation recipients aged 35 years and older.
**Endocrine evaluation includes serum thyroid-stimulating hormone, thyroxine, follicle-stimulating hormone (in males), and estradiol levels (in females).
††Monitoring at office visits for original malignancy as outlined in other chapters in this volume. Patients with chronic myelogenous leukemia have molecular studies for BCR/abl gene transcript and marrow cytogenetics for the Philadelphia chromosome annually for 5 years after transplantation.
‡‡Immunizations are detailed in Table 23-3.

Table 23-6 Follow-up of patients after stem cell transplantation (children in complete remission): University of Washington Medical Center/Fred Hutchinson Cancer Research Center

	YEAR 1	2	3	4	5
Office visit	9-18*	3-6	2-4	1-2	1-2
Lansky Play-Performance Scale evaluation	1	1	1	1	1
Ophthalmological evaluation†	1	1	1	1	1
Oral medicine evaluation	1	1	1	1	1
Engraftment status‡	1	1	1	1	1
Tanner Development Score§	1	1	1	1	1
Growth hormone testing¶	1	1	1	1	1
Endocrine evaluation**	1	1	1	1	1
Monitoring for malignancy††	1	1	1	1	1
Pulmonary function tests	1	0	0	0	1
Immunizations‡‡	1	0	0	0	0

*Performed between 3 and 12 months after transplantation and discharge home.
†Ophthalmological evaluation consists of a comprehensive examination, including slit lamp biomicroscopy and Schirmer's test.
‡Engraftment status assessment comprises complete blood count and markers for donor origin hematopoiesis, including DNA polymorphism studies for sex-matched donor/recipient pairs or cytogenetic or in situ hybridization studies for Y body determination in sex-mismatched pairs.
§Tanner Development Score includes breast, pubic, and axillary hair and external genital score.
¶Growth hormone testing includes 12-hour spontaneous and stimulated testing.
**Endocrine evaluation includes serum thyroid-stimulating hormone, thyroxine, follicle-stimulating hormone, and when patients are 8 years of age or older, testosterone levels (in males) and estradiol levels (in females).
††Monitoring at office visits for original malignancy as outlined in other chapters in this volume.
‡‡Immunizations are detailed in Table 23-3.

The study was confirmed in a larger comparison of patient self-ratings of health and concurrent performance ratings assigned by the primary care physician.[85] Self-assessments (see Appendix B at the end of the chapter) were given on an analog scale (1 = very poor, 10 = excellent) and included overall physical health, psychological health, memory and concentration, and symptom severity. Concurrent mailers to physicians (see Appendix A at the end of the chapter) rated patients' functional performance (Table 23-2) on scales tested for validity and reliability.[86,87] During the 3 years of the study, 3,361 questionnaires were returned by 1,452 patients, including 312 patients surviving 10 to 24 years after transplantation. Of the 1,452 patients, 407 (28%) were less than 20 years of age at the time of transplantation, 982 (68%) received greater than or equal to 920 cGy TBI, and 556 (38%) developed chronic graft-versus-host disease. As shown in Table 23-4, patient self-ratings and physician performance ratings showed improvements after the first year and stable ratings thereafter (data are given as mean values plus or minus the standard deviation). Among patients greater than 20 years of age at transplantation, there was no apparent difference in self-reports of memory and concentration between patients who did or did not receive TBI. Throughout the time periods patients rated symptom severity at 3.1 (10 = most severe). Although symptoms may persist after transplantation, the magnitude for most was judged not severe and overall health and performance were rated highly.

SUMMARY

After more than 25 years of marrow and blood cell transplantation, it is considered the treatment of choice for a variety of hematological and immunological disorders. In some patients the impact of delayed complications is noteworthy and efforts at preventing and minimizing these complications are vital. Tables 23-5 and 23-6 provide a summary of follow-up testing after stem cell transplantation. Continued observation and long-term follow-up are necessary to the well-being of the patient and the assessment of the success of the transplantation procedure.

REFERENCES

1. Bortin MM, Horowitz MM, Rimm AA. Increasing utilization of allogeneic bone marrow transplantation: results of the 1988-1990 survey. Ann Intern Med 1992;116:505-12.
2. Silberman G, Crosse MG, Peterson EA, et al. Availability and appropriateness of allogeneic bone marrow transplantation for chronic myeloid leukemia in 10 countries. N Engl J Med 1994;331:1063-7.
3. Sullivan KM. World transplant records, 1993: bone marrow. In: Terasaki PI, Cecka JM, editors. Clinical transplants 1993. Los Angeles: UCLA Tissue Typing Laboratory, 1994:588-96.
4. Sullivan KM, Mori M, Sanders J, et al. Late complications of allogeneic and autologous transplantation. Bone Marrow Transplant 1992;10:127-34.
5. Nims JW. Late effects of bone marrow transplantation: a nursing perspective. In: Kasprisin CA, Snyder EL, editors. Bone marrow transplantation: a nursing perspective. Arlington, Va: American Association of Blood Banks, 1990:45-57.
6. Peters WP, Ross M, Vredenburgh JJ, et al. The use of intensive clinic support to permit outpatient autologous bone marrow transplantation for breast cancer. Semin Oncol 1994;21:25-31.
7. Flowers ME, Sullivan KM. Preadmission procedures, marrow transplant hospitalization, and posttransplant outpatient monitoring. In: Atkinson K, editor. Textbook on bone marrow transplantation. London: Cambridge University Press, 1992:75-86.
8. Rowe JM, Ciobanu N, Ascensao J, et al. Recommended guidelines for the management of autologous and allogeneic bone marrow transplantation: a report from the Eastern Cooperative Oncology Group (ECOG). Ann Intern Med 1994;120:143-58.
9. Phillips G, Armitage J, Bearman S, et al. American society for blood and marrow transplantation guidelines for clinical centers. Biol Blood Marrow Transplant. In press, 1995.
10. Jones RB, Shpall EJ. Dissemination and commercialization of hematopoietic progenitor cell transplantation [editorial]. Hematotherapy 1994;3:93-4.
11. Buckner CD. Reply to editorial "Dissemination and commercialization of hematopoietic progenitor cell transplantation." Hematotherapy 1994;3:249-50.
12. Clift R, Goldman J, Gratwohl, Horowitz M. Proposals for standardized reporting of results of bone marrow transplantation for leukaemia. Bone Marrow Transplant 1989;4:445-8.
13. Bearman SI, Appelbaum FR, Buckner CD, et al. Regimen-related toxicity in patients undergoing bone marrow transplantation. J Clin Oncol 1988;6:1562-8.
14. Benyunes MC, Sullivan KM, Deeg HJ, et al. Cataracts after bone marrow transplant: long-term follow-up of adults with fractionated total body irradiation. Int J Radiat Oncol Biol Phys 1995;32:661-70.
15. Thompson CB, Sanders JE, Flournoy N, Buckner CD, Thomas ED. The risks of central nervous system relapse and leukoencephalopathy in patients receiving marrow transplants for acute leukemia. Blood 1986;67:195-9.
16. Sullivan KM, Storb R, Shulman HM, et al. Immediate and delayed neurotoxicity after mechlorethamine preparation for bone marrow transplantation. Ann Intern Med 1982;27:182-9.
17. Atkinson K, Biggs J, Darveniza P, et al. Cyclosporine-associated central nervous system toxicity after allogeneic bone marrow transplantation. Transplantation 1984;38:34-7.
18. De Groen PC, Aksammit AJ, Rakela J, et al. Central nervous system toxicity after liver transplantation: the role of cyclosporine and cholesterol. N Engl J Med 1987;317:861-6.
19. Sanders JE. Endocrine problems in children after bone marrow transplant for hematologic malignancies. Bone Marrow Transplant 1991; 8(Suppl 1):2-4.
20. Sklar CA, Kim TH, Ramsay NK. Thyroid dysfunction among long-term survivors of bone marrow transplantation. Am J Med 1982;73: 688-94.
21. Serafino L, Arcese W, Papa G, D'Armiento M. Thyroid and pituitary function following allogeneic bone marrow transplant. Arch Intern Med 1988;148:1066-71.
22. Sanders JE. The impact of marrow transplant preparative regimens on subsequent growth and development. Semin Hematol 1991;28:244-9.
23. Wingard JR, Plotnick LP, Freemer CS, et al. Growth in children after bone marrow transplantation: busulfan plus cyclophosphamide versus cyclophosphamide plus total body irradiation. Blood 1992;79:1068-73.
24. Sanders JE. Growth and development after bone marrow transplant. In: Forman SJ, Blume KJ, Thomas ED, editors. Bone marrow transplantation. Boston: Blackwell Scientific Publishers, 1994:527-37.
25. Sanders JE, Pritchard S, Mahoney P, et al. Growth and development following marrow transplantation for leukemia. Blood 1986;68:1129-35.
26. Sanders JE, Buckner CD, Amos D, et al. Ovarian function following marrow transplantation for aplastic anemia of leukemia. J Clin Oncol 1988;6:813-8.
27. Sanders JE, Buckner CD, Leonard JM, et al. Late effects on gonadal function of cyclophosphamide, total-body irradiation, and marrow transplantation. Transplantation 1983;36:252-5.
28. Tanner JM, Whitehouse RH. Clinical longitudinal standards for height, weight, height velocity, weight velocity and stages of puberty. Arch Dis Child 1976;51:170-9.

29. Schubert MA, Sullivan KM, Schubert MM, et al. Gynecological abnormalities following allogeneic bone marrow transplantation. Bone Marrow Transplant 1990;5:425-30.
30. Hinterberger-Fischer M, Kier P, Kalhs P, et al. Fertility, pregnancies and offspring complications after bone marrow transplantation. Bone Marrow Transplant 1991;7:5-9.
31. Sanders JE, Hawley L, Levy W, et al. Pregnancies following high-dose cyclophosphamide with or without high-dose busulfan or total body irradiation and bone marrow transplantation. Blood 1996;87:3045-52.
32. Witherspoon RP, Lum LG, Storb R. Immunologic reconstitution after human marrow grafting. Semin Hematol 1984;21:2-10.
33. Olsen GA, Gockerman JP, Bast RC Jr, Borowitz M, Peters WP. Altered immunologic reconstitution after standard-dose chemotherapy or high-dose chemotherapy with autologous bone marrow support. Transplantation 1988;46:57-60.
34. Atkinson K, Farewell V, Storb R, et al. Analysis of late infections after human bone marrow transplantation: role of genotypic nonidentity between marrow donor and recipient and of nonspecific suppressor cells in patients with chronic graft-versus-host disease. Blood 1982;60:714-20.
35. Paulin T, Ringdén O, Nilsson B. Immunological recovery after bone marrow transplantation: role of age, graft-versus-host disease, prednisolone treatment and infections. Bone Marrow Transplant 1987;1: 317-28.
36. Aucouturier P, Barra A, Intrator L, et al. Long lasting IgG subclass and antibacterial polysaccharide antibody deficiency after allogeneic bone marrow transplantation. Blood 1987;70:779-85.
37. Sullivan KM, Kopecky KJ, Jocom J, et al. Immunomodulatory and antimicrobial efficacy of intravenous immunoglobulin in bone marrow transplantation. N Engl J Med 1990;323:705-12.
38. Bass EB, Powe NR, Goodman SN, et al. Efficacy of immune globulin in preventing complications of bone marrow transplantation: a meta-analysis. Bone Marrow Transplant 1993;12:273-82.
39. Agosti JM, Sprenger JD, Lum LG, et al. Transfer of allergen-specific IgE-mediated hypersensitivity with allogeneic bone marrow transplantation. N Engl J Med 1988;319:1623-8.
40. Ljungman P, Fridell E, Lönnqvuist B, et al. Efficacy and safety of vaccination of marrow transplant recipients with a live attenuated measles, mumps, and rubella vaccine. J Infect Dis 1989;159:610-5.
41. Winston DJ, Gale RP, Meyer DV, Young LS. Infectious complications of human bone marrow transplantation. Medicine 1979;58:1-31.
42. Atkinson K, Storb R, Prentice RL, et al. Analysis of late infections in 89 long-term survivors of bone marrow transplantation. Blood 1979; 53:720-31.
43. Bowden RA. Infections in patients with graft-versus-host disease. In: Burakoff SJ, Deeg HJ, Ferrarra J, Atkinson K, editors. Graft-versus-host disease: immunology, pathophysiology, and treatment. New York: Marcel Dekker, 1990:525-38.
44. Winston DJ, Schiffman G, Wang DC, et al. Pneumococcal infections after human bone marrow transplantation. Ann Intern Med 1979; 91:835-41.
45. Locksley RM, Flournoy N, Sullivan KM, Meyers JD. Infection with varicella-zoster virus after marrow transplantation. J Infect Dis 1985;152:1172-81.
46. Schuchter LM, Wingard JR, Piantadosi S, Burns WH, Santos GW, Saral R. Herpes zoster infection after autologous bone marrow transplantation. Blood 1989;74:1424-7.
47. Sullivan KM, Agura E, Anasetti C, et al. Chronic graft-versus-host disease and other late complications of bone marrow transplantation. Semin Hematol 1991;28:250-9.
48. Sullivan KM. Graft-versus-host disease. In: Forman SJ, Blume KJ, Thomas ED, editors. Bone marrow transplantation. Boston: Blackwell Scientific Publishers, 1994:339-62.
49. Sullivan KM, Shulman HM, Storb R, et al. Chronic graft-versus-host disease in 52 patients: adverse natural course and successful treatment with combination immunosuppression. Blood 1981;57:267-76.
50. Wingard JR, Piantadosi S, Vogelsang GB, et al. Predictors of death from chronic graft-versus-host disease after bone marrow transplantation. Blood 1989;74:1428-35.
51. Atkinson K. Chronic graft-versus-host disease [review]. Bone Marrow Transplant 1990;5:69-82.
52. Sullivan KM, Witherspoon RP, Storb R, et al. Prednisone and azathioprine compared with prednisone and placebo for treatment of chronic graft-versus-host disease: prognostic influence of prolonged thrombocytopenia after allogeneic marrow transplantation. Blood 1988;72:546-54.
53. Sullivan KM, Witherspoon RP, Storb R, et al. Alternating-day cyclosporine and prednisone for treatment of high-risk graft-versus-host disease. Blood 1988;72:555-61.
54. Vogelsang GB, Farmer ER, Hess AD, et al. Thalidomide for the treatment of chronic graft versus host disease. N Engl J Med 1992; 326:1055-8.
55. Hymes SR, Morison WL, Farmer ER, Walters LL, Tutschka PJ, Santos GW. Methoxalen and ultraviolet A radiation in treatment of chronic cutaneous graft-versus-host reaction. Acad Dermatol 1985; 12:30-7.
56. Fried RH, Murakami CS, Fisher LD, Willson RA, Sullivan KM, McDonald GB. Ursodeoxycholic acid treatment of refractory chronic graft-versus-host of the liver. Ann Intern Med 1992;116:624-9.
57. Clark JG, Schwartz DA, Flournoy N, Sullivan KM, Crawford SW, Thomas ED. Risk factors for airflow obstruction in recipients of bone marrow transplants. Ann Intern Med 1987;107:648-56.
58. Holland HK, Wingard JR, Beschorner WE, Saral R, Santos GW. Bronchiolitis obliterans in bone marrow transplantation and its relationship to chronic graft-v-host disease and low serum IgG. Blood 1988;72:621-7.
59. Sheridan JF, Tutschka PJ, Sedmak DD, Copelan EA. Immunoglobulin G subclass deficiency and pneumococcal infection after allogeneic bone marrow transplantation. Blood 1990;75:1583-6.
60. Sullivan KM, Storek J, Kopecky KJ, et al. A controlled trial of long-term administration of intravenous immunoglobulin to prevent late infection and chronic graft-versus-host disease following marrow transplantation: clinical outcome and effect on subsequent immune recovery. Biol Blood Marrow Transplant 1996;2:44-53.
61. Kelly PJ, Atkinson K, Ward RL, Sambrook PN, Biggs JC, Eisman JA. Reduced bone mineral density in men and women with allogeneic bone marrow transplantation. Transplantation 1990;50:881-3.
62. Stern JM, Chestnut CH 3d, Bruemmer B, et al. Bone density loss during treatment of chronic GVHD. Bone Marrow Transplant 1996;17:395-400.
63. Penn I. Tumors after renal and cardiac transplantation. In: Antin JH, Shulman LN, editors. Hematology/oncology clinics of North America, Vol 7. Philadelphia: WB Saunders Company, 1993:431.
64. Witherspoon RP, Fischer LD, Schoch G, et al. Secondary cancers after bone marrow transplantation for leukemia or aplastic anemia. N Engl J Med 1989;321:784-9.
65. Witherspoon RP, Deeg HJ, Storb R. Secondary malignancies after marrow transplantation for leukemia or aplastic anemia. Transplantation 1994;57:1413-8.
66. Curtis RE, Rowlings PA, Deeg HJ, et al. Solid cancers after bone marrow transplantation. N Engl J Med 1997;336:897.
67. Witherspoon RP, Storb R, Pepe M, Longton G, Sullivan KM. Cumulative incidence of secondary solid malignant tumors in aplastic anemia patients given marrow grafts after conditioning with chemotherapy alone [letter]. Blood 1992;79:289.
68. Socié G, Henry-Amar M, Bacigalupo A, et al. Malignant tumors occurring after treatment of aplastic anemia. N Engl J Med 1993; 329:1152-7.
69. Deeg, HJ, Socié G, Schoch G, et al. Malignancies after marrow transplantation for aplastic anemia and Fanconi anemia: a joint Seattle and Paris analysis of results in 700 patients. Blood 1996;87:386-92.
70. Mortimer J, Blinder MA, Schulman S, et al. Relapse of acute leukemia after marrow transplantation: natural history and results of subsequent therapy. J Clin Oncol 1989;7:50-7.

71. Radich JP, Sanders JE, Buckner CD, et al. Second allogeneic marrow transplantation for patients with recurrent leukemia after initial transplant with total-body irradiation-containing regimens. J Clin Oncol 1993;11:304-13.
72. Radich JP, Gehly G, Gooley T, et al. Polymerase chain reaction detection of the bcr-abl fusion transcript after allogeneic marrow transplantation for chronic myeloid leukemia: results and implications in 346 patients. Blood 1995;85:2632-8.
73. Higano CS, Raskind WH, Singer JW. Use of alpha interferon for treatment of relapse of chronic myelogenous leukemia in chronic phase after allogeneic bone marrow transplantation. Blood 1992;80:1437-42.
74. Weiden PL, Sullivan KM, Flournoy N, Storb R, Thomas ED. Antileukemic effect of chronic graft-versus-host disease: contribution to improved survival after allogeneic marrow transplantation. N Engl J Med 1981;304:1529-33.
75. Sullivan KM, Storb R, Buckner CD, et al. Graft-versus-host disease as adoptive immunotherapy in patients with advanced hematologic neoplasms. N Engl J Med 1989;320:828-34.
76. Kolb HJ, Mittermüller J, Clemm C, et al. Donor leukocyte transfusions for treatment of recurrent chronic myelogenous leukemia in marrow transplant patients. Blood 1990;76:2462-5.
77. Papadopoulos EB, Ladanyi M, Emanuel D, et al. Infusions of donor leukocytes to treat Epstein-Barr virus–associated lymphoproliferative disorders after allogeneic bone marrow transplantation. N Engl J Med 1994;330:1185-91.
78. Andrykowski MA, Altmaier EM, Barnett RL, Otis ML, Gingrich R, Henslee-Downey PJ. The quality of life in adult survivors of allogeneic bone marrow transplantation: correlates and comparison with matched renal transplant recipients. Transplantation 1990;50:399-406.
79. Wingard JR, Curbow B, Baker F, Piantadosi S. Health, functional status, and employment of adult survivors of bone marrow transplantation. Ann Intern Med 1991;114:113-8.
80. Chao NJ, Tierney DK, Bloom JR, et al. Dynamic assessment of quality of life after autologous bone marrow transplantation. Blood 1992;80:825-30.
81. Wingard JR, Curbow B, Gaker F, Zabora J, Piantadosi S. Sexual satisfaction in survivors of bone marrow transplantation. Bone Marrow Transplant 1992;9:185-90.
82. Schmidt GM, Niland JC, Forman SJ, et al. Extended follow-up in 212 long-term allogeneic bone marrow transplant survivors: issues of quality of life. Transplantation 1993;55:551-7.
83. Syrjala KL, Chapko MK, Vitaliano PP, Cummings C, Sullivan KM. Recovery after allogeneic marrow transplantation: prospective study of predictors of long-term physical and psychosocial functioning. Bone Marrow Transplant 1993;11:319-27.
84. Bush NE, Haberman M, Donaldson G, Sullivan KM. Quality of life in 125 adults surviving 6-18 years after bone marrow transplantation. Soc Sci Med 1995;40:479-90.
85. Campbell J, Sullivan KM, Leisenring W, et al. Quality of life as self reported by 1452 bone marrow transplant recipients spanning 24 years [abstract]. Blood 1995;86:620a.
86. Mor V, Laliberte L, Morris JN, Wiemann M: The Karnofsky performance status scale: an examination of its reliability and validity in a research setting. Cancer 1984;53:2002-7.
87. Schag CC, Heinrich RL, Ganz PA. Karnofsky performance status revisited: reliability, validity, and guidelines. J Clin Oncol 1984;2:187-93.
88. Lansky SB, List MA, Lansky LL, Ritter-Sterr C, Miller DR. The measurement of performance in childhood cancer patients. Cancer 1987;60:1651-6.
89. Karnofsky DA, Burchenal, JH. The clinical evaluation of chemotherapeutic agents in cancer. In: MacLeod CM, editor. Evaluation of chemotherapeutic agents. New York: Columbia University Press, 1949:199-205.
90. Armitage JO. Research potential of the ABMTR Database. Autologous Blood and Marrow Registry Newsletter. November 1994, p 2.

➢ COUNTERPOINT

Memorial Sloan-Kettering Cancer Center

DAVID J. STRAUS

Sullivan and Siadak provide an excellent review of the complications of bone marrow and peripheral blood progenitor transplantation and of the policies for follow-up of patients undergoing those procedures at Fred Hutchinson Cancer Research Center. Physicians at the center pioneered the procedures, and their experience and resultant policies have evolved over the past two decades. This review for the most part reflects that experience.

Table 23-7 Follow-up of patients after stem cell transplantation (Hodgkin's lymphoma in complete remission)*: Memorial Sloan-Kettering Cancer Center

	YEAR				
	1	2	3	4	5
Office visit	4	3	3	2	1
Complete blood count	4	3	3	2	1
Chest x-ray	4	3	3	2	1
Liver function tests	4	3	3	2	1
Erythrocyte sedimentation rate	4	3	3	2	1
Thyroid profile	2	2	2	2	1
Abdominal computed tomography	2	2	2	2	1
Pelvic computed tomography	2	2	2	2	1
Mammography†	0	1	1	1	1

*The follow-up strategy recommended here is identical to the strategy I recommended for the follow-up of patients treated for Hodgkin's lymphoma in Chapter 22.
†Performed for female patients over the age of 30 who have received mantle irradiation.

Table 23-8 Follow-up of patients after stem cell transplantation (intermediate- or high-grade non-Hodgkin's lymphoma in complete remission)*: Memorial Sloan-Kettering Cancer Center

	YEAR				
	1	2	3	4	5
Office visit	4†	3	3	2	1
Complete blood count	4†	3	3	2	1
Chest x-ray	4†	3	3	2	1
Liver function tests	4†	3	3	2	1
Abdominal computed tomography	2-3	2	2	2	1
Pelvic computed tomography	2-3	2	2	2	1

*The follow-up strategy recommended here is identical to the strategy I recommended for the follow-up of patients treated for intermediate- or high-grade non-Hodgkin's lymphoma in Chapter 22.
†Performed every 2 months for patients with high-grade non-Hodgkin's lymphoma.

Table 23-9 Follow-up of patients after stem cell transplantation (low-grade non-Hodgkin's lymphoma in complete remission)*: Memorial Sloan-Kettering Cancer Center

	YEAR				
	1	2	3	4	5
Office visit	4	3	3	2	2
Complete blood count	4	3	3	2	2
Chest x-ray	4	3	3	2	2
Liver function tests	4	3	3	2	2
Abdominal computed tomography	2	2	2	2	2
Pelvic computed tomography	2	2	2	2	2

*The follow-up strategy recommended here is identical to the strategy I recommended for the follow-up of patients treated for low-grade non-Hodgkin's lymphoma in Chapter 22.

The policies that have been developed for the follow-up of patients after high-dose chemotherapy or radiation therapy with bone marrow or peripheral blood progenitor support, which has been mostly autologous, for the treatment of patients with Hodgkin's disease and non-Hodgkin's lymphoma at Memorial Sloan-Kettering Cancer Center reflect the relapse risk, which seems to be similar to that of patients after primary conventional treatment.[1-4] For patients with Hodgkin's disease and intermediate- or high-grade non-Hodgkin's lymphoma, the greatest risk for recurrence is within the first 3 to 5 years. Patients with intermediate-grade lymphomas have a lesser risk until 7 to 8 years after treatment. For patients with low-grade non-Hodgkin's lymphoma there remains a risk for recurrence even at 10 years. Follow-up of patients with low-grade non-Hodgkin's lymphoma suggests that a similar relapse pattern might be seen, although the duration of follow-up is limited.[5] For that reason the follow-up policies employed at Memorial Sloan-Kettering Cancer Center are the same as those developed for patients with lymphomas after primary treatment (Tables 23-7 through 23-9).

REFERENCES

1. Gulati SC, Shank B, Black P, et al. Autologous bone marrow transplantation for patients with poor-prognosis lymphoma. J Clin Oncol 1988;6:1303-13.
2. Yahalom J, Gulati SC, Toia M, et al. Accelerated hyperfractionated total-lymphoid irradiation, high-dose chemotherapy, and autologous bone marrow transplantation for refractory and relapsing patients with Hodgkin's disease. J Clin Oncol 1993;11:1062-70.
3. Anderson JE, Litzow MR, Appelbaum FR, et al. Allogeneic, syngeneic, and autologous marrow transplantation for Hodgkin's disease: the 21-year Seattle experience. J Clin Oncol 1993;11:2342-50.
4. Horning SJ, Negrin RS, Chao NJ, Long GD, Hoppe RT, Blume KG. Fractionated total-body irradiation, etoposide, and cyclophosphamide plus autografting in Hodgkin's disease and non-Hodgkin's lymphoma. J Clin Oncol 1994;12:2552-8.
5. Freedman AS, Nadler LM. Which patients with relapsed non-Hodgkin's lymphoma benefit from high-dose therapy and hematopoietic stem-cell transplantation? J Clin Oncol 1993;11:1841-3.

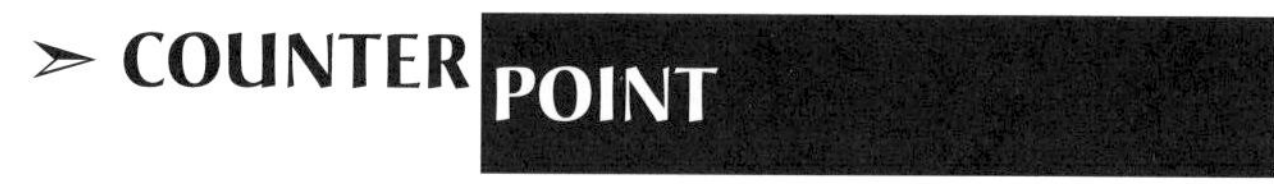

National Kyushu Cancer Center, Japan

JUN OKAMURA

Sullivan and Siadak cover every aspect of possible late sequelae after stem cell transplantation based on their 25 years of experience. They indicate the importance of establishing a long-term follow-up monitoring system with a broad-based approach performed by various individuals in addition to the transplant physicians. I essentially agree with each subject discussed. From a practical point of view, however, the system of providing long-term care for patients receiving stem cell transplantation must be modified to consider the differences in medical systems among countries.

CHARACTERISTICS OF STEM CELL TRANSPLANTATION IN JAPAN

According to data from the National Registry for Bone Marrow Transplantation, which was established for children in 1983 and activated for adults in 1993, the annual number of transplantations has dramatically increased during the past few years in Japan.[1,2] Before 1990 fewer than 200 cases per year were reported in both adults and children. Introduction of autologous transplantation of either bone marrow or peripheral blood stem cells has created a new therapeutic modality for patients who need allogeneic transplantation but are not eligible for various reasons. Bone marrow transplantation using unrelated donors was initiated through the Japanese Marrow Donor Program in 1992, and national health insurance began covering autologous transplantation costs in 1994. Both these factors have contributed to an accelerated increase in the annual number of stem cell transplantations performed in Japan. As of mid-1995 the cumulative number of stem cell transplantations (including both allogeneic and autologous) in Japan is 2,686 for children and 2,793 for adults, according to the registry.

Japan is unique in the number of transplant teams. Currently there are more than 200 transplant teams throughout the nation (126 teams for children and 104 for adults). They are all involved in stem cell transplantation and report their results to the registry. The number of transplantations performed by a single team is extremely small compared with those of other countries. A team that performs more than 20 transplantations a year is rare in Japan.

Since most stem cell transplantations are performed at the institution nearest the patient's home (usually within a few hours by public transportation), the same physicians who perform the transplantation examine the patient at each clinical visit for months and even years. Therefore close relationships develop between the patients and transplant physicians and often last long after the patient's discharge from the hospital. One benefit of these close relationships is that most transplant physicians can easily obtain accurate

Table 23-10 Follow-up of patients after stem cell transplantation (in complete remission): National Kyushu Cancer Center, Japan

	YEAR				
	1	2	3	4	5
Office visit	8-9	8-9	8-9	8-9	8-9
Neurological evaluation*	8-9	8-9	8-9	8-9	8-9
Cardiovascular evaluation†	8-9	8-9	8-9	8-9	8-9
Pulmonary function tests	8-9	8-9	8-9	8-9	8-9
Ophthalmological evaluation‡	1§	1§	1§	1§	1§
Endocrine evaluation¶	1§	1§	1§	1§	1§
Gynecological evaluation**	1§	1§	1§	1§	1§

*Neurological evaluation includes electroencephalography and evaluation by computed tomography or magnetic resonance imaging of the brain. Magnetic resonance imaging is selected over computed tomography to detect any change in the white matter of the brain after stem cell transplantation.
†Cardiovascular evaluation includes chest x-ray, electrocardiography, and echocardiography.
‡Ophthalmological evaluation consists of a comprehensive examination including slit lamp biomicroscopy and Schirmer's test.
§Performed annually or more frequently as clinically indicated.
¶Endocrine evaluation includes serum thyroid-stimulating hormone, thyroxine, follicle-stimulating hormone (in males), and estradiol levels (in females).
**Gynecological evaluation includes pelvic examination, Papanicolaou smear, breast examination, and endocrine evaluation, which involves the tests listed above.

information regarding transplantation-related long-term effects directly from the patients at the clinic. However, because the number of transplantations performed at a single institution is so small, the long-term follow-up system for patients after transplantation may not be well organized at the majority of institutions owing to lack of experience. The necessity of establishing large referral transplant centers throughout the country is being widely discussed, although it will take time because of the complicated medical system in Japan.

FOLLOW-UP SYSTEM AT NATIONAL KYUSHU CANCER CENTER

Since 1977 physicians at National Kyushu Cancer Center have performed 130 stem cell transplantations, including 94 allogeneic transplantations, primarily for children but for a few adults as well. The average number of transplantations performed annually during the past few years has been between 20 and 30. Although results of transplantation were miserable for the first few years, survivors are now rapidly increasing in number, with one patient alive at 11 years after syngeneic transplantation. Approximately 60% of transplant patients are still alive. As at the majority of institutions in Japan, all patients at National Kyushu Cancer Center visit the clinic regularly (Table 23-10). On-site examinations are performed monthly for the first 6 months and every 2 to 3 months thereafter. Beyond approximately 5 years after transplantation, patients usually return to the clinic at 6-month intervals. At each clinical visit careful physical examination and laboratory studies, including neurological, cardiovascular, and respiratory function tests, are performed in addition to the routine workup to evaluate possible late effects after transplantation. Ophthalmological, endocrinological, and gynecological consultations are performed at each anniversary or when indicated.

LONG-TERM EFFECTS OF TRANSPLANTATION

As Sullivan and Siadak indicate, the development of cataracts has been a main concern as one of the late effects of transplantation, especially among children receiving TBI for control of their leukemias.[3] However, physicians at National Kyushu Cancer Center have not encountered a patient developing symptomatic cataracts after TBI who required further treatment. This is probably because of the change in the use of the TBI method since 1989; patients are now receiving a total of 13.2 Gy hyperfractionated TBI (11 fractions). In addition, physicians now routinely shield the lens during TBI. Patients who received a single dose of TBI (10 Gy) before 1989 all died of disease recurrence or complications.

Physicians at National Kyushu Cancer Center have not seen development of a second malignancy in a single patient, although this is probably due to the small size of the patient population and the short observation period.[4] Lymphoproliferative disorders have been reported with increasing frequency among patients who received bone marrow from unrelated donors through the Japanese Marrow Donor Program, in which more immunosuppressive drugs such as antithymocyte globulin are used.

As has been observed in large cohorts of children receiving stem cell transplantation, endocrine and growth deterioration is a serious concern.[5] Patients are regularly seen by endocrinologists for the diagnosis of problems and the initiation of hormone replacement therapy as soon as possible when such deterioration is indicated. As the number of survivors of transplantation increases, gonadal dysfunction, fertility, and gynecological and obstetrical care are becoming other issues of concern.[6] Although rare successful deliveries among adult transplant recipients in certain Japanese institutions have been reported, physicians at National Kyushu Cancer Center have not encountered such a case, probably because of the overall younger age and small size of the patient population.

Another important subject associated with stem cell transplantation is the psychological impact. Patients are usually strictly isolated in the protected environment and are forced to take various kinds of drugs to prevent serious infections. These procedures produce tremendous psychological pressure on the patients, and psychiatric symptoms such as anxiety, depression, and hallucinations frequently occur.[7] Although children seem to adapt better than adults to the environment, some children, especially when having difficulty in cooperating with the procedures, exhibit severe psychosomatic symptoms. These problems usually resolve once the patient leaves the protected environment after engraftment. However, the speed of recovery from psychological symptoms differs from patient to patient and some patients continue to have difficulty even after discharge from the hospital. Because of limited experience, physicians at National Kyushu Cancer Center do not know the depth of the psychiatric injuries or their duration. Certainly a more systematic long-term investigation of this problem is needed.

SUMMARY

Because of the increase in stem cell transplantations performed in Japan, physicians at smaller institutions are certain to encounter late complications like those already seen in large transplant centers as described by Sullivan and Siadak. By learning from their experience, physicians can establish a long-term follow-up system that is applicable to all smaller transplant institutions in Japan.

REFERENCES

1. Bone Marrow Transplantation Committee of the Japanese Society of Pediatric Hematology. National registry of bone marrow transplantation in children–1995. Jpn J Pediatr Hematol 1996;10:29-41.
2. Hamashima N. National survey for hematopoietic cell transplantation in adults. 1995 Annual Report, Society of Japan Hemopoietic Cell Transplantation 1996;March:1-10.
3. Benyunes MC, Sullivan KM, Deeg HJ, et al. Cataracts after bone marrow transplantation: long-term follow-up of adults treated with fractionated total body irradiation. Int J Radiat Oncol Biol Phys 1995;32:661-70.
4. Deeg HJ, Socie G, Schoch G, et al. Malignancies after marrow transplantation for aplastic anemia: a joint Seattle and Paris analysis of results in 700 patients. Blood 1996;87:386-92.
5. Sanders JE. Endocrine problems in children after bone marrow transplant for hematologic malignancies: the long-term follow-up team. Bone Marrow Transplant 1991,8(Suppl 1).2-4.
6. Sanders JE, Buckner CD, Amos D, et al. Ovarian function following marrow transplantation for aplastic anemia or leukemia. J Clin Oncol 1988;6:813-8.
7. Kellman J, Rigler D, Siegel SE. Psychological effects of isolation in protected environments. Am J Psychiatry 1977;134:563-5.

➢ COUNTERPOINT

Royal Liverpool University Hospital, UK

RICHARD E. CLARK

Over the past two decades the transplantation of hemopoietic stem cells has evolved into an important treatment modality for many forms of cancer. In the 1970s and early 1980s the vast majority of transplantation procedures used allogeneic stem cells obtained from a suitable family donor. Although siblings with fully matched human lymphocyte antigen remain the most commonly used allogeneic stem cell donors, the more recent development of national panels of volunteer marrow donors has permitted allogeneic transplantation for patients who lack a suitable family donor. Allogeneic transplantation remains the only curative modality for several leukemias, notably chronic myeloid leukemia and advanced acute leukemia and myeloma, as well as for several nonmalignant conditions such as hemoglobinopathy and severe combined immunodeficiency. The annual number of allogeneic transplantations performed in Europe continues to increase steadily.[1]

Over the past decade there has been a steady increase in the number of transplantation procedures carried out using the patient's own stem cells. More properly termed high-dose chemotherapy with hemopoietic stem cell rescue (since the effective therapy is the high-dose chemotherapy rather than the transplantation), the colloquialism "autologous transplantation" is in general use. In the past 5 years transplantation of stem cells obtained from peripheral blood after chemotherapy and myeloid growth factor priming has also become increasingly popular. Nomenclature has become somewhat confused, since autologous transplantations using peripheral blood–derived stem cells are often referred to simply as stem cell transplantations. Hematological recovery (especially of the platelet lineage) may be more rapid after transplantation with peripheral blood stem cells than with conventional autologous bone marrow. Furthermore, in many hematooncology centers leukapheresis of peripheral blood–derived stem cells is considerably easier from a practical point of view than bone marrow harvest, since the latter requires general anesthesia and operating theater time. Because of these advantages, 65% of autografts carried out in Europe in 1994 used exclusively peripheral blood stem cells and only 29% used exclusively bone marrow–derived material; this is a reverse of the position in 1990.[1] An additional initial theoretical hope was that peripheral blood stem cells might be less contaminated with malignant cells than conventional bone marrow harvests. However, recent data suggest that the stem cell–mobilizing procedure may recruit some malignant cells into the peripheral blood.[2-4]

Of 3,502 allogeneic transplantations carried out in Europe in 1994, 2,737 (78%) were for leukemia or a related disorder, 609 (17.4%) were for a nonmalignant disease, and only 156 (4.4%) were for a nonleukemic malignancy (principally non-Hodgkin's lymphoma).[1] Since the follow-up of patients with leukemia or myeloma is outside the scope of this book, a detailed discussion of the particular problems of allograft recipients (such as graft-versus-host disease) is inappropriate. This counterpoint therefore concentrates principally on the follow-up of autograft recipients.

Sullivan and Siadak provide an authoritative review of the follow-up of the stem cell recipient, drawing on examples from the practice at Fred Hutchinson Cancer Research Center. The Seattle practice differs little from the way stem cell recipients are followed up in the United Kingdom. However, there are some aspects of follow-up in which the philosophy or practice of physicians in the United Kingdom may differ from those in the United States, and these are discussed.

INFECTION AND ITS PROPHYLAXIS

On discharge from the bone marrow transplant unit most patients will have achieved a neutrophil count greater than

Table 23-11 Dietary advice given on discharge after hematopoietic stem cell transplantation at Royal Liverpool University Hospital

ADVICE

The following advice is given to help you make a good recovery with minimal complications.

AVOID INFECTION

Avoid large crowds of people, public transport, public places, people who have colds or other signs of infection.
Avoid extremities of temperature, either hot or cold.
If you have chills, rigors, or pain, contact the ward.
If you are bruising or bleeding, contact the ward.
If you feel unwell for any reason, contact the ward.
Continue to take all your medication until told otherwise.
Discuss care of your Hickman line with your primary/associate nurse.

SKIN CARE

It is not unusual for your skin to remain dry for a time after your transplant.
You may feel that your skin is sensitive to certain products.
If you develop a rash or your skin is itchy or sore, contact the ward.

MOUTH CARE

Your mouth will be dry and still at risk of infection for a few months. It is important to continue with your mouth care.

DIETARY ADVICE

Drinks

You may now use pasteurized milk from a fresh bottle/carton, kept for 24 hours only.
You may use tap water. Cartons of juice should be fresh daily.
Large bottles of fizzy drinks and squash should be avoided.
Cans of beer/lager and wine may be taken but check with your doctor first.
Continue to use Complan, Build Up, etc. to supplement your diet.

Hot Food

It is not necessary to microwave your food.
All food should be cooked properly, eaten immediately, and not reheated.
Fresh meat/fish should be cooked on the day of purchase.
Fresh/frozen/tinned vegetables may be taken if cooked thoroughly.
Avoid jacket potatoes.

Cold Food

Raw vegetables and salads should be avoided.
Avoid cold meat and fish unless tinned or individually packed.
Fresh fruit must be washed and skinned.
Prepacked cheese, bought fresh and eaten within 48 hours, may be taken.
Avoid blue-veined cheeses.
Bread should be fresh daily.
Individually boxed cereals are preferable to the larger boxes.

Eating Out

For the first few months after your transplant, avoid restaurants unless you can be sure of the quality of the food preparation.
Avoid "take-away" food.

EXERCISE

Expect to feel tired and "strange" to be at home. Take things easy, do as much or as little as you are able.
Increase your activities gradually. Take plenty of rest.
If you have had total body irradiation, it is not unusual 5 to 10 weeks after treatment to feel more lethargic and depressed than usual. These symptoms will ease.

0.5×10^9/L. Standard neutropenic prophylaxis is usually discontinued at this level, although occasional patients with significant residual oral mucositis or candidiasis may be given an azole antifungal agent for a little longer.[5] The gastrointestinal tract may remain abnormally permeable to microorganisms for some weeks after high-dose treatment,[6] and accordingly many units recommend avoidance of foods high in microorganisms for some time after peripheral blood neutrophil recovery.[7] Patients in the bone marrow transplant program at Royal Liverpool University Hospital continue with minor dietary restrictions until 3 months after transplantation (Table 23-11).

The effect of high-dose chemotherapy on the immune system is not limited to the granulocyte, megakaryocyte, and erythroid lineages, whose end cells are readily assessed in the complete blood count. Profound suppression of both T and B lymphocyte number and function occurs after high-dose conditioning therapy.[8] For some weeks after discharge from the unit the stem cell recipient suffers from iatrogenic severe combined immune deficiency, and the peripheral blood neutrophil or lymphocyte count is a poor guide to the degree of this immunosuppression.

Hemopoietic stem cell recipients are particularly at risk for *Pneumocystis carinii* pneumonia. Co-trimoxasole is effective in preventing this infection,[9] although it may also suppress hematological recovery after stem cell transplantation. For patients who remain significantly cytopenic, inhalations of nebulized pentamidine are an alternative. There is also an increased risk of reactivation of herpes simplex and varicella-zoster virus infection, the latter clinically manifesting as shingles that is not necessarily strictly confined to a given dermatome distribution. Reactivation of cytomegalovirus infection may also occur. In recipients of autografts (unlike allogeneic stem cells), cytomegalovirus disease is rarely a serious clinical problem.

Prophylaxis against infection varies among different units. In Europe co-trimoxasole and acyclovir prophylaxis are typically given for 3 to 6 months after transplantation. At

Royal Liverpool University Hospital all autograft recipients commence acyclovir at a dose of 200 mg orally every 6 hours the day before transplantation and remain on this schedule until 3 months after transplantation. This schedule is doubled or quadrupled if herpes or varicella infection or contact is suspected. *P. carinii* pneumonia prophylaxis is begun at 28 days after transplantation when, if patients are independent of platelet transfusion and have achieved a peripheral blood platelet and neutrophil count greater than 30×10^9/L and 1×10^9/L, respectively, they commence co-trimoxasole at a dose of 960 mg 3 times weekly until 3 months after transplantation. Patients who have not achieved this level of hemopoietic engraftment receive inhaled nebulized pentamidine 150 mg weekly (after preliminary bronchodilation with nebulized salbutomol) until they are able to receive oral co-trimoxasole.

REVACCINATION

Permanent loss of long-term immunity is less common after autologous than after allogeneic stem cell transplantation, although abnormal T cell responses to mitogens have been reported several months after an autograft.[10] Extensive revaccination is therefore less widely practiced in autograft stem cell recipients. A recent survey showed that 37% of European bone marrow transplant centers routinely revaccinated autograft recipients, in contrast to 65% of centers in which routine revaccination of allograft recipients was advised. The principal immunizations were with tetanus and diphtheria toxoid and the inactivated form of poliovirus and influenza virus.[11]

The practice for autograft recipients at Royal Liverpool University Hospital is to advise revaccination (with diphtheria and tetanus toxoid and inactivated poliovirus) at 6 to 12 months only in patients whose conditioning regimen included TBI. Physicians also recommend recombinant hepatitis B in patients at occupational or other risk but do not advise use of live attenuated vaccines. Prophylactic intravenous immunoglobulin infusions are restricted to allograft recipients with serum immunoglobulin gamma G levels less than 5 g/L.

PULMONARY FUNCTION

Interstitial pneumonitis is a common complication after allogeneic stem cell transplantation and indeed is the most common cause of transplantation-related mortality. Interstitial pneumonitis may also occur after autografting in 5% to 11% of patients.[12,13] Evidence of more subtle degrees of lung dysfunction may be seen on pulmonary function tests, particularly the transfer coefficient.[14] Pulmonary impairment after autografting is related to pretransplantation pulmonary dysfunction and to previous treatment,[14,15] although conditioning therapy that includes TBI may increase the probability of pulmonary function test abnormalities.[13]

SUMMARY

As well as the problems discussed previously, the autologous stem cell recipient is at risk of cataracts, endocrine and gonadal dysfunction, impairment of fertility, secondary malignancy, and (perhaps most important) relapse of the underlying malignancy. However, for many of these potential complications evidence is lacking that a routine surveillance strategy is of clinical benefit. For example, abnormal pulmonary function tests after autografting in the absence of overt respiratory symptoms have little clinical significance,[13] and accordingly, routine pulmonary function monitoring after stem cell transplantation is not widely practiced. Because of differences in the delivery and financing of health care between countries, the routine monitoring of the autologous stem cell recipient in the United Kingdom is more reactive to patient symptoms than in the United States.

Table 23-12 Follow-up of patients after stem cell transplantation (in complete remission): Royal Liverpool University Hospital, UK

	YEAR				
	1	2	3	4	5
Office visit*	6-8	4	4	2-3	2-3
Complete blood count	6-8	4	4	2-3	2-3
Endocrine evaluation†	1-2	1-2	1-2	1-2	1-2
Reimmunization	1‡	0	0	0	0

*Frequency of visits for cytopenic patients may increase, especially if they are dependent on blood products.
†Endocrine evaluation includes serum thyroid-stimulating hormone, thyroxine, follicle-stimulating hormone, and estradiol levels (in females) and is performed once every 6 months for ovarian failure and annually for thyroid failure.
‡Performed at 6 to 12 months after transplantation.

Table 23-12 gives the routine investigations performed or advised for adult stem cell recipients at Royal Liverpool University Hospital. Physicians at this institution do not perform routine ophthalmological or oral medicine review unless the patient gives a history of relevant symptoms. Mammographic screening is not carried out any more frequently than for healthy women at equivalent risk for breast cancer (in the United Kingdom this is currently at 3-year intervals for women ages 50 to 64). Routine monitoring of graft status is more appropriate to allogeneic stem cell recipients, and physicians do not routinely examine the bone marrow in autograft recipients with a normal complete blood count unless marrow involvement by relapse of the underlying disease is strongly suspected. Conversely, physicians would not wait until the annual follow-up to perform assessments of gonadal and endocrine function, and assays of follicle-stimulating hormone, luteinizing hormone, and estrogens in women at risk of premature menopause are performed more than once annually.

FUTURE PROSPECTS

A major component of the follow-up of stem cell recipients is the detection of relapse of the underlying disease. This aspect of follow-up of stem cell recipients is covered in detail elsewhere in this book. In the context of the minimal residual disease that exists in many stem cell recipients there is considerable interest in the use of molecular monitoring.

The level or proportion of an abnormal DNA or mRNA transcript may be monitored in a semiquantitative fashion, and a consistently rising level may correlate with and precede overt relapse.[16] This early detection of emerging relapse may be clinically useful in the case of allograft recipients with underlying chronic myeloid leukemia, since leukocyte infusions from the original donor may produce complete molecular remissions in most patients. Preliminary evidence suggests that donor leukocyte infusions may be more effective if given before overt hematological relapse in chronic myeloid leukemia.[17] In diseases other than chronic myeloid leukemia, no information is available on whether molecular monitoring of a tumor-specific mutation yields information that will influence the treatment of stem cell recipients. However, current studies are examining the prognostic significance of molecular monitoring in a number of settings, especially in acute leukemia and lymphoproliferative disease. At present, then, routine molecular monitoring of underlying disease in autograft recipients is not justified outside of a research protocol. This may well change in the light of current prospective studies of molecular monitoring after stem cell transplantation.

REFERENCES

1. Gratwohl A, Hermans J, Baldomero H. Hematopoietic precursor cell transplants in Europe: activity in 1994. Report from the European Group for Blood and Marrow Transplantation (EBMT). Bone Marrow Transplant 1996;17:137-48.
2. Lemoli RM, Fortuna A, Motta MR, et al. Concomitant mobilization of plasma cells and hematopoietic progenitors into peripheral blood of multiple myeloma patients: positive selection and transplantation of enriched CD34+ cells to remove circulating tumor cells. Blood 1996;87:1625-34.
3. Ross AA, Cooper BW, Lazarus HM, et al. Detection and viability of tumor cells in peripheral blood stem cell collections from breast cancer patients using immunocytochemical and clonogenic assay techniques. Blood 1993;82:2605-10.
4. Brugger W, Bross KJ, Glatt M, Weber F, Mertelsmann R, Kanz L. Mobilization of tumor cells and hematopoietic progenitor cells into peripheral blood of patients with solid tumors. Blood 1994;83:636-40.
5. Uzun O, Anaissie EJ. Antifungal prophylaxis in patients with hematologic malignancies: a reappraisal. Blood 1995;86:2063-72.
6. Fegan C, Poynton CH, Whittaker JA. The gut mucosal barrier in bone marrow transplantation. Bone Marrow Transplantation 1990; 5:373-7.
7. Bibbington A, Wilson P, Jones M. Audit of nutritional advice given to bone marrow transplant patients in the United Kingdom and Eire. Clinical Nutrition 1993;12:230-5.
8. Atkinson K. Reconstruction of the hemopoietic and immune systems after marrow transplantation. Bone Marrow Transplant 1990;5:209-26.
9. Garaventa A, Rondelli R, Castagnola E, et al. Fatal pneumopathy in children after bone marrow transplantation—report from the Italian Registry. Italian Association of Pediatric Hematology-Oncology BMT Group. Bone Marrow Transplant 1995;16:669-74.
10. Takaue Y, Okamoto Y, Kawano Y, et al. Regeneration of immunity and varicella-zoster virus infection after high-dose chemotherapy and peripheral blood stem cell autografts in children. Bone Marrow Transplant 1994;14:219-23.
11. Ljungman P, Cordonnier C, de Bock R, et al. Immunisations after bone marrow transplantation: results of a European survey and recommendations from the infectious diseases working party of the European Group for Blood and Marrow Transplantation. Bone Marrow Transplant 1995;15:455-60.
12. Granena A, Carreras E, Rozman C, et al. Interstitial pneumonitis after BMT: 15 years experience in a single institution. Bone Marrow Transplant 1993;11:453-8.
13. Carlson K, Bäcklund L, Smedmyr B, Öberg G, Simonsson B. Pulmonary function and complications subsequent to autologous bone marrow transplantation. Bone Marrow Transplant 1994;14:805-11.
14. Badier M, Guillot C, Delpierre S, Vanuxem P, Blaise D, Maraninchi D. Pulmonary function changes 100 days and one year after bone marrow transplantation. Bone Marrow Transplant 1993;12:457-61.
15. Nenadov Beck M, Meresse V, Hartmann O, Gaultier C. Long-term pulmonary sequelae after autologous bone marrow transplantation in children without total body irradiation. Bone Marrow Transplant 1995;16:771-5.
16. Lion T, Henn T, Gaiger A, Kahls P, Gadner H. Early detection of relapse after bone marrow transplantation in patients with chronic myelogenous leukaemia. Lancet 1993;341:275-6.
17. van Rhee F, Lin F, Cullis JO, et al. Relapse of chronic myeloid leukaemia after allogeneic bone marrow transplant: the case for giving donor leucocyte transfusions before the onset of hematologic relapse. Blood 1994;83:3377-83.

➢ COUNTERPOINT

Roswell Park Cancer Institute

Myron S. Czuczman

Sullivan and Siadak provide a succinctly written, thoroughly referenced set of guidelines for the long-term follow-up of patients after hematopoietic stem cell transplantation. Fred Hutchinson Cancer Research Center is one of the leading centers for transplantation in the world, and the authors' recommendations are based on actual long-term, posttransplantation follow-up in a large number of patients. I agree with their follow-up methodology, and this counterpoint largely serves to reemphasize certain important points made by Sullivan and Siadak.

Until infused stem cells are successfully engrafted, patients require close monitoring for acute toxicities, including acute graft-versus-host disease, venoocclusive disease, secondary organ toxicity associated with the type of preparative regimen used, infection, and bleeding. Once acute toxicities have been treated or resolved, patients are still at risk for late complications. Late complications include chronic graft-versus-host disease, late cardiopulmonary or other organ toxicities associated with high-dose chemotherapy and total body irradiation, gonadal dysfunction, immunological deficiency, bone disease, infection, and recrudescence of primary cancer or development of secondary malignancy.

The majority of transplant recipients at Roswell Park Cancer Institute have primary hematological disorders, but recently the percentage of patients with solid tumors undergoing hematopoietic stem cell transplantation has been increasing. Patient follow-up after transplantation at Roswell Park Cancer Institute is similar to that conducted at Fred Hutchinson Cancer Research Center and provides essentially the same information. In addition to medical,

Table 23-13 Follow-up of patients after stem cell transplantation (in complete remission): Roswell Park Cancer Institute

	YEAR				
	1	2	3	4	5
Office visit	3*	2-4	2	2	1-2
Karnofsky Performance Scale evaluation	1	1	1	1	1
Ophthalmological evaluation†	1	1	1	1	1
Engraftment status‡	1	1	1	1	1
Gynecological evaluation§	1	1	1	1	1
Mammogram¶	1	1	1	1	1
Endocrine evaluation**	1	1	1	1	1
Monitoring for malignancy††	1	1	1	1	1
Pulmonary function tests	1	0	0	0	1
Immunizations‡‡	1	0	0	0	0

*Performed between 3 and 12 months after transplantation and discharge home.
†Ophthalmological evaluation consists of a comprehensive examination including slit lamp biomicroscopy and Schirmer's test.
‡Engraftment status assessment includes complete blood count and markers for donor origin hematopoiesis, including DNA polymorphism studies for sex-matched donor/recipient pairs or cytogenetic or in situ hybridization studies for Y body determination in sex-mismatched pairs.
§Gynecological evaluation includes pelvic examination, Papanicolaou smear, breast examination, and endocrine evaluation, which involves the tests listed below.
¶For total body irradiation recipients aged 35 years and older.
**Endocrine evaluation includes serum thyroid-stimulating hormone, thyroxine, follicle-stimulating hormone, estradiol levels (in females), and testosterone levels (in males).
††Monitoring at office visits for original malignancy as outlined in other chapters in this volume. Patients with chronic myelogenous leukemia have molecular studies for BCR/abl gene transcript and marrow cytogenetics for the Philadelphia chromosome annually for 5 years after transplantation.
‡‡Immunizations are detailed in Table 23-3.

hematological, and immunological status, a patient's functional and psychological status should be monitored.

After hematopoietic stem cell transplantation, long-term follow-up studies are largely disease specific. The follow-up studies recommended by Sullivan and Siadak serve as good general templates (Tables 23-5 and 23-6), but the actual timing of diagnostic tests may change because of abnormal physical findings, laboratory studies, or subjective patient complaints (Table 23-13).

Sensitive, disease-specific assays to monitor minimal residual disease and evaluate its relationship to clinical relapse are being evaluated after transplantation. Polymerase chain reaction assays for bcl-2 in non-Hodgkin's lymphoma, BCR/abl in chronic myeloid leukemia, and promyelocytic leukemia–retinoic acid receptor in acute promyelocytic leukemia after transplantation are being evaluated at Roswell Park Cancer Institute and other transplant centers. Physicians at this institution are also studying multicolor flow cytometry and fluorescent in situ hybridization techniques as possible ways of detecting early recurrence.

Nonintensive therapeutic interventions are being studied for early relapsed disease after transplantation. In addition to decreasing immunosuppressive medications, donor leukocyte infusions are being used to treat relapsed leukemia after allogeneic bone marrow transplantation. In the autologous transplant setting the study of immunomodulatory agents such as cyclosporine (with or without interferon),[1-8] monoclonal antibodies,[9,10] and low-dose interleukin-2[11,12] is ongoing, with the goal of enhancing host immune function and immunosurveillance to clear minimal residual disease and improve disease-free survival rates.

Largely to cut medical costs, an increasing number of patients are undergoing hematopoietic stem cell transplantation in less expensive outpatient and community settings.

Nevertheless, the recommended follow-up of Sullivan and Siadak and the monitoring of patients after transplantation should not be mitigated because of financial constraints. Rather, they should continue so that late complications will be detected in time to allow intervention that will ensure patients' overall well-being and quality of life.

REFERENCES

1. Santos GW. Autologous graft vs. host disease. Exp Hematol 1991;19:25a.
2. Hess AD, Jones RC, Santos GW. Autologous graft-vs-host disease: mechanisms and potential therapeutic effect. Bone Marrow Transplant 1993:12(Suppl 3):S65-9.
3. Kennedy MJ. Induced autologous graft-versus-host disease for the treatment of cancer. Cancer Treat Rev 1994;20:97-103.
4. Weisdorf DJ, Anderson PM, Blazar BR, Uckun FM, Kersey JH, Ramsay NK. Interleukin 2 immediately after autologous bone marrow transplantation for acute lymphoblastic leukemia—a phase I study. Transplantation 1993;55:61-6.
5. Ratanatharathorn V, Uberti J, Karanes C, et al. Phase I study of alpha-interferon augmentation of cyclosporine-induced graft versus host disease in recipients of autologous bone marrow transplantation. Bone Marrow Transplant 1994;13:625-30.
6. Yeager AM, Vogelsang GB, Jones RJ, et al. Induction of cutaneous graft-versus-host disease by administration of cyclosporine to patients undergoing autologous bone marrow transplantation for acute myeloid leukemia. Blood 1992;79:3031-5.
7. Kennedy MJ, Vogelsang GB, Bevreidge RA, et al. Phase I trial of intravenous cyclosporine to induce graft-versus-host disease in women undergoing autologous bone marrow transplantation for breast cancer. J Clin Oncol 1993;11:478-84.
8. Kennedy MJ, Vogelsang GB, Jones RJ, et al. Phase I trial of interferon gamma to potentiate cyclosporine-induced graft-versus-host disease in women undergoing autologous bone marrow transplantation for breast cancer. J Clin Oncol 1994;12:249-57.
9. Grossbard ML, Gribben JG, Freedman AS, et al. Adjuvant immunotoxin therapy with anti-B4-blocked ricin after autologous bone marrow transplantation for patients with B-cell non-Hodgkin's lymphoma. Blood 1993;81:2263-2271.
10. Grossbard ML, O'Day S, Gribben JG, et al. A phase II study of anti-B4-blocked ricin (anti-B4-bR) therapy following autologous bone marrow transplantation (ABMT) for B-cell non-Hodgkin's lymphoma (B-NHL). J Clin Oncol 1994;13:951a.
11. Meloni G, Foa R, Tosti S, et al. Autologous bone marrow transplantation followed by interleukin-2 in children with advanced leukemia: a pilot study. Leukemia 1992;6:780-5.
12. Tiberghien P. Racadot E, Fest T, et al. IL-2 treatment after autologous bone marrow transplantation in poor prognosis Hodgkin's disease: defective IL-2 induced LAK activity? Bone Marrow Transplant 1991;7(Suppl 2):145.

Table 23-14 Follow-up of patients after stem cell transplantation by institution

YEAR/PROGRAM	OFFICE VISIT	KARNOF	OPHTHAL	GRAFT	GYN	MAMM	ENDO	MALIG	PFT	IMMUN	CBC
Year 1											
Memorial Sloan-Kettering I[a,b]	4					[c]					4
Memorial Sloan-Kettering II[d,e]	4[f]										4[f]
Memorial Sloan-Kettering III[g,h]	4										4
Roswell Park	3[i]	1	1[j]	1[k]	1[l]	1[m]	1[n]	1[o]	1	1[p]	
Univ Washington/ Fred Hutchinson I[q]	9-18[i]	1	1[j]	1[k]	1[l]	1[n]	1[n]	1[o]	1	1[p]	
Univ Washington/ Fred Hutchinson II[r]	9-18[i]		1[j]	1[k]		1[s]	1[s]	1[t]	1	1[p]	
Japan: National Kyushu	8-9		1[j,w]		1[l,w]		1[w,y]		8-9		
UK: Royal Liverpool	6-8[bb]						1-2[cc]				6-8
Year 2											
Memorial Sloan-Kettering I[a,b]	3					1[c]					3
Memorial Sloan-Kettering II[d,e]	3										3
Memorial Sloan-Kettering III[g,h]	3										3
Roswell Park	2-4	1	1[j]	1[k]	1[l]	1[m]	1[n]	1[o]			
Univ Washington/ Fred Hutchinson I[q]	3-6	1	1[j]	1[k]	1[l]	1[m]	1[n]	1[o]			
Univ Washington/ Fred Hutchinson II[r]	3-6		1[j]	1[k]			1[s]	1[t]			
Japan: National Kyushu	8-9		1[j,w]		1[l,w]		1[w,y]		8-9		
UK: Royal Liverpool	4[bb]						1-2[cc]				4

ABD CT abdominal computed tomography
CBC complete blood count
CV cardiovascular evaluation
CXR chest-ray
ENDO endocrine evaluation
ESR erythrocyte sedimentation rate
GH growth hormone testing
LFT liver function test
GRAFT engraftment status
GYN gynecological evaluation
IMMUN immunizations
KARNOF Karnofsky Performance Scale evaluation
LANSKY Lansky Play Performance Score evaluation
MALIG monitoring for malignancy
MAMM mammogram
NEUROL neurological evaluation
OPHTHAL ophthalmological evaluation
ORAL MED oral medical evaluation
PFT pulmonary function tests
REIMMUN reimmunization
TANNER Tanner Development Score
THYROID thyroid profile

CXR	LFT	ESR	THYROID	ABD CT	PELVIC CT	NEUROL	CV	REIMMUN	ORAL MED	LANSKY	TANNER	GH
4	4	4	2	2	2							
4[f]	4[f]			2-3	2-3							
4	4			2	2							
									1			
									1	1	1[u]	1[v]
						8-9[z]	8-9[aa]					
								1[dd]				
3	3	3	2	2	2							
3	3			2	2					2	2	
3	3			2	2							
									1			
									1	1	1[u]	1[v]
						8-9[z]	8-9[aa]					

a Patients with Hodgkin's lymphoma.
b The follow-up strategy recommended here is identical to the strategy this author recommended for the follow-up of patients treated for Hodgkin's lymphoma in Chapter 22.
c Performed for female patients over the age of 30 who have received mantle irradiation.
d Patients with intermediate- or high-grade non-Hodgkin's lymphoma.
e The follow-up strategy recommended here is identical to the strategy this author recommended for the follow-up of patients treated for intermediate- or high-grade non-Hodgkin's lymphoma in Chapter 22.
f Performed every 2 months for patients with high-grade non-Hodgkin's lymphoma.
g Patients with low-grade non-Hodgkin's lymphoma.
h The follow-up strategy recommended here is identical to the strategy this author recommended for the follow-up of patients treated for low-grade non-Hodgkin's lymphoma in Chapter 22.
i Performed between 3 and 12 months after transplantation and discharge home.
j Ophthalomological cvaluation consists of a comprehensive examination including slit lamp biomicroscopy and Schirmer's test.
k Engraftment status assessment comprises complete blood count and markers for donor origin hematopoiesis, including DNA polymorphism studies for sex-matched donor/recipient pairs or cytogenetic or in situ hybridization studies for Y body determination in sex-mismatched pairs.
l Gynecological evaluation includes pelvic examination, Papanicolaou smear, breast examination, and endocrine evaluation.
m For total body irradiation recipients aged 35 years and older.
n Endocrine evaluation includes serum thyroid-stimulating hormone, thyroxine, follicle-stimulating hormone, and estradiol levels (in females).
o Monitoring at office visits for original malignancy as outlined in other chapters in this volume. Patients with chronic myelogenous leukemia have molecular studies for BCR/abl gene transcript and marrow cytogenetics for the Philadelphia chromosome annually for 5 years after transplantation.
p Immunizations are detailed in Table 23-3.
q For adult patients.
r For patients who are children.
s Endocrine evaluation includes serum thyroid-stimulating hormone, thyroxine, and follicle-stimulating hormone, and when patients are 8 years of age or older, testosterone levels (in males) and estradiol levels (in females).
t Monitoring at office visits for original malignancy as outlined in other chapters in this volume.
u Tanner Development Score includes breast, pubic, and axillary hair and external genital score.
v Growth hormone testing incudes 12-hour spontaneous and stimulated testing.
w Performed annually or more frequently as clinically indicated.
y Endocrine evaluation includes serum thyroid-stimulating hormone, thyroxine, follicle-stimulating hormone (in males), and estradiol levels (in females).
z Neurological evaluation includes electroencephalography and evaluation by computed tomography or magnetic resonance imaging of the brain. Magnetic resonance imaging is selected over computed tomography to detect any change in the white matter of the brain after stem cell transportation.
aa Cardiovascular evaluation includes chest x-ray, electrocardiography, and echocardiography.
bb Frequency of visits for cytopenic patients may increase, especially if they are dependent on blood products.
cc Endocrine evaluation includes serum thyroid-stimulating hormone, thyroxine, follicle-stimulating hormone, and estradiol levels (in females) and is performed once every 6 months for ovarian failure and annually for thyroid failure.
dd Performed at 6 to 12 months after transplantation.

Continued.

Table 23-14 Follow-up of patients after stem cell transplantation by institution—cont'd

YEAR/PROGRAM	OFFICE VISIT	KARNOF	OPHTHAL	GRAFT	GYN	MAMM	ENDO	MALIG	PFT	IMMUN	CBC
Year 3											
Memorial Sloan-Kettering I[a,b]	3					1[c]					3
Memorial Sloan-Kettering II[d,e]	3										3
Memorial Sloan-Kettering III[g,h]	3										3
Roswell Park	2	1	1[j]	1[k]	1[l]	1[m]	1[n]	1[o]			
Univ Washington/ Fred Hutchinson I[q]	2-4	1	1[j]	1[k]	1[l]	1[m]	1[n]	1[o]			
Univ Washington/ Fred Hutchinson II[r]	2-4		1[j]	1[k]			1[s]	1[t]			
Japan: National Kyushu	8-9		1[j,w]		1[l,w]		1[w,y]		8-9		
UK: Royal Liverpool	4[bb]						1-2[cc]				4
Year 4											
Memorial Sloan-Kettering I[a,b]	2					1[c]					2
Memorial Sloan-Kettering II[d,e]	2										2
Memorial Sloan-Kettering III[g,h]	2										2
Roswell Park	2	1	1[j]	1[k]	1[l]	1[m]	1[n]	1[o]			
Univ Washington/ Fred Hutchinson I[q]	1-2	1	1[j]	1[k]	1[l]	1[m]	1[n]	1[o]			
Univ Washington/ Fred Hutchinson II[r]	1-2		1[j]	1[k]			1[s]	1[t]			
Japan: National Kyushu	8-9		1[j,w]		1[l,w]		1[w,y]		8-9		
UK: Royal Liverpool	2-3[bb]						1-2[cc]				2-3
Year 5											
Memorial Sloan-Kettering I[a,b]	1					1[c]					1
Memorial Sloan-Kettering II[d,e]	1										1
Memorial Sloan-Kettering III[g,h]	2										2
Roswell Park	1-2	1	1[j]	1[k]	1[l]	1[m]	1[n]	1[o]	1		
Univ Washington/ Fred Hutchinson I[q]	1-2	1	1[j]	1[k]	1[l]	1[m]	1[n]	1[o]	1		
Univ Washington/ Fred Hutchinson II[r]	1-2		1[j]	1[k]			1[s]	1[t]	1		
Japan: National Kyushu	8-9		1[j,w]		1[l,w]		1[w,y]		8-9		
UK: Royal Liverpool	2-3[bb]						1-2[cc]				2-3

CXR	LFT	ESR	THYROID	ABD CT	PELVIC CT	NEUROL	CV	REIMMUN	ORAL MED	LANSKY	TANNER	GH
3	3	3	2	2	2							
3	3			2	2							
3	3			2	2							
									1			
									1	1	1[u]	1[v]
						8-9[z]	8-9[aa]					
2	2	2	2	2	2							
2	2			2	2							
2	2			2	2							
									1			
									1	1	1[u]	1[v]
						8-9[z]	8-9[aa]					
1	1	1	1	1	1							
1	1			1	1							
2	2			2	2							
									1			
									1	1	1[u]	1[v]
						8-9[z]	8-9[aa]					

FRED HUTCHINSON CANCER RESEARCH CENTER
CLINICAL RESEARCH DIVISION LONG-TERM FOLLOW-UP EVALUATION

DATE: RE:

TO: REF NO:
STUDY DATE:
STUDY INTERVAL:
LAST FOLLOW-UP DATE:

- Are your name and mailing address correct as shown above? No Yes
  (Please enclose changes or corrections.)
- Have you had contact with this patient since ? No Yes
- If you are no longer following this patient, would you please provide us with the complete name and address of the physician who is currently following him/her?

SURVIVAL STATUS

☐ ALIVE - Date of your most recent contact with patient: __/__/__

PERFORMANCE SCORE at most recent contact date:
[see enclosure for **Karnofsky Performance Score** (KPS) and **Lansky Play-Performance Score** (LPPS) scales.]

Current **KPS** *(for ages ≥ 17 years old)* ______%

Current **LPPS** *(for ages < 17 years old)* ______%

☐ DEAD - Date of Death: __/__/__

Autopsy performed? No Yes
(If yes, please send copies of death summary and/or autopsy report)

Cause of Death: ____________________

DISEASE STATUS

☐ No evidence of original disease

☐ Persistent disease
☐ Recurrence
☐ New malignancy
☐ Benign tumor
☐ B-Cell lymphoproliferative disorder
☐ Other hematologic, oncologic, immunologic disorder

If you checked one or more of the six items above, please complete the following information for each item checked:

Date documented: __/__/__ Diagnosis: ____________________

Site(s) involved: ____________________

Rx: ____________________

Appendix A Physician form.

DATE: REF NO:
RE: STUDY INTERVAL:

INTERIM EVENTS

HOSPITALIZATIONS: NO YES
Date(s) Reason(s)

OTHER MEDICAL PROBLEMS: NO YES
Date(s) Description

INFECTIONS: NO YES
Date(s) Type of Infection(s)

Cataracts: None OD OS Both

	OD	OS
Date developed:	__/__/__	__/__/__
Date of surgical repair:	__/__/__	__/__/__

TRANSFUSIONS: NO YES
Date of last RBC transfusion: __/__/__
Date of last platelet transfusion: __/__/__

Avascular necrosis: No Yes
Date diagnosed: __/__/__
Site(s): ____________________

VACCINATIONS: NO YES
Type of vacination:

CURRENT DATA

PHYSICAL EXAM

Date of Exam: __/__/__

Ht(cm): ________ Wt(kg): ________

BP: __/__/__

General Appearance:
HEENT:
Oral:
Skin/Hair:
Cardiac:
Lungs:
GI/Liver:
GU:
Joints/Contractures:
Neuro:

Tanner score:
Menarche:

MEDICATIONS

Continued.

DATE: REF NO:
RE: STUDY INTERVAL:

CURRENT LABS

Date blood collected: __/__/__
Hgb/Hct ______/______
MCV ____________
MCH/MCHC ______/______
WBC ____________
Polys ______
Bands ______
Lymphs ______
Monos ______
Eos ______
Baso ______
Meta ______
Myelo ______
Blasts ______
Other ______

Abs. retic ____________
Platelets ____________

Date blood collected: __/__/__
Creat./BUN ______/______
Tot. Bilirubin ____________
SGOT ____________
Alk. Phos. ____________

Date blood collected: __/__/__
IgG ______
IgA ______
IgM ______
IgE ______

Date blood collected: __/__/__
T3 ______
T4 - Thyroxine ______
TSH ______

Date blood collected: __/__/__
FSH, serum ______
LH, serum ______
Testosterone, serum ______
Estradiol, serum ______

Date of most recent bone marrow exam: __/__/__
Results:

Date of most recent cytogenetics: __/__/__
Results:

If aplastic, was PNH screen done? None done Neg Pos

Date PNH screen done: __/__/__

Completed by: ____________________________ Date completed: __/__/__

Appendix A, cont'd. Physician form.

FRED HUTCHINSON CANCER RESEARCH CENTER
CLINICAL RESEARCH DIVISION LONG-TERM FOLLOW-UP EVALUATION

DATE:

TO:

STUDY DATE:

FOLLOW-UP INTERVAL:

Telephone Number(s):

Are your name and mailing address correct as noted? [If no, please make corrections above] Yes No

Please provide us with the complete name and address of your current physician(s):

CURRENT PHYSICAL ACTIVITY

- Are you going to school? No Yes Grade/Level ______
- Do you have a home tutor? No Yes
- Are you working? No Yes Occupation ______

  Check all that apply:

  ______Full-time

  ______Part-time

  ______Outside the home

  ______Inside the home

- Do you participate in recreational activities? No Yes

  What types of activities: How often?

  ______ ______

  ______ ______

  ______ ______

- Are your daily or recreational activities restricted? No Yes

  How are they restricted?______

  ______

HOW WOULD YOU RATE YOUR OVERALL PHYSICAL HEALTH DURING THE PAST TWO WEEKS?

(Circle appropriate rating below)

1 2 3 4 5 6 7 8 9 10

Very Poor Excellent

Appendix B Patient form.

Continued.

DATE:
TO:
Page: 2

WHAT ARE YOUR CURRENT MEDICAL PROBLEMS?

(Continue on reverse or attach additional sheet if necessary)

Please describe problems, infections and hospitalizations along with date of onset:

Date	Problem

HOW SEVERELY DO YOUR CURRENT SYMPTOMS AFFECT YOUR DAILY LIFE?

(Circle appropriate rating below)

1 2 3 4 5 6 7 8 9 10

Not at all severe — Extremely severe

WHAT MEDICATIONS ARE YOU CURRENTLY TAKING?

(Continue on reverse or attach additional sheet if necessary)

Please provide names of drugs, amounts and frequency taken:

HOW WOULD YOU RATE YOUR PSYCHOLOGICAL HEALTH DURING THE PAST TWO WEEKS?

(Circle appropriate rating below)

1 2 3 4 5 6 7 8 9 10

Very Poor — Excellent

HOW WOULD YOU RATE YOUR SOCIAL INTERACTIONS WITH YOUR FAMILY AND FRIENDS DURING THE PAST TWO WEEKS?

(Circle appropriate rating below)

1 2 3 4 5 6 7 8 9 10

Very Poor — Excellent

HOW WOULD YOU RATE YOUR MEMORY AND CONCENTRATION DURING THE LAST TWO WEEKS?

(Circle appropriate rating below)

1 2 3 4 5 6 7 8 9 10

Very Poor — Excellent

Completed by: ______________________ Date completed: __/__/__

Appendix B, cont'd. Patient form.

SECTION III

Horizons

CHAPTER 24

How Molecular Genetics Can Affect Cancer Surveillance Strategies

Washington University Medical Center

Paul J. Goodfellow and Diane M. Radford

CONCEPTS

Cancer Is Genetic Disease

Cancers arise and progress as the result of accumulated genetic damage or mutations. The genes that are mutated in cancers include those that function in the control of cellular proliferation and cell-cell interactions and in the regulation of replication of genetic material. "Cancer genes" are usually categorized as either oncogenes or tumor suppressor genes. The terms "oncogene" and "tumor suppressor gene" relate to genes' normal cellular functions. Oncogenes positively regulate cell growth. Tumor suppressor genes normally serve to negatively regulate cell growth. In cancers oncogenes are altered so that the positive growth signals are enhanced (expressed in tissues or cells in which they would not normally function). Mutation in a tumor suppressor gene can lead to a reduced level or complete loss of its normal growth-slowing activities.

Some Cancers Are the Result of an Inherited Gene Defect

A small proportion of all cancers represent inherited genetic disease. An inherited mutation in a particular predisposition gene can dramatically increase an individual's risk for cancer. Among the best-known examples of inherited cancers are the heritable forms of colorectal and breast cancers. Typically in any given inherited cancer the predisposition to tumor development is restricted to a limited number of tissues or organ systems. Features of inherited cancers include a family history of cancer, early age of onset relative to the population at large, multiple primary tumors, and frequent bilaterality. It is important to bear in mind that the inherited mutation is not, in and of itself, sufficient for cancer development and that additional genetic events are required before cancers arise.

Most Cancers Arise as the Result of Mutations That Occur in Somatic Tissues

The vast majority of tumors are sporadic (the result of a series of mutations in somatic cells). Features of sporadic cancers include a negative family history for cancers, a single primary tumor, and late age of onset or an age of onset consistent with the normal range for similar tumors in the population. The absence of any family history relates to the fact that all of the mutations are acquired in somatic cells and as such are unique to the tumor cells. By definition, they were not inherited and cannot be passed on to the cancer patient's progeny. Late age of onset is a function of the stochastic nature of mutational events. Epidemiological studies suggest that three to eight mutations are usually required for cancer formation.[1] In inherited cancers one mutation is present in every body cell. In sporadic cancers all the mutations associated with tumor formation are acquired in somatic cells. With each cell division there is some chance for a mutation that will contribute to tumor formation. If n mutational events are required for the development of a given type of cancer, sporadic forms of the cancer are the result of n somatic mutations, while the inherited forms require $n - 1$ somatic events. Single primary tumors are most likely for sporadic cancers because the chance of a single cell and its progeny acquiring all of the genetic alterations necessary for cancer formation is small.

CURRENT APPLICATIONS OF MOLECULAR GENETICS TO THE MANAGEMENT OF CANCER PATIENTS

Inherited Cancers

Molecular genetics plays a unique role in the care of patients with inherited forms of cancer and their at-risk family members. In the past a diagnosis of inherited cancer was based solely on clinical findings (such as positive family history, multiple primary tumors, and early age of onset). For a number of cancers DNA studies can now be performed to confirm or refute a clinical diagnosis of inherited disease.

A molecular genetic diagnosis can have a real impact on the further surveillance of the cancer patient and on the surveillance of the patient's family members. Molecular genetic techniques are used to identify family members who have inherited the disease allele and as a result are at high risk for cancer. Conversely, molecular diagnostic tools can serve to determine which family members did not inherit the disease allele and therefore do not need the intense level of surveillance that might be recommended for their genetically affected relatives. A molecular diagnosis of inherited cancer can also heighten the health care team's awareness of the risk for additional primary tumors and the need for increased surveillance for such tumors. With some inherited forms of cancer, presymptomatic genetic diagnosis offers the opportunity for prophylactic surgery. There is hope that, in the future, chemoprevention and gene therapy of these cancers will be possible.

If the defective gene has been isolated for an inherited form of cancer, direct testing for a mutation that predisposes to tumor development can be performed. The predisposition gene has not been cloned, but its position in the genome has been precisely determined; indirect genetic testing can be performed. In indirect testing the DNA from affected family members (those with the inherited cancers) is demonstrated to share a common region of the genome that includes the mutated predisposition gene. Family members of unknown genetic status are assessed to determine whether they share the disease gene region that is common to their affected family members. Schematic representations of direct and indirect genetic testing are presented in Figure 24-1. Both direct and indirect testing methods are currently used for genetic testing in cancer families. Both approaches have limitations. Direct genetic testing (identifying the mutation causally associated with disease) is generally expensive and is not currently possible for all inherited cancers. Indirect testing for a shared region of the genome that includes the disease gene depends on the availability of DNA specimens from multiple affected and unaffected family members and is based on probabilities, rather than a simple test for the mutation's presence or absence.

Molecular diagnosis is now possible for a number of inherited cancers and cancer syndromes. For each the molecular genetic diagnosis has implications for the care of patients.

Colorectal cancers

Familial clustering of colorectal cancers has long been recognized. Because closely related family members have in common not only their genes, but also the environment in which they live, the relative contributions that genetics and the environment make to the predisposition to cancer have been difficult to determine. Careful evaluation of pedigree data has led to the suggestion that as many as 15% of colorectal cancers result from single-gene defects that predispose to colorectal cancer. In any given family with inherited colorectal cancer, one of several predisposition genes exerts its deleterious effect.

FAMILIAL ADENOMATOUS POLYPOSIS

Among the inherited forms of colorectal cancer, familial adenomatous polyposis is the best understood. Familial adenomatous polyposis is an autosomal dominant trait with high penetrance and variable expressivity. Describing familial adenomatous polyposis as highly penetrant means that cancer will develop in the vast majority of individuals inheriting the predisposing mutation. Variable expressivity refers to the many phenotypic or clinical manifestations that can result from the mutant familial adenomatous polyposis gene but that are not necessarily seen in all patients. Familial adenomatous polyposis comprises only a small proportion (approximately 1%) of colorectal cancers, yet patients with this disease represent a group that can benefit from genetic investigations.

The hallmark of familial adenomatous polyposis is multiple adenomatous polyps (usually more than 100) in the colon and rectum. The polyps have a marked propensity to progress to carcinoma, and if left untreated, all patients with familial adenomatous polyposis would be expected to develop carcinomas. The mean age at diagnosis of colorectal cancers in patients with familial adenomatous polyposis is approximately 40 years. It is important to bear in mind that familial adenomatous polyposis is not only a disease of the colon and rectum. Some patients have polyps in the upper gastrointestinal tract, which can give rise to periampullary adenocarcinomas. Patients are also at increased risk for a variety of extracolonic tumors, including osteomas, fibromas, desmoids, papillary thyroid carcinomas, and, less frequently, adrenal cortical tumors and hepatoblastomas. Other manifestations of familial adenomatous polyposis include sebaceous cysts, dental anomalies, and congenital hypertrophy of the retinal epithelium. The clinical features of familial adenomatous polyposis have been reviewed numerous times, and many of the pertinent references relating clinical and genetic findings can be found by accessing entry 175100 in *Online Mendelian Inheritance in Man* (OMIM).[2]

The genetics of familial adenomatous polyposis is both simple and complex. The phenotype of multiple adenomatous polyps is striking and on its own is suggestive of genetic disease. Seventy-five percent or more of patients with familial adenomatous polyposis have similarly affected relatives. In 1987, DNA marker linkage studies in familial adenomatous polyposis families localized the predisposition gene to band q21 on the long arm of chromosome 5.[3,4] Linkage studies in families with Gardner's syndrome (polyposis plus extraintestinal features) proved that the predisposition gene for Gardner's syndrome mapped to the same region as familial adenomatous polyposis.[5] The gene for familial adenomatous polyposis, termed *APC,* was cloned in 1991,[6,7] and mutations were identified both in patients with familial adenomatous polyposis and in those with Gardner's syndrome.[8] The discovery that both disorders were associated with mutations in the *APC* gene meant that familial adenomatous polyposis and Gardner's syndrome are allelic (variants of the same gene). Many different mutations within the *APC* gene have been identified in association with familial adenomatous polyposis and Gardner's syndrome. The clinical heterogeneity of the two disorders is paralleled by allelic heterogeneity (multiple forms of the same gene). The vast majority of familial adenomatous polyposis and

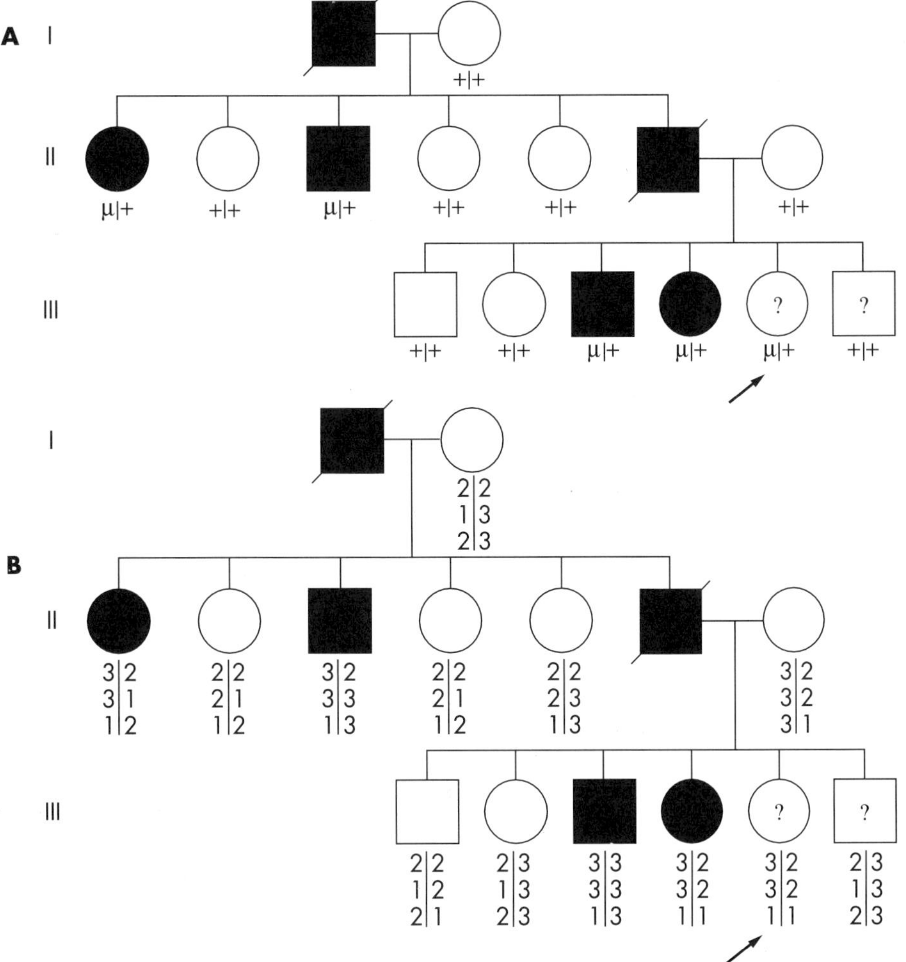

Figure 24-1 Direct and indirect genetic testing in a family with inherited cancer. **A**, Direct detection of a mutation that predisposes to cancer development.
+ : normal form of the predisposition gene
μ : cancer predisposition mutation
B, Indirect testing for a cancer susceptibility allele. DNA polymorphisms in the region of the cancer susceptibility gene are assayed, and the pattern that marks the mutation-bearing chromosome determined. All affected family members have a 3 3 1 polymorphism pattern. In both pedigree **A** and **B** the female of unknown disease status in generation III is shown to have inherited the predisposition to cancer development. Her brother, on the other hand, inherited the normal form of the gene.

■ ● : affected male, affected female

□ ○ : unaffected male, unaffected female

■ : deceased affected male

? ? : at-risk family member of unknown clinical status

↗ : at-risk family member demonstrated to carry the cancer susceptibility allele

Gardner's syndrome families show evidence of involvement of a chromosome 5q21 gene, and for some time the disorders were assumed to be genetically homogeneous (all caused by mutation in one gene). Recently a few families in which the predisposition to disease appears not to involve the chromosome 5 *APC* gene have been reported.[9,10] These are, however, likely to represent rare exceptions.

Approximately one fourth of patients with familial adenomatous polyposis have no family history of disease[11,12] and as such represent new mutations in the *APC* gene. The new germline mutants pass on the predisposition allele to 50% of their progeny, as expected for any mendelian trait.

APC mutations have been detected with a variety of techniques.[6,8,13] All the current methodologies are based on analysis of genetic material isolated from peripheral white blood cells. The *APC* gene is very large, and the number of mutations identified to date is considerable. Most mutations lead to premature truncation of the 2,843 amino acid protein.[14] The enormous size of the *APC* gene and its complex organization mean that a direct search for mutation is labor intensive. Since most mutations result in a truncated protein, the premature protein truncation test[13,15] may prove an effective means for identifying mutations in affected and at-risk family members. *APC* mutation testing using a range of methods is now performed in a number of medical centers and is also commercially available. A direct DNA test can be used to determine with almost 100% accuracy who has inherited the predisposition allele. In most instances direct DNA testing would be expected to be undertaken if the mutation is identified in one or more family members known to be affected with familial adenomatous polyposis and the DNA of other members of unknown or uncertain status tested specifically for the mutation that is being inherited in the family. How this information might be used will be discussed with similar information obtained using indirect genetic testing.

Indirect genetic testing for familial adenomatous polyposis began almost immediately after the gene was localized. Normal DNA variation (polymorphism) in the region of the *APC* gene is evaluated in affected family members, and the pattern of polymorphism that marks the chromosome with the disease mutation is noted. The DNA from family members at risk for familial adenomatous polyposis is then assessed for its pattern of variation in the *APC* gene region. If an at-risk individual does not have the collection of normal DNA variants that are shared by affected family members, that individual is at low risk of having inherited the familial adenomatous polyposis predisposition mutation. Conversely, demonstration that an individual inherited from an affected parent the normal polymorphisms that mark the mutation-bearing chromosome means that the at-risk individual probably inherited the familial adenomatous polyposis predisposition mutation. These indirect analyses depend on DNA comparisons of affected family members, unaffected family members, unaffected parents, and unknown family members. The analyses cannot be applied to all familial adenomatous polyposis patients and families. DNA must be available from key individuals, and there are certain constraints on family structure. Nonetheless, indirect genetic testing has been reported as having 99.9% accuracy in examining specific DNA variants in the ideal family structure.[16] A more conservative estimate of 90% probability for assigning correctly the *APC* mutation status based on indirect DNA typing was reported by Cachon-Gonzalez et al.[17] New DNA analysis methods, including investigation of DNA from archived pathology specimens from deceased family members, make possible accurate indirect testing.

One of the biggest benefits of presymptomatic genetic testing for familial adenomatous polyposis is identification of at-risk individuals who did not inherit the predisposition mutation. The genetically negative family members, in principle, are no longer required to participate in frequent clinical screening programs. Presymptomatic identification of individuals who, based on their genotype, are destined to have disease could improve compliance with screening programs. With better screening in patients with familial adenomatous polyposis, decisions regarding the nature and timing of surgeries are based on what is known about disease progression in the individual and not on how the disease can be expected to behave in the population as a whole. An additional benefit associated with presymptomatic genetic diagnoses is that caregivers know which members of a family benefit most from their attention.

In a recent review on the clinical application of genetic investigations of familial adenomatous polyposis, Petersen[18] outlined recommendations for clinical screening for familial adenomatous polyposis family members who have had presymptomatic genetic testing. Mutation carriers should begin annual, flexible sigmoidoscopy before puberty, at age 10 or 11. Disease surveillance for the genetically negative family members can be greatly reduced.[18] A positive genetic diagnosis should also lead to increased surveillance for extracolonic tumors in familial adenomatous polyposis gene carriers. Molecular genetic diagnosis plays an important role for families in which, for example, histories are uncertain or at-risk family members died before disease might have been detected. A genetic diagnosis can remove virtually all uncertainty and, by doing so, help both patient and physician make appropriate decisions about surveillance. Both direct and indirect testing can have a negative psychosocial impact on patients with familial adenomatous polyposis as well as their families. Medical geneticists continue to attempt to develop appropriate means of dealing with genetic testing for familial adenomatous polyposis.

Hereditary nonpolyposis colorectal carcinoma

Hereditary nonpolyposis colorectal carcinoma (HNPCC) is the term used to describe a group of disorders recognized clinically as dominantly inherited colorectal cancers. Colorectal cancers develop at a young age in affected members of HNPCC kindreds (at least one family member below 45 years of age). Patients with HNPCC do not have multiple premalignant lesions. The absence of polyps or multiple adenomas distinguishes HNPCC from familial adenomatous polyposis. Colon cancers in HNPCC tend to be right sided. Multiple primary and metachronous colorectal cancers are not infrequent in patients with HNPCC. HNPCC is like familial adenomatous polyposis in that it is a multisystem disease. There is an increased risk for other types of tumors, including carcinomas of the endometrium, stomach, urinary tract, hepatobiliary tract, and other sites.[19]

At present the definition of HNPCC is based solely on clinical findings.[20] A minimum of three family members over two or more generations must have documented colorectal cancers. At least one family member must have had the disease diagnosed before age 45. One affected individual must be a first-degree relative (sibling, parent, or child) of two other affected family members. Such a restrictive definition of disease could exclude many kindreds that are, at the gene level, HNPCC families. In fact, clear mendelian inheritance of a predisposition to colorectal cancer outside of the familial adenomatous polyposis syndrome has been difficult to prove.[21,22] Houlston et al.,[23] however, presented data suggesting that at least 13% of colorectal cancers were associated with a dominant predisposition gene distinct from familial adenomatous polyposis.

HNPCC is genetically heterogeneous. The discovery that more than one gene could result in HNPCC came with successes in mapping the predisposition loci in large HNPCC families and in identifying mutations in candidate genes. In any given HNPCC family one predisposition gene is mutated. At present four genes are known, and possibly other genes are yet to be identified.

DNA marker linkage studies in large HNPCC families served to map genes for nonpolyposis colorectal cancer to two distinct chromosomal regions. In 1993 Peltolomaki et al.[24] mapped a predisposition gene to the short arm of chromosome 2 in the region of bands p16-p15. Aaltonen et al.[25] studied additional families, some providing further evidence for the existence of a predisposition gene on the short arm of chromosome 2, and others showing clearly that the inherited predisposition to colorectal cancers mapped elsewhere. Lindblom et al.[26] found that in some HNPCC families the predisposition gene mapped to the short arm of chromosome 3 in the region of bands p23-p21. Both groups discovered that the DNA of colorectal cancers from members of the HNPCC families investigated was characterized by an unusual form of genetic instability.[25,26] The tumor DNAs were marked by what appeared to be numerous replication errors involving simple repeat sequences, consistent with a defect in DNA mismatch repair. For many of the DNA sequences evaluated, the tumor DNA makeup was recognizably different from the normal (nontumor) DNA of the same patient. Similar errors in tumor DNA were also identified in 12% to 28% of sporadic colorectal cancers investigated by other groups.[27,28] The DNA instability phenotype, dubbed replication error, microsatellite instability, or ubiquitous somatic mutation, is suggestive of the effects of a mutation in a mutator gene. The vast majority of colorectal cancers from patients with HNPCC display the DNA replication error phenotype.[29]

The mapping of HNPCC predisposition genes was quickly followed by gene cloning and the identification of mutations in families.[30-33] The genes were identified rapidly in part because there was a hint as to the normal function of the HNPCC predisposition genes. Because HNPCC tumors appeared to exhibit defective DNA mismatch repair, it was reasonable to assume that defects in mismatch repair genes might underlie the disease phenotype. Gene sequences from bacterial and yeast DNA mismatch repair genes were used to isolate the human equivalents. One gene, termed *MSH2*, mapped to the chromosome 2 region known to contain an HNPCC predisposition gene, was proved to be mutated in disease kindreds.[30,31] Another, *MLH1*, mapped to the chromosome 3 HNPCC region, was similarly mutant in families.[32] Other families with HNPCC appeared to have normal *MSH2* and *MLH1* genes, which led to a search for mutations in other DNA mismatch repair genes. Two more genes, *PMS1* on chromosome 2 and *PMS2* on chromosome 7, were identified and demonstrated to be mutated in HNPCC kindreds.

Clearly, HNPCC is much more complex at the gene level than familial adenomatous polyposis. Allelic heterogeneity (different mutations in the same gene that can result in HNPCC) has been demonstrated. Each of the four possible HNPCC genes is large. Even when it is known which gene *(MSH2, MLH1, PMS1,* or *PMS2)* is likely to be involved, the prospect of undertaking a search for mutations is daunting. Presymptomatic identification of HNPPC disease allele carriers is, however, possible and is being undertaken in many centers. Both direct and indirect testing is in use. Commercially available direct mutation testing is on the horizon. Much work is needed before issues of sensitivity and reliability of either type of testing can be addressed adequately.

How a molecular genetic diagnosis of HNPCC might be used in cancer surveillance is unknown. Houlston et al.[23] estimate, based on investigation of 203 pedigrees derived from a consecutive series of colorectal cancers, that dominant genes predisposing to colorectal cancer have a frequency of six in 1,000 and a lifetime penetrance of 63%. This means that more than one in 200 individuals in the population has a predisposition gene, which 63% of the time will result in the development of colorectal cancer. Not all of the genetic predisposition measured by Houlston et al.[23] is expected to manifest as HNPCC. Nonetheless, mutations in HNPCC genes could account for a significant proportion of the population's risk of developing colorectal cancer, and genetic testing may be valuable in some situations.

Lynch[34] recently presented a well-thought-out plan for the integration of molecular genetic testing and cancer surveillance in HNPCC. The article is also an excellent source for references to important papers that address procedures and recommendations for managing patients with HNPCC and their families that were developed before the identification of the disease genes. The care plan begins with taking a family history and categorizing a patient as at risk or not at risk for HNPCC, based on family history. The recommended surveillance for colorectal cancers is then determined by how strong the family history is. For unequivocal HNPCC it is suggested that colonoscopy begin at age 20 to 25 and be repeated at 3-year intervals. For individuals at lower but clearly increased risk (one first-degree relative with colorectal cancer diagnosed at less than 50 years of age or two affected first-degree relatives), colonoscopy or flexible sigmoidoscopy and barium enema should be performed at age 35. Repeat evaluation at 5- to 10-year intervals is suggested. Clearly, molecular genetic tests for HNPCC genes should lead to increased surveillance for at-risk individuals who inherit the predisposition gene and to possible testing of additional family members. At present no clear guidelines have been established for surgical intervention in patients with HNPCC.

It is important to bear in mind that HNPCC involves an increased risk for tumors outside the colon and rectum. Surveillance for endometrial and other HNPCC-related cancers may be warranted for some individuals. The management plan presented by Lynch[34] does not emphasize the fact that an individual's medical history can dramatically increase the level of suspicion that genetic disease is present. Even in the absence of a family history of colorectal cancers, multiple primary tumors and early onset are suggestive of an inherited predisposition to cancer. At present the proportion of HNPCC patients who have a de novo mutation in the predisposition genes is unknown. Molecular genetic studies may be warranted for individuals whose history prompts suspicion. Demonstrating that tumors from such patients have DNA replication errors characteristic of HNPCC might further increase the suspicion of genetic disease. In HNPCC, molecular genetic studies of both the tumor DNA and cellular DNA could play a role in determining a strategy for cancer surveillance.

Multiple endocrine neoplasia type 2 and familial medullary thyroid carcinoma

Medullary thyroid carcinoma comprises approximately 10% of all thyroid cancers,[35] and it is estimated that as many as 25% of medullary thyroid carcinomas represent inherited disease.[36] Medullary thyroid carcinoma is a feature common to three clinically distinct, dominantly inherited disorders.[37,38] Multiple endocrine neoplasia (MEN) 2A is characterized by medullary thyroid carcinomas, pheochromocytomas, and occasionally parathyroid adenomas. MEN 2B includes the clinical features of medullary thyroid carcinomas, pheochromocytomas, mucosal neuromas, ganglioneuromas, and additional skeletal and ophthalmic abnormalities. Familial medullary thyroid carcinoma, on the other hand, is characterized by medullary thyroid carcinoma and no additional endocrine abnormalities. All three disorders are associated with inherited mutation in the *RET* protooncogene.[39-43] *RET* mutations associated with MEN 2 and familial medullary thyroid carcinoma are highly penetrant and show variable expressivity. In all three disorders medullary thyroid carcinoma is preceded by hyperplasia of the calcitonin-secreting thyroid C cells,[44] and as a consequence an elevated serum calcitonin level is a very good marker for C cell hyperplasia or medullary thyroid carcinoma. In its inherited forms medullary thyroid carcinoma tends to be multifocal and to arise at an early age relative to sporadic cases. The age at onset of medullary thyroid carcinoma is less in MEN 2B than in MEN 2A, often occurring in the first or second decade of life. In MEN 2A the thyroid cancers frequently develop in early to middle adulthood. The age at onset of medullary thyroid carcinoma is later in familial medullary thyroid carcinoma than in either MEN 2A or MEN 2B.

The genetics of MEN 2 and familial medullary thyroid carcinoma is relatively straightforward. The MEN 2A gene was mapped to chromosome 10 in 1987. In 1990 the inherited predisposition to MEN 2B was mapped to the same region of chromosome 10 as MEN 2A, and the following year the gene predisposing to familial medullary thyroid carcinoma was also mapped to the region. Gene identification came in 1993 and 1994 with the demonstration that all three disorders result from *RET* mutation.[45]

MEN 2A is characterized by considerable allelic heterogeneity. The mutations associated with the MEN 2A phenotype are restricted to five cysteine codons in the *RET* gene. All are missense mutations (resulting in substitution of another amino acid). A recent compilation of data for an international consortium for the study of *RET* mutation showed that 95% of MEN 2A families studied to date have a *RET* mutation, and of those, 87% are in codon 634.[46] MEN 2B, on the other hand, appears to be a relatively homogeneous disorder. Of 64 unrelated patients with MEN 2B investigated, 60 had the same single-base substitution in codon 918, in a region of *RET* demonstrated to be unaltered in the DNA of patients with MEN 2A.[46] Familial medullary thyroid carcinoma shows a level of allelic heterogeneity comparable to that seen in MEN 2A. A surprising observation was that some familial medullary thyroid carcinoma kindreds share the same mutations as MEN 2A kindreds. Despite an apparently identical genotype the clinical phenotypes in even large families with many affected members can differ. A strong correlation exists between the codon 918 mutation and the MEN 2B genotype[41-43] and to a lesser extent between substitution of an arginine for a cysteine at residue 634 and an increased likelihood of developing hyperparathyroidism.[47]

The role that genetics can play in the management of MEN 2A and familial medullary thyroid carcinoma family members is well documented. Indirect genetic testing was implemented shortly after the demonstration that the inherited predisposition locus mapped to chromosome 10.[48] With the identification of mutations in the *RET* gene associated with MEN 2A and familial medullary thyroid carcinoma, direct DNA testing became possible. By use of either direct or indirect genetic testing, disease allele carriers can be identified presymptomatically, long before the development of the C cell hyperplasia that precedes medullary thyroid carcinoma. Two groups have reported on the use of direct DNA screening tests to direct treatment of asymptomatic MEN 2A mutation carriers.[49,50] No clear guidelines for prophylactic thyroidectomy exist at present. Thyroidectomy in a MEN 2A gene carrier amounts to a curative procedure. Removal of the gland before development of cancer eliminates the possibility of medullary thyroid carcinoma and is a form of cancer prevention.[51] In MEN 2A the risk for pheochromocytomas and parathyroid hyperplasia, however, remains. A genetic diagnosis can be used to better direct screening for other tumors in family members. Family members who do not inherit the disease allele need not be screened for tumors.

Molecular genetics can also play a role in cancer surveillance of patients with medullary thyroid carcinoma and a negative family history of MEN 2A, MEN 2B, or familial medullary thyroid carcinoma. Not all patients with *RET* mutation and medullary thyroid carcinoma have a clear history of similar cancers in their family. Approximately 50% of patients with MEN 2B have de novo mutation in the *RET* gene and a negative family history.[52,53] Patients with MEN 2B have a striking phenotype and are easily recognized as having genetic disease. New mutations that result in MEN 2A and familial medullary thyroid carcinoma are much less frequent than those associated with MEN 2B. Medullary thyroid carcinoma at an early age might, however, be suggestive of an inherited *RET* defect, even in the absence of a positive family history. One way of determining whether a patient with medullary thyroid carcinoma has an inherited form of the cancer would be to search for mutations in the *RET* gene in the patient's constitutional DNA. Identification of a mutation would confirm the diagnosis of genetic disease and would alter surveillance for the patient and family members. Conversely, a failure to identify a *RET* mutation would make the diagnosis of genetic disease less likely. A negative mutation test, however, is not definitive. As many as 13% of medullary thyroid carcinoma families do not have recognizable *RET* mutations.[46] In such instances, study of *RET* sequences in the medullary thyroid carcinoma DNA and comparison with the patient's constitutional (blood or other tissue) DNA could prove helpful. Approximately 30% of sporadic medullary thyroid carcinomas have a tumor-specific mutation involving *RET* codon 918.[41,43] The identification of the *RET* codon 918 mutation in the tumor DNA and demonstration that the mutation is not in the normal cellular DNA could be taken as further proof that a tumor arose as the result of somatic, not inherited, mutation. If an individual is known to have sporadic medullary thyroid carcinoma, there is no need for surveillance for development of the other tumors associated with MEN 2. The risk for recurrence of medullary thyroid carcinoma, however, remains. Widespread use of direct testing for *RET* mutation in medullary thyroid carcinoma tumor DNA is unlikely. Such analyses are expensive, are available in only a few research centers, and have small relative benefits to the patient and family.

Multiple endocrine neoplasia type 1

MEN 1 is an autosomal dominant disorder in which, as the name suggests, there is a predisposition to a variety of endocrine neoplasms. The target organs most frequently involved are the parathyroid glands, the pituitary, and the pancreas. Patients with MEN 1 are at increased risk for a variety of other tumors. Variable expressivity is a well-recognized feature of MEN 1. In the past, and to a lesser extent today, MEN 1 was referred to as Wermer's syndrome, multiple endocrine adenoma, multiple endocrine adenomatosis, and pluriglandular syndrome. Most patients with MEN 1 (over 90%) have parathyroid hyperplasia or adenomas and biochemically detectable hyperparathyroidism. Testing for elevated levels of parathyroid hormone and for hypercalcemia has in fact been used routinely as part of disease screening in MEN 1 families. The next most frequently observed neoplasms in MEN 1 are pancreatic tumors, followed by pituitary tumors.[54] Entry 31100 in OMIM[2] includes a description of the clinical features of MEN 1 and a large list of references relating clinical and genetic findings. The incidence of MEN 1 is unknown. Patients with hyperparathyroidism, Zollinger-Ellison syndrome, pituitary tumors, or insulinomas, however, frequently have features of MEN 1.[54] MEN 1 may actually be more prevalent than suggested by clear family histories alone.

In 1988 the gene that predisposes to MEN 1 was mapped to the long arm of chromosome 11.[55] Despite enormous effort the MEN 1 gene had not yet been identified at the time this chapter was prepared. Molecular genetic testing for MEN 1 is restricted at present to indirect or linkage-based analyses. The disease gene region was refined to the band q13 region, and tightly linked markers for use in presymptomatic detection of carriers were discovered.[56] Larsson et al.[57] devised indirect tests that they estimated to be more than 99% accurate for predicting inheritance of the MEN 1 predisposition. In a recent publication they reviewed the use of indirect testing in screening for MEN 1.[58] As is the case for all indirect testing the ability to determine the MEN 1 genotype of an at-risk family member depends on the availability of DNA specimens from other family members, both affected and unaffected. A clinical diagnosis of MEN 1 is not always straightforward, and the accuracy of a molecular genetic diagnosis is directly related to the certainty of clinical diagnosis for all of the family members included in the analyses.

Predictive testing alters cancer surveillance for MEN 1 gene carriers. By knowing who in a family has inherited the predisposition allele, physicians can focus screening on the individuals who will most benefit from it. Skogseid et al.[59] recently reviewed how genetic screening and biochemical screening for MEN 1 could be integrated. Both biochemical and radiological investigations are required. Screening and tumor surveillance should begin between ages 10 and 15 and continue, essentially, for the rest of the patient's life. As is the case for any autosomal dominant trait, half of the progeny of a gene carrier will not inherit the disease allele and do not benefit from disease screening. Surveillance of an at-risk member of an MEN 1 family is costly, and knowing who in a family did not inherit the predisposition has real economic benefits.

Inherited breast cancer

As is the case for many cancers, breast cancer can occur either in the context of an inherited syndrome or as sporadic disease. Only 5% to 9% of cases of breast cancer fall into the category of inherited disease.[60] The chance that breast cancer is due to some inherited predisposition is higher if it is diagnosed at a younger age. It is important to bear in mind, however, that even in women whose breast cancer is diagnosed before the age of 30 years, the chance that disease is due to some inherited gene defect is no more than 40%.[61] The term "familial breast cancer," as distinct from "inherited breast cancer," is reserved for families in which at least two first-degree relatives are affected but for which there is insufficient evidence to establish autosomal dominant transmission of disease.

Inherited breast cancers show considerable genetic heterogeneity. Breast cancer is a feature of Li-Fraumeni syndrome (also referred to as SBLA syndrome), hereditary early-onset breast cancer syndrome (also known as site-specific breast cancer syndrome), breast-ovarian cancer syndrome, Cowden's disease, Muir-Torre syndrome, and Peutz-Jeghers syndrome. Heterozygous carriers of the ataxia telangiectasia gene are also predisposed to breast cancer. In several of these conditions the responsible genes have been identified. The susceptibility to breast cancer associated with each of these syndromes varies.

Li-Fraumeni syndrome was first described in 1969. The syndrome is characterized by a much increased risk for the development of soft tissue sarcoma, osteosarcoma, breast cancer, brain tumors, laryngeal cancer, leukemia, and adrenocortical cancer.[62] (See OMIM[2] entry 151623 for additional references.) Two research groups working independently reported inherited (constitutional) mutations in the *TP53* gene on the short arm of chromosome 17p, band p13.1, segregating in Li-Fraumeni families. The majority of Li-Fraumeni families harbor germline mutations of *TP53*. The probability of invasive cancer in individuals with an inherited *TP53* mutation has been reported to be 50% by age 30 and 90% by age 70.[63] Breast cancer is the most frequent manifestation of Li-Fraumeni syndrome, developing in 89% of females by age 50.[63] The proportion of all breast cancer in the population caused by germline *TP53* mutations is small, however, on the order of 1%.

The hereditary early-onset breast cancer syndrome also demonstrates autosomal dominant inheritance. In 1990 Hall et al.[64] reported linkage between markers from the long arm of chromosome 17, in the region 17q12-21, and the predisposition to breast cancer in 45% of families in which multiple members were affected. The linkage was not seen, however, in families in which the average age at diagnosis was greater than 50 years. Narod et al.[65] subsequently confirmed linkage of the same region with the predisposition to cancer development in families in which both breast and ovarian cancer segregated. The predisposition gene at 17q12-21 was termed *BRCA1*. It is estimated that up to 94% of families in which there are multiple cases of breast and ovarian cancer have constitutional mutations in the *BRCA1* gene.[66] Over a 4-year period the localization of the *BRCA1* region on chromosome 17 was further and further refined, culminating in the cloning of *BRCA1* in 1994.[67-70] The *BRCA1* gene is large. The predicted protein is 1,863 amino acids and includes a zinc finger motif that may be involved in transcriptional regulation. Mutation in *BRCA1* is estimated to account for 4% to 5% of breast cancers, with as many as one in 150 to one in 2,000 individuals in the population carrying disease alleles.[70-74] The penetrance of *BRCA1* is high. Female carriers of the mutated *BRCA1* have an 85% to 87% lifetime risk of breast cancer. The risk that *BRCA1* mutations confer for ovarian cancer is more variable. Easton et al.[74,75] have calculated the risk to be 11% by age 60 in some families and 42% by age 60 in others. *BRCA1* is a tumor-suppressor gene and conforms to the "two-hit hypothesis."[76] It is generally accepted that two mutations (hits) in the *BRCA1* are required before tumors develop. In inherited breast cancer associated with *BRCA1* mutation the first mutation is carried in the germline and therefore is present in every cell in the individual. The second mutation occurs in the breast epithelial cells later in life. As with most inherited cancers, these cancers occur at a younger age than their sporadic counterparts and are more frequently bilateral.[77] It is thought that 28% of breast cancers diagnosed before the age of 30 are due to germline *BRCA1* mutations.[78] In a Dutch series of hereditary breast cancer families the cumulative risk of contralateral breast cancer was 37% after 20 years.[79] The age at diagnosis differs between individuals and between families, reflecting the variable expressivity of the mutated gene. The mutated *BRCA1* gene also confers a higher risk of colon and prostate cancers. Lifetime risks of prostate cancer and colon cancer are 6% and 8%, respectively.[74] Tonin et al.[66] have reported that in families linked to *BRCA1,* higher incidences of primary peritoneal cancer, cancer of the fallopian tube, and melanoma are also found.

Hall et al.[64] pointed out that only 45% of the families they investigated showed linkage to 17q markers and that another gene might account for the disease in the remainder of hereditary early-onset breast cancer families. In 1994 Wooster et al.[80] reported on the discovery of linkage of a region on the long arm of chromosome 13 with hereditary early-onset breast cancer in families demonstrated not to show linkage between 17q markers and disease predisposition. The region (including the gene termed *BRCA2*) maps to 13q12-13, proximal to the retinoblastoma gene. The size of the region containing the gene is at present too large to consider an immediate search for genes, but over the next few years it will be refined and the gene cloned in the same manner as *BRCA1*. In contrast to *BRCA1* families, males who carry the mutated *BRCA2* gene also develop breast cancer but not with the same frequency as their female family members.[80,81] Ovarian cancer is not a feature of *BRCA2* inheritance. The penetrance of *BRCA2* mutations in females is comparable to that of *BRCA1,* on the order of 80%. Currently, predictive testing for *BRCA2* can only be performed by indirect means in the research setting, since the gene has not been cloned. Mutations in *BRCA2* probably account for 70% of the hereditary early-onset cases that do not show linkage with *BRCA1*. It is possible that other genes not yet located are involved in predisposition in the remainder of inherited early-onset cases.

Cowden's disease (multiple hamartoma syndrome), named after the patient in whom it was first described, comprises bilateral breast cancer, multiple facial trichilemmomas, acral keratoses, oral papillomatoses, gastrointestinal polyposis, female genital tract tumors, and benign and malignant thyroid tumors. The risk of breast cancer is 30% to 50% by age 50.[71] The gene responsible for this syndrome has yet to be identified. Williard et al.[82] reported that there was no amplification or rearrangement of the *HER-2/neu* oncogene, the *ras* oncogene, or *pS-2* in tumors from these patients. Predictive testing is not yet possible in Cowden's disease families.

In Muir-Torre syndrome an association is found among a variety of skin tumors and internal malignancies. The skin tumors reported include sebaceous adenomas, epitheliomas, sebaceous gland carcinomas, and squamous carcinomas. An assortment of internal malignancies have been described, including colorectal cancer, endometrial cancer, and ovarian cancer. Breast cancer is found in 12% of females.[83] It has been determined that Muir-Torre syndrome is probably an allelic variant of HNPPC. Hall et al.[84,85] have found linkage between Muir-Torre inheritance and the *MSH2* gene, and DNA from these tumors contains multiple replication errors.

Peutz-Jeghers syndrome also confers a higher risk of breast cancer development at a young age. The majority of these patients exhibit a characteristic phenotype in which melanin spots are found on lips and buccal mucosa and hamartomatous polyps are found in the gastrointestinal tract.[86] The risk of breast cancer associated with this syndrome is unclear from the literature. However, breast cancer is found in patients less than 40 years of age and is frequently bilateral.

The disease ataxia-telangiectasia (AT) is an autosomal recessive disorder in which female carriers of the mutations have an increased risk of breast cancer. Swift et al.[87,88] reported that the carrier frequency of *AT* mutation in the population is 1.4% and the relative risk of breast cancer is 6.8 times that of the general population. It has been calculated that at least 7% of patients with breast cancer in the United States are heterozygous carriers of *AT* mutations.[89] The *AT* gene is required for the transcription of *TP53* in response to the damage caused by radiation.[90] The carriers have an increased sensitivity to irradiation, and thus mammograms in these women may actually be to their detriment. The gene responsible for *AT* was cloned recently.[91] Genetic screening for *AT* mutations is not being carried out at this time.

The main use of molecular biology in the surveillance of breast cancer will be in those high-risk families in which there appears to be autosomal dominant inheritance. The surveillance will likely begin with a careful and detailed family history, including second- and third-degree relatives. Since all these syndromes can be transmitted through males in the family, the history should include the paternal line. Hoskins et al.[92] have summarized guidelines for pedigree assessment by the clinician. Study of breast cancer families is confounded by the frequent, sporadic occurrence of the disease in family members who do not carry the mutation. These tumors are likely to occur at a later age than the inherited tumors and are more likely to be unilateral.

Predictive testing for inherited breast cancer can be performed by indirect or direct means. Indirect testing involves linkage analysis using a set of highly informative, closely linked, flanking markers. Once the pattern of markers that is coinherited with the disease allele has been established, the physician can predict which unaffected family members carry the mutation. Linkage analysis is possible only in large families with multiple affected individuals. Whether a pedigree is informative depends on the age of certain family members, that is, whether they are truly unaffected or are simply going to develop the disease at a later age.

After a gene has been cloned, the way is open for direct testing by mutational analysis. The *BRCA1* gene is large, covering more than 100,000 bases of DNA. It contains 24 exons, of which 22 code for RNA. The predicted protein is 1,863 amino acids and includes a zinc finger motif that may be involved in transcriptional regulation. Miki et al.[69] reported five predisposing mutations in eight kindreds. Since the original report, several groups have discovered other mutations coinherited with the phenotype.[93-95] Shattuck-Eidens et al.[96] summarized the known mutations in February 1995. At that time 38 distinct mutations were recognized, the majority of which result in premature termination of the *BRCA1* protein. Although no definite correlation could be found between mutation position and phenotype, mutations at the 3' end tend to confer a lower risk of ovarian cancer. The large size of this gene and the multiplicity of mutations make the application of wide-scale predictive testing in the screening setting difficult. Guidelines as to who should be tested for germline *BRCA1* mutations have yet to be developed. Cornelis et al.[77] consider that testing should be offered only to families with a strong history of early-onset breast or breast/ovarian cancer. *BRCA1* testing is not yet available commercially and should be performed in the research setting. The sensitivity and specificity of *BRCA1* testing have not been defined. Because of the legal and ethical ramifications of predictive testing, guidelines establishing who should be tested will be required. Recommendations have been published for *TP53* mutation testing.[97] Sidransky et al.[98] analyzed the DNA of 126 patients below the age of 40 who had breast cancer. Only one was found to have a constitutional *TP53* mutation, indicating that routine screening of the population for *TP53* mutations is unlikely to be cost effective. The same may be true for *BRCA1* testing. Hogervorst et al.[99] have described a protein truncation test for *BRCA1* that shows promise and would not be as labor intensive as direct sequencing.

As with all genetic testing the individuals being investigated should be adequately protected. Counseling should precede testing to ensure that the family understands the implications of the test. There should be no coercion, and the individual should retain the right to decide whether to be tested. The confidentiality of the test results should be ensured, and third parties denied access to the results unless the patient consents. The results of the test should not put the individual at risk for discrimination, such as from insurance carriers. The testing should be of benefit to the patient.[97]

The current options for high-risk patients are either close clinical surveillance or prophylactic surgery. A main advantage of being able to predict inheritance of *BRCA1* and *BRCA2* mutations will be to identify women who perceive themselves to be at very high risk but do not in fact carry the mutation. If they carry the mutation, the risk of breast cancer is more than 80%, whereas if they do not, it is in the order of 10% or less (the lifetime risk of breast cancer in the general female population). Women in high-risk families are under extreme psychological stress and often perceive their risk to be higher than it actually is. Despite their levels of anxiety they are less likely to comply with current surveillance recommendations, such as breast self-examination and screening mammography.[100,101] If an at-risk family member is found not to be a carrier, she may be spared unnecessary prophylactic surgery, although she should be informed that breast cancer can still develop from other causes. Current screening recommendations for high-risk women include mammography every 6 to 12 months beginning 5 to 10 years before the earliest breast cancer in the family, breast examination by a physician beginning in the patient's twenties and repeated every 6 months, and adherence to monthly breast self-examinations. The efficacy of mammography in decreasing mortality from breast cancer in the under-40 age group is unknown. Individuals who do not carry the mutation would not require this intensive level of surveillance. Instead the recommendations for the general female population could be followed, that is, a yearly breast examination by a physician beginning in the twenties and mammography every 1 to 2 years from ages 40 to 49 and annually from 50 onward.

The option of bilateral prophylactic mastectomy should be discussed with high-risk women from inherited breast cancer families, and they should be informed of the current level of information about this operation. Unlike prophylactic thyroidectomy, mastectomy does not completely remove the risk of subsequent cancer. Patients considering this option should be advised that cases of breast cancer have been seen after prophylactic mastectomy, with the incidence ranging from 1.5% to 18%.[102,103] Subcutaneous mastectomy, sparing the nipple and areola complex, leaves behind 10% to 15% of breast tissue and is not recommended for prophylaxis; thus the total or simple mastectomy is preferable. Breast epithelium can be found in the dermis of the inferior skin flap, the pectoralis major fascia and muscle, and high in the axilla, areas not commonly excised even with prophylactic total mastectomy. It has not been proved that prophylactic surgery is any better than close follow-up in these high-risk patients or that the volume of breast tissue removed reduces breast cancer risk proportionately. Struewing et al.[104] have studied the impact of availability of testing in families linked to *BRCA1*. Two thirds of the individuals stated that they would want to be tested so they could decide whether to have prophylactic oophorectomy, and one third would want to be tested in order to aid in a decision about prophylactic mastectomy. Similarly, prophylactic oophorectomy does not completely protect the patient from the development of ovarian cancer, since peritoneal carcinomatosis has been seen after this operation.[105] The optimal management of these patients is unknown; however, if the patient decides to undergo surgery, she should be supported emotionally by the management team.

The role of chemoprevention and dietary and life-style changes in altering risk in high-risk individuals is unknown. Tamoxifen is being assessed as a chemopreventive agent through the National Surgical Adjuvant Breast Project P-1 trial.

Widespread DNA Testing for Cancer Predisposition

At present the potential role of genetic testing in the early detection and prevention of cancers is not well understood. The risks and benefits associated with DNA testing for cancer predisposition are likely to vary enormously depending on the particular predisposition gene being investigated and the center or environment in which testing is being performed. The National Advisory Council for Human Genome Research recently attempted to identify the major questions that need to be addressed before widescale DNA testing for cancer predisposition can be brought into place. It recognized several areas of deficiency in genetic testing for cancer risk. The population frequency of mutations in known cancer predisposition genes such as *BRCA1* and *MSH2* remains to be determined. The lifetime risk for the development of cancers for those individuals carrying a given *MSH2* or *MLH1* mutation is not known. These problems are not unique to the *BRCA1* or *MSH2* genes. The council also raised questions concerning technical problems that are associated with genetic testing. The reliability, sensitivity, and specificity of each DNA test must be determined before widespread testing can be undertaken. The effectiveness of genetic testing in reducing cancer morbidity and mortality must be considered, as must the psychological impact of testing. If a test does not improve patient survival or reduce disease, is it valuable? If a test result increases the patient's level of anxiety or makes the patient uninsurable, is it justifiable? The report from the National Advisory Council for Human Genome Research stated that "it is premature to offer DNA testing or screening for cancer predisposition outside a carefully monitored research environment."[106] Public awareness that "DNA tests" for cancer risk are available is increasing dramatically. As a consequence, health care professionals can expect an increasing number of requests for cancer predisposition testing. Caution and more research are needed to establish how genetic information can best be used to benefit the individual and society as a whole.

Sporadic Cancers

Recent advances in molecular biology may make possible the detection of cancers well before they could be diagnosed by conventional means. In theory, mutations that result in tumor formation can be detected long before the gross tumor is apparent.[107] Polymerase chain reaction provides the sensitivity required to identify mutations in cell populations derived from exfoliative cytology specimens. The case of Vice-President Hubert Humphrey is an example of the application of molecular genetic techniques to the detection of mutations in specimens that appear normal by conventional criteria. Hruban et al.[108] were able to find a specific *TP53* mutation in a "negative" urine cytology specimen taken from Mr. Humphrey in 1967. Cystoscopy at that time was negative for cancer, but in situ bladder cancer was diagnosed in 1969 and invasive cancer in 1976. The primary invasive tumor was found to have a *TP53* mutation in codon 227. Analysis of the DNA from cells from the archived cytology slides revealed that the same mutation was present at low frequency in the specimen taken 2 years before the diagnosis of cancer in situ and 9 years before the diagnosis of invasive cancer.

Enriched polymerase chain reaction can detect one copy of a mutant *KRAS2* allele oncogene in 10,000 normal alleles. Such mutations have been found in colonic effluent as long as 4 years before the development of colon cancer.[109] *KRAS2* mutations have also been found in gastric aspirates and stool specimens of patients with pancreatic cancer.[110] Mao et al.[107] analyzed the sputum samples of patients entered into the Johns Hopkins Lung Project. Lung cancer later developed in 15 patients from this trial of lung cancer screening. Of these, 10 were demonstrated to have either *KRAS2* or *TP53* mutations in their primary tumor. In eight cases the specific mutation could be detected in the sputum samples collected before the clinical diagnosis of cancer.

The real value of molecular genetic tests will be their ability to alter the course of disease. In some cases increasing the lead time for detection of cancer will improve survival. Polymerase chain reaction–based detection of mutation has, to a limited extent, been applied to the surveillance of high-risk conditions, such as cervical dysplasia,[111-113] Barrett's esophagus,[114,115] and ulcerative colitis,[116,117] in which early intervention is associated with improved survival.

Molecular genetic investigations of tumors may also improve disease staging and thus stratify patients into groups at high versus low risk for recurrence. In a recent study of allelic loss of chromosome 18q sequences, Jen et al.[118] demonstrated that the status of chromosome 18q has significant prognostic value in patients with stage II colorectal cancer. The authors present data suggesting that the prognosis of patients who have stage II colorectal cancers with loss of 18q sequences is similar to that of patients with stage III disease. Given that patients with stage III colorectal cancer are a group that might benefit from adjuvant therapy, it seems logical that stratifying patients based on the molecular genetic characteristics of their tumors would lead to improved treatment and patient survival.

TP53 mutations in saliva have been used to detect recurrence of head and neck cancers at an early stage. Similarly, histologically negative surgical margins of head and neck cancer resections have been found to contain a small percentage of cancer cells by polymerase chain reaction analysis.[119,120] Both polymerase chain reaction and fluorescence in situ hybridization techniques are used to detect recurrent and minimal residual disease in patients with hematological malignancies.[121,122] Early detection of cancer recurrence may lead to improved survival if and when the appropriate therapies become available.

Molecular genetics will be an advantage in cancer surveillance only if it provides more information than can be obtained using the methods currently available. DNA tests used in cancer surveillance need to have comparable or greater levels of sensitivity and specificity than those in current use. This is clearly the case for the DNA-based, presymptomatic identification of individuals inheriting cancer predisposition genes. At present there are no "universal" genetic markers for the detection of sporadic cancers. Some critics have suggested that molecular genetics is all promise and no product. This is changing. New markers for cancer cells continue to be developed, and with them, improved technologies for the analysis of clinical specimens are certain to appear.

Recently the gene for multiple endocrine neoplasia type 1 (MEN 1) was identified.[123] The chromosome 13 breast cancer susceptibility gene, *BRCA2,* was identified,[124,] as was the Cowden's disease gene.[125]

REFERENCES

1. Klein G, Klein E. Evolution of tumours and the impact of molecular oncology. Nature 1985;315:190-5.
2. Online mendelian inheritance in man (OMIM). http:gdbwww.gdb.org/omim/docs/ in_brief.html. Baltimore: Johns Hopkins University Medical School.
3. Bodmer WF, Bailey CJ, Bodmer J, et al. Localization of the gene for familial adenomatous polyposis on chromosome 5. Nature 1987; 328:614-8.
4. Leppert M, Dobbs M, Scambler P, et al. The gene for familial polyposis coli maps to the long arm of chromosome 5. Science 1987; 238:1411-3.
5. Nakamura Y, Lathrop M, Leppert M, et al. Localization of the genetic defect in familial adenomatous polyposis within a small region of chromosome 5. Am J Hum Genet 1988;43:638-44.
6. Groden J, Thliveris A, Samowitz W, et al. Identification and characterization of the familial adenomatous polyposis coli gene. Cell 1991;66:589-600.
7. Kinzler KW, Nilbert MC, Vogelstein B, et al. Identification of a gene located at chromosome 5q21 that is mutated in colorectal cancers. Science 1991;251:1366-70.
8. Nishisho I, Nakamura Y, Miyoshi Y, et al. Mutations of chromosome 5q21 genes in FAP and colorectal cancer patients. Science 1991; 253:665-9.
9. Tops CM, van der Klift HM, van der Luijt RB, et al. Non-allelic heterogeneity of familial adenomatous polyposis. Am J Med Genet 1993;47:563-7.
10. Stella A, Resta N, Gentile M, et al. Exclusion of the APC gene as the cause of a variant form of familial adenomatous polyposis (FAP). Am J Hum Genet 1993;53:1031-7.
11. Maher ER, Barton DE, Slatter R, et al. Evaluation of molecular genetic diagnosis in the management of familial adenomatous polyposis coli: a population based study. J Med Genet 1993;30:675-8.
12. Bisgaard ML, Fenger K, Bulow S, Niebuhr E, Mohr J. Familial adenomatous polyposis (FAP): frequency, penetrance, and mutation rate. Hum Mutat 1994;3:121-5.

13. Powell SM, Petersen GM, Krush AJ, et al. Molecular diagnosis of familial adenomatous polyposis. N Engl J Med 1993;329:1982-7.
14. Nagase H, Nakamura Y. Mutations of the APC (adenomatous polyposis coli) gene. Hum Mutat 1993;2:425-34.
15. van der Luijt R, Khan PM, Vasen H, et al. Rapid detection of translation-terminating mutations at the adenomatous polyposis coli (APC) gene by direct protein truncation test. Genomics 1994;20:1-4.
16. Tops CMJ, Wijnen JT, Griffioen G, et al. Presymptomatic diagnosis of familial adenomatous polyposis by bridging DNA markers. Lancet 1989;2:1361-3.
17. Cachon-Gonzalez MB, Delhanty JD, Burn J, et al. Linkage analysis in adenomatous polyposis coli: the use of four closely linked DNA probes in 20 UK families. J Med Genet 1991;28:681-5.
18. Petersen GM. Knowledge of the adenomatous polyposis coli gene and its clinical application. Ann Med 1994;26:205-8.
19. Lynch HT, Smyrk TC, Watson P, et al. Genetics, natural history, tumor spectrum, and pathology of hereditary nonpolyposis colorectal cancer: an updated review. Gastroenterology 1993;104:1535-49.
20. Vasen HF, Mecklin JP, Khan PM, Lynch HT. The international collaborative group on hereditary non-polyposis colorectal cancer (ICG-HNPCC). Dis Colon Rectum 1991;34:424-5.
21. Bailey-Wilson JE, Elston RC, Schuelke GS, et al. Segregation analysis of hereditary nonpolyposis colorectal cancer. Genet Epidemiol 1986;3:27-38.
22. Cannon-Albright LA, Skolnick MH, Bishop DT, Lee RG, Burt RW. Common inheritance of susceptibility to colonic adenomatous polyps and associated colorectal cancers. N Engl J Med 1988;319:533-7.
23. Houlston RS, Collins A, Slack J, Morton NE. Dominant genes for colorectal cancer are not rare. Ann Hum Genet 1992;56:99-103.
24. Peltolomaki P, Aaltonen LA, Sistonen P, et al. Genetic mapping of a locus predisposing to human colorectal cancer. Science 1993;260: 810-2.
25. Aaltonen LA, Peltomaki P, Leach FS, et al. Clues to the pathogenesis of familial colorectal cancer. Science 1993;260:812-5.
26. Lindblom A, Tannergard P, Werelius B, Nordenskjold M. Genetic mapping of a second locus predisposing to hereditary non-polyposis colon cancer. Nat Genet 1993;5:279-82.
27. Thibodeau SN, Bren G, Schaid D. Microsatellite instability in cancer of the proximal colon. Science 1993;260:816-9.
28. Ionov Y, Peinado MA, Malkhosyan S, Shibata D, Perucho M. Ubiquitous somatic mutations in simple repeated sequences reveal a new mechanism for colonic carcinogenesis. Nature 1993;363:558-61.
29. Aaltonen LA, Peltomaki P, Mecklin JP, et al. Replication errors in benign and malignant tumors from hereditary nonpolyposis colorectal cancer patients. Cancer Res 1994;54:1645-8.
30. Fishel R, Lescoe MK, Rao MR, et al. The human mutator gene homolog *MSH2* and its association with hereditary nonpolyposis colon cancer. Cell 1993;75:1027-38.
31. Leach FS, Nicolaides NC, Papadopoulos N, et al. Mutations of a *mutS* homolog in hereditary nonpolyposis colorectal cancer. Cell 1993;75:1215-25.
32. Papadopoulos N, Nicolaides NC, Wei YF, et al. Mutation of a *mutL* homolog in hereditary colon cancer. Science 1994;263:1625-9.
33. Nicolaides NC, Papadopoulos N, Liu B, et al. Mutations of two *PMS* homologues in hereditary nonpolyposis colon cancer. Nature 1994; 371:75-80.
34. Lynch PM. Hereditary nonpolyposis colorectal carcinoma (HNPCC): clinical application of molecular diagnostic testing. Ann Med 1994; 26:221-8.
35. Rasmusson B. Bone abnormalities in patients with medullary carcinoma of the thyroid. Acta Radiol Oncol 1980;19:461-5.
36. Saad MF, Ordonez NG, Rashid RK, et al. Medullary carcinoma of the thyroid: a study of the clinical features and prognostic factors in 161 patients. Medicine 1984;63:319-42.
37. Schimke RN. Genetic aspects of multiple endocrine neoplasia. Annu Rev Med 1984;35:25-31.
38. Farndon JR, Leight GS, Dilley WG, et al. Familial medullary thyroid carcinoma without associated endocrinopathies: a distinct clinical entity. Br J Surg 1986;73:278-81.
39. Mulligan LM, Kwok JB, Healey CS, et al. Germ-line mutations of the *RET* proto-oncogene in multiple endocrine neoplasia type 2A. Nature 1993;363:458-60.
40. Donis-Keller H, Dou S, Chi D, et al. Mutations in the *RET* proto-oncogene are associated with MEN 2A and FMTC. Hum Mol Genet 1993;2:851-6.
41. Hofstra RM, Landsvater RM, Ceccherini I, et al. A mutation in the *RET* proto-oncogene associated with multiple endocrine neoplasia type 2B and sporadic medullary thyroid carcinoma. Nature 1994; 367:375-6.
42. Carlson KM, Dou S, Chi D, et al. Single missense mutation in the tyrosine kinase catalytic domain of the *RET* proto-oncogene is associated with multiple endocrine neoplasia type 2B. Proc Natl Acad Sci U S A 1994;91:1579-83.
43. Eng C, Smith DP, Mulligan LM, et al. Point mutation within the tyrosine kinase domain of the *RET* proto-oncogene in multiple endocrine neoplasia type 2B and related sporadic tumours. Hum Mol Genet 1994;3:237-41.
44. Wolfe HJ, Melvin KE, Cervi-Skinner SJ, et al. C-cell hyperplasia preceding medullary thyroid carcinoma. N Engl J Med 1973;289:437-41.
45. Goodfellow PJ. Inherited cancers associated with the *RET* proto-oncogene. Curr Opin Genet Dev 1994;4:446-52.
46. Mulligan LM, Marsh DJ, Robinson BG, et al. Genotype-phenotype correlation in MEN2: report of the international *RET* mutation consortium. J Intern Med 1995;284:343-6.
47. Mulligan LM, Eng C, Healey CS, et al. Specific mutations of the *RET* proto-oncogene are related to disease phenotype in MEN 2A and FMTC. Nat Genet 1993;6:70-4.
48. Sobol H, Narod SA, Nakamura Y, et al. Screening for multiple endocrine neoplasia type 2A with DNA-polymorphism analysis. N Engl J Med 1989;321:996-1001.
49. Lips CJ, Landsvater RM, Hoppener JW, et al. Clinical screening as compared with DNA analysis in families with multiple endocrine neoplasia type 2A. N Engl J Med 1994;331:828-35.
50. Wells SA, Chi DD, Toshima K, et al. Predictive DNA testing and prophylactic thyroidectomy in patients at risk for multiple endocrine neoplasia type 2A. Ann Surg 1994;220:237-50.
51. Uttiger RD. Medullary thyroid carcinoma, genes, and the prevention of cancer. N Engl J Med 1994;331:870-1.
52. Norum RA, Lafreniere RG, O'Neal LW, et al. Linkage of the multiple endocrine neoplasia type 2B gene (MEN2B) to chromosome 10 markers linked to MEN2A. Genomics 1990;8:313-7.
53. Carlson KM, Bracamontes J, Jackson CE, et al. Parent-of-origin effects in multiple endocrine neoplasia type 2B. Am J Hum Genet 1994;55:1076-82.
54. Brandi ML, Marx SJ, Aurbach GD, Fitzpatrick LA. Familial multiple endocrine neoplasia type 1: a new look at pathophysiology. Endocr Rev 1987;8:391-405.
55. Larsson C, Skogseid B, Oberg K, Nakamura Y, Nordenskjold M. Multiple endocrine neoplasia type 1 gene maps to chromosome 11 and is lost in insulinoma. Nature 1988;332:85-7.
56. Nakamura Y, Larsson C, Julier C, et al. Localization of the genetic defect in multiple endocrine neoplasia type 1 within a small region of chromosome 11. Am J Hum Genet 1989;44:751-5.
57. Larsson C, Shepherd J, Nakamura Y, et al. Predictive testing for multiple endocrine neoplasia type 1 using DNA polymorphisms. J Clin Invest 1992;89:1344-9.
58. Larsson C, Nordenskjold M. Family screening in multiple endocrine neoplasia type 1 (MEN1). Ann Med 1994;26:191-8.
59. Skogseid B, Rastad J, Oberg K. Multiple endocrine neoplasia type 1: clinical features and screening. Endocrinol Metab Clin North Am 1994;23:1-18.
60. Lynch HT, Lynch J, Conway T, et al. Hereditary breast cancer and family cancer syndromes. World J Surg 1994;18:21-31.
61. Eng C, Stratton M, Ponder B, et al. Familial cancer syndromes. Lancet 1994;343:709-13.
62. Lynch HT, Watson P, Conway TA, Lynch JF. Natural history and age at onset of hereditary breast cancer. Cancer 1992;69:1404-7.

63. Birch JM, Hartley AL, Tricker KJ, et al. Prevalence and diversity of constitutional mutations in the p53 gene among 21 Li-Fraumeni families. Cancer Res 1994;54:1298-1304.
64. Hall JM, Lee ML, Newman B, et al. Linkage of early-onset familial breast cancer to chromosome 17q21. Science 1990;250:1684-9.
65. Narod SA, Fuenteun J, Lynch HT, et al. Familial breast-ovarian cancer locus on chromosome 17q12-q23. Lancet 1991;338:82-3.
66. Tonin P, Moslehi R, Green R, et al. Linkage analysis of 26 Canadian breast and breast ovarian cancer families. Hum Genet 1995;95:544-50.
67. Hall JM, Friedman L, Guenther C, et al. Closing in on a breast cancer gene on chromosome 17q. Am J Hum Genet 1992;50:1235-42.
68. Easton DF, Bishop DT, Ford D, Crockford GP. Genetic linkage analysis in familial breast and ovarian cancer: results from 214 families: the breast cancer linkage consortium. Am J Hum Genet 1993;52:678-701.
69. Miki Y, Swensen J, Shattuck-Eidens D, et al. A strong candidate for the breast and ovarian cancer susceptibility gene *BRCA1*. Science 1994;266:66-71.
70. Bowcock AM. Molecular cloning of *BRCA1:* a gene for early-onset familial breast and ovarian cancer. Breast Cancer Res Treat 1993; 28:121-35.
71. Easton DF, Ford D, Peto J. Inherited susceptibility to breast cancer. Cancer Surveys 1993;18:95-113.
72. Easton DF, Ford D, Bishop DT, the Breast Cancer Linkage Consortium. Breast and ovarian cancer incidence in *BRCA1*-mutation carriers. Am J Hum Genet 1995;56:265-71.
73. Easton DF. Inherited component of cancer: genetics of malignant disease. Br Med Bull 1994;50:527-35.
74. Easton DF, Narod SA, Ford D, Steel M. The genetic epidemiology of *BRCA1:* breast cancer linkage consortium [letter]. Lancet 1994; 344:761.
75. Ford D, Easton DF, Bishop DT, Narod SA, Goldgar DE. Risks of cancer in *BRCA1*-mutation carriers: breast cancer linkage consortium. Lancet 1994;343:692-5.
76. Knudson AG. Mutation and cancer: statistical study of retinoblastoma. Proc Natl Acad Sci U S A 1971;68:820-3.
77. Cornelis RS, Vasen HF, Meijers-Hijhboer H, et al. Age at diagnosis as an indicator for eligibility for *BRCA1* DNA testing in familial breast cancer. Hum Genet 1995;95:539-44.
78. Narod SA. Genetics of breast and ovarian cancer: genetics of malignant disease. Br Med Bull 1994;50:656-76.
79. Vasen HF. Screening in breast cancer families: is it useful? Ann Med 1994;26:185-90.
80. Wooster R, Neuhausen SL, Mangion J, et al. Localization of a breast cancer susceptibility gene, *BRCA2,* to chromosome 13q12-13. Science 1994;265:2088-90.
81. Stratton MR, Ford D, Neuhasen S, et al. Familial male breast cancer is not linked to the *BRCA1* locus on chromosome 17q. Nat Genet 1994;7:103-7.
82. Williard W, Borgen P, Bol R, Tiwari R, Osborne M. Cowden's disease: a case report with analyses at the molecular level. Cancer 1992;69:2969-74.
83. Cruz VF, Pardo R, Saenz D, Fernandez T, Leiva O. Muir-Torre syndrome with multiple neoplasia. Br J Surg 1992;79:1161.
84. Hall NR, Murday VA, Chapman P, et al. Genetic linkage in Muir-Torre syndrome to the same chromosomal region as cancer family syndrome. Eur J Cancer 1994;30A:180-2.
85. Hall NR, Williams MA, Murday VA, Newton JA, Bishop DT. Muir-Torre syndrome: a variant of the cancer family syndrome. J Med Genet 1994;31:627-31.
86. Trau H, Schewach-Millet M, Fisher BK, Tsur H. Peutz-Jeghers syndrome and bilateral breast carcinoma. Cancer 1982;50:788-92.
87. Swift M, Morrell D, Massey RB, Chase CL. Incidence of cancer in 161 families affected by ataxia-telangiectasia. N Engl J Med 1991; 325:1831-6.
88. Swift M, Reitnauer PJ, Morrell D, Chase CL. Breast and other cancers in families with ataxia-telangiectasia. N Engl J Med 1987; 316:1289-94.
89. Eeles RA, Stratton MR, Goldgar DE, Easton DF. The genetics of familial breast cancer and their practical implications. Eur J Cancer 1994;30A:1383-90.
90. Kastan M, Zhan Q, el-Deiry WS, et al. A mammalian cell cycle checkpoint pathway utilizing p53 and *GADD45* is defective in ataxia-telangiectasia. Cell 1992;71:587-97.
91. Savitsky K, Var-Shira A, Gilad S, et al. A single ataxia telangiectasia gene with a product similar to PI-3 kinase. Science 1995; 268:1749-53.
92. Hoskins KF, Stopfer JE, Calzone KA, et al. Assessment and counseling for women with a family history of breast cancer. JAMA 1995;273:577-85.
93. Castilla LH, Couch FJ, Erdos MR. Mutations in the *BRCA1* gene in families with early-onset breast and ovarian cancer. Nat Genet 1994;8:387-91.
94. Simard J, Tonin P, Durocher F, et al. Common origins of *BRCA1* mutations in Canadian breast and ovarian cancer families. Nat Genet 1994;8:392-8.
95. Friedman L, Ostermeyer EA, Szabo CI, et al. Confirmation of *BRCA1* by analysis of germline mutations linked to breast and ovarian cancer in ten families. Nat Genet 1994;8:399-404.
96. Shattuck-Eidens D, McClure M, Simard J, et al. A collaborative survey of 80 mutations in the *BRCA1* breast and ovarian cancer susceptibility gene. JAMA 1995;273:535-41.
97. Li F, Garber JE, Friend SH. Recommendations on predictive testing for germline p53 mutations among cancer-prone individuals. J Natl Cancer Inst 1992;84:1156-60.
98. Sidransky D, Tokino T, Helzlsouer K, et al. Inherited p53 gene mutations in breast cancer. Cancer Res 1992;52:2984-6.
99. Hogervorst FB, Cornelis RS, Bout M, et al. Rapid detection of *BRCA1* mutations by the protein truncation test. Nat Genet 1995; 10:208-12.
100. Lerman C, Schwartz M. Adherence and psychological adjustment among women at high risk for breast cancer. Breast Cancer Res Treat 1993;28:145-55.
101. Thirlaway K, Fallowfield L. The psychological consequences of being at risk of developing breast cancer. Eur J Cancer Prev 1993; 2:467-71.
102. Temple WJ, Lindsay RL, Magi E, Urbanski SJ. Technical considerations for prophylactic mastectomy in patients at high risk for breast cancer. Am J Surg 1991;161:413-5.
103. Ziegler LD, Kroll SS. Primary breast cancer after prophylactic mastectomy. Am J Clin Oncol 1991;14:451-4.
104. Struewing JP, Lerman C, Kase RG, et al. Anticipated uptake and impact of genetic testing in hereditary breast and ovarian cancer families. Cancer Epid Biomark Prev 1995;4:169-73.
105. Gallion HH, Smith SA. Hereditary ovarian carcinoma. Semin Surg Oncol 1994;10:249-54.
106. National Advisory Council for Human Genome Research. Statement on use of DNA testing for presymptomatic identification of cancer risk. JAMA 1994;271:785.
107. Mao L, Hruban RH, Boyle JO, Tockman M, Sidransky D. Detection of oncogene mutations in sputum precedes diagnosis of lung cancer. Cancer Res 1994;54:1634-7.
108. Hruban RH, van der Riet P, Erozan YS, Sidransky D. Brief report: molecular biology and the early detection of carcinoma of the bladder—the case of Hubert H. Humphrey. N Engl J Med 1994; 330:1276-8.
109. Tobi M, Luo FC, Ronai Z. Detection of K-ras mutation in colonic effluent samples from patients without evidence of colorectal carcinoma. J Natl Cancer Inst 1994;86:1007-10.
110. Sidransky D. Molecular screening—how long can we afford to wait? [editorial; comment]. J Natl Cancer Inst 1994;86:955-6.
111. Das BC, Gopalkrishna V, Das DK, Sharma JK, Singh V, Luthra UK. Human papillomavirus DNA sequences in adenocarcinoma of the uterine cervix in Indian women. Cancer 1993;72:147-53.
112. Sheets EE, Crum CP. Current status and future clinical potential of human papillomavirus infection and intraepithelial neoplasia. Curr Opin Obstet Gynecol 1993;5:63-6.
113. Pasetto N, Sesti F, De Santis L, Piccione E, Novelli G, Dallapiccola B. The prevalence of *HPV16DNA* in normal and pathological cervical scrapes using the polymerase chain reaction. Gynecol Oncol 1992;46:33-6.

114. Blount PL, Metzler SJ, Yin J, Huang Y, Krasna MJ, Reid BJ. Clonal ordering of 17p and 5q allelic losses in Barrett dysplasia and adenocarcinoma. Proc Natl Acad Sci U S A 1993;90: 3221-5.
115. Casson AG, Manolopoulos B, Troster M, et al. Clinical implications of p53 gene mutation in the progression of Barrett's epithelium to invasive esophageal cancer. Am J Surg 1994;167:52-7.
116. Yin J, Harpaz N, Tong Y, et al. p53 point mutations in dysplastic and cancerous ulcerative colitis lesions. Gastroenterology 1993; 104:1633-9.
117. Brentnall TA, Crispin DA, Rabinovitch PS, et al. Mutations in the p53 gene: an early marker of neoplastic progression in ulcerative colitis. Gastroenterology 1994;107:369-78.
118. Jen J, Kim H, Piantadosi S, et al. Allelic loss of chromosome 18q and prognosis in colorectal cancer. N Engl J Med 1994;331:213-21.
119. Sidransky D, Boyle J, Koch W. Molecular screening: prospects for a new approach. Arch Otolaryngol Head Neck Surg 1993;119:1187-90.
120. Koch WM, Boyle JO, Mao L, Hakim J, Hruban RH, Sidransky D. p53 gene mutations as markers of tumor spread in synchronous oral cancers. Arch Otolaryngol Head Neck Surg 1994;120:943-7.
121. Maeda Y, Horiuchi F, Morita S, et al. Detection of minimal residual disease using colon-specific primers for CDRIII in patients with acute B lymphocytic leukemia with or without Philadelphia chromosome: possibility of clinical application as a tool for improving prognosis. Exp Hematol 1994;22:881-7.
122. Amiel A, Yarkoni S, Slavin S, et al. Detection of minimal residual disease state in chronic myelogenous leukemia patients using fluorescence in situ hybridization. Cancer Genet Cytogenet 1994;76:59-64.
123. Chandrasekharappa SC, Guru SC, Manickam P, et al. Positional cloning of the gene for multiple endocrine neoplasia-Type 1. Science 1997;276:404-7.
124. Wooster R, Bignell G, Lancaster J, et al. Identification of the breast cancer susceptibility gene BRCA2. Nature 1995;378:789-92.
125. Liaw D, Marsh DJ, Li J, et al. Germline mutations of the PTEN gene in Cowden disease, an inherited breast and thyroid cancer syndrome. Nat Genet 1997;16:64-7.

CHAPTER 25

Decision Analysis of Cancer Patient Follow-Up

David J. Bruinvels and Job Kievit

In Chapter 2 the epidemiological principles for evaluating diagnostic test performance in cancer patient follow-up and the principles of follow-up evaluation were discussed. However, to combine these principles and apply them in clinical practice may not be as straightforward as expected. This chapter provides a method to combine the epidemiological and economic tools introduced earlier by the use of decision analysis models. The goal of the chapter is to offer a basic insight into the techniques of medical decision making and to provide readers with tools to construct their own decision models.

Decision analysis is a collective term describing methods and techniques used to aid clinicians in medical practice. A decision analysis can be divided into four basic steps: problem identification, problem structure, data acquisition, and evaluation.[1]

The first step (problem identification) is to identify the clinical problem. What is the problem? Which outcomes are of clinical importance? What are the characteristics of patients? Which options are available? Which arguments are against and in favor of each option? Only after these questions are answered should the physician continue to the second step.

The second step (problem structure) is to structure the clinical problem of interest. The problem should be defined textually by writing a descriptive algorithm. All actions and outcomes should be stated in a logical and chronological order. The clinician should start with a simple algorithm and gradually increase realism and detail, or start exhaustively and remove options that offer no clear benefit over alternative options.

The problem should also be defined graphically by constructing a decision tree. A tree structure can be drawn from left to right, with actions, events, and outcomes represented using accepted conventions for creating a decision tree (decision nodes, chance nodes, terminal nodes); the quantitative aspects of the structure should not be considered at this point.

The descriptive algorithm and the decision tree should be checked to be sure they match. The descriptive algorithm and decision tree should sufficiently take into account the various options and arguments brought forward in the problem identification. The various aspects of problem identification must still represent a sufficient inventory of the problem, considering the descriptive algorithm and decision tree.

The third step (data acquisition) is to assess the various quantitative data to solve the problem. This is done by quantifying the various aspects of the problem represented in the algorithm and decision tree. Data can be grouped into four categories: disease, diagnosis, therapy, and outcome. Data are expressed as numerical values of the probabilities and utilities of potential events during cancer patient follow-up. Probabilities may be extracted from studies published in the medical literature or from data in a hospital information system. Utilities can be assessed by using some of the tools introduced in Chapter 4 such as the standard gamble, visual analog scales, and time trade-off methods.

The fourth step (evaluation) is to evaluate the results of the decision analysis by calculating (various) expected value(s), performing sensitivity analysis, interpreting the results, and drawing conclusions. Dividing the process of decision analysis into four steps may give the impression that conducting an analysis is always straightforward. Although an analysis always starts with the problem structure and ends with an evaluation, the intermediate process is characterized by jumps back and forth between the different steps. The development of a successful decision analysis often requires considerable time and perseverance. In the next section of this chapter the different types of decision analysis models are introduced.

After a successful decision analysis the results have to be implemented in clinical practice. In cancer patient follow-up this may lead to a routine follow-up schedule that can be used for a certain category of cancer patients. Often decision analysts have a hard time convincing clinicians to change their current follow-up schedule based on a decision analysis alone. This skepticism can be overcome by conducting randomized controlled trials that compare follow-up schedules based on decision analysis with schedules currently in use.

The way by which cancer patient follow-up may be translated into a decision tree is demonstrated later in this chapter. A decision tree not only must reflect the complexity of the cancer patient follow-up itself, but also has to take into account all the actions that may follow a positive or negative test result. Therefore it has to consider the natural course of

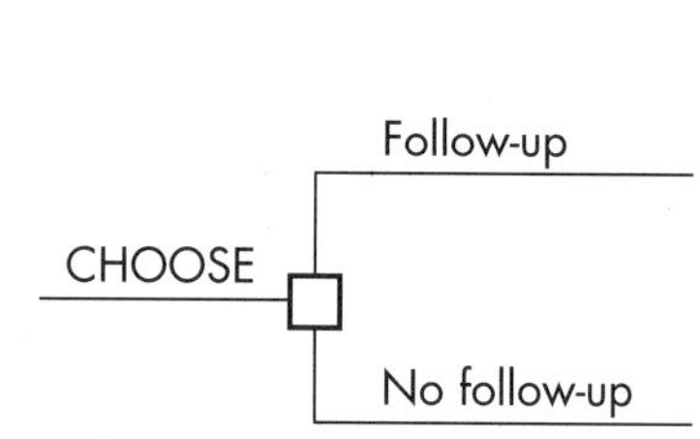

Figure 25-1 Example tree: decision node.

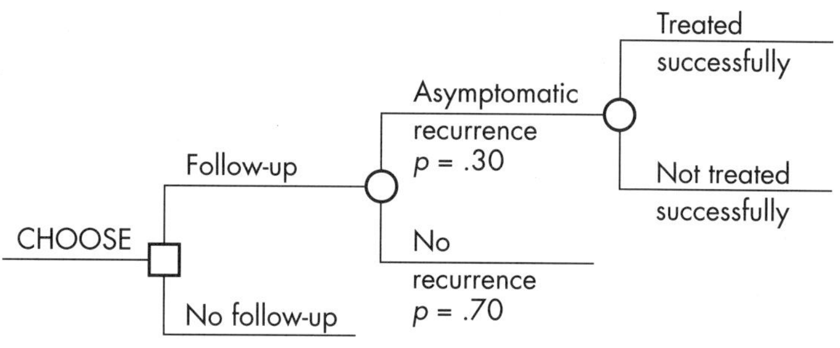

Figure 25-3 Example tree: two chance nodes.

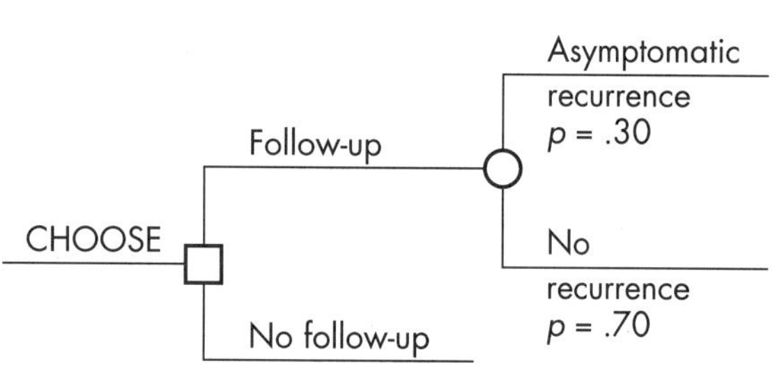

Figure 25-2 Example tree: chance node.

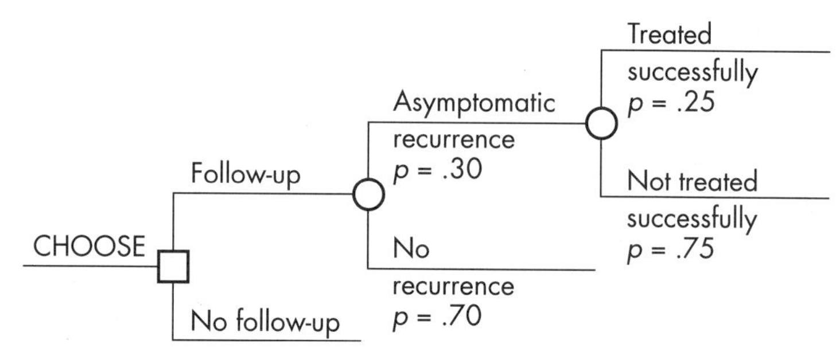

Figure 25-4 Example tree: probabilities.

the disease and all the events associated with it, making it a more complex task than might have been anticipated.

DECISION MODELS

The fundamental analytical tool for decision analysis is the decision tree. It is a way of displaying the proper temporal and logical sequence of a clinical decision problem.[2] There are many ways to model a decision tree. This section of the chapter describes the two most frequently used types of decision analysis models: conventional decision models and Markov models.

A decision tree uses branches and nodes to structure a clinical problem. The basic structure of a decision tree is analogous to the structure of a living tree. Both start with a single stem that splits into branches at different levels of the tree. A simple decision tree has only a few ending branches; a complex tree may have several hundred. The point where a branch of a decision tree splits is called a node. Three types of nodes are recognized: decision nodes stand for the branching of diagnostic and therapeutic actions that physicians can control; chance nodes stand for the branching of events not controlled by physicians, who may only influence the probability of these events; and terminal nodes represent the point of the tree where a branch ends.

By convention a decision tree is built from left to right and contains the three basic types of nodes: decision nodes, chance nodes, and terminal nodes. Decision nodes are placed at the beginning of the tree, and chance nodes are placed at all the subsequent levels of branches. For instance, a decision tree used to determine whether to perform cancer patient follow-up should begin with a decision node saying, "Do I perform follow-up, or do I not perform follow-up?" This choice becomes the first branching point of the decision tree (Figure 25-1). Such a decision or choice node can depict two or more alternative courses of action. It is conventionally represented in a decision tree as a small square. Decision nodes may be followed by other decision nodes, chance nodes, or terminal nodes. For instance, the decision in the example tree to perform follow-up may reveal an asymptomatic tumor recurrence or may not reveal a recurrence (Figure 25-2). The occurrence of this event is uncertain and beyond the control of the decision maker. A chance node can denote two or more possible outcomes of a situation. It is conventionally represented in a decision tree as a small circle. Chance nodes should, for practical purposes, be followed only by other chance nodes or by terminal nodes. For instance, an asymptomatic recurrence may be treated successfully or may not be treated successfully (Figure 25-3). In the example tree the first (diagnostic) chance node is followed by a second (therapeutic) chance node.

Each chance node in a decision tree represents an element of uncertainty. These uncertainties or probabilities might be derived from clinical or epidemiological studies or from informed guesses. In the example tree the probabilities of detection and treatment of a recurrence can be filled in. The probability of detecting a recurrence is estimated to be 30% and the probability of successfully treating an asymptomatic recurrence to be 25% (Figure 25-4).

The outcome of a branch in the decision tree is represented by a terminal node. The outcome may be manifold,

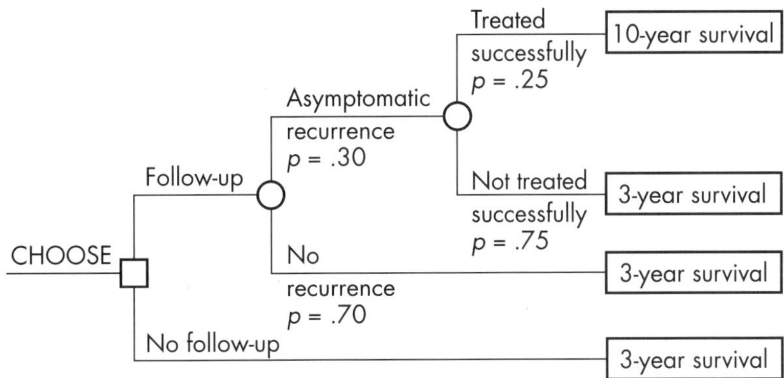

Figure 25-5 Example tree: outcomes.

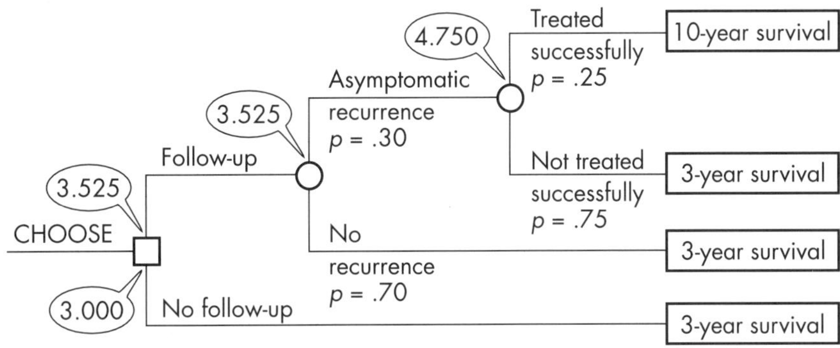

Figure 25-6 Example tree: foldback.

such as average life expectancy or quality of life of patients in the corresponding branch of the decision tree. In the example tree the life expectancy of a patient with a successfully treated recurrence will be longer (10 years) than the life expectancy of an untreated patient (3 years) as shown in Figure 25-5. The outcome of all branches of the tree, also known as the expected utility, is calculated by folding back the decision tree from right to left, as in Figure 25-6. In the example tree the expected utility of this conventional decision model would be a life expectancy of 3.525 years for patients with follow-up and 3 years for patients without follow-up. Based on this decision tree alone and disregarding other considerations such as costs and hazards of follow-up, cancer patient follow-up would be preferable to no follow-up.

Conventional decision models like the example tree are the most basic type of decision analysis models. Although these decision models are easy to construct and to fold back, they often require unrealistic simplifications. A more convincing decision model of cancer patient follow-up should include the events after primary tumor resection as a function of the elapsed follow-up time. Time-dependent variables that would be used in such a decision model are recurrence rates, mortality rates, and cancer detection rates.

In 1983 Markov models were introduced as a way to include time-dependent variables in decision trees.[3] In contrast to conventional decision models, Markov models provide a far more convenient way of modeling prognosis for clinical problems with ongoing risk. The model assumes that the patient is always in one of a finite number of health states referred to as Markov states. For instance, in a cancer patient follow-up decision tree there could be three health states: *NED* (no evidence of disease), *REC* (recurrence), and *DEAD* (Figure 25-7). The Markov states are preceded by a Markov node, which is conventionally represented in a decision tree as a small square containing an "M" or two small circles. All events of interest are modeled as transitions from one health state to another. In the example tree in Figure 25-8, patients in the *NED* state can have a recurrence *(REC)* or stay without evidence of disease *(NED)*. Patients with a recurrence *(REC)* can die of their recurrence *(DEAD)* or stay alive *(REC)*. Deceased patients remain *DEAD*.

In contrast to conventional decision trees, which are folded back only once, Markov trees are folded back continuously. This is because a Markov analysis is divided into equal increments of time, referred to as Markov cycles. During each Markov cycle, patients may make a transition from one state to another. For instance, a patient could go for 3 years without evidence of disease *(NED)*, live with a symptomatic recurrence for 2 years *(REC)*, and finally die of cancer-related causes *(DEAD)*. If the chosen cycle length is half a year, the patient would reside six cycles (3 years) in

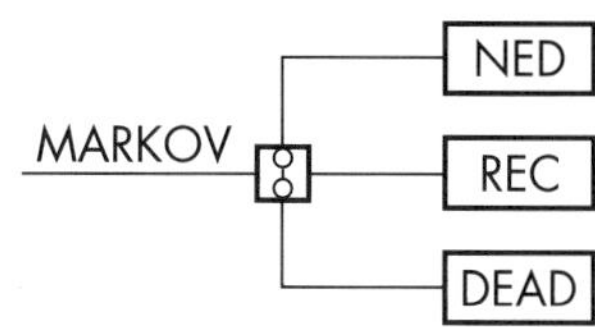

Figure 25-7 Example tree: three health states.

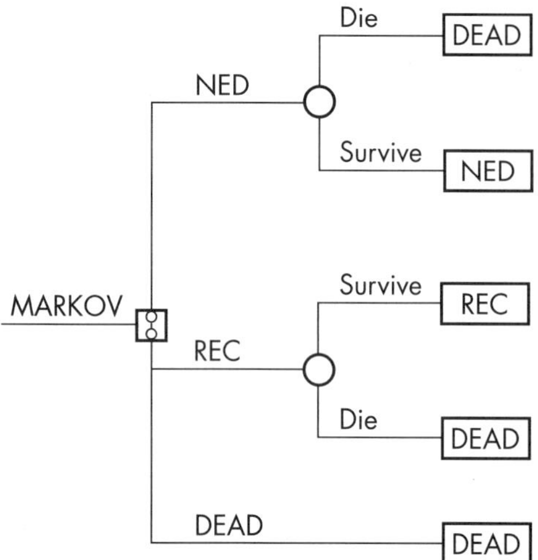

Figure 25-8 Example tree: simple Markov model with three health states.

NED, spend four cycles (2 years) in *REC,* and end in the *DEAD* state for the remainder of the analysis. When the Markov states *NED* and *REC* are assigned a utility of 1 (alive) and the state *DEAD* is assigned a utility of 0 (dead), the expected utility for this patient would be 10 Markov cycles, corresponding to a 5-year life expectancy.

Markov models may be evaluated by matrix algebra, cohort simulation, or Monte Carlo simulation.[4] These methods of folding back a Markov analysis are beyond the scope of this book, but fortunately decision-making computer software can be used in the evaluation of these models. The following decision-making software is available at this writing (in alphabetical order): Continuous Risk 2.0 by Nevada simulations (e-mail: NEVSIM@aol.com); DATA 3.0 by TreeAge software (e-mail: TREEAGE@aol.com); Decision Maker 7.0 by S. Pauker & F. Sonnenberg (e-mail: Sonnenbe@cs.rutgers.edu); and SMLtree 3.0 by J. Hollenberg (address: 445 E. 68th St., Box 20, New York, NY 10021).

MODELING CANCER PATIENT FOLLOW-UP

In this section of the chapter the basics of a decision model of cancer patient follow-up are discussed. It by no means provides a complete decision tree ready for use. As outlined earlier, decision analysis is a process of repeating the same steps over and over until a satisfactory decision model emerges. Before starting with the construction of a complex decision tree on cancer patient follow-up, the reader is advised to consult the excellent books on decision analysis by Weinstein et al.[2] and Sox et al.[5] and a paper on Markov analysis by Sonnenberg et al.[4] A thorough overview of published medical decision analysis of cancer patients is given by Smith et al.[6]

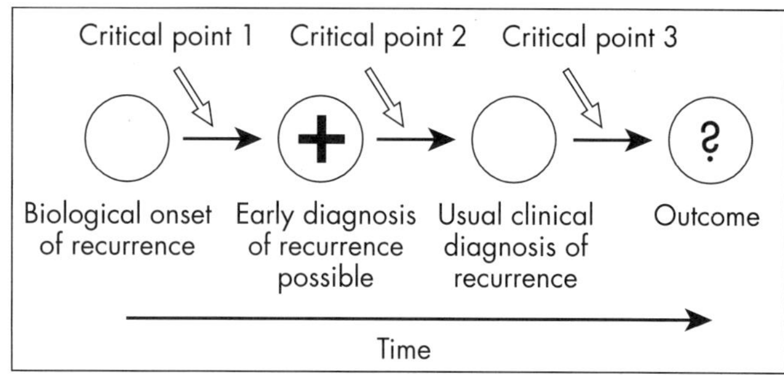

Figure 25-9 Natural history of recurrence.

A cancer patient follow-up schedule should take into account the natural history of disease. A useful schedule of this natural history was given by Sackett et al.[7] A version of this schedule modified for cancer recurrences is shown in Figure 25-9. Four key points in the natural history of patients with colorectal cancer are recognized:

1. Biological onset of recurrence. Many recurrences originate from the primary tumor. Most of these recurrences are already present at primary tumor resection but are often too small to be detected.
2. Early diagnosis of recurrence possible. With the passage of time, recurrences progress and may be detected if the correct test is applied. At this point early diagnosis becomes possible by means of follow-up.
3. Usual clinical diagnosis of recurrence. Recurrences progress to the point at which symptoms appear and the patient seeks clinical help.
4. Outcome. Finally the malignant disease runs its course and arrives at its outcome of complete remission after intervention, death by cancer, or death with cancer by other causes.

The time between the onset of recurrence and the clinical diagnosis is often referred to as the preclinical phase. The time after clinical diagnosis is often referred to as the clinical phase of recurrence.[8]

There are certain critical points in the natural history of a disease before which therapy is either more effective or easier to apply than afterward. If the only critical point of a cancer recurrence were in position 1, detection of asymptomatic recurrence by follow-up would be too late to be useful (Figure 25-9). Similarly, if the only critical point of a cancer recurrence were in position 3, early detection would be a waste of time and money. Only when the critical point of a cancer recurrence is at position 2 does early detection by follow-up lead to a better outcome. Each type of cancer recurrence has its unique critical points. Recurrences of colorectal cancer, for instance, may have critical points at posi-

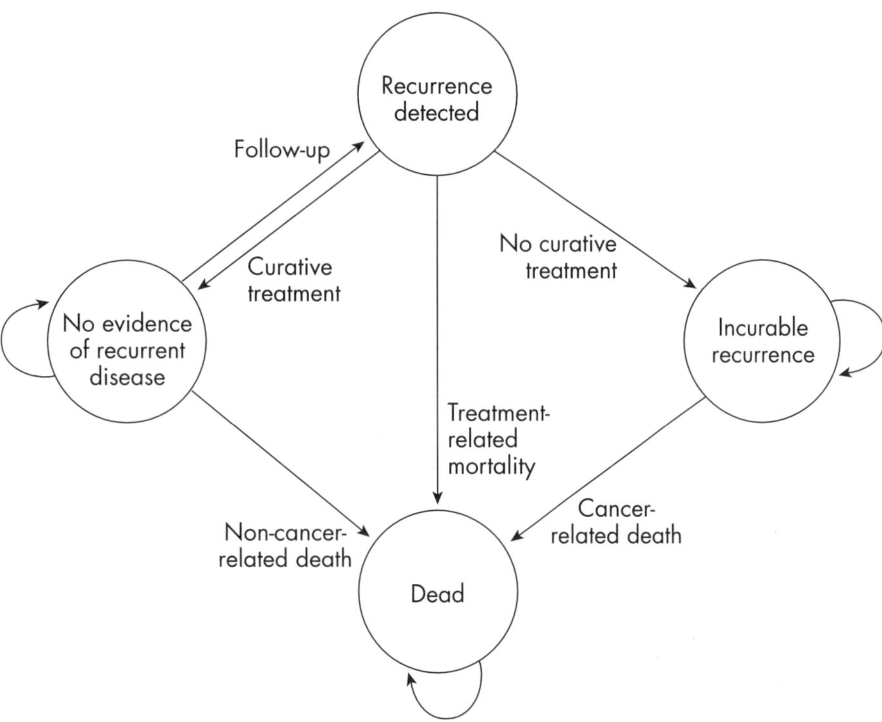

Figure 25-10 Markov model of cancer patient follow-up.

tions 2 and 3 and may be treated with curative intent. It is speculated that this specific behavior is caused by metastatic inefficiency.[9] Although many cells from the primary tumor enter the vascular system, relatively few metastases develop. Therefore solitary liver metastases of colorectal origin may be treated for cure, whereas, for instance, solitary liver metastases of breast cancer virtually always herald disseminated disease.

Because of the diverse nature of oncological disease, many categories of cancer patients, each with its own critical point, are recognized. Follow-up is beneficial only to those categories of patients with a critical point between the moment of early diagnosis and clinical diagnosis. Therefore not only the primary organ site of a cancer patient, but also the characteristics of the primary tumor and the probability of developing a second cancer, are important. The physical condition and coexisting disease, such as cardiovascular disease or diabetes mellitus, also influence the natural history of cancer in these patients. Finally, the recurrence site may determine the position of a critical point. Follow-up should therefore focus on locations where recurrences can be treated for cure or for markedly improved quality of life.

To reflect reality more or less accurately, a decision analysis model should take into account the natural history of oncological disease. Upon this oncological framework various follow-up scenarios may be placed as overlays. The most effective way to build a decision tree that compares two or more cancer patient follow-up strategies is to structure the natural history using a Markov model, like the one in Figure 25-10. It is necessary to start with a number of simplifying assumptions:

1. Not all cancer patients will die because of recurrences. Therefore in the model all patients are subject to two types of mortality: cancer-related mortality and age- and sex-specific mortality not related to cancer.
2. The characteristics of the primary tumor and recurrences determine the prognosis of a patient with cancer. This is approximated in the model by directly relating cancer-related mortality to location, size, and number of recurrences.
3. In most types of cancer the chance of recurrence is related to the nature of the primary tumor. In the model the cancer recurrence rate is determined by the primary tumor characteristics, such as primary tumor stage and location.
4. Follow-up is aimed at detecting asymptomatic recurrences in patients with primary tumors who are treated for cure and who are without evidence of recurrent disease. In the model most recurrences are present at the time of primary tumor resection but are too small (<0.5 cm) to be detected.
5. The model recognizes only recurrences at predefined tumor sites, such as local recurrences, hepatic metastases, or pulmonary metastases. These metastatic locations depend on the location and type of the primary tumor.

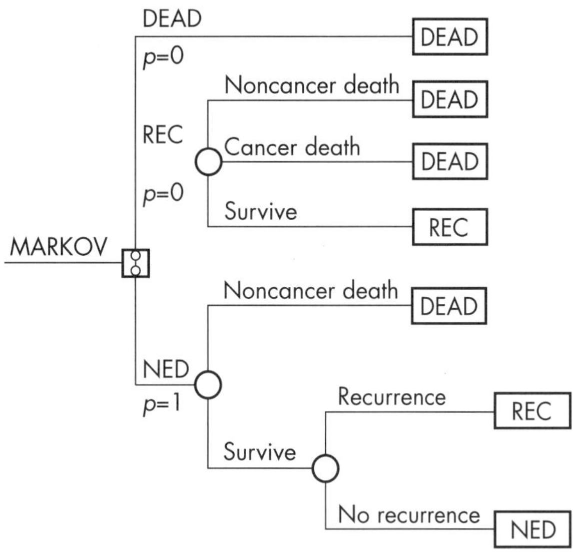

Figure 25-11 Example tree: Markov model of cancer recurrence.

6. Recurrences do not grow in a linear or exponential fashion. The growth of recurrences for each tumor site can be approximated by a mathematical growth curve. Gompertz equations are currently most often used for modeling cancer growth.[10] Gompertzian growth is characterized by an exponential growth phase followed by a phase of decreasing growth resulting in an S-shaped growth curve.
7. Tumor growth is not unlimited. The maximum tumor size often depends on the blood supply of the tumor and the amount of necrosis in the tumor. The model assumes that the maximum size of a recurrence, when allowed to grow undisturbed, is on average 17 cm, which is based on a spherical tumor with a maximum of 2.4×10^{12} cells.[11] This estimate is constant regardless of the location and type of the primary tumor.

In the decision model all cancer patients enter the analysis without evidence of disease *(NED)*. Some are completely cured of their disease, and others have microscopic metastases, the risk of which varies with factors such as the primary tumor stage and site. In time these occult deposits grow and eventually are detected or lead to symptoms. In the model this is simulated by the Markov process, which allows time to pass and gives undetected recurrences the opportunity to grow and eventually become detectable or symptomatic *(REC)*. Death is also accounted for in the model. In every Markov cycle a patient may die of either cancer-related or non-cancer-related causes. Cancer-related causes are based on the location, number, and size of the recurrences. Non-cancer-related causes are based on age- and sex-related mortality. In the cycle following death, deceased patients are transferred to the death state *(DEAD)*. An example of a tree structure that may be used to model the natural history of cancer recurrence is shown in Figure 25-11.

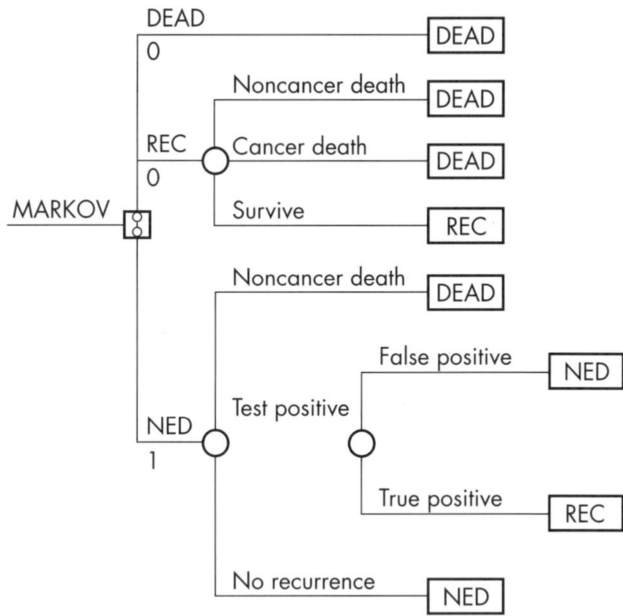

Figure 25-12 Example tree: Markov model of cancer patient follow-up.

For most types of cancer there is no agreement on which follow-up schedule is best. Therefore another important element of the decision analysis should be the evaluation of various follow-up strategies. Each diagnostic test in follow-up has different test characteristics, as discussed in Chapter 2. The probability of a positive test depends on the location, number, and size of recurrences. Therefore, as recurrences grow, test characteristics such as sensitivity and specificity vary over time. The decision model has to simulate these changing test characteristics. Again, a few extra assumptions are necessary:

1. When a cancer patient follow-up test indicates the presence of recurrence, the diagnosis is always assessed with additional diagnostic testing.
2. In the model these additional diagnostic tests in general find a recurrence larger than 0.5 cm and miss smaller recurrences.
3. In the model symptoms are regarded as if they were a follow-up test, meaning that they also have a sensitivity and specificity that depend on location and size of recurrence.
4. Because recurrences less than 0.5 cm remain undetected, no mortality is associated with these recurrences in the model.

The primary goal of cancer patient follow-up is to detect asymptomatic recurrences that can still be cured. The decision model determines whether a recurrence can be detected during each Markov cycle. Recurrences are detected either by symptoms or by abnormal follow-up test results. The probability of true-positive symptoms and abnormal test results depends on the location, number, and size of the recurrences. Symptoms and test results may also be false

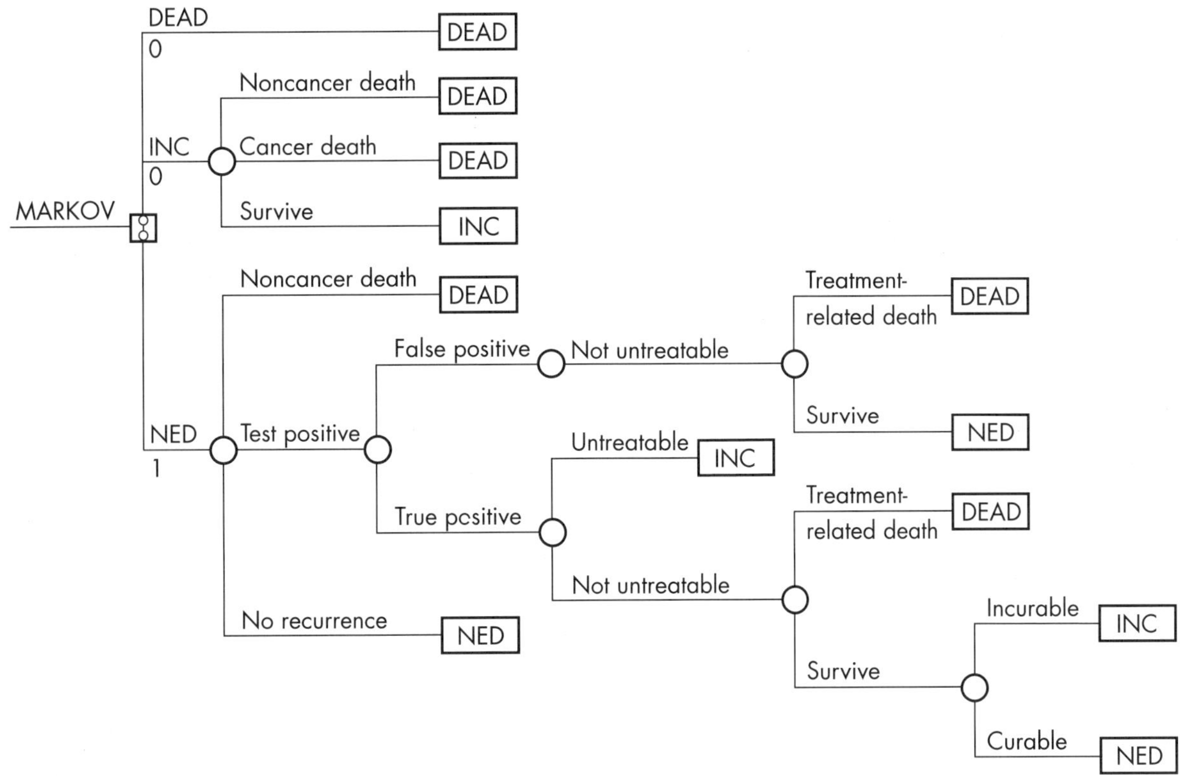

Figure 25-13 Example tree: Markov model of cancer patient follow-up and treatment of recurrence.

positive in patients without recurrences. However, symptoms and abnormal test results are always followed by additional diagnostic testing to assess the exact nature of a possible recurrence and, eventually, chances for curative treatment. With a decision model based on these assumptions it is possible to assess the effects and costs of cancer patient follow-up strategies with different follow-up tests and different test frequencies (Figure 25-12).

After confirmation of a recurrence, two options are available to a patient: the patient is cured and is without evidence of disease, or the patient is incurable. To incorporate this into the decision model, two assumptions are made. The model assumes that cancer-related mortality is directly related to the tumor size or volume. Thus the resection of recurrences reduces or eliminates cancer-related mortality. It is assumed that patients without recurrence after treatment are at risk only for non-cancer-related mortality and for mortality associated with second primary tumors.

If recurrence cannot be treated, patients are told and are transferred by the model to the incurable health state *(INC)* of the Markov tree (Figure 25-13). For patients with less advanced recurrences the model suggests curative treatment. During the treatment some recurrences regress or are resected and other recurrences are resistant to treatment. Patients with therapy-resistant recurrences are transferred to the incurable health state *(INC)*. After successful treatment the patient is cured and will never have a recurrence at the same location. Alternatively the patient is not cured because of missed tumor cells. Probabilities of attempting curative treatment, effect of treatment, and complete remission or resection of recurrence depend on its location. Some patients, however, die of age- and sex-related mortality caused by the treatment and are transferred to the death state *(DEAD)*. Patients with asymptomatic recurrences less than 0.5 cm or without recurrences remain with no clinical evidence of recurrent disease *(NED)*.

At this point it is possible to estimate the effects on life expectancy (LE) for various follow-up strategies with the decision model. However, it would also be useful to determine the role of quality of life in cancer patient follow-up. With a few changes to the decision model it is possible to calculate the quality-adjusted life expectancy (QALE). Instead of assigning a utility of 1 to all Markov states in which patients are alive *(NED, INC)*, patients with incurable disease *(INC)* can, for instance, be given a utility of 0.75. The expected utility then reflects the QALE rather than the LE.

Finally, the costs related to cancer patient follow-up can be included into the decision model. A second utility can be assigned to each health state. It then is possible to calculate the costs related to the follow-up strategy, analogous to the QALE. Such a model, when rolled back, presents both the QALE and the costs, making it possible to conduct a cost-effectiveness analysis. The basic principles of cost-effectiveness analysis are discussed in Chapter 2.

DISCUSSION

This chapter provides a review of the basic techniques needed to construct a decision tree on cancer patient follow-up. The reader should not try to use all techniques at once to construct a decision model for the first time but rather should begin with a simple decision model. Decision models, like living trees, tend to grow and must be pruned continuously to prevent them from becoming too complex or too large to be contained by the available computer software.

Clinical decision analysis may play an important role in the future of cancer patient follow-up. The use of decision models has provided insight into the complex structure of the follow-up of patients with cancer. As with most scientific research, these decision analyses may lead to more unanswered questions than solutions. Although decision models are useful tools in the assessment of existing or new technologies, decision models of a disease are only an approximation of reality. Decision models of cancer patient follow-up may never be able to predict the outcome of follow-up in individual patients because it is impossible to account for all the unique patient characteristics. In this respect decision analysis provides no improvement over conventional clinical decision making. The strength of decision analysis is the identification of categories of patients who may benefit from follow-up and treatment of early detected recurrences, which will lead to a more effective use of existing and new technologies. Furthermore, clinical decision analysis provides for an inexpensive, safe provisional assessment of the expected outcome of controlled randomized trials. It may thus help to assess whether a trial is feasible and may lead to valid results at an acceptable price.

REFERENCES

1. Kievit J, Lubsen J. The Erasmus Summer Programme 1995. Clinical and public health research methods: section clinical decision analysis. Rotterdam, The Netherlands: Erasmus University, 1995.
2. Weinstein MC, Fineberg HV, Elstein AS, et al. Clinical decision analysis. Philadelphia: WB Saunders Company, 1980.
3. Beck JR, Pauker SG. The Markov process in medical prognosis. Med Decis Making 1983;3:419-58.
4. Sonnenberg FA, Beck JR. Markov models in medical decision making: a practical guide. Med Decis Making 1993;13:322-38.
5. Sox HC, Blatt MA, Higgins MC, Marton KI. Medical decision making. Stoneham, Mass: Butterworth-Heinemann, 1988.
6. Smith TJ, Hillner BE, Desch CE. Efficacy and cost-effectiveness of cancer treatment: rational allocation of resources based on decision analysis. J Natl Cancer Inst 1993;85:1460-74.
7. Sackett DL, Haynes RB, Guyatt GH, Tugwell P. Clinical epidemiology. 2nd ed. Boston: Little, Brown & Company, 1991.
8. Vandenbroucke JP, Hofman A. Grondslagen der epidemiologie. 4th ed. Utrecht: Wetenschappelijke uitgeverij Bunge, 1990.
9. Sugarbaker PH. Metastatic inefficiency: the scientific basis for resection of liver metastases from colorectal cancer. J Surg Oncol 1993;3(Suppl):158-60.
10. Norton L, Simon R, Brereton HD, Bodgen AE. Predicting the course of Gompertzian growth. Nature 1976;264:542-5.
11. Brunton GF, Wheldon TE. Characteristic species dependent growth patterns of mammalian neoplasms. Cell Tissue Kinet 1978;11:161-75.

Index

M

Q

R